Encyclopedia of

HUMAN NUTRITION

SECOND EDITION

ENCYCLOPEDIA OF HUMAN NUTRITION

SECOND EDITION

Editor-in-Chief
BENJAMIN CABALLERO

Editors
LINDSAY ALLEN
ANDREW PRENTICE

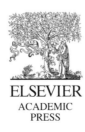

ELSEVIER
ACADEMIC
PRESS

Amsterdam   Boston   Heidelberg   London   New York   Oxford
Paris   San Diego   San Francisco   Singapore   Sydney   Tokyo

DISCARD
Magale Library
Southern Arkansas University
Magnolia, Arkansas 71753

Elsevier Ltd., The Boulevard, Langford Lane, Kidlington, Oxford, OX5 1GB, UK

© 2005 Elsevier Ltd.

The following articles are US Government works in the
public domain and not subject to copyright:

CAROTENOIDS/Chemistry, Sources and Physiology

FOOD FORTIFICATION/Developed Countries

FRUCTOSE

LEGUMES

TEA

TUBERCULOSIS/Nutrition and Susceptibility

TUBERCULOSIS/Nutritional Management

VEGETARIAN DIETS

*All rights reserved. No part of this publication may be reproduced or transmitted in any form or by any
means, electronic, or mechanical, including photocopy, recording, or any information storage and
retrieval system, without permission in writing from the publishers.*

*Permissions may be sought directly from Elsevier's Rights Department in Oxford, UK:
phone (+44) 1865 843830, fax (+44) 1865 853333, e-mail permissions@elsevier.com.*

Requests may also be completed on-line via the homepage (http://www.elsevier.com/locate/permissions).

Second edition 2005

Library of Congress Control Number: 2004113614

A catalogue record for this book is available from the British Library

ISBN 0-12-150110-8 (set)

This book is printed on acid-free paper
Printed and bound in Spain

EDITORIAL ADVISORY BOARD

EDITOR-IN-CHIEF

Benjamin Caballero
Johns Hopkins University
Maryland
USA

EDITORS

Lindsay Allen
University of California
Davis, CA, USA

Andrew Prentice
London School of Hygiene & Tropical Medicine
London, UK

Christopher Bates
MRC Human Nutrition Research
Cambridge, UK

Carolyn D Berdanier
University of Georgia
Athens, GA, USA

Bruce R Bistrian
Harvard Medical School
Boston, MA, USA

Johanna T Dwyer
Frances Stern Nutrition Center
Boston, MA, USA

Paul Finglas
Institute of Food Research
Norwich, UK

Terrence Forrester
Tropical Medicine Research Institute
University of the West Indies,
Mona Campus, Kingston, Jamaica

Hedley C Freake
University of Connecticut
Storrs, CT, USA

Catherine Geissler
King's College London
London, UK

Susan A Jebb
MRC Human Nutrition Research
Cambridge, UK

Rachel Johnson
University of Vermont
Burlington, VT, USA

Janet C King
Children's Hospital Oakland Research Institute
Oakland, CA, USA

Anura Kurpad
St John's National Academy of Health Sciences
Bangalore, India

Kim Fleisher Michaelson
The Royal Veterinary and Agricultural University
Frederiksberg, Denmark

Carlos Monteiro
University of Sâo Paulo
Sâo Paulo, Brazil

John M Pettifor
University of the Witwatersrand & Chris
  Hani-Baragwanath Hospital
Johannesburg, South Africa

Barry M Popkin
University of North Carolina
Chapel Hill, NC, USA

Michele J Sadler
MJSR Associates
Ashford, UK

Ricardo Uauy
London School of Hygiene and Tropical Medicine
  UK and INTA University of Chile, Santiago, Chile

David York
Pennington Biomedical Research Center
Baton Rouge, LA, USA

FOREWORD

Why an encyclopedia? The original Greek word means 'the circle of arts and sciences essential for a liberal education', and such a book was intended to embrace all knowledge. That was the aim of the famous Encyclopedie produced by Diderot and d'Alembert in the middle of the 18th century, which contributed so much to what has been called the Enlightenment. It is recorded that after all the authors had corrected the proofs of their contributions, the printer secretly cut out whatever he thought might give offence to the king, mutilated most of the best articles and burnt the manuscripts! Later, and less controversially, the word 'encyclopedia' came to be used for an exhaustive repertory of information on some particular department of knowledge. It is in this class that the present work falls.

In recent years the scope of Human Nutrition as a scientific discipline has expanded enormously. I used to think of it as an applied subject, relying on the basic sciences of physiology and biochemistry in much the same way that engineering relies on physics. That traditional relationship remains and is fundamental, but the field is now much wider. At one end of the spectrum epidemiological studies and the techniques on which they depend have played a major part in establishing the relationships between diet, nutritional status and health, and there is greater recognition of the importance of social factors. At the other end of the spectrum we are becoming increasingly aware of the genetic determinants of ways in which the body handles food and is able to resist adverse influences of the environment. Nutritionists are thus beginning to explore the mechanisms by which nutrients influence the expression of genes in the knowledge that nutrients are among the most powerful of all influences on gene expression. This has brought nutrition to the centre of the new 'post-genome' challenge of understanding the effects on human health of gene-environment interactions.

In parallel with this widening of the subject there has been an increase in opportunities for training and research in nutrition, with new departments and new courses being developed in universities, medical schools and schools of public health, along with a greater involvement of schoolchildren and their teachers. Public interest in nutrition is intense and needs to be guided by sound science. Governments are realizing more and more the role that nutrition plays in the prevention of disease and the maintenance of good health, and the need to develop a nutrition policy that is integrated with policies for food production.

The first edition of the Encyclopaedia of Human Nutrition established it as one of the major reference works in our discipline. The second edition has been completely revised to take account of new knowledge in our rapidly advancing field. This new edition is as comprehensive as the present state of knowledge allows, but is not overly technical and is well supplied with suggestions for further reading. All the articles have been carefully reviewed and although some of the subjects are controversial and sensitive, the publishers have not exerted the kind of political censorship that so infuriated Diderot.

John Waterlow.

J.C. Waterlow
Emeritus Professor of Human Nutrition
London School of Hygiene and Tropical Medicine
February 2005

INTRODUCTION

The science of human nutrition and its applications to health promotion continue to gain momentum. In the relatively short time since the release of the first edition of this Encyclopedia, a few landmark discoveries have had a dramatic multiplying effect over nutrition science: the mapping of the human genome, the links between molecular bioenergetics and lifespan, the influence of nutrients on viral mutation, to name a few.

But perhaps the strongest evidence of the importance of nutrition for human health comes from the fact that almost 60% of the diseases that kill humans are related to diet and lifestyle (including smoking and physical activity). These are all modifiable risk factors. As individuals and organizations intensify their efforts to reduce disease risks, the need for multidisciplinary work becomes more apparent. Today, an effective research or program team is likely to include several professionals from fields other than nutrition. For both nutrition and non-nutrition scientists, keeping up to date on the concepts and interrelationships between nutrient needs, dietary intake and health outcomes is essential. The new edition of the Encyclopedia of Human Nutrition hopes to address these needs. While rigorously scientific and up to date, EHN provides concise and easily understandable summaries on a wide variety of topics. The nutrition scientist will find that the Encyclopedia is an effective tool to "fill the void" of information in areas beyond his/her field of expertise. Professionals from other fields will appreciate the ease of alphabetical listing of topics, and the presentation of information in a rigorous but concise way, with generous aid from graphs and diagrams.

For a work that involved more than 340 authors requires, coordination and attention to detail is critical. The editors were fortunate to have the support of an excellent team from Elsevier's Major Reference Works division. Sara Gorman and Paula O'Connell initiated the project, and Tracey Mills and Samuel Coleman saw it to its successful completion.

We trust that this Encyclopedia will be a useful addition to the knowledge base of professionals involved in research, patient care, and health promotion around the globe.

Benjamin Caballero, Lindsay Allen and Andrew Prentice
Editors
April 2005

GUIDE TO USE OF THE ENCYCLOPEDIA

Structure of the Encyclopedia

The material in the Encyclopedia is arranged as a series of entries in alphabetical order. Most entries consist of several articles that deal with various aspects of a topic and are arranged in a logical sequence within an entry. Some entries comprise a single article.

To help you realize the full potential of the material in the Encyclopedia we have provided three features to help you find the topic of your choice: a Contents List, Cross-References and an Index.

1. Contents List

Your first point of reference will probably be the contents list. The complete contents lists, which appears at the front of each volume will provide you with both the volume number and the page number of the entry. On the opening page of an entry a contents list is provided so that the full details of the articles within the entry are immediately available.

Alternatively you may choose to browse through a volume using the alphabetical order of the entries as your guide. To assist you in identifying your location within the Encyclopedia a running headline indicates the current entry and the current article within that entry.

You will find 'dummy entries' where obvious synonyms exist for entries or where we have grouped together related topics. Dummy entries appear in both the contents lists and the body of the text.

Example
If you were attempting to locate material on food intake measurement via the contents list:

FOOD INTAKE *see* DIETARY INTAKE MEASUREMENT: Methodology; Validation. DIETARY SURVEYS. MEAL SIZE AND FREQUENCY

The dummy entry directs you to the Methodology article, in The Dietary Intake Measurement entry. At the appropriate location in the contents list, the page numbers for articles under Dietary Intake Measurement are given.

If you were trying to locate the material by browsing through the text and you looked up Food intake then the following information would be provided in the dummy entry:

Food Intake *see* **Dietary Intake Measurement**: Methodology; Validation. **Dietary Surveys. Meal Size and Frequency**

Alternatively, if you were looking up Dietary Intake Measurement the following information would be provided:

DIETARY INTAKE MEASUREMENT

Contents
Methodology
Validation

2. Cross-References

All of the articles in the Encyclopedia have been extensively cross-referenced.

The cross-references, which appear at the end of an article, serve three different functions. For example, at the end of the ADOLESCENTS/Nutritional Problems article, cross-references are used:

i. To indicate if a topic is discussed in greater detail elsewhere.

> *See also*: **Adolescents**: Nutritional Requirements of Adolescents. **Anemia**: Iron-Deficiency Anemia. **Calcium**: Physiology. **Eating Disorders**: Anorexia Nervosa; Bulimia Nervosa; Binge Eating. **Folic Acid**: Physiology, Dietary Sources, and Requirements. **Iron**: Physiology, Dietary Sources, and Requirements. **Obesity**: Definition, Aetiology, and Assessment. **Osteoporosis**: Nutritional Factors. **Zinc**: Physiology.

ii. To draw the reader's attention to parallel discussions in other articles.

> *See also*: **Adolescents**: Nutritional Requirements of Adolescents. **Anemia**: Iron-Deficiency Anemia. **Calcium**: Physiology. **Eating Disorders**: Anorexia Nervosa; Bulimia Nervosa; Binge Eating. **Folic Acid**: Physiology, Dietary Sources, and Requirements. **Iron**: Physiology, Dietary Sources, and Requirements. **Obesity**: Definition, Aetiology, and Assessment. **Osteoporosis**: Nutritional Factors **Zinc**: Physiology.

iii. To indicate material that broadens the discussion.

> *See also*: **Adolescents**: Nutritional Requirements of Adolescents. **Anemia**: Iron-Deficiency Anemia. **Calcium**: Physiology. **Eating Disorders**: Anorexia Nervosa; Bulimia Nervosa; Binge Eating. **Follic Acid**: Physiology, Dietary Sources, and Requirements. **Iron**: Physiology, Dietary Sources, and Requirements. **Obesity**: Definition, Aetiology, and Assessment. **Osteoporosis**: Nutritional Factors. **Zinc**: Physiology.

3. Index

The index will provide you with the page number where the material is located, and the index entries differentiate between material that is a whole article, is part of an article or is data presented in a figure or table. Detailed notes are provided on the opening page of the index.

4. Contributors

A full list of contributors appears at the beginning of each volume.

CONTRIBUTORS

E Abalos
Centro Rosarino de Estudios Perinatales
Rosario, Argentina

A Abi-Hanna
Johns Hopkins School of Medicine
Baltimore, MD, USA

L S Adair
University of North Carolina
Chapel Hill, NC, USA

A Ahmed
Obetech Obesity Research Center
Richmond, VA, USA

B Ahrén
Lund University
Lund, Sweden

J Akré
World Health Organization, Geneva, Switzerland

A J Alberg
Johns Hopkins Bloomberg School of Public Health
Baltimore, MD, USA

L H Allen
University of California at Davis
Davis, CA, USA

D Anderson
University of Bradford
Bradford, UK

J J B Anderson
University of North Carolina
Chapel Hill, NC, USA

R A Anderson
US Department of Agriculture
Beltsville, MD, USA

L J Appel
Johns Hopkins University
Baltimore, MD, USA

A Ariño
University of Zaragoza
Zaragoza, Spain

M J Arnaud
Nestle S.A.
Vevey, Switzerland

E W Askew
University of Utah
Salt Lake City, UT, USA

R L Atkinson
Obetech Obesity Research Center
Richmond, VA, USA

S A Atkinson
McMaster University
Hamilton, ON, Canada

L S A Augustin
University of Toronto
Toronto, ON, Canada

D J Baer
US Department of Agriculture
Beltsville, MD, USA

A Baqui
Johns Hopkins Bloomberg School of Public Health
Baltimore, MD, USA

Y Barnett
Nottingham Trent University
Nottingham, UK

G E Bartley
Agricultural Research Service
Albany, CA, USA

C J Bates
MRC Human Nutrition Research
Cambridge, UK

J A Beltrán
University of Zaragoza
Zaragoza, Spain

A E Bender
Leatherhead, UK

D A Bender
University College London
London, UK

I F F Benzie
The Hong Kong Polytechnic University
Hong Kong SAR, China

C D Berdanier
University of Georgia
Athens, GA, USA

R Bhatia
United Nations World Food Programme
Rome, Italy

Z A Bhutta
The Aga Khan University
Karachi, Pakistan

J E Bines
University of Melbourne
Melbourne, VIC, Australia

J Binkley
Vanderbilt Center for Human Nutrition
Nashville, TN, USA

R Black
Johns Hopkins Bloomberg School of Public Health
Baltimore, MD, USA

J E Blundell
University of Leeds
Leeds, UK

A T Borchers
University of California at Davis
Davis, CA, USA

C Boreham
University of Ulster at Jordanstown
Jordanstown, UK

F Branca
Istituto Nazionale di Ricerca per gli Alimenti e la Nutrizione
Rome, Italy

J Brand-Miller
University of Sydney
Sydney, NSW, Australia

A Briend
Institut de Recherche pour le Développement
Paris, France

P Browne
St James's Hospital
Dublin, Ireland

I A Brownlee
University of Newcastle
Newcastle-upon-Tyne, UK

H Brunner
Centre Hospitalier Universitaire Vaudois
Lausanne, Switzerland

A J Buckley
University of Cambridge
Cambridge, UK

H H Butchko
Exponent, Inc.
Wood Dale, IL, USA

J Buttriss
British Nutrition Foundation
London, UK

B Caballero
Johns Hopkins Bloomberg School of Public Health and
   Johns Hopkins University
Baltimore, MD, USA

E A Carrey
Institute of Child Health
London, UK

A Cassidy
School of Medicine
University of East Anglia
Norwich, UK

G E Caughey
Royal Adelaide Hospital
Adelaide, SA, Australia

J P Cegielski
Centers for Disease Control and Prevention
Atlanta, GA, USA

C M Champagne
Pennington Biomedical Research Center
Baton Rouge, LA, USA

S C Chen
US Department of Agriculture
Beltsville, MD, USA

L Cheskin
Johns Hopkins University
Baltimore, MD, USA

S Chung
Columbia University
New York, NY, USA

L G Cleland
Royal Adelaide Hospital
Adelaide, SA, Australia

L Cobiac
CSIRO Health Sciences and Nutrition
Adelaide, SA, Australia

G A Colditz
Harvard Medical School
Boston, MA, USA

T J Cole
Institute of Child Health
London, UK

L A Coleman
Marshfield Clinic Research Foundation
Marshfield, WI, USA

S Collier
Children's Hospital, Boston, Harvard Medical School,
   and Harvard School of Public Health
Boston, MA, USA

M Collins
Muckamore Abbey Hospital
Antrim, UK

K G Conner
Johns Hopkins Hospital
Baltimore, MD, USA

K C Costas
Children's Hospital Boston
Boston, MA, USA

R C Cottrell
The Sugar Bureau
London, UK

W A Coward
MRC Human Nutrition Research
Cambridge, UK

J M Cox
Johns Hopkins Hospital
Baltimore, MD, USA

S Cox
London School of Hygiene and Tropical Medicine
London, UK

P D'Acapito
Istituto Nazionale di Ricerca per gli Alimenti e la Nutrizione
Rome, Italy

S Daniell
Vanderbilt Center for Human Nutrition
Nashville, TN, USA

O Dary
The MOST Project
Arlington, VA, USA

T J David
University of Manchester
Manchester, UK

C P G M de Groot
Wageningen University
Wageningen, The Netherlands

M de Onis
World Health Organization
Geneva, Switzerland

M C de Souza
Universidad de Mogi das Cruzes
São Paulo, Brazil

R de Souza
University of Toronto
Toronto, ON, Canada

C H C Dejong
University Hospital Maastricht
Maastricht, The Netherlands

L Demeshlaira
Emory University
Atlanta, GA, USA

K G Dewey
University of California at Davis
Davis, CA, USA

H L Dewraj
The Aga Khan University
Karachi, Pakistan

C Doherty
MRC Keneba
The Gambia

C M Donangelo
Universidade Federal do Rio de Janeiro
Rio de Janeiro, Brazil

A Dornhorst
Imperial College at Hammersmith Hospital
London, UK

E Dowler
University of Warwick
Coventry, UK

J Dowsett
St Vincent's University Hospital
Dublin, Ireland

A K Draper
University of Westminster
London, UK

M L Dreyfuss
Johns Hopkins Bloomberg School of Public Health
Baltimore, MD, USA

R D'Souza
Queen Mary's, University of London
London, UK

C Duggan
Harvard Medical School
Boston, MA, USA

A G Dulloo
University of Fribourg
Fribourg, Switzerland

E B Duly
Ulster Hospital
Belfast, UK

J L Dupont
Florida State University
Tallahassee, FL, USA

J Dwyer
Tufts University
Boston, MA, USA

J Eaton–Evans
University of Ulster
Coleraine, UK

C A Edwards
University of Glasgow
Glasgow, UK

M Elia
University of Southampton
Southampton, UK

P W Emery
King's College London
London, UK

J L Ensunsa
University of California at Davis
Davis, CA, USA

C Feillet-Coudray
National Institute for Agricultural Research
Clermont-Ferrand, France

J D Fernstrom
University of Pittsburgh
Pittsburgh, PA, USA

M H Fernstrom
University of Pittsburgh
Pittsburgh, PA, USA

F Fidanza
University of Rome Tor Vergata
Rome, Italy

P Fieldhouse
The University of Manitoba
Winnipeg, MB, Canada

N Finer
Luton and Dunstable Hospital NHS Trust
Luton, UK

J Fiore
University of Westminster
London, UK

H C Freake
University of Connecticut
Storrs, CT, USA

J Freitas
Tufts University
Boston, MA, USA

R E Frisch
Harvard Center for Population and Development Studies
Cambridge, MA, USA

G Frost
Imperial College at Hammersmith Hospital
London, UK

G Frühbeck
Universidad de Navarra
Pamplona, Spain

D Gallagher
Columbia University
New York, NY, USA

L Galland
Applied Nutrition Inc.
New York, NY, USA

C Geissler
King's College London
London, UK

M E Gershwin
University of California at Davis
Davis, CA, USA

H Ghattas
London School of Hygiene and Tropical Medicine
London, UK

E L Gibson
University College London
London, UK

T P Gill
University of Sydney
Sydney, NSW, Australia

W Gilmore
University of Ulster
Coleraine, UK

G R Goldberg
MRC Human Nutrition Research
Cambridge, UK

J Gómez-Ambrosi
Universidad de Navarra
Pamplona, Spain

J M Graham
University of California at Davis
Davis, CA, USA

J Gray
Guildford, UK

J P Greaves
London, UK

M W Green
Aston University
Birmingham, UK

R Green
University of California
Davis, CA, USA

R F Grimble
University of Southampton
Southampton, UK

M Grønbæk
National Institute of Public Health
Copenhagen, Denmark

J D Groopman
Johns Hopkins University
Baltimore MD, USA

S M Grundy
University of Texas Southwestern Medical Center
Dallas, TX, USA

M A Grusak
Baylor College of Medicine
Houston, TX, USA

M Gueimonde
University of Turku
Turku, Finland

C S Gulotta
Johns Hopkins University and Kennedy
  Krieger Institute
Baltimore, MD, USA

P Haggarty
Rowett Research Institute
Aberdeen, UK

J C G Halford
University of Liverpool
Liverpool, UK

C H Halsted
University of California at Davis
Davis, CA, USA

J Hampsey
Johns Hopkins School of Medicine
Baltimore, MD, USA

E D Harris
Texas A&M University
College Station, TX, USA

Z L Harris
Johns Hopkins Hospital and School of Medicine
Baltimore, MD, USA

P J Havel
University of California at Davis
Davis, CA, USA

W W Hay Jr
University of Colorado Health Sciences Center
Aurora, CO, USA

R G Heine
University of Melbourne
Melbourne, VIC, Australia

R Heinzen
Johns Hopkins Bloomberg School of Public Health
Baltimore, MD, USA

A Herrera
University of Zaragoza
Zaragoza, Spain

B S Hetzel
Women's and Children's Hospital
North Adelaide, SA, Australia

A J Hill
University of Leeds
Leeds, UK

S A Hill
Southampton General Hospital
Southampton, UK

G A Hitman
Queen Mary's, University of London
London, UK

J M Hodgson
University of Western Australia
Perth, WA, Australia

M F Holick
Boston University Medical Center
Boston, MA, USA

C Hotz
National Institute of Public Health
Morelos, Mexico

R Houston
Emory University
Atlanta, GA, USA

H-Y Huang
Johns Hopkins University
Baltimore, MD, USA

J R Hunt
USDA-ARS Grand Forks Human Nutrition Research Center
Grand Forks, ND, USA

R Hunter
King's College London
London, UK

P Hyland
Nottingham Trent University
Nottingham, UK

B K Ishida
Agricultural Research Service
Albany, CA, USA

J Jacquet
University of Geneva
Geneva, Switzerland

M J James
Royal Adelaide Hospital
Adelaide, SA, Australia

W P T James
International Association for the Study of Obesity/
International Obesity Task Force Offices
London, UK

A G Jardine
University of Glasgow
Glasgow, UK

S A Jebb
MRC Human Nutrition Research
Cambridge, UK

K N Jeejeebhoy
University of Toronto
Toronto, ON, Canada

D J A Jenkins
University of Toronto
Toronto, ON, Canada

G L Jensen
Vanderbilt Center for Human Nutrition
Nashville, TN, USA

I T Johnson
Institute of Food Research
Norwich, UK

P A Judd
University of Central Lancashire
Preston, UK

M A Kalarchian
University of Pittsburgh
Pittsburgh, PA, USA

R M Katz
Johns Hopkins University School of Medicine and Mount
  Washington Pediatric Hospital
Baltimore, MD, USA

C L Keen
University of California at Davis
Davis, CA, USA

N L Keim
US Department of Agriculture
Davis, CA, USA

E Kelly
Harvard Medical School
Boston, MA, USA

C W C Kendall
University of Toronto
Toronto, ON, Canada

T W Kensler
Johns Hopkins University
Baltimore, MD, USA

J E Kerstetter
University of Connecticut
Storrs, CT, USA

M Kiely
University College Cork
Cork, Ireland

P Kirk
University of Ulster
Coleraine, UK

S F L Kirk
University of Leeds
Leeds, UK

P N Kirke
The Health Research Board
Dublin, Ireland

G L Klein
University of Texas Medical Branch at Galveston
Galveston TX, USA

R D W Klemm
Johns Hopkins University
Baltimore, MD, USA

D M Klurfeld
US Department of Agriculture
Beltville, MD, USA

P G Kopelman
Queen Mary's, University of London
London, UK

J Krick
Kennedy–Krieger Institute
Baltimore, MD, USA

D Kritchevsky
Wistar Institute
Philadelphia, PA, USA

R Lang
University of Teeside
Middlesbrough, UK

A Laurentin
Universidad Central de Venezuela
Caracas, Venezuela

A Laverty
Muckamore Abbey Hospital
Antrim, UK

M Lawson
Institute of Child Health
London, UK

F E Leahy
University of Auckland
Auckland, New Zealand

A R Leeds
King's College London
London, UK

J Leiper
University of Aberdeen
Aberdeen, UK

M D Levine
University of Pittsburgh
Pittsburgh, PA, USA

A H Lichtenstein
Tufts University
Boston MA, USA

E Lin
Emory University
Atlanta, GA, USA

L Lissner
Sahlgrenska Academy at Göteborg University
Göteborg, Sweden

C Lo
Children's Hospital, Boston, Harvard Medical School, and
Harvard School of Public Health
Boston, MA, USA

P A Lofgren
Oak Park, IL, USA

B Lönnerdal
University of California at Davis
Davis, CA, USA

M J Luetkemeier
Alma College
Alma, MI, USA

Y C Luiking
University Hospital Maastricht
Maastricht, The Netherlands

P G Lunn
University of Cambridge
Cambridge, UK

C K Lutter
Pan American Health Organization
Washington, DC, USA

A MacDonald
The Children's Hospital
Birmingham, UK

A Maqbool
The Children's Hospital of Philadelphia
Philadelphia, PA, USA

M D Marcus
University of Pittsburgh
Pittsburgh, PA, USA

E Marietta
The Mayo Clinic College of Medicine
Rochester, MN, USA

P B Mark
University of Glasgow
Glasgow, UK

V Marks
University of Surrey
Guildford, UK

D L Marsden
Children's Hospital Boston
Boston, MA, USA

R J Maughan
Loughborough University
Loughborough, UK

K C McCowen
Beth Israel Deaconess Medical Center and Harvard
Medical School
Boston, MA, USA

S S McDonald
Raleigh, NC, USA

S McLaren
London South Bank University
London, UK

J L McManaman
University of Colorado
Denver, CO, USA

D N McMurray
Texas A&M University
College Station, TX, USA

D J McNamara
Egg Nutrition Center
Washington, DC, USA

J McPartlin
Trinity College
Dublin, Ireland

R P Mensink
Maastricht University
Maastricht, The Netherlands

M Merialdi
World Health Organization
Geneva, Switzerland

A R Michell
St Bartholomew's Hospital
London, UK

J W Miller
UC Davis Medical Center
Sacramento, CA, USA

P Miller
Kennedy–Krieger Institute
Baltimore, MD, USA

D J Millward
University of Surrey
Guildford, UK

D M Mock
University of Arkansas for Medical Sciences
Little Rock, AR, USA

N Moore
John Hopkins School of Medicine
Baltimore, MD, USA

J O Mora
The MOST Project
Arlington, VA, USA

T Morgan
University of Melbourne
Melbourne, VIC, Australia

T A Mori
University of Western Australia
Perth, WA, Australia

J E Morley
St Louis University
St Louis, MO, USA

P A Morrissey
University College Cork
Cork, Ireland

M H Murphy
University of Ulster at Jordanstown
Jordanstown, UK

S P Murphy
University of Hawaii
Honolulu, HI, USA

J Murray
The Mayo Clinic College of Medicine
Rochester, MN, USA

R Nalubola
Center for Food Safety and Applied Nutrition,
US Food and Drug Administration, MD, USA

J L Napoli
University of California
Berkeley, CA, USA

V Nehra
The Mayo Clinic College of Medicine
Rochester, MN, USA

B Nejadnik
Johns Hopkins University
Baltimore, MD, USA

M Nelson
King's College London
London, UK

P Nestel
International Food Policy Research Institute
Washington, DC, USA

L M Neufeld
National Institute of Public Health
Cuernavaca, Mexico

M C Neville
University of Colorado
Denver, CO, USA

F Nielsen
Grand Forks Human Nutrition Research Center
Grand Forks, ND, USA

N Noah
London School of Hygiene and Tropical Medicine
London, UK

K O O'Brien
Johns Hopkins University
Baltimore, MD, USA

S H Oh
Johns Hopkins General Clinical Research Center
Baltimore, MD, USA

J M Ordovas
Tufts University
Boston, MA, USA

S E Ozanne
University of Cambridge
Cambridge, UK

D M Paige
Johns Hopkins Bloomberg School of Public Health
Baltimore, MD, USA

J P Pearson
University of Newcastle
Newcastle-upon-Tyne, UK

S S Percival
University of Florida
Gainesville, FL, USA

T Peters
King's College Hospital
London, UK

B J Petersen
Exponent, Inc.
Washington DC, USA

J C Phillips
BIBRA International Ltd
Carshalton, UK

M F Picciano
National Institutes of Health
Bethesda, MD, USA

A Pietrobelli
Verona University Medical School
Verona, Italy

S Pin
Johns Hopkins Hospital and School of Medicine
Baltimore, MD, USA

B M Popkin
University of North Carolina
Chapel Hill, NC, USA

E M E Poskitt
London School of Hygiene and Tropical Medicine
London, UK

A D Postle
University of Southampton
Southampton, UK

J Powell-Tuck
Queen Mary's, University of London
London, UK

V Preedy
King's College London
London, UK

N D Priest
Middlesex University
London, UK

R Rajendram
King's College London
London, UK

A Raman
University of Wisconsin–Madison
Madison, WI, USA

H A Raynor
Brown University
Providence, RI, USA

Y Rayssiguier
National Institute for Agricultural Research
Clermont-Ferrand, France

L N Richardson
United Nations World Food Programme
Rome, Italy

F J Rohr
Children's Hospital Boston
Boston, MA, USA

A R Rolla
Harvard Medical School
Boston, MA, USA

P Roncalés
University of Zaragoza
Zaragoza, Spain

A C Ross
The Pennsylvania State University
University Park, PA, USA

R Roubenoff
Millennium Pharmaceuticals, Inc.
Cambridge, MA, USA and Tufts University
Boston, MA, USA

D Rumsey
University of Sheffield
Sheffield, UK

C H S Ruxton
Nutrition Communications
Cupar, UK

J M Saavedra
John Hopkins School of Medicine
Baltimore, MD, USA

J E Sable
University of California at Davis
Davis, CA, USA

M J Sadler
MJSR Associates
Ashford, UK

N R Sahyoun
University of Maryland
College Park, MD, USA

S Salminen
University of Turku
Turku, Finland

M Saltmarsh
Alton, UK

J M Samet
Johns Hopkins Bloomberg School of Public Health
Baltimore, MD, USA

C P Sánchez-Castillo
National Institute of Medical Sciences and Nutrition
Salvador Zubirán, Tlalpan, Mexico

M Santosham
Johns Hopkins Bloomberg School of Public Health
Baltimore, MD, USA

C D Saudek
Johns Hopkins School of Medicine
Baltimore, MD, USA

A O Scheimann
Johns Hopkins School of Medicine
Baltimore, MD, USA

B Schneeman
University of California at Davis
Davis, CA, USA

D A Schoeller
University of Wisconsin–Madison
Madison, WI, USA

L Schuberth
Kennedy Krieger Institute
Baltimore, MD, USA

K J Schulze
Johns Hopkins Bloomberg School of Public Health
Baltimore, MD, USA

Y Schutz
University of Lausanne
Lausanne, Switzerland

K B Schwarz
Johns Hopkins School of Medicine
Baltimore, MD, USA

J M Scott
Trinity College Dublin
Dublin, Ireland

C Shaw
Royal Marsden NHS Foundation Trust
London, UK

J Shedlock
Johns Hopkins Hospital and School of Medicine
Baltimore, MD, USA

S M Shirreffs
Loughborough University
Loughborough, UK

R Shrimpton
Institute of Child Health
London, UK

H A Simmonds
Guy's Hospital
London, UK

A P Simopoulos
The Center for Genetics, Nutrition and Health
Washington, DC, USA

R J Smith
Brown Medical School
Providence, RI, USA

P B Soeters
University Hospital Maastricht
Maastricht, The Netherlands

N Solomons
Center for Studies of Sensory Impairment, Aging and
   Metabolism (CeSSIAM)
Guatemala City, Guatemala

J A Solon
MRC Laboratories Gambia
Banjul, The Gambia

K Srinath Reddy
All India Institute of Medical Sciences
New Delhi, India

S Stanner
British Nutrition Foundation
London, UK

J Stevens
University of North Carolina at Chapel Hill
Chapel Hill, NC, USA

J J Strain
University of Ulster
Coleraine, UK

R J Stratton
University of Southampton
Southampton, UK

R J Stubbs
The Rowett Research Institute
Aberdeen, UK

C L Stylianopoulos
Johns Hopkins University
Baltimore, MD, USA

A W Subudhi
University of Colorado at Colorado
Colorado Springs, CO, USA

J Sudagani
Queen Mary's, University of London
London, UK

S A Tanumihardjo
University of Wisconsin-Madison
Madison, WI, USA

J A Tayek
Harbor–UCLA Medical Center
Torrance, CA, USA

E H M Temme
University of Leuven
Leuven, Belgium

H S Thesmar
Egg Nutrition Center
Washington, DC, USA

B M Thomson
Rowett Research Institute
Aberdeen, UK

D I Thurnham
University of Ulster
Coleraine, UK

L Tolentino
National Institute of Public Health
Cuernavaca, Mexico

D L Topping
CSIRO Health Sciences and Nutrition
Adelaide, SA, Australia

B Torun
Center for Research and Teaching in Latin
   America (CIDAL)
Guatemala City, Guatemala

M G Traber
Oregon State University
Corvallis, OR, USA

T R Trinick
Ulster Hospital
Belfast, UK

K P Truesdale
University of North Carolina at Chapel Hill
Chapel Hill, NC, USA

N M F Trugo
Universidade Federal do Rio de Janeiro
Rio de Janeiro, Brazil

P M Tsai
Harvard Medical School
Boston, MA, USA

K L Tucker
Tufts University
Boston, MA, USA

O Tully
St Vincent's University Hospital
Dublin, Ireland

E C Uchegbu
Royal Hallamshire Hospital
Sheffield, UK

M C G van de Poll
University Hospital Maastricht
Maastricht, The Netherlands

W A van Staveren
Wageningen University
Wageningen, The Netherlands

J Villar
World Health Organization
Geneva, Switzerland

M L Wahlqvist
Monash University
Victoria, VIC, Australia

A F Walker
The University of Reading
Reading, UK

P A Watkins
Kennedy Krieger Institute and Johns Hopkins
   University School of Medicine
Baltimore, MD, USA

A A Welch
University of Cambridge
Cambridge, UK

R W Welch
University of Ulster
Coleraine, UK

K P West Jr
Johns Hopkins University
Baltimore, MD, USA

S Whybrow
The Rowett Research Institute
Aberdeen, UK

D H Williamson
Radcliffe Infirmary
Oxford, UK

M-M G Wilson
St Louis University
St Louis, MO, USA

R R Wing
Brown University
Providence, RI, USA

C K Winter
University of California at Davis
Davis, CA, USA

H Wiseman
King's College London
London, UK

M Wolraich
Vanderbilt University
Nashville, TN, USA

R J Wood
Tufts University
Boston, MA, USA

X Xu
Johns Hopkins Hospital and School of Medicine
Baltimore, MD, USA

Z Yang
University of Wisconsin-Madison
Madison, WI, USA

A A Yates
ENVIRON Health Sciences
Arlington, VA, USA

S H Zeisel
University of North Carolina at Chapel Hill
Chapel Hill, NC, USA

X Zhu
University of North Carolina at Chapel Hill
Chapel Hill, NC, USA

S Zidenberg-Cherr
University of California at Davis
Davis, CA, USA

T R Ziegler
Emory University
Atlanta, GA, USA

CONTENTS

VOLUME 1

B

C

G

K

L

M

N

VOLUME 4

R

S

Acids *see* **Electrolytes**: Acid-Base Balance

ADIPOSE TISSUE

G Frühbeck and J Gómez-Ambrosi, Universidad de Navarra, Pamplona, Spain

© 2005 Elsevier Ltd. All rights reserved.

Introduction

The role of white adipose tissue (WAT) in storing and releasing lipids for oxidation by skeletal muscle and other tissues became so firmly established decades ago that a persistent lack of interest hindered the study of the extraordinarily dynamic behavior of adipocytes. However, disentangling the neuroendocrine systems that regulate energy homeostasis and adiposity has jumped to a first-priority challenge, with the recognition of obesity as one of the major public health problems. Strictly speaking, obesity is not defined as an excess of body weight but as an increased adipose tissue accretion, to the extent that health may be adversely affected. Therefore, in the last decades, adipose tissue has become the research focus of biomedical scientists for epidemiological, pathophysiological, and molecular reasons. Although the primary role of adipocytes is to store triglycerides during periods of caloric excess and to mobilize this reserve when expenditure exceeds intake, it is now widely recognized that adipose tissue lies at the heart of a complex network that participates in the regulation of a variety of quite diverse biological functions (**Figure 1**).

Development

Adipose tissue develops extensively in homeotherms with the proportion to body weight varying greatly among species. Adipocytes differentiate from stellate or fusiform precursor cells of mesenchymal origin. There are two processes of adipose tissue formation. In the primary fat formation, which takes place relatively early (in human fetuses the first traces of a fat organ are detectable between the 14th and 16th weeks of prenatal life), gland-like aggregations of epitheloid precursor cells, called lipoblasts or preadipocytes, are laid down in specific locations and accumulate multiple lipid droplets becoming brown adipocytes. The secondary fat formation takes place later in fetal life (after the 23rd week of gestation) as well as in the early postnatal period, whereby the differentiation of other fusiform precursor cells that accumulate lipid to ultimately coalesce into a single large drop per cell leads to the dissemination of fat depots formed by unilocular white adipocytes in many areas of connective tissue. Adipose tissue may be partitioned by connective tissue septa into lobules. The number of fat lobules remains constant, while in the subsequent developmental phases the lobules continuously increase in size. At the sites of early fat development, a multilocular morphology of adipocytes predominates, reflecting the early developmental stage. Microscopic studies have shown that the second trimester may be a critical period for the development of obesity in later life. At the beginning of the third trimester, adipocytes are present in the main fat depots but are still relatively small. During embryonic development it is important to emphasize the temporospacial tight coordination of angiogenesis with the formation of fat cell clusters. At birth, body fat has been reported to

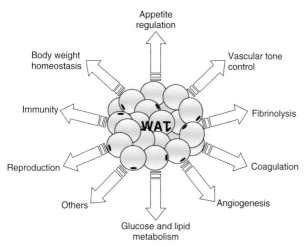

Figure 1 Dynamic view of white adipose tissue based on the pleiotropic effects on quite diverse physiological functions.

account for approximately 16% of total body weight (with brown fat constituting 2–5%) with an increase in body fat of around 0.7–2.8 kg during the first year of life.

Adipogenesis, i.e., the development of adipose tissue, varies according to sex and age. Furthermore, the existence of sensitive periods for changes in adipose tissue cellularity throughout life has been postulated. In this regard, two peaks of accelerated adipose mass enlargement have been established, namely after birth and between 9 and 13 years of age. The capacity for cell proliferation and differentiation is highest during the first year of life, while it is less pronounced in the years before puberty. Thereafter, the rate of cell proliferation slows down during adolescence and, in weight stable individuals, remains fairly constant throughout adulthood. In case of a maintained positive energy balance adipose mass expansion takes places initially by an enlargement of the existing fat cells. The perpetuation of this situation ends up in severe obesity where the total fat cell number can be easily trebled. Childhood-onset obesity is characterized by a combination of fat cell hyperplasia and hypertrophy, whereas in adult-onset obesity a hypertrophic growth predominates. However, it has been recently shown that adult humans are capable of new adipocyte formation, with fat tissue containing a significant proportion of cells with the ability to undergo differentiation. Interestingly, the hyperplasic growth of fat cells in adults does not take place until the existing adipocytes reach a critical cell size.

Initially, excess energy storage starts as hypertrophic obesity resulting from the accumulation of excess lipid in a normal number of unilocular adipose cells. In this case, adipocytes may be four times their normal size. If the positive energy balance is maintained, a hyperplasic or hypercellular obesity characterized by a greater than normal number of cells is developed. Recent observations regarding the occurrence of apoptosis in WAT have changed the traditional belief that acquisition of fat cells is irreversible. The adipose lineage originates from multipotent mesenchymal stem cells that develop into adipoblasts (**Figure 2**). Commitment of these adipoblasts gives rise to preadipose cells (preadipocytes), which are cells that have expressed early but not late markers and have yet to accumulate triacylglycerol stores (**Figure 3**). Multipotent stem cells and adipoblasts, which are found during embryonic development, are still present postnatally. The relationship between brown and white fat during development has not been completely solved. Brown adipocytes can be detected among all white fat depots in variable amounts depending on species, localization, and environmental temperature. The transformation of characteristic brown adipocytes into white fat cells can take place rapidly in numerous species and depots during postnatal development.

The morphological and functional changes that take place in the course of adipogenesis represent a shift in transcription factor expression and activity leading from a primitive, multipotent state to a final phenotype characterized by alterations in cell shape and lipid accumulation. Various redundant signaling pathways and transcription factors directly influence fat cell development by converging in the upregulation of PPARγ, which embodies a common and essential regulator of adipogenesis as well as of adipocyte hypertrophy. Among the broad panoply of transcription factors, C/EBPs and the basic helix-loop-helix family (ADD1/SREBP-1c) also stand out together with their link with the existing nutritional status. The transcriptional repression of adipogenesis includes both active and passive mechanisms. The former directly interferes with the transcriptional machinery, while the latter is based on the binding of negative regulators to yield inactive forms of known activators.

Hormones, cytokines, growth factors, and nutrients influence the dynamic changes related to adipose tissue mass as well as its pattern of distribution (**Figure 4**). The responsiveness of fat cells to neurohumoral signals may vary according to peculiarities in the adipose lineage stage at the moment of exposure. Moreover, the simultaneous presence of some adipogenic factors at specific threshold concentrations may be a necessary requirement to trigger terminal differentiation.

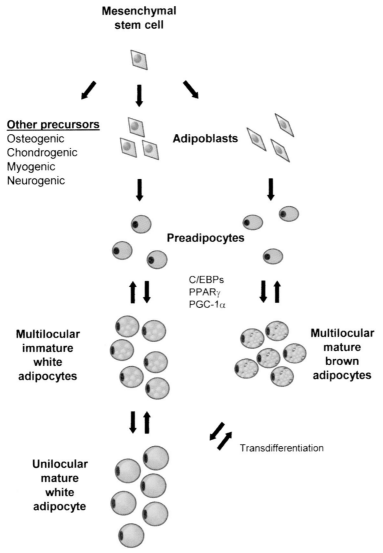

Figure 2 Schematic diagram of the histogenesis of white and brown adipocytes. C/EBPs, CCAAT/enhancer binding proteins; PGC-1α, peroxisome proliferator-activated receptor-γ coactivator-1; PPARγ, peroxisome proliferator-activated receptor-γ.

Structure

Adipose tissue is a special loose connective tissue dominated by adipocytes. The name of these cells is based on the presence of a large lipid droplet with 'adipo' derived from the Latin *adeps* meaning 'pertaining to fat.' In adipose tissue, fat cells are individually held in place by delicate reticular fibers clustering in lobular masses bounded by fibrous septa surrounded by a rich capillary network. In adults, adipocytes may comprise around 90% of adipose mass accounting only for roughly 25% of the total cell population. Thus, adipose tissue itself is composed not only of adipocytes, but also other cell types called the stroma-vascular fraction, comprising blood cells, endothelial cells, pericytes, and adipose precursor cells among others (**Figure 5**);

these account for the remaining 75% of the total cell population, representing a wide range of targets for extensive autocrine-paracrine cross-talk.

Adipocytes, which are typically spherical and vary enormously in size (20–200 μm in diameter, with variable volumes ranging from a few picoliters to about 3 nanoliters), are embedded in a connective tissue matrix and are uniquely adapted to store and release energy. Surplus energy is assimilated by adipocytes and stored as lipid droplets. The stored fat is composed mainly of triacylglycerols (about 95% of the total lipid content comprised principally of oleic and palmitic acids) and to a smaller degree of diacylglycerols, phospholipids, unesterified fatty acids, and cholesterol. To accommodate the lipids adipocytes are capable of changing their

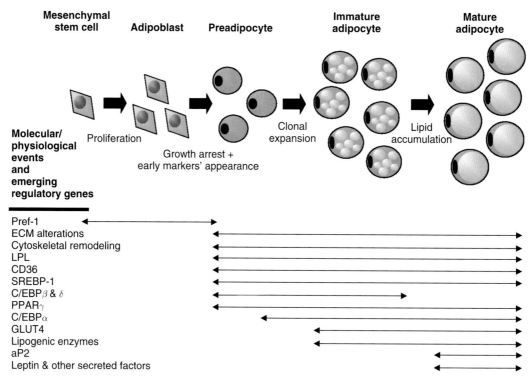

Figure 3   Multistep process of adipogenesis together with events and participating regulatory elements. aP2, adipocyte fatty acid binding protein; C/EBPα, CCAAT/enhancer binding protein α; C/EBPβ & δ, CCAAT/enhancer binding protein β & δ; CD36, fatty acid translocase; ECM, extracellular matrix; GLUT4, glucose transporter type 4; LPL, lipoprotein lipase; PPARγ, peroxisome proliferator-activated receptor-γ; Pref-1, preadipocyte factor-1; SREBP-1, sterol regulatory element binding protein-1.

diameter 20-fold and their volumes by several thousand-fold. However, fat cells do not increase in size indefinitely. Once a maximum capacity is attained, which in humans averages 1000 picoliters, the

formation of new adipocytes from the precursor pool takes place.

Histologically, the interior of adipocytes appears unstained since the techniques of standard tissue

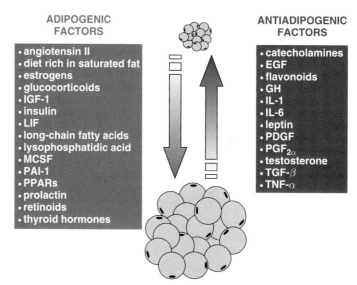

Figure 4   Factors exerting a direct effect on adipose mass. EGF, epidermal growth factor; GH, growth hormone; IGF-1, insulin-like growth factor-1; IL-1, interleukin-1; IL-6, interleukin-6; LIF, leukemia inhibitory factor; MCSF, macrophage colony stimulating factor; PAI-1, plasminogen activator inhibitor-1; PDGF, platelet-derived growth factor; PGF$_{2\alpha}$, prostaglandin F$_{2\alpha}$; PPARs, peroxisome proliferator-activated receptors; TGF-β, transforming growth factor-β; TNF-α, tumor necrosis factor-α.

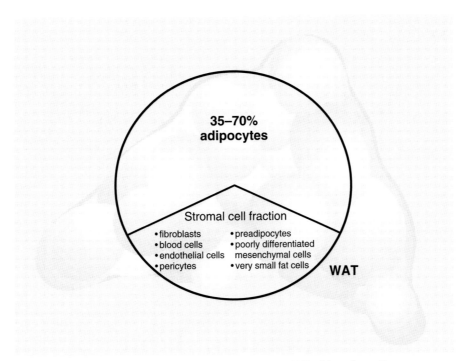

Figure 5 Schematic representation of cell types present in adipose tissue. WAT, white adipose tissue.

preparation dissolve out the lipids, leaving a thin rim of eosinophilic cytoplasm that typically loses its round shape during tissue processing, thus contributing to the sponge-like appearance of WAT in routine preparations for light microscopy (**Figure 6** and **Figure 7**). Owing to the fact that about 90% of the cell volume is a lipid droplet, the small dark nucleus becomes a flattened semilunar structure pushed against the edge of the cell and the thin cytoplasmic rim is also pushed to the periphery of the adipocytes. Mature white adipose cells contain a single large lipid droplet and are described as unilocular. However, developing white adipocytes are transiently multilocular containing multiple lipid droplets before these finally coalesce into a single large drop (**Figure 8**). The nucleus is round or oval in young fat cells, but is cup-shaped and peripherally displaced in mature adipocytes. The cytoplasm is stretched to form a thin sheath around the fat globule, although a relatively large volume is concentrated around the nucleus. A thin external lamina called basal lamina surrounds the cell. The smooth cell membrane shows no microvilli but has abundant smooth micropinocytotic invaginations that often fuse to form small vacuoles appearing as rosette-like configurations (**Figure 9**). Mitochondria are few in number with loosely arranged membranous cristae. The Golgi zone is small and the cytoplasm is filled with free ribosomes, but contains only a limited number of short profiles of the

granular endoplasmic reticulum. Occasional lysosomes can be found. The coalescent lipid droplets contain a mixture of neutral fats, triglycerides, fatty acids, phospholipids, and cholesterol. A thin interface membrane separates the lipid droplet from the cytoplasmic matrix. Peripheral to this membrane is a system of parallel meridional thin filaments. Because of the size of these cells, relative to the thickness of the section, the nucleus (accounting for only one-fortieth of the cell volume) may not always be present in the section. Unilocular adipocytes usually appear in clumps near blood vessels, which is reasonable since the source and dispersion of material stored in fat cells depends on transportation by the vascular system.

Brown fat is a specialized type of adipose tissue that plays an important role in body temperature regulation. In the newborn brown fat is well developed in the neck and interscapular region. It has a limited distribution in childhood, and occurs only to a small degree in adult humans, while it is present in significant amounts in rodents and hibernating animals. The brown color is derived from a rich vascular network and abundant mitochondria and lysosomes. The individual multilocular adipocytes are frothy appearing cells due to the fact that the lipid, which does not coalesce as readily as in white fat cells and is normally stored in multiple small droplets, has been leached out during tissue

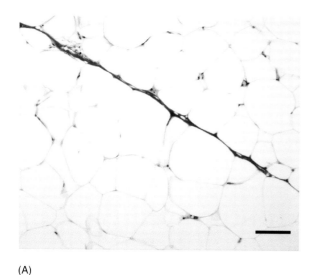

(A)

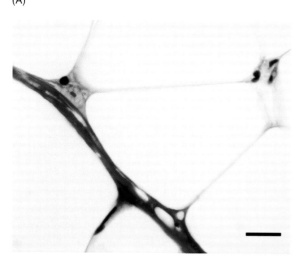

(B)

Figure 6 (A) Human subcutaneous white adipose tissue with Masson trichrome staining (10×; bar = 100 μm). (B) Same tissue at a higher magnification (40×; bar = 25 μm). (Courtesy of Dr. M A Burrell and M Archanco, University of Navarra, Spain.)

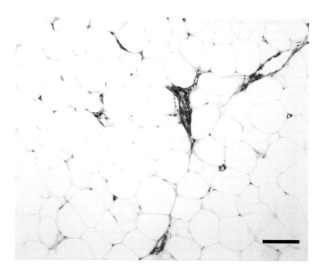

(A)

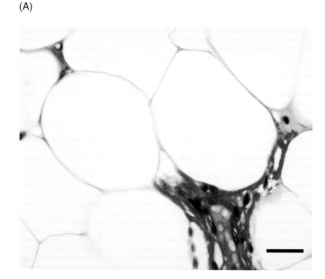

(B)

Figure 7 (A) Human omental white adipose tissue with Masson trichrome staining (10×; bar = 100 μm). (B) Same tissue at a higher magnification (40×; bar = 25 μm). (Courtesy of Dr. M A Burrell and M Archanco, University of Navarra, Spain.)

processing (**Figure 10**). The spherical nuclei are centrally or eccentrically located within the cell. Compared to the unilocular white adipocytes, the cytoplasm of the multilocular brown fat cell is relatively abundant and strongly stained because of the numerous mitochondria present. The mitochondria are involved in the oxidation of the stored lipid, but because they exhibit a reduced potential to carry out oxidative phosphorylation, the energy produced is released in the form of heat due to the uncoupling activity of UCP and not captured in adenosine triphosphate (ATP). Therefore, brown adipose tissue is extremely well vascularized so that the blood is warmed when it passes through the active tissue.

Distribution

White adipose tissue may represent the largest endocrine tissue of the whole organism, especially in overweight and obese patients. The anatomical distribution of individual fat pads dispersed throughout the whole body and not connected to each other contradicts the classic organ-specific localization. WAT exhibits clear, regional differences in its sites of predilection (**Table 1**). The hypodermal region invariably contains fat, except in a few places such as the eyelids and the scrotum. Adipocytes also accumulate around organs like the kidneys and adrenals, in the coronary sulcus of the heart, in bone marrow, mesentery, and omentum. Unilocular fat is

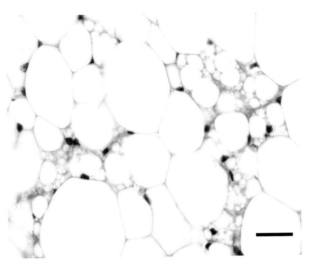

Figure 8 Paraffin section of rat abdominal white adipose tissue with a hematoxylin and eosin stain showing the simultaneous presence of uni- and multilocular adipocytes (40×; bar = 25 µm). (Courtesy of Dr. M A Burrell and M Archanco, University of Navarra, Spain.)

widely distributed in the subcutaneous tissue of humans but exhibits quantitative regional differences that are influenced by age and sex. In infants and young children there is a continuous subcutaneous fat layer, the panniculus adiposus, over the whole body. This layer thins out in some areas in adults but persists and grows thicker in certain other regions. The sites differ in their distribution among sexes, being responsible for the characteristic body form of males and females, termed android and ginecoid fat distribution. In males, the main regions include the nape of the neck, the subcutaneous area over the deltoid and triceps muscles, and the lumbosacral region. In females, subcutaneous fat is most abundant in the buttocks, epitrochanteric region, anterior and lateral aspects of the thighs, as well as the breasts. Additionally, extensive fat depots are found in the omentum, mesenteries, and the retroperitoneal area of both sexes. In well-nourished, sedentary individuals, the fat distribution persists and becomes more obvious with advancing age with males tending to deposit more fat in the visceral compartment. Depot-specific differences may be related not only to the metabolism of fat cells but also to their capacity to form new adipocytes. Additionally, regional differences may result from variations in hormone receptor distribution as well as from specific local environmental characteristics as a consequence of differences in innervation and vascularization.

Regional distribution of body fat is known to be an important indicator for metabolic and cardiovascular alterations in some individuals.

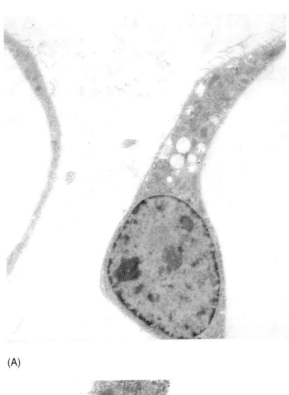

(A)

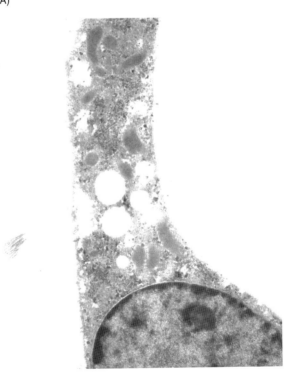

(B)

Figure 9 (A) Transmission electron micrographs with the characteristically displaced nucleus to one side and slightly flattened by the accumulated lipid. The cytoplasm of the fat cell is reduced to a thin rim around the lipid droplet (7725×). (B) The cytoplasm contains several small lipid droplets that have not yet coalesced. A few filamentous mitochondria, occasional cisternae of endoplasmic reticulum, and a moderate number of free ribosomes are usually visible (15 000×). (Courtesy of Dr. M A Burrell and M Archanco, University of Navarra, Spain.)

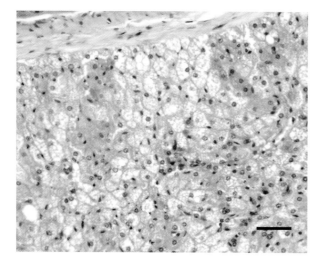

(A)

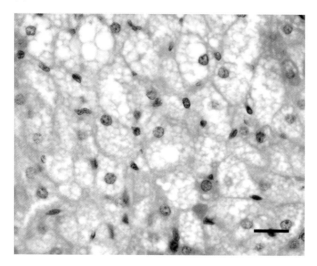

(B)

Figure 10 (A) Paraffin section of rat brown adipose tissue with a hematoxylin and eosin stain (20×; bar = 50 μm). (B) Same tissue at a higher magnification (40×; bar = 25 μm). (Courtesy of Dr. M A Burrell and M Archanco, University of Navarra.)

The observation that the topographic distribution of adipose tissue is relevant to understanding the relation of obesity to disturbances in glucose and lipid metabolism was formulated before the 1950s. Since then numerous prospective studies have revealed that android or male-type obesity correlates more often with an elevated mortality and risk for the development of diabetes mellitus type 2, dyslipidemia, hypertension, and atherosclerosis than gynoid or female-type obesity. Obesity has been reported to cause or exacerbate a large number of health problems with a known impact on both life expectancy and quality of life. In this respect, the association of increased adiposity is accompanied by important pathophysiological

Table 1 Distribution of main human adipose tissue depots

Subcutaneous (approx. 80%; deep + superficial layers)
Truncal
– Cervical
– Dorsal
– Lumbar
Abdominal
Gluteofemoral
Mammary

Visceral (approx. 20%; thoracic-abdominal-pelvic)
Intrathoracic (extra-intrapericardial)
Intra-abdominopelvic
– Intraperitoneal
    Omental (greater and lesser omentum)
    Mesenteric (epiplon, small intestine, colon, rectum)
    Umbilical
– Extraperitoneal
    Peripancreatic (infiltrated with brown adipocytes)
    Perirenal (infiltrated with brown adipocytes)
– Intrapelvic
    Gonadal (parametrial, retrouterine, retropubic)
    Urogenital (paravesical, para-retrorectal)

Intraparenchymatous (physiologically or pathologically)
Inter-intramuscular and perimuscular (inside the muscle fascia)
Perivascular
Paraosseal (interface between bone and muscle)
Ectopic (steatosis, intramyocardial, lypodystrophy, etc.)

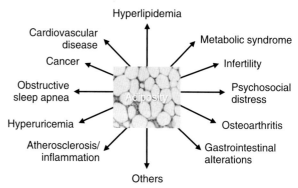

Figure 11 Main comorbidities associated with increased adiposity.

alterations, which lead to the development of a wide range of comorbidities (**Figure 11**).

Function

Although many cell types contain small reserves of carbohydrate and lipid, the adipose tissue is the body's most capacious energy reservoir. Because of the high energy content per unit weight of fat as well as its hydrophobicity, the storage of energy in the form of triglycerides is a highly efficient biochemical phenomenon (1 g of adipose tissue contains around 800 mg triacylglycerol and only about 100 mg of water). It represents quantitatively the most variable component of the organism, ranging from a few per cent of body weight in top athletes to more than half of the total body weight in severely obese patients. The normal range is about 10–20% body fat for males and around 20–30% for females, accounting approximately for a 2-month energy reserve. During pregnancy most species accrue additional reserves of adipose tissue to help support the development of the fetus and to further facilitate the lactation period.

Energy balance regulation is an extremely complex process composed of multiple interacting homeostatic and behavioral pathways aimed at maintaining constant energy stores. It is now evident that body weight control is achieved through highly orchestrated interactions between nutrient selection, organoleptic influences, and neuroendocrine responses to diet as well as being influenced by genetic and environmental factors. The concept that circulating signals generated in proportion to body fat stores influence appetite and energy expenditure in a coordinated manner to regulate body weight was proposed almost 50 years ago. According to this model, changes in energy balance sufficient to alter body fat stores are signaled via one or more circulating factors acting in the brain to elicit compensatory changes in order to match energy intake to energy expenditure. This was formulated as the 'lipostatic theory' assuming that as adipose tissue mass enlarges, a factor that acts as a sensing

hormone or 'lipostat' in a negative feedback control from adipose tissue to hypothalamic receptors informs the brain about the abundance of body fat, thereby allowing feeding behavior, metabolism, and endocrine physiology to be coupled to the nutritional state of the organism. The existing body of evidence gathered in the last decades through targeted expression or knockout of specific genes involved in different steps of the pathways controlling food intake, body weight, adiposity, or fat distribution has clearly contributed to unraveling the underlying mechanisms of energy homeostasis. The findings have fostered the notion of a far more complex system than previously thought, involving the integration of a plethora of factors.

The identification of adipose tissue as a multifunctional organ as opposed to a passive organ for the storage of excess energy in the form of fat has been brought about by the emerging body of evidence gathered during the last few decades. This pleiotropic nature is based on the ability of fat cells to secrete a large number of hormones, growth factors, enzymes, cytokines, complement factors, and matrix proteins, collectively termed adipokines or adipocytokines (**Table 2, Figure 12**), at the same time as expressing receptors for most of these factors (**Table 3**), which warrants extensive cross-talk at a local and systemic level in response to specific external stimuli or metabolic changes. The vast majority of adipocyte-derived factors have been shown to be dysregulated in alterations accompanied by changes

Table 2 Relevant factors secreted by adipose tissue into the bloodstream

Molecule	Function/effect
Adiponectin/ACRP30/AdipoQ/ apM1/GBP28	Plays a protective role in the pathogenesis of type 2 diabetes and cardiovascular diseases
Adipsin	Possible link between the complement pathway and adipose tissue metabolism
Angiotensinogen	Precursor of angiotensin II; regulator of blood pressure and electrolyte homeostasis
ASP	Influences the rate of triacylglycerol synthesis in adipose tissue
FFA	Oxidized in tissues to produce local energy. Serve as a substrate for triglyceride and structural molecules synthesis. Involved in the development of insulin resistance
Glycerol	Structural component of the major classes of biological lipids and gluconeogenic precursor
IGF-I	Stimulates proliferation of a wide variety of cells and mediates many of the effects of growth hormone
IL-6	Implicated in host defense, glucose and lipid metabolism, and regulation of body weight
Leptin	Signals to the brain about body fat stores. Regulation of appetite and energy expenditure. Wide variety of physiological functions
NO	Important regulator of vascular tone. Pleiotropic involvement in pathophysiological conditions
PAI-1	Potent inhibitor of the fibrinolytic system
PGI_2 & $PGF_{2\alpha}$	Implicated in regulatory functions such as inflammation and blood clotting, ovulation, menstruation, and acid secretion
Resistin	Putative role in insulin resistance May participate in inflammation
TNF-α	Interferes with insulin receptor signaling and is a possible cause of the development of insulin resistance in obesity
VEGF	Stimulation of angiogenesis

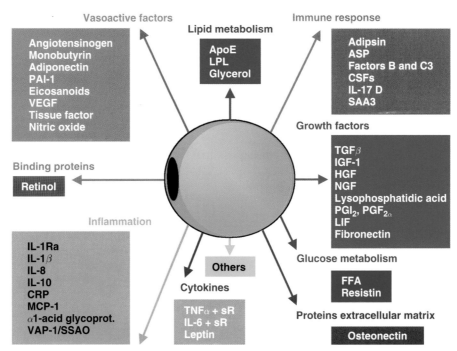

Figure 12 Factors secreted by white adipose tissue, which underlie the multifunctional nature of this endocrine organ. Although due to their pleiotropic effects some of the elements might be included in more than one physiological role, they have been included only under one function for simplicity reasons. apoE, apolipoprotein E; ASP, acylation-stimulating protein; CRP, C-reactive protein; CSFs, colony-stimulating factors; FFA, free fatty acids; HGF, hepatocyte growth factor; IGF-1, insulin-like growth factor-1; IL-10, interleukin-10; IL-17 D, interleukin-17 D; IL-1Ra, interleukin-1 receptor antagonist; IL-1β, interleukin-1β; IL-6, interleukin, 6; IL-8, interleukin-8; LIF, leukemia inhibitory factor; LPL, lipoprotein lipase; MCP-1, monocyte chemoattractant protein-1; NGF, nerve growth factor; PAI-1, plasminogen activator inhibitor -1; PGF$_{2\alpha}$, prostaglandin F$_{2\alpha}$; PGI$_2$, prostacyclin; SAA3, serum amyloid A3; sR, soluble receptor; TGF-β, transforming growth factor-β; TNF-α, tumor necrosis factor-α; VAP-1/SSAO, vascular adhesion protein-1/semicarbazide-sensitive amine oxidase; VEGF, vascular endothelial growth factor.

in adipose tissue mass such as overfeeding and lipodystrophy, thus providing evidence for their implication in the etiopathology and comorbidities asssociated with obesity and cachexia.

WAT is actively involved in cell function regulation through a complex network of endocrine, paracrine, and autocrine signals that influence the response of many tissues, including hypothalamus, pancreas, liver, skeletal muscle, kidneys, endothelium, and immune system, among others. Adipose tissue serves the functions of being a store for reserve energy, insulation against heat loss through the skin, and a protective padding of certain organs. A rapid turnover of stored fat can take place, and with only a few exceptions (orbit, major joints as well as palm and foot sole), the adipose tissue can be used up almost completely during starvation. Adipocytes are uniquely equipped to participate in the regulation of other functions such as reproduction, immune response, blood pressure control, coagulation, fibrinolysis, and angiogenesis, among others. This multifunctional nature is based on the existence of the full complement of enzymes, regulatory proteins, hormones, cytokines, and receptors needed to

carry out an extensive cross-talk at both a local and systemic level in response to specific external stimuli or neuroendocrine changes. This secretory nature has prompted the view of WAT as an extremely active endocrine tissue. Interestingly, the high number and ample spectrum of genes found to be expressed in WAT together with the changes observed in samples of obese patients substantiates the view of an extraordinarily active and plastic tissue. The complex and complementary nature of the expression profile observed in adipose tissue from obese organisms reflects a plethora of adaptive changes affecting crucial physiological functions that may need to be further explored through genomic and proteomic approaches.

The endocrine activity of WAT was postulated almost 20 years ago when the tissue's ability for steroid hormone interconversion was alluded to. In recent years, especially since the discovery of leptin, the list of adipocyte-derived factors has been increasing at a phenomenal pace. Another way of addressing the production of adipose-derived factors is by focusing on the function they are implicated in (**Figure 12**). One of the best known

Table 3 Main receptors expressed by adipose tissue

Receptor	Main effect of receptor activation on adipocyte metabolism
Hormone-cytokine receptors	
Adenosine	Inhibition of lipolysis
Adiponectin (AdipoR1 & AdipoR2)	Regulation of insulin sensitivity and fatty acid oxidation
Angiotensin II	Increase of lipogenesis
	Stimulation of prostacyclin production by mature fat cells.
	Interaction with insulin in regulation of adipocyte metabolism
GH	Induction of leptin and IGF-I expression. Stimulation of lipolysis
IGF-I & -II	Inhibition of lipolysis. Stimulation of glucose transport and oxidation
IL-6	LPL activity inhibition. Induction of lipolysis
Insulin	Inhibition of lipolysis and stimulation of lipogenesis. Induction of glucose uptake and oxidation. Stimulation of leptin expression
Leptin (OB-R)	Stimulation of lipolysis. Autocrine regulation of leptin expression
NPY-Y1 & Y5	Inhibition of lipolysis. Induction of leptin expression
Prostaglandin	Strong antilypolitic effects (PGE_2). Modulation of preadipocyte differentiation ($PGF_{2\alpha}$ and PGI_2)
TGF-β	Potent inhibition of adipocyte differentiation
TNF-α	Stimulation of lipolysis. Regulation of leptin secretion. Potent inhibition of adipocyte differentiation. Involvement in development of insulin resistance
VEGF	Stimulation of angiogenesis
Catecholamine-nervous system receptors	
Muscarinic	Inhibition of lipolysis
Nicotinic	Stimulation of lipolysis
α_1-AR	Induction of inositol phosphate production and PKC activation
α_2-AR	Inhibition of lipolysis. Regulation of preadipocyte growth
β_1-, β_2- & β_3-AR	Stimulation of lipolysis. Induction of thermogenesis. Reduction of leptin mRNA levels
Nuclear receptors	
Androgen	Control of adipose tissue development (antiadipogenic signals). Modulation of leptin expression
Estrogen	Control of adipose tissue development (proadipogenic signals). Modulation of leptin expression
Glucocorticoids	Stimulation of adipocyte differentiation
PPARδ	Regulation of fat metabolism. Plays a central role in fatty acid-controlled differentiation of preadipose cells
PPARγ	Induction of adipocyte differentiation and insulin sensitivity
RAR/RXR	Regulation of adipocyte differentiation
T_3	Stimulation of lipolysis. Regulation of leptin secretion. Induction of adipocyte differentiation. Regulation of insulin effects
Lipoprotein receptors	
HDL	Clearance and metabolism of HDL
LDL	Stimulation of cholesterol uptake
VLDL	Binding and internalization of VLDL particles. Involvement in lipid accumulation

Abbreviations: ACRP30, adipocyte complement-related protein of 30 kDa; apM1, adipose most abundant gene transcript 1; ASP, acylation-stimulating protein; FFA, free fatty acids; GBP28, gelatin-binding protein 28; GH, growth hormone; HDL, high density lipoprotein; IGF, insulin-like growth factor; IL-6, interleukin 6; LDL, low density lipoprotein; LPL, lipoprotein lipase; NO, nitric oxide; NPY-Y1 & -Y5, neuropeptide receptors Y-1 & -5; OB-R, leptin receptor; PAI-1, plasminogen activator inhibitor -1; PGE_2, prostaglandin E_2; $PGF_{2\alpha}$, prostaglandin $F_{2\alpha}$; PGI_2, prostacyclin; PPAR, peroxisome proliferator-activated receptor; RAR, retinoic acid receptor; RXR, retinoid x receptor; T3, triiodothyronine; TGF-β, transforming growth factor-β; TNF-α, tumor necrosis factor-α; VEGF, vascular endothelial growth factor; VLDL, very low-density lipoprotein; α_1- & α_2-AR, α_1- & α_2-adrenergic receptors; β_1-, β_2- & β_3-AR, β_1-, β_2- & β_3 adrenergic receptors.

aspects of WAT physiology relates to the synthesis of products involved in lipid metabolism such as perilipin, adipocyte lipid-binding protein (ALBP, FABP4, or aP2), CETP (cholesteryl ester transfer protein), and retinol binding protein (RBP). Adipose tissue has also been identified as a source of production of factors with immunological properties participating in immunity and stress responses, as is the case for ASP (acylation-simulating protein) and metallothionein. More recently, the pivotal role of adipocyte-derived factors in cardiovascular function control such as angiotensinogen, adiponectin, peroxisome proliferator-activated receptor γ angiopoietin related protein/fasting-induced adipose factor (PGAR/FIAF), and C-reactive protein (CRP) has been established. A further subsection of proteins produced by adipose tissue concerns other factors with an autocrine-paracrine function like

PPAR-γ (peroxisome proliferator-activated receptor), IGF-1, monobutyrin, and the UCPs.

It is generally assumed that under normal physiological circumstances adult humans are practically devoid of functional brown adipose tissue. As is the case in other larger mammals the functional capacity of brown adipose tissue decreases because of the relatively higher ratio between heat production from basal metabolism and the smaller surface area encountered in adult animals. In addition, clothing and indoor life have reduced the need for adaptive nonshivering thermogenesis. However, it has been recently shown that human WAT can be infiltrated with brown adipocytes expressing UCP-1.

Regulation of Metabolism

The control of fat storage and mobilization has been marked by the identification of a number of regulatory mechanisms in the last few decades. Isotopic tracer studies have clearly shown that lipids are continuously being mobilized and renewed even in individuals in energy balance. Fatty acid esterification and triglyceride hydrolysis take place continuously. The half-life of depot lipids in rodents is about 8 days, meaning that almost 10% of the fatty acid stored in adipose tissue is replaced daily by new fatty acids. The balance between lipid loss and accretion determines the net outcome on energy homeostasis.

The synthesis of triglycerides, also termed lipogenesis, requires a supply of fatty acids and glycerol. The main sources of fatty acids are the liver and the small intestine. Fatty acids are esterified with glycerol phosphate in the liver to produce triglycerides. Since triglycerides are bulky polar molecules that do not cross cell membranes well, they must be hydrolyzed to fatty acids and glycerol before entering fat cells. Serum very low-density lipoproteins (VLDLs) are the major form in which triacylglycerols are carried from the liver to WAT. Short-chain fatty acids (16 carbons or less) can be absorbed from the gastrointestinal tract and carried in chylomicra directly to the adipocyte. Inside fat cells, glycerol is mainly synthesized from glucose. In WAT, fatty acids can be synthesized from several precursors, such as glucose, lactate, and certain amino acids, with glucose being quantitatively the most important in humans. In the case of glucose, GLUT4, the principal glucose transporter of adipocytes, controls the entry of the substrate into the adipocyte. Insulin is known to stimulate glucose transport by promoting GLUT4 recruitment as well as increasing its activity. Inside the adipocyte, glucose is initially phosphorylated and then metabolized both in the cytosol and in the mitochondria to produce cytosolic

acetyl-CoA with the flux being influenced by phosphofructokinase and pyruvate dehydrogenase. Glycerol does not readily enter the adipocyte, but the membrane-permeable fatty acids do. Once inside the fat cells, fatty acids are re-esterified with glycerol phosphate to yield triglycerides. Lipogenesis is favored by insulin, which activates pyruvate kinase, pyruvate dehydrogenase, acetyl-CoA carboxylase, and glycerol phosphate acyltransferase. When excess nutrients are available insulin decreases acetyl-CoA entry into the tricarboxylic acid cycle while directing it towards fat synthesis. This insulin effect is antagonized by growth hormone. The gut hormones glucagon-like peptide 1 and gastric inhibitory peptide also increase fatty acid synthesis, while glucagon and catecholamines inactivate acetyl-CoA carboxylase, thus decreasing the rate of fatty acid synthesis.

The release of glycerol and free fatty acids by lipolysis plays a critical role in the ability of the organism to provide energy from triglyceride stores. In this sense, the processes of lipolysis and lipogenesis are crucial for the attainment of body weight control. For this purpose adipocytes are equipped with a well-developed enzymatic machinery, together with a number of nonsecreted proteins and binding factors directly involved in the regulation of lipid metabolism. The hydrolysis of triglycerides from circulating VLDL and chylomicrons is catalyzed by lipoprotein lipase (LPL). This rate-limiting step plays an important role in directing fat partitioning. Although LPL controls fatty acid entry into adipocytes, fat mass has been shown to be preserved by endogenous synthesis. From observations made in patients with total LPL deficiency it can also be concluded that fat deposition can take place in the absence of LPL. A further key enzyme catalyzing a rate-limiting step of lipolysis is HSL (hormome sensitive lipase), which cleaves triacylglycerol to yield glycerol and fatty acids. Some fatty acids are re-esterified, so that the fatty acid: glycerol ratio leaving the cell is usually less than the theoretical 3:1. Increased concentrations of cAMP activate HSL as well as promote its movement from the cytosol to the lipid droplet surface. Catecholamines and glucagon are known inducers of the lipolytic activity, while the stimulation of lipolysis is attenuated by adenosine and protaglandin E_2. Interestingly, HSL deficiency leads to male sterility and adipocyte hypertrophy, but not to obesity, with an unaltered basal lipolytic activity suggesting that other lipases may also play a relevant role in fat mobilization.

The lipid droplets contained in adipocytes are coated by structural proteins, such as perilipin, that stabilize the single fat drops and prevent triglyceride hydrolysis in the basal state. The phosphorylation of perilipin following adrenergic stimulation or other hormonal inputs induces a structural change of the lipid droplet that allows the hydrolysis of triglycerides. After hormonal stimulation, HSL and perilipin are phosphorylated and HSL translocates to the lipid droplet. ALBP, also termed aP2, then binds to the N-terminal region of HSL, preventing fatty acid inhibition of the enzyme's hydrolytic activity.

The function of CETP is to promote the exchange of cholesterol esters of triglycerides between plasma lipoproteins. Fasting, high-cholesterol diets as well as insulin stimulate CETP synthesis and secretion in WAT. In plasma, CETP participates in the modulation of reverse cholesterol transport by facilitating the transfer of cholesterol esters from high-density lipoprotein (HDL) to triglyceride-rich apoB-containing lipoproteins. VLDLs, in particular, are converted to low-density lipoproteins (LDLs), which are subjected to hepatic clearance by the apoB/E receptor system. Adipose tissue probably represents one of the major sources of CETP in humans. Therefore, WAT represents a cholesterol storage organ, whereby peripheral cholesterol is taken up by HDL particles, acting as cholesterol efflux acceptors, and is returned for hepatic excretion. In obesity, the activity and protein mass of circulating CETP is increased showing a negative correlation with HDL concentrations at the same time as a positive correlation with fasting glycemia and insulinemia suggesting a potential link with insulin resistance.

Synthesis and secretion of RBP by adipocytes is induced by retinoic acid and shows that WAT plays an important role in retinoid storage and metabolism. In fact, RBP mRNA is one of the most abundant transcripts present in both rodent and human adipose tissue. Hepatic and renal tissues have been regarded as the main sites of RBP production, while the quantitative and physiological significance of the WAT contribution remains to be fully elucidated.

The processes participating in the control of energy balance, as well as the intermediary lipid and carbohydrate metabolism, are intricately linked by neurohumoral mediators. The coordination of the implicated molecular and biochemical pathways underlies, at least in part, the large number of intracellular and secreted proteins produced by WAT with autocrine, paracrine, and endocrine effects. The finding that WAT secretes a plethora of pleiotropic adipokines at the same time as expressing receptors for a huge range of compounds has led to the development of new insights into the functions of adipose tissue at both the basic and clinical level. At this early juncture in the course of adipose tissue research, much has been discovered. However, a great deal more remains to be learned about its physiology and clinical relevance. Given the adipocyte's versatile and ever-expanding list of secretory proteins, additional and unexpected discoveries are sure to emerge. The growth, cellular composition, and gene expression pattern of adipose tissue is under the regulation of a large selection of central mechanisms and local effectors. The exact nature and control of this complex cross-talk has not been fully elucidated and represents an exciting research topic.

Abbreviations

ACRP30/apM1/ GBP28	adipocyte complement-related protein of 30 kDa/adipose most abundant gene transcript 1/gelatin-binding protein 28
ADD1/SREBP-1C	adipocyte determination and differentiation factor-1/sterol regulatory element binding protein-1c
ALBP/FABP4/aP2	adipocyte fatty acid binding protein
apoE	apolipoprotein E
ASP	acylation-stimulating protein
ATP	adenosine triphosphate
cAMP	cyclic adenosin monophosphate
CD36	fatty acid translocase
C/EBPs	CCAAT/enhancer binding proteins
CETP	cholesteryl ester transfer protein
CRP	C-reactive protein
CSF	colony-stimulating factor
ECM	extracellular matrix
EGF	epidermal growth factor
FFA	free fatty acids
FGF	fibroblast growth factor
GH	growth hormone
GLP-1	glucagon-like peptide-1
GLUT4	glucose transporter type 4
HDL	high density lipoprotein
HGF	hepatocyte growth factor
HSL	hormone-sensitive lipase
IGF	insulin-like growth factor
IL	interleukin
IL-1Ra	interleukin-1 receptor antagonist
LDL	low density lipoprotein
LIF	leukemia inhibitory factor
LPL	lipoprotein lipase
MCP-1	monocyte chemoattractant protein-1
MCSF	macrophage colony stimulating factor
MIF	macrophage migration inhibitory factor
MIP-1α	macrophage inflammatory protein-1α

NGF	nerve growth factor
NO	nitric oxide
NPY-Y1 & -Y5	neuropeptide receptors Y-1 & -5
OB-R	leptin receptor
PAI-1	plasminogen activator inhibitor-1
PDGF	platelet-derived growth factor
PGAR/FIAF	peroxisome proliferator-activated receptor angiopoietin related protein/fasting-induced adipose factor
PGC-1α	peroxisome proliferator-activated receptor-γ coactivator-1α
PGE$_2$	prostaglandin E$_2$
PGF$_{2\alpha}$	prostaglandin F$_{2\alpha}$
PGI$_2$	prostacyclin
PPAR	peroxisome proliferator-activated receptor
Pref-1	preadipocyte factor-1
RAR	retinoic acid receptor
RBP	retinol binding protein
RXR	retinoid x receptor
SAA3	serum amyloid A3
T$_3$	triiodothyronine
TGF-β	transforming growth factor-β
TNF-α	tumor necrosis factor-α
UCP	uncoupling protein
VAP-1/SSAO	vascular adhesion protein-1/semicarbazide-sensitive amine oxidase
VEGF	vascular endothelial growth factor
VLDL	very low density lipoprotein
WAT	white adipose tissue
α_1- & α_2-AR	α_1- & α_2-adrenergic receptors
β_1-, β_2- & β_3-AR	β_1-, β_2- & β_3 adrenergic receptors

See also: **Cholesterol**: Sources, Absorption, Function and Metabolism; Factors Determining Blood Levels. **Diabetes Mellitus**: Etiology and Epidemiology; Classification and Chemical Pathology; Dietary Management. **Fatty Acids**: Metabolism; Monounsaturated; Omega-3 Polyunsaturated; Omega-6 Polyunsaturated; Saturated; *Trans* Fatty Acids. **Hypertension**: Etiology. **Lipids**: Chemistry and Classification; Composition and Role of Phospholipids. **Lipoproteins**. **Obesity**: Definition, Etiology and Assessment; Fat Distribution; Childhood Obesity; Complications; Prevention; Treatment. **Pregnancy**: Safe Diet for Pregnancy.

Further Reading

Ailhaud G and Hauner H (2004) Development of white adipose tissue. In: Bray GA and Bouchard C (eds.) *Handbook of Obesity. Etiology and Pathophysiology*, 2nd edn, pp. 481–514. New York: Marcel Dekker, Inc.

Frayn KN, Karpe F, Fielding BA, Macdonald IA, and Coppack SW (2003) Integrative physiology of human adipose tissue. *International Journal of Obesity* 27: 875–888.

Fried SK and Ross RR (2004) Biology of visceral adipose tissue. In: Bray GA and Bouchard C (eds.) *Handbook of Obesity. Etiology and Pathophysiology*, 2nd edn, pp. 589–614. New York: Marcel Dekker, Inc.

Frühbeck G (2004) The adipose tissue as a source of vasoactive factors. *Current Medicinal Chemistry (Cardiovascular & Hematological Agents)* 2: 197–208.

Frühbeck G and Gómez-Ambrosi J (2003) Control of body weight: a physiologic and transgenic perspective. *Diabetologia* 46: 143–172.

Frühbeck G, Gómez-Ambrosi J, Muruzábal FJ, and Burrell MA (2001) The adipocyte: a model for integration of endocrine and metabolic signaling in energy metabolism regulation. *American Journal of Physiology* 280: E827–E847.

Gómez-Ambrosi J, Catalán V, Diez-Caballero A, Martínez-Cruz A, Gil MJ, García-Foncillas J, Cienfuegos JA, Salvador J, Mato JM, and Frühbeck G (2004) Gene expression profile of omental adipose tissue in human obesity. *The FASEB Journal* 18: 215–217.

Lafontan M and Berlan M (2003) Do regional differences in adipocyte biology provide new pathophysiological insights? *Trends in Pharmacological Sciences* 24: 276–283.

Langin D and Lafontan M (2000) Millennium fat-cell lipolysis reveals unsuspected novel tracks. *Hormone and Metabolic Research* 32: 443–452.

Pond CM (1999) Physiological specialisation of adipose tissue. *Progress in Lipid Research* 38: 225–248.

Rosen ED, Walkey CJ, Puigserver P, and Spiegelman BM (2000) Transcriptional regulation of adipogenesis. *Genes and Development* 14: 1293–1307.

Shen W, Wang Z, Punyanita M, Lei J, Sinav A, Kral JG, Imielinska C, Ross R, and Heymsfield SB (2003) Adipose quantification by imaging methods: a proposed classification. *Obesity Research* 11: 5–16.

Trayhurn P and Beattie JH (2001) Physiological role of adipose tissue: white adipose tissue as an endocrine and secretory organ. *Proceedings of the Nutrition Society* 60: 329–339.

Unger RH (2003) The physiology of cellular liporegulation. *Annual Review of Physiology* 65: 333–347.

Wajchenberg BL (2000) Subcutaneous and visceral adipose tissue: their relation to the metabolic syndrome. *Endocrine Reviews* 21: 697–738.

ADOLESCENTS

Contents
Nutritional Requirements
Nutritional Problems

Nutritional Requirements

C H S Ruxton, Nutrition Communications, Cupar, UK
J Fiore, University of Westminster, London, UK

© 2005 Elsevier Ltd. All rights reserved.

Introduction

Adolescence is the period of transition between childhood and adulthood. This reflects not only the physical and emotional changes experienced by the adolescent, but the development of dietary behaviors. Whereas younger children are characterized by their resistance to new experiences, the adolescent may use food to assert their independence, not always in a beneficial way. This section will cover development in adolescence and highlight nutrients that are important during this time. Information on adolescent energy and nutrient intakes from a broad range of countries will be presented. The findings will be put in context with dietary recommendations.

Physical Changes During Adolescence

Adolescence is generally assumed to be the period of human development from 10 to 18 years of age, a time during which rapid growth and physical maturity take place.

Growth

During prepubescent childhood, the growth of boys and girls follows a similar trajectory, although boys may be slightly taller and heavier than girls. Around the 9th year, the pubertal growth spurt, which can last up to 3.5 years, will occur in girls with boys beginning 2 years later. Girls reach their full height approximately 2 years before boys and are, therefore, the taller of the two sexes for a period of time. Current UK standards for height and weight during adolescence are presented in **Table 1**.

Maximum height velocity is generally seen in the year preceding menarche for girls and at around 14 years for boys. On average, weight velocity peaks at 12.9 years for girls and 14.3 years for boys. Annual growth rates during adolescence can be as much as 9 cm/8.8 kg in girls and 10.3 cm/9.8 kg in boys. Energy and protein intakes per kilogram body weight have been observed to peak during maximal growth, suggesting increased requirements during adolescence. Undernutrition in this crucial window of development can result in a slow height increment, lower peak bone mass, and delayed puberty. On the other hand, overnutrition is not without its risks. It is believed that obesity in young girls can bring about an early menarche, which then increases the risk of breast cancer in later adulthood. Menarche is deemed precocious if it occurs before the age of eight. Rising childhood obesity levels in Western countries have resulted in a rise in the proportion of girls displaying precocious menarche.

Table 1 Percentiles for height, weight, and body mass index

Age (years)	Height (cm)			Weight (kg)			Body mass index		
	3rd	50th	97th	3rd	50th	97th	2nd	50th	99.6th
(a) Boys									
11	130.8	143.2	155.8	26.1	34.5	50.9	14	17	26
16	158.9	173.0	187.4	44.9	60.2	83.2	16	20	30
18	163.3	176.4	189.7	52.0	66.2	87.9	17	21	32
(b) Girls									
11	130.9	143.8	156.9	26.0	35.9	53.6	14	17	27
16	151.6	163.0	174.6	42.8	55.3	74.1	16	20	31
18	152.3	163.6	175.0	44.7	57.2	76.3	17	21	32

It is not fully known when growth ceases. Certainly, height gains of up to 2 cm can still occur between 17 and 28 years. Important nutrients for growth include protein, iron, calcium, vitamin C, vitamin D, and zinc. Calcium, in particular, has a key role in bone development, and huge increments in bone density are seen during adolescence under the influence of sex hormones. Bone density peaks in the early twenties and a low bone density at this time is related to increased osteoporosis risk in later life, especially for women. Studies have suggested that body mass index in adolescence is the best predictor of adult bone density, explaining why children who experience anorexia nervosa are likely to have a higher risk of osteoporosis.

Adipose stores

There are few differences in body fat between boys and girls in the prepubertal stage. However, during puberty, girls develop adipose tissue at a greater rate than boys, laying down stores in the breast and hip regions. The pattern for boys is rather different and tends towards a more central deposition. Methods for estimating fatness in adolescents include weight for height, body mass index (weight in kilograms/height in meters^2), skinfold thickness measures, bioelectrical impedance analysis, densitometry, magnetic resonance imaging, dual energy X-ray absorptiometry, and computer tomography. Waist circumference is gaining popularity as a useful proxy of fatness in the field. Many researchers argue that it is a better predictor than body mass index (BMI) of the central adipose stores, which place the individual most at risk from later obesity, diabetes, and coronary heart disease.

Current UK standards for BMI and waist circumference are outlined in **Table 1**. The 90th percentile is viewed as the lower cut-off point for classification of overweight and can identify those at risk of chronic disease. In a Norwegian longitudinal survey, adolescents with a mean baseline BMI above the 95th centile increased their risk of early mortality by 80–100% compared with adolescents whose mean baseline BMI was between 25th and 75th centiles. Despite this intriguing data, it is notoriously difficult to establish which adolescents will persist with an excess body weight into adulthood. This is partly because adolescents have yet to reach their full height and partly because the etiology of obesity is related to lifestyle factors that may change with time. Attempts to track fatness from childhood to adulthood have produced contradictory results, with some authors claiming that certain ages, such as 7 years and adolescence, are 'risk' points for the development of later obesity and others finding that only the adiposity of older adolescents tracks

to adulthood. Thus, there is no guarantee that the overweight adolescent will remain so in later life.

Sexual Development

In girls, the onset of menarche at around 13 years is triggered by the attainment of a specific level of body fat, with taller, heavier girls more likely to experience an early menarche. Vigorous exercise, e.g., gymnastics and endurance running, can delay the menarche, due both to the physiological effects of regular training and the depletion of body fat. Iron becomes more important for girls as menstrual periods become regular and heavier, and there is evidence that the iron status of many girls may be inadequate. Low iron status in this age group is, in part, due to higher requirements, but it is also linked to nutritional practices such as missing breakfast, avoiding red meat, and dieting.

Dietary Recommendations

There are, of course, a variety of national recommendations for nutritional intake, which, for adolescents, are normally based on a combination of deficiency studies and extrapolations from adult studies. In the UK, US, and Canada, guidelines have evolved from a simple recommended dietary intake (RDI) to a more complex bell-shaped distribution with a mean representing the intake likely to satisfy the needs of 50% of the population. The upper extreme, at the 97.5th centile, represents the intake likely to meet the needs of the majority of the population, while the lower extreme, at the 2.5th centile, represents the lowest acceptable intake. Current UK reference nutrient intakes (RNIs), presented in **Table 2**, cover a range of nutrients from fats and sugars to the main micronutrients. Dietary guidelines are an important reference point for nutrition scientists and dietitians, but it must also be borne in mind that they relate to the average needs of populations, rather than individuals.

Instead of numerical recommendations, many nations have adopted more conceptual ways of representing the ideal diet. This makes sense as recommended nutrient intakes are poorly understood by the public and need to be put into context by health professionals. Communication tools such as the plate model, pyramid system, food groups, and traffic light system can help to get healthy eating messages across to adolescents.

Dietary Intakes

There is a lay belief that most adolescents have a nutritionally inadequate diet yet, despite reported

Table 2 UK Dietary guidelines for adolescents

(a) Dietary reference values macronutrients

Age group (years)	Sex	Energy (MJ)	Protein (g)	NSP (g)	Fat (% energy)	Starch/intrinsic sugars (% energy)	Nonmilk extrinsic sugars (% energy)
11–14	M	9.27	42.1	18	35	39	11
	F	7.92	41.2	18	35	39	11
15–18	M	11.51	55.2	18	35	39	11
	F	8.83	45.0	18	35	39	11

(b) Reference nutrient intakes vitamins and minerals

Age group (years)	Sex	Vit. B_2 (mg)	Vit. B_2 (mg)	Niacin (mg)	Vit. B_6 (mg)	Vit. B_{12} (μg)	Folate (μg)	Vit. C (mg)	Vit. A (μg)	Ca (mg)	Fe (mg)	Zn (mg)
11–14	M	0.9	1.2	15	1.2	1.2	200	35	600	1000	11.3	9.0
	F	0.7	1.1	12	1.0	1.2	200	35	600	800	14.8	9.0
15–18	M	1.1	1.3	18	1.5	1.5	200	40	700	1000	11.3	9.5
	F	0.8	1.1	14	1.2	1.5	200	40	600	800	14.8	7.0

NSP, nonstarch polysaccharide.

low intakes of some micronutrients in surveys, there is little evidence of widespread clinical deficiencies, or indications that adolescents are failing to achieve appropriate heights and weights. Iron is the exception, where mean intakes are low and clinical markers suggest deficiency in some age groups. There is justifiable concern about the general healthiness of diets eaten by 'at risk' subgroups such as dieters, smokers, strict vegetarians, and adolescents who drink excess amounts of alcohol.

Dietary surveys

Mean daily intakes of energy and selected micronutrients from a selection of major international surveys of adolescents are presented in **Table 3**. Caution should be exercised when interpreting data from dietary surveys because under-reporting of energy is widespread in adolescent and adult populations. Selective under-reporting, often focused on energy-dense or high-fat foods, can partially explain low reported intakes of energy and certain micronutrients. It is also complex to make comparisons between the data from different countries given the range of dietary assessment methods used. There is normally a trade-off between sample size and methodology, which sees the larger surveys favoring less precise methods such as 24-h recalls or food frequency questionnaires in order to make data collection more economical. The results of the most recent UK National Diet and Nutrition Survey (NDNS) of 2672 young people aged 4–18 years (adolescent values given in **Table 4**) will be discussed in detail as this represents a survey with particularly strong dietary methodology (i.e., 7-day weighed inventory).

Energy and Protein

Despite mean height and weight data, which are consistent with expected results, energy intakes in UK adolescents remain below estimated average requirements (EARs). Mean energy intakes for boys and girls were 77–89% of EARs; a similar finding to that demonstrated by surveys of younger children and adults. Girls aged 15–18 years had the lowest energy intakes as a proportion of EARs and, apart from under-reporting, this could be due to smoking, slimming, or indeed lower than anticipated energy expenditure. It is well documented that physical activity is particularly low in adolescent girls. Indeed, the NDNS reported that 60% of girls (and 40% of boys) failed to perform the recommended amount of 1 h moderate physical activity per day. Popular sources of energy in the UK adolescent diet included cereal products (one third of energy), savory snacks, potatoes, meat/meat products, white bread, milk/dairy products, biscuits/cakes, spreading fats, and confectionery. Soft drinks contributed on average 6% of energy intakes.

Figure 1 gives a comparison of energy intakes across a range of countries; mainly in Europe. The values represent the mean of reported energy intakes for children aged 9–18 years in these countries, with the majority of surveys focusing on intakes of 11–18 year olds. It is interesting that a large number of countries display similar results (around 10 000 kJ day^{-1}), with a handful of countries, namely Germany, Greece, Portugal, Sweden, and the UK displaying intakes closer to 8000 kJ. For these countries, under-reporting, lower energy requirements, or conscious energy restriction prompted by weight concerns could be reasons for the apparent low intakes.

Table 3 Key international surveys of adolescent dietary intakes

Country	Sex (age in years)	Energy (mJ)	Energy (kcal)	Protein (% energy)	CHO (% energy)	Sugars (g)	Fat (% energy)	Fe (mg)	Ca (mg)	Vit. A (µg)	Vit. B1 (mg)	Vit. B2 (mg)	Vit. B6 (µg)	Vit. B12 (µg)	Niacin (mg)	Folate (µg)	Vit. C (mg)
Australia 24HR 1995	M (12–15)	11.59	2777	15.1	50.9	33.5	24.7	16.1	1093	1296	2.4	3.0	–	–	46.0	271	121
	M (16–18)	13.53	3233	15.4	49.6	32.9	24.5	17.9	1280	1186	2.3	3.0	–	–	53.5	313	154
	F (12–15)	8.53	2038	8.5	51.1	33.1	25.6	11.0	784	1130	1.5	2.0	–	–	33.4	206	124
	F (16–18)	8.69	2076	8.7	50.1	32.1	24.0	11.1	801	877	1.5	1.8	–	–	35.3	217	126
Austria 7dUR, 24HR 1991, 2002	M (11–14)	9.49	2268	13.2	48.2	–	35.2	13.0	903	–	1.4	1.6	1.5	5.7	–	229	113
	M (15–18)	11.65	2784	12.9	50.0	–	37.2	15.4	1002	–	1.4	1.7	1.5	–	–	247	140
	F (10–14)	9.49	2268	12.6	49.4	–	35.8	10.2	834	–	1.1	1.4	1.3	5.0	–	217	132
	F (15–18)	8.49	2029	12.7	49.5	–	33.5	13.4	784	–	1.0	1.2	1.2	4.0	–	201	99
Belgium 3dUR, FFQ 1991, 1995	M (11–12)	11.49	2746	11.6	–	–	–	–	–	–	–	–	–	–	–	–	–
	M (12–18)	13.06	3122	13.0	48.6	149	37.2	13.4	913	–	1.5	1.7	1.6	–	–	–	83
	F (11–12)	11.72	2802	11.6	–	–	–	–	–	–	1.0	–	–	–	–	–	–
	F (1–18)	9.44	2256	14.9	48.8	112	36.7	8.2	805	–	1.2	1.3	1.2	–	–	–	78
Canada 24HR, 1993	M (13–15)	9.71	2321	15.0	51.0	–	34.0	15.8	1299	1191	1.7	2.2	1.6	5.1	–	205	110
	F (13–15)	7.09	1695	15.0	54.0	–	32.0	10.5	954	892	1.2	1.6	1.1	3.4	–	155	118
Denmark 7dUR 1995	M (11–14)	10.90	2605	–	51.0	–	35.0	–	1286	–	1.5	2.2	1.7	6.7	27.0	304	79
	M (15–18)	12.15	2903	14.0	–	–	35.0	–	1362	–	1.5	2.3	–	7.1	30.0	295	80
	F (11–14)	8.70	2079	–	51.0	–	34.0	–	1061	–	1.1	1.7	1.4	5.1	23.0	238	72
	F (15–18)	9.70	2318	14.0	–	–	34.0	–	1121	–	1.2	1.8	1.5	5.5	23.0	266	79
Finland 24HR, 4dUR, 3DUR 1996–97	M (12–13)	10.2	2437	–	47.0	–	–	–	1230	–	1.8	2.2	–	–	28.0	–	81
	M (12–18)	–	–	–	–	–	40.0	19.7	–	–	–	–	–	–	17.0	–	–
	M (15–16)	11.8	2820	15.0	–	–	–	–	–	–	–	–	–	–	–	–	–
	F (12–13)	8.5	2031	–	–	–	–	–	–	–	1.7	–	–	–	–	–	–
	F (12–18)	–	–	–	50.0	–	37.0	13.5	–	–	–	–	–	–	–	–	–
	F (15–16)	8.6	2055	14.0	–	–	–	–	–	–	1.9	–	–	–	–	–	–
France DH, 1dWR 1988, 1993–94	M (10–13)	–	–	–	47.8	142.5	–	–	–	–	1.2	2.1	1.7	11.0	–	–	88
	M (11–14)	10.83	2587	15.4	–	–	36.5	12.6	1250	–	1.4	1.8	1.8	5.6	–	253	91
	M (11–18)	–	–	15.7	–	–	–	–	835	–	1.0	2.2	–	–	–	–	–
	M (13–18)	12.10	2892	14.9	48.8	126.8	36.0	12.5	1300	–	1.4	1.8	2.0	7.0	–	–	127
	F (10–13)	–	–	–	47.7	113.3	–	–	1100	–	1.0	1.8	1.5	7.5	–	–	99
	F (11–14)	8.84	2112	15.9	–	–	–	11.4	835	–	–	1.8	1.8	5.6	17.0	253	91
	F (11–18)	–	–	16.1	–	–	–	–	–	–	1.3	–	–	–	–	–	–
	F (13–18)	9.16	2188	16.1	45.7	98.2	–	10.4	1100	–	–	1.7	1.4	7.0	–	–	112

Continued

Table 3 Continued

Country	Sex (age in years)	Energy (mJ)	Energy (kcal)	Protein (% energy)	CHO (% energy)	Sugars (g)	Fat (% energy)	Fe (mg)	Ca (mg)	Vit. A (μg)	Vit. B_1 (mg)	Vit. B_2 (mg)	Vit. B_6 (μg)	Vit. B_{12} (μg)	Niacin (mg)	Folate (μg)	Vit. C (mg)
Germany DH, 3-d/7-d	M (10–12)	9.08	2170	12.9	46.0	–	38.0	12.4	795	–	1.1	1.2	1.3	4.4	24.0	221	87
Recall, 1dWR	M (13–14)	10.41	2487	13.2	45.6	–	37.5	14.3	893	–	1.3	1.5	1.4	5.5	28.6	245	98
1985–95, 1998	M (15–18)	11.14	2661	13.2	46.9	–	38.3	14.8	902	–	1.4	1.7	1.6	5.7	30.4	263	97
	F (10–12)	7.78	1860	12.9	47.6	–	36.4	11.1	681	–	1.0	1.2	1.1	4.0	20.4	203	87
	F (13–14)	8.49	2028	12.6	45.1	–	39.2	12.2	754	–	1.1	1.1	1.2	4.2	24.1	210	98
	F (15–18)	8.59	2052	13.1	46.5	–	37.0	12.3	728	–	1.0	1.3	1.5	4.4	24.6	216	92
Greece 1dWR, 24HR	M (10–11)	–	–	15.7	44.0	–		11.0	963	–	–	–	–	–	–	–	119
1993–94, 1999	M (12–14)	8.90	2126	15.6	45.0	97	40.0	13.5	1011	–	1.7	2.1	1.8	4.7	18.0	226	112
	M (14–16)	9.00	2151	15.0	47.2	–	–	13.8	871	–	2.5	2.0	1.9	4.3	19.2	251	123
	F (10–11)	–	–	15.6	44.0	–		10.0	851	–	–	–	–	–	–	–	108
	F (12–14)	9.70	2318	14.7	48.0	88	41.8	10.1	748	–	1.4	1.6	1.3	4.1	13.2	212	108
	F (14–16)	7.08	1692	14.5	46.0	–	–	9.4	771	–	2.4	1.5	–	3.2	–	217	118
Ireland DH 1988	M (11–14)	11.3	2700	–	50.3	–	36.3	14.7	1208	–	1.8	2.5	2.2	4.9	40.2	246	76
	M (15–17)	14.0	3346	14.2	49.3	–	36.0	19.3	1549	–	2.2	3.1	2.6	7.2	51.7	306	95
	F (11–14)	9.10	2174	–	50.2	–	36.0	–	962	–	–	1.9	1.7	3.9	32.0	198	76
	F (12–15)	–	–	–	–	–	–	12.4	–	–	1.4	–	–	–	–	–	–
	F (15–17)	8.90	2127	13.9	48.9	–	37.1	11.6	950	–	1.3	1.8	1.6	4.0	32.0	182	79
Japan UR n/a	M (15–19)	10.6	2545	14.4	51.9	–	28.3	8.6	633	978	1.2	1.4	1.3	8.1	16.6	303	89
	F (15–19)	8.0	1918	15.1	50.4	–	29.7	7.4	516	875	0.9	1.2	1.1	6.4	13.2	268	91
Netherlands 2dUR	M (13–16)	10.9	2605	13.1	51.2	188	35.5	10.9	1045	778	1.2	1.6	1.6	3.9	–	–	79
1997–98	M (16–19)	11.6	2772	13.3	49.5	184	35.4	11.5	1095	972	1.3	1.6	1.8	4.4	–	–	71
	F (13–16)	8.7	2079	13.7	50.3	146	35.9	9.0	904	724	1.0	1.4	1.3	3.4	–	–	81
	F (16–19)	9.1	2175	13.4	50.3	152	35.5	9.9	908	754	1.2	1.4	1.4	3.4	–	–	81
New Zealand 24HR,	M (15–18)	12.4	2963	15.0	49.0	82	35.0	15.2	957	505	1.8	2.1	1.8	4.9	43.0	280	155
FFQ 1997	F (15–18)	8.86	2117	14.0	51.0	69	34.0	10.4	783	342	1.3	1.5	1.1	3.2	28.0	203	120
Norway 1dWR,	M (11–14)	–	–	–	–	–	31.1	–	–	–	–	–	–	–	–	–	–
FFQ n/a	M (13–14)	15.0	3585	–	–	–	–	–	1625	–	2.1	2.8	–	–	–	–	110
	M (13–15)	–	–	13.4	–	–	–	–	–	–	–	–	–	–	–	–	–
	F (11–14)	10.9	2605	–	54.9	–	28.9	–	–	–	1.6	–	–	–	–	–	–
	F (13–14)	–	–	–	–	–	–	–	1142	–	–	2.1	–	–	–	–	104
	F (13–15)	–	–	13.7	–	–	–	–	–	–	–	–	–	–	–	–	–

Continued

Table 3 Continued

Country	Sex (age in years)	Energy (mJ)	Energy (kcal)	Protein (% energy)	CHO (% energy)	Sugars (g)	Fat (% energy)	Fe (mg)	Ca (mg)	Vit. A (µg)	Vit. B_1 (mg)	Vit. B_2 (mg)	Vit. B_6 (µg)	Vit. B_{12} (µg)	Niacin (mg)	Folate (µg)	Vit. C (mg)
Portugal 24HR 1995	M (12–18)	8.86	2117	–	49.1	–	–	–	890	–	–	–	–	–	–	–	–
	M (13–17)	9.41	2248	17.6	–	–	–	–	–	–	–	–	–	–	–	–	77
	F (12–18)	9.40	2248	–	53.4	–	33.3	–	853	–	–	–	–	–	–	–	–
	F (13–17)	8.14	1945	17.8	–	–	–	–	–	–	–	–	–	–	–	–	99
Spain 24HR, FFQ	M (10–12)	11.50	2747	15.4	51.8	–	40.3	11.3	713	749	1.4	1.4	–	4.7	28.0	128	71
1989–92	M (13–15)	12.54	2997	17.8	47.7	–	40.1	16.5	746	691	2.1	1.8	–	7.2	40.0	159	68
	F (10–12)	10.89	2602	13.5	43.9	–	40.8	–	666	1088	1.3	1.3	–	7.2	25.0	138	96
	F (13–15)	1052	2514	16.1	42.0	–	42.1	13.2	653	982	1.9	1.6	–	9.6	36.0	168	84
	F (17–18)	–	–	–	–	–	–	13.3	–	–	–	–	–	–	–	–	–
Sweden 7dUR	M (13–14)	–	–	–	–	–	–	17.4	1279	–	–	–	–	–	–	–	–
1989–90, 1993–94	M (14–16)	8.90	2127	–	52.6	–	32.1	18.2	1406	–	1.8	2.4	2.0	6.6	33.5	178	68
	M (17–18)	10.50	2509	14.7	49.4	–	–	–	1472	–	1.8	2.8	2.2	8.7	36	138	77
	F (13–14)	–	–	–	–	–	–	–	1061	–	–	–	–	–	–	–	–
	F (14–15)	7.21	1722	–	–	–	–	13.4	1046	–	1.4	1.8	1.5	4.9	24.9	144	68
	F (17–18)	7.88	1884	14.2	54.1	–	–	13.3	966	–	1.2	1.8	1.5	5.5	23.0	105	77
Switzerland 7dUR	M (11–12)	–	–	13.3	46.1	–	–	–	–	–	–	–	–	–	–	–	–
1994–95	M (13–14)	11.98	2863	–	–	–	40.1	16.0	1311	–	1.5	2.2	–	–	–	–	185
	M (15–18)	12.56	3001	–	–	–	35.0	–	1157	–	1.3	1.8	–	–	–	–	163
	F (11–12)	–	–	–	49.4	–	–	–	–	–	–	–	–	–	–	–	–
	F (13–15)	7.90	1887	–	–	–	37.4	9.3	819	–	–	1.3	–	–	–	–	110
	F (15–18)	8.12	1939	–	–	–	35.8	–	832	–	1.5	1.3	–	–	–	–	146
Turkey 24HR 2003	M (11–14)	9.92	2372	15.0	50.9	–	34.1	13.3	1030	1151	1.2	2.0	1.7	4.0	13.1	179	127
	F (11–14)	9.41	2250	14.6	48.2	–	37.2	11.8	1060	1386	1.1	2.0	1.7	3.9	12.6	163	135
USA 24HR 1999–2000	M (12–19)	11.24	2686	13.9	54.2	–	32.0	18.3	1081	–	–	–	–	–	–	421	–
	F (12–19)	8.34	1993	13.4	55.5	–	31.1	13.4	793	–	–	–	–	–	–	323	–

24HR refers to '24 hour' recall. WR, weighed record; FFQ, food intake questionnaire; UR, unweighed record; DH, diet history.
Vitamin A = micrograms retinol equivalent.
Dates of actual surveys are given where available. Data from more than one survey are presented for some countries.

Table 4 Average daily dietary intakes of UK adolescents from the National Diet and Nutrition Survey (2000)

Sex (age in years) Sample size	Energy (MJ)	Protein (% energy)	CHO (% energy)	NMES (% energy)	Fat (% energy)	NSP (g)	Fe (mg)	Ca (mg)	Vit. A (µg)	Vit. B₁ (mg)	Vit. B₂ (mg)	Vit. B₆ (µg)	Vit. B₁₂ (µg)	Niacin (mg)	Folate (µg)	Vit. C (mg)
M (11–14) N = 234	8.28 89% EAR	13.1 152% RNI	51.7	16.9	35.2	11.6	10.8 96% RNI	799 80% RNI	577 96% RNI	1.71 190% RNI	1.74 145% RNI	2.2 183% RNI	4.5 375% RNI	30 200% RNI	247 124% RNI	78.4 224% RNI
M (15–18) N = 179	9.69 83% EAR	13.9 139% RNI	50.5	15.8	35.9	13.3	12.6 112% RNI	878 88% RNI	628 90% RNI	1.93 175% RNI	1.95 150% RNI	2.7 180% RNI	5.0 333% RNI	36.8 204% RNI	309 154% RNI	86.5 216% RNI
F (11–14) N = 238	7.03 89% EAR	12.7 128% RNI	51.2	16.2	36.1	10.2	9.1 61% RNI	641 80% RNI	482 80% RNI	1.42 203% RNI	1.35 123% RNI	1.9 190% RNI	3.3 275% RNI	24.8 207% RNI	210 105% RNI	73.7 210% RNI
F (15–18) N = 210	6.82 77% EAR	13.9 121% RNI	50.6	15.3	35.9	10.6	8.9 60% RNI	653 82% RNI	562 94% RNI	1.41 176% RNI	1.34 122% RNI	2.0 167% RNI	3.4 227% RNI	25.6 183% RNI	215 108% RNI	81.2 203% RNI

Study conducted January to December 1997 with a sample size of 2672.
EAR, estimated average requirement; RNI, reference nutrient intake; NMES, Nonmilk extrinsic sugars (similar to added sugars); NSP, nonstarch polysaccharide.

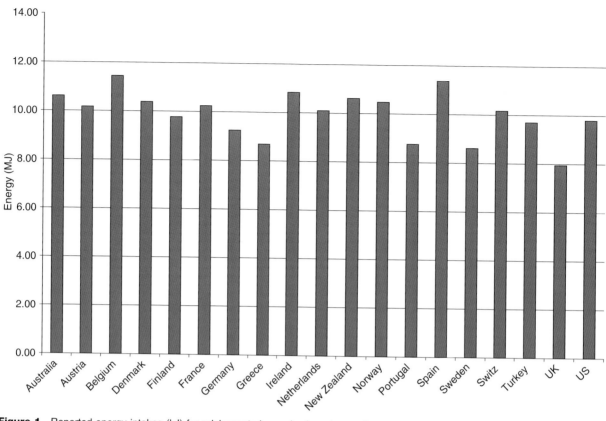

Figure 1 Reported energy intakes (kJ) for adolescents in a selection of countries.

In the NDNS, mean protein intakes were considerably in excess of requirements, as assessed by RNI, for all ages and both sexes. The main sources were meat and meat products (which contributed 30% of overall protein), cereals, bread, and milk products. It is believed that protein requirements in adolescents are between 0.8 and 1.0 g per kg body mass, although this fails to take into account any additional needs related to regular exercise (which are likely to be minor for most sports and be covered by normal protein intakes). As a proportion of energy, protein intakes were higher in Southern European countries, Australia, and New Zealand compared with intakes in the US and Northern European countries.

Fat

Mean total fat intake as a proportion of energy in the NDNS was around 35%, corresponding to the UK dietary reference value (DRV). This is lower than the intakes (38–40% energy from fat) found in previous studies. However, intakes of saturated fat, at 14% energy, still exceeded the DRV of 11% energy. Of more concern was the subgroup of adolescents in the highest percentile of intakes who consumed around 17% energy from saturated fat.

This emphasizes the view that, although mean intakes may look acceptable when compared with dietary guidelines, there may be 'at risk' groups whose dietary habits predispose them to a greater risk of chronic disease. Main sources of saturated fat in the adolescent diet included meat and meat products (around 20%), savory snacks, and fried foods. In most other countries, fat intakes were 36–38% energy with the highest fat intake reported in Finland, Greece, Belgium, Germany, Switzerland, and Spain at around 38% energy. In the US, where the dietary guideline is 30%, intakes were around 32% energy from fat.

Carbohydrates

Average total carbohydrate intake in the NDNS was close to the DRV of 50% energy. The main sources were cereals, bread, savory snacks, vegetables, and potatoes. Fiber intakes, expressed as nonstarch polysaccharide (NSP), were 10–13 g day^{-1}, which approached 70% of the adult guideline. Vegetables, potatoes, and savory snacks together contributed 40% of NSP. Interesting, there was no clear relationship between NSP and bowel movements, although it was noted that adolescents who experienced less than one bowel movement per day tended to have NSP intakes at the lowest end of the distribution spectrum. The mean intake of nonmilk extrinsic sugars (a proxy for added sugars) was 16% of energy, around 4 percentage points higher than the DRV of 11% food energy. Key sources were soft drinks (providing 42% of sugars), sugar preserves, and confectionery, particularly chocolate. Children from lower income households tended to have lower intakes of total carbohydrate, nonmilk extrinsic sugars, and NSP compared with children from higher income households.

Recommendations to reduce fat are often accompanied by those urging a decrease in added sugars due to concerns about obesity, dental health, and micronutrient dilution. However, an inverse relationship between fat and sugars is evident in the majority of dietary surveys, suggesting that concurrent reductions in fat and sugar may neither be realistic nor totally beneficial. A previous survey found a difference of 4% energy from fat between children in the lowest and highest thirds of sugar intake. Observational studies, including the latest NDNS, have also found an inverse relationship between body mass index and sugar intake. Explanations for this include self-imposed sugar restrictions amongst heavier people, and food choices in favor of higher sugar, low-fat foods, which could be less obesigenic. With respect to the potential impact of added sugars on micronutrient dilution, studies in the UK, Germany, and the US have found that a broad range of sugar intake is consistent with adequate micronutrient intakes. This may be partly due to fortification of sugar-containing foods, e.g., breakfast cereals. Lower levels of vitamins and minerals tend to be seen only at the upper and lower extremes of sugar consumption, suggesting that these diets lack variety.

Micronutrients

Main sources of micronutrients are breakfast cereals, milk, bread, chips/potatoes, and eggs. Surveys that report comparisons between intakes and recommendations have found satisfactory intakes for most micronutrients when means are considered. Intakes of vitamins B_1, B_2, B_6, B_{12} C, and niacin greatly exceeded RNIs in the NDNS, perhaps reflecting high protein intakes and the fortification of popular foods such as breakfast cereals, bread, and beverages. Even folate, a problem nutrient in earlier studies, was consumed at an acceptable level.

Nutrient intakes that remain at lower than expected levels were iron and zinc for both sexes,

and calcium and vitamin A for girls. Mean iron intake was particularly low in 11–18-year-old girls at 60% of the RNI (see **Table 4**). Mean iron intakes often fail to meet recommended levels in the majority of studies reported, particularly in women and girls. This may reflect avoidance of iron-containing foods, e.g., red meat, for reasons of perceived health, food safety, or dislike. Iron status is also hampered by absorption rates, which can be as low as 10%. It is important to reverse this trend as increasing numbers of young girls are now demonstrating clinical evidence of poor iron status, e.g., more than a quarter of 15–18-year-old girls in the NDNS. A New Zealand survey reported that 4–6% of adolescents were anemic. Good sources of iron are meat/meat products, breakfast cereals, bread, chips/potatoes, chocolate, and crisps. Around 25% of iron intakes are from fortified foods, which supply non-heme iron. The latter four food groups are not particularly rich in iron but, nevertheless, contribute over 10% due to the significant amounts eaten.

Poor intakes of calcium are of concern due to the rising incidence of osteoporosis in later life, especially amongst women. While average calcium intakes were around 80% of the RNI in the NDNS, there was a considerable proportion of adolescents with intakes below the lower RNI (the bottom end of the acceptable spectrum). In 11–14-year-old children, 12% of boys and 24% of girls fell into this category, while in 15–18 year olds, the figures were 9% and 19%, respectively. Good sources of calcium are milk, cheese, yogurt, tinned fish, and, in many countries, fortified grain products. Concern has been expressed that the rise in soft drink consumption has displaced milk from the diets of adolescents and this could be contributing to the low calcium intakes found in many surveys. Fluid milk consumption has fallen dramatically over the last decade in Western countries and this is due to a range of factors including preference for other beverages, dieters' concerns about calories, and attitude of adolescents towards milk. It should not be forgotten that physical activity is an important aspect in the prevention of osteoporosis. Some life-style practices, such as smoking and drinking alcohol, are related to a higher requirement for micronutrients, suggesting that specific groups of adolescents may be more at risk from a poor nutrient status.

Impact of Lifestyle on Dietary Intakes

Young people consume particular foods and diets for a variety of reasons, often completely unrelated to their nutritional content. These can include:

slimming or weight control (whether justified or not); peer group pressure to consume certain foods or brands; the development of personal ideology, such as the use of vegetarian diets; following a specific diet to enhance sporting prowess; or even convenience. Energy and nutrient intakes are influenced by specialized eating patterns, thus it is important to consider life-style choices when interpreting dietary survey data.

Breakfast Consumption

Breakfast is identified in many studies as a nutrient-dense, low-fat meal, yet is often omitted by adolescents. Around 10% of younger children miss breakfast, rising to 20% as adulthood is approached. Boys omit breakfast less than girls and favor cereals rather than bread or a cooked breakfast. Data on breakfast habits have revealed higher intakes of sugars, fiber, and micronutrients, such as folate, niacin, iron, calcium and zinc, amongst high breakfast cereal consumers. Fat intakes, as a proportion of energy, are inversely related to breakfast cereal intake, probably due to the higher carbohydrate intakes of breakfast consumers. Previous surveys of adolescents have found an inverse relationship between breakfast cereal consumption and body mass index.

Consumption of School Lunches

Although the popularity of school lunches has diminished over the last 10 years, they are still eaten regularly by almost 40% of children, particularly those from lower socioeconomic groups. School lunches have been found to contribute 30–40% of total energy and are often criticized for containing a high proportion of fat and low levels of key micronutrients such as vitamin C and calcium. Older children often prefer to eat lunch at cafes and take-aways rather than consider school meals and this practice has been found to relate to lower nutrient-dense diets, particularly in the case of iron. Initiatives have been taken forward in many schools to improve the quality and perception of school meals including action groups involving pupils, caterers, and teachers. There have also been efforts at government level to integrate the production of school meals with classroom-based topics around nutrition, health, and life style. It is too early to say whether these efforts have had a significant impact on the nutrition of adolescents.

Snacking and Soft Drink Consumption

There has been a general shift over the last decade towards fewer meals eaten at home and more eaten in restaurants and cafes combined with an increase in snacking. Snacks, including soft drinks, now contribute a significant proportion of the daily energy intake of adolescents. Concerns about the possible impact of snacks on measures of overweight and nutrient composition have not been borne out by the evidence, although it is acknowledged that data collection in this area is complicated by the myriad of definitions for 'snack.' A number of observational studies have found that frequent snackers have similar nutrient intakes to those who snack infrequently. With respect to body size, snacking tends to relate to a lower body mass index rather than one that is high. Intervention studies also provide valuable evidence on the effects of snacking. A study in adults, which attempted to increase consumption of snacks to around 25% of daily energy using a variety of low- and high-fat products, found that the subjects compensated for the additional energy by reducing the amount eaten at meals. While these data suggest that snacking is more benign than was previously thought, it is important to emphasize the concept of balance. Common snack foods amongst adolescents are potato crisps, carbonated drinks, biscuits, and confectionery. While these foods certainly have a role in creating variety and enjoyment in the diet, no one would argue that they should represent the primary sources of energy for young people. In the case of soft drinks, evidence from short-term intervention studies suggests that higher intakes (in excess of two cans per day) are linked with higher energy intakes and lower intakes of micronutrients. Yet most epidemiological studies show an inverse correlation between sugar consumption (a proxy for soft drink consumption) and mean body mass index. Further work is needed to determine optimal cut-offs for soft drink intakes, particularly for adolescents who tend to be major consumers.

Smoking

The proportion of adolescent smokers rises with age and is between 8% and 20% with an average exposure, in older children, of around 40 cigarettes per week. Since the 1980s, smoking has decreased in adolescent boys but not in girls. Smokers tend to have different dietary habits from nonsmokers and this is reflected in their nutrient intakes. Studies have found that smokers consume less dairy foods, wholemeal bread, fruit and breakfast cereals, and more coffee, alcohol and chips. Smokers' diets tend to be lower in fiber, vitamin B_1, and vitamin C compared with nonsmokers. In a study of 18 year olds, male smokers had higher percentage energy from fat and lower intakes of sugars and iron. Contrary to evidence from adult surveys, smoking has not been found to relate to body size in adolescents, although the opposite is believed to be true for teenage girls who use smoking as a misguided means to control energy intake. As would be expected, dietary restraint is more common amongst female smokers.

Consumption of Alcohol

In the NDNS, alcohol was consumed by 10% of 11–14 year olds and 37–46% of 15–18 year olds with older boys most likely to drink alcohol. Other European surveys have found higher proportions (60–90% in 14–18-year-old males), while US surveys have found similar proportions to the UK. The average contribution of alcohol to energy intakes in the NDNS was just over 1%, with higher contributions reported by Danish and Irish studies (around 2–5% energy). Excess alcohol intake can increase micronutrient requirements but few younger adolescents fall into this category. However, binge drinking in the 15–18-year-old age group is a concern. One US study found that 20% of adolescents could be classed as problem drinkers, while 7% could be classed as alcoholics. Regular moderate consumption of alcohol can contribute to obesity since the energy provided by alcoholic drinks rarely displaces energy from other food sources. This is likely to increase overall daily energy intakes and could lead to a positive energy balance.

Other Factors that Impact on Dietary Intakes

Comparisons between boys and girls often reveal differences in dietary patterns, yet these are seldom consistent between surveys. On the whole, boys eat more meat and dairy products, while girls favor fruit, salad vegetables, and artificially sweetened drinks. The dietary practices of girls are more likely to be influenced by a desire to limit energy intakes. Lower intakes of dairy products, meat, and breakfast cereals seen in older adolescent girls explain their typically poor intakes of iron and calcium.

Differences in diet are sometimes seen between children from different social classes or income groups. In the NDNS, children from a lower socioeconomic background were less likely to consume low-fat dairy foods, fruit juice, salad vegetables, high-fiber cereals, fruit juices, and fruit than children from a higher socioeconomic background. This impacted on mean daily nutrient intakes with lower socioeconomic children consuming less protein, total sugars, total carbohydrate, and fiber. There was a similar trend for micronutrients, particularly vitamin C. Some surveys have found higher fat intakes in children from lower socioeconomic backgrounds. Such a dietary pattern, characterized by lower than optimal levels of protective nutrients, combined with a higher prevalence of smoking, may partly explain the higher burden of chronic disease experienced by people from lower socioeconomic groups.

Promoting Optimal Diets

The findings of the studies shown in **Tables 3** and **4** reveal that most adolescents in the developed world are likely to be receiving adequate energy and protein to support growth. The intakes of micronutrients found in subgroups of the population may not be high enough to ensure optimal health but it is difficult to interpret the effects of these without appropriate biochemical data. For iron, there is good evidence of clinical deficiency in low iron consumers, particularly girls but for other nutrients, biochemical evidence is scarce. Longitudinal studies that attempt to link early diet with the incidence of later disease are a valuable tool and seem to suggest that high intakes of fruit, vegetables, folate, and n-3 polyunsaturated fatty acids (present in oily fish) are dietary indicators that relate to important aspects of health later in life. Despite these scientific findings, health messages relating to fruit and vegetables seem to have fallen on deaf ears. The NDNS showed that 70% of children had eaten no citrus fruit during the week of the dietary survey. Around 60% had eaten no green leafy vegetables or tomatoes, valuable sources of vitamins and minerals.

Since energy intake is the main predictor of micronutrient intakes, it makes sense to ensure that adolescents avoid restricting energy. Yet this finding needs to be considered against a background of rising obesity in the adolescent population. There is strong evidence that adolescence is the time when substantial reductions in physical activity are seen and such a trend, combined with lower energy intakes, could result in larger numbers of children failing to meet their individual nutrient requirements.

The key to tackling this lies as much with physical activity as it does with dietary intervention. Energy intakes need to be maintained at a level suitable for optimal micronutrient uptake while, at the same time, energy expenditure should be increased to ensure energy balance. A wide range of foods encompassing the main food groups will ensure a nutrient-dense diet. Special conditions in adolescence, such as pregnancy, lactation, and sports training, may increase requirements above normal and merit manipulation of the diet to favor food groups known to be important sources of certain nutrients.

Conclusions

Diets of adolescents in developed countries meet the macronutrient requirements of the majority of individuals resulting in appropriate rates of growth. While fat intakes, as a proportion of energy, have continued to decline towards dietary guidelines, concern remains over the intakes of iron, calcium, zinc, and vitamin A in many subgroups of adolescents, particularly older girls. Maintaining adequate energy intakes and encouraging consumption of fruit, vegetables, lean meat, and oily fish may be a key route to achieving an optimal intake of micronutrients. Present recommendations for adolescents include a continuing reduction in dietary fat to help prevent later diseases of affluence. This should be combined with encouragement to increase physical activity in order to address the rising incidence of obesity in most developed countries.

See also: **Adolescents**: Nutritional Problems. **Alcohol**: Absorption, Metabolism and Physiological Effects; Disease Risk and Beneficial Effects; Effects of Consumption on Diet and Nutritional Status. **Calcium**. **Dietary Surveys**. **Osteoporosis**.

Further Reading

Alexy U, Sichert-Hellert W, and Kersting M (2003) Associations between intake of added sugars and intakes of nutrients and food groups in the diets of German children and adolescents. *British Journal of Nutrition* **90**: 441–447.

Cruz JA (2000) Dietary habits and nutritional status in adolescents over Europe–Southern Europe. *European Journal of Clinical Nutrition* **54**(supplement 1): S29–S35.

Deckelbaum RJ and Williams CL (2001) Childhood obesity: the health issue. *Obesity Research* **9**(supplement 4): 239S–243S.

Frary CD, Johnson RK, and Wang MQ (2004) Children and adolescents' choices of foods and beverages high in added sugars are associated with intakes of key nutrients and food groups. *Journal of Adolescent Health* **34**: 56–63.

Gregory JR, Lowe S, Bates CJ et al. (2000) *National Diet and Nutrition Survey: Young People Aged 4 to 18 Years*. London: The Stationery Office.

Lambert J, Agostoni C, Elmadfa I et al. (2004) Diet intake and nutritional status of children and adolescents in Europe. *British Journal of Nutrition* **92**(supplement 2): S147–S211.

Ruxton CHS, Storer H, Thomas B, and Talbot D (2000) Teenagers and young adults. In: Thomas B (ed.) *Manual of Dietetic Practice*, 2nd ed, pp. 256–262. UK: Blackwells: Oxford.

Serra-Majem L (2001) Vitamin and mineral intakes in European children. Is food fortification needed? *Public Health Nutrition* **4**: 101–107.

Nutritional Problems

C Lo, Childrens' Hospital Boston, Harvard Medical School and Harvard School of Public Health, Boston, MA, USA

© 2005 Elsevier Ltd. All rights reserved.

Introduction: Normal Adolescent Growth and Diets

Adolescence is a unique time of rapid growth, with half of eventual adult weight and 45% of peak bone mass accumulated during adolescence. Adolescence is a time when peak physical muscular development and exercise performance is reached. However, adolescent diets are often notorious for their reliance on snacks and 'junk foods' that are high in calories, sugar, salt, and saturated fat, which could provide extra energy for high-activity demands of teenagers, but often risk becoming part of bad habits leading to obesity and increased risk of atherosclerotic heart disease in later life. Although most studies have been on older subjects, it is now clear that many Western diseases, especially heart disease, stroke, diabetes, hypertension, and many cancers, are diet related, and that diets high in saturated fat and low in fruits, vegetables, and fiber may increase risks of heart disease.

Indeed, autopsy reports of atherosclerotic plaques already present in adolescents who died accidentally suggests that prevention of heart disease should start quite early in life. Epidemiologic evidence from large cohort studies have concluded that a striking 80% reduction of heart disease and diabetes might be achieved in those with diets lower in saturated and trans fat and higher in fruits, vegetables, folate, fiber, and n-3 fish oils. Other factors include regular exercise, moderate alcohol use, and avoidance of obesity and smoking.

Nutrient Requirements

About every 10 years, the Institute of Medicine convenes several committees of nutrition scientists to review the scientific literature and recommend levels of daily dietary nutrients that would keep 95% of the population from developing deficiencies.

In the past, the dietary reference intakes (DRIs) or recommended dietary allowances (RDAs) concentrated on ensuring that nutrient deficiencies were minimized by specifying lower limits of intakes. However, it is now clear that many Western diets provide too much of some nutrients such as total calories, simple carbohydrates, saturated fats, and salt. Therefore, recent editions of DRIs (see **Table 1** to **5**) have

Table 1 Recommended dietary allowances and adequate intakes

Life stage group	Vitamin A (μg day⁻¹)	Vitamin C (mg day⁻¹)	Vitamin D (μg day⁻¹)	Vitamin E (μg day⁻¹)	Vitamin K (μg day⁻¹)	Thiamin (mg day⁻¹)	Riboflavin (mg day⁻¹)	Niacin (μg day⁻¹)	Vitamin B_6 (mg day⁻¹)	Folate (μg day⁻¹)	Vitamin B_{12} (μg day⁻¹)	Pantothenic Acid (mg day⁻¹)	Biotin (μg day⁻¹)	Choline (μg day⁻¹)
Males														
9–13 years	**600**	**45**	5*	**11**	60*	**0.9**	**0.9**	**12**	**1.0**	**300**	**1.8**	4*	20*	375*
14–18 years	**900**	**75**	5*	**15**	75*	**1.2**	**1.3**	**16**	**1.3**	**400**	**2.4**	5*	25*	550*
19–30 years	**900**	**90**	5*	**15**	120*	**1.2**	**1.3**	**16**	**1.3**	**400**	**2.4**	5*	30*	550*
Females														
9–13 years	**600**	**45**	5*	**11**	60*	**0.9**	**0.9**	**12**	**1.0**	**300**	**1.8**	4*	20*	375*
14–18 years	**700**	**65**	5*	**15**	75*	**1.0**	**1.0**	**14**	**1.2**	**400**	**2.4**	5*	25*	400*
19–30 years	**700**	**75**	5*	**15**	90*	**1.1**	**1.1**	**14**	**1.3**	**400**	**2.4**	5*	30*	425*

Food and Nutrition Board, Institute of Medicine, The National Academies. Copyright 2001 by the National Academy of Sciences. All rights reserved.
This table (taken from the DRI reports, see http://www.nap.edu) presents recommended dietary allowances (RDAs) in **bold type** and adequate intakes (AIs) in ordinary type followed by an asterisk (*). RDAs and AIs may both be used as goals for individual intake. RDAs are set to meet the needs of almost all (97–98%) individuals in a group. For healthy breast-fed infants, the AI is the mean intake. The AI for other life-stage and gender groups is believed to cover needs of all individuals in the group, but lack of data or uncertainty in the data prevent being able to specify with confidence the percentage of individuals covered by this intake.

Table 2 Recommended dietary allowances and adequate intakes

Life stage group	Calcium (mg day⁻¹)	Chromium (µg day⁻¹)	Copper (µg day⁻¹)	Fluoride (mg day⁻¹)	Iodine (µg day⁻¹)	Iron (mg day⁻¹)	Magnesium (mg day⁻¹)	Manganese (mg day⁻¹)	Molybdenum (µg day⁻¹)	Phosphorus (mg day⁻¹)	Selenium (µg day⁻¹)	Zinc (mg day⁻¹)
Males												
9–13 years	1300*	25*	700	2*	120	8	240	1.9*	34	1250	40	8
14–18 years	1300*	35*	890	3*	150	11	410	2.2*	43	1250	55	11
19–30 years	1000*	35*	900	4*	150	8	400	2.3*	45	700	55	11
Females												
9–13 years	1300*	21*	700	2*	120	8	240	1.6*	34	1250	40	8
14–18 years	1300*	24*	890	3*	150	15	360	1.6*	43	1250	55	9
19–30 years	1000*	25*	900	3*	150	18	310	1.8*	45	700	55	8

Food and Nutrition Board, Institute of Medicine, National Academies. Copyright 2001 by the National Academy of Sciences. All rights reserved.

This table presents recommended dietary allowances (RDAs) in **bold type** and adequate intakes (AIs) in ordinary type followed by an asterisk (*). RDAs and AIs may both be used as goals for individual intake. RDAs are set to meet the needs of almost all (97–98%) individuals in a group. For healthy breast-fed infants, the AI is the mean intake. The AI for other life-stage and gender groups is believed to cover needs of all individuals in the group, but lack of data or uncertainty in the data prevent being able to specify with confidence the percentage of individuals covered by this intake.

Sources: *Dietary Reference Intakes for Calcium, Phosphorous, Magnesium, Vitamin D, and Fluoride* (1997); *Dietary Reference Intakes for Thiamin, Riboflavin, Niacin, Vitamin B₆, Folate, Vitamin B₁₂, Pantothenic Acid, Biotin, and Choline* (1998); *Dietary Reference Intakes for Vitamin C, Vitamin E, Selenium, and Carotenoids* (2000); and *Dietary Reference Intakes for Vitamin A, Vitamin K, Arsenic, Boron, Chromium, Copper, Iodine, Iron, Manganese, Molybdenum, Nickel, Silicon, Vanadium, and Zinc* (2001). These reports may be accessed via http://www.nap.edu

Table 3 Dietary reference intakes (DRIs): tolerable upper intake levels (UL)[a], vitamins

Life stage group	Vitamin A (μg day^{-1})	Vitamin C (mg day^{-1})	Vitamin D (μg day^{-1})	Vitamin E (μg day^{-1})	Vitamin K	Thiamin	Riboflavin	Niacin (μg day^{-1})	Vitamin B$_6$ (mg day^{-1})	Folate (μg day^{-1})	Vitamin B$_{12}$	Pantothenic acid	Biotin	Choline (g day^{-1})	Carotenoids
Males, females															
9–13 years	1700	1200	50	600	ND	ND	ND	20	60	600	ND	ND	ND	2.0	ND
14–18 years	2800	1800	50	800	ND	ND	ND	30	80	800	ND	ND	ND	3.0	ND
19–70 years	3000	2000	50	1000	ND	ND	ND	35	100	1000	ND	ND	ND	3.5	ND

[a]UL = The maximum level of daily nutrient intake that is likely to pose no risk of adverse effects. Unless otherwise specified, the UL represents total intake from food, water, and supplements. Owing to lack of suitable data, ULs could not be established for vitamin K, thiamin, riboflavin, vitamin B$_{12}$, pantothenic acid, biotin, or carotenoids. In the absence of ULs, extra caution may be warranted in consuming levels above recommended intakes.

Food and Nutrition Board, Institute of Medicine, National Academies. Copyright 2001 by the National Academy of Sciences. All rights reserved.

Sources: *Dietary Reference Intakes for Calcium, Phosphorous, Magnesium, Vitamin D, and Fluoride* (1997); *Dietary Reference Intakes for Thiamin, Riboflavin, Niacin, Vitamin B$_6$, Folate, Vitamin B$_{12}$, Pantothenic Acid, Biotin, and Choline* (1998); *Dietary Reference Intakes for Vitamin C, Vitamin E, Selenium, and Carotenoids* (2000); and *Dietary Reference Intakes for Vitamin A, Vitamin K, Arsenic, Boron, Chromium, Copper, Iodine, Iron, Manganese, Molybdenum, Nickel, Silicon, Vanadium, and Zinc* (2001). These reports may be accessed via http://www.nap.edu

Table 4 Dietary reference intakes (DRIs): tolerable upper intake levels (UL)[a], Elements

Life stage group	Arsenic	Boron (mg day⁻¹)	Calcium (g day⁻¹)	Chromium	Copper (μg day⁻¹)	Fluoride (mg day⁻¹)	Iodine (μg day⁻¹)	Iron (mg day⁻¹)	Magnesium (μg day⁻¹)	Manganese (mg day⁻¹)	Molybdenum (μg day⁻¹)	Nickel (mg day⁻¹)	Phosphorus (g day⁻¹)	Selenium (μg day⁻¹)	Silicon	Vanadium (μg day⁻¹)	Zinc (mg day⁻¹)
Males, females																	
9–13 years	ND	11	2.5	ND	5000	10	600	40	350	6	1100	0.6	4	280	ND	ND	23
14–18 years	ND	17	2.5	ND	8000	10	900	45	350	9	1700	1.0	4	400	ND	ND	34
19–50 years	ND	20	2.5	ND	10 000	10	1100	45	350	11	2000	1.0	4	400	ND	1.8	40

[a]UL = The maximum level of daily nutrient intake that is likely to pose no risk of adverse effects. Unless otherwise specified, the UL represents total intake from food, water, and supplements. Owing to lack of suitable data, ULs could not be established for arsenic, chromium, and silicon. In the absence of ULs, extra caution may be warranted in consuming levels above recommended intakes.

Food and Nutrition Board, Institute of Medicine, National Academies. Copyright 2001 by the National Academy of Sciences. All rights reserved.

Sources: Dietary Reference Intakes for Calcium, Phosphorous, Magnesium, Vitamin D, and Fluoride (1997); Dietary Reference Intakes for Thiamin, Riboflavin, Niacin, Vitamin B₆, Folate, Vitamin B₁₂, Pantothenic Acid, Biotin, and Choline (1998); Dietary Reference Intakes for Vitamin C, Vitamin E, Selenium, and Carotenoids (2000); and Dietary Reference Intakes for Vitamin A, Vitamin K, Arsenic, Boron, Chromium, Copper, Iodine, Iron, Manganese, Molybdenum, Nickel, Silicon, Vanadium, and Zinc (2001). These reports may be accessed via http://www.nap.edu

Table 5 Dietary reference intakes (DRIs): estimated average requirements

Life stage group	Vit A (μg day⁻¹)[a]	Vit C (mg day⁻¹)	Vit E (μg day⁻¹)[b]	Thiamin (mg day⁻¹)	Riboflavin (mg day⁻¹)	Niacin (μg day⁻¹)[c]	Vit B_6 (mg day⁻¹)	Folate (μg day⁻¹)[d]	Vit B_{12} (μg day⁻¹)	Copper (μg day⁻¹)	Iodine (μg day⁻¹)	Iron (mg day⁻¹)	Magnesium (mg day⁻¹)	Molybdenum (μg day⁻¹)	Phosphorus (mg day⁻¹)	Selenium (μg day⁻¹)	Zinc (mg day⁻¹)
Males																	
9–13 years	445	39	9	0.7	0.8	9	0.8	250	1.5	540	73	5.9	200	26	1055	35	7.0
14–18 years	630	63	12	1.0	1.1	12	1.1	330	2.0	685	95	7.7	340	33	1055	45	8.5
19–30 years	625	75	12	1.0	1.1	12	1.1	320	2.0	700	95	6	330	34	580	45	9.4
Females																	
9–13 years	420	39	9	0.7	0.8	9	0.8	250	1.5	540	73	5.7	200	26	1055	35	7.0
14–18 years	485	56	12	0.9	0.9	11	1.0	330	2.0	685	95	7.9	300	33	1055	45	7.3
19–30 years	500	60	12	0.9	0.9	11	1.1	320	2.0	700	95	8.1	255	34	580	45	6.8

[a] As retinol activity equivalents (RAEs). 1 RAE = 1 Tg retinol, 12 Tg ϑ-carotene, 24 Tg l-carotene, or 24 Tg ϑ-cryptoxanthin. The RAE for dietary provitamin A carotenoids is twofold greater than retinol equivalents (RE), whereas the RAE for preformed vitamin A is the same as RE.

[b] As α-tocopherol. α-Tocopherol includes RRR-α-tocopherol, the only form of α-tocopherol that occurs naturally in foods, and the 2R-stereoisomeric forms of α-tocopherol (RRR-, RSR-, RRS-, and RSS-α-tocopherol) that occur in fortified foods and supplements. It does not include the 2S-stereoisomeric forms of α-tocopherol (SRR-, SSR-, SRS-, and SSS-α-tocopherol), also found in fortified foods and supplements.

[c] As niacin equivalents (NE). 1 mg of niacin = 60 mg of tryptophan.

[d] As dietary folate equivalents (DFE). 1 DFE = 1 μg food folate = 0.6 μg of folic acid from fortified food or as a supplement consumed with food = 0.5 μg of a supplement taken on an empty stomach.

Food and Nutrition Board, Institute of Medicine, National Academies. Copyright 2001 by the National Academy of Sciences. All rights reserved.

This table presents estimated average requirements (EARs), which serve two purposes: for assessing adequacy of population intakes, and as the basis for calculating recommended dietary allowances (RDAs) for individuals for those nutrients. EARs have not been established for vitamin D, vitamin K, pantothenic acid, biotin, choline, calcium, chromium, fluoride, manganese, or other nutrients not yet evaluated via the DRI process.

specified estimated average requirements (EARs), adequate intakes (AIs), and upper limits (ULs).

Obesity

Obesity has recently become an epidemic in the US, with 31% of American adults classified as obese (body mass index $>30\,kg\,m^{-2}$) and 68% classified as overweight (body mass index $>25\,kg\,m^{-2}$) in 2000. The prevalence of obesity in childhood tripled from 5% in 1980 to 15% in 2000 according to National Health and Nutrition Examination Surveys (NHANES). There is every indication that the developed countries of Western Europe are not far behind. Indeed, obesity is becoming a worldwide problem, rapidly increasing in many developing countries including China and India, and overtaking undernutrition as the major nutritional problem.

Although obesity affects children in all socioeconomic classes, it is more prevalent in those of lower socioeconomic status in the US and developed countries, whereas it tends to affect the well-off in developing countries. This suggests that food insecurity and poor food choices are more the problem than lack of availability because of poverty. Although only 30% of obesity begins in adolescence, some estimate that 80% of obese adolescents will become obese adults, and obese adolescents are at much more risk for diabetes and major medical complications later in life. Since long-term weight loss is usually very difficult to achieve and is often unsuccessful despite widespread attempts at dieting, efforts to prevent obesity in early life are important.

Ultimately, weight gain results from dietary energy intake exceeding metabolic basal needs and activity. Only rarely is this due to some identifiable disorder of basal metabolic requirements such as hypothyroidism. However, it is difficult to measure either dietary intake or activity with enough accuracy to detect the relatively small mismatch necessary to add weight. For example, a small increase in dietary intake of $200\,kcal\,day^{-1}$, without a corresponding increase in activity could theoretically result in a weight gain of 8 kg over the course of a year.

Although the heritability of obesity has been estimated to be on the order of 60–80% on the basis of twin studies and family histories, the genetics of obesity are complex and just beginning to be understood. Adult weight is much more reflective of biological parents rather than adoptive parents in twin studies. Known genetic syndromes producing obesity in humans are rare (on the order of 1–2% of obese patients) but should be considered, such as trisomy 21 (Down's syndrome), Prader-Willi,

Bardet-Biedl and Beckwith-Wiedemann syndromes, hypothyroidism, and polycystic ovary syndrome.

The adipose fat cell is not only a passive storage site but an endocrinologically active secretor of many substances like leptin, adiponectin, and cytokines, which participate in an inflammatory response and may mediate a host of adverse consequences, including insulin resistance and diabetes. Obesity is related to an increased risk of developing type 2 insulin-resistance diabetes mellitus, hyperlipidemia, heart disease, obstructive sleep apnea, asthma and other respiratory problems, back pain and orthopedic problems, fatty liver (nonalcoholic steato-hepatitis or NASH), gallstones, and depression. The increasing incidence of type 2 diabetes in obese adolescents is already being noticed, with estimates of 200 000 diabetics under age 20 years in the US predicted to rise to a lifetime risk of developing diabetes of 33–39% for those born in the year 2000.

The rapid increase in obesity has made standards based on population percentiles meaningless as medical obesity involved more than just the top 5% of weight-for-age. Instead of just relying on cross-sectional height- and weight-for-age graphs (see **Figures 1** and **2**), there has developed a need for a more valid indicator of obesity. The body mass index (BMI) charts recently released by the Centers for Disease Control allow for tracking of BMI standards for adolescents, who should have a BMI lower than the $20–25\,kg\,m^{-2}$ expected for adults. Although long-term validation data is not as available as in adults, in adolescents obesity is considered above the 95th percentile for age, with risk for obesity defined as above 85th percentile for age.

Body mass index is defined as weight (in kilograms) divided by height (in meters) squared, and is considered the best anthropometric surrogate for body composition (see **Figures 3** and **4**). Waist size may be an easier measurement to follow in adults, and particularly identifies central adiposity. Measurements by tape and caliper of mid-arm circumference and triceps skinfolds have a fairly good correlation (0.7–0.8) with more expensive research methods of underwater weighing and dual-energy X-ray absorptiometry (DEXA), and can be made even more accurate by including biceps, subscapular, and suprailiac skinfold measurements. Bioelectric impedance measures the difference in resistance between adipose and lean body tissue, but can be affected by fluid shifts especially in ill patients.

Physical examination should include blood pressure measurement because of the high percentage of comorbidity of the metabolic syndrome (obesity, hypertension, dyslipidemia, and/or diabetes).

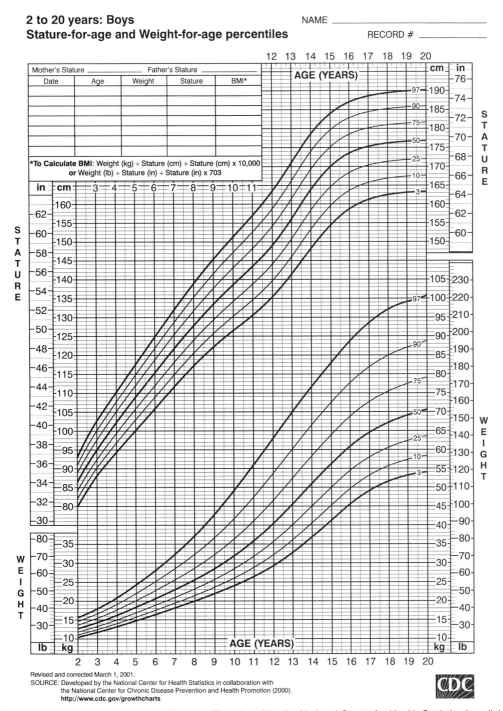

2 to 20 years: Boys
Stature-for-age and Weight-for-age percentiles

NAME _____

RECORD # _____

*To Calculate BMI: Weight (kg) ÷ Stature (cm) ÷ Stature (cm) x 10,000
or Weight (lb) ÷ Stature (in) ÷ Stature (in) x 703*

Revised and corrected March 1, 2001.
SOURCE: Developed by the National Center for Health Statistics in collaboration with
the National Center for Chronic Disease Prevention and Health Promotion (2000).
http://www.cdc.gov/growthcharts

Figure 1 Weight-for-age percentiles: boys, 2–20 years. (Developed by the National Center for Health Statistics in collaboration with the National Center for Chronic Disease Prevention and Health Promotion 2000: http://www.cdc.gov/growthcharts)

The metabolic syndrome is defined as three or more of the following: abdominal obesity (waist circumference greater than 40 inches (100 cm) in men or 35 inches (90 cm) in women), fasting hypertriglyceridemia ($<150 \, \text{mg dl}^{-1}$), high fasting glucose greater than $110 \, \text{mg dl}^{-1}$, low high-density cholesterol ($<40 \, \text{mg dl}^{-1}$), and high blood pressure ($>135/$ $85 \, \text{mm Hg}$). So far, it is mostly seen in later life ($>40\%$ of those over 60), but is increasingly seen at younger ages (7% of 20–29 years old). Acanthosis nigricans is a skin hyperpigmentation, chiefly around the neck, seen in about 20% of obese patients, especially African-Americans, which reflects insulin resistance and this finding should

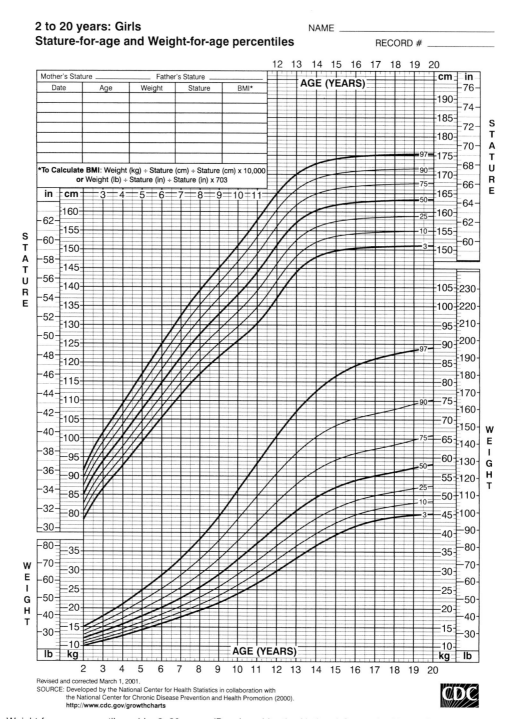

2 to 20 years: Girls
Stature-for-age and Weight-for-age percentiles

NAME _____

RECORD # _____

Revised and corrected March 1, 2001.
SOURCE: Developed by the National Center for Health Statistics in collaboration with
the National Center for Chronic Disease Prevention and Health Promotion (2000).
http://www.cdc.gov/growthcharts

Figure 2 Weight-for-age percentiles: girls, 2–20 years. (Developed by the National Center for Health Statistics in collaboration with the National Center for Chronic Disease Prevention and Health Promotion 2000: http://www.cdc.gov/growthcharts)

provoke screening tests for type 2 diabetes. Laboratory screening tests might include thyroid-stimulating hormone for hypothyroidism, fasting glucose, insulin, and glycosylated hemoglobin (HbA1C) for type 2 diabetes.

Diet histories and diet recalls are particularly important in nutritional assessments, but quantitative calorie counts are particularly unreliable in obese patients because of widespread conscious and subconscious underreporting of 20% or more. Regular meetings with a dietician should involve counseling on healthy eating choices. The recommendations regarding daily activity should include hours of television watching per day or per week because this is

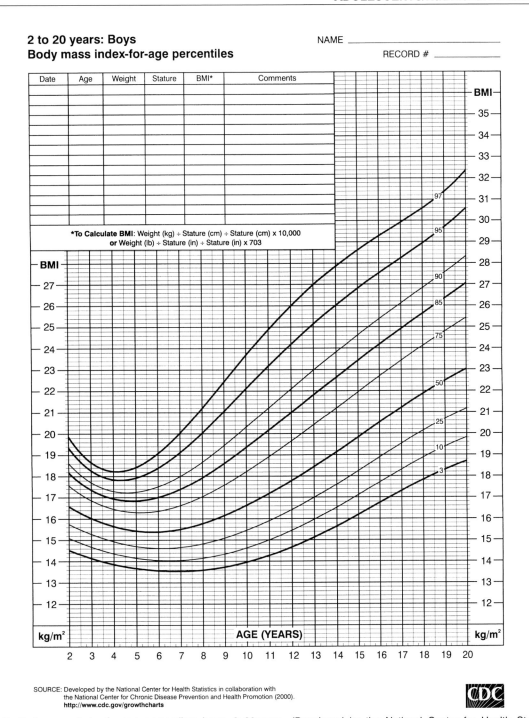

2 to 20 years: Boys
Body mass index-for-age percentiles

NAME _____

RECORD # _____

*To Calculate BMI: Weight (kg) ÷ Stature (cm) ÷ Stature (cm) x 10,000
or Weight (lb) ÷ Stature (in) ÷ Stature (in) x 703

SOURCE: Developed by the National Center for Health Statistics in collaboration with the National Center for Chronic Disease Prevention and Health Promotion (2000).
http://www.cdc.gov/growthcharts

Figure 3 Body mass index-for-age percentiles: boys, 2–20 years. (Developed by the National Center for Health Statistics in collaboration with the National Center for Chronic Disease Prevention and Health Promotion 2000: http://www.cdc.gov/growthcharts)

well correlated with obesity, not only because of decreased activity but also because of the influence of commercial snack food advertising.

Treatment should ideally involve a multidisciplinary team with a dietician, social worker, physical therapist, and physician, concentrating on lifestyle modification, moderate caloric restriction and regular exercise, with frequent follow-up and compliance being a good indicator of likelihood of success. Recent success with low-carbohydrate diets rather than the traditional low-fat diet advice suggests the importance of the role of satiety in maintaining caloric restriction. Most commercial diet plans promise short-term weight loss, but very few long-term studies have shown these to keep weight off for more than 6–12 months. As adolescents naturally

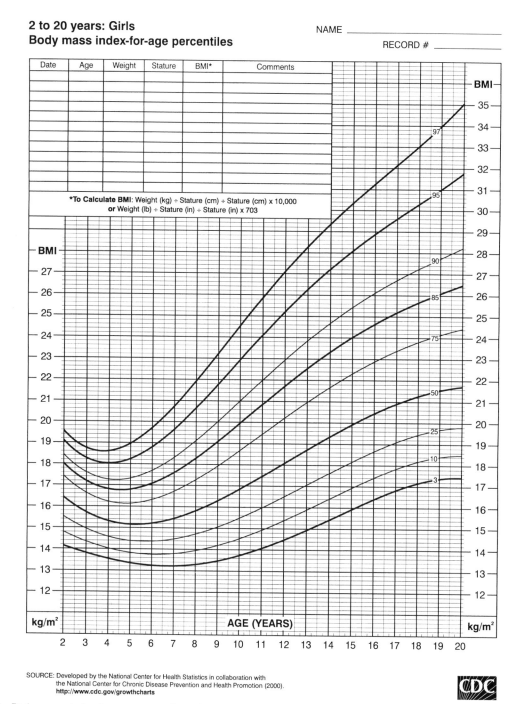

2 to 20 years: Girls
Body mass index-for-age percentiles

NAME _____

RECORD # _____

*To Calculate BMI: Weight (kg) ÷ Stature (cm) ÷ Stature (cm) x 10,000
or Weight (lb) ÷ Stature (in) ÷ Stature (in) x 703

SOURCE: Developed by the National Center for Health Statistics in collaboration with
the National Center for Chronic Disease Prevention and Health Promotion (2000).
http://www.cdc.gov/growthcharts

Figure 4 Body mass index-for-age percentiles: girls, 2–20 years. (Developed by the National Center for Health Statistics in collaboration with the National Center for Chronic Disease Prevention and Health Promotion 2000: http://www.cdc.gov/growthcharts)

gain weight with height as they progress through puberty, it is probably more important that they learn healthy eating and activity habits over the long term rather than losing weight quickly only to gain it back within a few months.

Medications such as phenteramine-fenfluramine and stimulants have gained recent notoriety with unforeseen side effects. Possible treatment with leptin and other hormones or antagonists has much future promise, but so far has been effective only in rare patients with specific defects. Surgical gastroplasty has proven the most successful long-term therapy for massively obese adults, possibly because of suppression of ghrelin, increased satiety, and reduced hunger, but morbidity and mortality is variable and the option of major surgery should be carefully considered only as a last resort before offering it to any adolescents.

Eating Disorders

Eating disorders affect 3–5 million in the US; 86% are diagnosed before the age of 20 and up to 11% of high-school students are affected. More than 90% are female, 95% Caucasian, and 75% have an onset in adolescence. Eating disorders are probably the most frequent causes of undernutrition in adolescents in developed countries, but only a relatively small percentage meet the full Diagnostic and Statistical Manual (DSM) IV criteria for anorexia nervosa (see **Table 6**), while most cases fall into the more general category eating disorder NOS (not otherwise specified). Bulimia, binge eating, and/or purging are probably much more common than full-blown anorexia nervosa, with some estimates of up to 20–30% of college women in the US, and often occur surreptitiously without telltale weight loss. Lifetime prevalence estimates range from 0.5% to 3% for anorexia nervosa and 1–19% for bulimia. So far eating disorders are considered rare in developing countries, but prevalence often increases dramatically when Western influences such as television advertising are introduced, as was the experience in the South Pacific Islands.

The pathophysiology of anorexia nervosa is not well understood, and there is probably a combination of environmental and psychological factors with a biochemical imbalance of neurotransmitters, especially serotonin and its precursor 5-hyroxyindole acetic acid, which tends to be reduced. There is a substantial biologic predisposition to run in families with heritability in twin studies of 35–90%.

Eating disorders should be suspected in any adolescent below normal weight ranges or with recent weight loss, but other medical conditions such as intestinal malabsorption, inflammatory bowel disease, and malignancy should also be considered. It is important to realize that most height and weight charts represent cross-sectional population norms, which may not be as sensitive as longitudinal tracking or height velocity of individuals, since puberty occurs at different ages. For example, a 12-year-old who does not gain weight for 6 months may just be entering puberty, or might be severely affected by growth failure due to a malignancy or inflammatory bowel disease.

Physical signs and symptoms of inadequate caloric intake may include amenorrhea, cold hands and feet, dry skin and hair, constipation, headaches, fainting, dizziness, lethargy, hypothermia, bradycardia, orthostatic hypotension, and edema. There is no specific laboratory diagnosis, but there are often endocrine and electrolyte abnormalities especially hypokalemia, hypophosphatemia, and hypochloremic metabolic alkalosis from vomiting, which often require careful supplementation.

Treatment may be very difficult and prolonged, often involving behavior therapy and occasionally long inpatient stays in a locked unit with threats of forced nasogastric feeding to maintain weight. There is a high risk of refeeding syndrome with edema, possible arrhythmias, and sudden death from electrolyte abnormalities, so protocols have been developed to provide a slow increase of calories, supplemented by adequate amounts of phosphorus and potassium. The anorexic patient's persistent distorted view of body image reality is very resistant to casual counseling.

The consequences of anorexia nervosa can be quite severe and include menstrual dysfunction, cardiovascular disease, arrhythmias, anemia, liver disease, swollen joints, endocrinopathies, cerebral atrophy, and even sudden death. There is a significant bone loss or osteopenia associated with amenorrhea and lack of estrogen stimulation, which is not completely reversed even with hormone replacement. Anorexia nervosa is well associated with other psychiatric diagnoses such as depression, anxiety, personality disorders, obsessive-compulsive disorder, and substance abuse, and psychiatric problems often continue to remain an issue even when normal weight is maintained. Prognosis is relatively poor compared to other adolescent medical illnesses,

Table 6 DSM-IV criteria for anorexia nervosa

A. Refusal to maintain body weight at or above a minimally normal weight for age and height (e.g., weight loss leading to maintenance of body weight less than 85% of that expected or failure to make expected weight gain during period of growth, leading to body weight less than 85% of that expected)
B. Intense fear of gaining weight or becoming fat, even though underweight
C. Disturbance in the way in which one's body weight or shape is experienced; undue influence of body weight or shape on self-evaluation, or denial of the seriousness of the current low body weight
D. In postmenarchal females, amenorrhea, that is, the absence of at least three consecutive menstrual cycles

Specify types
Restricting type: during the episode of anorexia nervosa, the person does not regularly engage in binge eating or purging behavior (i.e., self-induced vomiting or the misuse of laxatives or diuretics)
Binge-eating-purging type: during the episode of anorexia nervosa, the person has regularly engaged in binge eating or purging behavior (i.e., self-induced vomiting or the misuse of laxatives or diuretics)

with 33% persistence at 5 years and 17% at 11 years. Six per cent die within 5 years and 8.3% by 11 years.

Other Nutritional Diseases

In many countries of the world, HIV infection and acquired immunodeficiency syndrome (AIDS) has become one of the leading causes of undernutrition and cachexia, especially in younger patients. Indeed, many of the syndromes and consequences of protein-energy malnutrition are also seen in AIDS cachexia, such as frequent respiratory and other infections, diarrhea, malabsorption, and rashes. Weight loss is an AIDS-defining symptom, and weight loss of a third of usual weight usually signifies terminal illness. Fortunately, new generations of protease inhibitors and other medications have dramatically slowed the progression of HIV infection in many patients, as well as reducing the vertical transmission rate. Indeed, some studies have suggested that multivitamin supplementation of pregnant mothers may itself reduce vertical transmission rates in developing countries where antivirals are difficult to obtain. Proper attention to nutrition, with early enteral energy and micronutrient supplementation, is an important part of care, which is best instituted long before weight loss becomes manifest.

Specific Nutrients

Calcium

Calcium is the major component of bone, providing structural skeletal support to the human body (see 00033). The approximately 2–3 kg of bone calcium in each person also provides a storage reservoir for the small percentage of ionized calcium that allows muscle to contract, nerves to communicate, enzymes to function, and cells to react. The body has developed several hormonal mechanisms, including vitamin D, parathyroid hormone, and calcitonin, to protect the small amount of ionized calcium in the blood from changing drastically. Tight control of blood calcium levels is needed because unduly low blood calcium might result in uncontrolled tetanic muscle contractions and seizures, while high blood calcium levels may cause kidney stones and muscle calcifications. To increase blood calcium levels, vitamin D and its metabolites increase calcium absorption from the intestinal tract, parathyroid hormone increases calcium reabsorption from the kidney, and both increase resorption of calcium from the bone.

During the early years of life, calcium is deposited in the bone as it grows, but after about the 3rd decade, there is a steady decline in bone calcium. This is especially marked after menopause in women, when estrogen declines, and often leads to bone loss (osteopenia) to below a threshold that predisposes women in particular to fractures (osteoporosis). Osteoporosis is not just a disease of the elderly, and may occur in much younger patients, especially athletic young women, those with anorexia nervosa, those on steroids and other medications, and in anyone on prolonged bed rest, including astronauts experiencing long periods of weightlessness.

Dietary calcium is often seen as the most limiting factor in the development of peak bone mass, and strategies to increase dietary calcium have been promoted. Other factors in the development of bone mineral include height, weight, racial background and inheritance, gender, activity, vitamin D deficiency, parathyroid hormone deficiency, vitamin A, vitamin K, growth hormone, calcium, phosphorus, and magnesium. Phosphorus, the other major component of bone mineral, is relatively common in the diet.

In the 1997 DRIs, AIs of calcium were raised from 800 to 1300 mg in 9–18 year olds. Only a small percentage of the population takes in the RDA for calcium. The estimated average calcium intake in American women is only about 500–600 mg a day, and is much lower in the developing world (as low as 200 mg a day). From calcium tracer studies performed since the 1950s, intestinal calcium absorption ranges from 10% to 40% of ingested calcium, with a higher percentage absorption with lower calcium intakes. A large percentage (usually 70–80%) of dietary calcium is from milk and dairy products, which provides about 250 mg calcium per 8 oz (240 ml) glass of milk, and most studies show better absorption from dairy products than from vegetable sources. However, many people, especially non-Caucasians, develop relative lactose intolerance after childhood, and are reluctant to increase their dairy food intake.

Thus, attention has focused on whether supplementation or fortification with calcium, especially during adolescence, will ensure achievement of peak bone mass. Calcium supplementation in adolescent females has shown short-term increases in bone mineral density, but this may be because it increases mineralization in a limited amount of trabecular bone, and it remains to be seen whether this leads to long-term improvement or protection against future fractures. Also, most studies still assume that increased bone mineral density is synonymous with reduced fracture risk, although fractures may depend on many other factors such as optimal bone architecture and lack of falls. Although the majority of scientific opinion probably favors increased dietary calcium intake in adolescence, the factors that control bone mineralization are not yet completely understood, and long-term protection against eventual bone loss and fractures remains to be demonstrated by randomized clinical trials.

Iron

Iron deficiency is one of the most common vitamin or mineral deficiencies in the world, affecting 20% or more of women and children especially in developing countries. Adolescent women who have started menses or who are pregnant are particularly at risk for developing iron deficiency, which may ldevelop long before iron stores are exhausted and anemia ensues. Anemia (low hemoglobin or red cell volume) may lead to reduced school and work performance and may affect cognitive function, as well as leading to cardiovascular and growth problems. Diagnosis is made most simply by hemoglobin level or packed red cell volume (hematocrit) and red cell morphology, or alternatively by transferrin saturation, serum ferritin, or serum iron level. Microscopic examination of a red cell smear typically shows red cells that are small (microcytic) and pale (hypochromic).

Folate

Folate is a vitamin that is responsible for one-carbon methyl transfer in a variety of cellular reactions, including formation of purines and pyrimidines, which make up DNA and RNA. Folate deficiency may result in megaloblastic anemia, as forming red cells fail to divide. As the best source of folate is in green leafy vegetables, folate nutrition may be marginal in many adolescents. Recent epidemiologic evidence suggests that folate supplementation, at levels that are higher than usual dietary intake ($200–400\,\mu g\,day^{-1}$), reduced the incidence of neural tube defects (anencephaly and spina bifida) in newborns. Supplementation needs to be started early in pregnancy, within the first 8 weeks and before most pregnancies are apparent, so should involve most women of child-bearing age. The recent decision to fortify grains and cereals with folic acid in the US will also reduce serum homocysteine levels, lowering the risk of cardiovascular disease.

Zinc and Other Minerals

Zinc is a component of many metalloenzymes including those needed for growth, pancreatic enzymes, and intestinal secretions. Although it is unusual to find a documented case of clinical zinc deficiency apart from occasional cases of acrodermatitis enteropathica, there has been recent concern over the possibility of relative zinc deficiency, especially among chronically ill patients with excessive intestinal secretions. Zinc deficiency could lead to impaired taste (hypogeusia) and appetite and immunodeficiency as well as affecting growth. A large group of adolescents in Shiraz, Iran was described to be of very short stature because of dietary zinc deficiency. Similarly, a group of people in Keshan, China was found to develop cardiomyopathy because of a selenium deficiency in the soil. Iodine deficiency is surprisingly common worldwide, perhaps involving up to half of the world population or 3 billion people, especially in areas of Southeast Asia where it is not supplemented in salt. It may cause hypothyroidism, goiter (neck masses), cretinism, or impaired intelligence if severe.

See also: **Adolescents**: Nutritional Requirements. **Anemia**: Iron-Deficiency Anemia. **Calcium**. **Eating Disorders**: Anorexia Nervosa; Bulimia Nervosa; Binge Eating. **Folic Acid**. **Iron**. **Obesity**: Definition, Etiology and Assessment. **Osteoporosis**. **Zinc**: Physiology.

Further Reading

(2002) Adolescent Nutrition: a springboard for health. *Journal of the American Dietetic Association* Supplement March.

Cheung LWY and Richmond JB (eds.) (1995) *Child Health, Nutrition, and Physical Activity*, Human Kinetics. Windsor, Ontario.

Ebbeling CB, Pawlak DB, and Ludwig DS (2002) Childhood obesity: public health crisis, common sense cure. *Lancet* 360: 473–482.

Grand R, Sutphen J, and Dietz W (eds.) (1987) *Pediatric Nutrition*. London: Butterworth.

Heald F (1969) In *Adolescent Nutrition and Growth*. New York: Appleton Century Croft.

Hu FB, Manson JE, Stampfer MJ *et al.* (2001) Diet, lifestyle, and the risk of type 2 diabetes mellitus in women. *New England Journal of Medicine* 345(11): 790–797.

Kleinman R (ed.) (2004) *Pediatric Nutrition Handbook*, 5th edn. Elk Grove Village, Illinois American Academy of Pediatrics.

Koletzko B, girardet JP, Klish W, and Tabacco O (2002) Obesity in children and adolescents worldwide. *Journal of Pediatric Gastroenterology and Nutrition* 202: S205–S212.

McKigney J and Munro H (eds.) (1973) *Nutrient Requirements in Adolescents*. Cambridge: MIT Press.

Rickert VI (ed.) (1996) *Adolescent Nutrition: Assessment and Management*. Boston, MA: Jones and Bartlett.

Styne DM (2001) Childhood and adolescent obesity. *Pediatric Clinics of North America* 48: 823–854.

Walker WA, Watkins J, and Duggan C (eds.) (2003) *Nutrition in Pediatrics*, 3rd edn. London: BC Decker.

AGING

P Hyland and Y Barnett, Nottingham Trent University, Nottingham, UK

© 2005 Elsevier Ltd. All rights reserved.

Introduction

The aging processes, and interventions to ameliorate them, have fascinated humans since the dawn of civilization. Research into aging is now a vital area of human endeavor, as our species reaches the limits of its longevity and faces the prospect of an aging population.

This article aims to highlight the processes involved with aging and how they affect the entire hierarchical structure of living organisms, from molecules to cells, tissues, organs, and systems. Accordingly, many theories have evolved to explain the aging processes at each of these levels. A brief overview of these theories will highlight the framework for investigations into the aging processes with the ultimate aim of reducing their deleterious effects, such as age-related disease, perhaps with nutritional and molecular biological intervention strategies.

The term 'aging' can have a wide variety of different meanings in different circumstances. For example, the normal processes from birth, through growth and maturation, an extended period of adulthood, and on to senescence can be thought of as aging.

The term is used here to describe a progressive sequence of detrimental age-related changes that are observed to occur in every individual of a given species, although they may appear at different rates. These changes lead to a breakdown in the normal homeostatic mechanisms, with the result that the functional capacity of the body and its ability to respond to a wide variety of extrinsic and intrinsic agents is often decreased. This causes the degradation of structural elements within the cells, tissues, and organs of the body, leading eventually to the onset of age-related disorders and ultimately death.

Social and Demographic Considerations

An individual's life expectancy is contributed to by the interaction of intrinsic (genetic and epigenetic) factors with extrinsic (environmental and life style) factors (**Figure 1**). In the world's more developed countries (MDCs) the life expectancy at birth in the 1900s was around 47 years. By the end of the twentieth century this rose to a mean of 78 and 76 years in western Europe and north America, respectively, with many individuals living much longer. This dramatic increase in average life expectancy has been largely due to improvements in environmental conditions such as nutrition, housing, sanitation, and medical and social services, and has resulted in a large increase in the number of older people around the world. This change in the age structure of society is compounded by the decreasing fertility levels in the world's populations leading to large gains in worldwide median population ages. Our aging populations have a growing number and proportion of older people and, importantly, a growing number and proportion of very elderly people.

Based on the current rates and trends in population growth it has been predicted that by the year 2025 the elderly population (aged 65 and above) in the world's MDCs will increase by more than 50%, and will more than double worldwide. The elderly population itself is aging with the very elderly (aged 80 and above) being the fastest growing section of the elderly population. This

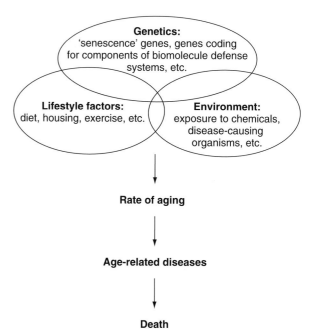

Figure 1 Interactive factors that contribute to the aging process. (Reproduced with permission from Barnett YA (1994) Nutrition and the ageing process. *British Journal of Biomedical Sciences* **51**: 278–287.)

changing demographic picture will result in a large increased prevalence worldwide of long-term illness, disability, and the degenerative diseases associated with aging. These alterations in the proportions of the population of working age and those beyond working age will have a significant impact on the funding and costs of healthcare for all nations, making research into aging of critical international importance.

Theories of Aging

The human body has a hierarchy of structure and function, ranging from cellular biomolecules, through to organelles and cells, and on to tissues, organs, and the body's various systems. The biological manifestations that occur with aging affect the entire hierarchical structure of living systems. Age-related effects are seen in the accumulation of damaged cellular biomolecules (e.g., advanced glycosylation end products, lipid peroxidation products, genetic damage, and mutation), damaged organelles (mitochondria), and loss of cellular function, which contributes to dysfunction of the body's tissues, organs, and systems. These hierarchical changes have paved the way for over 300 theories in an attempt to explain how and why aging occurs. These theories have previously been broadly categorized into: (1) programed or genetic theories; and (2) damage accumulation (stochastic) theories.

However, with ongoing research these categories have not proven to be entirely comprehensive or mutually exclusive and it is more likely that there is a shifting range throughout the life span that reflects a decreasing influence of genetic factors and an increasing influence of stochastic events.

Programed and Genetic Theories

Programed and genetic theories propose that the process of aging follows a biological timetable, perhaps a continuation of the one that regulates childhood growth and development. There are a number of lines of evidence supporting these theories.

Longevity genes It is clear that aging is controlled to some extent by genetic mechanisms. The distinct differences in life span among species are a direct indication of genetic control, at least at the species level. A number of genes have been identified in yeast, nematode worms (*Caenorhabditis elegans*), and fruit flies (*Drosophila melanogaster*) that significantly increase the organism's potential maximum life span. The products of these genes act in a diverse number of ways and are involved in stress response and resistance, development, signal transduction, transcriptional regulation, and metabolic activity.

However, the genetics of longevity have not been as revealing in mammalian studies. In mouse systems genes involved with immune response have been implicated in longevity, as has the 'longevity gene' $p66^{shc}$, which is involved in signal transduction pathways that regulate the cellular response to oxidative stress. In humans, a number of mitochondrial DNA polymorphisms are associated with longevity. Linkage analysis in humans systems has associated certain genes on chromosome 4 with exceptional longevity. Further support for human longevity genes may be provided by the observation that siblings and parents of centenarians live longer. The major histocompatibility complex (MHC), the master genetic control of the immune system, may also be one of the gene systems controlling aging, since a number of genetic defects that cause immunodeficiency shorten the life span of humans. Certain MHC phenotypes have also been associated with malignancy, autoimmune disease, Alzheimer's disease, and xeroderma pigmentosum in humans.

Accelerated aging syndromes No distinct phenocopy exists for normal aging, but there are several genetic diseases/syndromes that display some features of accelerated aging, including Hutchinson-Gilford syndrome (classic early onset Progeria), Werner's syndrome, and Down's syndrome. Patients with these syndromes suffer from many signs of premature aging including hair loss, early greying, and skin atrophy, and also suffer from premature age-related diseases such as atherosclerosis, osteoporosis, and glucose intolerance. The defined genetics involved in these syndromes provide strong evidence for the genetic basis of aging.

Neuroendocrine theories These theories propose that functional decrements in neurons and their associated hormones are pivotal to the aging process. An important version of this theory suggests that the hypothalamic-pituitary-adrenal (HPA) axis is the key regulator of mammalian aging. The neuroendocrine system regulates early development, growth, puberty, the reproductive system, metabolism, and many normal physiological functions. Functional changes to this system could exert effects of aging throughout an organism. However, the cells of the neuroendocrine system are subject to the normal cellular aging processes found in all cells, and the changes occurring in the neuroendocrine system may be secondary expressions of the aging phenotype.

Immunologic theory and immunosenescence
Deterioration of the immune system with aging ('immunosenescence') may contribute to morbidity and mortality due to decreased resistance to infection and, possibly, certain cancers in the aged. T-cell function decreases and autoimmune phenomena increase in elderly individuals.

Although the immune system obviously plays a central role in health status and survival, again the cells of the immune system are subject to the normal cellular aging processes found in all cells. Changes to the immune system may be secondary expressions of the aging phenotype.

Cellular senescence At the cellular level, most, if not all, somatic cell types have a limited replicative capacity *in vitro* before they senesce and die. The number of cell population doublings *in vitro* is inversely correlated with donor age. This is called the 'Hayflick phenomenon' after the scientist credited with its discovery. This limit in the capacity of a cell type or tissue to divide and replenish itself would have major repercussions *in vivo*. There is evidence that replicative senescence is related to *in vivo* aging, but definitive evidence that senescent cells accumulate *in vivo* is lacking to date. Many alterations to normal cellular physiology are exhibited with the senescent phenotype, indicating that senescent cells exist in a growth state that is quite distinct from that of young cells and are subject to a complex alteration to their cellular physiology.

A number of possible explanations for limiting the number of cell population doublings have been proposed, including a tumor suppressive mechanism. One proposal is that the shortening of telomeres, the sequences of noncoding DNA located at the end of chromosomes, is a measure of the number of cell divisions that a cell has experienced. These telomeres may act as specialized regions of the genome, a sacrificial 'sentinel' zone, for the detection of DNA damage being noncoding, more prone to damage, and less prone to repair than the genome as a whole. Damage to telomeres transposes to telomere shortening, and loss of telomere higher order structure may trigger senescence and/or apoptosis.

Studies involving fusion of normal cells (subject to senescence) with immortal cell lines *in vitro* have clearly demonstrated that the senescent phenotype is dominant, and that unlimited division potential results from changes in normal growth control mechanisms. These fusion studies have also revealed the existence of several dominant genes associated with the process of cellular senescence. These genes reside on a number of chromosomes, including 1,4, and X.

Disposable soma theory The disposable soma theory suggests that aging is due to stochastic background damage to the organism, i.e., damage that is not repaired efficiently because the energy resources of the somatic cells are limited. So, instead of wasting large amounts of energy in maintaining the whole body in good condition, it is far more economical to simply repair the heritable stem cell genetic material, in order to ensure the survival of the species. In this way the future of the species is secured at the expense of individual lives. When the somatic energy supply is exhausted, the body ages and dies, but the genetic material survives (in the next generation).

Damage Accumulation (Stochastic) Theories

The 'damage' or 'error' theories emphasize intrinsic and environmental insults to our cellular components that accumulate throughout life and gradually cause alterations in biological function and the physiological decline associated with aging.

Somatic mutation and DNA repair Damage to DNA occurs throughout the lifetime of a cell. If this damage is not repaired or removed then mutations may result. Mutations may result in the synthesis of aberrant proteins with altered or absent biological function; alterations to the transcriptional and translational machinery of a cell; and deregulation of gene control. The accumulation of mutations on their own, or in combination with other age-related changes, may lead to alterations in cellular function and ultimately the onset of age-related disease.

Error catastrophe This theory suggests that damage to mechanisms that synthesize proteins results in faulty proteins, which accumulate to a level that causes catastrophic damage to cells, tissues, and organs. Altered protein structure has been clearly demonstrated to occur with age; however, most of these changes are posttranslational in nature, and hence do not support this theory of aging. Such changes to protein structure may result in progressive loss of 'self-recognition' by the cells of the immune system and thus increase the likelihood that the immune system would identify self-cells as foreign and launch an immune attack. Indeed, the incidence of autoimmune episodes is known to increase with age.

Cross-linking   The cross-linking theory states that an accumulation of cross-linked biomolecules caused by a covalent or hydrogen bond damages cellular and tissue function through molecular aggregation and decreased mobility. The modified malfunctional biomolecules accumulate and become increasingly resistant to degradation processes and may represent a physical impairment to the functioning of organs. There is evidence *in vitro* for such cross-linking over time in collagen and in other proteins, and in DNA. Many agents exist within the body that have the potential to act as cross-linking agents, e.g., aldehydes, antibodies, free radicals, quinones, citric acid, and polyvalent metals, to name but a few.

Free radicals   The most popular, widely tested and influential of the damage accumulation theories of aging is the 'free radical' theory, first proposed by Harman in 1956. Free radicals from intrinsic and extrinsic sources (**Table 1**) can lead to activation of cytoplasmic and/or nuclear signal transduction pathways, modulation of gene and protein expression, and also alterations to the structure and ultimately the function of biomolecules. Free radicals may thus induce alterations to normal cell, tissue, and organ functions, which may result in a breakdown of homeostatic mechanisms and lead to the onset of age-related disorders and ultimately death. It can

be predicted from this theory that the life span of an organism may be increased by slowing down the rate of initiation of random free radical reactions or by decreasing their chain length. Studies have demonstrated that it is possible to increase the life span of cells *in vitro* by culturing them with various antioxidants or free radical scavengers. Antioxidant supplementation with a spin-trapping agent has been demonstrated to increase the lifespan of the senescence accelerated mouse, although as yet there is little evidence for increasing the life span of a normal mammalian species by such strategies.

Mitochondrial DNA damage   This hypothesis combines elements of several theories, covering both the stochastic and genetic classes of aging theories. It is proposed that free radical reactive oxygen species generated in the mitochondria contribute significantly to the somatic accumulation of mitochondrial DNA mutations. This leads to a downward spiral wherein mitochondrial DNA damage results in defective mitochondrial respiration that further enhances oxygen free radical production, mitochondrial DNA damage, and mutation. This leads to the loss of vital bioenergetic capacity eventually resulting in aging and cell death.

The absence of evidence that exclusively supports any one theory leaves no doubt that aging is due to many processes, interactive and interdependent, that determine life span and death.

Table 1   Extrinsic and intrinsic sources of free radicals

Extrinsic sources	Intrinsic sources
Radiation: ionizing, ultraviolet	Plasma membrane: lipoxygenase, cycloxygenase, NADPH oxidase
Drug oxidation: paracetamol, carbon tetrachloride, cocaine	Mitochondria: electron transport, ubiquinone, NADH dehydrogenase
Oxidizing gases: oxygen, ozone, nitrogen dioxide	Microsomes: electron transport, cytochrome p450, cytochrome b_5
Xenobiotic elements: arsenic (As), lead (Pb), mercury (Hg), cadmium (Cd)	Peroxisomes: oxidases, flavoproteins
Redox cycling substances: paraquat, diquat, alloxan, doxorubicin	Phagocytic cells: neutrophils, macrophytes, eosinophils, endothelial cells
Heat shock	Auto-oxidation reactions: Metal catalyzed reactions
Cigarette smoke and combustion products	Other: hemoglobin, flavins, xanthine oxidase, monoamine oxidase, galactose oxidase, indolamine dioxygenase, tryptophan dioxygenase
	Ischemia – reperfusion

Age-Related Diseases

Regardless of the molecular mechanisms that underlie the aging process, a number of well-characterized changes to the structure and therefore the function of the major cellular biomolecules (lipids, proteins, carbohydrates, and nucleic acids) are known to occur with age (**Table 2**). The age-related alterations to the structure and therefore the function of cellular biomolecules have physiological consequences and may directly cause or lead to an increased susceptibility to the development of a number of diseases (**Figure 2**).

Cellular biomolecules are constantly exposed to a variety of extrinsic and intrinsic agents that have the potential to cause damage. A number of defense systems exist, e.g., antioxidant enzymes and DNA repair systems, which aim to reduce, remove, or repair damaged biomolecules. These defense systems are not perfect, however, and biomolecular damage may still occur. Such damage can result in the degradation of structural elements within the cells, tissues, and organs of the body, leading to a decline in biological function and eventually to disease and death.

Table 2 Major age-related alterations in biomolecule structure and the resultant physiological consequences of such structural changes

Biomolecule	Alteration	Physiological consequence
Lipids	Lipid peroxidation	Oxidized membranes become rigid, lose selective permeability and integrity. Cell death may occur
		Peroxidation products can act as cross-linking agents and may play a role in protein aggregation, the generation of DNA damage and mutations, and the age-related pigment lipofuscin
Proteins	Racemization, deamination, oxidatation, and carbamylation	Alterations to long-lived proteins may contribute to aging and/or pathologies. For example, modified crystallins may aggregate in the lens of the eye thus leading to the formation of cataracts
		Cross-linking and formation of advance glycosylation end-products (AGEs), which can severely affect protein structure and function
		Effects on the maintenance of cellular homeostasis
Carbohydrates	Fragmentation, depolymerization Glucose auto-oxidation	Alters physical properties of connective tissue. Such alteration may be involved in the etiology and pathogenesis of osteoarthritis and other age-related joint disorders
		Glycosylation of proteins *in vivo* with subsequent alteration of biological function; for example, glycosylation of insulin in patients with diabetes may result in altered biological function of insulin and so contribute to the pathogenesis of the disease
Nucleic acids	Strand breaks Base adducts Loss of 5-methyl cytosine from DNA	Damage could be expected to interfere with the processes of transcription, translation, and DNA replication. Such interference may reduce a cell's capacity to synthesize vital polypeptides/proteins. In such circumstances cell death may occur. The accumulation of a number of hits in critical cellular genes associated with the control of cell growth and division has been shown to result in the process of carcinogenesis
		Dedifferentiation of cells (5-methylcytosine plays an important role in switching off genes as part of gene regulation)
		If viable, such dedifferentiated cells may have altered physiology and may contribute to altered tissue/organ function

The physiological alterations with age proceed at different rates in different individuals. Some of the common changes seen in humans are: the function of the immune system decreases by the age of 30 years of age, reducing defenses against infection or tumor establishment and increasing the likelihood of autoimmune disorders; metabolism starts to slow down at around 25 years of age; kidney and liver function decline; blood vessels lose their elasticity; bone mass peaks at age 30 years and drops about 1% per year thereafter; the senses fade; the epidermis becomes dry and the dermis thins; the quality of and need for sleep diminish; and the brain loses 20% of its weight, slowing recall and mental performance. A number of age-related diseases may develop as a consequence of the tissue, organ, and system deterioration (**Table 3**).

Modification of the Aging Process

Can the adverse consequences of aging be prevented? Down through the ages many have pursued the elixir of life. Attempts to increase the average life expectancy and quality of life in the elderly can only succeed by slowing the aging process itself. In humans, the rate of functional decline associated with aging may be reduced through good nutrition, exercise, timely health care, and avoidance of risk factors for age-related disease.

Nutritional Modification

It is clear that diet contributes in substantial ways to the development of age-related diseases and that modification of the diet can contribute to their prevention and thus help to improve the quality of life in old age. Macronutrient intake levels can play a significant part in the progression of age-related diseases and affect the quality of life. For example, the total and proportional intakes of polyunsaturated fatty acids and saturated fatty acids in the Western diet may have an effect on the incidence of atherosclerosis and cardiovascular diseases.

Our dietary requirements also change as we age and if such changes are not properly addressed this could lead to suboptimal nutritional status. This challenge is compounded by a decrease in the body's ability to monitor food and nutrient intakes. Dietary intake and requirements are complex issues, intertwined with many health and life style issues. However, most research points towards the need for

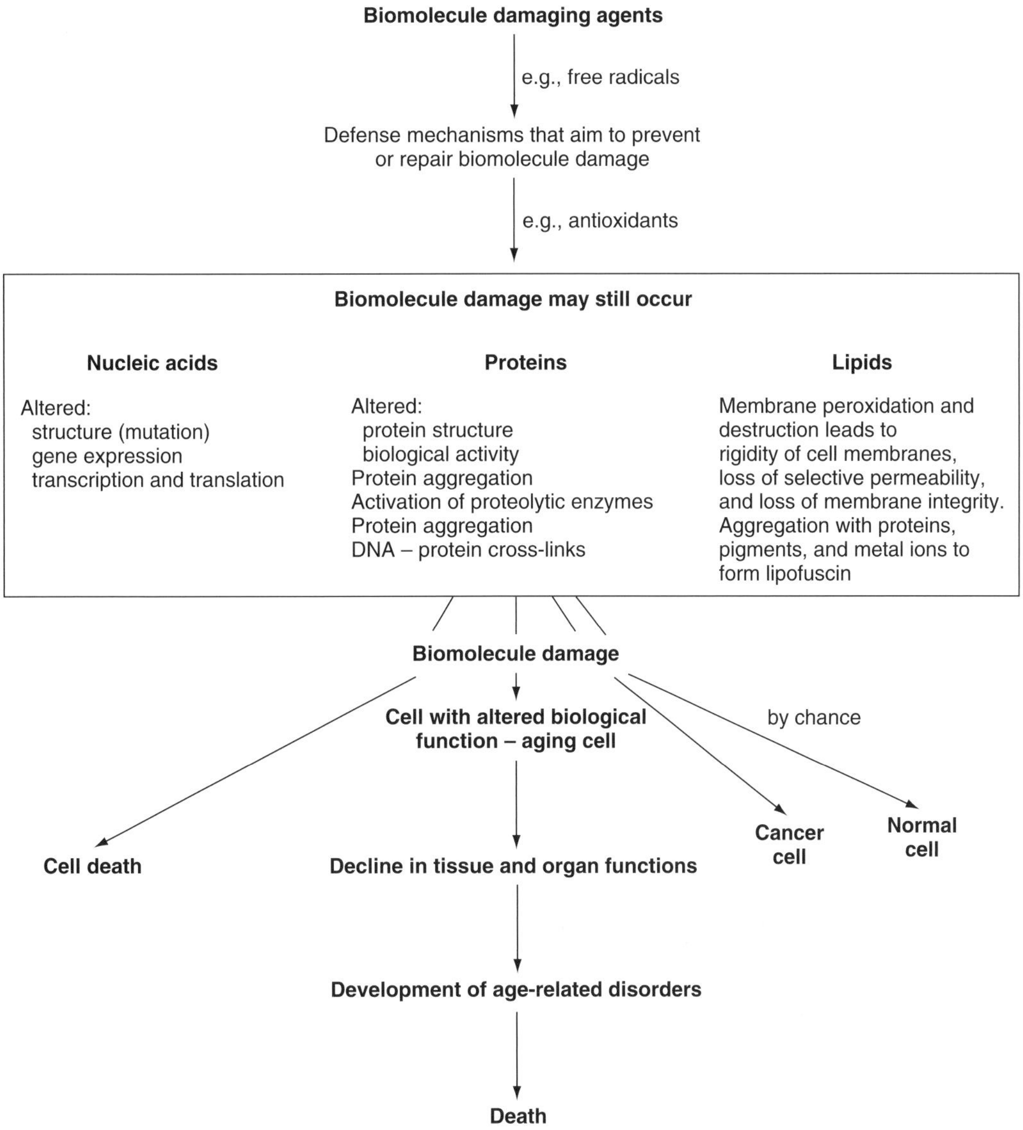

Figure 2 Biomolecule damage and the aging process. (Reproduced with permission from Barnett YA (1994) Nutrition and the aging process. *British Journal of Biomedical Sciences* **51**: 278–287.)

a varied diet as we age, with an increased emphasis on micronutrient intake levels.

An exemplary diet for healthy aging can be found in the traditional diet of Okinawa, Japan. Okinawans are the longest-living population in the world according to the World Health Organization, with low disability rates and the lowest frequencies of coronary heart disease, stroke, and cancer in the world. This has been attributed to healthy life style factors such as regular physical activity, minimal tobacco use, and developed social support networks as antistress mechanisms, all of which are underpinned by a varied diet low in salt and fat (with monosaturates as the principal fat) and high levels of micronutrient and antioxidant consumption.

Vitamins and micronutrients The mechanisms by which certain vitamins and micronutrients mediate their protective effect in relation to a number of age-related disorders is based in large part upon their abilities to prevent the formation of free radicals or scavenging them as they are formed, either directly (e.g., vitamins C, E, and β-carotene) or indirectly (e.g., copper/zinc superoxide dismutase, manganese-dependent superoxide dismutase, selenium-dependent glutathione peroxidase). **Table 4** summarizes the effects that a variety of vitamins and micronutrients can have on age-related disease. Only by exploring more fully the underlying molecular mechanisms of aging and the major classes of antioxidants will it be possible to establish the role

Table 3 Major age-related alterations *in vivo* and the resultant pathological conditions

Body system	Pathological changes
Cardiovascular	Atherosclerosis, coronary heart disease, hypertension
Central nervous system	Reduction of cognitive function, development of various dementias (e.g., Alzheimer's disease and Parkinson's disease)
Endocrine	Noninsulin-dependent diabetes, hypercortisolemia
Hemopoietic	Anemia, myelofibrosis
Immune	General decline in immune system function, particularly in T cells
Musculoskeletal	Osteoporosis, osteoarthritis, skeletal muscle atrophy
Renal	Glomerulosclerosis, interstitial fibrosis
Reproductive	Decreased spermatogenesis, hyalinization of semeniferous tubules
Respiratory	Interstitial fibrosis, decreased vital capacity, chronic obstructive pulmonary disease
Sense organs	Cataracts, senile macular degeneration, diabetic retinopathy
All systems	Cancer

Table 4 Effects of vitamins and micronutrients on age-related disorders

Vitamin or micronutrient	Possible effect on age-related disorder
Vitamins B_6, E copper, zinc, and selenium	Impairment of immune function in older humans if inadequate amounts
Vitamins C, E, and carotenoids	Increased amount in the diet is associated with delayed development of various forms of cataract
	Protective effect against the development of lung cancer in smokers
Carotenoids and zinc	Dietary supplementation associated with a decreased risk of age-related macular degeneration
Selenium	Absolute or relative deficiency associated with development of a number of cancers (not breast cancer)
Vitamin C, β-carotene, α-tocopherol, and zinc	Dietary supplementation may decrease the rate of development of atherosclerosis
Selenium, copper, zinc, lithium, vanadium, chromium, and magnesium	Dietary deficits are associated with an increased risk of cardiovascular disease
Vitamins B_{12}, B_6, and folate	Adequate levels throughout a lifetime may prevent some of the age-related decrease in cognitive function
Chromium	Deficiency is associated with an increased risk of the development of type 2 diabetes mellitus

of, and develop strategies for using various classes of antioxidants to reduce the effects of aging. Other dietary components may also have a beneficial effect in preventing or delaying the onset of age-related disease. For example, as a deterrent against the onset of osteoporosis, adults should ensure adequate calcium and vitamin D intakes.

Dietary energy restriction The effect of caloric restriction on life span has only been convincingly demonstrated in rodents to date. Feeding mice and rats diets that are severely deficient in energy (about 35% of that of animals fed ad libitum, after the initial period of growth) retards the aging of body tissues, inhibits the development of disease and tumors, and prolongs life span significantly. The exact mechanism of action of dietary energy restriction remains to be elucidated, but may involve modulation of free radical metabolism, or the reduced hormone excretion that occurs in dietary restricted animals may lower whole body metabolism resulting in less 'wear and tear' to body organs and tissues.

Current investigations into the effects of dietary energy restriction (of about 30%) on the life spans of primates, squirrels, and rhesus monkeys continue. Caloric restriction in rhesus monkeys leads to reductions in body temperature and energy expenditure consistent with the rodent studies. These investigations should have direct implications for a dietary energy restriction intervention aimed at slowing down the aging process in humans, should any humans wish to extend their life span at such a cost. Once the mechanisms of effects of caloric restriction on longevity are understood it may be possible to develop drugs that act through these mechanisms directly, mitigating the need for diets that interfere with the quality of life.

Molecular Biological Interventions and the Aging Process

Accelerated aging syndromes show degenerative characteristics similar to those appearing during normal aging. The mutations leading to these disorders are being identified and their roles in the aging process are being elucidated. Examining differences in the genetic material from normal elderly people and those with progeria should help to give a better understanding of the genetic mechanisms of aging. Identification of a control gene or genes that inhibit the action of the genes producing the progeroid phenotype might make it possible to slow down aberrant protein production in normal people as well.

As an example, the genetic defect that predisposes individuals to the development of Werner's syndrome has now been elucidated. Individuals with this disease carry two copies of a mutant gene that codes for a helicase enzyme (helicases split apart or unwind the two strands of the DNA double helix). DNA helicases play a role in DNA replication and repair.

In light of the biological function of these enzymes it has been proposed that the reason for the premature aging in Werner's syndrome is that the defective helicase prevents DNA repair enzymes from removing background DNA damage, which thus becomes fixed as mutations, with consequent deleterious effects on cellular function. It remains to be determined whether increasing the fidelity or activity of helicases in cells will extend their life span.

Since it appears that the loss of telomeric DNA sequences can lead to replicative senescence in dividing cells, in theory by preventing such telomere loss the life span of the cell could be extended. A naturally occurring enzyme, telomerase, exists to restore telomeric DNA sequences lost by replication. Telomerase is normally only functional in germ cells. Manipulating certain cell types (e.g., cells of the immune system) to regulate the expression telomerase may extend their functional life span. Drugs that enhance telomerase activity in somatic cells are currently being developed. However, cellular senescence has been implicated as a tumor suppressor mechanism and it has been found that cancer cells express telomerase. An uncontrolled expression of this enzyme in somatic cells may lead to the onset of malignancy through uncontrolled cell proliferation. Thus, any intervention aiming to increase life span based on the cellular expression of telomerase must strike a balance between maintaining controlled cell division and uncontrolled proliferation.

A number of single gene mutations have been identified that affect metabolic function, hormonal signaling, and gene silencing pathways. In the future it may be possible to develop drugs to mimic the antiaging effects that these genes exert.

See also: **Antioxidants**: Diet and Antioxidant Defense; Observational Studies; Intervention Studies. **Cancer**: Epidemiology and Associations Between Diet and Cancer. **Coronary Heart Disease**: Lipid Theory; Prevention. **Fats and Oils. Fatty Acids**: Monounsaturated; Saturated. **Growth and Development, Physiological Aspects. Lipids**: Chemistry and Classification; Composition and Role of Phospholipids. **Nucleic Acids. Nutrient Requirements, International Perspectives. Older People**: Nutritional Requirements; Nutrition-Related Problems; Nutritional Management of Geriatric Patients. **Protein**: Synthesis and Turnover; Requirements and Role in Diet; Digestion and Bioavailability. **Supplementation**: Role of Micronutrient Supplementation.

Further Reading

Barnett YA (1994) Nutrition and the ageing process. *British Journal of Biomedical Sciences* 51: 278–287.

Bellamy D (ed.) (1995) *Ageing: A Biomedical Perspective.* Chichester: Wiley.

Esser K and Martin GM (1995) *Molecular Aspects of Ageing* Chichester: Wiley.

Finch CE (1991) *Longevity, Senescence and the Genome* Chicago: University of Chicago Press.

Hayflick L (1993) Aspects of cellular ageing. *Reviews in Clinical Gerontology* 3: 207–222.

Kanungo MS (1994) In *Genes and Ageing*. Cambridge: Cambridge University Press.

Kirkland JL (2002) The biology of senescence: potential for the prevention of disease. *Clinics in Geriatric Medicine* 18: 383–405.

Kirkwood TBL (1992) Comparative lifespans of species: why do species have the lifespans they do? *American Journal of Clinical Nutrition* 55: 1191S–1195S.

Mera SL (1992) Senescence and pathology in ageing. *Medical Laboratory Sciences* 4: 271–282.

(1995) Somatic mutations and ageing: cause or effect? *Mutation Research, DNAging* (special issue) 338: 1–234.

Tominaga K, Olgun A, Smith JR, and Periera-Smith OM (2002) Genetics of cellular senescence. *Mechanisms of Ageing and Development* 123: 927–936.

Troen BR (2003) The biology of ageing. *The Mount Sinai Journal of Medicine* 70(1): 3–22.

US Bureau of the Census (1999) Report WP/98, World Population Profile. Washington, DC: US Government Printing Office.

von Zglinicki T, Bürkle A, and Kirkwood TBL (2001) Stress, DNA damage and ageing – an integrated approach. *Experimental Gerontology* 36: 1049–1062.

ALCOHOL

Contents

Absorption, Metabolism and Physiological Effects

R Rajendram, R Hunter and V Preedy, King's College London, London, UK
T Peters, King's College Hospital, London, UK

© 2005 Elsevier Ltd. All rights reserved.

After caffeine, ethanol is the most commonly used recreational drug worldwide. 'Alcohol' is synonymous with 'ethanol,' and 'drinking' often describes the consumption of beverages containing ethanol.

In the United Kingdom, a unit of alcohol (standard alcoholic drink; **Table 1**) contains 8 g of ethanol. The Department of Health (United Kingdom) and several of the medical Royal Colleges have recommended sensible limits for alcohol intake based on units of alcohol. However, because the amount of ethanol in one unit varies throughout the world (**Tables 2 and 3**), the unit system does not allow international comparisons.

Despite these guidelines, the quantity of alcohol consumed varies widely. Many enjoy the pleasant psychopharmacological effects of alcohol. However, some experience adverse reactions due to genetic variation of enzymes that metabolize alcohol. Misuse of alcohol undoubtedly induces pathological changes in most organs of the body. Some questionable data have suggested that alcohol may be beneficial in the reduction of ischaemic heart disease.

Many of the effects of alcohol correlate with the peak concentration of ethanol in the blood during a drinking session. It is therefore important to understand the factors that influence the blood ethanol concentration (BEC) achieved from a dose of ethanol.

Physical Properties of Ethanol

Ethanol is produced from the fermentation of glucose by yeast. Ethanol (**Figure 1**) is highly soluble in water due to its polar hydroxyl (OH) group. The nonpolar (C_2H_5) group enables ethanol to dissolve lipids and thereby disrupt biological membranes. As a relatively uncharged molecule, ethanol crosses cell membranes by passive diffusion.

Absorption and Distribution of Alcohol

The basic principles of alcohol absorption from the gastrointestinal (GI) tract and subsequent distribution are well understood. Beverages containing ethanol pass down the oesophagus into the stomach. The endogenous flora of the GI tract can also transform food into a mixture of alcohols including ethanol. This is particularly important if there are anatomical variations in the upper GI tract (e.g., diverticulae).

Alcohol continues down the GI tract until absorbed. The ethanol concentration therefore

Table 1 Unit system of ethanol content of alcoholic beverages[a]

Beverage containing ethanol	Units of ethanol
Half pint of low-strength beer (284 ml)	1
Pint of beer (568 ml)	2
500 ml of high-strength beer	6
Pint of cider	2
One glass of wine (125 ml)	1
Bottle of wine (750 ml)	6
One measure of spirits (e.g., whisky, gin, vodka)	1
Bottle of spirits (e.g., vodka; 750 ml)	36

[a]The unit system is a convenient way of quantifying consumption of ethanol and offers a suitable means to give practical guidance. However, there are several problems with the unit system. The ethanol content of various brands of alcoholic beverages varies considerably (for example, alcohol content of beers/ales is 0.5–9.0%—a pint may contain 2–5 units) and the amounts of alcohol consumed in homes bear little in common with standard measures.

Table 2 Geographical variation in the amount of ethanol in one unit[a]

Country	Amount of alcohol (g)
Japan	14
United States	12
Australia and New Zealand	10
United Kingdom	8

[a]The unit system does not permit international comparisons.

Table 3 Guidelines for the consumption of alcohol[a]

	Men (units)		Women (units)	
	Weekly[b]	Daily[c]	Weekly[b]	Daily[c]
Low risk	0–21	3–4	0–14	2–3
Hazardous	22–50	≥4	15–35	≥3
Harmful	>50		>35	≥1–2[d]

[a]Guidelines regarding the consumption of alcohol are designed to reduce harm. The Royal Colleges' (1995) guidelines are for weekly consumption rates, and the Department of Health's (1995) guidelines are for daily consumption.
[b]Recommendations of the Working Group of the Royal Colleges of Physicians, Psychiatrists and General Practitioners (UK).
[c]Recommendations of the Department of Health (UK).
[d]When pregnant or about to become pregnant, consumption of more than 1 or 2 units of alcohol, one or two times per week, is harmful.

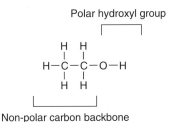

Figure 1 Chemical structure of ethanol.

decreases down the GI tract. There is also a concentration gradient of ethanol from the lumen to the blood. The concentration of ethanol is much higher in the lumen of the upper small intestine than in plasma (**Table 4**). Alcohol diffuses passively across the cell membranes of the mucosal surface into the submucosal space and then the submucosal capillaries.

Absorption occurs across all of the GI mucosa but is fastest in the duodenum and jejunum. The rate of

Table 4 Approximate ethanol concentrations in the gastrointestinal tract and in the blood after a dose of ethanol[a]

Site	Ethanol concentration	
	g/dl	mmol/l
Stomach	8	1740
Jejunum	4	870
Ileum	0.1–0.2	22–43
Blood (15–120 minutes after dosage)	0.1–0.2	22–43

[a]Ethanol appears in the blood as quickly as 5 minutes after ingestion and is rapidly distributed around the body. A dose of 0.8 g ethanol/kg body weight (56 g ethanol (7 units) consumed by a 70 kg male) should result in a blood ethanol concentration of 100–200 mg/dl (22–43 mmol/l) between 15 and 120 minutes after dosage. Highest concentrations occur after 30–90 minutes.

gastric emptying is the main determinant of absorption because most ethanol is absorbed after leaving the stomach through the pylorus.

Alcohol diffuses from the blood into tissues across capillary walls. Ethanol concentration equilibrates between blood and the extracellular fluid within a single pass. However, equilibration between blood water and total tissue water may take several hours, depending on the cross-sectional area of the capillary bed and tissue blood flow.

Ethanol enters most tissues but its solubility in bone and fat is negligible. Therefore, in the postabsorption phase, the volume of distribution of ethanol reflects total body water. Thus, for a given dose, BEC will reflect lean body mass.

Metabolism of Alcohol

The rate at which alcohol is eliminated from the blood by oxidization varies from 6 to 10 g/h. This is reflected by the BEC, which falls by 9–20 mg/dl/h after consumption of ethanol. After a dose of 0.6–0.9 g/kg body weight without food, elimination of ethanol is approximately 15 mg/dl blood/h. However, many factors influence this rate and there is considerable individual variation.

Absorbed ethanol is initially oxidized to acetaldehyde (**Figure 2**) by one of three pathways (**Figure 3**):

1. Alcohol dehydrogenase (ADH)—cystosol
2. Microsomal ethanol oxidizing system (MEOS)—endoplasmic reticulum
3. Catalase—peroxisomes

Alcohol Dehydrogenase

ADH couples oxidation of ethanol to reduction of nicotinamide adenine dinucleotide (NAD^+) to NADH. ADH has a wide range of substrates and functions, including dehydrogenation of steroids and oxidation of fatty acids.

Alcohol Dehydrogenase Isoenzymes

ADH is a zinc metalloprotein with five classes of isoenzymes that arise from the association of eight different subunits into dimers (**Table 5**). A genetic model accounts for these five classes of ADH as

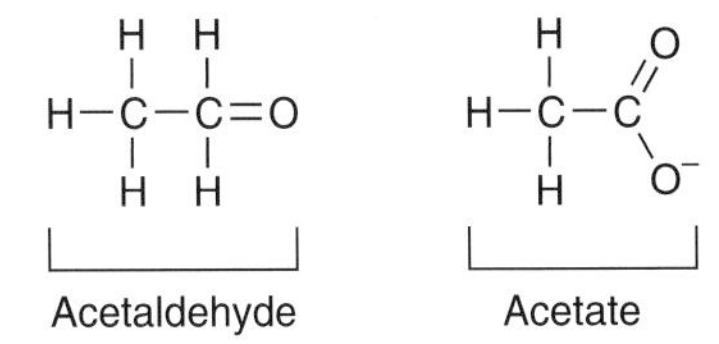

Figure 2 Chemical structures of acetaldehyde and acetate, the products of ethanol metabolism.

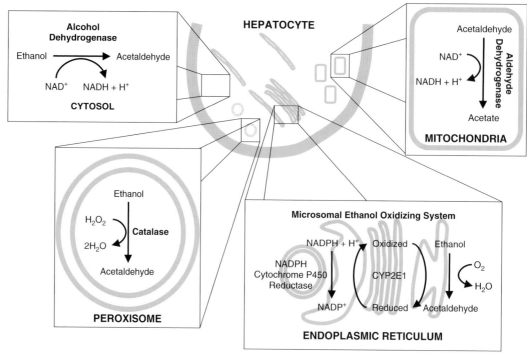

Figure 3 Pathways of ethanol metabolism.

products of five gene loci (ADH1–5). Class 1 iso-enzymes generally require a low concentration of ethanol to achieve 'half-maximal activity' (low K_m), whereas class 2 isoenzymes have a relatively high K_m. Class 3 ADH has a low affinity for ethanol and does not participate in the oxidation of ethanol in the liver. Class 4 ADH is found in the human stomach and class 5 has been reported in liver and

Table 5 Classes of alcohol dehydrogenase isoenzymes

Class	Subunit	Location	K_m (mmol/l)[a]	V_{max}
1				
ADH1	α	Liver	4	54
ADH2	β	Liver, lung	0.05–34	
ADH3	γ	Liver, stomach	0.6–1.0	
2				
ADH4	π	Liver, cornea	34	40
3				
ADH5	χ	Most tissues	1000	
4				
ADH7	σ, μ	Stomach, oesophagus, other mucosae	20	1510
5				
ADH6	—	Liver, stomach	30	

[a]K_m supplied is for ethanol; ADH also oxidizes other substrates. Adapted with permission from Kwo PY and Crabb DW (2002) Genetics of ethanol metabolism and alcoholic liver disease. In: Sherman DIN, Preedy VR and Watson RR (eds.) *Ethanol and the Liver. Mechanisms and Management*, pp. 95–129. London: Taylor & Francis.

stomach. Whereas the majority of ethanol metabolism occurs in the liver, gastric ADH is responsible for a small portion of ethanol oxidation.

Catalase

Peroxisomal catalase, which requires the presence of hydrogen peroxide (H_2O_2), is of little significance in the metabolism of ethanol. Metabolism of ethanol by ADH inhibits catalase activity because H_2O_2 production is inhibited by the reducing equivalents produced by ADH.

Microsomal Ethanol Oxidizing System

Chronic administration of ethanol with nutritionally adequate diets increases clearance of ethanol from the blood. In 1968, the MEOS was identified. The MEOS has a higher K_m for ethanol (8–10 mmol/l) than ADH (0.2–2.0 mmol/l) so at low BEC, ADH is more important. However, unlike the other pathways, MEOS is highly inducible by chronic alcohol consumption. The key enzyme of the MEOS is cytochrome P4502E1 (CYP2E1). Chronic alcohol use is associated with a 4- to 10-fold increase of CYP2E1 due to increases in mRNA levels and rate of translation.

Acetaldehyde Metabolism

Acetaldehyde is highly toxic but is rapidly converted to acetate. This conversion is catalyzed by aldehyde

Table 6   Classes of aldehyde dehydrogenase isoenzymes

Class	Structure	Location	K_m ($\mu mol/l$)[a]
1 ALDH1	$\alpha 4$	**Cytosolic** Many tissues: highest in liver	30
2 ALDH2	$\alpha 4$	**Mitochondrial** Present in all tissues except red blood cells Liver > kidney > muscle > heart	1

[a]K_m supplied is for acetaldehyde; ALDH also oxidizes other substrates.
Adapted with permission from Kwo PY and Crabb DW (2002) Genetics of ethanol metabolism and alcoholic liver disease. In: Sherman DIN, Preedy VR and Watson RR (eds.) *Ethanol and the Liver. Mechanisms and Management*, pp. 95–129. London: Taylor & Francis.

dehydrogenase (ALDH) and is accompanied by reduction of NAD^+ (**Figure 3**). There are several isoenzymes of ALDH (**Table 6**). The most important are ALDH1 (cytosolic) and ALDH2 (mitochondrial). The presence of ALDH in tissues may reduce the toxic effects of acetaldehyde.

In alcoholics, the oxidation of ethanol is increased by induction of MEOS. However, the capacity of mitochondria to oxidize acetaldehyde is reduced. Hepatic acetaldehyde therefore increases with chronic ethanol consumption. A significant increase of acetaldehyde in hepatic venous blood reflects the high tissue level.

Metabolism of Acetate

The final metabolism of acetate derived from ethanol remains unclear. However, some important principles have been elucidated:

1. The majority of absorbed ethanol is metabolized in the liver and released as acetate. Acetate release from the liver increases $2\frac{1}{2}$ times after ethanol consumption.
2. Acetyl-CoA synthetase catalyzes the conversion of acetate to acetyl-CoA via a reaction requiring adenosine triphosphate. The adenosine monophosphate produced is converted to adenosine in a reaction catalyzed by 5′-nucleosidase.
3. Acetyl-CoA may be converted to glycerol, glycogen, and lipid, particularly in the fed state. However, this only accounts for a small fraction of absorbed ethanol.
4. The acetyl-CoA generated from acetate may be used to generate adenosine triphosphate via the Kreb's cycle.

5. Acetate readily crosses the blood–brain barrier and is actively metabolized in the brain. The neurotransmitter acetylcholine is produced from acetyl-CoA in cholinergic neurons.
6. Both cardiac and skeletal muscle are very important in the metabolism of acetate.

Based on these observations, future studies on the effects of ethanol metabolism should focus on skeletal and cardiac muscle, adipose tissue, and the brain.

Blood Ethanol Concentration

The relationship between BEC and the effects of alcohol is complex and varies between individuals and with patterns of drinking. Many of the effects correlate with the peak concentration of ethanol in the blood and organs during a drinking session. Other effects are due to products of metabolism and the total dose of ethanol ingested over a period of time. These two considerations are not entirely separable because the ethanol concentration during a session may determine which pathways of ethanol metabolism predominate.

It is of considerable clinical interest to understand what factors increase the probability of higher maximum ethanol concentrations for any given level of consumption.

Factors Affecting Blood Ethanol Concentration

Gender Differences in Blood Ethanol Concentration

Women achieve higher peak BEC than men given the same dose of ethanol per kilogram of body weight. The volume of distribution of ethanol reflects total body water. Because the bodies of women contain a greater proportion of fat, it is not surprising that the BEC is higher in women. However, gender differences in the gastric metabolism of ethanol may also be relevant.

Period over which the Alcohol Is Consumed

Rapid intake of alcohol increases the concentration of ethanol in the stomach and small intestine. The greater the concentration gradient of alcohol, the faster the absorption of ethanol and therefore peak BEC. If alcohol is consumed and absorbed faster than the rate of oxidation, then BEC increases.

Effects of Food on Blood Ethanol Concentration

The peak BEC is reduced when alcohol is consumed with or after food. Food delays gastric emptying into

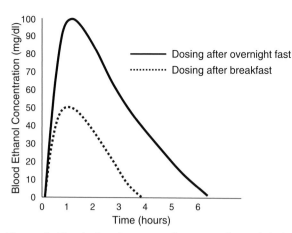

Figure 4 Blood ethanol concentration curve after oral dosing of ethanol. A subject injected 0.8 g/kg ethanol over 30 minutes either after an overnight fast or after breakfast. The peak blood ethanol concentration and the area under the curve are reduced if ethanol is consumed with food.

the duodenum and reduces the sharp early rise in BEC seen when alcohol is taken on an empty stomach. Food also increases elimination of ethanol from the blood. The area under the BEC/time curve (AUC) is reduced (**Figure 4**). The contributions of various nutrients to these effects have been studied, but small, often conflicting, differences have been found. It appears that the caloric value of the meal is more important than the precise balance of nutrients.

In animal studies ethanol is often administered with other nutrients in liquid diets. The AUC is less when alcohol is given in a liquid diet than with the same dose of ethanol in water. The different blood ethanol profile in these models may affect the expression of pathology.

However, food increases splanchnic blood flow, which maintains the ethanol diffusion gradient in the small intestine. Food-induced impairment of gastric emptying may be partially offset by faster absorption of ethanol in the duodenum.

Beverage Alcohol Content and Blood Ethanol Concentration

The ethanol concentration of the beverage consumed (**Table 7**) affects ethanol absorption and can affect BEC. Absorption is fastest when the concentration is 10–30%. Below 10%, the low ethanol concentration in the GI tract reduces diffusion and the greater volume of liquid slows gastric emptying. However, concentrations above 30% irritate the GI mucosa and the pyloric sphincter, increasing secretion of mucous and delaying gastric emptying.

Table 7 Alcohol content of selected beverages

Beverage	Alcohol content		
	g/dl (%)	mmol/l	mol/l
Low-strength beers	3–4	650–870	0.65–0.87
High-strength beers	8–9	1740–1960	1.74–1.96
Wine	7–14	1520–3040	1.52–3.04
Brandy	35–45	7610–9780	7.61–9.78
Vodka	35–50	7610–10870	7.61–10.87
Gin	35–50	7610–10870	7.61–10.87
Whisky	35–75	7610–16300	7.61–16.30

First-Pass Metabolism of Ethanol

The AUC is significantly lower after oral dosing of ethanol than after intravenous or intraperitoneal administration. The total dose of intravenously administered ethanol is available to the systemic circulation. The difference between AUC_{oral} and AUC_{iv} represents the fraction of the oral dose that was either not absorbed or metabolized before entering the systemic circulation (first-pass metabolism (FPM)). The ratio of AUC_{oral} to AUC_{iv} reflects the oral bioavailability of ethanol.

The investigation of ethanol metabolism has primarily focused on the liver and its relationship to liver pathology. However, gastric metabolism accounts for approximately 5% of ethanol oxidation and 2–10% is excreted in the breath, sweat, or urine. The rest is metabolized by the liver.

After absorption, ethanol is transported to the liver in the portal vein. Some is metabolized by the liver before reaching the systemic circulation. However, hepatic ADH is saturated at a BEC that may be achieved in an average-size adult after consumption of one or two units. If ADH is saturated by ethanol from the systemic blood via hepatic artery, ethanol in the portal blood must compete for binding to ADH. Although hepatic oxidation of ethanol cannot increase once ADH is saturated, gastric ADH can significantly metabolize ethanol at the high concentrations in the stomach after initial ingestion. If gastric emptying of ethanol is delayed, prolonged contact with gastric ADH increases FPM. Conversely, fasting, which greatly increases the speed of gastric emptying, virtually eliminates gastric FPM.

Physiological Effects of Alcohol

Ethanol or the products of its metabolism affect nearly all cellular structures and functions.

Effects of Alcohol on the Central Nervous System

Ethanol generally decreases the activity of the central nervous system. In relation to alcohol, the most important neurotransmitters in the brain are glutamate, gamma-aminobutyric acid (GABA), dopamine, and serotonin.

Glutamate is the major excitatory neurotransmitter in the brain. Ethanol inhibits the N-methyl-D-aspartate (NMDA) subset of glutamate receptors. Ethanol thereby reduces the excitatory effects of glutamate. GABA is the major inhibitory neurotransmitter in the brain. Alcohol facilitates the action of the GABA-a receptor, increasing inhibition. Changes to these receptors seem to be important in the development of tolerance of and dependence on alcohol.

Dopamine is involved in the rewarding aspects of alcohol consumption. 'Enjoyable' activities such as eating or use of other recreational drugs also release dopamine in the nucleus accumbens of the brain. Serotonin is also involved in the in reward processes and may be important in encouraging alcohol use.

The most obvious effects of ethanol intoxication on the central nervous system begin with behavior modification (e.g., cheerfulness, impaired judgment, and loss of inhibitions). These 'excitatory' effects result from the disinhibition described previously (inhibition of cells in the brain that are usually inhibitory). As a result of these effects, it is well recognized that driving under the influence of ethanol is unsafe. However, the definition of what is safe or acceptable varies between countries (**Table 8**) and often changes.

The effects of ethanol are dose dependent (**Table 9**) and further intake causes agitation, slurred speech, memory loss, double vision, and loss of coordination. This may progress to depression of consciousness and loss of airway protective reflexes, with danger of aspiration, suffocation, and death.

Table 8 Legal limits of blood ethanol concentrations for driving[a]

Legal limit[b]	Blood ethanol concentration	
	mg/dl	mmol/l
Norway and Sweden	20	4.3
France, Germany, Italy, and Australia	50	11
United Kingdom, United States, and Canada	80	17
Russia	"Drunkenness"	

[a]Ethanol impairs judgment and coordination. It is well recognized that driving under the influence of ethanol is unsafe. However, the definition of what is safe or acceptable varies between countries and can change as a result of social, political, or scientific influences.
[b]Legislation regarding legal limits of blood ethanol for driving may change.

Table 9 Relationship between amount of ethanol consumed, blood ethanol concentration (BEC), and effect of ethanol on the central nervous system

Alcohol consumed (units)	Possible BEC	Effect
1–5	10–50 mg/dl 2–11 mmol/l	No obvious change in behavior
2–7	30–100 mg/dl 7–22 mmol/l	Increased self-confidence; loss of inhibitions
		Impaired judgment, attention, and control
	Euphoria	Mild sensorimotor impairment, delayed reaction times
	Sociability	Legal limits for driving generally fall within this range (see **Table 8**)
8–15	90–250 mg/dl 20–54 mmol/l	Loss of critical judgment
		Impairment of perception, memory, and comprehension
		Reduced visual acuity
		Reduced coordination, impaired balance
		Drowsiness
11–20	180–300 mg/dl 39–65 mmol/l	Disorientation
		Exaggerated emotional states
		Disturbances of vision and perception of color, form, motion, and depth
	Confusion	Increased pain threshold
		Further reduction of coordination, staggering gait, slurred speech
15–25	250–400 mg/dl 54–87 mmol/l	Loss of motor functions
		Markedly reduced response to stimuli
		Marked loss of coordination, inability to stand/walk
	Stupor	Incontinence
		Impaired consciousness
22–30	350–500 mg/dl 76–108 mmol/l	Unconsciousness
		Reduced or abolished reflexes
		Incontinence
	Coma	Cardiovascular and respiratory depression (death possible)
38	>600 mg/dl >130 mmol/l	Respiratory arrest
	Death	

[a]Approximate amounts of alcohol required by a 70 kg male to produce the corresponding blood ethanol concentration and intoxicating effects of ethanol. One unit of alcohol contains 8g of ethanol.
Adapted with permission from Morgan MY and Ritson B (2003) *Alcohol and Health: A Handbook for Students and Medical Practitioners*, 4th edn. London: Medical Council on Alcohol.

This sequence of events is particularly relevant in the hospital setting, where patients may present intoxicated with a reduced level of consciousness. It is difficult to determine whether there is coexisting pathology such as an extradural hematoma or overdose of other drugs in addition to ethanol. Although measurement of BEC is helpful (**Table 9**), it is safest to assume that alcohol is not responsible for any disturbance in consciousness and to search for another cause.

Neuroendocrine Effects of Alcohol

Alcohol activates the sympathetic nervous system, increasing circulating catecholamines from the adrenal medulla. Hypothalamic–pituitary stimulation results in increased circulating cortisol from the adrenal cortex and can, rarely, cause a pseudo-Cushing's syndrome with typical moon-shaped face, truncal obesity, and muscle weakness. Alcoholics with pseudo-Cushing's show many of the biochemical features of Cushing's syndrome, including failure to suppress cortisol with a 48-h low-dose dexamethasone suppression test. However, they may be distinguished by an insulin stress test. In pseudo-Cushing's, the cortisol rises in response to insulin-induced hypoglycemia, but in true Cushing's there is no response to hypoglycemia.

Ethanol affects hypothalamic osmoreceptors, reducing vasopressin release. This increases salt and water excretion from the kidney, causing polyuria. Significant dehydration may result particularly with consumption of spirits containing high concentrations of ethanol and little water. Loss of hypothalamic neurons (which secrete vasopressin) has also been described in chronic alcoholics, suggesting long-term consequences for fluid balance. Plasma atrial natriuretic peptide, increased by alcohol consumption, may also increase diuresis and resultant dehydration.

Alcoholism also affects the hypothalamic–pituitary–gonadal axis. These effects are further exacerbated by alcoholic liver disease. There are conflicting data regarding the changes observed. Testosterone is either normal or decreased in men, but it may increase in women. Estradiol is increased in men and women, and it increases as hepatic dysfunction deteriorates. Production of sex hormone-binding globulin is also perturbed by alcohol.

The development of female secondary sexual characteristics in men (e.g., gynaecomastia and testicular atrophy) generally only occurs after the development of cirrhosis. In women, the hormonal changes may reduce libido, disrupt menstruation, or even induce premature menopause. Sexual dysfunction is also common in men with reduced libido and impotence. Fertility may also be reduced, with decreased sperm counts and motility.

Effects of Alcohol on Muscle

Myopathy is common, affecting up to two-thirds of all alcoholics. It is characterized by wasting, weakness, and myalgia and improves with abstinence. Histology correlates with symptoms and shows selective atrophy of type II muscle fibers. Ethanol causes a reduction in muscle protein and ribonucleic acid content. The underlying mechanism is unclear, but rates of muscle protein synthesis are reduced, whereas protein degradation is either unaffected or inhibited. Attention has focused on the role of acetaldehyde adducts and free radicals in the pathogenesis of alcoholic myopathy.

Alcohol and Nutrition

The nutritional status of alcoholics is often impaired. Some of the pathophysiological changes seen in alcoholics are direct consequences of malnutrition. However, in the 1960s, Charles Lieber demonstrated that many alcohol-induced pathologies, including alcoholic hepatitis, cirrhosis, and myopathy, are reproducible in animals fed a nutritionally adequate diet. Consequently, the concept that all alcohol-induced pathologies are due to nutritional deficiencies is outdated and incorrect.

Myopathy is a direct consequence of alcohol or acetaldehyde on muscle and is not necessarily associated with malnutrition. Assessment of nutritional status in chronic alcoholics using anthropometric measures (e.g., limb circumference and muscle mass) may be misleading in the presence of myopathy.

Acute or chronic ethanol administration impairs the absorption of several nutrients, including glucose, amino acids, biotin, folate, and ascorbic acid. There is no strong evidence that alcohol impairs absorption of magnesium, riboflavin, or pyridoxine, so these deficiencies are due to poor intakes. Hepatogastrointestinal damage (e.g., villous injury, bacterial overgrowth of the intestine, pancreatic damage, or cholestasis) may impair the absorption of some nutrients such as the fat-soluble vitamins (A, D, E, and K). In contrast, iron stores may be adequate as absorption is increased.

Effects of Alcohol on the Cardiovascular System

Alcohol affects both the heart and the peripheral vasculature. Acutely, alcohol causes peripheral vasodilatation, giving a false sensation of warmth that can be dangerous. Heat loss is rapid in cold weather or when swimming, but reduced awareness leaves people vulnerable to hypothermia. The main adverse effect of acute alcohol on the cardiovascular system is the induction of arrhythmias. These are often harmless and experienced as palpitations but can rarely be fatal. Chronic ethanol consumption can cause systemic hypertension and congestive cardiomyopathy. Alcoholic cardiomyopathy accounts for up to one-third of dilated cardiomyopathies but may improve with abstinence or progress to death.

The beneficial, cardioprotective effects of alcohol consumption have been broadcast widely. This observation is based on population studies of mortality due to ischemic heart disease, case–control studies, and animal experiments. However, there is no evidence from randomised controlled trials. The apparent protective effect of alcohol may therefore result from a confounding factor. Furthermore, on the population level, the burden of alcohol-induced morbidity and mortality far outweighs any possible cardiovascular benefit.

Effects of Alcohol on Liver Function

Central to the effects of ethanol is the liver, in which 60–90% of ethanol metabolism occurs. Ethanol displaces many of the substrates usually metabolized in the liver. Metabolism of ethanol by ADH in the liver generates reducing equivalents. ALDH also generates NADH with conversion of acetaldehyde to acetate. The NADH/NAD+ ratio is increased, with a corresponding increase in the lactate/pyruvate ratio. If lactic acidosis combines with a β-hydroxybutyrate predominant ketoacidosis, the blood pH can fall to 7.1 and hypoglycemia may occur. Severe ketoacidosis and hypoglycemia can cause permanent brain damage. However, in general the prognosis of alcohol-induced acidosis is good. Lactic acid also reduces the renal capacity for urate excretion. Hyperuricemia is exacerbated by alcohol-induced ketosis and acetate-mediated purine generation. Hyperuricemia explains, at least in part, the clinical observation that alcohol misuse can precipitate gout.

The excess NADH promotes fatty acid synthesis and inhibits lipid oxidation in the mitochondria, resulting in fat accumulation. Fatty changes are usually asymptomatic but can be seen on ultrasound or computed tomography scanning, and they are associated with abnormal liver toxicity tests (e.g., raised activities of serum γ-glutamyl transferase, aspartate aminotransferase, and alanine transaminases).

Progression to alcoholic hepatitis involves invasion of the liver by neutrophils with hepatocyte necrosis. Giant mitochondria are visible and dense cytoplasmic lesions (Mallory bodies) are seen. Alcoholic hepatitis can be asymptomatic but usually presents with abdominal pain, fever, and jaundice, or, depending on the severity of disease, patients may have encephalopathy, ascites, and ankle oedema.

Continued alcohol consumption may lead to cirrhosis. However, not all alcoholics progress to cirrhosis. The reason for this is unclear. It has been suggested that genetic factors and differences in immune response may play a role.

In alcoholic cirrhosis there is fibrocollagenous deposition, with scarring and disruption of surrounding hepatic architecture. There is ongoing necrosis with concurrent regeneration. Alcoholic cirrhosis is classically said to be micronodular, but often a mixed pattern is present. The underlying pathological mechanisms are complex and are the subject of debate. Induction of the MEOS and oxidation of ethanol by catalase result in free radical production. Glutathione (a free radical scavenger) is reduced in alcoholics, impairing the ability to dispose of free radicals. Mitochondrial damage occurs, limiting their capacity to oxidize fatty acids. Peroxisomal oxidation of fatty acids further increases free radical production. These changes eventually result in hepatocyte necrosis, and inflammation and fibrosis ensue. Acetaldehyde also contributes by promoting collagen synthesis and fibrosis.

Alcohol and Facial Flushing

Genetic variations in ADH and ALDH may explain why particular individuals develop some of the pathologies of alcoholism and others do not. For example, up to 50% of Orientals have a genetically determined reduction in ALDH2 activity ('flushing' phenotype). As a result, acetaldehyde accumulates after ethanol administration, with plasma levels up to 20 times higher in people with ALDH2 deficiency. Even small amounts of alcohol produce a rapid facial flush, tachycardia, headache, and nausea. Acetaldehyde partly acts through catecholamines, although other mediators have been implicated, including histamine, bradykinin, prostaglandin, and endogenous opioids.

This is similar to the disulfiram reaction due to the rise of acetaldehyde after inhibition of ALDH. Disulfiram is used therapeutically to encourage abstinence in alcohol rehabilitation programs. The aversive effects of acetaldehyde may reduce the development of alcoholism and the incidence of cirrhosis in 'flushers.' However, some alcoholics with ALDH2 deficiency and, presumably, higher hepatic acetaldehyde levels develop alcoholic liver disease at a lower intake of ethanol than controls.

Effects of Acetaldehyde

Acetaldehyde is highly toxic and can bind cellular constituents (e.g., proteins including CYP2E1, lipids, and nucleic acids) to produce harmful acetaldehyde adducts (**Figure 5**). Adduct formation changes

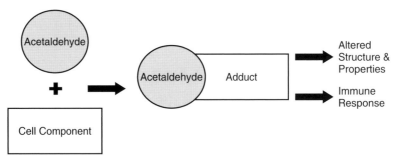

Figure 5 Formation of acetaldehyde adducts.

the structure and the biochemical properties of the affected molecules. The new structures may be recognized as foreign antigens by the immune system and initiate a damaging response.

Adduct formation leads to retention of protein within hepatocytes, contributing to the hepatomegaly, and several toxic manifestations, including impairment of antioxidant mechanisms (e.g., decreased glutathione (GSH)). Acetaldehyde thereby promotes free radical-mediated toxicity and lipid peroxidation. Binding of acetaldehyde with cysteine (one of the three amino acids that comprise GSH) and/or GSH also reduces liver GSH content. Chronic ethanol administration significantly increases rates of GSH turnover in rats. Acute ethanol administration inhibits GSH synthesis and increases losses from the liver. Furthermore, mitochondrial GSH is selectively depleted and this may contribute to the marked disruption of mitochondria in alcoholic cirrhosis.

Effects of Acetate

The role of acetate in alcohol-induced pathology is not well understood. The uptake and utilization of acetate by tissues depend on the activity of acetyl-CoA synthetase. Acetyl-CoA and adenosine are produced from the metabolism of acetate. Acetate crosses the blood–brain barrier easily and is actively metabolized in the brain. Many of the central nervous system depressant effects of ethanol may be blocked by adenosine receptor blockers. Thus, acetate and adenosine may be important in the intoxicating effects of ethanol.

Ethanol increases portal blood flow, mainly by increasing GI tract blood flow. This effect is reproduced by acetate. Acetate also increases coronary blood flow, myocardial contractility, and cardiac output. Acetate inhibits lipolysis in adipose tissue and promotes steatosis in the liver. The reduced circulating free fatty acids (a source of energy for many tissues) may have significant metabolic consequences. Thus, many of the effects of alcohol may be due to acetate.

Summary

Ethanol is probably the most commonly used recreational drug worldwide. Taken orally, alcohol is absorbed from the GI tract by diffusion and is rapidly distributed throughout the body in the blood before entering tissues by diffusion. Ethanol is metabolized to acetaldehyde mainly in the stomach and liver. Acetaldehyde is highly toxic and binds cellular constituents, generating harmful acetaldehyde adducts. Acetaldehyde is further oxidized to acetate, but the fate of acetate and its role in the effects of ethanol are much less clear. Ethanol and the products of its metabolism affect nearly every cellular structure or function and are a significant cause of morbidity and mortality.

See also: **Alcohol**: Disease Risk and Beneficial Effects; Effects of Consumption on Diet and Nutritional Status. **Liver Disorders**.

Further Reading

Department of Health (1995) *Sensible Drinking: The Report of an Inter-Departmental Working Group*. London: Department of Health.

Gluud C (2002) Endocrine system. In: Sherman DIN, Preedy VR, and Watson RR (eds.) *Ethanol and the Liver. Mechanisms and Management*, pp. 472–494. London: Taylor & Francis.

Haber PS (2000) Metabolism of alcohol by the human stomach. *Alcoholism: Clinical & Experimental Research* 24: 407–408.

Henderson L, Gregory J, Irving K and Swan G (2003) The National Diet and Nutrition Survey: adults aged 19–64 years. Volume 2: Energy, protein, carbohydrate, fat and alcohol intake. London: TSO.

Israel Y, Orrego H, and Carmichael FJ (1994) Acetate-mediated effects of ethanol. *Alcoholism: Clinical & Experimental Research* 18(1): 144–148.

Jones AW (2000) Aspects of in-vivo pharmacokinetics of ethanol. *Alcoholism: Clinical & Experimental Research* 24: 400–402.

Kwo PY and Crabb DW (2002) Genetics of ethanol metabolism and alcoholic liver disease. In: Sherman DIN, Preedy VR, and Watson RR (eds.) *Ethanol and the Liver. Mechanisms and Management*, pp. 95–129. London: Taylor & Francis.

Lader D and Meltzer H (2002) *Drinking: Adults' Behaviour and Knowledge in 2002*. London: Office for National Statistics.

Lieber CS (1996) The metabolism of alcohol and its implications for the pathogenesis of disease. In: Preedy VR and Watson RR (eds.) *Alcohol and the Gastrointestinal Tract*, pp. 19–39. New York: CRC Press.

Lieber CS (2000) Alcohol: Its metabolism and interaction with nutrients. *Annual Review of Nutrition* 20: 395–430.

Mezey E (1985) Effect of ethanol on intestinal morphology, metabolism and function. In: Seitz HK and Kommerell B (eds.) *Alcohol Related Diseases in Gastroenterology*, pp. 342–360. Berlin: Springer-Verlag.

Morgan MY and Ritson B (2003) *Alcohol and Health: A Handbook for Students and Medical Practitioners*, 4th edn. London: Medical Council on Alcohol.

Peters TJ and Preedy VR (1999) Chronic alcohol abuse: Effects on the body. *Medicine* 27: 11–15.

Preedy VR, Adachi J, Ueno Y *et al.* (2001) Alcoholic skeletal muscle myopathy: Definitions, features, contribution of neuropathy, impact and diagnosis. *European Journal of Neurology* 8: 677–687.

Preedy VR, Patel VB, Reilly ME *et al.* (1999) Oxidants, antioxidants and alcohol: Implications for skeletal and cardiac muscle. *Frontiers in Bioscience* 4: 58–66.

Royal Colleges (1995) Alcohol and the heart in perspective. Sensible limits reaffirmed. A Working Group of the Royal Colleges of Physicians, Psychiatrists and General Practitioners. *Journal of the Royal College of Physicians of London* 29: 266–271.

Disease Risk and Beneficial Effects

M Grønbæk, National Institute of Public Health, Copenhagen, Denmark

© 2005 Elsevier Ltd. All rights reserved.

Alcohol has for hundreds of years been part of the diet for many people. When enjoyed in small amounts and together with meals, alcohol may have positive effects on health, especially on the prevention of coronary heart disease. In larger amounts, and especially drunk in binges, alcohol is a toxic and dependence-inducing substance, with many short- and long-term detrimental effects. The latter, combined with the high alcohol intake in subsets of the population, implies that alcohol has a major impact on public health in most Western countries. A higher alcohol intake results in higher rates of certain cancer, cirrhosis, suicide, traffic accidents, abuse, and a number of socioeconomic conditions.

Alcohol and Mortality

Amount of Alcohol

Several large prospective population studies from many countries have described the impact of alcohol intake on mortality as J-shaped, indicating both the beneficial effect of a light to moderate alcohol intake and a detrimental effect of a high alcohol intake (**Figure 1**).

Some have explained the J shape as an artefact due to misclassification or confounding. Prevailing beliefs among these researchers is that abstainers comprise a mix of former heavy drinkers, underreporting drinkers, ill people who have stopped drinking, and people with an especially unhealthy lifestyle apart from abstaining. However, most researchers attribute the 'J' to a combination of beneficial and harmful effects of ethanol. This is based on findings from population studies of alcohol-related morbidity and cause-specific mortality that show a decreased relative risk of coronary heart disease, and an increased risk of certain cancers and cirrhosis, with increased alcohol intake. Further evidence derives from studies in which people who were ill at baseline were excluded, and these confirmed the previously mentioned findings.

Benefits—Coronary Heart Disease

A large number of investigators have studied the relation between alcohol intake and coronary heart disease. Studies indicate that the descending leg of the curve is mainly attributable to death from coronary heart disease, as mentioned previously. The lowest risk seems to be among subjects reporting an

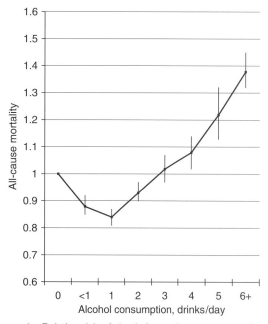

Figure 1 Relative risk of death from all causes according to total alcohol intake. Relative risk is set at 1.00 among nondrinkers (0 drinks/week). (Reproduced with permission from Boffetta P and Garfinkel L (1990) Alcohol drinking and mortality among men enrolled in an American Cancer Society prospective study. *Epidemiology* 1: 342–348.)

average intake of one to four drinks daily. Several studies have found plausible mechanisms for the apparent cardioprotective effect of a light to moderate intake of alcohol. Subjects with a high alcohol intake have a higher level of high-density lipoprotein, which has been found to be a mediator of the effect of alcohol on coronary heart disease. Thus, 40–60% of the effect of alcohol on coronary heart disease is likely to be attributable to the effect on high-density lipoprotein. Furthermore, drinkers have a lower low-density lipoprotein. Also, alcohol has a beneficial effect on platelet aggregation, and thrombin level in blood is higher among drinkers than among nondrinkers. Ultimately, a few small-scale intervention studies have indicated that alcohol has a beneficial effect on fibronolytic factors.

Risks—Large Number of Somatic Diseases

At the other end of the range of intake, the ascending leg has been explained by the increased risk of cirrhosis and development of certain types of cancers with a high alcohol intake. The mechanisms by which alcohol induces cirrhosis have been intensively studied but sparsely enlightened. It is well documented that women, most likely due to smaller size and different distribution of body fat and water, are at higher risk of developing cirrhosis than men, but other risk factors for alcoholic cirrhosis are not well established (**Figure 2**).

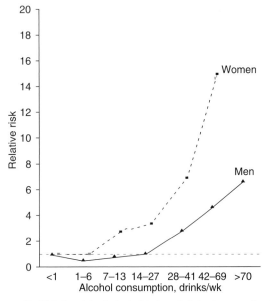

Figure 2   Relative risk of alcohol-induced cirrhosis according to sex and alcohol intake. Relative risk is set at 1.00 among nondrinkers (<1 drink/week). (Reproduced with permission from Becker U *et al.* (1996) Prediction of risk of liver disease in relation to alcohol intake, sex and age: A prospective population study. *Hepatology* **23**: 1025–1029.)

The types of cancer related to a high alcohol intake are those in direct contact with the alcohol; those of the oropharynx and oesophagus and those related to cirrhosis (liver cancer). There is a strong dose-dependent increase in risk of upper digestive tract cancer with increasing alcohol intake. Heavy drinkers of alcohol (5–10 drinks per day) have a 10–15 times higher risk of these relatively rare cancers. Of larger public health relevance are the more frequent cancers—breast and colorectal cancer, which have both been suggested to be related to alcohol. Hence, the risk of breast cancer is doubled for heavy drinking women compared to that for nondrinking women. It is controversial whether a small, frequent daily intake implies an increased risk, although meta-analyses have suggested a 7–9% increased risk per drink per day. Also, the risk of colon cancer is increased among heavy drinkers. The relative risk is twice as high for heavy drinkers compared to nondrinkers, but it is very likely that only colorectal cancer risk is increased, and newer studies have suggested that the risk is mainly increased among beer drinkers. Although not directly related to somatic diseases, other more frequent causes of death among heavy alcohol drinkers, such as traffic accidents, violence, and suicides, substantially add to the ascending leg of the J-shaped curve.

Modifiers of the J Shape

During the past decade, a number of factors that may influence the shape of the curve describing the relation between alcohol and morbidity and mortality have been identified.

Age and Risk Factor Profile

A few studies have indicated that subjects already at high risk of coronary disease experience a greater beneficial effect of drinking alcohol moderately; conversely, only in those with a high risk level is coronary heart disease prevented. Hence, the large Nurses Health Study found that the J-shaped relation was significant only in women older than 50 years of age, whereas younger women who had a light alcohol intake did not differ from abstainers with regard to mortality. Fuchs *et al.* found that women at high risk for coronary heart disease (due to risk factors such as older age, diabetes, family history of coronary heart disease, high cholesterol, and hypertension) who had a light alcohol intake were at a lower risk of death than women who were at the same risk level but did not drink alcohol. In a study by the American Cancer Society, the finding by Fuchs *et al.* was confirmed among men, and the different mortality risk functions for different age groups were emphasized.

Drinking Pattern

It seems quite obvious that a small, frequent intake (steady) of alcohol has different health implications than a high, irregular (binge) one, and that many of the results from studies measuring only average weekly intake, for example, are imprecise. A few studies have been able to distinguish between frequency and amount of intake, and these studies have supported the previous statement both with regard to all-cause mortality and with regard to the apparent beneficial effect of alcohol on coronary heart disease.

A very large study on all-cause mortality confirmed the J-shaped relation but also clearly showed that those who had an infrequent high alcohol intake had a higher risk of death than those with a similar average intake who had a frequent pattern (**Figure 3**).

One of the mechanisms by which alcohol is assumed to exert its beneficial effect on coronary heart disease is by lowering high-density lipoprotein. Studies in rats have shown that a steady small intake of alcohol implies an increase in high-density lipoprotein level, whereas a peak intake of the same average amount of alcohol does not. Australian and US studies have shown that drinking pattern— steady versus binge drinking—plays a role in the apparent cardioprotective effect of alcohol.

Drinking with Meals

Drinking with meals has been shown to positively affect fribronolysis and lipids. The issue has been sparsely studied in free-living populations, and the results are not consistent. An Italian study showed that drinkers of wine outside meals exhibited higher death rates from all causes, noncardiovascular diseases, and cancer compared to drinkers of wine with meals. However, a larger US study could not confirm these results.

Type of Alcohol

Correlational studies suggest that there may be different effects of the different types of alcoholic beverages. They have shown that mortality from coronary heart disease is lower in countries where wine is the predominant type of alcohol than in countries where beer or spirits are the beverages mainly ingested. These results have been supported from population studies from many countries, suggesting that wine drinkers are at lower risk of death from all causes, including coronary heart disease and cancer, than beer and spirits drinkers (**Figures 4–6**).

One way in which the different types of beverages may exert their different effects on the development of coronary heart disease is via abdominal obesity. It has been suggested that beer drinkers are at a higher risk of developing abdominal obesity than wine drinkers (**Figure 7**). These beverage-specific differences may be explained by either the traits of the drinker or the different substances in the different beverages. Wine consumption in many populations is related to higher socioeconomic status, higher education, and more optimal health behaviour in general compared with beer and spirits consumption. Because these factors are negatively associated

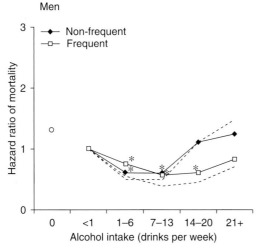
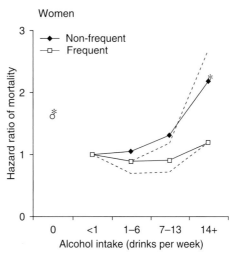

Figure 3 Hazard ratios for all-cause mortality according to quantity and frequency of alcohol intake in men and women (∗ = P<0.05 compared to reference, frequent = at least 2 drinking days per week; nonfrequent = less than 2 drinking days per week). Adjusted for education, smoking, body mass index, physical activity, diet, and diseases before baseline. Reference category is drinkers of less than one but more than zero drinks per week. (Reproduced with permission from Tolstrup J *et al.* (2004) Drinking pattern and mortality in middle-aged men and women. *Addiction* **99**: 323–330.)

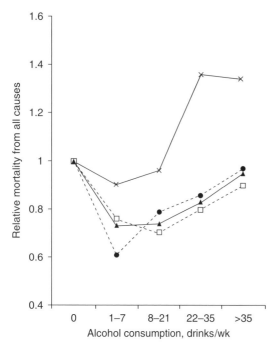

Figure 4 Relative risk of death from all causes according to type of alcohol intake. Data pertain to non-wine drinkers (crosses), wine drinkers (triangles), drinkers for whom wine made up 1–30% of their total alcohol consumption (circles), and drinkers for whom wine made up more than 30% of their total alcohol intake (squares). Relative risk is set at 1.00 among nondrinkers (<1 drink/week). Estimates were adjusted for age, sex, educational level, smoking status, body mass index, and physical activity. (Reproduced with permission from Grønbæk M *et al.* (2000) Type of alcohol consumed and mortality from all causes, coronary heart disease, and cancer. *Annals of Internal Medicine* **133**: 411–419.)

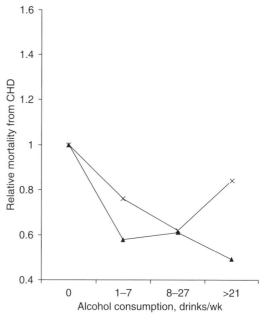

Figure 5 Relative risk of death from coronary heart disease (CHD) according to type of alcohol intake. Data pertain to non-wine drinkers (crosses) and wine drinkers (triangles). Relative risk is set at 1.00 among nondrinkers (<1 drink/week). Estimates were adjusted for age, sex, educational level, smoking status, body mass index, and physical activity. (Reproduced with permission from Grønbæk M *et al.* (2000) Type of alcohol consumed and mortality from all causes, coronary heart disease, and cancer. *Annals of Internal Medicine* **133**: 411–419.)

with mortality, it has been proposed that an unequal distribution according to beverage type may explain the beverage-specific differences in mortality observed in some studies. Several of the components in wine may have antioxidant properties. Hence, flavonoids such as quercetin, rutin, catechin, and epicatechin are present in red wine, responsible for the color of the wine. These compounds have been found to inhibit eicosanoid synthesis and platelet aggregation *in vitro*. Frankel *et al.* found flavonoids to be 10–20 times more potent than vitamin E, and they found an inhibition of low-density lipoprotein oxidation in humans by these phenolic substances. Hertog *et al.* found a preventive effect of dietary flavonoids on risk of developing ischemic heart disease. A high intake of fruits, vegetables, and fish and a low intake of saturated fat have been suggested to reduce the risk of cardiovascular disease. The Mediterranean diet, which includes fruits and vegetables, has been found to have a weak protective effect on cardiovascular disease in 6 of 10 cohort studies. Therefore, diet may play a role in the complex

relation between alcoholic beverage type and coronary heart disease mortality. In the Danish Diet Cancer and Health Study, preference of wine was associated with a higher intake of fruit, fish, vegetables, and salad and a higher frequency of use of olive oil for cooking compared with preference of beer or spirits in both men and women. However, sensitivity analysis of the effect of a potential confounder shows that such a confounder, or conglomerate of confounders, should be very strong to explain the previous findings.

Abstainers

Abstainers may have stopped drinking due to ill health. Empiric evidence for the argument is sparse, but it does seem reasonable that some subjects may stop drinking when they are seriously ill. Another reason to quit drinking is alcoholic dependence; some alcoholics can only keep away from drinking by total abstinence. These people will be more ill and thus more likely to die than others. Both situations will confound the relation between alcohol intake and mortality; ill health is the confounder, unequally distributed among intake groups and associated with mortality. A large number of

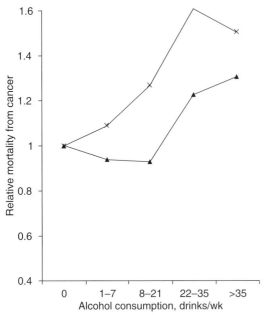

Figure 6   Relative risk of death from cancer according to type of alcohol intake. Data pertain to non-wine drinkers (crosses) and wine drinkers (triangles). Relative risk is set at 1.00 among nondrinkers (<1 drink/week). Estimates were adjusted for age, sex, educational level, smoking status, body mass index, and physical activity. (Reproduced with permission from Grønbæk M *et al.* (2000) Type of alcohol consumed and mortality from all causes, coronary heart disease, and cancer. *Annals of Internal Medicine* **133**: 411–419.)

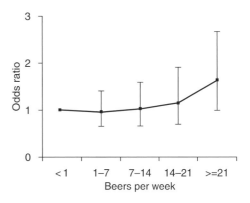

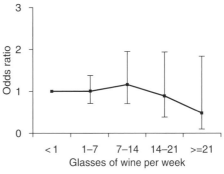

Figure 7   Odds ratio for developing abdominal obesity (waist measure >102 cm) among men. (Reproduced with permission from Vadstrup E *et al.* (2003) Waist circumference in relation to history of amount and type of alcohol: Results from the Copenhagen City Heart Study. *International Journal of Obesity* **27**: 238–246.)

studies, however, have tried to exclude such subjects from analyses, without notable differences; that is, abstainers, or nondrinkers, still seem to be at a higher risk of death than light to moderate drinkers.

Validity of Alcohol Intake

Reporting bias by high-intake or low-intake consumers could, to some extent, explain the apparent lower mortality among light to moderate drinkers. In the type of studies included in this review,– with an emphasis on prospective population studies, one obvious source of bias is misclassification of subjects according to their self-reported alcohol intake. Studies of the validity of self-reported total alcohol intake have mainly concentrated on validating total alcohol intake in suspected alcoholics, whereas intake validity among low-intake consumers in the general population is poorly studied. No reference of alcohol intake (sales reports, collateral information, biological markers, etc.) has been identified. Some biochemical markers of alcohol intake have been suggested, such as γ-glutamyl transferase, high-density lipoprotein, and carbohydrate-deficient transferrin, the latter being one of the most promising. However, in a study from Copenhagen, it was shown that carbohydrate-deficient transferrin was

an invalid marker of self-reported alcohol intake in a general population. With regard to information on alcohol intake from the general population, the need for any such marker can further be questioned. First, participants in prospective cohort studies sampled from the general population have less reason to underreport, or deny, their alcohol intake than alcoholics or insurance populations. Second, in a study on alcoholic cirrhosis, it was found that self-reported alcohol intake in the questionnaire used in most of the studies included in the overview was a reliable measure of 'true alcohol intake' since self-reported alcohol intake is a valid predictor of this outcome (**Figure 2**).

Beverage-Specific Reporting Bias

Differential beverage-specific reporting bias by high-intake or low-intake consumers using the frequency questionnaire may, to some extent, explain the apparent lower mortality among wine drinkers than among beer and spirits drinkers. A few validation studies have shown the correlation between total alcohol consumption reported by questionnaire and interview to be 0.8. With regard to type of beverage, there was an overall agreement between frequency questionnaire and dietary interview. Thus, most subjects in one consumption category of any type of beverage according to the frequency questionnaire also responded to this category in the interview. Mean differences between intake of all three types of beverages were very small or zero, and there were no systematic differences at different levels of average intakes of any of the types of beverages. These are not true validation studies because neither of the two methods can be considered as reference or 'gold standard.' Thus, alcohol intake may have been underreported, and subjects may have reported intake of the three types of beverages differentially. Nevertheless, the close agreement for most individuals suggests that in the range of a small to moderate intake of different types of beverages, the more simple questionnaire approach is not disadvantageous to the expensive and time-consuming personal interview.

Conclusions

The risks and benefits of alcohol on health describe a J-shaped relation. This relation between alcohol intake and all-cause mortality is influenced by several factors, including age, since the J shape seems to persist among the elderly but not among young subjects; sex, since the ascending leg of the curve seems to be steeper for women than for men; drinking pattern, since a small daily intake seems to imply a decreased mortality from cardiovascular disease, whereas binge drinking does not; and type of alcohol, since wine drinkers in some studies seem to be at a lower risk than beer and spirits drinkers.

See also: **Alcohol**: Absorption, Metabolism and Physiological Effects; Effects of Consumption on Diet and Nutritional Status. **Cancer**: Epidemiology and Associations Between Diet and Cancer; Effects on Nutritional Status. **Cholesterol**: Sources, Absorption, Function and Metabolism. **Coronary Heart Disease**: Prevention. **Diabetes Mellitus**: Etiology and Epidemiology; Classification and Chemical Pathology. **Hypertension**: Dietary Factors. **Obesity**: Definition, Etiology and Assessment; Complications. **Older People**: Nutrition-Related Problems.

Further Reading

Becker U *et al.* (1996) Prediction of risk of liver disease in relation to alcohol intake, sex and age: A prospective population study. *Hepatology* **23**: 1025–1029.

Criqui MH and Rigel BL (1994) Does diet or alcohol explain the French paradox? *Lancet* **344**: 1719–1723.

Fagrell B *et al.* (1999) The effects of light to moderate drinking on cardiovascular diseases. *Journal of International Medicine* **246**: 331–340.

Fuchs CS *et al.* (1995) Alcohol consumption and mortality among women. *New England Journal of Medicine* **332**: 1245–1250.

Grønbæk M *et al.* (1994) Influence of sex, age, body mass index, and smoking on alcohol and mortality. *British Medical Journal* **308**: 302–306.

Grønbæk M *et al.* (1998) Population based cohort study of the association between alcohol intake and cancer of the upper digestive tract. *British Medical Journal* **317**: 844–848.

Grønbæk M *et al.* (2000) Type of alcohol consumed and mortality from all causes, coronary heart disease, and cancer. *Annals of Internal Medicine* **133**: 411–419.

Hendriks HF *et al.* (1994) Effect of moderate dose of alcohol with evening meal on fibrinolytic factors. *British Medical Journal* **308**: 1003–1006.

McElduff P and Dobson AJ (1997) How much alcohol and how often? Population based case–control study of alcohol consumption and risk of a major coronary event. *British Medical Journal* **314**: 1159–1164.

Mukamal KJ *et al.* (2003) Roles of drinking pattern and type of alcohol consumed in coronary heart disease in men. *New England Journal of Medicine* **348**: 109–118.

Thun MJ *et al.* (1997) Alcohol consumption and mortality among middle-aged and elderly U.S. adults. *New England Journal of Medicine* **337**: 1705–1714.

Tolstrup J *et al.* (2004) Drinking pattern and mortality in middle-aged men and women. *Addiction* **99**: 323–330.

Vadstrup E *et al.* (2003) Waist circumference in relation to history of amount and type of alcohol: Results from the Copenhagen City Heart Study. *International Journal of Obesity* **27**: 238–246.

Wannamethee SG and Shaper AG (1999) Type of alcoholic drink and risk of major coronary heart disease events and all-cause mortality. *American Journal of Public Health* **89**: 685–690.

Effects of Consumption on Diet and Nutritional Status

C H Halsted, University of California Davis, Davis, CA, USA

© 2005 Elsevier Ltd. All rights reserved.

Introduction

Alcohol is a component of the diet that provides 7.1 kcal per gram and on average 5.6% of total dietary energy in the US. When consumed in moderation, alcoholic beverages protect against cardiovascular disease, but when alcohol is consumed in excess it can become an addictive drug with potential for displacement of beneficial components of the diet, damage to several organ systems including the liver, brain, and heart, and increased risk of several cancers. The consumption of excessive amounts of alcohol contributes to generalized malnutrition, with particular effects on the availability and metabolism of both water- and fat-soluble vitamins including folate, thiamine, pyridoxine, and vitamins A and D. All of the effects of alcoholism on nutritional status are magnified in the presence of alcoholic liver disease. This entry will address the benefits and risks of alcohol consumption and the effects of drinking alcohol on human nutritional status.

Effects of Alcohol Consumption on the Diet

Alcohol is consumed by about two-thirds of adult Americans, and the estimated per capita annual consumption of alcohol exceeds 2 gallons for each US citizen over age 14 years. In the US, young adults between 18 and 25 years of age consume more alcohol than any other age group, and the preferred beverages are wine, beer, and spirits in that order. Men and teenage boys consume about 3 times more alcohol than teenage girls and adult women. Among alcohol consumers, most are moderate drinkers, while about 10% are heavy drinkers at risk of addiction and organ damage. Moderate drinking can be defined as no more than 2 drinks per day for men or 1 drink per day for women, where 1 drink is equivalent to 12–15 g of alcohol. Heavy drinking is defined as consuming more than 5 drinks on any given day per week in men or 4 drinks on any given day per week for women. Chronic alcoholics are addicts who typically consume excessive amounts of alcohol on a daily basis. Binge drinkers are chronic alcoholics who escalate their alcohol intake over weeks or months, typically to the exclusion of the essential components of their regular diets. Alcoholic beverages differ in their alcohol content, such that spirits contain about 40 g/100 ml, wine about 12 g/100 ml, and beer about 4.5 g/100 ml. Thus, the amount of alcohol in 12 oz of beer (16 g) is roughly equivalent to the amount found in 5 oz wine or 1.5 oz spirits.

The effects of alcohol on the diet depend upon the amount consumed each day and changes in overall eating behavior. Although alcohol contains 7.1 kcal per gram, it is rapidly metabolized to acetaldehyde in the liver at rates up to $50 \, g \, h^{-1}$, and none is stored as energy equivalents in the body. Furthermore, the metabolism of alcohol influences the metabolism of dietary fat and carbohydrate. There are three metabolic routes for the disposal of alcohol by the body: two in the liver and one in the stomach. Alcohol dehydrogenase (ADH) is present in the cytosol of hepatocytes and metabolizes the relatively low levels of alcohol that would be expected after moderate drinking. The metabolism of alcohol by ADH causes a redox change that promotes lipid synthesis in the liver as well as reduced gluconeogenesis and increased lactate production. Thus, even moderate drinking can cause fatty liver with elevated serum triglyceride levels and, in the absence of dietary carbohydrate, may result in low blood glucose levels that impair concentration and even consciousness. The second liver enzyme, CYP2E1, is part of the cytochrome P450 family, and metabolizes alcohol at levels to be expected after heavy drinking. During metabolism of high levels of alcohol, CYP2E1 utilizes adenosine triphosphate (ATP) energy units and thus 'wastes' stored calories, with resultant potential for weight loss. Another form of this enzyme, gastric CYP2E1, exists in the stomach and, as the first of the three alcohol-metabolizing enzymes to encounter alcohol, accounts for about 30% of all alcohol metabolism in men, but only 10% in women. This gender difference may explain why women's tolerance to alcohol is much less than men's, hence the recognized lower 'safe' level for moderate drinking in women.

The Potential Benefits of Moderate Alcohol Consumption

In 1992, French scientists published a report that indicated that cardiovascular mortality was much less among predominantly wine-drinking residents of the Mediterranean southern provinces of France than in northern provinces where wine is less frequently preferred, in spite of similar overall dietary components and rates of consumption of alcoholic beverages (Table 1). This report on the 'French paradox' was assumed to confer specific cardioprotective benefit to wine, but was soon tempered by in vitro studies, which showed that the protective effect of wine on the oxidation of low-density lipoprotein could be mimicked by constitutive antioxidant flavonoids present not only in grapes but in many other fruits and vegetables. Another epidemiological study concluded that the lower mortality risk among wine drinkers compared to non-wine drinkers could be attributed in large part to a better life style, including less smoking, more exercise, and better diet. Subsequent population studies defined J-shaped curves for alcohol-related mortality, where mortality is increased in abstainers and progressively increased in those who consume more than one (women) or two (men) drinks per day. It can now be concluded that the benefits of moderate drinking are confined to reductions in incidences of coronary vessel occlusions and ischemic strokes, but not to hemorrhagic

Table 1 Benefits and risks of alcohol consumption

	Minimal amount or duration (drink units per day)	Mechanism
Benefits		
Coronary disease protection	1–2 (women),	Flavonoid antioxidants
Cerebrovascular disease (nonhemorrhagic) protection	2–4 (men)	Elevated HDL lipoprotein Reduced platelet adhesiveness
Risks		
Cancer		
Oropharynx and esophagus	>2 (women), >4 (men)	Unknown; higher risk in smoking alcoholics
Breast (women)	>2	Increases estrogen production
Colon	>2 (women), >4 (men)	Risk increases with low folate
Alcoholic liver disease		
Fatty liver	>2	Increased liver fat synthesis
Alcoholic hepatitis	>3 (women) × 10 years >6 (men) × 15 years	Toxicity of alcohol metabolism
Alcoholic cirrhosis	>3 (women) × 15 years >6 (men) × 20 years	Increased collagen synthesis
Pancreas		
Pancreatitis	~10 years	Acute inflammation of pancreas
Pancreatic insufficiency	~10–15 years	Loss of exocrine and endocrine pancreatic cells
Cardiomyopathy	Binge drinking	Mitochondrial damage of muscle cells or thiamine deficiency
Neurological		
Acute trauma, e.g., motor vehicle accidents	1–2 in social setting	Legal intoxication
Coma and death	10–20 in rapid succession	Severe toxicity
Withdrawal syndrome	Follows binge	Neuronal hyperexcitability
Wernicke-Korsokoff syndrome	10–15 years	Thiamine deficiency
Anemia	5–10 years	Combinations of iron, folate and pyridoxal deficiencies

strokes. Whereas red and white wine both contain protective antioxidant flavonoids, moderate amounts of alcohol also improve the circulating lipid profile by increasing levels of high-density lipoprotein and tissue plasminogen activator while reducing platelet adhesiveness.

The risks of Excessive Alcohol Consumption

Unlike other abused drugs, chronic alcohol in excess affects many different organ systems, which include the liver, pancreas, heart, and brain (**Table 1**). Excessive chronic alcohol use also increases the risk of certain cancers. While these risks are apparent among the 7% of US citizens over aged 14 who abuse alcohol, their prevalence is generally no less in countries such as France, Italy, and Spain where drinking wine with meals is considered part of the culture. The organ damage from chronic alcoholism may impact on processes of nutrient assimilation and metabolism, as is the case with chronic liver and pancreatic disease, or may be modulated in large part by nutrient deficiencies, as with thiamine and brain function. This section will consider specific effects of alcohol abuse on certain organs as a

background for consideration of specific effects on nutritional status.

Alcoholic Liver Disease

Alcoholic liver disease is among the top ten causes of mortality in the US with somewhat higher mortality rates in western European countries where wine is considered a dietary staple, and is a leading cause of death in Russia. Among the three stages of alcoholic liver disease, fatty liver is related to the acute effects of alcohol on hepatic lipid metabolism and is completely reversible. By contrast, alcoholic hepatitis usually occurs after a decade or more of chronic drinking, is associated with inflammation of the liver and necrosis of liver cells, and carries about a 40% mortality risk for each hospitalization. Alcoholic cirrhosis represents irreversible scarring of the liver with loss of liver cells, and may be associated with alcoholic hepatitis. The scarring process greatly alters the circulation of blood through the liver and is associated with increased blood pressure in the portal (visceral) circulation and shunting of blood flow away from the liver and through other organs such as the esophagus. The potentially lethal complications of portal hypertension include rupture of esophageal varices, ascites or accumulation of fluid in the abdominal cavity, and the syndrome of hepatic encephalopathy, which is due to inadequate hepatic detoxification of substances in the visceral blood that is shunted around the liver. The risk of developing alcoholic cirrhosis is dependent upon the amount of alcohol exposure independent of the presence or absence of malnutrition. For example, a study of well-nourished German male executives found that the incidence of alcoholic cirrhosis was directly related to the daily amount and duration of alcohol consumption, such that daily ingestion of 160 g alcohol, equivalent to that found in a pint of whisky, over a 15-year period predicted a 50% risk of cirrhosis on liver biopsy. Other worldwide demographic data indicate that mortality rates from cirrhosis of the liver can be related to national per capita alcohol intake. These studies have defined the threshold risk for eventual development of alcoholic cirrhosis as 6 drinks per day for men, and about half that for women.

Pancreatitis and Pancreatic Insufficiency

Pancreatitis occurs less frequently than liver disease in chronic alcoholics, and is characterized by severe attacks of abdominal pain due to pancreatic inflammation, while pancreatic insufficiency is due to the eventual destruction of pancreatic cells that secrete digestive enzymes and insulin. This destructive process is associated with progressive scarring of the pancreas together with distortion and partial blockage of the pancreatic ducts, which promote recurrent episodes of acute inflammatory pancreatitis. Since the pancreas is the site of production of proteases and lipases for protein and lipid digestion, destruction of more than 90% of the pancreas results in significant malabsorption of these major dietary constituents, as well as diabetes secondary to reduced insulin secretion. Consequently, patients with pancreatic insufficiency exhibit severe loss of body fat and muscle protein. Since the absorption of fat-soluble vitamins is dependent upon pancreatic lipase for solubilization of dietary fat, these patients are also at risk for deficiencies of vitamins A, D, and E.

Cancers

Chronic alcoholics are at increased risk for cancer of the oro-pharynx and esophagus, colon, and breast. The risk of oro-pharyngeal cancer is greatest when heavy smoking is combined with excessive daily alcohol. Increased risk of squamous cell cancer of the esophagus is also compounded by smoking and may be associated with deficiencies of vitamin A and zinc. Breast cancer in women may be mediated through increased estrogen production during heavy alcohol intake. Colon cancer risk is greatest among alcoholics with marginal folate deficiency.

Heart

Although coronary disease risk is decreased by alcohol consumption, excessive alcohol use also impairs cardiac muscle function. Episodic heavy drinking bouts can lead to arrhythmias in the 'holiday heart' syndrome. Chronic alcoholics are prone to left-sided heart failure secondary to decreased mitochondrial function of cardiac muscle cells, possibly mediated by abnormal fatty acid metabolism. A specific form of high output heart failure, or 'wet beriberi,' occurs in association with thiamine deficiency.

Neurological Effects

The many neurological effects of acute and chronic alcohol abuse can be categorized as those related directly to alcohol, those secondary to chronic liver disease, and those mediated by thiamine deficiency. The stages of acute alcohol toxicity progress upward from legal intoxication with reduced reaction time and judgment, as occurs with blood levels greater than $0.08\,g\,dl^{-1}$ that usually define legal intoxication, to coma and death with levels greater than $0.4\,g\,dl^{-1}$. While mild intoxication is common with social drinking, coma and death have been described among college age males who consume excessive amounts of alcohol in a very short period of time. Automobile accidents, which account for a large portion of alcohol-related deaths, are more common in drunken pedestrians than drivers. Intoxication also leads to frequent falls and head trauma, and subdural hematoma can present with delayed but progressive loss of cognition, headaches, and eventual death. Chronic alcoholics are prone to episodes of alcohol withdrawal, which can be characterized according to stages of tremulousness, seizures, and delirium tremens with hyper-excitability and hallucinations at any time up to 5 days after the last drink. This state of altered consciousness is distinct from hepatic encephalopathy, which results from diversion of toxic nitrogenous substances around the scarred cirrhotic liver and is associated with progressive slowing of cerebral functions with stages of confusion, loss of cognition, and eventual coma and death. Progressive altered cognition and judgment can also result from cerebral atrophy following years of heavy drinking, and may also be mediated by thiamine deficiency as described in greater detail below.

Anemia

Chronic alcoholics who substitute large amounts of alcohol for other dietary constituents are at risk for developing anemia. The causes of anemia in chronic alcoholics are multifactorial, including iron deficiency secondary to bleeding from episodic gastritis or other gastrointestinal sites, folate deficiency from inadequate diet or malabsorption, and deficiency of pyridoxine (vitamin B_6) due to abnormal effects on its metabolism. Consequently, the bone marrow may demonstrate absent iron and mixtures of megaloblastosis from folate deficiency and sideroblastosis from pyridoxine deficiency.

The Effects of Alcohol Consumption on Nutritional Status

Body Weight and Energy Balance

The effects of alcohol on body weight are dependent upon the timing and amount of alcohol consumption in relation to meals and on the presence or absence of organ damage, in particular alcoholic liver disease (**Table 2**). Whereas body weight is usually unaffected by moderate alcohol consumption, chronic alcoholics who drink daily while substituting alcohol for other dietary constituents lose weight due to the energy neutral effect of alcohol in the diet. Moderate drinkers on weight loss regimens are less likely to lose weight while consuming alcohol with their meals since one effect of alcohol is to decrease restraint over food intake. At the same time, those who consume alcohol with high-fat meals are more likely to gain weight due to an acute effect of alcohol on reducing the oxidation of fat at the same time as it promotes its storage.

The presence of alcoholic liver disease results in significant changes in body composition and energy balance. Although fatty liver is fully reversible, progression to alcoholic hepatitis can have profound effects on nutritional status. According to large

Table 2 Effects of alcohol on body weight

Drinking behavior	Explanation
Moderate drinking	
Reduce weight	Substitution of carbohydrate by alcohol; more likely in women
Increase weight	Decreased dietary restraint
Heavy drinking	
Reduce weight	Substitution of nonalcohol calories by alcohol calories, which are 'wasted' during metabolism
Increase weight	Alcohol metabolism decreases lipid metabolism, promotes fat storage

multicenter studies, alcoholic hepatitis patients demonstrate universal evidence for protein calorie malnutrition, according to the physical findings of muscle wasting and edema, low levels of serum albumin and other visceral proteins, and decreased cell-mediated immunity, whereas their 6-month mortality is related in part to the severity of malnutrition. Anorexia is a major cause of weight loss in alcoholic liver disease, and may be caused by increased circulating levels of leptin. Furthermore, active alcoholic hepatitis contributes to increased resting energy expenditure as another cause of weight loss. On the other hand, resting energy expenditure is normal in stable alcoholic cirrhotics who are also typically underweight or malnourished in part due to preferential metabolism of endogenous fat stores. At the same time, the digestion of dietary fat is decreased in cirrhotic patients due to diminished secretion of bile salts and pancreatic enzymes.

Micronutrient Deficiencies

The chronic exposure to excessive amounts of ethanol is associated with deficiencies of multiple nutrients, in particular thiamine, folate, pyridoxine, vitamin A, vitamin D, and zinc (**Table 3**). The frequency of these deficiencies is increased in the presence of alcoholic liver disease, which results in decreased numbers of hepatocytes for vitamin storage and metabolism. Many of the clinical signs of alcoholic liver disease are related to vitamin deficiencies.

Thiamine

Low circulating levels of thiamine have been described in 80% of patients with alcoholic cirrhosis. Thiamine pyrophosphate is a coenzyme in the intermediary metabolism of carbohydrates, in particular for transketolases, which play a role in cardiac and neurological functions. While alcoholic beverages are essentially devoid of thiamine, acute exposure to alcohol decreases the activity of intestinal transporters required for thiamine absorption. The major neurological signs and symptoms of thiamine deficiency in alcoholics include peripheral neuropathy, partial paresis of ocular muscles, widebased gait secondary to cerebellar lesions, cognitive defects, and severe memory loss. The presence of peripheral neuropathy is sometimes referred to as 'dry beriberi,' while the other symptoms constitute the Wernicke-Korsokoff syndrome. Whereas abnormal eye movements can be treated acutely by thiamine injections, the other signs are often permanent and contribute to the dementia that often afflicts

Table 3 Micronutrient deficiencies in chronic alcoholic patients

Deficiency	Cause	Effect
Thiamine	• Poor diet • Intestinal malabsorption	• Peripheral neuropathy • Wernicke-Korsokoff syndrome • High output heart failure
Folate	• Poor diet • Intestinal malabsorption • Decreased liver storage • Increase urine excretion	• Megaloblastic anemia • Hyperhomocysteinemia • Neural tube defect • Altered cognition
Pyridoxine (vitamin B$_6$)	• Poor diet • Displacement from circulating albumin promotes urine excretion	• Peripheral neuropathy • Sideroblastic anemia
Vitamin A	• Malabsorption • Increased biliary secretion	• Night blindness • May promote development of alcoholic liver disease
Vitamin D	• Malabsorption • Decteased sun exposure	• Calcium deficiency • Metabolic bone disease
Zinc	• Poor diet • Increaded urine excretion	• Night blindness • Decreased taste • Decreased immune funtion
Iron	• Gastrointestinal bleeding	• Anemia

alcoholics after years of drinking. 'Wet beriberi' refers to the high-output cardiac failure that can also occur in thiamine-deficient alcoholics, and is responsive to thiamine therapy in addition to conventional treatment. Since endogenous thiamine is used during carbohydrate metabolism, acute cardiac failure can be precipitated by the administration of intravenous glucose to malnourished and marginally thiamine-deficient patients by depletion of remaining thiamine stores. This process can be prevented by the addition of soluble vitamins including thiamine to malnourished chronic alcoholic patients who are undergoing treatment for medical emergencies.

Folate

Folates are polyglutamylated in their dietary forms and circulate in the methylated and reduced monoglutatate form. Folates function in DNA synthesis and cell turnover, and play a central role in methionine metabolism as substrate for the enzyme methionine synthase in the conversion of homocysteine to methionine. While originally recognized as a cause of megaloblastic anemia, the expanding consequences of folate deficiency are related to elevated circulating homocysteine and include increased risk for neural tube defects and other congenital abnormalities in newborns and altered cognition in the elderly. Prior to folate fortification in the US, the incidence of low serum folate levels in chronic alcoholics was at about 80%. Megaloblastic anemia, due to the negative effects of folate deficiency on DNA synthesis, has been described in about one-third of patients with alcoholic liver disease. Excessive alcohol use is associated with reversible hyperhomocysteinemia in chronic alcoholics because of the inhibitory effect of alcohol or its metabolite acetaldehyde on methionine synthase. Furthermore, folate deficiency may play a role in the pathogenesis of alcoholic liver disease by exacerbating abnormalities in the metabolism of S-adenosylmethionine.

The causes of folate deficiency in chronic alcoholism are multiple. With the exception of beer, all alcoholic beverages are devoid of folate, and the typical diet of the chronic alcoholic does not include its fresh vegetable sources. Chronic alcoholism is associated with intestinal folate malabsorption, decreased liver folate uptake, and accelerated folate excretion in the urine. In addition, alcoholic liver disease results in decreased liver stores of folate, so the duration of time for development of folate deficiency with marginal diet is shortened.

Pyridoxine Deficiency

Pyridoxine (vitamin B$_6$) is required for transamination reactions, including the elimination of homocysteine. Pyridoxine deficiency in chronic alcoholism is caused by poor diet, whereas displacement of pyridoxal phosphate from circulating albumin by the alcohol metabolite acetaldehyde increases its urinary excretion. Low serum levels of pyridoxal phosphate are common in chronic alcoholics, and pyridoxine deficiency is manifest by peripheral neuropathy and sideroblastic anemia. In alcoholic hepatitis, the serum level of alanine transaminase (ALT) is disproportionately low compared to aspartate transaminase (AST), due to the requirement of pyridoxine for ALT activity.

Vitamin B₁₂

The incidence of vitamin B_{12} deficiency in chronic alcoholism is undefined, since serum levels are often normal or increased due to the presence of B_{12} analogs in alcoholic liver disease. Nevertheless, the intestinal absorption of vitamin B_{12} is decreased in chronic alcoholics due to defective uptake at the ileum. Presumed low levels of vitamin B_{12} in the liver may contribute to abnormal hepatic methionine metabolism with elevated serum homocysteine, since this vitamin is a cofactor for methionine synthase.

Vitamin A

Although serum levels of vitamin A are usually normal in chronic alcoholics, liver retinoids are progressively lowered through the stages of alcoholic liver disease.

Retinoids may play a central role in hepatic function, where vitamin A is stored as retinyl esters in fat-storing transitional Ito cells. The process of transformation of Ito cells to collagen-producing, hepatic stellate cells is associated with depletion of retinyl esters, which may be implicated in the development of alcoholic liver disease. The causes of vitamin A deficiency in alcoholic liver disease include malabsorption, which is due to decreased secretion of bile and pancreatic enzymes necessary for the digestion of dietary retinyl esters and their incorporation into water-soluble micelles prior to intestinal transport. In addition, the transport of retinol is impaired due to decreased hepatic production of retinol-binding protein. Thirdly, the metabolism of alcohol induces microsomal enzymes that promote the production of polar retinol metabolites, which are more easily excreted in the bile. The signs of vitamin A deficiency include night blindness with increased risk of automobile accidents and increased risk of esophageal cancer due to abnormal squamous cell cycling. Conversely, patients with alcoholic liver disease are more susceptible to vitamin A hepatotoxicity so that supplemental doses should be used with caution.

Vitamin D and Calcium

Chronic alcoholic patients are at increased risk for metabolic bone disease due to low vitamin D and hence decreased absorption of calcium. Alcoholic liver disease increases the likelihood of low circulating levels of 25-hydroxy vitamin D because of decreased excretion of bile required for absorption of this fat-soluble vitamin, poor diet, and often decreased sun exposure. Calcium deficiency results from low levels of vitamin D that are required to regulate its absorption, and also because the fat malabsorption that often accompanies alcoholic liver disease results in increased binding of calcium to unabsorbed intestinal fatty acids.

Zinc

Zinc is a cofactor for many enzymatic reactions including retinol dehydrogenase, is stored in the pancreas, and circulates in the blood bound mainly to albumin. Chronic alcoholic patients are frequently zinc deficient because of poor diet, deficiency of pancreatic enzymes, and increased urine excretion due to low zinc-binding albumin in the circulation. The consequences of zinc deficiency include night blindness from decreased production of retinal, decreased taste, and hypogonadism, which may result in lowered testosterone levels and increased risk of osteoporosis in men. Since zinc is required for cellular immunity, its deficiency may contribute to increased infection risk in alcoholic patients.

Iron

Chronic alcoholic patients are often iron deficient because of increased frequency of gastrointestinal bleeding, typically due to alcoholic gastritis or esophageal tears from frequent retching and vomiting, or from rupture of esophageal varices in patients with cirrhosis and portal hypertension. The major consequence of iron deficiency is anemia, which may be compounded by the concurrent effects of folate and pyridoxine deficiencies. Conversely, increased exposure to iron, e.g., from cooking in iron pots, increases the likelihood and severity of alcoholic liver disease, since the presence of iron in the liver promotes oxidative liver damage during the metabolism of alcohol.

See also: **Ascorbic Acid**: Deficiency States. **Calcium. Cancer**: Epidemiology and Associations Between Diet and Cancer. **Folic Acid. Iron. Liver Disorders. Thiamin**: Physiology. **Vitamin A**: Biochemistry and Physiological Role. **Vitamin B₆. Vitamin E**: Metabolism and Requirements. **Zinc**: Physiology.

Further Reading

Halsted CH (2004) Nutrition and alcoholic liver disease. *Seminars in Liver Diseases* **24**: 289–304.

Halsted CH (1995) Alcohol and folate interactions: clinical implications. In: Bailey LB (ed.) *Folate in Health and Disease*, pp. 313–327. New York: M. Decker, Inc.

Klatsky AL (2002) Alcohol and cardiovascular diseases: a historical overview. *Annals of the New York Academy of Science* **957**: 7–15.

Lieber CS (1992) In *Medical and Nutritional Complications of Alcoholism: Mechanisms and Management*. New York and London: Plenum Medical Book Company.

Lieber CS (2000) ALCOHOL: its metabolism and interaction with nutrients. *Annual Review of Nutrition* **20**: 395–430.

Lieber CS (2004) New concepts of the pathogenesis of alcoholic liver disease lead to novel treatments. *Current Gastroenterology Reports* **6**: 60–65.

McClain CJ, Hill DB, Song Z, Chawla R, Watson WH, Chen T, and Barve S (2002) S-Adenosylmethionine, cytokines, and alcoholic liver disease. *Alcohol* **27**: 185–192.

Mendenhall C, Roselle GA, Gartside P, and Moritz T (1995) Relationship of protein calorie malnutrition to alcoholic liver disease: a reexamination of data from two Veterans Administration Cooperative Studies. *Alcoholism: Clinical and Experimental Research* **19**: 635–641.

Mezey E (1991) Interaction between alcohol and nutrition in the pathogenesis of alcoholic liver disease. *Seminars in Liver Disease* **11**: 340–348.

Nanji A (1993) Role of eicosanoids in experimental alcoholic liver disease. *Alcohol* **10**: 443–446.

Secretary of Health and Human Services (2000) *Tenth Special Report to the U.S. Congress on Alcohol and Health*. US Department of Health and Human Services, National Institute of Alcohol Abuse and Alcoholism.

ALUMINUM

N D Priest, Middlesex University, London, UK

© 2005 Elsevier Ltd. All rights reserved.

Occurrence in Food and the Environment

Properties and Natural Occurrence

Aluminum was discovered in 1825 by the Danish chemist Oersted. It is a soft, ductile, malleable, silvery metal. Its atomic number is 13, and it has one stable isotope, ^{27}Al. Aluminum belongs to group 3a of the periodic table, along with boron, indium, gallium, and thallium. It most commonly forms trivalent ionic (Al^{3+}) compounds, but it has some covalent characteristics. Aluminum is the most common metal in the earth's crust and is the third most common element. It is too reactive to occur in nature as the free metal.

Aluminum occurs in natural systems as the trivalent ion and in these it has no oxidation-reduction chemistry. In aqueous solution, the chemistry is complicated by the formation of several pH-dependent complex ions. These ions—$Al(OH)^{2+}$, $Al(OH)_2^+$, and $Al(OH)_4^-$—compete with Al^{3+} and $Al(OH)_3$ within aquatic systems. Aluminum is minimally soluble in water at approximately pH 6, when the $Al(OH)_2^+$ ion dominates, but solubility increases at lower and higher pH values. At pH 7 and higher, the most important ion is $Al(OH)_4^-$, whereas at low pH values Al^{3+} dominates.

In contrast to its abundance in the earth's crust, most natural waters contain very little dissolved aluminum (often $<10\,\mu g\,l^{-1}$), reflecting the low solubility of minerals and the deposition of Al^{3+} in sediments as the hydroxide. Seawater contains only $1\,\mu g\,l^{-1}$ of aluminum, and much of this is thought to be bound within the skeletons of diatoms. Where natural waters have either been acidified by acid rain or treated with aluminum sulfate to produce drinking water, the levels of the metal are higher. Concentrations in acidified lakes and rivers (up to $700\,\mu g\,l^{-1}$) commonly exceed levels toxic to fish. In acidic well water, concentrations $>1\,mg\,l^{-1}$ may occur. Aluminum concentrations in tap water should not exceed $200\,\mu g\,l^{-1}$ a guideline specified by the World Health Organization (WHO) on esthetic grounds.

Air concentrations of aluminum range from less than $1\,\mu g\,m^{-3}$ in rural environments to as high as $10\,\mu g\,m^{-3}$ in urban, industrialized areas. The higher levels in the latter result from the dust-creating activities of urban man.

Nonfood Uses

Aluminum compounds are widely utilized by industry. They are used in the paper industry, for water purification, in the dye industry, in missile fuels, in paints and pigments, in the textile industry, as a catalyst in oil refining, in the glass industry, and as components of cosmetic and pharmaceutical preparations. Of these, the uses within the cosmetic/pharmaceutical industry are of particular significance since they provide the most likely sources of aluminum uptake by the body.

The following are major cosmetic/pharmaceutical uses of aluminum compounds:

- Aluminum hydroxide as an antacid, particularly for patients suffering from peptic and duodenal ulcers
- Aluminum hydroxide as an effective, nonabsorbed phosfate binder for patients with long-standing kidney failure

- As a component of buffered aspirin
- Aluminum hydroxide and monostearates as components of some vaccines/injection solutions
- Aluminum chloride, aluminum zirconium glycine complex, and aluminum chlorohydrate as the active ingredients of antiperspirants

Many of these applications are under review and their use is discouraged where alternatives of equal efficacy are available and where the potential for high aluminum uptakes exists. For example, both calcium carbonate and lanthanum sulfate are possible alternatives to the long-term use of aluminum hydroxide as a phosfate binder.

Food Uses of Aluminum Compounds

Aluminum compounds that may be employed as food additives are listed in **Table 1**. Although most are present in foods as trace components, others may be present in significant quantities. For example, aluminum-based baking powders, employing sodium aluminum phosfate (SALP), may contain more than $10\,mg\,g^{-1}$ of aluminum, and bread or cake made with these may contain 5–15 mg of the element per slice. American processed cheese may contain as much as 50 mg of aluminum per slice due to the addition of Kasel, an emulsifying agent. Pickled cucumbers may contain 10 mg of aluminum per fruit when alum has been employed as a firming agent. Aluminum anticaking agents may also be present in significant quantities in common table salt.

Table 1 Permitted aluminum-containing food additives and uses

Compound	Use
Aluminum	Metallic color for surface treatment
Aluminum ammonium sulfate (ammonium alum)	Acidic compound used as a neutralizing agent and as a buffer
Aluminum potassium sulfate (potassium alum)	Acidic compound used as a neutralizing agent, a buffer, and a firming agent
Aluminum sodium sulfate (soda/sodium alum)	Buffer, neutralizing agent, and firming agent
Aluminum sulfate (alum)	Firming agent in pickling
Aluminum calcium silicate	Anticaking agent for powders
Aluminum sodium silicate	Anticaking agent for powders
Sodium calcium aluminosilicate	Anticaking agent for powders
Kaolin (contains aluminum oxide)	Anticaking agent for powders
Sodium aluminum phosphate (acidic), SALP	Acid, raising (leavening) agent for flour
Sodium aluminum phosphate (basic), Kasel	Emulsifying salt

Natural Aluminum in Food

Even though concentrations of aluminum in soil are high (3–10%), most food plants contain little aluminum. Reports describe diverse levels in different foods and reported values vary for similar foods. Much of this variation results from either the inadequate removal of soil and/or contamination of foods with soil prior to analysis or the use of poor analytical techniques. A selection of results for plant foods is given in **Table 2**. This shows that most uncooked plant foods contain $<5\,\mu g\,g^{-1}$. However, reported concentrations in herbs and spices are higher due to their dehydrated state and their content of aluminum-containing grinding materials.

The concentration of natural aluminum in animal-derived foods is influenced by the low concentration of aluminum in animal feeds, the poor biological uptake of 'food aluminum' by food animals, and the limited ability of body aluminum to transfer to products such as eggs and milk. Consequently, most animal-based foods contain $<1\,\mu g\,g^{-1}$ of aluminum (**Table 3**).

Of the remaining miscellaneous foods in common usage, few contain significant aluminum. Beer stored in aluminum cans for up to 1 year contains $<29\,\mu g\,cm^{-3}$ and the maximum level recorded in beverages within aluminum cans is 1.5 mg per $375\text{-}cm^3$ can. Tea, which when dry contains large quantities of aluminum ($1.28\,mg\,g^{-1}$), contains relatively little when steeped ($2.8\,\mu g\,cm^{-3}$). For comparison, brewed coffee contains less than $0.4\,\mu g\,cm^{-3}$.

The aluminum concentration of acidic foods may be increased by cooking in aluminum vessels. In one study the increment to the aluminum content of an average-sized serving of rhubarb was 25 mg. Onions boiled in aluminum saucepans similarly accumulate the metal. In contrast, the cooking of nonacidic food products in aluminum utensils has little effect on their aluminum content. Similarly, the use of aluminum foil for wrapping foods adds little to their metal content.

Total Dietary Intake of Aluminum

Regarding measurements of the aluminum content of individual foods, the measurement of total daily diets is complicated by problems of analysis and sample contamination. However, relatively reliable data are available for some countries. In a Finnish study, daily intake of aluminum from food was calculated to be 6.7 mg. Studies performed by the US Food and Drug Administration suggest average daily intake values of between 9 and 14 mg

Table 2 Concentrations of natural aluminum in plant foods

Food	Concentration ($\mu g\,g^{-1}$)
Cereals	
Barley	5.0–7.0
Maize (corn)	0.4–3.1
Oats	5.1
Wheat	4.0–16
Rye	4.8
Whole wheat bread	5.4
Cheerios	4.7
Corn Flakes	<2
Macaroni	<2
Rolled oats	<2–5.0
Rice Krispies	<2
Spaghetti	<2
Vegetables	
Asparagus	1.7–9.0
Green beans	8.0
Cabbage, inner leaf	5.7
Carrots	3.8
Cauliflower head	4.0
Leek	15
Onions	5.0–10
Potatoes	<1–20
Spinach	6.9
Tomatoes	0.2–1.1
Fruit	
Apples	0.2–0.9
Bananas	<0.4
Grapes	<0.5
Honeydew melon	0.2
Oranges	<0.4
Plums	<0.3–0.5
Rhubarb	0.8–4.8
Pineapples	<0.3
Herbs and spices	
Allspice	51–101
Basil	167–450
Cinnamon	48–115
Marjoram	>500–1000
Mustard	5–10
Nutmeg	5–11
Paprika	49–700
Black pepper	48–237
Sesame seed	5–<10
Thyme	>500–<1000
Nuts	
Peanuts	<2
Walnuts	<2
Oils	
Olive	0.1–0.4
Sugars	
White sugar	<2
Brown sugar	<2
Cuban raw	5.3
Molasses	110

Table 3 Concentration of natural aluminum in animal foods

Food	Concentration ($\mu g\,g^{-1}$)
Milk	0.1–0.7
Cottage cheese	<2
Swiss cheese	19
Beef	<1
Steak	2.3–8.4
Bovine kidney	0.4–1.0
Bovine liver	<2
Lamb	<1
Pork	<1
Bacon	<2
Veal	<1
Chicken	<1
Eggs	0.2–1.4
Turkey	<1
Carp	0.7–1.0
Haddock	<1
Salmon (canned)	8.2
Sole	<1

Table 4 Sources of dietary aluminum intake

Food component	Al content (mg/standard serving)
US male and female mean Al intake	9–14/day
Cornbread (homemade)	18
Processed cheese, yellow cake (iced)	10–11
Fish sticks, muffins, hamburger	4–6
Pancakes, spinach	2–3
Lasagne	1

Bioavailability and Metabolism

Given the ubiquitous nature of aluminum in the environment, it is surprising that the human body contains little and that it has no function as an essential trace mineral. To a large extent, this level reflects the integrity of the body's barriers to metal ion intake.

Bioavailability of Ingested Aluminum

Metal ions enter the body by one of three main routes: via the gut wall, by inhalation, and through wounds. For most individuals, the important route of aluminum uptake is through the gut wall. This is true even though the bioavailability of aluminum may be higher by other routes.

Like most polyvalent metal ions, most ingested aluminum passes through the intestinal tract without being absorbed. An estimate of the daily aluminum uptake by the body from all sources, based on an estimate of average daily intake and the level of

(**Table 4**). In general, it is likely that daily intakes of aluminum in North America are higher than in Europe due to a higher utilization of SALP and Kasel in the preparation of processed foods.

excreted aluminum, indicated an absorbed fraction of 0.001.

More precise measurements of absorption have been made using the isotope ^{26}Al. The first reported study utilizing ^{26}Al indicated that in the presence of excess citrate, 1% of the metal was absorbed. This result was considered consistent with the ability of citrate to complex metal ions, holding them in solution at physiological pH values, but unrepresentative because of the large amount of citrate employed. Moreover, the study estimated aluminum uptake from the results of single blood analyses, which may not provide a true measure of uptake. Later studies employing this method have indicated lower uptake values, typically 0.0005. They have also shown that some subpopulations, including those suffering from Alzheimer's disease and some 'normal' individuals, absorb more aluminum than average members of the population and that the coingestion of silicic acid inhibits aluminum absorption by a factor of approximately 3.

Complete balance studies using the ^{26}Al tracer have been undertaken to determine bioavailability. These showed that the fractional uptake of aluminum following administration as a citrate solution was 0.005 and following its intake as hydroxide was 0.0001. The coadministration of citrate with aluminum hydroxide enhanced aluminum uptake by a factor of approximately 10. A later study measured the bioavailability of aluminum in drinking water, and a fractional uptake of 0.002 was determined. It follows that at a maximum concentration of aluminum in drinking water of $200 \, \mu g \, l^{-1}$, this source will normally account for approximately 6% of total (nonmedical) aluminum uptake.

In addition to the concentration of citrate in ingested food, other factors have been shown to affect the bioavailability of aluminum: age—metal uptake in milk-fed infants is higher than average and uptake may also be greater in the elderly; gut contents reduce metal bioavailability; silicic acid binds strongly to aluminum, reducing its bioavailability; and local gut conditions affect the ability of the gut wall to sequester aluminum, changing the time available for its uptake. Overall, results suggest that aluminum bioavailability varies between approximately 0.01 and 0.0001.

Biokinetics of Aluminum in Blood

The biochemistry of aluminum is, to a large extent, determined by its valency, ion size, and redox chemistry. The effective ionic radius of Al^{3+} is $54 \, pm$. This is sufficiently similar to that of Fe^{3+} ($65 \, pm$) for it to follow some of its metabolic pathways.

However, its progress through these is halted at stages where iron is transformed to its divalent, Fe^{2+} state. Aluminum is also sufficiently similar to calcium to codeposit in the skeleton. In addition, aluminum binds particularly strongly to phosfates, giving it the potential to bind with DNA, ATP, and many other biomolecules.

Within the blood, transferrin, the iron-transport protein, binds aluminum most avidly. However, compared to Fe^{3+} ions, the strength of this affinity is low. Consequently, aluminum will not displace iron from transferrin. Aluminum also binds with low-molecular-weight proteins and citrate. Aluminum complexes with low-molecular-weight species may leak from blood vessels into surrounding tissue fluids. The extent of binding to low-molecular-weight molecules is uncertain, but studies indicate that 50% or less of blood aluminum may be bound to them. It has also been suggested that silicic acid in blood may also bind aluminum to form aluminosilicate colloidal particles, which would then deposit within reticuloendothelial organs.

Aluminum is initially rapidly lost from the blood to other body fluids and to excretion, reflecting the weakness/kinetics of the binding of the Al^{3+} ion to proteins. Subsequently, the rate of loss slows. Volunteer studies showed that more than half of the ion had left the blood by 15 minutes postadministration, and that by 1 h an average of 68% had been lost. At 1 day, approximately 2% remained in the blood and by 5 days only 0.4% remained. These variations make the interpretation of isolated blood and serum aluminum levels particularly difficult. At 1 h after uptake, little or no aluminum in the blood is associated with red blood cells. However, at 880 days after intake 14% is associated with these cells. Unlike those in plasma, aluminum deposits in red blood cells are cleared with a long half-life and they may provide a basis for an aluminum assay.

Aluminum Excretion and Body Retention

^{26}Al studies have shown that most aluminum entering blood is excreted in the urine, with only approximately 1% lost in feces. In these studies, intersubject variability was conspicuous, such that 1 and 5 days after intake the range of fractional aluminum excretions was 0.5–0.8 and 0.6–0.9, respectively. In another study employing a single volunteer, the long-term retention of aluminum was determined. At early times this volunteer showed a retention pattern consistent with the mean of that found in the short-term study. However, approximately 4% of injected aluminum was retained for years. This finding indicates that under conditions of continuous intake, aluminum is accumulated by the body, even in subjects with normal kidney function.

From a retention equation, and assuming daily systemic uptakes of 15 µg of aluminum, terminal body burdens of the metal were predicted. The calculations suggested that 50 years of continuous uptake of aluminum should give rise to body burdens of 2–7 mg. This estimate is lower than others based on the results of chemical analyses (35–60 mg). It is suggested that the most likely reasons for this discrepancy are errors in the extrapolation of body burden from the results of the chemical analysis of small pieces of tissue and errors due to the measurement of samples that have become contaminated with environmental aluminum (i.e., dust).

Aluminum Deposition in Tissues

Most metals are deposited to a much greater extent than average in a few organs: liver, kidneys, and skeleton. However, the proportion of the total body burden deposited in these is variable and depends on many factors, including the chemical properties of the ion and the age, sex, and metabolic status of the individual. The major site of deposition of aluminum is the skeleton. Skeletal deposits of aluminum have been demonstrated in normal bone using chemical analysis and are easily detected in bone from renal failure patients using histochemical staining techniques.

The levels of aluminum deposited in the liver are uncertain. Published measurements of total liver aluminum suggest values of 6–9 mg for normal adults, indicating that a significant fraction of the aluminum body burden is present in this organ. However, external counting of [26]Al did not indicate large liver deposits. Moreover, a comparative failure of aluminum to deposit in the normal liver would be consistent with the low levels of fecal excretion seen and with the low concentrations of aluminum found in the livers of some dialyzed renal patients. Also, at least in rats, the relative depositions of trivalent metals in the skeleton and liver have been shown to be a function of ion size, with appreciable liver deposition occurring only where the ion size is large. The ion size of aluminum is very small. However, the observation that with time aluminum levels build up in red blood cells may indicate the presence of a delayed pathway of aluminum accumulation by the liver since this organ is involved in the breakdown of hemoglobin.

Within the skeleton, aluminum, in common with most other polyvalent metal ions, initially deposits as a very thin layer on bone surfaces. The mechanisms of deposition have not been investigated, but one report suggests that three may be involved: entrapment of aluminum ions within the hydration shell of existing bone mineral; incorporation of aluminum into new bone mineral at sites of bone apposition; and binding of the metal to acidic organic components of the bone matrix, such as phosphoproteins.

Subsequently, aluminum remains on bone surfaces until it back-exchanges into tissue fluids, the bone surface is removed by osteoclasts, or the bone surface is buried by the apposition of new bone. These processes will result in the gradual loss of bone aluminum and in a transfer of aluminum from bone surfaces to the volume of the bone matrix. Such volume deposits are clearly seen in stained biopsy sections from dialysis patients.

The back-exchange of deposited aluminum, from bone surfaces to blood, may occur relatively quickly and its rate will be an important determinant of the rate of early loss of aluminum from the body. At longer times after deposition, more aluminum will be removed by bone turnover. Given that in adult man the rate of bone turnover is very low (3–20% per year), most firmly deposited metal may be expected to be retained in the body for tens of years. This accounts for the reported body retention of 2% of the injected [26]Al at 5 years postinjection and its low rate of loss at this time (equivalent retention half-time greater than 5 years). In children, who exhibit high rates of bone growth and turnover, aluminum is lost more rapidly.

Toxicity of Systemic Aluminum

The toxicity of aluminum has been extensively reviewed both by WHO and by the US Department of Health and Human Services. Exposure to aluminum at environmental levels produces no known adverse effects in man. There is little evidence to suggest that aluminum may produce adverse effects under conditions of chronic, excess, occupational exposure. Under conditions of high medical exposure, resulting in large aluminum body burdens, the metal is toxic. Aluminum intoxication is characterized by aluminum-induced bone disease (AIBD), microcytic anemia, and encephalopathy. Most information concerning these has been obtained by the study of dialyzed renal failure patients. These patients had lost their ability to excrete aluminum and accumulated large body burdens of aluminum by transfer of the metal from contaminated dialyzates (most commonly tap water) during hemodialysis. The amount of transfer, and resultant body burdens, depended on the duration of treatment and the concentration of aluminum in the dialyzate.

In addition, toxic effects of aluminum have been demonstrated in four groups of patients with normal kidney function: patients supported by total parenteral feeding, patients with hepatic insufficiency receiving aluminum antacids, premature infants receiving prolonged intravenous therapy, and other patients receiving parenteral therapy. Aluminum-induced toxicity has also been claimed in some occupationally exposed groups, but evidence supporting these claims is not conclusive.

Studies on developing mice and rats that had been exposed to aluminum either during gestation or during lactation indicate that this metal may have an adverse effect on the development of some regions of the brain. In such animals, adverse effects on reflexes and simple motor behaviors, but not consistently on learning and memory, have been demonstrated.

Aluminum-Induced Bone Disease

AIBD is characterized either by a low turnover osteomalacia or by an aplastic disease. Chemical analyses have shown these conditions to be present when bone aluminum levels are between 12 and $500 \mu g g^{-1}$. High levels of the metal in diseased bones have also been demonstrated using aluminum-specific histochemical bone stains.

Aluminum-induced osteodystrophic osteomalacia develops in the absence of hypophosphatemia. The condition does not respond to vitamin D therapy, but it may be prevented by hyperparathyroidism. The disease is progressive and produces a variety of symptoms, including severe bone pain, muscle pains, and multiple nontraumatic fractures. It is normal for AIBD patients to remain asymptomatic for many years before physical signs of the disease, including funnel chest deformity, sternal bowing, and loss of height, become evident.

At the histological level, AIBD is characterized by a low rate of bone formation. The disease is variable, but bone removed from most patients show an increased amount of unmineralized osteoid; an increase in bone volume; a very low rate of bone apposition; a patchy, irregular pattern of calcification; a reduction in the number of active osteoblasts and osteoclasts; and irregular, misshaped bone trabeculae.

Although the causation of AIBD is not firmly established, it seems likely that it is produced by impaired bone matrix mineralization and by decreased osteoclastic activity. The progress of AIBD may be halted, and even reversed, by repeated administration of the chelating agent desferrioxamine.

Microcytic Anemia

Microcytic anemia, a disease characterized by the presence of small red blood cells in blood, has been described in renal patients. This disease occurs in the absence of iron deficiency and is reversed following the use of purified dialyzate. The mechanism by which aluminum induces microcytic anemia is uncertain, but it has been suggested that a disturbance in the hem biosynthetic pathway may be involved. In this context, the red blood cells of intoxicated dialysis patients may contain a considerable fraction of the total blood aluminum content.

Encephalopathy

Several neurological effects have been attributed to aluminum intoxication. In weanling rats, dietary aluminum fed at high levels to their dams has been demonstrated to delay brain maturation. This effect has not been described in man.

Aluminum-induced impairment of cognitive function following the occupational exposure of gold miners to inhaled aluminum, the exposure of members of the general public to ingested aluminum sulfate, and, recently, exposure of workers and ex-workers in the aluminum industry has been claimed but not proven. No convincing evidence has been produced to either support or refute the existence of neurological effects at low levels of aluminum uptake. However, there is sufficient evidence that such effects may occur in man at some levels of uptake. For example, dialysis patients exposed to lower than average levels of aluminum sometimes demonstrate disturbed cerebral function compared to controls.

In one study of dialysis patients, correlations were sought between cognitive function and exposure to aluminum in both dialysis source water and administered oral gut phosfate binders. The results of the study were confusing since it found negative correlations between the cognitive measures and source water aluminum but positive correlations with the level of orally administered phosfate binder. Again, in a gold miner study, some results indicated cognitive impairment, whereas others were less conclusive. It has been noted that most studies performed to date are flawed, because they have failed to include normal aging controls. Attempts to improve cognitive scores by chelation therapy have met with very limited success.

The most important neurological effects produced by aluminum occur at large body burdens. These include ataxia, dysarthria, dysphagia, myoclonia, convulsions, and dementia. Epidemiological studies have shown that aluminum-induced encephalopathy (dialysis dementia) was absent at dialysis centers using water with aluminum concentrations less than $50 \mu g l^{-1}$. In contrast, encephalopathy was common in those that employed water with aluminum concentrations greater than $200\,\mu g\,l^{-1}$. At these centers, the prevalence of the disease increased significantly with increasing cumulative exposure to aluminum and was often a direct cause of death. In terminal cases, facial grimacing, myotonic spasms, and dysphagia interfere with eating and lead to inhalation pneumonia and death. The recorded concentrations of aluminum in the brains of such patients are highly variable, but values of $15–100\,mg\,kg^{-1}$ are typical. Experience has shown that chelation therapy with desferrioximine is effective in reversing neurological effects in renal patients.

The mechanisms of encephalopathy are not clear. Most evidence suggests that aluminum likely crosses the blood–brain barrier by a transferrin-mediated mechanism. Imaging secondary ion mass spectrometry has shown aluminum to be deposited within the brain cortex as focal deposits at sites known to be rich in transferrin receptors. These sites, corresponding to the distribution of pyramidal neurones, have a high demand for iron in the synthesis of respiratory chain enzymes. It is suggested that damage at these sites results in the neuropathy.

Evidence for a Role in Alzheimer's Disease

Alzheimer's disease (AD) is a progressive, often insidious, dementing disease occurring in mid- to late life. Its incidence increases with age, such that at age 85+ approximately 20% of people suffer from the condition. AD causes neurone death and a reduction in brain volume. The progression of the disease (which in most cases means approximately 7 years of intellectual and personal decline until death) cannot be arrested and eventually patients become bedridden. At this stage, concomitant bedsores, feeding difficulties, and pneumonia result in death.

The diagnosis of AD in made on the basis of the histological examination of brain tissues. These show the presence of widespread accumulations of β-amyloid senile plaques and neurofibrillary tangles throughout the limbic system and in parts of the cerebral isocortex and brain stem. β-Amyloid plaque formation occurs in the majority of nondemented elderly individuals, but neurofibrillary tangles are rare. Consequently, it has been suggested that in AD plaque formation precedes and may predispose to neurofibrillary tangle formation.

The etiology of the disease is complex and incompletely understood. Two risk factors for the disease have been identified and confirmed: old age and family history. 'Familial' AD is genetically variable but mutations in chromosome 21 are often involved.

These cases show a marked tendency toward early onset and can be positively identified to represent only a small proportion of the total AD population.

The etiology of nonfamilial, sporadic AD is unknown. However, cases have been attributed to head injury and environmental factors, including aluminum. Involvement of aluminum in AD has been suggested because (1) of the similar symptomologies of AD and dialysis dementia; (2) the administration of aluminum to animals produces histological changes within the brain that are, in some respects, similar to those seen in the brains of AD patients; (3) of some reports indicating the presence of aluminum within the cores of senile plaques; (4) of the results of some epidemiological studies that have linked AD incidence either with aluminum levels in drinking water or with its consumption as medicines; and (5) a disease similar to AD is prevalent in some Pacific islands (Guam), where the levels of aluminum in soils and water are high.

However, (1) the pathologies of AD and dialysis dementia are different; (2) the histomorphological changes seen in experimental animals differ, in important respects, from those seen in the brains of AD patients; (3) not all studies have indicated the presence of aluminum within the cores of senile plaques, and attempts to demonstrate enhanced levels of aluminum in the brain of AD patients have mostly failed; (4) the results of the epidemiological studies are conflicting and have been criticised on methodological and logical grounds; and (5) Guam disease and AD are clinically different.

It follows that it is now generally accepted that in the absence of a clear association between exposure to aluminum and the disease and/or an identified mechanism for disease induction by the metal, there is insufficient evidence to suggest that aluminum is causative with respect to AD.

See also: **Aging**. **Bone**. **Food Safety**: Heavy Metals.

Further Reading

Ackrill P and Day JP (1993) The use of desferrioximine in dialysis-associated aluminium disease. *Contributions to Nephrology* **102**: 125–134.

Day JP, Drumm PV, Edwardson JA *et al.* (1994) Biological chemistry of aluminium studied using ^{26}Al and accelerator mass spectrometry. *Nuclear Instruments and Methods in Physics Research B* **92**: 463–468.

Doll R (1993) Review: Alzheimer's disease and environmental aluminium. *Age and Ageing* **22**: 138–153.

Edwardson JA, Moore PB, Ferrier IN *et al.* (1993) Effect of silicon on gastrointestinal absorption of aluminium. *Lancet* **342**: 211–212.

Gardner MJ and Gunn AM (1995) Speciation and bioavailability of aluminium in drinking water. *Chemical Speciation and Bioavailability* **7**: 9–16.

National Research Council (2003) *Food and Nutrition Board: Food Chemicals Codex, 5th edn* Washington, DC: National Academy Press.

Nieboer E and Gibson BL (1993) In *Health Effects of Aluminum: A Critical Review with Emphasis on Aluminum in Drinking Water*. Toronto: Ontario Ministry of Health.

Pennington JAT and Schoen SA (1995) Estimates of dietary exposures to aluminium. *Food Additives and Contaminants* **5**: 119–128.

Powell JJ and Thompson RPH (1993) The chemistry of aluminium in the intestinal lumen and its uptake and absorption. *Proceedings of the Nutrition Society* **52**: 241–253.

Priest ND (1993) The bioavailability and metabolism of aluminium compounds in man. *Proceedings of the Nutrition Society* **52**: 231–240.

Priest ND (2004) The biological behaviour and bioavailability of aluminium in man, with special reference to studies employing aluminium-26 as a tracer: Review and study update. *Journal of Environmental Monitoring* **6**: 1–30.

Priest ND, Newton D, Day JP *et al.* (1995) Human metabolism of aluminium-26 and gallium-67 injected as citrates. *Human & Environmental Toxicology* **14**: 287–293.

Priest ND, Talbot RJ, Austin JG *et al.* (1996) The bioavailability of aluminium-26 labelled aluminium citrate and aluminium hydroxide in volunteers. *Biometals* **9**: 221–228.

Rowan MJ (1993) Recent research on the causes of Alzheimer's disease. *Proceedings of the Nutrition Society* **52**: 255–262.

Talbot RJ, Newton D, Priest ND *et al.* (1995) Intersubject variability in the metabolism of aluminium following intravenous injection as citrate. *Human & Experimental Toxicology* **14**: 595–599.

US Department of Health and Human Services (1999) *Toxicological Profile for Aluminum*. Atlanta: US Department of Health and Human Services, Agency for Toxic Substances and Disease Registry, Public Health Service.

World Health Organization (1997) *Environmental Health Criteria 194: Aluminum*. Geneva: World Health Organization, International Programme on Chemical Safety.

AMINO ACIDS

Contents
Chemistry and Classification
Metabolism
Specific Functions

Chemistry and Classification

P W Emery, King's College London, London, UK

© 2005 Elsevier Ltd. All rights reserved.

Amino acids are a series of small organic molecules whose prime importance lies in the fact that they are the monomers from which proteins are made. The form and functions of proteins depend on the sequence in which the amino acids are joined together since each amino acid has specific chemical and physical properties. In this article, the structures and chemical properties of each amino acid are outlined, with an indication of how this affects the metabolic role of the free amino acid and how it affects the behavior of the amino acid residue within a protein. These chemical properties also form the basis for methods of analysis of amino acids. Some amino acids can be synthesized within the body from other molecules, whereas others cannot, so the final section explains the basis of the classification into essential and nonessential amino acids.

Chemical Structures and Nomenclature

Amino acids are small organic molecules with the general formula shown in **Figure 1**.

The central carbon atom in this structure is called the α-carbon, and the amino and carboxyl groups attached to it are known as the α-amino group and the α-carboxyl group, respectively. The R groups of the 20 amino acids that can be incorporated into proteins are shown in **Table 1**; these R groups give the different amino acids their specific chemical and physical properties.

The α-amino group acts as a weak base and is always protonated at physiological pH; similarly, the α-carboxyl group acts as weak acid and at physiological pH is always ionized. Thus, free amino acids in biological material exist as zwitterions, as shown in **Figure 2**.

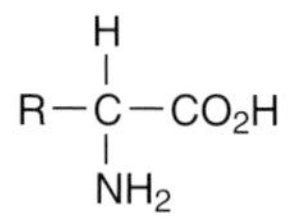

$$R - \overset{\overset{\displaystyle H}{|}}{\underset{\underset{\displaystyle NH_2}{|}}{C}} - CO_2H$$

Figure 1 Amino acid structure.

Table 1 Amino acid characteristics

Name (3 letter code; 1 letter code)	Structure	Molecular weight	pK$_a$
Small neutral amino acids Glycine (Gly; G)		75	2.35 9.78
Alanine (Ala; A)		89	2.35 9.87
Branched-chain amino acids Valine (Val; V)		117	2.29 9.74
Isoleucine (Ile; I)		131	2.32 9.76
Leucine (Leu; L)		131	2.33 9.74
Aromatic amino acids Tryptophan (Trp; W)		204	2.43 9.44
Tyrosine (Tyr; Y)		181	2.20 9.11 10.13
Phenylalanine (Phe; F)		165	2.16 9.18
Hydroxyl-containing amino acids Serine (Ser; S)		105	2.19 9.21
Threonine (Thr; T)		119	2.09 9.10
Sulfur-containing amino acids Cysteine (Cys; C)		121	1.92 8.35 10.46
Methionine (Met; M)		149	2.13 9.28

Continued

Table 1　Continued

Name (3 letter code; 1 letter code)	Structure	Molecular weight	pK_a
Imino acid Proline (Pro; P)		115	1.95 10.64
Acidic side chains Aspartic acid (Asp; D)		133	1.99 3.90 9.90
Glutamic acid (Glu; E)		147	2.10 4.07 9.47
Amides Asparagine (Asn; N)		132	2.10 8.84
Glutamine (Gln; Q)		146	2.17 9.13
Basic side chains Histidine (His; H)		155	1.80 6.04 9.76
Lysine (Lys; K)		146	2.16 9.18 10.79
Arginine (Arg; R)		174	1.83 8.99 12.48
Nonprotein amino acids Ornithine		132	1.71 8.69 10.76
Citrulline		175	Not determined
γ-Aminobutyric acid (GABA)		103	4.03 10.56
Homocysteine		117	2.22 8.87 10.86

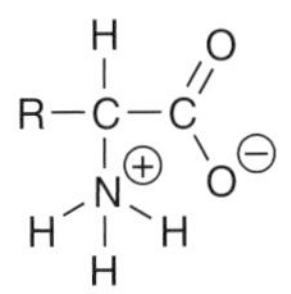

Figure 2 Zwitterionic structure of an amino acid.

The α-carbon atom is asymmetric so that amino acids show stereoisomerism; the exception to this is glycine, in which the R group is a second hydrogen atom. Most of the amino acids found in nature are in the L form, and only L-amino acids can be used for protein synthesis in higher organisms. However, D-amino acids may be ingested from bacterial sources, and if high concentrations accumulate they may be toxic. The human body has a D-amino acid oxidase enzyme, found in the liver and the kidney, that disposes of these molecules by oxidative deamination.

The most important common chemical property of the amino acids is their ability to form peptide bonds with one another. The α-amino group of one amino acid reacts with the α-carboxyl group of another to form a peptide bond with the elimination of water (**Figure 3**). The results of this process are conventionally known as peptides or oligopeptides if they contain 2–20 amino acid residues or as polypeptides, which may contain 21 to several thousand amino acid residues. The polypeptides may undergo further processing, including chemical modification, before taking up their final conformation as proteins.

Each amino acid also has specific chemical properties that depend on the nature of the R group. This affects the behavior of the free amino acids and the corresponding amino acid residues in peptides and polypeptides. For convenience, the amino acids may be considered in groups according to some common properties.

Small Neutral Amino Acids: Glycine and Alanine

The small side chains, a hydrogen atom and a methyl group, respectively, have little effect on the shape of a peptide chain. The free amino acids tend to be heavily involved as metabolic intermediates. Glycine is a precursor of purines, porphyrins, bile

acids, and creatine; it acts as a neurotransmitter and as a conjugating substance that aids the excretion of xenobiotics by making them more water-soluble. Alanine is the transamination product of pyruvic acid and is thus closely associated with the metabolism of carbohydrates, acting as a major precursor for gluconeogenesis.

Branched-Chain Amino Acids: Valine, Leucine, and Isoleucine

These have bulky, nonpolar side chains, so they are often found within the hydrophobic core of proteins. Isoleucine has an extra chiral center, so four optical isomers are theoretically possible, but only L-isoleucine (and not L-allo-isoleucine) is found in proteins. Branched-chain amino acids are metabolized initially in muscle and adipose tissue rather than liver, where most of the other amino acids are metabolized.

Aromatic Amino Acids: Tryptophan, Tyrosine, and Phenylalanine

These are also bulky and nonpolar, and they may interact with other hydrophobic molecules. The phenolic hydrogen of tyrosine is weakly acidic and can form hydrogen bonds to create cross-links or can be donated during catalysis. Tyrosine residues on certain membrane-bound receptors become phosphorylated by tyrosine kinase domains, thereby initiating a signal transduction cascade. Tryptophan is important as a precursor of the neurotransmitter 5-hydroxytryptamine (serotonin) and of the nicotinamide-containing coenzymes NAD and NADP. Phenylalanine can be converted to tyrosine in the body, but not vice versa. Tyrosine is a precursor of the catecholamines and the thyroid hormones and also the pigment melanin.

Hydroxyl-Containing Amino Acids: Serine and Threonine

These are polar, very weakly acidic molecules but uncharged at neutral pH. They can form hydrogen bonds and are thus quite soluble. Threonine has an additional chiral centre, but again only L-threonine is found in proteins. Serine is found at the active centre of some enzymes. It is also the usual site of

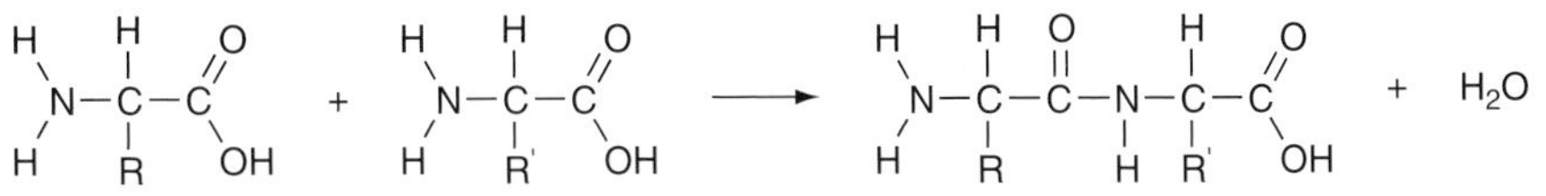

Figure 3 Peptide bond formation.

attachment for the carbohydrate residues in glycoproteins and for the phosphoryl groups in phosphoproteins.

Sulfur-Containing Amino Acids: Cysteine and Methionine

Methionine is nonpolar, but cysteine is polar. Cysteine can form weak hydrogen bonds with oxygen and nitrogen; it is also weakly acidic and is sometimes found at the active site of enzymes. Cysteine also acts as a reducing agent within the cell, both as the free amino acid and in the form of the antioxidant tripeptide glutathione. The sulfydril groups of two cysteine residues can be oxidized to form the double amino acid cystine, and this is the predominant form of the amino acid in extracellular fluid. When the same reaction occurs between cysteine residues in adjacent polypeptide chains, a strong, covalent disulfide bond is formed that gives the protein a rigid structure. This appears to be particularly important in stabilizing extracellular or secreted proteins. Methionine can be converted to *S*-adenosyl-methionine, the donor of methyl groups in transmethylation reactions. Methionine can be converted to cysteine in the body, but not vice versa. Selenium can replace sulfur in some cysteine and methionine residues, particularly when selenium intake is high. The antioxidant protein glutathione peroxidase requires a selenocysteine residue at its active site.

Imino Acid: Proline

Since its structure contains a secondary amine rather than a primary amine, proline is actually an imino acid rather than an amino acid, but it forms peptide bonds and is incorporated into proteins just like an amino acid. It causes an abrupt and rigid change of direction in the polypeptide chain, and this has a major effect on the final conformation of the protein. The carbon at the 4 position can be hydroxylated to form hydroxyproline. Every third residue of the structural protein collagen is a hydroxyproline residue.

Acidic Side Chains: Aspartic Acid and Glutamic Acid

These are dicarboxylic acids, although at physiological pH they exist almost entirely in the anionic form and so should be referred to as aspartate and glutamate. They are mainly found on the surfaces of proteins. The free amino acids play a central role in transamination reactions, equilibrating rapidly with their corresponding keto acids oxaloacatate and

2-oxoglutarate. Glutamate is a precursor for the inhibitory neurotransmitter γ-aminobutyric acid (GABA). The monosodium salt of glutamate is used in the food industry as a flavor enhancer.

Amides: Asparagine and Glutamine

Although they are uncharged, these molecules are strongly polar. They are often found on the surface of proteins, where they can form hydrogen bonds with water or with other polar molecules. The conversion of glutamate to glutamine is central to the disposal of ammonia and to the maintenance of acid–base balance. Glutamine is a precursor for the synthesis of purines and pyrimidines. It is also a precursor for gluconeogenesis, and it is the main source of energy for enterocytes and leucocytes. There is evidence that glutamine may play a role in the control of protein metabolism and that it may be beneficial in augmenting the immune response in critically ill patients.

Basic Side Chains: Histidine, Lysine, and Arginine

These are hydrophilic amino acids that are positively charged at neutral pH. The imidazole group of histidine has a pK_a just below 7, so it is weakly ionized at physiological pH, giving it some buffering capacity and making it useful at the active site of many enzymes. Histidine is also a precursor for the physiologically active amine histamine. Arginine is an intermediate in the urea cycle and a precursor for polyamine synthesis. It is also the precursor for nitric oxide, which appears to have many physiologically important properties, including that of an endothelial-derived relaxing factor and a cell signaling molecule in the coordination of the inflammatory response. Although arginine, like glutamine, is a nonessential amino acid, there is evidence that increasing the dietary supply of arginine can improve clinical outcome in critically ill patients. Lysine is the limiting amino acid in cereals and cereal-based diets.

Posttranslational Modification

Some amino acid residues may become chemically modified after they have been incorporated into polypeptide chains. They will thus be present when the protein is degraded but cannot be reutilized for protein synthesis.

Hydroxylation of proline to hydroxyproline is mainly associated with collagen. Hydroxylysine is also found in collagen.

The side chain nitrogen atoms of the dibasic amino acids (histidine, arginine, and lysine) can all be methylated. For example, N^T-methylhistidine (3-methylhistidine) is found mainly in the contractile proteins actin and myosin so that detection of N^T-methylhistidine in a food sample usually indicates the presence of meat. It has also been suggested that measurement of the urinary excretion of N^T-methylhistidine could provide an index of the rate of breakdown of myofibrillar proteins in skeletal muscle, although interpretation is complicated by the presence of N^T-methylhistidine derived from other tissues.

The hydroxyl groups of serine, threonine, and tyrosine can all be phosphorylated. Phosphoserine residues bind calcium and are found in proteins such as casein. Another calcium-binding residue is γ-carboxyglutamic acid, which is found in prothrombin.

The hydroxyl groups of serine can also be glycosylated to form glycoproteins and proteoglycans. The amide group of asparagine can also be glycosylated.

The ε-N of certain lysine residues can be oxidized by the copper-containing enzyme lysyl oxidase to form allysine. Four allysine residues in adjacent polypeptide chains may then condense to form desmosine (**Figure 4**). This covalent link gives considerable strength and elasticity to the connective tissue protein elastin.

The ε-N of lysine residues is also susceptible to chemical reactions within food systems. It undergoes the Maillard reaction with carbonyl groups of carbohydrates to form a series of brown and slightly bitter products. This is an integral part of the baking process when producing bread, cakes, and biscuits, although there is evidence that large quantities of some Maillard products may be toxic or carcinogenic. On the other hand, since the lysine in Maillard products is not biologically available when the food is ingested, this can seriously reduce the protein quality of heat-treated animal feedstuffs.

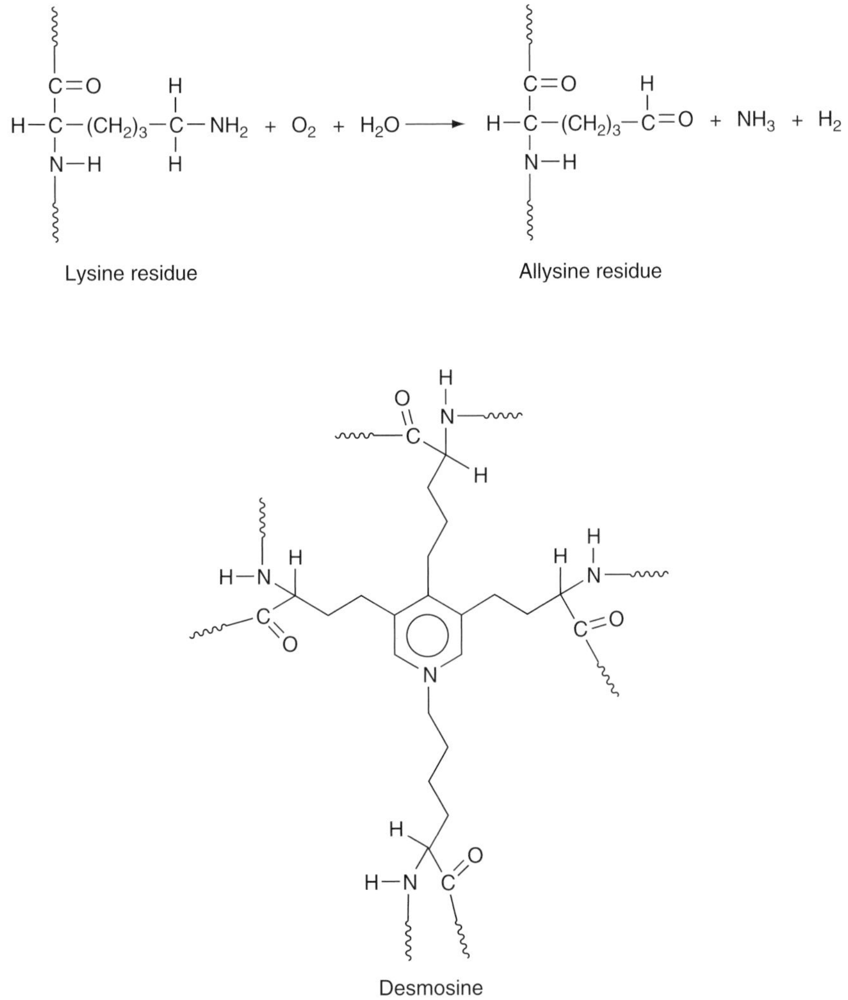

Figure 4 Formation of allysine and structure of desmosine.

Proteins within living systems can also be damaged by covalent binding to other molecules (usually reactive biochemicals) to form adducts, thereby rendering the protein inoperative or immunogenic. Adducts can be formed by the reaction of an aldehyde function with a receptive nucleophilic centre in the protein, particularly the ε-amino groups on lysine residues but also the α-amino terminus, the thiol groups on cysteine residues, the imidazole groups on histidine residues, and the phenolic groups on tyrosine residues. The aldehydes that may be involved in adduct formation include malondialdehyde and 4-hydroxy-2-nonenal, which are produced by free radical damage to polyunsaturated fatty acids in cell membranes, and acetaldehyde, which is produced when alcohol is metabolized. Adduct formation may play a role in the pathological processes leading to diseases such as alcoholic cirrhosis and coronary heart disease.

Nonprotein Amino Acids

There are several amino acids found in biological systems that are not incorporated into proteins. Ornithine and citrulline, for example, are intermediates of the urea cycle; GABA is a neurotransmitter.

Homocysteine is an intermediate in the transulphuration pathway for the conversion of methionine to cysteine. Homocystinuria is an inborn error of metabolism that is characterized by the accumulation of high concentrations of homocysteine, and this leads to severe cardiovascular disease at an early age. However, there is a much more common mutation in the enzyme 5,10-methylenetetrahydrofolate reductase that causes a moderate increase in plasma homocysteine concentration in more than 10% of the population. A high plasma homocysteine concentration appears to be an independent risk factor for cardiovascular disease in the population as a whole, although the mechanism is not known. Supplementing the diet with folic acid is often effective in reducing plasma homocysteine concentration because methyltetrahydrofolate is a substrate for the remethylation of homocysteine by the vitamin B_{12}-dependent enzyme methionine synthase. An inverse relationship has been observed between plasma homocysteine concentration and folate status in many studies, and this has led to the proposal that plasma homocysteine concentration may be used as a biomarker of folate intake.

Peptides

In addition to free amino acids and proteins, significant amounts of amino acids are present in physiological systems as small peptides. One of the most important is the tripeptide glutathione (γ-glutamylcysteinylglycine), which acts as an intracellular antioxidant.

Dipeptides found within the cell include carnosine (β-alanylhistidine) and its methylated derivatives anserine and balenine. These may act as buffers; no other physiological role has been identified.

Peptides are also used in food systems. For example, cysteine-containing peptides, or cysteine itself, are used as improvers in bread making to speed up the cross-linking that is required to give the bread its texture.

Another peptide used in the food industry is aspartame, which is composed of aspartic acid and phenylalanine. It is a very powerful sweetener that does not have the bitter aftertaste of some other intense sweeteners.

Analysis

The analysis of amino acids is based on chromatographic techniques. Traditional amino acid analyzers involved separation of the amino acid mixture on a column of ion-exchange resin using a series of sodium or lithium citrate buffers of increasing pH. The column effluent was then reacted with ninhydrin and passed through a spectrophotometer that would detect and quantify a series of peaks. This method is still used, although high-performance liquid chromatography (HPLC) hardware is usually employed. Other postcolumn detection systems can be used, replacing the ninhydrin reagent with orthophthalaldehyde (OPA) or fluorescamine and detecting the product fluorimetrically, thereby increasing the sensitivity.

Amino acids can also be separated by HPLC on a reversed-phase column. The mobile phase is usually based on an aqueous buffer with a gradient of increasing concentration of acetonitrile. In this case, the amino acids are usually converted to a fluorimetrically detectable (or ultraviolet-absorbing) form before being injected onto the column. A wide variety of derivatizing agents can be used for this, including OPA, 1-fluoro-2,4-dinitrobenzene, dansyl chloride, phenylisothiocyanate, and 9-fluorenyl-methyl chloroformate.

It is also possible to measure amino acids using gas–liquid chromatography, but this has never been popular, perhaps because the sample cleanup and derivatization steps are more laborious. The amino acids have to be converted to volatile derivatives before analysis, commonly either N-trifluoroacetyl-n-butyl or N-heptafluorobutyl-isobutyl esters. Gas–liquid chromatography is potentially a very sensitive method. It can also be coupled with mass spectrometry for identification of unknown compounds or for measurement of tracer enrichment when carrying out metabolic studies with stable isotopes.

These analytical methods can be applied equally to the measurement of amino acids in proteins, after hydrolysis, or free amino acids in physiological fluids such as plasma, urine, or tissue extracts. For physiological fluids, the protein must first be removed, and this is usually accomplished by precipitating with an acid such as sulfosalicylic acid or an organic molecule such as acetonitrile. The chromatographic requirements for physiological fluids are more demanding than for protein hydrolysates because there are many more contaminating substances producing extra peaks from which the amino acid peaks must be resolved, so the run time is generally longer.

Proteins have to be hydrolyzed before their amino acid composition can be measured. This is done by heating to 110 °C with an excess of 6 M HCl, either under nitrogen or in a vacuum. Proteins are usually hydrolyzed for 24 h, but this actually represents a compromise since some amino acids, including valine and isoleucine, may take longer than 24 h to liberate completely, whereas others, including tyrosine, threonine, and serine, are progressively destroyed. Thus, for complete accuracy a protein should be hydrolysed for different lengths of time (usually between 16 and 72 h) and appropriate extrapolations made to the analytical values for each amino acid.

Acid hydrolysis destroys tryptophan, so a separate alkaline hydrolysis is needed to measure this amino acid. The sulfur-containing amino acids are also partially oxidized during acid hydrolysis, so the protein may be oxidized with performic acid before hydrolysis and the oxidation products of cysteine and methionine measured. Finally, acid hydrolysis converts the amides glutamine and asparagine to their parent dicarboxylic acids, so values are often reported as total [glutamic acid plus glutamine] and [aspartic acid plus asparagine]. If separate values are required for the amides, the protein must be subjected to enzymic hydrolysis.

Classification

From a nutritional standpoint, the most important classification of amino acids is the division between those that are essential (or indispensable) and those that are nonessential (or dispensable). Essential amino acids may be defined as those that the body cannot synthesize in sufficient quantities.

This classification is based on work carried out by W. C. Rose in the 1930s. Young, rapidly growing rats were fed purified diets from which one amino acid was removed. For some of the amino acids, this made

Table 2 Essential amino acids for the rat

Valine
Isoleucine
Leucine
Tryptophan
Phenylalanine
Threonine
Methionine
Histidine
Lysine
(Arginine)

no difference to the rats' growth rate—these are the nonessential amino acids shown in **Table 2**. For the essential amino acids removal from the diet resulted in immediate cessation of growth, followed by loss of weight, decline in food intake, and eventual death of the rats. The response to the removal of arginine was less dramatic because the rats continued to grow, but at a reduced rate. Thus, it appeared that the rat can synthesize arginine, but not at a high enough rate to support maximal growth.

It has subsequently been shown that the reason why certain amino acids are essential is that their carbon skeletons cannot be synthesized in mammalian cells. As long as the carbon skeletons are present, all amino acids except threonine and lysine can be formed by transamination. It should be noted, however, that tyrosine can only be synthesized from phenylalanine, and cysteine can only be synthesized from methionine.

Rose also determined which amino acids are essential for man by carrying out nitrogen balance experiments on healthy young adult volunteers. He showed that nitrogen balance could be maintained on a diet in which the only source of nitrogen was a mixture of the 10 amino acids that are essential for the rat. He then found that histidine and arginine could also be removed without affecting nitrogen balance. Thus, the 8 amino acids that are essential for adult man are shown in **Table 3**.

More recent work has identified certain circumstances, usually associated with disease or recovery from malnutrition, in which the addition of particular nonessential amino acids to an otherwise

Table 3 Essential amino acids for man

Valine
Isoleucine
Leucine
Phenylalanine
Tryptophan
Threonine
Methionine
Lysine

adequate diet appears to cause an unexpected improvement in either nitrogen balance or growth rate. It is hypothesized that the rate at which the body can synthesize these particular amino acids is limited, and that in extreme circumstances the requirement for them becomes greater than the rate at which they can be synthesized. These amino acids are thus sometimes called conditionally essential amino acids, and these include glycine, arginine, histidine, and glutamine.

See also: **Amino Acids**: Metabolism; Specific Functions. **Protein**: Synthesis and Turnover; Requirements and Role in Diet; Digestion and Bioavailability; Quality and Sources; Deficiency.

Further Reading

Bender DA (1985) *Amino Acid Metabolism*, 2nd edn. Chichester, UK: John Wiley & Sons.

Bigwood EJ (ed.) (1972) Protein and amino acid functions. In *International Encyclopaedia of Food and Nutrition*. Oxford: Pergamon Press.

Gehrke CW and Zumwalt RW (1987) Symposium on chromatography of amino acids. *Journal of the Association of Official Analytical Chemists* 70: 146–147.

Laidlaw SA and Kopple JD (1987) Newer concepts of the indispensable amino acids. *American Journal of Clinical Nutrition* 46: 593–605.

Metzler DE (1977) *Biochemistry* New York: Academic Press.

Reeds PJ (2000) Dispensable and indispensable amino acids for humans. *Journal of Nutrition* 130: 1835S–1840S.

Rose WC (1957) The amino acid requirements of adult man. *Nutrition Abstracts and Reviews* 27: 631–647.

Williams AP (1988) Determination of amino acids. In: Macrae R (ed.) *HPLC in Food Analysis*, 2nd edn., pp. 441–470. London: Academic Press.

Metabolism

P W Emery, King's College London, London, UK

© 2005 Elsevier Ltd. All rights reserved.

Amino acids are generated within the body from three different sources. They enter the body from protein in the diet, and nonessential (dispensable) amino acids are synthesized from other metabolic intermediates, but by far the largest quantities of free amino acids arise from the breakdown of tissue proteins. Similarly, there are three metabolic fates for amino acids. Amino acid disposal is dominated by protein synthesis, but amino acids are also oxidized to carbon dioxide, water, and urea, or they may be metabolized to other small molecules. The pathways involved in each of these processes are considered, followed by a

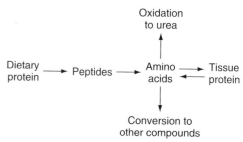

Figure 1 Overview of amino acid metabolism.

discussion of the movement of amino acids between different compartments within the body (**Figure 1**).

Amino Acid Supply

Dietary Intake

Protein is digested in the stomach by pepsins and in the small intestine by proteolytic enzymes from the pancreas. The products of digestion are mainly small peptides, which are then taken up by the intestinal epithelium and hydrolyzed to free amino acids. The portal circulation transports these amino acids to the liver, where approximately 75% of the amino acids are metabolized. The remaining 25% then enter the systemic circulation for transport to other tissues.

Amino Acid Biosynthesis

The essential (indispensable) amino acids must be supplied in the diet because their carbon skeletons cannot be synthesized in the human body, whereas the nonessential amino acids can be synthesized from common intermediates of the central metabolic pathways within the cell (i.e., glycolysis, the pentose phosphate pathway and the TCA cycle). As long as the keto-analogs are present, almost all amino acids can be generated by the process of transamination. The exceptions are threonine and lysine. Threonine is a poor substrate for mammalian transaminase enzymes, whereas the keto-analog of lysine, α-oxo-ε-aminocaproate, is unstable and cyclizes spontaneously to pipecolic acid.

Glutamic acid, glutamine, proline, and arginine
Glutamic acid is synthesized by transamination of 2-oxoglutarate, a TCA cycle intermediate. This reaction represents the first stage in the catabolism of many other amino acids, particularly the branched-chain amino acids. Vitamin B_6 is a cofactor for all transamination (aminotransferase) reactions. Glutamine is made from glutamic acid and ammonium in an energy-requiring reaction catalyzed by glutamine synthetase. The synthesis of glutamine plays an important role in the removal of the ammonium

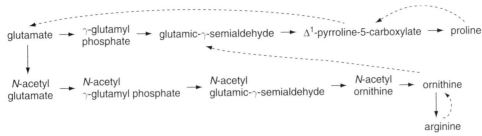

Figure 2 Synthesis and catabolism of proline and arginine. Solid lines indicate biosynthetic pathways; broken lines indicate catabolic pathways.

formed in peripheral tissues by deamination of amino acids as it is transported to the liver and used for urea synthesis.

Glutamic acid can be phosphorylated to γ-glutamyl phosphate by ATP, and this can then be dephosphorylated to glutamic-γ-semialdehyde. This undergoes nonenzymic cyclization to Δ^1-pyroline-5-carboxylate, which can then be reduced to proline (**Figure 2**).

Arginine is made from ornithine via the reactions of the urea cycle. Ornithine can theoretically be made by transamination of glutamic-γ-semialdehyde, but as mentioned previously this cyclizes spontaneously to pyroline-5-carboxylate. Thus, in practice glutamate is first acetylated by acetyl CoA to N-acetyl glutamate so that when this is converted to N-acetyl glutamic-γ-semialdehyde the amino group is blocked and cannot cyclize. The N-acetyl glutamic-γ-semialdehyde is then transaminated to N-acetyl ornithine, and this is deacetylated to ornithine (**Figure 2**).

Aspartic acid and asparagine Aspartic acid is derived from transamination of oxaloacetic acid, a TCA cycle intermediate. As with glutamic acid synthesis, this represents a common mechanism for removing amino groups from many other amino acids. Asparagine is made from aspartic acid by transfer of the amide group from glutamine.

Alanine Alanine is made by transamination of pyruvic acid, which is generated by glycolysis.

Serine and glycine Serine and glycine are readily interconvertible via methylene tetrahydrofolate, which either condenses with a glycine molecule to yield serine or is cleaved to yield glycine and tetrahydrofolate (**Figure 3**). However, there are also separate biosynthetic pathways for both molecules. Glycine can be synthesized by transamination of glyoxylate, which arises from the pentose phosphate pathway. Serine can be made by dephosphorylation of 3-phosphoserine, which is made by sequential

dehydrogenation and transamination of 3-phosphoglycerate, a glycolytic intermediate (**Figure 3**).

Histidine Histidine is synthesized by a relatively long pathway that has no branch points and does not lead to the formation of any other important intermediates. The main precursors are phosphoribosyl pyrophosphate and ATP, with the α-amino group arising by transamination from glutamate (**Figure 4**).

Cysteine In man and other animals, cysteine can only be synthesized from the essential amino acid methionine. Methionine reacts with ATP to form S-adenosylmethionine, an important methylating agent within the cell. Transfer of the methyl group results in the formation of S-adenosylhomocysteine, which is then converted to homocysteine. Homocysteine can condense with serine to form cystathionine, which is then cleaved by cystathionase to yield cysteine (**Figure 5**).

An alternative fate for homocysteine is remethylation to methionine. The methyl donor for this reaction can be either methyltetrahydrofolate, in a

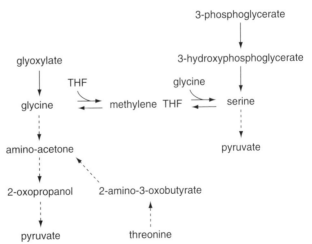

Figure 3 Synthesis and catabolism of glycine, serine, and threonine. Solid lines indicate biosynthetic pathways; broken lines indicate catabolic pathways. THF, tetrahydrofolate.

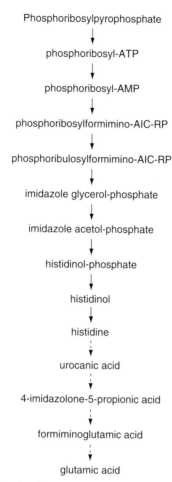

Phosphoribosylpyrophosphate

↓

phosphoribosyl-ATP

↓

phosphoribosyl-AMP

↓

phosphoribosylformimino-AIC-RP

↓

phosphoribulosylformimino-AIC-RP

↓

imidazole glycerol-phosphate

↓

imidazole acetol-phosphate

↓

histidinol-phosphate

↓

histidinol

↓

histidine

↓

urocanic acid

↓

4-imidazolone-5-propionic acid

↓

formiminoglutamic acid

↓

glutamic acid

Figure 4 Synthesis and catabolism of histidine. Solid lines indicate biosynthetic pathways; broken lines indicate catabolic pathways.

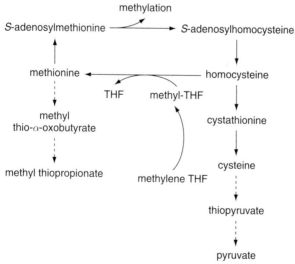

Figure 5 Synthesis and catabolism of methionine and cysteine. Solid lines indicate biosynthetic pathways; broken lines indicate catabolic pathways. THF, tetrahydrofolate.

reaction for which vitamin B_{12} is a cofactor, or betaine. Remethylation seems to be quite sensitive to folate status, and plasma homocysteine is becoming accepted as a biomarker of nutritional status with respect to folate.

Homocystinuria is an important inborn error of metabolism that is caused by impaired activity of cystathionine synthetase, the enzyme that catalyzes the condensation of homocysteine with serine. One of the consequences of homocystinuria is premature cardiovascular disease. There is considerable evidence that milder elevations of plasma homocysteine, caused by poorly active variants of the methylenetetrahydrofolate reductase enzyme (which is required to make the methyl donor methyltetrahydrofolate) or by low folic acid status, may be an important risk factor for cadiovascular disease throughout the population.

Tyrosine In mammals, including man, tyrosine can only be formed by hydroxylation of the essential amino acid phenylalanine. The inborn error of metabolism phenylketonuria is caused by a failure of the enzyme phenylalanine hydroxylase.

Protein Breakdown

Amino acids are continuously released by the hydrolysis of proteins. This occurs by several different mechanisms. Much intracellular proteolysis occurs within lysosomes, which provide the acidic environment within which enzymes such as cathepsins operate. However, there are also cytosolic proteolytic enzymes that operate at neutral or alkaline pH. These include the enzymes that hydrolyze proteins bound to ubiquitin. There are also extracellular proteinases that degrade extracellular proteins such as collagen.

Disposal of Amino Acids

Protein Synthesis

Protein synthesis represents the major route of disposal of amino acids. Amino acids are activated by binding to specific molecules of transfer RNA and assembled by ribosomes into a sequence that has been specified by messenger RNA, which in turn has been transcribed from the DNA template. Peptide bonds are then formed between adjacent amino acids. Once the polypeptide chain has been completed, the subsequent folding, posttranslational amino acid modifications, and protein packaging are all determined by the primary sequence of amino acids. The rate of protein synthesis is controlled by the rate of transcription of specific genes, the number and state of aggregation of ribosomes, and modulation of the rate of initiation of peptide synthesis.

Amino Acid Catabolism

Many amino acids can be converted to other useful molecules within the cell, and the same pathways may also lead to oxidation of the amino acid. It is therefore convenient to consider these metabolic fates together.

Glycine, serine, and threonine   The interconversion of glycine and serine has already been mentioned (**Figure 3**), and this can act as a mechanism for disposal of either amino acid. In quantitative terms, however, the main tendency is for both to be converted to the common intermediate methylene tetrahydrofolate, which acts as a methyl donor in many important biosynthetic reactions, including the conversion of dUMP to dTMP for DNA synthesis.

An alternative pathway for serine catabolism is deamination to pyruvate. However, the K_m of this enzyme is relatively high, so the pathway would only operate at high serine concentrations (**Figure 3**).

Another pathway of glycine catabolism is by condensation with acetyl CoA to form amino-acetone. This is then transaminated and dehydrogenated to yield carbon dioxide and pyruvate. Amino-acetone is also formed by the NAD-linked dehydrogenation of threonine, followed by the spontaneous decarboxylation of the unstable intermediate 2-amino-3-oxo-butyrate, and this appears to be the main pathway of catabolism of threonine in mammals (**Figure 3**).

Glycine is also an important precursor for several larger molecules. Purines are synthesized by a pathway that begins with the condensation of glycine and phosphoribosylamine. Porphyrins, including hem, are synthesized from glycine and succinyl CoA via δ-aminolaevulinic acid. Creatine synthesis involves the addition of the guanidino nitrogen from arginine to glycine. Glycine is also used to conjugate many foreign compounds, allowing them to be excreted in the urine. Glycine also conjugates with cholic acid to form the major bile acid glycocholic acid.

Glutamic acid, glutamine, proline, and arginine
Glutamic acid can be transaminated to 2-oxoglutarate, which can enter the TCA cycle. The amino group would be tranferred to aspartate, which would then enter the urea cycle. Alternatively, glutamate can be deaminated by glutamate dehydrogenase, with the resulting ammonium entering the urea cycle as carbamoyl phosphate. Decarboxylation of glutamate yields γ-aminobutyric acid, an important inhibitory neurotransmitter.

Glutamine is deaminated to glutamic acid in the kidney; this process is central to the maintenance of acid–base balance and the control of urine pH. Glutamine also acts as a nitrogen donor in the synthesis of purines and pyrimidines.

Proline is metabolized by oxidation to glutamic acid, although the enzymes involved are not the same as those that are responsible for the synthesis of proline from glutamic acid (**Figure 2**).

Arginine is an intermediate of the urea cycle and is metabolized by hydrolysis to ornithine. Ornithine can transfer its δ-amino group to 2-oxoglutarate, forming glutamic-γ-semialdehyde, which can then be metabolized to glutamate (**Figure 2**). Ornithine can also be decarboxylated to putrescine, which in turn can be converted to other polyamines such as spermidine and spermine.

Arginine can also be oxidized to nitric oxide and citrulline. Nitric oxide appears to be an important cellular signaling molecule that has been implicated in numerous functions, including relaxation of the vascular endothelium and cell killing by macrophages. In the vascular endothelium, nitric oxide is made by two different nitric oxide synthase isozymes, one of which is inducible and the other acts constitutitively.

Aspartic acid and asparagine   Aspartic acid can be transaminated to oxaloacetic acid, a TCA cycle intermediate. Alternatively, when aspartic acid feeds its amino group directly into the urea cycle, the resulting keto acid is fumarate, another TCA cycle intermediate. Aspartic acid is also the starting point for pyrimidine synthesis. Asparagine is metabolized by deamidation to aspartic acid.

Lysine   In mammals, lysine is catabolized by condensing with 2-oxoglutarate to form saccharopine, which is then converted to α-aminoadipic acid and glutamate. The α-aminoadipic acid is ultimately converted to acetyl CoA. In the brain, some lysine is metabolized via a different pathway to pipecolic acid (**Figure 6**). Lysine is also the precursor for the synthesis of carnitine, which carries long-chain fatty acids into the mitochondrion for oxidation. In mammals this process starts with three successive methylations of a lysine residue in a protein. The trimethyl lysine is then released by proteolysis before undergoing further reactions to form carnitine.

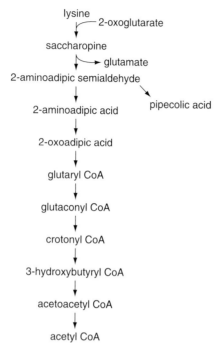

Figure 6 Metabolism of lysine.

Methionine and cysteine   The conversion of methionine to cysteine via the so-called transsulfuration pathway has already been mentioned (**Figure 5**). This pathway appears to act mainly as a biosynthetic pathway for the synthesis of cysteine. There is an alternative pathway for methionine catabolism that involves transamination to methyl thio-α-oxobutyrate and then to methyl thiopropionate.

Cysteine can be transaminated to thiopyruvate, which then undergoes desulfuration to pyruvate and hydrogen sulfide (**Figure 5**). Cysteine can also be oxidized to cysteine sulfinic acid, which can then be decarboxylated to hypotaurine, and this is then oxidized to taurine. High concentrations of taurine are found within most cells of the body, although its role is far from clear. In the liver the main fate of taurine is the production of taurocholic acid, which acts as an emulsifier in the bile. Another key role for cysteine is in the synthesis of the tripeptide glutathione, which is an important intracellular antioxidant.

Leucine, isoleucine, and valine   The branched-chain amino acids are unusual in that the first step in their metabolism occurs in muscle rather than liver. This step is transamination, producing α-oxoisocaproic acid, α-oxo-β-methyl valeric acid, and α-oxoisovaleric acid. These ketoacids are then transported to the liver for decarboxylation and dehydrogenation. Subsequent catabolism yields acetyl CoA and acetoacetate in the case of leucine, acetyl CoA and propionyl CoA from isoleucine, and succinyl CoA from valine (**Figure 7**).

Histidine   The first step in histidine metabolism is deamination to urocanic acid. Subsequent metabolism of this compound can follow several different pathways, but the major pathway is the one that involves formiminoglutamic acid (FIGLU), which is demethylated by a terahydrofolic acid-dependent

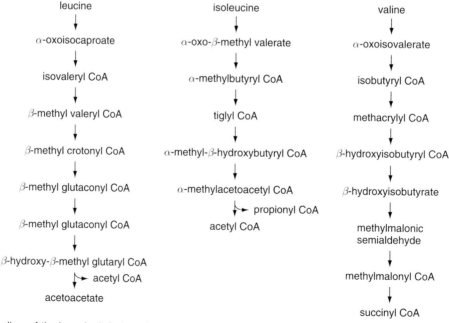

Figure 7 Metabolism of the branched-chain amino acids.

reaction to glutamic acid (**Figure 4**). This forms the basis of the FIGLU test for folate status. Another physiologically important pathway of histidine metabolism is decarboxylation to histamine, for which vitamin B_6 is a cofactor.

Phenylalanine and tyrosine Since mammalian enzymes cannot break open the benzene ring of phenylalanine, the only important pathway for catabolism of this amino acid is through hydroxylation to tyrosine. If the phenylalanine hydroxylase enzyme is lacking, as in phenylketonuria, a high concentration of phenylalanine accumulates and it is converted to phenylpyruvate, phenyllactate, and phenylacetate, which are toxic.

Tyrosine is transaminated to *p*-hydroxyphenylpyruvate, which is then decarboxylated to homogentisic acid. This is subsequently metabolized to acetoacetic acid and fumaric acid (**Figure 8**). Small amounts of tyrosine are hydroxylated to 3,4-dihydroxyphenylalanine (DOPA), which is then decarboxylated to the catecholamines dopamine, noradrenaline, and adrenaline. DOPA can also be converted to the pigment melanin. In the thyroid gland, protein-bound tyrosine is iodinated to the thyroid hormones tri-iodothyronine and thyroxine.

Tryptophan Tryptophan is oxidized by the hormone-sensitive enzyme tryptophan oxygenase to *N*-formyl kynurenine, which then follows a series of steps to yield amino-carboxymuconic semialdehyde. Most of this undergoes enzymic decarboxylation, leading ultimately to acetyl CoA. However, a small proportion undergoes nonenzymic cyclization to quinolic acid, which leads to the formation of NAD. This is why excess dietary tryptophan can meet the requirement for the vitamin niacin (**Figure 9**).

One of the steps in the catabolism of tryptophan is catalyzed by the vitamin B_6-dependent enzyme kynureninase. If vitamin B_6 status is inadequate

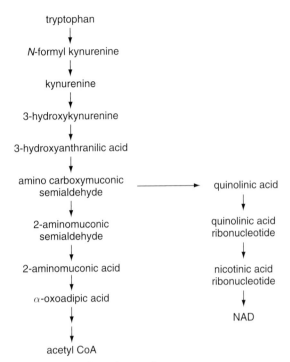

Figure 9 Metabolism of tryptophan.

and a large dose of tryptophan is administered, much of the tryptophan will be metabolized by an alternative pathway to kynurenic and xanthurenic acids, which will be excreted in the urine. This is the basis of the tryptophan load test for vitamin B_6 status.

A small amount of tryptophan undergoes hydroxylation to 5-hydroxytryptophan, which is then decarboxylated to the physiologically active amine 5-hydroxytryptamine (serotonin).

Alanine Alanine is metabolized by transamination to pyruvate.

Urea Cycle

From the previous discussion, it can be seen that the metabolism of most amino acids involves removal of the amino groups by transamination. 2-oxoglutarate is the main acceptor of these amino groups, being converted to glutamate, which can then be deaminated to release ammonium. However, ammonium is highly toxic and cannot be allowed to accumulate, so it is converted to urea, which is the form in which most of the nitrogen derived from protein is excreted from the body. Urea is formed in the liver by the cyclic series of reactions shown in **Figure 10**. It can be seen that only one of the nitrogen atoms in the urea molecule is actually derived from ammonium, via carbamyl phosphate. The other nitrogen atom comes from

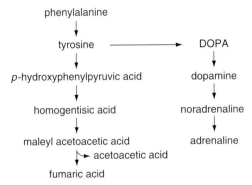

Figure 8 Metabolism of phenylalanine and tyrosine.

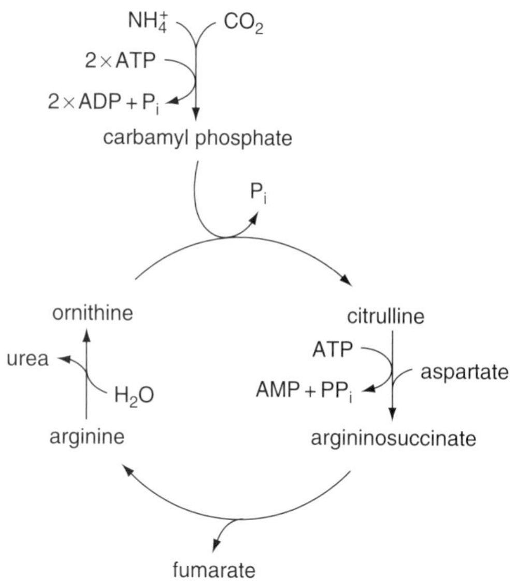

$$NH_4^+ \quad CO_2$$
$$2 \times ATP$$
$$2 \times ADP + P_i$$
carbamyl phosphate

P_i

ornithine   citrulline

urea   ATP
H_2O $AMP + PP_i$ aspartate

arginine   argininosuccinate

fumarate

Figure 10   The urea cycle.

aspartic acid, which is formed by transamination of oxaloacetic acid.

The rate of production of urea by the liver is normally greater than the rate of urea excretion in the urine. This is because some of the urea diffuses into the colon, where it is hydrolyzed to ammonia by bacteria. The ammonia can be absorbed and taken up by the liver, where it can be reincorporated into amino acids, thereby augmenting the net supply of nonessential amino acids. The colonic bacteria can also use ammonia to synthesize essential amino acids, and there is evidence that some of these essential amino acids can also be absorbed and utilized by the human body. However, the rate at which this happens is clearly not sufficient to meet the body's requirements for essential amino acids.

Glucogenic and Ketogenic Amino Acids

The carbon skeletons that are left after amino acids have been transaminated are converted to common intermediates of the central metabolic pathways of the cell and so are ultimately used to provide energy. Clearly, for an adult in energy and nitrogen balance, energy will be derived from amino acids in the same proportion as protein is present in the diet, and for most human diets this is 10–15% of energy.

In certain circumstances, such as starvation, diabetes, or a high-fat diet, the body may need to synthesize glucose from amino acids rather than oxidize them directly. Experiments with diabetic dogs fed on single amino acids have shown that most of the amino acids can be converted to glucose and are therefore classified as glucogenic. However, leucine and lysine cannot be converted to glucose, and in these circumstances they give rise to acetoacetic acid, so they are classified as ketogenic. This classification can be related to the catabolic pathways outlined previously. The ketogenic amino acids are those that are metabolized only to acetyl CoA, whereas those that are metabolized to pyruvate or TCA cycle intermediates are glucogenic. Tryptophan, phenylalanine, tyrosine, isoleucine, methionine, and cysteine are both glucogenic and ketogenic.

Interorgan Exchange of Amino Acids

Amino Acid Pools

Free amino acids make up only approximately 2% of the total amino acid content of the body, with the rest being present as protein. The concentrations of free amino acids are regulated largely by modulation of their catabolic pathways, although in the case of nonessential amino acids there is also some regulation of the rate at which they are synthesized. There is evidence that the rates of protein synthesis and degradation are regulated by amino acid supply, and that this is another homeostatic mechanism acting to maintain free amino acid concentrations within safe limits. Protein degradation is suppressed following a meal containing protein, and the rate of protein synthesis may be increased so that there is net storage of amino acids as protein. Subsequently, in the postabsorptive state the changes in the rates of protein synthesis and breakdown are reversed so that there is net release of amino acids from protein. In nongrowing adults these changes balance out over a 24-h period so that there is no net change in body protein content. The amplitude of these diurnal changes in the rates of protein synthesis and degradation appears to vary in direct proportion to the amount of protein that an individual habitually consumes.

Free amino acids are found in all cells of the body and in extracellular fluid. They are transported between tissues in the plasma and into cells by a variety of transport mechanisms that are relatively specific for particular groups of amino acids. Amino acids are also present in red blood cells, but their role in interorgan transport appears to differ from that of plasma. For example, the plasma amino acid concentration increases as blood traverses the gastrointestinal tract after a meal, whereas the amino acid content of blood cells actually decreases.

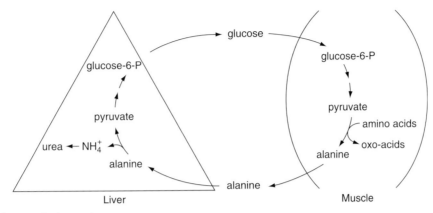

Figure 11 The glucose–alanine cycle.

Metabolism in Different Organs

The liver is responsible for most of the deamination of amino acids, except for the branched-chain amino acids, which are transaminated in muscle. Oxidation of amino acids is one of the main sources of energy for the liver. The liver is also the main site of gluconeogenesis, extracting large amounts of glutamine and alanine from the plasma for this purpose. The liver is the only site of urea synthesis.

Skeletal and cardiac muscle and adipose tissue are the main sites for transamination of the branched-chain amino acids, and the resulting ketoacids are transported to the liver for oxidation. However, in fasting and diabetes the capacity of muscle to oxidize branched-chain ketoacids increases markedly. In the postabsorptive state there is a net loss of amino acids from muscle, whereas in the fed state there is net uptake, reflecting the changes in net protein deposition and loss. However, at all times there is net output of alanine and glutamine from muscle, representing the disposal of the amino groups from the branched-chain amino acids. Muscle also takes up glucose, which is metabolized to supply the carbon skeletons for alanine and glutamine. Thus, there is a well-recognized glucose–alanine cycle between muscle and liver (**Figure 11**).

The kidney is a prime site of glutamine deamidation, producing ammonium to maintain acid–base balance and regulate the pH of the urine. Glutamine also serves as a substrate for gluconeogenesis in the kidney.

Glutamine is the major energy source for the small intestine, and at least part of the glutamine is derived from the lumen of the gut. Much of the glutamine is metabolized to pyruvate, which is then transaminated and exported to the liver as alanine. Some glutamine is also converted by the gut to citrulline, which then circulates to the kidney to be converted to arginine. Glutamine is also a major energy source for lymphocytes and monocytes when the immune system is activated.

See also: **Amino Acids**: Chemistry and Classification; Specific Functions. **Folic Acid**. **Inborn Errors of Metabolism**: Classification and Biochemical Aspects; Nutritional Management of Phenylketonuria. **Niacin**. **Protein**: Synthesis and Turnover; Digestion and Bioavailability. **Vitamin B$_6$**.

Further Reading

Bender DA (1985) *Amino Acid Metabolism*, 2nd edn. Chichester, UK: John Wiley and Sons.

Finkelstein JD (1990) Methionine metabolism in mammals. *Journal of Nutritional Biochemistry* 1: 228–237.

McCully KS (1996) Homocysteine and vascular disease. *Nature Medicine* 2: 386–389.

Millward DJ (2003) An adaptive metabolic demand model for protein and amino acid requirements. *British Journal of Nutrition* 90: 249–260.

Munro HN and Allison JB (1964 and 1970) *Mammalian Protein Metabolism*, vols. 1–4. London: Academic Press.

Newsholme EA and Leech AR (1983) *Biochemistry for the Medical Sciences* Chichester, UK: John Wiley and Sons.

Waterlow JC and Stephen JML (1981) *Nitrogen Metabolism in Man* London: Applied Science.

Specific Functions

M C G van de Poll, Y C Luiking, C H C Dejong and P B Soeters, University Hospital Maastricht, Maastricht, The Netherlands

© 2005 Elsevier Ltd. All rights reserved.

Introduction

Apart from being the building blocks of proteins, many amino acids are indispensable for certain vital functions or have specific functions of their own. They can function as neurotransmitters, as precursors for neurotransmitters and other important metabolites, including crucial oligo- and polypeptides, as a stimulus for hormonal release, and in inter-organ nitrogen transport and nitrogen excretion. Consequently, manipulation of free amino acid levels by dietary or topical supplementation may support and modulate these specific functions.

Amino Acid Flux, Concentration, and Function

Many amino acids have specific functions or support specific functions by serving as precursors or substrates for reactions in which vital end products are produced. The availability of amino acids to serve these purposes is determined by the rate at which they are released into the plasma and other pools in which these reactions take place, as well as by the rate of disappearance through excretion, protein synthesis, or conversion to other amino acids. The rate of this release, referred to as amino acid flux, is determined by the breakdown of (dietary) proteins or the conversion from other amino acids. Increased demand for one or more amino acids generally leads to an increased flux of the required amino acids across specific organs. Since it is the flux of an amino acid that determines its availability for metabolic processes, the flux is far more important for maintenance of specific functions than the plasma concentration. In fact it is striking that fluxes of some amino acids can double without significantly affecting plasma levels despite the fact that the plasma pool may be quantitatively negligible compared to the flux per hour. Plasma amino acid concentrations must therefore be subject to strong regulatory mechanisms. Increased demand and utilization of a specific amino acid may lead to decreased plasma and tissue concentrations, which may act as a signal to increase flux. Thus, a low plasma concentration in itself does not necessarily imply that the supply of the amino acid in question is inadequate, but it may indicate that there is increased turnover of the amino acid and that deficiencies may result when dietary or endogenous supply is inadequate. Other factors determining amino acid concentration are induction of enzymes and stimulation or blocking of specific amino acid transporters affecting the exchange and distribution of amino acids between different compartments. The regulation of plasma and tissue concentrations of specific amino acids may also be executed by the fact that release of the amino acid by an organ (e.g., muscle) and the uptake of that amino acid by another organ (e.g., liver) are subject to a highly integrated network including the action of cytokines and other hormones.

By repeated conversion of one amino acid to another, metabolic pathways arise by which (part of) the carbon backbone of a single amino acid can pass through a succession of different amino acids. Because of this interconvertibility, groups of amino acids rather than one specific amino acid contribute to specific functions. Apart from the rate at which these amino acids interconvert, the rate at which they gain access to the tissue where the specific end products exert their functions is also an important determinant of deficiencies of amino acids.

Amino acid Deficiencies and Supplementation

In many diseases and during undernutrition diminished turnover of amino acids can occur. These deficiencies may concern specific amino acids in certain diseases or a more generalized amino acid deficiency. The resulting functional deficits can contribute to the symptoms, severity, and progress of the disease. In some instances these deficits can be counteracted by simple supplementation of the deficient amino acids. Amino acid supplementation is also applied to enhance turnover and improve amino acid function in nondeficient patients. However, amino acid supplementation in nondeficient states does not necessarily lead to an increased function since the organism utilizes what is programed by regulating hormones and cytokines. An additional factor to consider is that metabolic processes can be subject to counterregulatory feedback mechanisms. Some important metabolic processes served by a specific amino acid require only a marginal part of the total flux of that amino acid. The question may be raised whether true shortages may arise in such pathways, and supplemented amino acids may be

AMINO ACIDS/Specific Functions 93

Table 1 Specific functions of amino acids and their intermediate products

Amino acid	Intermediate products	Function	Supplementation efficacy
Alanine	Pyruvate	Gluconeogenesis Nitrogen transport	Data too limited
Arginine	Nitric oxide	Vasodilation Immunomodulation Neurotransmission	Positive effects of arginine-containing immunonutrition on morbidity in surgical and trauma patients suggested; further research required
	Urea Creatine Agmatine	Ammonia detoxification Muscle constituent/fuel Cell signaling Ornithine precursor	
Citrulline Ornithine	Arginine production Polyamines	Cell differentiation Proline precursor	Improves healing of burns (ornithine α-ketoglutarate)
Proline	Hydroxyproline	Hepatocyte DNA, protein synthesis Collagen synthesis	
Asparagine		Aspartic acid precursor	(Asparaginase-induced asparagine depletion is therapeutic in leukemia)
Aspartic acid **Methionine**	Oxaloacetate, fumarate Creatine	Gluconeogenesis Cysteine precursor (*see* arginine)	
Cysteine (Cystine)	Glutathione Taurine	Antioxidant Bile acid conjugation, neuronal cell development, regulation of membrane potential, calcium transport, antioxidant	Improves antioxidant status in undernutrition, inflammatory diseases Reduces contrast-induced nephropathy in renal failure Mucolysis, symptom reduction in COPD Hepatoprotective in acetaminophen intoxication
Glutamic acid	Glutamine α-ketoglutarate Glutathione γ-aminobutyric acid	Ammonia disposal Gluconeogenesis Antioxidant Inhibition CNS Excitation CNS (NMDA receptor)	
Glutamine	Ammonia	Inter-organ nitrogen transport Renal HCO_3^- production	Reduces infectious morbidity in trauma patients, burn patients, and surgical patients
	Purines, pyrimidines	RNA synthesis, DNA synthesis Glutamic acid precursor	
Glycine		Inhibition CNS (glycine receptor) Excitation CNS (NMDA receptor)	Adjuvant to antipsychotics, probably reduces negative symptoms of schizophrenia
	Glutathione Creatine	Antioxidant (*see* arginine) Serine precursor	
Serine	D-serine	Excitation CNS (NMDA receptor) Glycine precursor Cysteine precursor	Adjuvant to antipsychotics, probably reduces negative symptoms of schizophrenia
Threonine	Glycine Serine	Brain development	
Histidine	Histamine	Immunomodulation Gastric acid secretion	
Lysine	Carnitine Glutamate	Mitochondrial oxidation of long-chain fatty acids	Reduces chronic stress-induced anxiety
Branched chain amino acids			
Isoleucine	α-keto-β-methylvaleric acid		Upper gastrointestinal hemorrhage
Leucine	α-ketoisocaproic acid	Important in regulation of energy and protein metabolism Substrate for glutamine synthesis	Improve protein malnutrition and restore amino acid and neurotransmitter balance in hepatic failure and hepatic encephalopathy (supplemented BCAA)
Valine	α-ketoisovaleric acid		

Continued

Table 1 Continued

Amino acid	Intermediate products	Function	Supplementation efficacy
Aromatic amino acids			
Phenylalanine		Tyrosine precursor	
Tyrosine	L-dopa	Dopamine synthesis	Possible slight improvement of cognitive functions after physical or mental exhaustion. Metabolites are powerful pharmacotherapeutic drugs
	Dopamine	Movement, affect on pleasure, motivation	
	Noradrenaline, adrenaline	Activation of sympathetic nervous system (fight-or-flight response)	
	Tri-iodothyronine, thyroxine	Regulation of basal metabolic rate	
Tryptophan	Kynureninic acid	CNS inhibition	No scientific evidence for beneficial effects of supplementation
	Quinolinic acid	CNS excitation	
	Serotonin	Mood regulation Sleep regulation Intestinal motility	
	Melatonin	Regulation of circadian rhythms	

Different fonts indicate: nonessential amino acids, **essential amino acids**, and *conditionally essential amino acids*.

disposed of in pathways other than those serving to improve a specific function.

Assessment of Amino Acid Function

The effectiveness of amino acid supplementation, particularly with respect to clinical effectiveness, can be assessed at four levels. First, the intervention should lead to an increased local or systemic concentration of the amino acid in question. The conversion of amino acids in (interorgan) metabolic pathways can lead to an increase in the levels of amino acids other than the one supplemented, increasing or mediating its functionality. Alternatively, supplementation of one amino acid may decrease the uptake of other amino acids because they compete for a common transporter. Second, the metabolic process for which the supplemented amino acid forms the substrate should be stimulated or upregulated by this increased amino acid availability. Third, this enhanced metabolic activity must lead to physiological changes. Fourth, these changes must be clinically effective in a desirable fashion.

Alanine

Alanine and glutamine are the principal amino acid substrates for hepatic gluconeogenesis and ureagenesis. Alanine is produced in peripheral tissues in transamination processes with glutamate, branched chain amino acids, and other amino acids; following its release in the systemic circulation, alanine is predominantly taken up by the liver and to a lesser extent by the kidney. Here, alanine can be deaminated to yield pyruvate and an amino group, which can be used for transamination processes, ureagenesis, or can be excreted in urine. Thus, the alanine released from peripheral tissues may be converted to glucose in the liver or kidney and eventually become a substrate for peripheral (mainly muscular) glycolysis. This so-called glucose-alanine cycle may be especially relevant during metabolic stress and critical illness when the endogenous alanine release from peripheral tissues is increased. Simultaneously, alanine serves as a nitrogen carrier in this manner. Alanine is often used as the second amino acid in glutamine dipeptides that are applied to increase solubility and stability of glutamine in nutritional solutions.

Supplementation

No clinical benefits have been ascribed to supplementation with alanine, although it has never been considered whether the beneficial effects of the dipeptide alanine-glutamine, which are generally ascribed to glutamine, may also be due to alanine. In this context, it should be realized, however, that alanine itself constitutes the strongest drive for hepatic ureagenesis (leading to breakdown of alanine).

Arginine, Citrulline, Ornithine, and Proline (Figure 1)

Arginine is a nitrogen-rich amino acid because it contains three nitrogen atoms and is the precursor for nitric oxide (NO). The conversion to NO is catalyzed by the enzyme nitric oxide synthase (NOS), and results in coproduction of the amino acid citrulline. Depending on its site of release, NO exerts several functions including stimulation of the pituitary gland, vasodilation, neurotransmission, and immune modulation. Arginine is also a precursor for urea synthesis in the urea cycle, which has an important function in the detoxification of ammonia and excretion of waste nitrogen from the body. A full urea cycle is only present in the liver, but the arginase enzyme that converts arginine to urea and ornithine is to a limited extent also found in other tissues and cells, such as brain, kidney, small intestine, and red blood cells. Ornithine is utilized for the formation of proline, polyamines (putrescine, spermine, and spermidine), glutamic acid, and glutamine. Arginine is involved in collagen formation, tissue repair, and wound healing via proline, which is hydroxylated to form hydroxyproline. This role in wound healing may additionally be mediated by stimulation of collagen synthesis by NO, although this claim is still under investigation. It is currently thought that arginine availability is regulated by the balance between NOS and arginase enzyme activity, which subsequently determines substrate availability for NO and ornithine production. Proline also stimulates hepatocyte DNA and protein synthesis. Polyamines are potent inducers of cell differentiation.

In addition to synthesis of NO, urea, and ornithine, arginine is used for synthesis of creatine, which is an important constituent of skeletal muscle and neurons and acts as an energy source for these tissues. Furthermore, arginine may be catabolized to agmatine, which acts as a cell-signaling molecule. Arginine not only acts as an intermediate in the synthesis of functional products, but also is a potent stimulus for the release of several hormones, such as insulin, glucagon, somatostatin, and growth hormone, illustrating its pharmacological characteristics.

Arginine can be synthesized by the body from citrulline. However, since virtually all arginine produced in the liver is trapped within the urea cycle, the kidney is the only arginine-synthesizing organ that significantly contributes to the total body pool of free arginine. Diminished renal arginine synthesis has been found in patients with renal failure and in highly catabolic conditions, like sepsis, burn injury, or trauma (which may be related to concomitant renal failure). In these situations arginine may be considered a conditionally essential amino acid and it has been suggested that arginine supplementation can become useful in these situations.

Citrulline is formed from glutamine, glutamic acid, and proline in the intestine. Plasma citrulline concentration reflects intestinal metabolic function and has recently been introduced as a potential marker for (reduced) enterocyte mass.

Supplementation

Based on its pluripotent functions, arginine has been widely used in supplemental nutrition for surgical patients, patients with burns, and patients with sepsis and cancer in order to modify the inflammatory response, to enhance organ perfusion, and to stimulate wound healing. However, the benefits of arginine supplementation in these conditions are not uniformly proven and accepted. Moreover, arginine is never given alone but is always provided in a mixture of amino acids and other nutrients. The use of NO donors that have vasodilatory actions is an established therapeutic modality in coronary artery disease and for erectile dysfunction. Given this fact it remains worthwhile to clarify the need for arginine supplementation as the natural substrate for NO synthesis in other conditions.

Using citrulline as an arginine-delivering substrate has been suggested, but has not been applied clinically. Ornithine is supplied as part of the ornithine-α-ketoglutarate molecule (see glutamine). Creatine is widely used by professional and recreational athletes as a nutritional supplement, although the ascribed performance-enhancing effects have not been proven.

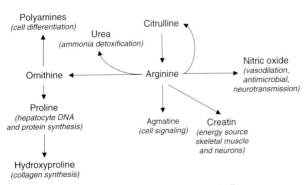

Figure 1 Specific functions of arginine metabolism.

Asparagine and Aspartic Acid

Asparagine can be converted by asparaginase to ammonia and aspartic acid, which is the precursor of the citrate cycle intermediates oxaloacetate and fumarate; this reaction is reversible. In fasting humans asparagine and aspartic acid are utilized as precursors for *de novo* synthesis of glutamine and alanine in muscle.

Supplementation

The claim that asparagine or aspartic acid supplementation improves endurance has not been confirmed in human studies. Asparaginase, which degrades asparagine, is widely used in the treatment of pediatric leukemia since the resulting asparagine depletion leads to apoptosis of leukemic cells.

Cysteine, Cystine, Methionine, and Taurine (Figure 2)

Methionine is converted to cysteine and its dipeptide cystine. In addition methionine is a precursor for creatine (see arginine). The potential for formation of disulfide bonds between its thiol (-SH) groups makes protein-bound cysteine important in the folding and structural assembly of proteins. Reduced cysteine thiol groups are found in protein (albumin), free cysteine, and in the principal intracellular antioxidant tripeptide glutathione (see glycine, glutamic acid) for which free cysteine is the synthesis rate-limiting constituent. Through the formation of disulfides (e.g., cystine, cysteinyl-glutathione, glutathione disulfide, mercaptalbumin) thiol-containing molecules can scavenge oxygen-derived free radicals. The ratio between oxidized and reduced thiol groups reflects the cellular redox state. Owing to its small pool size cysteine deficiencies rapidly occur during malnutrition.

Cysteine is also the precursor for taurine, which is abundant in all mammalian cells, particularly in neuronal cells and lymphocytes, but is not a true amino acid and is not incorporated in proteins. Taurine is involved in the conjugation of bile acids

and may act as an antioxidant. Moreover, taurine is an osmolyte by virtue of the fact that through its transporter its intracellular concentrations are between 50 and 100-fold higher than in the extracellular compartment. This gradient contributes to the maintenance of the cellular hydration state. Similarly, it has been proposed that taurine is involved in stabilization of cell membrane potential and regulation of Ca^{2+} transport through several calcium-ion channels. Based upon these characteristics it has been suggested that taurine is involved in the control of cardiac muscle cell contraction, which has led to the addition of taurine to commercially available energy drinks. Its high level in lymphocytes suggests an important role in immunological resistance to infections. Taurine plays an important part in the development and maintenance of neuronal and especially retinal cells.

Supplementation

Although methionine is the only sulfur-containing essential amino acid, it has not been considered as part of supplementation regimes. Since cysteine easily oxidizes to cystine, which has a poor solubility, it is generally supplemented in the form of *n*-acetylcysteine (NAC). Both directly and indirectly, as a precursor for glutathione, NAC has attracted attention as a potentially protective agent against oxidative injury in numerous conditions including endurance exercise, ischemia reperfusion injury, adult respiratory distress syndrome (ARDS), and cystic fibrosis. In addition, NAC has mucolytic properties in chronic obstructive pulmonary disease (COPD) patients by reducing disulfide bonds of polymers in mucus, blocking their reactivity. Currently, only robust evidence exists for the usefulness of NAC supplementation in the protection against nephropathy, induced by administration of iodine-containing contrast agents for radiological imaging in patients with chronic renal failure, in the reduction of the number of exacerbations and disability in COPD patients, and in the treatment of liver injury induced by acetaminophen intoxication. On the other hand it has been suggested that glutathione depletion by buthionine sulfoximine administration potentiates the effect of radiotherapy by increasing the susceptibility of tumor cells to radiation-induced oxidative injury.

In a few studies it has been demonstrated that taurine supplementation improves retinal development in premature babies receiving parenteral nutrition. Human data on the efficacy of taurine supplementation in so-called energy drinks are very limited. In the absence of taurine supplementation in

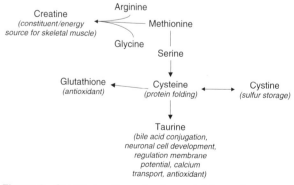

Figure 2 Specific functions of sulfur-containing amino acids.

children taurine concentrations drop, suggesting its conditional indispensability also in the postneonatal period. This has led to the addition of taurine to standard feeding formulas for infants and growing children.

Glutamine, Glutamic acid, and Ornithine α-Ketoglutarate (Figure 3)

Glutamine is the most abundant amino acid in plasma and in tissue. In glutamine-consuming cells it is readily converted by the enzyme glutaminase to form ammonia and glutamic acid, which is the primary intermediate in almost all routes of glutamine degradation. In the presence of ammonia this process can occur in reverse, catalyzed by the enzyme glutamine synthetase. In contrast to glutamic acid, glutamine can easily pass through the cellular membrane, thus exporting waste nitrogen out of the cell and serving as an inter-organ nitrogen carrier. In the kidney glutamine donates NH_3, which is the acceptor for protons released from carbonic acid, to form NH_4^+ and thus facilitates the formation of HCO_3^-, which is essential in plasma pH regulation.

Following conversion to glutamic acid and subsequently α-ketoglutarate, glutamine may supplement intermediates of the citrate cycle. In this manner glutamine serves as the preferred fuel for rapidly dividing cells of, for example, the immune system cells and intestinal mucosa. In the brain glutamic acid is the most abundant excitatory neurotransmitter and the precursor for gamma-aminobutyric acid, which is an important inhibitory neurotransmitter. Glutamine is a direct precursor for purine and pyrimidine and therefore is involved in RNA and DNA synthesis and cell proliferation. In addition it is a constituent of the tripeptide glutathione, which is the principal intracellular antioxidant in eukaryotes (see also sections on cysteine and glycine).

Supplementation

Of all the compounds discussed above glutamine is the most extensively applied in clinical and experimental amino acid supplementation, often in the form of the more soluble and stable dipeptides alanyl- and glycyl-glutamine. Glutamic acid and α-ketoglutarate are less ideally suited for use in feeding formulas because of poor inward transport of glutamic acid and poor solubility and stability of α-ketoglutarate. Moreover, glutamic acid has been related to the 'Chinese restaurant syndrome,' characterized by light-headiness and nausea after consumption of Chinese food containing glutamic acid for flavor improvement. However, scientific evidence is weak. Numerous experimental and clinical studies have suggested that glutamine supplementation has positive effects on immune function, intestinal mucosal integrity, nitrogen balance, and glutathione concentration in a wide variety of conditions. Nevertheless, the true benefit of glutamine supplementation is difficult to quantify in clinical practice. Its benefit has especially been claimed in the critically ill and surgical patients in whom clinical outcome is multifactorial. Recent meta-analyses support the view that glutamine supplementation is safe and may reduce infectious morbidity and hospital stay in surgical patients. A positive effect of glutamine supplementation on morbidity and mortality in critical illness, trauma patients, and burn patients has been demonstrated in a few well-designed clinical trials. However, due to the paucity of such trials reliable meta-analyses are not possible in these latter patient categories. It has been demonstrated in some small clinical series that supplementation with ornithine α-ketoglutarate may improve wound healing in burn patients, benefiting from the combined actions of both α-ketoglutarate and ornithine (see sections on arginine and ornithine).

Glycine, Serine, and Threonine

Threonine is an essential amino acid, which can be converted to glycine in the liver and subsequently to serine. Glycine is a constituent of glutathione (see also sections on cysteine and glutamic acid) and is a versatile neurotransmitter in the central nervous system. Through the glycine receptor it has a direct inhibitory neurotransmitter function but it is also a ligand for the glycine site at the N-methyl-D-aspartate (NMDA) glutamic acid receptor. Activation of this glycine site is needed for NMDA activation, which makes glycine a mediator in the excitatory neurotransmitter effects of glutamic acid. Besides a role in the central nervous system, glycine is also

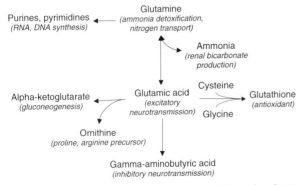

Figure 3 Specific functions of glutamine and glutamine degradation products.

thought to possess anti-inflammatory properties, but to date these properties have only been demonstrated in the test tube. Furthermore, glycine can react with arginine and methionine to form creatine (see section on arginine). Finally, glycine, like taurine, is a conjugate for bile acids.

Glycine is convertible to serine in a reversible reaction, which can be converted to its stereoisomeric form D-serine; this is also a ligand for the glycine site at the NMDA receptor. Furthermore, serine is an intermediate in the pathway from methionine to cysteine and a precursor for pyrimidines and purines and as such is involved in cell proliferation. It is also a precursor for gluconeogenesis, albeit of lesser importance than glutamine and alanine.

Supplementation

Based upon their excitatory effects on the central nervous system both glycine and D-serine have been implicated in the treatment of schizophrenia. As adjuvant therapy to standard psychopharmacological treatment they may reduce the negative symptoms of the disease.

High doses of threonine in adults have been used as tentative therapy for spastic syndromes, a therapy that probably acts through increased glycine formation. A negative effect of excessive threonine, which is abundant in bovine infant formula nutrition, has been considered in experimental studies on brain development, and it has been suggested that this happens through its conversion to glycine and serine, or through competition of amino acid transport across the blood–brain barrier.

Histidine

Histidine is the precursor for histamine, which is important for the immune system by mediating growth and functionality of immune cells. Excessive release of histamine from mast cells induces the clinical signs of allergy (dilation of capillaries and larger blood vessels, increased capillary permeability and swelling, itching, and anaphylactic shock). These phenomena are effected via the H_1 receptor, which is found in smooth muscle cells of the vascular wall and bronchi, among others. Furthermore, histamine acts as a neurotransmitter and mediates gastric acid production. The latter occurs via the H_2 receptor found in gastric mucosa. There is no literature available on the potential relationship between histidine availability and histamine production and action.

Supplementation

H_1 receptor antagonists are applied in the treatment of allergy and H_2 receptor antagonists have been shown to be very effective in the inhibition of gastric acid secretion and have greatly improved the treatment of individuals with peptic ulcer disease and acid reflux esophagitis. Histamine is present in abundance in many dietary sources; no beneficial effects of supplementation of either histidine or histamine are known.

Branched Chain Amino Acids (Isoleucine, Leucine, Valine)

Branched chain amino acids (BCAAs) are essential amino acids, which together compose approximately a third of the daily amino acid requirement in humans. BCAAs, and especially leucine, play an important role in the regulation of energy and protein metabolism. BCAAs are primarily oxidized in skeletal muscle and not in the liver. BCAAs donate their amino groups to furnish glutamic acid in muscle in transamination reactions yielding the α-ketoacids α-ketoisocaproic acid, α-keto-β-methylvaleric acid, and α-ketoisovaleric acid. These transamination products of BCAAs can enter the citrate cycle and contribute to ATP production by aerobic substrate oxidation, which is important during the change from rest to exercise. After consumption of protein-containing meals, a large part of the BCAA passes through the liver and is taken up by muscle where it primarily contributes to protein synthesis and the synthesis of glutamine, which accounts for about 70% of the amino acid release from muscle. The importance of the essential branched chain amino acids for protein synthesis is strikingly exemplified by the negative nitrogen balance and catabolism that follows upper gastrointestinal bleeding caused by ingestion of large amounts of hemoglobin (which lacks isoleucine). Leucine has been suggested to regulate the turnover of protein in muscle cells by inhibiting protein degradation and enhancing protein synthesis. This has led to a worldwide interest in the possible use of BCAAs in general, and leucine in particular, for metabolic support.

In liver failure the plasma concentrations of the aromatic amino acids (AAAs) tyrosine, phenylalanine, and tryptophan increase, probably because they are predominantly broken down in the liver, whereas the plasma levels of BCAAs decrease while they are degraded in excess in muscle as a consequence of hepatic failure-induced catabolism. As AAAs and BCAAs are all neutral amino acids and share a common transporter across the blood–brain barrier (system L carrier), changes in their plasma ratio are reflected in the brain, subsequently disrupting the neurotransmitter profile of the catecholamines and indoleamines (see sections on tyrosine and tryptophan). It has been hypothesized that this disturbance contributes to the multifactorial pathogenesis of hepatic encephalopathy. In line with this hypothesis it has been suggested that normalization of the amino acid pattern by supplementing extra BCAAs counteracts hepatic encephalopathy.

Supplementation

Specialized formulas that are widely used for hepatic failure and hepatic encephalopathy are based on a high content of BCAAs to improve protein malnutrition and restore the amino acid and neurotransmitter balance. Although BCAA-enriched formulas have been proven to improve neurological status in comatose liver patients it is not certain that this is achieved by the addition of BCAAs specifically, because of a lack of adequate control groups.

Since BCAAs compete with tryptophan for uptake by the brain, they have (in line with the ascribed benefits in hepatic encephalopathy) been applied as competitive antagonists for tryptophan transport, reducing tryptophan-induced cognitive impairment (see also section on tryptophan).

Isoleucine, which is absent in the hemoglobin molecule, can be supplemented to patients with upper gastrointestinal bleeding to restore the balance of amino acids that are taken up by the splanchnic organs. This has been demonstrated to improve mainly protein synthesis in liver and muscle in small observational studies. Prospective randomized clinical trials are, however, still lacking.

Lysine

Lysine is an essential amino acid that is mainly provided by meat products and is therefore limited in diets where wheat is the primary protein source. Lysine is also the first rate-limiting amino acid in milk-fed newborns for growth and protein synthesis. Lysine is catabolized to glutamate and acetyl-CoA and is also the precursor for the synthesis of carnitine, which is needed for mitochondrial oxidation of long-chain fatty acids.

Supplementation

Lysine supplementation in patients with renal failure is contraindicated, as the amino acid shows some degree of nephrotoxicity.

Phenylalanine and Tyrosine

Phenylalanine is hydroxylated to tyrosine by the enzyme phenylalanine hydroxylase. The inborn disease phenylketonuria is characterized by a deficiency of this enzyme.

Tyrosine is the precursor for dihydroxyphenylalanine (dopa), which can successively be converted to the catecholamines dopamine, noradrenaline (norepinephrine) and adrenaline (epinephrine). Although only a small proportion of tyrosine is used in this pathway, this metabolic route is extremely relevant. Dopamine is an important neurotransmitter in different parts of the brain and is involved in movement and affects pleasure and motivation. Disruption of dopamine neurons in the basal ganglia is the cause of Parkinson's disease. Noradrenaline and ardrenaline are the most important neurotransmitters in the sympathetic nervous system. The sympathetic nervous system becomes activated during different forms of emotional and physical arousal, and results in the induction of phenomena such as increased blood pressure and heart rate, increased alertness, and decreased intestinal motility (fight-or-flight response). Besides acting as a precursor for catecholamines, tyrosine can be iodinated and as such is the precursor for the thyroid hormones triiodothyronine and thyroxine. These hormones are important regulators of general whole body rate of metabolic activity.

Supplementation

The processes described in the paragraph above quantitatively contribute only marginally to total tyrosine turnover and the limited data on tyrosine supplementation in phenylketonuria suggest that tyrosine deficiency is not causal in the development of cognitive dysfunction in the disease. In two studies tyrosine supplementation has been found to modestly increase mental status and cognitive performance following exhausting efforts such as prolonged wakefulness and intensive military training. In contrast, tyrosine derivatives (L-dopa, noradrenaline, adrenaline) have strong pharmacological properties. L-dopa is the direct precursor of dopamine synthesis and has been found to have strong beneficial effects in Parkinson's disease. The fact that administration of tyrosine as the physiological precursor of catecholamines has no or minor effects on catecholamine-induced sympathic activity, whereas the effects of the catecholamines or more direct precursors is very strong, suggests that tyrosine hydroxylation to L-dopa is not limited by substrate availability.

Tryptophan

Functional end products of the essential amino acid tryptophan arise mainly through two distinctive pathways. The major pathway is degradation of tryptophan by oxidation, which fuels the kynurenine pathway (See 00011). The second and quantitatively minor pathway is hydroxylation of tryptophan and its subsequent decarboxylation to the indoleamine 5-hydroxytryptamine (serotonin) and subsequently melatonin. The metabolites of the kynurenine pathway, indicated as kynurenines, include quinolic acid and kynurenic acid. Quinolinic acid is an agonist of the NMDA receptor (see also section on glutamic acid), while kynurenic acid is a nonselective NMDA-receptor antagonist with a high affinity for the glycine site of the NMDA receptor (see also section on glycine), and as such is a blocker of amino acid-modulated excitation of the central nervous system. Imbalance between kynurenic acid and quinolinic acid can lead to excitotoxic neuronal cell death and is believed to play a role in the development of several neurological diseases such as Huntington's chorea and epilepsy. In addition, an immuno-modulatory role is suggested for several metabolites of the kynurenine pathway.

Serotonin is synthesized in the central nervous system and is involved in the regulation of mood and sleep. In addition it is found in high quantities in neurons in the gastrointestinal tract where it is involved in regulation of gut motility. Tryptophan competes with BCAAs for transport across the blood–brain barrier and the ratio between trypto-phan and BCAAs therefore determines the uptake of both (groups of) amino acids by the brain (see section on BCAAs). Since albumin has a strong tryptophan-binding capacity, the plasma albumin concentration is inversely related to the plasma concentration of free tryptophan and as such influences the BCAA to tryptophan ratio and hence the brain uptake of both BCAAs and tryptophan. It has been suggested that increased plasma AAAs (tyrosine, phenylalanine, and tryptophan) levels in patients with liver failure are caused by the inability of the liver to degrade these amino acids. The resulting change in the ratio between AAA and BCAA plasma levels has been implied in the pathogenesis of hepatic encephalopa-thy since this may cause marked disturbances in transport of both AAAs and BCAAs across the blood–brain barrier, leading to disturbed release of indoleamines and catecholamines in the brain (see also section on BCAAs). High tryptophan concentrations have been associated with chronic fatigue disorders and hepatic encephalopathy while low tryptophan plasma concentrations have been implicated in the etiology of mood disorders, cognitive impairment, and functional bowel disorders. Melatonin, which is produced in the degradation pathway of serotonin during the dark period of the light-dark cycle, is an important mediator of circadian rhythms.

Supplementation

Inhibition of serotonin reuptake from the neuronal synapse and the subsequent increase in its functionality is one of the mainstays of the pharmacological treatment of depression. Like many amino acids, tryptophan is commercially available as a nutritional supplement or as a so-called smart drug, claiming to reduce symptoms of depression, anxiety, obsessive-compulsive disorders, insomnia, fibromyalgia, alcohol withdrawal, and migraine. However, no convincing clinical data are available to support these claims. In contrast tryptophan depletion induced by ingestion of a tryptophan-deficient amino acid mixture, is widely used in experimental psychiatry to study the biological background of various psychiatric disorders.

See also: **Amino Acids**: Chemistry and Classification; Metabolism. **Brain and Nervous System**. **Carbohydrates**: Regulation of Metabolism. **Cytokines**. **Electrolytes**: Acid-Base Balance; Water–Electrolyte Balance. **Glucose**: Metabolism and Maintenance of Blood Glucose Level. **Inborn Errors of Metabolism**: Classification and Biochemical Aspects; Nutritional Management of Phenylketonuria. **Protein**: Synthesis and Turnover; Requirements and Role in Diet; Quality and Sources. **Stomach**: Structure and Function.

Further Reading

Cynober LA (ed.) (2004) *Metabolic and Therapeutic Aspects of Amino Acids in Clinical Nutrition*, 2nd edn. Boca Raton: CRC Press.

Fürst P and Young V (2000) *Proteins, Peptides and Amino Acids in Enteral Nutrition*. Nestlé Nutrition Workshop Series Clinical & Performance Program, vol. 3. Vevey: Nestec Ltd and Basel: Karger.

Guyton AC and Hall JE (1996) *Textbook of Medical Physiology*, 9th edn. Philadelphia: W.B. Saunders.

Labadarios D and Pichard C (2002) *Clinical Nutrition: early Intention*. Nestlé Nutrition Workshop Series Clinical & Performance Program, vol. 7. Vevey: Nestec Ltd and Basel: Karger.

Newsholme P, Procopio J, Lima MMR, Ptihon-Curi TC, and Curi R (2003) Glutamine and glutamate – their central role in cell metabolism and function. *Cell Biochemistry and Function* 21: 1–9.

Wu G and Morris SM (1998) Arginine metabolism: nitric oxide and beyond. *Biochemical Journal* 336: 1–17.

Young V, Bier DM, Cynober L, Hayashi Y, and Kadowaki M (eds.) (2003) The third Workshop on the Assessment of adequate Intake of Dietary Amino Acids. *J Nutr Supplement* 134: 1553S–1672S.

ANEMIA

Contents

Iron-Deficiency Anemia

K J Schulze and M L Dreyfuss, Johns Hopkins
Bloomberg School of Public Health, Baltimore, MD,
USA

© 2005 Elsevier Ltd. All rights reserved.

Anemia is defined by abnormally low circulating hemoglobin concentrations. A variety of etiologies exist for anemia, including dietary deficiencies of folate or vitamin B_{12} (pernicious or macrocytic anemia), infections and inflammatory states (anemia of chronic disease), and conditions that result in insufficient production of red blood cells (aplastic anemia) or excessive destruction of red blood cells (hemolytic anemia). However, worldwide, the most prevalent form of anemia is that of iron deficiency, which causes anemia characterized by hypochromic and normo- or microcytic red blood cells. Iron deficiency anemia remains a health problem in both the developed and the developing world. This article discusses the metabolism of iron; the assessment of iron deficiency; iron requirements across the life span; and the consequences, prevention, and treatment of iron deficiency and iron deficiency anemia.

Iron Metabolism

The adult body contains 2.5–5 g of iron, approximately two-thirds of which is present in hemoglobin. Other essential iron-containing systems include muscle myoglobin (3%) and a variety of iron-containing enzymes (5–15%), including cytochromes. In addition to the role of iron in oxygen transfer via hemoglobin and myoglobin, iron is involved in energy metabolism and also affects neural myelination and neurotransmitter metabolism. Iron stores vary considerably but may represent up to 30% of body iron, and iron that circulates with transferrin represents less than 1% of body iron. Men have a higher concentration of iron per kilogram body weight than women because they have larger erythrocyte mass and iron stores.

More than 90% of body iron is conserved through the recycling of iron through the reticuloendothelial system (**Figure 1**). Iron is transported through the body by the protein transferrin, which carries up to two iron atoms. The distribution of iron to body tissues is mediated by transferrin receptors (TfRs), which are upregulated in the face of increased tissue demand for iron. The transferrin/TfR complex is internalized via cell invagination, iron is released into the cell cytosol, and transferrin is recycled back to the cell surface.

In hematopoietic cells, iron is used to produce hemoglobin through its combination with zinc protoporphyrin to form heme. Therefore, protoporphyrin accumulates relative to hemoglobin in red blood cells during iron deficiency. Mature red blood cells circulate in the body for approximately 120 days before being destroyed. Macrophage cells of the liver and spleen phagocytize senescent red blood cells and the iron released in this process is recycled back to the circulation or, when iron is readily available, incorporated with ferritin or hemosiderin for storage. A typical ferritin molecule may contain 2000 iron atoms. Hemosiderin is a less soluble variant of ferritin that may contain even greater amounts of iron.

The production of transferrin receptors and ferritin is regulated by iron response proteins (IRPs) that 'sense' intracellular iron concentrations and interact with iron response elements (IREs) of protein mRNA. When cellular iron concentrations are low, the IRP–IRE interaction works to prevent translation of mRNA to ferritin or to stabilize mRNA to enhance the translation of transferrin receptors. Identifying other proteins regulated through the IRP–IRE interaction is an area of particular interest. Although body iron is highly conserved, daily basal losses of iron of ~ 1 mg/day do occur even in healthy individuals. These basal losses occur primarily through the gastrointestinal tract (in bile, sloughing of ferritin-containing enterocytes, and via blood loss), and sweat and urine are additional minor sources of iron loss (**Figure 1**). Iron losses are not strictly regulated; rather, iron balance is achieved through the regulation of dietary iron absorption.

Dietary Iron Absorption

The efficiency of iron absorption depends on both the bioavailability of dietary iron and iron status.

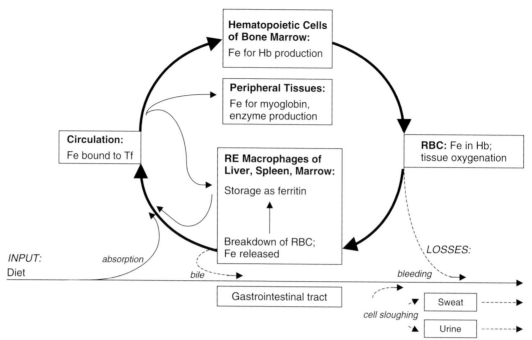

Figure 1   Iron metabolism and balance: inputs, losses, and recycling of iron through the reticuloendothelial system. Fe, iron; Tf, transferrin; Hb, hemoglobin; RBC, red blood cell; RE, reticuloendothelial.

Typically, 5–20% of the iron present in a mixed diet is absorbed. Dietary iron exists in two forms, heme and non-heme. Heme iron is derived from animal source food and is more bioavailable than non-heme iron, with approximately 20–30% of heme iron absorbed via endocytosis of the entire heme molecule. Iron is then released into the enterocyte by a heme oxidase.

Non-heme iron exists in plant products and its bioavailability is compromised by the concurrent ingestion of tannins, phytates, soy, and other plant constituents, that decrease its solubility in the intestinal lumen. Bioavailability of non-heme iron is increased by concurrent ingestion of ascorbic acid and meat products. Non-heme iron is reduced from the ferric to the ferrous form in the intestinal lumen and transported into enterocytes via the divalent metal transporter (DMT-1). Once inside the enterocyte, iron from heme and non-heme sources is similarly transported through the cell and across the basolateral membrane by the ferroportin transporter in conjunction with the ferroxidase hephaestin after which it can be taken up by transferrin into the circulation. The regulation of iron across the basolateral membrane of the enterocyte is considered the most important aspect of iron absorption.

The absorption efficiency of non-heme iron in particular is also inversely related to iron status. The factor responsible for communicating body iron status to the enterocyte to allow for the up- or downregulation of iron absorption remained elusive until recently,

when the hormone hepcidin was identified. Hepcidin declines during iron deficiency, and its decline is associated with an increased production of the DMT-1 and ferroportin transporters in a rat model, although its exact mode of action is unknown. Hepcidin may also regulate iron absorption and retention or release of iron from body stores during conditions of enhanced erythropoiesis and inflammation.

Iron Requirements

Iron requirements depend on iron losses and growth demands for iron across life stages. To maintain iron balance or achieve positive iron balance, therefore, the amount of iron absorbed from the diet must equal or exceed the basal losses plus any additional demands for iron attributable to physiologic state (e.g., growth, menstruation, and pregnancy) and/or pathological iron losses (e.g., excess bleeding). When iron balance is negative, iron deficiency will occur following the depletion of the body's iron reserves. Thus, ensuring an adequate supply of dietary iron is of paramount importance. The risk of iron deficiency and iron deficiency anemia varies across the life cycle as iron demand and/or the likelihood of consuming adequate dietary iron changes.

Basal Iron Loss

Because basal iron losses are due to cell exfoliation, these losses are relative to interior body surfaces, totaling an estimated 14 μg/kg body weight/day, and are approximately 0.8 mg/day for nonmenstruating women and 1.0 mg/day for men. Basal losses in infants and children have not been directly determined and are estimated from data available on adult men. Basal losses are reduced in people with iron deficiency and increased in people with iron overload. The absorbed iron requirement for adult men and nonmenstruating women is based on these obligate iron losses.

Infancy and Childhood

The iron content of a newborn infant is approximately 75 mg/kg body weight, and much of this iron is found in hemoglobin. The body iron of the newborn is derived from maternal–fetal iron transfer, 80% of which occurs during the third trimester of pregnancy. Preterm infants, with less opportunity to establish iron stores, have a substantially reduced endowment of body iron at birth than term infants.

During the first 2 months of life, there is a physiologic shift of body iron from hemoglobin to iron stores. For the first 6 months of life, the iron requirement of a term infant is satisfied by storage iron and breast milk iron, which is present in low concentrations but is highly bioavailable (50–100%) to the infant. However, by 6 months of age in term infants, and even earlier in preterm infants, iron intake and body stores become insufficient to meet the demands for growth (expanding erythrocyte mass and growth of body tissues), such that negative iron balance will ensue at this time without the introduction of iron supplements or iron-rich weaning foods.

A full-term infant almost doubles its body iron content and triples its body weight in the first year of life. Although growth continues through childhood, the rate of growth declines following the first year of life. Similarly, the requirement for iron expressed per kilogram body weight declines through childhood from a high of 0.10 mg/kg in the first 6 months to 0.03 mg/kg/d by 7–10 years of age until increasing again during the adolescent growth spurt. Throughout the period of growth, the iron concentration of the diet of infants and children must be greater than that of an adult man in order to achieve iron balance.

Adolescence

Adolescents have very high iron requirements, and the iron demand of individual children during periods of rapid growth is highly variable and may exceed mean estimated requirements. Boys going through puberty experience a large increase in erythrocyte mass and hemoglobin concentration. The growth spurt in adolescent girls usually occurs in early adolescence before menarche, but growth continues postmenarche at a slower rate. The addition of menstrual iron loss to the iron demand for growth leads to particularly high iron requirements for postmenarchal adolescent girls.

Menstruation

Although the quantity of menstrual blood loss is fairly constant across time for an individual, it varies considerably from woman to woman. The mean menstrual iron loss is 0.56 mg/day when averaged over a monthly cycle. However, menstrual blood losses are highly skewed so that a small proportion of women have heavy losses. In 10% of women, menstrual iron loss exceeds 1.47 mg/day and in 5% it exceeds 2.04 mg/day. Therefore, the daily iron requirement for menstruating women is set quite high to cover the iron needs of most of the population. Menstrual blood loss is decreased by oral contraceptives but increased by intrauterine devices. However, recent progesterone-releasing versions of the device lead to decreased menstrual blood loss or amenorrhea.

Pregnancy and Lactation

The body's iron needs during pregnancy are very high despite the cessation of menstruation during this period. Demand for iron comes primarily from the expansion of the red blood cell mass (450 mg), the fetus (270 mg), the placenta and cord (90 mg), and blood loss at parturition (150 mg). However, the requirement for iron is not spread evenly over the course of pregnancy, as depicted in **Figure 2**, with iron requirements actually reduced in the first trimester because menstrual blood loss is

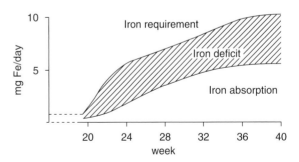

Figure 2 The discrepancy between iron requirements and availability of iron from dietary absorption in pregnant women beyond 20 weeks of gestation. The resulting iron deficit is maintained as pregnancy progresses into the second and third trimesters. (Reproduced with permission from the Food and Agriculture Organization of the United Nations (2001) Iron. In *Human Vitamin and Mineral Requirements: Report of a Joint FAO/WHO Expert Consultation, Bangkok, Thailand*, pp. 195–221. Rome: FAO.)

absent and fetal demand for iron is negligible. Iron requirements increase dramatically through the second and third trimesters to support expansion of maternal red blood cell mass and fetal growth. The maternal red cell mass expands approximately 35% in the second and third trimesters to meet increased maternal oxygen needs. When iron deficiency is present, the expansion of the red cell mass is compromised, resulting in anemia. Furthermore, an expansion of the plasma fluid that is proportionately greater than that of the red cell mass results in a physiologic anemia attributable to hemodilution.

To attempt to meet iron requirements during pregnancy, iron absorption becomes more efficient in the second and third trimesters. Iron absorption nearly doubles in the second trimester and can increase up to four times in the third trimester. Despite this dramatic increase in iron absorption, it is virtually impossible for pregnant women to acquire sufficient iron through diet alone because of the concurrent increase in iron requirements during the latter half of pregnancy (**Figure 2**).

There is also an iron cost of lactation to women of approximately 0.3 mg/day as iron is lost in breastmilk. However, this is compensated by the absence of menstrual iron losses and the gain in iron stores achieved when much of the iron previously invested in expansion of the red cell mass is recovered postpartum.

Pathological Losses

Conditions that cause excessive bleeding additionally compromise iron status. Approximately 1 mg of iron is lost in each 1 ml of packed red blood cells. Excessive losses of blood may occur from the gastrointestinal tract, urinary tract, and lung in a variety of clinical pathologies, including ulcers, malignancies, inflammatory bowel disease, hemorrhoids, hemoglobinuria, and idiopathic pulmonary hemosiderosis. In developing countries, parasitic infestation with hookworm and schistosomiasis can contribute substantially to gastrointestinal blood loss and iron deficiency.

Recommended Nutrient Intakes for Iron

Recommended intakes of dietary iron are based on the requirement for absorbed iron and assumptions about the bioavailability of iron in the diet. They are meant to cover the iron needs of nearly the entire population group. Thus, the amount of dietary iron necessary to meet an iron requirement depends in large part on the bioavailability of iron in the diet (**Figure 3**). Americans consume approximately 15 mg of iron daily from a diet that is considered moderately to highly bioavailable (10–15%) due to the meat and ascorbic acid content. Studies in European countries suggest that iron intake

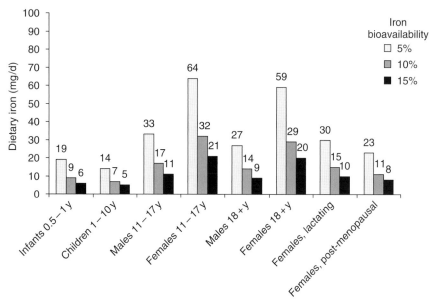

Figure 3 The Recommended Nutrient Intake (RNI) for iron given different levels of bioavailability of iron in the diet: 5%, low; 10%, moderate; and 15%, high. The RNI is based on the amount of iron necessary to meet requirements of 95% of the population for each age/sex group. Because typical iron intakes range from 10 to 15 mg/day, iron requirements are nearly impossible to meet on low-bioavailability diets. (Data from the Food and Agriculture Organization of the United Nations (2001) Iron. In *Human Vitamin and Mineral Requirements: Report of a Joint FAO/WHO Expert Consultation, Bangkok, Thailand*, pp. 195–221. Rome: FAO.)

averages 10 mg/day, representing a decline in dietary iron. Although estimates of total iron intake in developing countries are not substantially lower than that, iron is often consumed in plant-based diets that inhibit its absorption and contain few animal products to counterbalance that effect, such that the bioavailability of iron is closer to 5%. Thus, **Figure 3** demonstrates the total amount of dietary iron that would be necessary to meet the iron requirements of various population groups based on its bioavailability. Where intakes are sufficient and bioavailability adequate, dietary iron can meet the iron needs of adolescent boys and adult men and also lactating and postmenopausal women. However, regardless of bioavailability, iron requirements are not met by many adolescent girls and adult menstruating women who have above average menstrual blood loss. Few if any population groups can achieve iron intakes sufficient to meet iron requirements when bioavailability of iron is poor.

Dietary recommendations for infants are based on the iron content and bioavailability of human milk. The iron in infant formula is much less bioavailable (10%) than that of human milk and is thus present in greater concentrations than that of human milk. Infants who are not breast-fed should consume iron-fortified formula. Complementary foods offered after 6 months of age can potentially meet iron needs if they have a high content of meat and ascorbic acid. This is rarely the case in developing or developed countries, and fortified infant cereals and iron drops are often introduced at this time in developed countries. In developing countries where diets are poor in bioavailable iron, iron-fortified weaning foods are not commonly consumed, and iron supplements are rarely given to infants and children.

Pregnant women rarely have sufficient iron stores and consume diets adequate to maintain positive iron balance, particularly in the latter half of pregnancy, as previously discussed. They cannot meet their iron requirements through diet alone even in developed countries, where high iron content diets with high bioavailability are common. Supplementation is universally recommended for pregnant women, as discussed later.

Indicators of Iron Deficiency and Anemia

Indicators of iron deficiency can be used to distinguish the degree of iron deficiency that exists across the spectrum from the depletion of body iron stores to frank anemia (**Table 1**). Indicator cutoffs vary by age, sex, race, and physiologic state (e.g., pregnancy),

Table 1 Indicators for assessing the progression of iron deficiency from depletion of iron stores to iron deficiency anemia

Stage of iron deficiency	Consequence	Indicator
Depletion	Decline in storage iron	↓ Serum ferritin
Deficiency	Decreased circulating iron	↓ Serum iron ↑ Total iron binding capacity ↓ Transferrin saturation
	Insufficient tissue iron	↑ Transferrin receptor
	Impaired heme synthesis	↑ Protoporphyrin/ heme
Depletion	Impaired red blood cell production	↓ Hemoglobin ↓ Hematocrit ↓ Red blood cell indices

so using a proper reference is important when interpreting indicators of iron deficiency.

Serum ferritin is directly related to liver iron stores—a gold standard for iron deficiency that is infrequently used due to the invasive nature of the test. Different sources place the cutoff for serum ferritin concentrations indicative of depleted stores at 12 or 15 μg/l. Once iron stores are exhausted, serum ferritin is not useful for determining the extent of iron deficiency. Serum ferritin is also useful for diagnosing iron excess. A major limitation of serum ferritin is the fact that it acts as an acute phase reactant and therefore is mildly to substantially elevated in the presence of inflammation or infection, complicating its interpretation when such conditions exist.

Transferrin saturation is measured as the ratio between total serum iron (which declines during iron deficiency) and total iron binding capacity (which increases during iron deficiency). Typically, transferrin is approximately 30% saturated, and low transferrin saturation (<16%) is indicative of iron deficiency. Transferrin saturation concentrations higher than 60% are indicative of iron overload associated with hereditary hemochromatosis. The use of transferrin saturation to distinguish iron deficiency is limited because of marked diurnal variation and its lack of sensitivity as an indicator.

Elevated circulating TfRs are a sensitive indicator of the tissue demand for iron. Circulating TfR is not affected by inflammation, a limitation of other indicators of iron status. Furthermore, expressing TfR as a ratio with ferritin appears to distinguish with a great deal of sensitivity iron deficiency anemia from anemia of chronic disease, making this combined measure potentially very useful in settings in which these conditions coexist.

Elevated erythrocyte zinc protoporphyrin indicates iron-deficient erythropoiesis. Protoporphyrin concentrations may also be elevated by inflammation and lead exposure.

Finally, although hemoglobin concentrations or percentage hematocrit are not specific for iron deficiency, these measures are used most frequently as a proxy for iron deficiency in field settings because of their technical ease. Anemia is defined as a hemoglobin concentration of less than 110 g/l for those 6 months to 5 years old and for pregnant women, 115 g/l for those 5–11 years old, 120 g/l for nonpregnant females older than 11 years and for males 12–15 years old, or 130 g/l for males older than 15 years of age. Other measures of red blood cell characteristics include total red blood cell counts, mean corpuscular volume, and mean hemoglobin volume.

The choice of indicators and the strategy for assessment will depend on technical feasibility and whether a screening or survey approach is warranted. When more than 5% of a population is anemic, iron deficiency is considered a public health problem, and population-based surveys may be useful for assessing and monitoring the prevalence of iron deficiency. When anemia is less prevalent, screening for iron deficiency in high-risk groups or symptomatic individuals is a more efficient approach. Hemoglobin alone would be insufficient to diagnose iron deficiency in an individual, but hemoglobin distributions can offer clues as to the extent to which anemia is attributable to iron deficiency in a population. Preferred indicators, such as transferrin and/or ferritin, may not be feasible due to blood collection requirements, cost, or technical difficulty in a population survey, but they may be indispensable for characterizing iron status of a population subgroup or individual.

Prevalence of Iron Deficiency and Iron Deficiency Anemia

Although iron deficiency anemia is considered the most prevalent nutritional deficiency globally, accurate prevalence estimates are difficult to obtain. Worldwide, prevalence estimates for iron deficiency anemia have ranged from 500 million to approximately 2 billion people affected. However, most global prevalence estimates are based on anemia surveys, which will overestimate the amount of anemia attributable to iron deficiency but underestimate the prevalence of less severe iron deficiency. There is clearly a disparity in anemia prevalence between the developing and developed world, with ∼50% of children and nonpregnant women in the developing world considered anemic compared with ∼10% in the developed world. The prevalence of anemia increases during pregnancy, with ∼20% of US women anemic during pregnancy and estimates of anemia prevalence in some developing countries exceeding 60%.

Data from the US NHANES III (1988–1994) survey, which used a variety of indicators of iron status, showed that 9% of US toddlers were iron deficient and 3% had iron deficiency anemia. Eleven percent of adolescent females and women of reproductive age were iron deficient, and 3–5% of these women had iron deficiency anemia. Iron deficiency in the developed world is more common among low-income minorities.

Consequences of Iron Deficiency and Iron Deficiency Anemia

Iron deficiency anemia has been implicated in adverse pregnancy outcomes, maternal and infant mortality, cognitive dysfunction and developmental delays in infants and children, and compromised physical capacity in children and adults. However, data to support causal relationships with some of these outcomes is limited, and the extent to which outcomes are associated with iron deficiency specifically or more generally with anemia regardless of the etiology is the subject of debate.

A variety of observational studies demonstrate an association of maternal hemoglobin concentrations during pregnancy with birth weight, the likelihood of low birth weight and preterm birth, and perinatal mortality, such that adverse pregnancy outcomes are associated in a 'U-shaped' manner with the lowest and highest maternal hemoglobin concentrations. Anemia during pregnancy may not be specific to iron deficiency, and randomized trials utilizing a strict placebo to firmly establish a causal link between iron status per se and adverse pregnancy outcomes are rare because of ethical concerns about denying women iron supplements during pregnancy. However, two randomized trials, one conducted in a developed country and the other in a developing country, have shown a positive impact of iron supplementation during pregnancy on birth weight. In the developed country study, control women with evidence of compromised iron stores were offered iron supplements at 28 weeks of gestation after 8 weeks of randomized iron supplementation. In the developing country study, the control group received supplemental vitamin A and the intervention group received folic acid in addition to iron.

Mortality among pregnant women and infants and children also increases with severe anemia. However, most data showing this relationship are observational and clinic based. Anemia in such circumstances is unlikely to be attributable to iron deficiency alone; furthermore, the degree to which mild to moderate anemia influences mortality outcomes is not well established.

Iron deficiency and iron deficiency anemia have been associated with impaired cognitive development and functioning. These effects of iron deficiency may be mediated in part by the deprivation of functional iron in brain tissue, and the impact of iron deprivation may vary depending on its timing in relation to critical stages of brain development. Iron interventions in anemic school-age children generally result in improved school performance. The results of iron interventions in infants and pre-school-age children are less clear, perhaps in part because cognition is more difficult to measure in this age group.

Studies have shown a negative impact of iron deficiency anemia on work productivity among adult male and female workers in settings requiring both strenuous labor (rubber plantation) and less intensive efforts (factory work). The impact of iron deficiency anemia on performance may be mediated by a reduction in the oxygen-carrying capacity of blood associated with low hemoglobin concentration and by a reduction in muscle tissue oxidative capacity related to reductions in myoglobin and effects on iron-containing proteins involved in cellular respiration.

Interventions: Prevention and Treatment of Iron Deficiency Anemia

Supplementation

Iron supplementation is the most common intervention used to prevent and treat iron deficiency anemia. Global guidelines established by the International Nutritional Anemia Consultative Group, the World Health Organization, and UNICEF identify pregnant women and children 6–24 months of age as the priority target groups for iron supplementation because these populations are at the highest risk of iron deficiency and most likely to benefit from its control. However, recommendations are given for other target groups, such as children, adolescents, and women of reproductive age, who may also benefit from iron supplementation for the prevention of iron deficiency. The recommendations are given in **Table 2**. Recommended dose and/or duration of supplementation are increased for populations where the prevalence of anemia is 40% or higher. The recommended treatment for severe anemia (Hb <70 g/l) is to double prophylactic doses for 3 months and then to continue the preventive supplementation regimen.

Ferrous sulfate is the most common form of iron used in iron tablets, but fumarate and gluconate are also sometimes used. A liquid formulation is available for infants, but it is not used often in anemia control programs in developing countries because of the expense compared to tablets. Crushed tablets can be given to infants and young children as an alternative, but this has not been very successful programmatically.

Efforts to improve the iron status of populations worldwide through supplementation have met with mixed success. Given the frequency with which iron

Table 2 Guidelines for iron supplementation to prevent iron deficiency anemia

Target group	Dose	Duration
Pregnant women	60 mg iron + 400 µg folic acid daily	6 months in pregnancy[a,b]
Children 6–24 months (normal birth weight)	12.5 mg iron[c] + 50 µg folic acid daily	6–12 months of age[d]
Children 6–24 months (low birth weight)	12.5 mg iron + 50 µg folic acid daily	2–24 months of age
Children 2–5 years	20–30 mg iron[c] daily	
Children 6–11 years	30–60 mg iron daily	
Adolescents and adults	60 mg iron daily[e]	

[a]If 6-months' duration cannot be achieved during pregnancy, continue to supplement during the postpartum period for 6 months or increase the dose to 120 mg iron daily during pregnancy.
[b]Continue for 3 months postpartum where the prevalence of pregnancy anemia is ≥40%.
[c]Iron dosage based on 2 mg iron/kg body weight/day.
[d]Continue until 24 months of age where the prevalence of anemia is ≥40%.
[e]For adolescent girls and women of reproductive age, 400 µg folic acid should be included with iron supplementation.
Adapted with permission from Stoltzfus RJ and Dreyfuss ML (1998) *Guidelines for the Use of Iron Supplements to Prevent and Treat Iron Deficiency Anemia*. Washington, DC: International Nutritional Anemia Consultative Group.

tablets must be taken to be effective, a lack of efficacy of iron supplementation in research studies and programs has often been attributed to poor compliance and the presence of side effects such as nausea and constipation. Ensuring compliance in some settings also requires extensive logistical support. Although in developing countries the maximum coverage of iron supplementation programs for pregnant women is higher than 50%, other high-risk groups are less frequently targeted for iron supplementation.

Comparative trials have demonstrated that both weekly and daily iron supplementation regimens significantly increase indicators of iron status and anemia, but that daily supplements are more efficacious at reducing the prevalence of iron deficiency and anemia, particularly among pregnant women and young children who have high iron demands. Therefore, daily iron supplements continue to be the recommended choice for pregnant women and young children because there is often a high prevalence of iron deficiency anemia in these populations. Weekly supplementation in school-age children and adolescents holds promise for anemia prevention programs because it reduces side effects, improves compliance, and lowers costs. Further assessment of the relative effectiveness of the two approaches is needed to determine which is more effective in the context of programs.

Fortification

Iron fortification of food is the addition of supplemental iron to a mass-produced food vehicle consumed by target populations at risk of iron deficiency anemia. Among anemia control strategies, iron fortification has the greatest potential to improve the iron status of populations. However, its success has been limited by technical challenges of the fortification process: (i) the identification of a suitable iron compound that does not alter the taste or appearance of the food vehicle but is adequately absorbed and (ii) the inhibitory effect of phytic acid and other dietary components that limit iron absorption. Water-soluble iron compounds, such as ferrous sulfate, are readily absorbed but cause rancidity of fats and color changes in some potential food vehicles (e.g., cereal flours). In contrast, elemental iron compounds do not cause these sensory changes but are poorly absorbed and are unlikely to benefit iron status. Research on iron compounds and iron absorption enhancers that addresses these problems has yielded some promising alternatives. Encapsulated iron compounds prevent some of the sensory changes that occur in fortified food vehicles. The addition of ascorbic acid enhances iron absorption from fortified

foods, and NaFe–EDTA provides highly absorbable iron in the presence of phytic acid.

Many iron-fortified products have been tested for the compatibility of the fortificant with the food vehicle and for the bioavailability of the fortified iron, but few efficacy or effectiveness trials have been done. Iron-fortified fish sauce, sugar, infant formula, and infant cereal have been shown to improve iron status. In contrast, attempts to fortify cereal flours with iron have met with little success because they contain high levels of phytic acid and the characteristics of these foods require the use of poorly bioavailable iron compounds.

In the developed world, iron fortification has resulted in decreased rates of iron deficiency and anemia during the past few decades. Some debate remains, however, about the potential for the acquisition of excess iron, which has been associated with increased chronic disease risk in some studies. In Europe, Finland and Denmark have recently discontinued food fortification programs because of concerns of iron overload. Individuals with hereditary hemochromatosis, $\sim$5/1000 individuals in populations of European descent, are at particular risk of iron overload.

Control of Parasitic Infections

Because geohelminths such as hookworm also contribute to iron deficiency, programs that increase iron intakes but do not address this major source of iron loss are unlikely to be effective at improving iron status. Other infections and inflammation also cause anemia, as does malaria, and the safety of iron supplementation during infection or malaria has been debated. Where malaria and iron deficiency coexist, the current view is that iron supplementation is sufficiently beneficial to support its use. Ideally, however, where multiple etiologies of anemia coexist, these etiologies need to be recognized and simultaneously addressed.

Other Micronutrients

Other nutrients and their deficiencies that can impact iron status, utilization, or anemia include vitamin A, folate, vitamin B_{12}, riboflavin, and ascorbic acid (vitamin C). Improving iron status can also increase the utilization of iodine and vitamin A from supplements. On the other hand, it is increasingly recognized that simultaneous provision of iron and zinc in supplements may decrease the benefit of one or both of these nutrients. These complex micronutrient interactions and their implications for nutritional interventions are incompletely understood but have significant implications for population-based supplementation strategies.

Summary

Iron deficiency anemia exists throughout the world, and pregnant women and infants 6–24 months old are at highest risk because of their high iron requirements. Women of reproductive age, school-age children, and adolescents are also high-risk groups that may require attention in anemia control programs. Although numerous indicators exist to characterize the progression of iron deficiency to anemia, difficulties remain with their use and interpretation, particularly in the face of other causes of anemia. Despite the proven efficacy of iron supplementation and fortification to improve iron status, there are few examples of effective anemia prevention programs. More innovative programmatic approaches that aim to improve iron status, such as geohelminth control or prevention of other micronutrient deficiencies, deserve more attention. Challenges remain in preventing and controlling iron deficiency anemia worldwide.

See also: **Adolescents**: Nutritional Requirements. **Breast Feeding. Children**: Nutritional Requirements. **Folic Acid. Infants**: Nutritional Requirements. **Iron. Lactation**: Dietary Requirements. **Pregnancy**: Nutrient Requirements.

Further Reading

ACC/SCN (2001) Preventing and treating anaemia. In: Allen LH and Gillespie SR (eds.) *What Works? A Review of the Efficacy and Effectiveness of Nutrition Interventions.* Geneva: ACC/SCN in collaboration with the Asian Development Bank, Manila.

Anonymous (2001) Supplement II: Iron deficiency anemia: Reexamining the nature and magnitude of the public health problem. *Journal of Nutrition* 131: 563S–703S.

Anonymous (2002) Supplement: Forging effective strategies to combat iron deficiency. *Journal of Nutrition* 132: 789S–882S.

Bothwell TH, Charlton RW, Cook JD, and Finch CA (1979) *Iron Metabolism in Man.* Oxford: Blackwell Scientific.

Cook JD, Skikne BS, and Baynes RD (1994) Iron deficiency: The global perspective. *Advances in Experimental Medicine and Biology* 356: 219–228.

Eisenstein RS and Ross KL (2003) Novel roles for iron regulatory proteins in the adaptive response to iron deficiency. *Journal of Nutrition* 133: 1510S–1516S.

Fairbanks VP (1999) Iron in medicine and nutrition. In: Shils M, Olson JA, Shike M, and Ross AC (eds.) *Modern Nutrition in Health and Disease*, 9th edn, pp. 193–221. Philadelphia: Lippincott Williams & Wilkins.

Food and Agriculture Organization of the United Nations (2001) Iron. In: *Human Vitamin and Mineral Requirements: Report of a Joint FAO/WHO Expert Consultation, Bangkok, Thailand*, pp. 195–221. Rome: FAO.

Frazer DM and Anderson GJ (2003) The orchestration of body iron intake: How and where do enterocytes receive their cues? *Blood Cells, Molecules, and Diseases* 30(3): 288–297.

Koury MJ and Ponka P (2004) New insights into erythropoiesis: The roles of folate, vitamin B_{12}, and iron. *Annual Review of Nutrition* 24: 105–131.

Leong W-I and Lonnerdal B (2004) Hepcidin, the recently identified peptide that appears to regulate iron absorption. *Journal of Nutrition* 134: 1–4.

Roy CN and Enns CA (2000) Iron homeostasis: New tales from the crypt. *Blood* 96(13): 4020–4027.

Stoltzfus RJ and Dreyfuss ML (1998) *Guidelines for the Use of Iron Supplements to Prevent and Treat Iron Deficiency Anemia.* Washington, DC: International Nutritional Anemia Consultative Group.

World Health Organization (2001) *Iron Deficiency Anaemia Assessment, Prevention and Control: A Guide for Programme Managers.* Geneva: WHO.

Megaloblastic Anemia

J M Scott, Trinity College Dublin, Dublin, Ireland
P Browne, St James's Hospital, Dublin, Ireland

© 2005 Elsevier Ltd. All rights reserved.

Introduction

A major distinction in diagnosis and classification of anemias is whether the eventual red cells that appear in the circulation are smaller (microcytic) or larger (macrocytic) than the usual normal cell size (normocytic). The most important example of the former is iron deficiency anemia where it appears that the red cell precursors, during their replication in the bone marrow from an original pluripotent stem cell undergo a higher than normal number of divisions. Since each such division results in two daughter cells that are slightly smaller, an increase in the number of divisions in the marrow compartment will result in smaller red cells in the circulation. In iron deficiency this is thought to happen because the usual progressive inactivation of the nucleus after each division occurs at a slower than normal rate.

The most characteristic example of a macrocytic anemia occurs because there is an abnormally slow rate of DNA biosynthesis in the developing red cell. Such reduced synthesis delays the rate of development of the nucleus and with it the rate of cell division during replication in the bone marrow compartment. Thus, by the time such cells have differentiated to the point at which they receive a signal to leave the bone marrow, they have undergone fewer than usual cell divisions, resulting in cells that are larger than normal

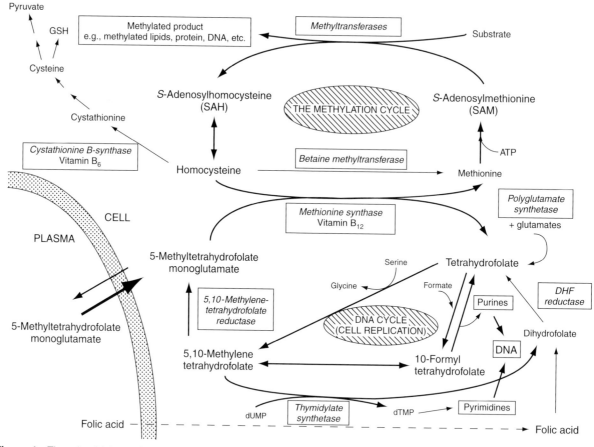

Figure 1 The role of folate cofactors in the DNA and methylation cycles.

or macrocytic. The other unique characteristic of such arrest in DNA biosynthesis is evidenced by the cells that are present in the bone marrow itself. The red cell precursors have a very different appearance from that of the normally developing red cell series (normoblasts). The nuclei are much larger than usual and are far less differentiated. These characteristic cells are called megaloblasts and only occur where there has been a slow down or arrest of DNA biosynthesis. This occurs in only three circumstances: folate deficiency, vitamin B_{12} deficiency, or during therapy with drugs that interfere directly or indirectly with DNA biosynthesis (**Figure 1**).

Definition

As the name suggests and as discussed above the unique feature that defines megaloblastic anemia is the presence of abnormal red cell precursors called megaloblasts in the bone marrow. Therefore, bone marrow examination by a competent hematologist remains the gold standard for diagnosis of megaloblastic anemia. As discussed below, such morphological examinations are no longer routinely part of

the diagnosis. However, despite the availability of other tests, the presence of megaloblasts in bone marrow aspirate remains the only way to achieve a definitive diagnosis and is still required if the patient fails to respond to treatment.

Biochemical Aspects of the Megaloblastic Anemias

The biochemical interrelationships between vitamin B_{12} and folate are described in **Figure 1** and discussed elsewhere in the chapters on cobalamins and folic acid. The folate cofactors are essential for the provision of so-called carbon one units for the biosynthesis of purines and pyrimidines and thus for DNA. Folate in the form of 5-methyltetrahydrofolate (5-methyl THF) is also needed to supply the methylation cycle with methyl groups (**Figure 1**). These are needed to regenerate methionine and S-adenosylmethionine (SAM) in cells, the latter being used to donate methyl groups to the three dozen or so methyltransferases present in all cells. In hepatocytes, part of the methylation cycle is used to degrade the 60% or so excess of methionine present in the diet over and above daily requirements. When folate status is reduced there will be a reduced capacity in cells to make DNA and thus to replicate. This will be most easily seen in rapidly dividing cells such as those of the bone marrow, hence the emergence of the very characteristic megaloblastic anemia with megaloblasts being seen in bone marrow aspirates. Clearly one would also expect to see a reduction in the methylation cycle, which could in turn reduce the activity of the numerous methyltransferases. The effects of such a reduction are less obvious and contrast sharply with what happens when the methylation cycle is interrupted by deficiency of vitamin B_{12} (see below). Vitamin B_{12} is involved in two enzymatic reactions in man, methylmalonyl CoA mutase and methionine synthase. As discussed later deficiency of the former leads to a raised level of methylmalonyl CoA in cells, which is seen in the circulation and the urine as methylmalonic acid (MMA). What is of very great interest is the clinical sequence of events during vitamin B_{12} deficiency and how they arise. There are two such sequences: the development of a megaloblastic anemia identical to that seen in folate deficiency and a neuropathy not usually associated with folate deficiency.

At a biochemical level, the explanation for the anemia is encapsulated in the methyl trap hypothesis, first put forward by Victor Herbert as early as 1961. The biosynthesis of 5-methyl THF by the enzyme 5,10-methylenetetrahydrofolate reductase (MTHFR) (**Figure 1**) is irreversible *in vivo*. Thus, once formed this folate cofactor can only be used by the vitamin B_{12}-dependent enzyme methionine synthase. The activity of the enzyme is reduced or absent in the bone marrow of patients with vitamin B_{12} deficiency. Progressively more and more of the folate cofactors become metabolically trapped as 5-methyl THF reducing the intracellular levels of 10-formyl THF and 5,10-methylene THF needed for the biosynthesis of purines and pyrimidines and thus for DNA and cell division. Although such cells contain folate, they are unable to use it and suffer from a kind of pseudo folate deficiency, thus producing an identical megaloblastic anemia to that seen in folate deficiency. One might question why cells do such an apparently destructive thing. The answer is that cells perceive vitamin B_{12} deficiency through an ever-reducing level of SAM. This essential methyl donor normally downregulates the amount of 5-methyl THF synthesized in cells by reducing the level of the enzyme MTHFR. Falling levels of SAM in vitamin B_{12} deficiency by contrast are met with an ever-increasing activity of MTHFR and diversion of the folate cofactors into the trapped form, namely 5-methyl THF, which, of course, cannot be regenerated into THF because of the absence of methionine synthase.

A very characteristic neuropathy is also associated with vitamin B_{12} deficiency. This neuropathy is due to a reduction or interruption of the methylation cycle. This is clear from two independent lines of evidence. Firstly, inactivation of methionine synthase in experimental animals (monkeys and pigs) leads to the classical so-called subacute combined degeneration of the spinal cord (SCD) seen in patients with severe vitamin B_{12} deficiency. Secondly, patients with genetically very rare dramatic reductions in the enzyme MTHFR have the classical signs and symptoms of SCD. The most plausible explanation is that as a result of reduced MTHFR levels they are unable to supply the methyl groups needed for the methylation cycle. It is of interest that such patients do not get megaloblastic anemia, presumably because while their folate metabolism is interfered with, there is no trapping of the folate cofactors metabolically as 5-methyl THF. It seems probable that a reduction in activity of one or more of the methyltransferases, the activity of which is compromised by an interruption of the methylation cycle, causes the characteristic neuropathy. It is unclear which specific methyltransferase is involved.

Diagnosis of Megaloblastic Anemia

As mentioned above the definitive diagnosis requires identification of the presence of megaloblasts in bone marrow aspirate. The taking of such an aspirate (usually from the hip bone) involves some discomfort for the patient and must be performed by an appropriately trained practitioner. Frequently, the routine diagnosis of unexplained macrocytic anemia falls to general physicians or general practitioners. In this situation, where there is clear evidence that the macrocytic anemia is due to deficiency of vitamin B_{12} or folate, it is not necessary to obtain a bone marrow aspirate to confirm megaloblastic changes. However, when bone marrow is not examined initially and a patient is treated for deficiency of vitamin B_{12} or folic acid, it is essential to verify that their response to treatment includes correction of anemia and macrocytosis. If there is any doubt, a bone marrow aspirate must be performed to exclude other possible underlying hematological disorders.

The first stage of diagnosis is based on the result of a full blood count (FBC) (also called complete blood count (CBC) in some countries) using an automatic instrument such as a Coulter counter. An FBC is done on virtually every patient admitted to hospital. Frequently, an FBC would also form part of an outpatient work-up or might be ordered by a GP through an associated hospital or laboratory. Where the hemoglobin level is below the reference value with respect to sex and age indicating anemia, the mean corpuscular volume (MCV) is assessed. This parameter essentially gives a mean of the size of red blood cells in the circulation. Megaloblastic anemia usually results in larger than normal red cells in the circulation and thus a raised MCV; however, sometimes quite advanced stages of megaloblastic anemia can be accompanied by a normal and, infrequently, even below normal MCV. This can arise because of the concomitant presence of iron deficiency. A raised MCV accompanying the anemia seen in the FBC (macrocytic anemia) moves the diagnosis to being one of megaloblastic anemia, although other causes of macrocytosis such as hypothyroidism or excess alcohol consumption may need to be considered also. Conventionally, the next step is to carry out a bone marrow aspirate to verify if megaloblasts are present, but, as mentioned earlier, this step can be omitted if the diagnosis of vitamin B_{12} or folate deficiency can be made rapidly and accurately. After a positive bone marrow aspirate, or in its absence if this step is omitted, the next analysis would be the determination of circulatory levels of folate and vitamin B_{12}. If only one of the vitamin levels is in the deficient range, most clinicians would embark upon the regimen of therapy discussed below. As mentioned above, antifolate or anti-DNA drugs, such as methotrexate, 5-fluorouracil, or cyclophosphamide, will also arrest DNA biosynthesis and cause megaloblastic anemia; however, it is usually known when patients are on such anticancer chemotherapy.

The circulating levels of folate and vitamin B_{12} can be measured in serum or plasma samples by a number of methods. Most regard microbiological assays using *Lactobacillus casei* for folate and *Lactobacillus leichmannii* for vitamin B_{12} as the 'gold standard.' However, these assays are difficult to perform and most laboratories use methods based on enzyme linked immunosorbent assays (ELISA) or competitive binding assays using a natural binder such as intrinsic factor for vitamin B_{12} or β-lactoglobulin for folate. While very low plasma or serum levels of $<2.0\,\mu g\,l^{-1}$ (4.5 nM) for folate and $<120\,ng\,l^{-1}$ (88 pM) for vitamin B_{12}, are considered as being diagnostic of deficiency, there is a gray area for both assays $2.0–2.7\,\mu g\,l^{-1}$ (4.5–6.1 nM) for serum folate and $120–200\,ng\,l^{-1}$ (88–148 pM) for vitamin B_{12} indicating possible deficiency. Values above $2.7\,\mu g\,l^{-1}$ (6.1 nM) for folate or $200\,ng\,l^{-1}$ (148 pM) for vitamin B_{12} usually indicate the absence of deficiency.

Some laboratories also offer red cell folate levels. The red cell during its maturation in the bone marrow incorporates a level of folate commensurate with what is present in the circulation during that period. When the red cell passes from the bone marrow into the circulation it can neither take up nor lose folate until the end of its life, usually 120 days later. Thus, the circulatory red cells give an average of the folate level over the previous 4 months. Unlike the plasma or serum level the red cell folate level is not influenced by recent fluctuation in dietary intake. Thus, low red cell folate levels of $<100\,\mu g\,l^{-1}$ (226 nM) are a very good indication of folate deficiency with a range of $100–150\,\mu g\,l^{-1}$ (226–340 nM) where there is possible deficiency and values above $150\,\mu g\,l^{-1}$ (340 nM) generally indicating the absence of folate deficiency. While red cell folate levels have significant advantages over serum folate levels they have one very significant drawback. Red cell folate levels are also significantly reduced in vitamin B_{12} deficiency. This is because the bone marrow cells take up the predominant circulating form of folate, namely 5-methyl THF. However, this form, which has just a single glutamate, is not retained by the cells unless it is converted into a predominant cellular form of folate with on average five glutamate residues. The enzyme that adds these glutamates does not use 5-methyl THF as a substrate; therefore, 5-methyl THF must be converted to THF before it can be converted to a polyglutamate. The only enzyme in the cell that converts 5-methyl THF to THF is the vitamin B_{12}-dependent methionine synthase. As mentioned above, its activity is reduced or absent in vitamin B_{12}-deficient bone marrow. Thus, such cells have an inability to conjugate and retain the circulating form of folate and as a result have reduced red cell folate levels. Thus, a low red cell folate level may lead to the misdiagnosis of vitamin B_{12} deficiency as folate deficiency, a circumstance which for the reasons discussed later must be avoided at all costs. Conseqently, it is always necessary to measure the level of plasma or serum folate . If it is also low or deficient and accompanied by a low red cell folate this is indicative of folate rather than vitamin B_{12} deficiency. This is because the circulating folate levels tends to back up in the serum resulting in higher rather than lower serum folate levels in vitamin B_{12} deficiency.

Before therapy, further investigations could be undertaken. These largely depend upon the availability of such tests in any particular clinical context. Elevated plasma homocysteine levels occur in both vitamin B_{12} and folate deficiency and raised homocysteine does not establish which vitamin is deficient. This is because such elevation is due to a reduction in the flux of homocysteine back to methionine as part of the methylation cycle (**Figure 1**). The enzyme that is compromised is methionine synthase, which uses vitamin B_{12} as a cofactor (**Figure 2**) and 5-methyltetrahydrofolate (**Figure 3**) and homocysteine as its substrates. This enzyme, and consequently the methylation cycle, thus requires both a normal folate and a normal vitamin B_{12} status for optimum activity. Thus reduction in the status of either vitamin is always accompanied by an elevation of plasma homocysteine. Homocysteine is also elevated in other circumstances, most notably in impaired renal function. This can, to some extent, be corrected for the creatinine level. Homocysteine is also elevated in vitamin B_6 deficiency and common C→T677 MTHFR polymorphism. Thus, while elevated plasma homocysteine confirms the presence of megaloblastic anemia, establishing which vitamin is deficient still relies on measurement of the circulating levels of the vitamins involved.

The measurement of plasma, serum, or urine MMA is very helpful in confirming a diagnosis of vitamin B_{12} deficiency. This analyte is elevated due to a reduction in the activity of methylmalonyl CoA mutase, the other vitamin B_{12}-dependent enzyme in man (**Figure 4**). It appears that it is not possible to be functionally deficient in vitamin B_{12} without a concomitant elevation in MMA, and so a false negative result is not really an issue. However, MMA like plasma homocysteine is also elevated during renal impairment, and while this can to some extent be corrected for by a raised creatinine, it cannot be assumed that elevation of MMA is due to vitamin B_{12} deficiency. While the estimation of plasma homocysteine is widely available the estimation of MMA requires gas chromatography mass spectroscopy (GC-MS) and has very limited availability in practice. Newer methods to measure vitamin B_{12} on its transport protein TC II are under development.

For the reasons given above, it is essential that vitamin B_{12} deficiency is not confused with folate deficiency. As mentioned previously, both conditions present with a morphologically indistinguishable megaloblastic anemia. The inappropriate treatment of vitamin B_{12} deficiency with folic acid is to be avoided at all costs (see below). Apart from using biochemical assays to measure circulatory levels of the two vitamins and looking for an elevation of the biomarkers plasma homocysteine and MMA, further tests can also implicate vitamin B_{12} malabsorption, the most common type of severe vitamin B_{12} deficiency. These include the Schilling test and the detection of antibodies against either intrinsic factor or the parietal cells that manufacture it.

In practice, if vitamin B_{12} deficiency cannot be ruled out, many clinicians will treat patients with vitamin B_{12} if uncertain about the diagnosis. If this is followed by a reticulocyte response and complete disappearance of the anemia, it confirms a diagnosis of vitamin B_{12} deficiency. The appropriate treatment regimen can then be implemented (see later). If treatment with vitamin B_{12} does not result in improvement of the anemia then the patient is treated for folic acid deficiency, but only after vitamin B_{12} deficiency has been excluded by all means at the clinician's disposal.

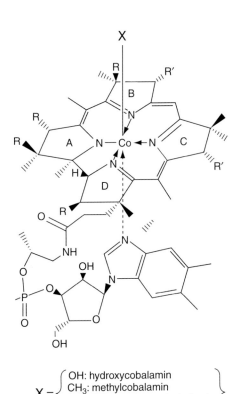

$$X = \begin{cases} \text{OH: hydroxycobalamin} \\ \text{CH}_3\text{: methylcobalamin} \\ \text{Ado: 5'deoxyadenosylcobalamin} \\ \text{CN: cyanocobalamin} \end{cases}$$

Figure 2 The structure of naturally occurring vitamin B_{12} (hydroxycobalamin), its synthetic form cyanocobalamin, and its two cofactor forms methylcobalamin and 5'deoxyadenosylcobalamin. Hydroxycobalamin, X = Co-hydroxide; cyanocobalamin, X = Co-cyanide; methylcobalamin, X = Co-CH$_3$; deoxyadenosylcobalamin, X = Co5'deoxyadenosyl.

Causes of Folate Deficiency

Dietary

The most common cause of folate deficiency is undoubtedly due to inadequate dietary intake. The naturally occurring folates, unlike the synthetic form of the vitamin folic acid, are chemically unstable (**Figure 3**). The folate in food after harvesting or during processing is subject to deterioration.

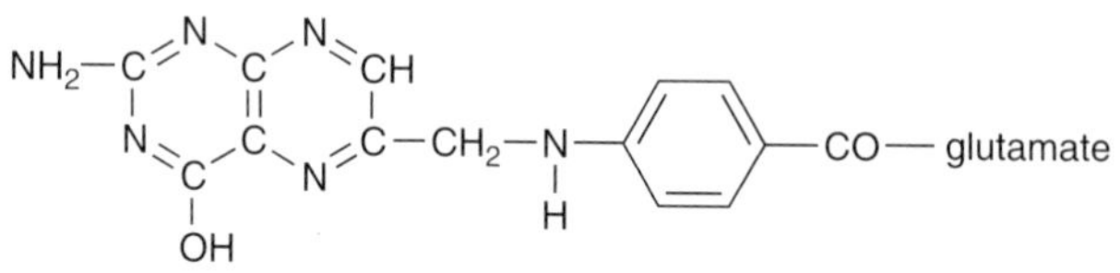

Folic acid

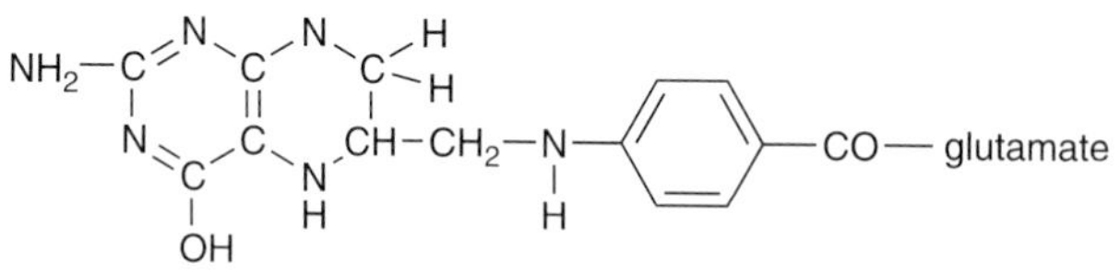

Tetrahydrofolate

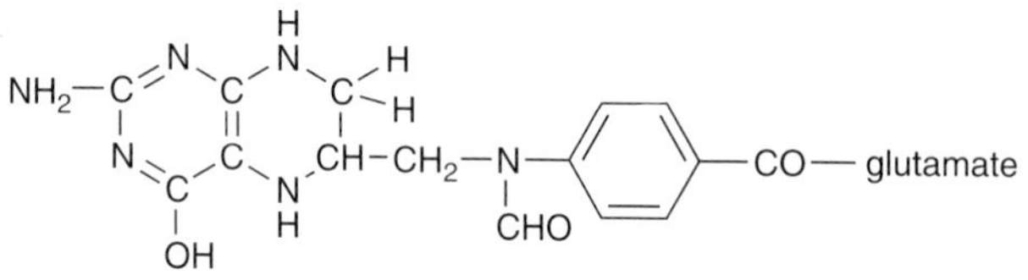

10-Formyltetrahydrofolate

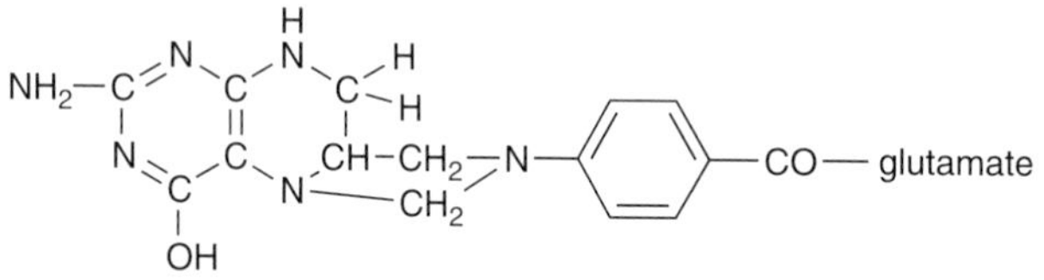

5,10-Methylenetetrahydrofolate

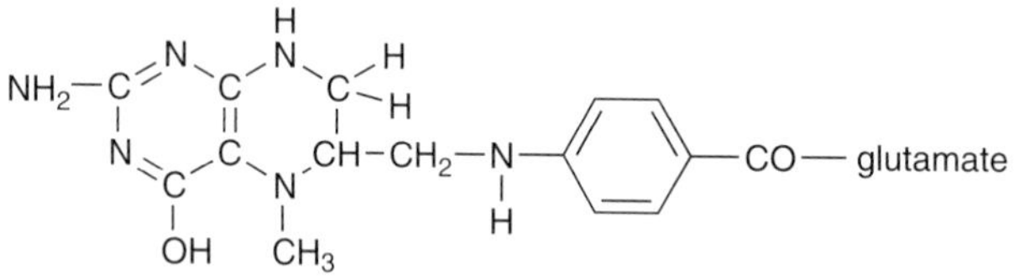

5-Methyltetrahydrofolate

Figure 3 The structure of synthetic folic acid and the naturally occurring forms of the vitamin.

Furthermore, folate can be lost from food during cooking. While the prevalence of overt folate deficiency in those on adequate mixed diets is relatively uncommon, it is now clear that many people have elevations of the biochemical marker homocysteine, which can be decreased by increased status of folic acid or folate, certainly where such diets are not fortified with folic acid. This has led many to conclude that more people than previously suspected are at increased risk of impaired folate function, such as might put them at increased risk of cardiovascular disease and other chronic diseases.

Malabsorption

Normally, the folate cofactors seem to be relatively bioavailable but in some circumstances malabsorption causing deficiency can occur, such as in celiac disease or tropical sprue.

Alcohol Abuse

Chronic alcoholics often have evidence of less than optimal folate status. It is unclear if this is due to inadequate dietary intake, some direct toxic effect of alcohol on folate metabolism in the bone marrow, or increased renal loss.

Drugs

Antifolate drugs such as methotrexate inhibit the enzyme dihydrofolate reductase, which is necessary for maintaining pyrimidine biosynthesis. A known side effect of methotrexate is megaloblastic anemia if given inappropriately.

Pregnancy

It is well established that many women are at risk of reduced folate status or even deficiency in their third trimester of pregnancy. This is probably due to an

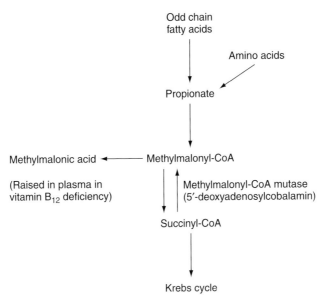

Figure 4 The role of vitamin B_{12} in the metabolism of propionates, odd chain fatty acids, and certain amino acids.

increased breakdown or catabolism of the vitamins associated with the rapid growth of the fetus/placenta rather than the transfer of maternal folate to the fetus, which is quantitatively small. Rapid cell division would result in an increased flux through tetrahydro and dihydrofolate forms of the vitamin, which are known to be the two most chemically unstable forms of the vitamin. In many countries folic acid is given in the latter stages of pregnancy to protect against this risk of megaloblastic anemia, the emergence of which very much depends upon the mother entering the pregnancy with poor stores. These events in the third trimester should not to be confused with the more recent incontrovertible evidence that the maternal periconceptional ingestion of folic acid prevents the majority of cases of spina bifida and other neural tube defects, which take place within the first 4 weeks postconception.

Causes of Vitamin B_{12} Deficiency

Dietary

No plant material can synthesize vitamin B_{12}. Apart from reports that some algae can synthesize vitamin B_{12} its origin in the food chain seems to be exclusively due to its biosynthesis by microorganisims. Thus, most vitamin B_{12} enters the human food chain from biosynthesis by microorganisms in herbivorous animals. Meat and products such as milk, cheese, or eggs introduce vitamin B_{12} into the human food chain. Chickens ingest food contaminated with microbes and introduce the vitamin via their meat and eggs. Vegetarians who have milk or

eggs (lacto ovo vegetarians) as part of their diet and thus a source of some, albeit reduced, dietary vitamin B_{12} still have reduced vitamin B_{12} status. Yet other communities who for religious or other reasons are strict vegetarians (vegans) have no source of vitamin B_{12} and are at high risk of deficiency. This risk can be reduced in some of these communities where fermented food is eaten, in which bacteria have introduced vitamin B_{12}; also, it has been suggested that in some circumstances the food is contaminated by bacteria. However, vegans and in particular babies born to and weaned by strict vegan women are established to be at risk of vitamin B_{12} deficiency and such babies have been reported on several occasions to show the signs and symptoms of the neuropathy associated with such deficiency.

Malabsorption

The majority of cases of vitamin B_{12} deficiency, particularly severe deficiency, are due to malabsorption. While vitamin B_{12} is a water-soluble vitamin it is extremely large and only between 1 and 3% of any specific dose will cross the intestinal wall by diffusion. Thus, the normal physiological absorption of vitamin B_{12} is dependent upon it forming a complex with a glycoprotein that is secreted by the parietal cells of the stomach called intrinsic factor (IF). The most classical case where IF is deficient or absent is in the autoimmune pernicious anemia (PA). The most usual presentation of this condition is where antibodies are produced against the parietal cells rendering them incapable of secretion not only of IF but also hydrochloric acid (HCl) leading to hypochlorhydria. Yet another form sees autoantibodies produced against IF itself rendering it incapable of binding vitamin B_{12} with consequent malabsorption of the IF-B_{12} complex in the ileum, where specific receptors are responsible for the active absorption of vitamin B_{12}. There is some evidence that many elderly people, perhaps even the majority, suffer to varying degrees from gastric atrophy. In such circumstances while they may still have an adequate supply of IF they lack a competent secretion of HCl. It is suggested that this acid and the accompanying action of pepsin is necessary to release vitamin B_{12} from the form in which it is present in food. The consequences would be varying degrees of malabsorption of food-bound vitamin B_{12} but an ability to absorb the free form of the vitamin present in foods fortified with vitamin B_{12} or from supplements. Other now infrequent causes of vitamin B_{12} malabsorption are resections of the stomach or removal of the ileum, the site of absorption.

Treatment of Folate Deficiency

If the deficiency is nutritional it is usually treated in the first instance with dietary supplements. In the past, daily supplements of $5.0\,\mathrm{mg\,day^{-1}}$ have been used but more recent evidence suggests that such high levels would only be appropriate for the immediate treatment of an overt deficiency. More long-term treatment would recommend dietary changes to improve folate intake. In practice, to achieve effective changes is very difficult so the recommendation might be to improve intake through foods fortified with the synthetic form of the vitamin, namely folic acid, or the use of supplements of folic acid. In both of these instances the aim is to achieve a maximum increased intake via folic acid of $400\,\mathrm{\mu g\,day^{-1}}$. Long-term ingestion of larger amounts are not recommended because of their ability to mask the diagnosis of vitamin B_{12} deficiencies (discussed above). Other causes of folate deficiency are treated by removing the cause, e.g., alcohol abuse.

Treatment of Vitamin B_{12} Deficiency

If the cause of the deficiency is nutritional, dietary supplements containing vitamin B_{12} (usually $2.0\,\mathrm{\mu g\,day^{-1})}$ should be taken.

If the deficiency is due to malabsorption, apart from where the vitamin B_{12} deficiency may be due to gastric atrophy, a dietary remedy is not effective because it will be malabsorbed. Such malabsorption conditions must be treated by regular monthly or bimonthly injections of $1000\,\mathrm{\mu g}$ of vitamin B_{12} for life. If these injections are discontinued a return to the vitamin B_{12} deficiency state is inevitable. This is not only due to malabsorption of dietary vitamin B_{12} but also the 1 or $2\,\mathrm{\mu g}$ of vitamin B_{12} secreted daily in the bile will be malabsorbed leading to negative balance. If the deficiency is due to gastric atrophy, supplements providing $500–1000\,\mathrm{\mu g\,day^{-1}}$ can replete stores and maintain B_{12} status.

Inappropriate Treatment of Vitamin B_{12} Deficiency with Folic Acid

As mentioned above, megaloblastic anemia caused by folate deficiency should not be confused with that caused by vitamin B_{12} deficiency. The subsequent inappropriate treatment with folic acid could have serious and frequently irreversible consequences.

Historically, before there was a clearer understanding of folate metabolism, in vitamin B_{12} deficiency, synthetic folic acid (**Figure 3**) was used in many instances to treat vitamin B_{12} deficiency. This at first appeared to be successful in that continued treatment with folic acid largely reversed the anemia. However, it became clear that at best this masked the underlying concomitant development of the neuropathy, and some data suggest that folic acid exacerbated the neuropathy. In any event, the inappropriate treatment of vitamin B_{12} with folic acid masks the emergence of the anemia. Historically, it appears that about one-third of patients with vitamin B_{12} deficiency present with anemia, one-third with the neuropathy, and one-third with both. In addition, the signs and symptoms associated with the anemia are easily recognizable while those of the neuropathy are less so. The earlier features of the neuropathy such as loss of balance, tingling of the fingers, and mild ataxia can easily be confused with advancing years, which coincides with the usual development of vitamin B_{12} deficiency. This masking of the presence of anemia in vitamin B_{12}-deficient patients by folic acid therapy, potentially causes an early diagnosis to be missed in up to two-thirds of patients. When the vitamin B_{12} deficiency is eventually recognized through the onward and progressive development of the neuropathy some of the pathological features may have reached the stage at which they are irreversible.

See also: **Alcohol**: Disease Risk and Beneficial Effects. **Anemia**: Iron-Deficiency Anemia. **Cobalamins**. **Celiac Disease**. **Folic Acid**.

Further Reading

Bailey LB (1995) *Folate in Health and Disease*. New York: Marcel Dekker.

Chanarin I (1979) *Megaloblastic Anaemias*, 2nd edn. Oxford: Blackwell Scientific.

Chanarin I (1990) *The Megaloblastic Anaemias*, 3rd edn. Oxford: Blackwell Scientific.

Cuskelly CJ, McNulty H, and Scott JM (1996) Effect of increasing dietary folate on red-cell folate; implications for prevention of neural tube defects. *Lancet* 347: 657–659.

Scott JM (1992) Folate-vitamin B_{12} interrelationships in the central nervous system. *Proceedings of the Nutrition Society* 51: 219–224.

Scott JM (1997) Bioavailability of vitamin B_{12}. *European Journal of Clinical Nutrition* 51(supplement 1): S49–S53.

Scott JM and Weir DG (1994) Folate vitamin B_{12} interrelationships. *Essays in Biochemistry* 28: 63–72.

Scott JM and Weir DG (1996) Homocysteine and cardiovascular disease. *Quarterly Journal of Medicine* 89: 561–563.

Wickramasinghe SM (1995) Megaloblastic anaemia. In *Baillière's Clinical Haematology*, vol. 8. London: Baillière Tindall.

ANTIOXIDANTS

Contents
Diet and Antioxidant Defense
Observational Studies
Intervention Studies

Diet and Antioxidant Defense

I F F Benzie, The Hong Kong Polytechnic University, Hong Kong SAR, China
J J Strain, University of Ulster, Coleraine, UK

© 2005 Elsevier Ltd. All rights reserved.

Introduction

Oxygen is an essential 'nutrient' for most organisms. Paradoxically, however, oxygen damages key biological sites. This has led to oxygen being referred to as a double-edged sword. The beneficial side of oxygen is that it permits energy-efficient catabolism of fuel by acting as the ultimate electron acceptor within mitochondria. During aerobic respiration, an oxygen atom accepts two electrons, forming (with hydrogen) harmless water. The less friendly side of oxygen is the unavoidable and continuous production of partially reduced oxygen intermediates within the body. These 'free radicals' (reactive oxygen species; ROS) are more reactive than ground-state oxygen and cause oxidative changes to carbohydrate, DNA, lipid, and protein. Such changes can affect the structures and functions of macromolecules, organelles, cells, and biological systems. This induces oxidant stress if allowed to proceed unopposed.

The human body is generally well equipped with an array of 'antioxidative' strategies to protect against the damaging effects of ROS. Our endogenous antioxidants are inadequate, however, as we are unable to synthesize at least two important antioxidant compounds, vitamin C and vitamin E. Ingestion of these, and perhaps other, antioxidants is needed to augment our defenses and prevent or minimize oxidative damage. In this article, the causes and consequences of oxidant stress and the types and action of antioxidants will be described, the source and role of dietary antioxidants will be discussed, and current evidence relating to dietary antioxidants and human health will be briefly reviewed.

Oxidant Stress

Oxidant, or oxidative, stress is a pro-oxidant shift in the oxidant–antioxidant balance caused by a relative or absolute deficiency of antioxidants (**Figure 1**). A pro-oxidant shift promotes damaging oxidative changes to important cellular constituents, and this may, in turn, lead to cellular dysfunction and, ultimately, to aging, disability, and disease.

Molecular oxygen is relatively unreactive in its ground state. However, molecular oxygen can be reduced in several ways within the body to produce more reactive species (**Table 1**). These species include radical and nonradical forms of oxygen, some of which contain nitrogen or chlorine. A 'free radical' is capable of independent existence and has a single (unpaired) electron in an orbital. Electrons

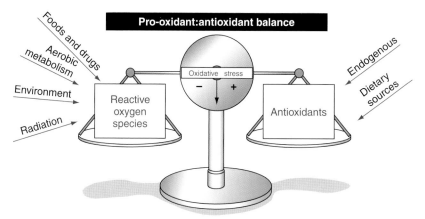

Figure 1 Antioxidant defenses balance reactive oxygen species load and oppose oxidant stress.

stabilize as pairs with opposing spins within an orbital. An unpaired electron seeks a partner for stability, and this increases the reactivity of the radical. A partner electron can be obtained by removing ('abstracting') an electron from another species or co-reactant. The result of this interaction may be either quenching by reduction (electron addition) of the radical with the production of a new radical by oxidation (electron loss) of the reductive ('antioxidant') co-reactant or quenching of two radicals if the co-reactant is also a radical (one quenched by reduction (electron addition) and one by oxidation (electron removal)).

Free radicals produced *in vivo* include superoxide, the hydroxyl radical, nitric oxide, oxygen-centered organic radicals such as peroxyl and alkoxyl radicals, and sulfur-centered thiyl radicals. Other oxygen-containing reactive species that are not radicals are also formed. These include hydrogen peroxide, peroxynitrite, and hypochlorous acid. While these are not radical species, they are actually or potentially damaging oxidants. The collective term ROS is often used to describe both radical and nonradical species.

What Causes Oxidant Stress?

Oxidant stress is caused by the damaging action of ROS. There are two main routes of production of ROS in the body: one is deliberate and useful; the other is accidental but unavoidable (**Figure 2**). Deliberate production of ROS is seen, for example,

Table 1 Reactive oxygen species found *in vivo* in general order of reactivity (from lowest to highest)

Name of species	Sign/formula	Radical (R) or nonradical (NR)	Comment
Molecular oxygen	O_2	R	Biradical, with two unpaired electrons; these are in parallel spins, and this limits reactivity
Nitric oxide	$NO^{\cdot}$	R	Important to maintain normal vasomotor tone
Superoxide	$O_2^{\cdot-}$	R	Single electron reduction product of O_2; large amounts produced *in vivo*
Peroxyl	$ROO^{\cdot}$	R	R is often a carbon of an unsaturated fatty acid
Singlet oxygen	$^1\Delta_g O_2$ $^1\Sigma_g^+ O_2$	NR	'Energized' nonradical forms of molecular oxygen; one unpaired electron is transferred to the same orbital as the other unpaired electron
Hydrogen peroxide	H_2O_2	NR	Small, uncharged, freely diffusible ROS formed by dismutation of superoxide
Hydroperoxyl	$HOO^{\cdot}$	R	Protonated, more reactive form of superoxide; formed at sites of low pH
Alkoxyl	$RO^{\cdot}$	R	R is carbon in a carbon-centered radical formed by peroxidation of unsaturated fatty acid
Hypochlorous	$HOCl$	NR	Formed in activated phagocytes to aid in microbial killing
Peroxynitrite	$HNOO^-$	NR	Highly reactive product of nitric oxide and superoxide
Hydroxyl	$^{\cdot}OH$	R	Fiercely, indiscriminately reactive radical

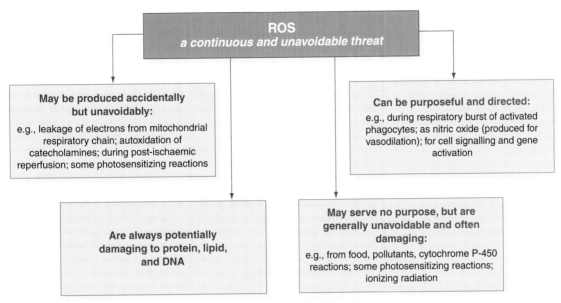

Figure 2 Sources of reactive oxygen species found *in vivo*.

during the respiratory burst of activated phagocytic white cells (macrophages, neutrophils, and monocytes). Activated phagocytes produce large amounts of superoxide and hypochlorous acid for microbial killing. The ROS nitric oxide is produced constitutively and inducibly, is a powerful vasodilator, and is vital for the maintenance of normal blood pressure. Nitric oxide also decreases platelet aggregability, decreasing the likelihood of the blood clotting within the circulation. Hydrogen peroxide is produced enzymatically from superoxide by the action of the superoxide dismutases (SODs) and is recognized increasingly as playing a central role in cell signalling and gene activation. Nonetheless, while some ROS are physiologically useful, they are damaging if they accumulate in excess as a result of, for example, acute or chronic inflammation or ischaemia.

Accidental, but unavoidable, production of ROS occurs during the passage of electrons along the mitochondrial electron transport chain. Leakage of electrons from the chain leads to the single-electron reduction of oxygen, with the consequent formation of superoxide. This can be regarded as a normal, but undesirable, by-product of aerobic metabolism. Around 1–3% of electrons entering the respiratory chain are estimated to end up in superoxide, and this results in a large daily ROS load *in vivo*. If anything increases oxygen use, such as exercise, then more ROS will be formed, and oxidant stress may increase owing to a pro-oxidant shift. Significant amounts of ROS are also produced during the metabolism of drugs and pollutants by the mixed-function cytochrome P-450 oxidase (phase I) detoxifying system

and as a consequence of the transformation of xanthine dehydrogenase to its truncated oxidase form, which occurs as a result of ischemia. This causes a flood of superoxide to be formed when the oxygen supply is restored. In addition, if free iron is present (as may happen in iron overload, acute intravascular hemolysis, or cell injury), there is a risk of a cycle of ROS production via iron-catalyzed 'autoxidation' of various constituents in biological fluids, including ascorbic acid, catecholamines, dopamine, hemoglobin, flavins, and thiol compounds such as cysteine or homocysteine. Preformed reactive species in food further contribute to the oxidant load of the body, and ROS are also produced by pathological processes and agents such as chronic inflammation, infection, ionizing radiation, and cigarette smoke. Breathing oxygen-enriched air results in enhanced production of ROS within the lungs, and various toxins and drugs, such as aflatoxin, acetaminophen, carbon tetrachloride, chloroform, and ethanol, produce reactive radical species during their metabolism or detoxification and excretion by the liver or kidneys. Clearly, all body tissues are exposed to ROS on a regular or even constant basis. However, sites of particularly high ROS loads within the human body include the mitochondria, the eyes, the skin, areas of cell damage, inflammation, and post-ischemic reperfusion, the liver, the lungs (especially if oxygen-enriched air is breathed), and the brain.

What does Oxidant Stress Cause?

A sudden and large increase in ROS load can overwhelm local antioxidant defenses and induce severe oxidant stress, with cell damage, cell death, and subsequent organ failure. However, less dramatic chronic oxidant stress may lead to depletion of defenses and accumulation of damage and ultimately cause physiological dysfunction and pathological change resulting in disability and disease. This is because oxidant stress causes oxidative changes to DNA, lipid, and protein. These changes lead in turn to DNA breaks, mutagenesis, changed phenotypic expression, membrane disruption, mitochondrial dysfunction, adenosine triphosphate depletion, intracellular accumulation of non-degradable oxidized proteins, increased atherogenicity of low-density lipoproteins, and crosslinking of proteins with subsequent loss of function of specialized protein structures, for example, enzymes, receptors, and the crystallins of the ocular lens. In addition, the aldehydic degradation products of oxidized polyunsaturated fatty acids (PUFAs) are carcinogenic and cytotoxic. Increased oxidant stress can also trigger apoptosis, or programed cell death, through a changed redox balance, damage to membrane ion-transport channels, and increased intracellular calcium levels (**Figure 3**).

Oxidant stress, through its effects on key biological sites and structures, is implicated in chronic noncommunicable diseases such as coronary heart disease, cancer, cataract, dementia, and stroke (**Figure 4**). Oxidant stress is also thought to be a key player in the aging process itself. A cause-and-effect relationship between oxidant stress and aging and disease has not been confirmed, however, and it is very unlikely that oxidant stress is the sole cause of aging and chronic degenerative disease. Nonetheless, there is evidence that oxidant stress contributes substantially to age-related physiological decline and pathological changes. Consequently, if it is accepted that oxidant stress is associated with aging and degenerative disease, then opposing oxidant stress by increasing antioxidant defense offers a potentially effective means of delaying the deleterious effects of aging, decreasing the risk of chronic disease, and achieving functional longevity. For this reason, there has been great interest in recent years in the source, action, and potential health benefits of dietary antioxidants.

Antioxidant Defense

An antioxidant can be described in simple terms as anything that can delay or prevent oxidation of a susceptible substrate. Our antioxidant system is complex, however, and consists of various intracellular and extracellular, endogenous and exogenous, and aqueous and lipid-soluble components that act in concert to prevent ROS formation (preventative antioxidants), destroy or inactivate ROS that are formed (scavenging and enzymatic antioxidants), and terminate chains of ROS-initiated peroxidation of biological substrates (chain-breaking antioxidants). In addition, metals and minerals (such as selenium, copper, and zinc) that are key components of antioxidant enzymes are often referred to as antioxidants.

There are many biological and dietary constituents that show 'antioxidant' properties *in vitro*. For an antioxidant to have a physiological role, however, certain criteria must be met.

1. The antioxidant must be able to react with ROS found at the site(s) in the body where the putative antioxidant is found.
2. Upon interacting with a ROS, the putative antioxidant must not be transformed into a more reactive species than the original ROS.
3. The antioxidant must be found in sufficient quantity at the site of its presumed action *in vivo* for it to make an appreciable contribution to defense at that site: if its concentration is very low, there must be some way of continuously recycling or resupplying the putative antioxidant.

Antioxidants Found Within the Human Body

The structures of the human body are exposed continuously to a variety of ROS. Humans have evolved an effective antioxidant system to defend against these damaging agents. Different sites of the body contain different antioxidants or contain the same antioxidants but in different amounts. Differences are likely to reflect the different requirements and characteristics of these sites.

Human plasma and other biological fluids are generally rich in scavenging and chain-breaking antioxidants, including vitamin C (ascorbic acid) and 'vitamin E.' Vitamin E is the name given to a group of eight lipid-soluble tocopherols and tocotrienols. In the human diet, γ-tocopherol is the main form of vitamin E, but the predominant form in human plasma is α-tocopherol. Bilirubin, uric acid, glutathione, flavonoids, and carotenoids also have antioxidant activity and are found in cells and/or plasma. Scavenging and chain-breaking antioxidants found *in vivo* are derived overall from both endogenous and exogenous sources. Cells contain, in addition, antioxidant enzymes, the SODs, glutathione peroxidase, and catalase. The transition

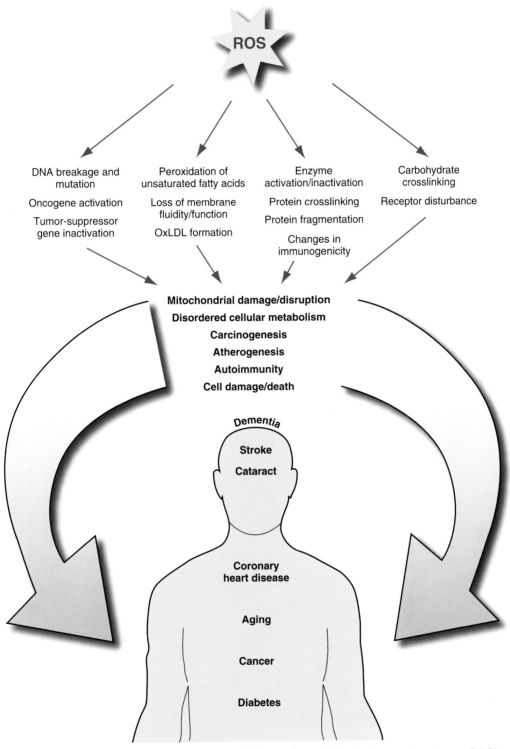

Figure 3 Possible involvement of reactive oxygen species (ROS) in ageing and chronic degenerative disease. OxLDL, oxidized low density lipoprotein.

metals iron and copper, which can degrade pre-existing peroxides and form highly reactive ROS, are kept out of the peroxidation equation by being tightly bound to, or incorporated within, specific proteins such as transferrin and ferritin (for iron) and caeruloplasmin (for copper). These proteins are regarded as preventive antioxidants. Caerulo-plasmin ferroxidase activity is also important for

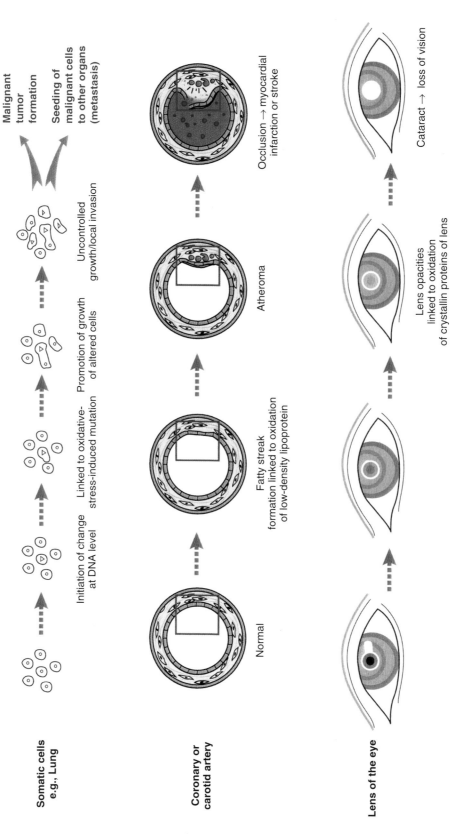

Figure 4 Antioxidants may help prevent the long-term oxidative changes to DNA, lipid, and protein that lead to age-related disease.

Table 2 Types of antioxidants

Physical barriers *prevent* ROS generation or ROS access to important biological sites; e.g., UV filters, cell membranes
Chemical traps or sinks 'absorb' energy and electrons and *quench* ROS; e.g., carotenoids, anthocyanidins
Catalytic systems *neutralize or divert* ROS, e.g., the antioxidant enzymes superoxide dismutase, catalase, and glutathione peroxidase
Binding and redox inactivation of metal ions *prevent generation* of ROS by inhibiting the Haber–Weiss reaction; e.g., ferritin, caeruloplasmin, catechins
Sacrificial and chain-breaking antioxidants *scavenge and destroy* ROS; e.g., ascorbic acid (vitamin C), tocopherols (vitamin E), uric acid, glutathione, flavonoids

ROS, reactive oxygen species.

the non-ROS-producing route of ferrous (Fe(II)) to ferric (Fe(III)) oxidation and for incorporating released iron into ferritin for 'safe' iron storage. Haptoglobin (which binds released hemoglobin), hemopexin (which binds released hem), and albumin (which binds transition-metal ions and localizes or absorbs their oxidative effects) can also be regarded as antioxidants in that they protect against metal-ion-catalyzed redox reactions that may produce ROS. An overview of the major types of antioxidants within the body and their interactions is given in **Table 2** and **Figure 5**.

Dietary Antioxidants

The human endogenous antioxidant system is impressive but incomplete. Regular and adequate dietary intakes of (largely) plant-based antioxidants, most notably vitamin C, vitamin E, and folic acid, are needed. Fresh fruits and vegetables are rich in antioxidants (**Figure 6**), and epidemiological evidence of protection by diets rich in fruits and vegetables is strong. To decrease the risk of cancer of various sites, five or more servings per day of fruits and vegetables are recommended. However, it is not known whether it is one, some, or all antioxidant(s) that are the key protective agents in these foods. Furthermore, it may be that antioxidants are simple co-travellers with other, as yet unidentified, components of antioxidant-rich foods. Perhaps antioxidants are not 'magic bullets' but rather 'magic markers' of protective elements. Nonetheless, the US recommended daily intakes (RDIs) for vitamin C and vitamin E were increased in 2000 in recognition of the strong evidence that regular high intakes of these antioxidant vitamins are associated with a decreased risk of chronic disease and with lower all-cause mortality.

To date, research on dietary antioxidant micronutrients has concentrated mainly on vitamin C and vitamin E. This is likely to be because humans have an undoubted requirement for these antioxidants, which we cannot synthesize and must obtain in regular adequate amounts from food. However, there are a plethora of other dietary antioxidants. Some or all of the thousands of carotenoids, flavonoids, and phenolics found in plant-based foods, herbs, and beverages, such as teas and wines, may also be important for human health, although there are currently no RDIs for these. Furthermore, while there are recommended intakes for vitamin C, vitamin E, and folic acid, these vary among countries, and there is currently no agreement as regards the 'optimal' intake for health. In addition, there is growing evidence that other dietary constituents with antioxidant properties, such as quercetin and catechins (found in teas, wines, apples, and onions), lycopene, lutein, and zeaxanthin (found in tomatoes, spinach, and herbs) contribute to human health. Zinc (found especially in lamb, leafy and root vegetables, and shellfish) and selenium (found especially in beef, cereals, nuts, and fish) are incorporated into the antioxidant enzymes SOD and glutathione peroxidase, and the elements are themselves sometimes referred to as antioxidants.

The levels of ascorbic acid, α-tocopherol, folic acid, carotenoids, and flavonoids within the body are maintained by dietary intake. While the role and importance of dietary antioxidants are currently unclear, antioxidant defense can be modulated by increasing or decreasing the intake of foods containing these antioxidants. There are a number of reasons for recommending dietary changes in preference to supplementation for achieving increased antioxidant status, as follows.

1. It is not clear which antioxidants confer protection.
2. The hierarchy of protection may vary depending on body conditions.
3. A cooperative mix of antioxidants is likely to be more effective than an increased intake of one antioxidant.
4. Antioxidants, including vitamin A, β-carotene, vitamin C, selenium, and copper, can be harmful in large doses or under certain circumstances.
5. Antioxidant status is likely to be affected by the overall composition of the diet, e.g., the fatty-acid and phytochemical mix.
6. The iron status of the body, environmental conditions, and lifestyle undoubtedly affect antioxidant demand.

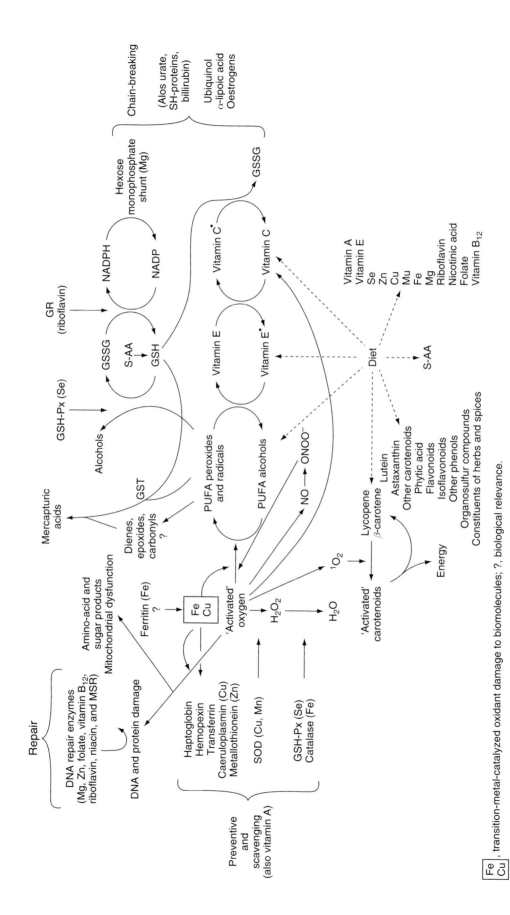

Figure 5 The integrated antioxidant defense system comprises both endogenous and dietary-derived antioxidants. GR, glutathione reductase (EC1.6.4.2); GSH, reduced glutathione; GSH-Px, glutathione peroxidase (EC1.11.1.9); GSSG, oxidized glutathione; GST, glutathione-S-transferase (EC 2.5.1.18); MSR, methionine sulfoxide reductase (EC1.8.4.5); NADPH and, NADP, are, respectively, the reduced and oxidized forms of the co-factor nicotinamide adenine dinucleotide phosphate; PUFA, polyunsaturated fatty acid; S-AA, sulfur amino-acids; SH, sulfydryl; SOD, superoxide dismutase (EC1.15.1.1).

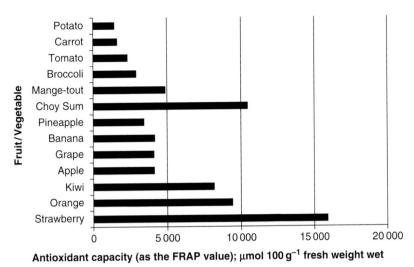

Figure 6 Antioxidant capacity varies among different fruits and vegetables. FRAP, Ferric Reducing/Anti-oxidant Power.

Antioxidant defense, therefore, is likely to be optimized through a balanced intake of a variety of antioxidants from natural sources rather than by pharmacological doses of one or a few antioxidants.

Dietary Recommendations for Increased Antioxidant Defense

Dietary recommendations that would result in increased antioxidant defense are not inconsistent with accepted recommendations for healthy eating. The recommendation to increase the consumption of plant-based foods and beverages is one that is widely perceived as health promoting, and the consistent and strong epidemiological links between high fruit and vegetable intake and the greater life expectancy seen in various groups worldwide whose diet is high in plant-based foods indicate that more emphasis should be given to this particular dietary recommendation. Vitamin C, vitamin E, various carotenoids, flavonoids, isoflavonoids, phenolic acids, organosulfur compounds, folic acid, copper, zinc, and selenium are all important for antioxidant defense, and these are found in plant-based foods and beverages such as fruits, vegetables, nuts, seeds, teas, herbs, and wines. Dietary strategies for health promotion should be directed towards optimizing the consumption of these items.

It is recommended generally that at least five servings of fruits and vegetables are eaten each day. This recommendation is based on a wealth of epidemiological evidence that, overall, indicates that 30–40% of all cancers can be prevented by diet. However, it is estimated that most individuals in developed countries eat less than half this amount of fruits and vegetables, and intake by people in developing nations is often very low. Furthermore, the antioxidant contents (both of individual antioxidants and in total) of foods vary widely among different food items and even within the same food item, depending on storage, processing, and cooking method. In addition, the issues of bioavailability and distribution must be considered, and it is of interest to see where dietary antioxidants accumulate (**Table 3**). Vitamin C is absorbed well at low doses and is concentrated in nucleated cells and in the eyes, but relative absorption within the gastrointestinal tract decreases as dose ingested increases. Of the eight isomers of 'vitamin E,' α-tocopherol and γ-tocopherol are distributed around the body and are found in various sites, including skin and adipose tissue. Vitamin E protects lipid systems, such as membranes and lipoproteins. While α-tocopherol is by far the predominant form in human lipophilic structures, there is limited information on the bioavailabilities and roles of the other isomers. Gastrointestinal absorption of catechins (a type of flavonoid found in high quantity in tea) is very low, and, although it has been shown that plasma antioxidant capacity increases after ingesting catechin-rich green tea, catechins appear to be excreted via the urine fairly rapidly. Some are likely to be taken up by membranes and cells, although this is not clear, but most of the flavonoids ingested are likely to remain within the gastrointestinal tract. However, this does not necessarily mean that they have no role to play in antioxidant defense, as the unabsorbed antioxidants may provide local defense to the gut lining (**Figure 7**).

With regard to plasma and intracellular distributions of dietary antioxidants, if it is confirmed that

Table 3 Dietary antioxidants: source, bioavailability, and concentrations in human plasma

	Dietary source	Bioavailability	Concentration	Comment
Ascorbic acid (vitamin C)	Fruits and vegetables, particularly strawberries, citrus, kiwi, Brussels sprouts, and cauliflower	100% at low doses (<100 mg) decreasing to <15% at >10 g	25–80 μmol l^{-1}	Unstable at neutral pH, concentrated in cells and the eye
'Vitamin E' (in humans mainly α-tocopherol)	Green leafy vegetables, e.g., spinach, nuts, seeds, especially wheatgerm, vegetable oils, especially sunflower	10–95%, but limited hepatic uptake of absorbed tocopherol	15–40 μmol l^{-1} (depending on vitamin supply and lipid levels)	Major tocopherol in diet is γ form, but α form is preferentially taken up by human liver
Carotenoids (hundreds)	Orange/red fruits and vegetables (carrot, tomato, apricot, melon, yam), green leafy vegetables	Unclear, dose and form dependent, probably <15%	Very low (<1 μmol l^{-1})	Lutein and zeaxanthin are concentrated in macula region of the eye
Flavonoids (enormous range of different types)	Berries, apples, onions, tea, red wine, some herbs (parsley, thyme), citrus fruits, grapes, cherries	Most poorly absorbed, quercetin absorption 20–50%, catechins <2%, dependent on form and dose	No data for most, likely <3 μmol l^{-1} in total	Quercetin and catechins may be most relevant to humans health as intake is relatively high, there is some absorption, possible gastrointestinal-tract protection by unabsorbed flavonoids

increasing defense by dietary means is desirable, frequent small doses of antioxidant-rich food may be the most effective way to achieve this. Furthermore, ingestion of those foods with the highest antioxidant contents may be the most cost-effective strategy. For example, it has been estimated that around 100 mg of ascorbic acid (meeting the recently revised US RDI for vitamin C) is supplied by one orange, a few strawberries, one kiwi fruit, two slices of pineapple, or a handful of raw cauliflower or uncooked spinach leaves. Interestingly, apples, bananas, pears, and plums, which are probably the most commonly consumed fruits in Western countries, are very low in vitamin C. However, these, and other, fruits contain a significant amount of antioxidant power, which is conferred by a variety of other scavenging and chain-breaking antioxidants (**Figure 6**).

Dietary Antioxidants and Human Health

Plants produce a very impressive array of antioxidant compounds, including carotenoids, flavonoids, cinnamic acids, benzoic acids, folic acid, ascorbic acid, tocopherols, and tocotrienols, and plant-based foods are our major source of dietary antioxidants. Antioxidant compounds are concentrated in the oxidation-prone sites of the plant, such as the oxygen-producing chloroplast and the PUFA-rich seeds and oils. Plants make antioxidants to protect their own structures from oxidant stress, and plants increase antioxidant synthesis at times of additional need and when environmental conditions are particularly harsh.

Humans also can upregulate the synthesis of endogenous antioxidants, but this facility is very limited. For example, production of the antioxidant enzyme SOD is increased with regular exercise, presumably as an adaptation to the increased ROS load resulting from higher oxygen use. However, an increase in other endogenous antioxidants, such as bilirubin and uric acid, is associated with disease, not with improved health. Increasing the antioxidant status of the body by purposefully increasing the production of these antioxidants, therefore, is not a realistic strategy. However, the concept that increased antioxidant intake leads to increased antioxidant defense, conferring increased protection against oxidant stress and, thereby, decreasing the risk of disease, is a simple and attractive one. Antioxidant defense can be modulated by varying the dietary intake of foods rich in natural antioxidants. It has been shown that following ingestion of an antioxidant-rich food, drink, or herb the antioxidant

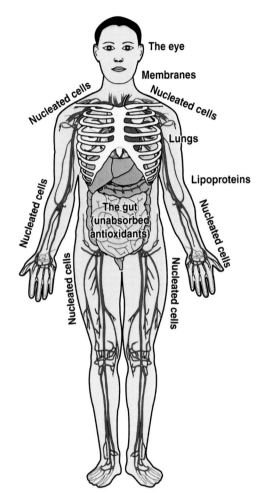

Figure 7 Dietary antioxidants are absorbed and distributed to various sites within the human body.

status of the plasma does indeed increase. The question remains, however, as to whether increasing the antioxidant defense of the body by dietary means, while achievable, is a desirable strategy to promote human health and well-being.

There are many age-related disorders that, in theory at least, may be prevented or delayed by increased antioxidant defense. These disorders include arthritis, cancer, coronary heart disease, cataract, dementia, hypertension, macular degeneration, the metabolic complications of diabetes mellitus, and stroke. The rationale for prevention of disease by antioxidants is based on the following facts.

1. Epidemiological evidence shows that a high intake of antioxidant-rich foods, and in some cases antioxidant supplements, is associated with a lower risk of these diseases.
2. Experimental evidence shows that oxidation of cells and structures (such as low-density lipoprotein, DNA, membranes, proteins, and mitochondria) is increased in individuals suffering from these disorders.
3. Experimental evidence shows that antioxidants protect protein, lipid, and DNA from oxidative damage.
4. Experimental evidence shows that biomarkers of oxidative damage to key structures are ameliorated by an increased intake of dietary antioxidants.

However, the following cautionary statements must be noted.

1. While there is a large body of observational evidence supporting a protective effect of dietary antioxidants, it has been suggested that the importance of this has been overstated, and recent studies are less supportive.
2. While phenomenological evidence is strong that oxidative damage does occur in aging and in chronic degenerative diseases, cause-and-effect relationships have not been confirmed.
3. While experimental evidence is quite strong, studies have generally been performed *in vitro* using very high concentrations of antioxidants, making their physiological relevance unclear.
4. Evidence from intervention trials is of variable quality and conflicting; animal studies have shown positive results but have often used very high does of antioxidants, and the relevance to human health is unclear; large human intervention trials completed to date, such as the α-Tocopherol β-Carotene Cancer Prevention Study, Gruppo Italiano per Io Studio Delia Sopravivenza nell'Infarto Miocardico, the Heart Protection Study, the Heart Outcomes Prevention Evaluation, and the Primary Prevention Project, have been largely disappointing in that they have not shown the expected benefits. These studies are summarized in **Table 4**.

Overall, observational data are supportive of beneficial effects of diets rich in antioxidants (**Figure 8**), and intervention trials have often used high-risk groups or individuals with established disease (**Table 4**). In addition, intervention trials have generally used antioxidant supplements (usually vitamin C or vitamin E) rather than antioxidant mixtures or antioxidant-rich foods. Therefore, while observational data support a role for antioxidant-rich food in health promotion, whether or not it is the antioxidants in the food that are responsible for the benefit remains to be confirmed.

Table 4 Summary of completed large antioxidant intervention trials

Name and aim of study	Subjects	Supplementation	Results/comments	Reference
The α-tocopherol β-carotene cancer prevention study (ATBC); primary prevention	29 133 high-risk subjects (male smokers, 50–69 years old; average of 20 cigarettes day^{-1} smoked for 36 years)	50 mg day^{-1} of α-tocopherol (synthetic) or 20 mg day^{-1} of β-carotene, or both, or placebo, for 5–8 years (median follow-up 6.1 years)	Supplementation with α-tocopherol had no effect on lung-cancer incidence; no evidence of interaction between α-tocopherol and β-carotene; significant increase in fatal coronary events in men with history of heart disease, and 18% increase in lung-cancer incidence in β-carotene supplemented men; follow-up showed significant (32%) decrease in risk of prostate cancer and nonsignificant (8%) decrease in fatal coronary heart disease in α-tocopherol supplemented subjects	The Alpha-tocopherol, Beta-carotene Cancer Prevention Study Group (1994) *Journal of the National Cancer Institute* 88: 1560–1570 Pryor WA (2000) *Free Radical Biology and Medicine* 28: 141–164
The Cambridge Heart Antioxidant Study (CHAOS); secondary prevention	2002 high-risk subjects (angiographically proven cardiovascular disease)	d-α-tocopherol 400 IU or 800 IU per day (median follow-up 510 days; results on different doses combined into one treatment group)	Significant decrease (77%) in non-fatal MI in treatment group; slight nonsignificant (18%) increase in fatal cardiovascular events in treatment group, but most (21/27) in noncompliant subjects	Stephens NG *et al.* (1996) *Lancet 347*: 781–786
Gruppo Italiano per lo Studio Delia Sopravivenza nell'Infarto Miocardico (GISSI); secondary prevention	11 324 survivors of MI within previous 3 months of enrollment	α-tocopherol (synthetic) 300 mg day^{-1} or omega 3 fatty acids (0.9 g day^{-1}) or both or neither for 3.5 years; subjects continued on normal medication (50% on statins)	Nonsignificant decrease (11%) in primary endpoints (death, nonfatal MI, and stroke) with vitamin E; high dropout rate (25%); open label study	Marchioli R (1999) *Lancet 354*: 447–455

Continued

Table 4 Continued

Name and aim of study	Subjects	Supplementation	Results/comments	Reference
Primary Prevention Project (PPP)	4495 subjects with ≥1 major cardiovascular risk factor	α-tocopherol (synthetic) 300 mg day^{-1} or aspirin 100 mg day^{-1} or both or neither, follow-up average of 3.6 years	Vitamin E had no significant effect on any primary endpoint (cardiovascular death, MI, or stroke)	Primary Prevention Project (2001) Lancet 357: 89–95
The Heart Outcomes Prevention Evaluation Study (HOPE); secondary prevention	9541 subjects (2545 women, 6996 men) aged ≥55 years, high-risk (cardiovascular disease or diabetes and ≥1 other CVD risk factor)	400 IU day^{-1} vitamin E (from 'natural sources') or Ramipril (angiotensin converting enzyme inhibitor) or both or neither; follow-up for 4–6 years	No significant effect of vitamin E on any primary endpoint (MI, stroke, or cardiovascular death)	The Heart Outcomes Prevention Evaluation Study Investigators (2000) New England Journal of Medicine 342: 154–160
Heart Protection Study	20 536 subjects, high-risk (diabetes, peripheral vascular disease or coronary heart disease)	Daily antioxidant cocktail (600 IU dl-α-tocopherol, 250 mg vitamin C, 20 mg β-carotene) or placebo for 5 years	No significant differences in hemorrhagic stroke or all-cause mortality between treatment and placebo groups	The Heart Protection Study Collaborative Group (2002) Lancet 360: 23–32

MI, myocardial infarction; CVD, cardiovascular disease.

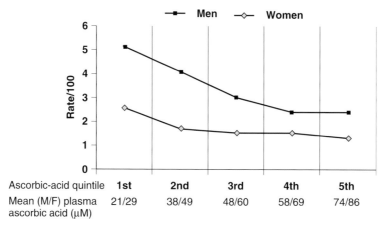

Figure 8 Age-adjusted rates of all-cause mortality by sex-specific ascorbic-acid quintiles in 8860 British men (squares) and 10 636 British women (diamonds).

Summary and Concluding Remarks

Our diet contains a multitude of antioxidants that we cannot synthesize, and most are plant-based. The available evidence supports a role for antioxidant-rich foods in the promotion of health, although it is not yet clear how many antioxidants and how much of each are needed to achieve an optimal status of antioxidant defense and minimize disease risk. Nor is it clear whether the benefit is of a threshold type or whether it continues to increase with the amount of antioxidant ingested. It is also not yet known whether those dietary antioxidants for which there is no absolute known requirement play a significant role in human antioxidant defense and health or whether they are merely coincidental co-travellers with other, as yet unknown, antioxidant or nonantioxidant dietary constituents that have beneficial effects. A reasonable recommendation is to eat a variety of antioxidant-rich foods on a regular basis. This is likely to be beneficial and is not associated with any harmful effects. However, further study is needed before firm conclusions can be drawn regarding the long-term health benefits of increasing antioxidant defense per se, whether through food or supplements. The challenge in nutritional and biomedical science remains to develop tools that will allow the measurement of biomarkers of functional and nutritional status and to clarify human requirements for dietary antioxidants, the goal being the design of nutritional strategies to promote health and functional longevity.

Acknowledgments

The authors thank The Hong Kong Polytechnic University and The University of Ulster for financially supporting this work.

See also: **Antioxidants**: Observational Studies; Intervention Studies. **Ascorbic Acid**: Physiology, Dietary Sources and Requirements. **Carotenoids**: Chemistry, Sources and Physiology; Epidemiology of Health Effects. **Copper. Folic Acid. Fruits and Vegetables. Iron. Riboflavin. Selenium. Vitamin E**: Physiology and Health Effects. **Zinc**: Physiology.

Further Reading

Ames BN and Wakimoto P (2002) Are vitamin and mineral deficiencies a major cancer risk? *Nature Reviews* 2: 694–704.

Asplund K (2002) Antioxidant vitamins in the prevention of cardiovascular disease: a systematic review. *Journal of Internal Medicine* 251: 372–392.

Benzie IFF (2003) Evolution of dietary antioxidants. *Journal of Comparative Biochemistry and Physiology* 136: 113–126.

Block G, Norkus E, Hudes M, Mandel S, and Helzlsouer K (2001) Which plasma antioxidants are most related to fruit and vegetable consumption? *American Journal of Epidemiology* 154: 1113–1118.

Chisholm GM and Steinberg D (2000) The oxidative modification hypothesis of atherogenesis: an overview. *Free Radical Biology and Medicine* 28: 1815–1826.

Clarkson PM and Thompson HS (2000) Antioxidants: what role do they play in physical activity and health? *American Journal of Clinical Nutrition* 72(Supplement 2): 637S–646S.

Cooke MS, Evans MD, Mistry N, and Lunec J (2002) Role of dietary antioxidants in the prevention of *in vivo* oxidative DNA damage. *Nutrition Research Reviews* 15: 19–41.

Halliwell B and Gutteridge JMC (1999) *Free Radicals in Biology and Medicine*, 3rd edn. Oxford: Clarendon Press.

Khaw KT, Bingham S, Welch A *et al.* (2001) Relation between plasma ascorbic acid and mortality in men and women in EPIC-Norfolk prospective study: a prospective population study. *Lancet* 357: 657–663.

Levine M, Wang Y, Padayatty SJ, and Morrow J (2001) A new recommended dietary allowance of vitamin C for healthy young women. *Proceedings of the National Academy of Science USA* 98: 9842–9846.

Lindsay DG and Clifford MN (eds.) (2000) Critical reviews produced within the EU Concerted Action 'Nutritional

Enhancement of Plant-Based Food in European Trade' (NEO-DIET). *Journal of the Science of Food Agriculture* 80: 793–1137.

McCall MR and Frei B (1999) Can antioxidant vitamins materially reduce oxidative damage in humans? *Free Radical Biology and Medicine* 26: 1034–1053.

Polidori MC, Stahl W, Eichler O, Niestrol I, and Sies H (2001) Profiles of antioxidants in human plasma. *Free Radical Biology and Medicine* 30: 456–462.

Pryor WA (2000) Vitamin E and heart disease: basic science to clinical intervention trials. *Free Radical Biology and Medicine* 28: 141–164.

Szeto YT, Tomlinson B, and Benzie IFF (2002) Total antioxidant and ascorbic acid content of fresh fruits and vegetables: implications for dietary planning and food preservation. *British Journal of Nutrition* 87: 55–59.

World Cancer Research Fund and the American Institute for Cancer Research (1997) *Food, Nutrition and the Prevention of Cancer: A Global Perspective*. Washington, DC: American Institute for Cancer Research.

Observational Studies

I F F Benzie, The Hong Kong Polytechnic University, Hong Kong, China

© 2005 Elsevier Ltd. All rights reserved.

Introduction

The study of temporal and geographical variation in disease prevalence in association with differences in environment, diet, and lifestyle helps identify possible factors that may modulate the risk of disease within and across populations. As such, observational epidemiology is a powerful, albeit blunt, tool that serves to inform and guide experimental studies and intervention trials. In the case of dietary antioxidants and chronic age-related disease, there is a logical biochemical rationale for the protective effect of antioxidants, and there is strong, and consistent observational evidence supportive of this. The way in which dietary antioxidants are believed to act is described in a separate chapter. In this chapter, observational evidence relating to dietary antioxidants and the risk of disease states is discussed.

Epidemiology: Setting the Scene

The risk of developing a disease can be increased by exposure to a disease-promoting factor or decreased by a protective factor. In terms of antioxidants, high risk is generally assumed to be associated with low intakes, plasma levels, or tissue concentrations of antioxidants. Epidemiological studies often express results in terms of the relative risk (RR) of mortality or disease. The RR is generally given as the mean and 95% confidence interval (CI). In general, an RR of 0.80 indicates an average reduction in risk of 20%; however, RR values must be interpreted with caution and the CI must be considered. If the CI spans 1.0, the RR is not statistically significant, regardless of its magnitude.

Different approaches are used in observational epidemiology. Cross-cultural studies compare standardized mortality rates (from all causes or from a specific disease) or disease prevalence and the factor of interest ('exposure variable') in different populations within or between countries. These can be regarded as 'snapshot' observational surveys. Case–control studies compare the factor of interest in people who have a disease (the cases) with that in those who do not (the controls). Prospective trials are longitudinal studies of apparently disease-free subjects whose health is monitored over years or decades; the exposure variable of interest is compared, retrospectively, between those who develop the disease of interest and those who do not.

The Observational View of Dietary Antioxidants

Cancer and cardiovascular disease (CVD) are the two leading causes of death worldwide, diabetes mellitus is reaching epidemic proportions, and dementia and maculopathy are largely untreatable irreversible disorders that are increasingly common in our aging population. The prevalence and standardized mortality rates of these diseases vary considerably between and within populations. Mortality from CVD varies more than 10-fold amongst different populations, and incidences of specific cancers vary 20-fold or more across the globe. This enormous variation highlights the multiple factors at play in the etiology of chronic age-related diseases. These factors include smoking habit, socioeconomic status, exposure to infectious agents, cholesterol levels, certain genetic factors, and diet. Dietary factors have long been known to play an important role in determining disease risk. Indeed, 30–40% of overall cancer risk is reported to be diet-related, and there is a wealth of compelling observational evidence that a lower risk of cancer, CVD, diabetes, and other chronic age-related disorders is associated with diets that are rich in antioxidants.

In terms of dietary antioxidants, the major research focus to date has been on the water-soluble vitamin C (ascorbic acid) and the lipophilic vitamin E. 'Vitamin E' is a group of eight lipid-soluble tocopherols and tocotrienols; however, the most widely studied form to date is α-tocopherol because it is the most abundant form in human plasma. Neither vitamin C nor vitamin E can be synthesized by humans, so they must be obtained in the diet, most coming from plant-based foods and oils. Deficiency of either of these vitamins is rare and can be prevented by the daily intake of a few milligrams of each. However, an adequate intake to prevent simple deficiency is unlikely to be sufficient for optimal health. Based on observational findings and experimental evidence that vitamin C and vitamin E protect key biological sites from oxidative damage *in vitro*, it has been suggested that there is a threshold of intake or plasma concentration for these antioxidants that confers minimum disease risk and promotes optimal health. The strength of the data supporting the health benefits of increased intakes of these vitamins was acknowledged in the US Food and Nutrition Board recommendation in 2000 to increase the daily intake of vitamin C to $75 \, \text{mg day}^{-1}$ for women and $90 \, \text{mg day}^{-1}$ for men and to increase that of vitamin E to $15 \, \text{mg day}^{-1}$ for both men and women. However, whether these new recommended intakes are 'optimal' is a contentious issue.

Supplementation trials with vitamin C or vitamin E have not to date shown the expected health benefits. The reasons for this mismatch between observational and supplementation data are not yet known, but some suggested reasons are outlined in **Table 1**. Nonetheless, despite the apparent lack of effect in supplementation trials, the variety and strength of observational findings, backed by a solid body of *in vitro* biochemical data, keep dietary antioxidants in the research spotlight, and in recent

years attention has focused on the influence of 'nonnutrient' dietary antioxidants, such as polyphenolic compounds, in addition to the effects of vitamin C and vitamin E. The current evidence for vitamin C, vitamin E, and non-nutrient dietary antioxidants in relation to the major causes of morbidity and mortality in developed countries is discussed briefly below.

Vitamin C

Low plasma ascorbic-acid concentrations have been reported to be strongly predictive of mortality, particularly in men. Results of a prospective trial in the UK (EPIC-Norfolk Prospective Study), in which 19 496 men and women aged 45–79 years were followed for 4 years, showed that men and women in the highest quintile of plasma ascorbic-acid concentration in samples collected within 1 year of entry into the study had significantly ($p < 0.0001$) lower all-cause mortality than those in the lowest quintile. Highest-quintile concentrations of plasma ascorbic acid (mean $\pm$ standard deviation) were $72.6 \pm 11.5 \, \mu\text{mol} \, l^{-1}$ for men and $85.1 \pm 13.7 \, \mu\text{mol} \, l^{-1}$ for women; lowest quintiles were $20.8 \pm 7.1 \, \mu\text{mol} \, l^{-1}$ and $30.3 \pm 10.1 \, \mu\text{mol} \, l^{-1}$, respectively, for men and women. In men and women in the highest quintile, RRs (CI) for all-cause mortality were, respectively, 0.48 (0.33–0.70) and 0.50 (0.32–0.81), relative to those in the lowest quintile. Mortality from ischemic heart disease was also significantly ($p < 0.001$) lower in the highest quintiles: for men the RR (CI) was 0.32 (0.15–0.75), and for women it was 0.07 (0.01–0.67). The relationship held for CVD and cancer in men ($p < 0.001$), but no significant difference in cancer mortality was seen in women, and CVD rates in women were affected less than those in men. The mean ascorbic-acid level in

Table 1 Possible reasons for the conflict in results between observational epidemiological and supplementation trials

- Antioxidants are likely to work in cooperation with each other; more of one may increase the need for another
- The action of an antioxidant within a heterogeneous food matrix may be different from that in pure supplemental form
- A high intake of antioxidants may help to promote health when taken regularly over decades but may have little discernable effect over a few months or years
- A high intake of antioxidants may slow or even prevent some of the deleterious age-related changes that lead to chronic disease, but antioxidants are unlikely to reverse established pathological changes
- Benefits of increased antioxidant intake may be seen only in those with marginal or depleted antioxidant status at baseline
- The effect of antioxidant supplementation may be seen only in subgroups of the study population, e.g., in those individuals with certain single-nucleotide polymorphisms
- The key players may not be the most widely studied antioxidants; for example, γ-tocopherol, rather than α-tocopherol, may play an important role in modulation of cancer risk but has been little studied to date
- Antioxidants can act as pro-oxidants under certain conditions, and the net effect of a dietary antioxidant may well depend on dose and conditions at its site of action
- Antioxidant action per se may not be the key mechanism of action of protection; for example, immunomodulatory, anti-inflammatory, anti-proliferative, and pro-apoptotic effects of dietary agents (antioxidants or otherwise) may be more relevant to overall effects in terms of disease risk

each quintile in women was around $10 \, \mu\text{mol} \, l^{-1}$ higher than that in men. Interestingly, the relationship between ascorbic-acid concentration and mortality was continuous throughout the range of plasma ascorbic-acid concentrations found. It was estimated that a $20 \, \mu\text{mol} \, l^{-1}$ increase in plasma ascorbic acid (achievable by one or two additional servings of fruit and vegetables each day) was associated with a 20% decrease in all-cause mortality, independent of age, blood pressure, cholesterol, smoking habit, and diabetes. Interestingly, also, mortality was not associated with supplement use, indicating that dietary sources of vitamin C are crucial.

In the Third National Health and Nutrition Examination Survey (NHANES III) in the USA, the plasma ascorbic-acid concentrations of 7658 men and women were not found to be independently associated with a history of cardiovascular disease in participants who reported no alcohol consumption; however, in 3497 participants who consumed alcohol a significantly lower prevalence of pre-existing angina was found in those with high plasma ascorbic acid ($>56 \, \mu\text{mol} \, l^{-1}$) than in those with 'low to marginal' levels ($<22 \, \mu\text{mol} \, l^{-1}$). No significant association was seen between plasma ascorbic acid and previous myocardial infarction or stroke in this cross-sectional survey. In the NHANES II prospective study, a 43% decrease in mortality was associated with higher plasma ascorbic-acid levels in more than 3000 men followed for up to 16 years. Plasma ascorbic-acid levels in the highest and lowest quartiles in this study were more than $73 \, \mu\text{mol} \, l^{-1}$ and less than $28.4 \, \mu\text{mol} \, l^{-1}$, respectively. The corresponding values in women were again higher, at more than $85 \, \mu\text{mol} \, l^{-1}$ and less than $39.7 \, \mu\text{mol} \, l^{-1}$, respectively, and no significant relationship between plasma ascorbic-acid levels and mortality was seen in women.

The Kuopio IHD (ischemic heart disease) Risk Factor Study followed 1605 men for 5 years and reported an RR (CI) of 0.11 (0.04–0.30) for acute myocardial infarction in those men with higher plasma ascorbic-acid concentrations. The Medical Research Council Trial of Assessment and Management of Older People in the Community, a prospective trial in the UK of 1214 elderly subjects followed for a median of 4.4 years, showed that those in the highest quintile of plasma ascorbic-acid level ($>66 \, \mu\text{mol} \, l^{-1}$) at entry had less than half the risk of dying in the follow-up period compared with those in the lowest quintile (plasma ascorbic-acid level of $<17 \, \mu\text{mol} \, l^{-1}$). Data on men and women were not analyzed separately, but there were fewer men (27%) in the highest quintile of ascorbic-acid

level. No relationship was seen between mortality and plasma levels or intake of β-carotene or lipid-standardized α-tocopherol. Interestingly, while the relationship between mortality and the concentration of plasma ascorbic acid was strong, there was no significant association between mortality and estimated dietary intake of vitamin C. This may reflect the difficulty in obtaining accurate dietary information, but it also suggests that different individuals may well need different intakes to achieve certain plasma levels of ascorbic acid.

There have been many case–control and cohort studies performed in Europe and the USA and published in the past 15 years, and some data from Asia have been gathered. In most case–control studies no significant relationship has been demonstrated between intake and/or plasma ascorbic-acid levels and the risk of cardiovascular events; however, the combination of findings from individual studies is revealing. In a detailed analysis of 11 cohort studies comparing high and low intakes of ascorbic acid in 50 000 subjects overall, with 2148 CVD events during follow-up, a Peto's Odds Ratio (95% CI) of 0.89 (0.79–0.99) for CVD was calculated, indicating a modest reduction in risk associated with a high intake of vitamin C. In an analysis of five cohort studies comparing high and low plasma ascorbic-acid levels, involving 13 018 subjects overall with 543 CVD events during follow-up, a Peto's Odds Ratio for CVD of 0.58 (0.47–0.72) was calculated. This was interpreted as showing high plasma ascorbic-acid levels to be a powerful predictor of freedom from CVD during follow-up.

The relationship between antioxidant-rich diets and protection from cancer is strong and clear; however, the influences of individual antioxidants are difficult to isolate. Cancer risk increases as total calorie intake increases, and this confounds prospective and retrospective dietary studies. Cancer causes many biochemical changes, and cancer treatment is harsh, and this confounds the results of studies comparing antioxidant levels in plasma in cases and controls unless the samples were collected and analysed before cancer developed (which may be a considerable time before diagnosis). Currently, the evidence for a cancer-opposing effect of high intakes or plasma concentrations of ascorbic acid is conflicting. To date, the strongest evidence of a role for vitamin C in lowering cancer risk is in relation to cancer of the stomach, with a low intake of vitamin C being associated with a two-to-three-fold increase in the risk of stomach cancer. A Spanish study showed a 69% lower risk of stomach cancer in those in the highest quintile of vitamin C intake, and low levels of ascorbic acid in gastric juice are found in patients with chronic atrophic gastritis or *Helicobacter pylori* infection, both of which are associated with a greatly increased risk of gastric cancer. Whether the decrease in ascorbic acid is directly related to the development of gastric cancer is not known, but it is known that ascorbic acid inactivates carcinogenic nitrosamines within the stomach. There is also evidence of a decreased risk of cancer of the mouth, pharynx, pancreas, lung, cervix, and breast in association with increased vitamin C intake, though not all studies find this. It has been estimated that if the diets of postmenopausal women were enriched with vitamin C, a 16% decrease in breast cancer in these women would result. No significant association was reported between vitamin C intake and the incidence of ovarian cancer in 16 years of follow-up of 80 326 women in the Nurses' Health Study. A study of 100 children with brain tumours showed a three-fold increase in risk in those children whose mothers had a low intake of vitamin C during pregnancy, suggesting that the dietary intake of vitamin C by pregnant women may help to determine the future cancer risk in their children. In a prospective study of 19 496 British men and women aged 45–79 years and followed for 4 years (the EPIC (European Prospective Investigation into Cancer and Nutrition) study), the RR (CI) of mortality from cancer for a $20 \, \mu mol \, l^{-1}$ increase in plasma ascorbic acid was 0.85 (0.74–0.99). In men there was a strong and continuous decrease in cancer risk with increasing plasma ascorbic-acid concentrations, with an RR (CI) in the highest quintile relative to the lowest quintile of 0.47 (0.27–0.88); i.e., the average risk in those with the highest plasma ascorbic-acid concentrations was less than half that of those in the lowest quintile. In women the decrease in RR did not reach statistical significance. The NHANES II study reported that men in the lowest quartile of ascorbic-acid level had a 62% higher risk of death from cancer during 12 years of follow-up than those in the highest quartile. However, this relationship was not seen in women. Of possible relevance here is the common finding in these studies that men, in general, had lower ascorbic-acid levels than women.

Vitamin C is concentrated in ocular tissues and fluids, particularly in the anterior aspect (cornea and lens). A case–control study in Spain reported a 64% reduction in the risk of cataract ($p < 0.0001$) in those with a plasma ascorbic-acid concentration of more than $49 \, \mu mol \, l^{-1}$; however, no significant association with the dietary intake of vitamin C was seen. In a case–control study in the Netherlands, the prevalence of age-related maculopathy was reported to be twice as high in those with low antioxidant intake (from fruits and vegetables); however

the data on vitamin C intake or plasma levels and maculopathy are conflicting. Lipid-soluble antioxidants, especially zeaxanthin and lutein (dietary-derived carotenoids that are highly concentrated in the lipid-rich fovea), may be more relevant in this condition than water-soluble vitamin C.

High plasma concentrations of ascorbic acid are reportedly associated with better memory performance, and lower plasma and cerebrospinal-fluid concentrations of ascorbic acid were found in patients with Alzheimer's disease than in non-demented controls. Individuals who took vitamin C supplements were reported to have a lower prevalence of Alzheimer's disease on follow-up after 4.3 years. However, not all studies have shown a significant association between vitamin C intake or plasma levels and cognitive decline or dementia.

Vitamin E

An extensive review noted that the data in relation to a connection between vitamin E and CVD risk are strong and convincing. In a large cross-cultural European (WHO/MONICA) observational study, a strong inverse relationship ($r^2 = 0.60$, $p < 0.005$) was found between plasma concentrations of lipid-standardized vitamin E and mortality from coronary heart disease (CHD) across 16 populations. In a detailed analysis, this relationship was found to be stronger than that between mortality and plasma cholesterol, smoking, and diastolic blood pressure combined ($r^2 = 0.44$, $p < 0.02$). In a case–control study in Scotland, patients with previously undiagnosed angina pectoris were found to have lower levels of plasma lipid-standardized vitamin E than controls. After adjustment for classical CHD risk factors, men in the highest quintile of lipid-standardized vitamin E level had an almost three-fold decrease in risk. Confusingly, some studies have reported a higher CVD risk in individuals with increased plasma total vitamin E, but these results are probably driven by elevated blood lipids. Vitamin E is carried in the lipoproteins, and it is important to lipid standardize plasma concentrations of this, and other, lipophilic antioxidants.

The Nurses' Health Study (women) and the Health Professionals Study (men) were initiated in the USA in 1980 and 1986, respectively, and recruited almost 200 000 subjects. It was found that women at the high end of vitamin E intake from diet alone had a small and non-significant decrease in CVD risk; however, those women in the highest quintile of vitamin E intake (more than $100 \, IU \, day^{-1}$) had an RR (CI) for CVD of 0.54 (0.36–0.82). It should be noted that an intake of

100 IU day^{-1} of vitamin E is achievable only by using supplements: intake from food alone is unlikely be more than 15 IU day^{-1}. In this study, protection against CVD was seen only in those women who had taken vitamin E supplements for at least 2 years. In the Health Professionals Follow-up Study the findings were very similar. Supplemental, but not dietary, intake of vitamin E (more than 100 IU day^{-1}) in men was associated with a significant decrease in CVD risk, averaging over 30%, but again the effect was seen only if supplements had been taken for at least 2 years. A separate study in the USA of more than 11 000 elderly subjects showed that the use of vitamin E supplements was associated with a significant decrease in the risk of heart disease (RR (CI) of 0.53 (0.34–0.84)). The results also showed a significant decrease in all-cause mortality in users of vitamin E supplements and suggested that long-term use was beneficial. A study in Finland of more than 5000 men and women showed an average of 40% lower CVD risk in the highest versus the lowest tertile of vitamin E intake. Interestingly, most (97%) of subjects in this study did not take supplements, indicating that the protective effect was due to higher intake from food. An inverse association between dietary vitamin E intake and heart disease was also seen in The Women's Iowa Health Study, which involved almost 35 000 postmenopausal women. In this study, an RR (CI) of 0.38 (0.18–0.80) for CVD mortality was seen in women in the highest quintile relative to those in the lowest quintile of vitamin E intake from food alone. However, the Medical Research Council Trial of Assessment and Management of Older People in the Community (UK) found no relation between either dietary intake of vitamin E or plasma concentration of lipid-standardized α-tocopherol and all-cause mortality or death from CVD in 1214 elderly participants followed for a median of 4.4 years.

Cancer is caused by mutations in key genes. Anything that protects DNA will, in theory, help to prevent cancer-causing mutations. Lipid peroxide degradation products are reported to be carcinogenic, and vitamin E opposes lipid peroxidation, possibly conferring indirect protection against cancer. Furthermore, by interacting with reactive species elsewhere in the cell, vitamin E may spare other antioxidants, thereby also indirectly protecting DNA. Vitamin E reportedly protects against cancer of the upper digestive tract, skin cancer, including melanoma, and lung cancer. Follow-up analysis of the placebo group of the Finnish ATBC (Alpha Tocopherol Beta Carotene) study (incidentally, a study that showed no protection against lung cancer

in a high-risk group supplemented with α-tocopherol and/or β-carotene) showed that there was a 36% higher incidence of lung cancer in those in the lowest quartile than in those in the highest quartile of diet-derived vitamin E. Vitamin E from dietary sources, but not supplements, has been reported to confer modest protection against breast cancer; however, as with vitamin C, no association was seen between vitamin E intake and the risk of ovarian cancer in the Nurses' Health Study follow-up.

Colorectal cancer is the second and third most common cancer in men and women, respectively. Dietary influences on the risk of colorectal cancer are currently unclear, and, based on recent findings of large prospective trials, it has been suggested that the influence of antioxidant-rich foods has been overstated. Nonetheless, there is evidence that vitamin E may be protective. In a case–control study in the USA of almost 1000 cases of rectal cancer, the risk was reported to be modestly decreased in women with a high vitamin E intake, but not in men. In a meta-analysis of five prospective nested case–control studies, there was a marginal decrease in the incidence of colorectal cancer in those in the highest quartile of plasma α-tocopherol, although no significant inverse association was seen in any of the studies individually. In the Iowa Women's Health Study, women with the highest risk of colon cancer were those with the lowest intake of vitamin E, although the relationship was significant only in women aged 55–59 years.

In addition to its antioxidant properties, vitamin E is reported to have immune-boosting and anti-inflammatory effects and to inhibit cell division, all of which may help explain the reported relationship between low intake or plasma concentrations of vitamin E and increased risk of various cancers. Currently, there is much interest in vitamin E in association with selenium in relation to the prevention of prostate, lung, and colon cancer. Indeed, the combination of vitamin E with other antioxidant micronutrients may be much more important than vitamin E alone. Furthermore, the different members of the vitamin E family may play cooperative or complementary roles in modulating the risk of disease. In terms of cancer prevention, γ-tocopherol is attracting much interest. Dietary intake of this form of vitamin E can be up to three times higher than that of α-tocopherol. Corn, canola, palm, soya bean, and peanut oils contain more γ-tocopherol than α-tocopherol. Despite a higher intake, however, our plasma levels of γ-tocopherol are only around 10% of those of α-tocopherol, owing to preferential placement of the α-form into very low-density lipoproteins. Interestingly, higher tissue levels of

α-tocopherol are reportedly found in animals fed both α-tocopherol and γ-tocopherol than in animals fed α-tocopherol alone, suggesting that intake of both forms may enhance the enrichment of tissues. Furthermore, the lower reaches of the gastrointestinal tract may contain high levels of γ-tocopherol, and this may help to destroy fecal mutagens. None of the epidemiological studies to date have estimated the dietary intake of γ-tocopherol, but the few studies that have measured plasma levels of γ-tocopherol show interesting results. In a nested case–control study of 6000 Japanese men, there was a statistically significant inverse relationship between the risk of cancer of the upper digestive tract and plasma levels of γ-tocopherol but not α-tocopherol. In a nested case–control study in the USA, a statistically significant protective effect against prostate cancer was found only when both plasma α-tocopherol and γ-tocopherol levels were high, with a five-fold decrease in prostate cancer in those in the highest quintile relative to those in the lowest quintile. Some of the putative effect of γ-tocopherol may be mediated through its antioxidant properties; however, γ-tocopherol has other properties relevant to cancer prevention, including effects on oncogenes and tumor suppressor genes and on cell cycle events, that the α-form does not have or demonstrates to a lesser extent. It is of interest that most vitamin E supplementation trials to date have used α-tocopherol. It may be that intake of both isomers is needed for optimal tissue uptake and effect. Furthermore, in view of the ability of α-tocopherol to displace bound γ-tocopherol, supplementation with the α-form alone may be counterproductive, in that it may deplete tissues of γ-tocopherol. Further studies are needed in this area.

The brain is rich in unsaturated fatty acids, and there is a reasonable rationale for the protection of lipid-rich neurones by vitamin E. Plasma and cerebrospinal α-tocopherol concentrations were found to be low in patients with Alzheimer's disease in some but not all studies. Cognitive function is reported to be directly correlated with plasma α-tocopherol levels. A high intake of vitamin E is associated with a decreased risk of the subsequent development of Alzheimer's disease, and an 8 month delay in significant worsening of Alzheimer's disease was reported in association with increased intakes of vitamin E. In the NHANES III study, better memory performance in elderly participants was reportedly found in those with higher plasma α-tocopherol levels. Based on data such as these, vitamin E (2000 IU day^{-1}) is currently being studied in relation to its possible ability to delay the onset of Alzheimer's disease in people with mild cognitive impairment.

'Non-Nutrient' Antioxidants

Plant-based foods contain a multitude of antioxidants other than vitamin C and vitamin E. The two major classes of these other dietary-derived antioxidants are the carotenoids and the polyphenolic flavonoids. There are hundreds of different carotenoids and thousands of flavonoids, and these compounds give fruits, vegetables, teas, and herbs their wonderful colors in shades of red, orange, yellow, and purple. These compounds are synthesized exclusively in plants and have no known function in human metabolism. No deficiency state for either class of compounds has been identified in humans. Consequently, there is no recommended daily intake or agreed requirement for any of these compounds, and they are regarded as 'non-nutrients.' Nonetheless, there is evidence that diets rich in carotenoids and flavonoids are beneficial to health. For example, in a study of 1299 elderly people in the USA, those with diets rich in carotenoid-containing fruits and vegetables were found to have a significantly decreased rate of CVD and fatal myocardial infarction: the RRs (CI) when the highest and lowest quartiles of intake were compared were 0.54 (0.34–0.86) for fatal CVD and 0.25 (0.09–0.67) for fatal myocardial infarction. The carotenoid lycopene has been reported to lower the risk of prostate cancer, but the evidence for a relationship between carotenoid intake and the risk of other cancers is conflicting. Increased intake of lutein and zeaxanthin may help to delay or prevent age-related maculopathy, because these carotenoids are concentrated in the macula and are likely to be very important in local protection of the lipid-rich retina. To date, however, epidemiological findings point to health benefits of foods containing carotenoids, and the influence, if any, of individual carotenoids remains to be established.

The same is true for the polyphenolic flavonoids, anthocyanins, and various other plant-based non-nutrient antioxidants in the diet. Many of these have antioxidant powers far higher than those of vitamin C and vitamin E when tested in *in vitro* systems. Dietary intake can be similar to that of vitamin C (100 mg day^{-1} or higher), but, as their bioavailability is low, plasma levels of individual flavonoids and other phenolic antioxidants are very low or undetectable. The major dietary polyphenolic compounds are quercetin, kaempferol, myricitin, and the catechins. These flavonoids are found in onions, apples, kale, broccoli, Brussels sprouts, teas, grapes, and wine. Moderate wine intake, especially of red wine (which is very rich in polyphenolic antioxidants), is associated with a significant

Table 2 Limitations of observational epidemiological studies of diet and disease

- Cross-cultural study has no power if rates of disease and/or population means of the exposure variable of interest do not vary significantly between the populations being compared
- Behavioral, genetic, and geographical, rather than dietary, variation may account for differences detected
- A 'snapshot' view of recent dietary habits or current status may not be representative of those in earlier or later life, and differences during these periods will confound and confuse the results
- In case–control studies, the disease process itself, drug treatment, or post-diagnosis changes in diet or lifestyle may cause or mask changes in the exposure variable
- Subclinical or undetected disease may be present in controls, decreasing contrast with cases
- Retrospective dietary recall may be unreliable, food tables may be out of date or incomplete, and analysis methods may be inaccurate
- In nested case–control studies, long-term follow-up is needed and may rely on a distant 'snapshot' measure of the exposure variable as a representative index of past and future levels
- Instability or inaccurate measurement of the exposure variable will lead to bias in the results
- Assessment methods and 'high' or 'low' thresholds may vary in different areas supplying data
- If protection is maximal above a 'threshold' level of the exposure variable, then no effect will be detectable if levels in most of the study population are below or above the threshold
- Prospective studies are very expensive, requiring a very large study group and years or decades of follow-up
- Prospective trials generally have disease or death as the measured outcome; this means that the participants in the trial cannot benefit from its findings

decrease in the risk of CHD. Tea consumption, especially a high intake of green tea, is associated with a lower risk of CVD and cancer. However, which of the myriad compounds contribute to the reported health benefits is not yet clear. It may be many; it may be none. It must be remembered that association does not prove causality. Equally, the lack of significant effects of supplementation trials in healthy subject does not mean that there is no effect. As outlined in **Table 1**, and further delineated in **Table 2**, observational studies have several limitations, and there are various reasons why a conflict may exist between what we observe and the outcome of supplementation trials.

Summary and Research Needs

Strong evidence from a variety of sources indicates that a high intake of vitamin C or something very closely associated with it in the diet is protective against cancer and CVD, the major causes of disability and death in our aging communities. Indeed, it may be that plasma ascorbic-acid concentration can predict overall mortality risk. This interesting concept remains to be confirmed. The evidence for the benefits of a high intake of vitamin E is also strong, but research is needed into which member(s) of the vitamin E family are most important. The evidence for the benefits of carotenoids and flavonoids stems largely from observational studies that show a decreased risk of disease in association with a high intake of foods or beverages rich in these non-nutrient antioxidants rather than the agents themselves. However, individuals who take these foods in large quantities are often more health

conscious, take fewer total calories, do not smoke, exercise more, and eat less red meat and saturated fat. The relationship between diet and health is clear, but diet is complex and dynamic, the underlying mechanisms of chronic diseases are uncertain, and the influence of individual dietary antioxidants is difficult to discern within the heterogeneous framework of the human diet and lifestyle. Antioxidants do appear to play a role in protecting key biological sites, but further study is needed to establish which, how, and where and to establish the doses needed to achieve optimal effect. To date there is no evidence that high intakes of antioxidants in the diet are harmful. It is not yet known, however, whether intake above a threshold level brings additional benefit or whether the benefit of increased intake is limited to those with initially poor or marginal antioxidant status. Furthermore, antioxidants are likely to act within a coordinated system, and more of one may require more of others for beneficial effects to be achieved. Achieving 'target thresholds' of several antioxidants may be critical to achieving the optimal effect of each, and threshold plasma concentrations of $50 \, \mu mol \, l^{-1}$ and $30 \, \mu mol \, l^{-1}$ for vitamin C and vitamin E, respectively, with a ratio of more than 1.3, have been proposed for minimizing the risk of CHD.

To establish cause and effect and to make firm recommendations about the type and dose of antioxidants needed to achieve optimal health requires much in the way of further study. Of particular interest and value in such study is the growing field of orthomolecular nutrition, in which advances in genomics and proteomics are used to determine gene–nutrient interaction and the influence of diet on epigenetic phenomena. Such molecular-based studies, guided by epidemiological data and incorporated into future supplementation trials, will help answer the questions about the mechanisms of action and which, if any, antioxidants are important, how much, and for whom. However, while many questions relating to dietary antioxidants and health remain unanswered, to understand how to obtain a mixture of antioxidants and promote health we need look only at the macro level of food rather than at the micro level of specific constituents or molecular level of response. Fruits, vegetables, teas, herbs, wines, juices, and some types of chocolate are rich in antioxidants. It is known that diets rich in a variety of such foods are beneficial to health. The results of molecular-based experimental studies will determine whether these two truths are linked in a cause-and-effect relationship.

Acknowledgments

The author thanks The Hong Kong Polytechnic University and The World Cancer Research Fund International for financially supporting this work.

See also: **Antioxidants**: Diet and Antioxidant Defense.

Further Reading

Ames BN and Wakimoto P (2002) Are vitamin and mineral deficiencies a major cancer risk? *Nature Reviews* 2: 694–704.

Asplund K (2002) Antioxidant vitamins in the prevention of cardiovascular disease: a systematic review. *Journal of Internal Medicine* 251: 372–392.

Benzie IFF (2003) Evolution of dietary antioxidants. *Journal of Comparative Biochemistry and Physiology* 136A: 113–126.

Block G, Norkus E, Hudes M, Mandel S, and Helzlsouer K (2001) Which plasma antioxidants are most related to fruit and vegetable consumption? *American Journal of Epidemiology* 154: 1113–1118.

Brigelius-Flohé R, Kelly FJ, Salonen JT et al. (2002) The European perspective on vitamin E: current knowledge and future research. *American Journal of Clinical Nutrition* 76: 703–716.

Clarkson PM and Thompson HS (2000) Antioxidants: what role do they play in physical activity and health? *American Journal of Clinical Nutrition* 72: 637S–646S.

Duthie GG, Gardner PT, and Kyle JAM (2003) Plant polyphenols: are they the new magic bullet? *Proceedings of the Nutrition Society* 62: 599–603.

Gey KF (1998) Vitamins E plus C and interacting co-nutrients required for optimal health: a critical and constructive review of epidemiology and supplementation data regarding cardiovascular disease and cancer. *Biofactors* 7: 113–175.

Grundman M and Delaney P (2002) Antioxidant strategies for Alzheimer's disease. *Proceedings of the Nutrition Society* 61: 191–202.

Khaw KT, Bingham S, Welch A et al. (2001) Relation between plasma ascorbic acid and mortality in men and women in EPIC-Norfolk prospective study: a prospective population study. *Lancet* 357: 657–663.

Lindsay DG and Clifford MN (eds.) (2000) Critical reviews within the EU Concerted Action 'Nutritional enhancement of plant-based food in European trade' ('NEODIET') *Journal of the Science of Food and Agriculture* 80: 793–1137.

McCall MR and Frei B (1999) Can antioxidant vitamins materially reduce oxidative damage in humans? *Free Radical Biology and Medicine* 26: 1034–1053.

Mensink RP and Plat J (2002) Post-genomic opportunities for understanding nutrition: the nutritionist's perspective. *Proceedings of the Nutrition Society* 61: 404–463.

Padayatty SJ, Katz A, Wang Y et al. (2003) Vitamin C as an antioxidant: evaluation of its role in disease prevention. *Journal of the American College of Nutrition* 22: 18–35.

Pryor WA (2000) Vitamin E and heart disease: basic science to clinical intervention trials. *Free Radical Biology and Medicine* 28: 141–164.

World Cancer Research Fund and the American Institute for Cancer Research (1997) *Food, Nutrition and the Prevention of Cancer: A Global Perspective.* Washington DC: American Institute for Cancer Research.

Intervention Studies

S Stanner, British Nutrition Foundation, London, UK

© 2005 Elsevier Ltd. All rights reserved.

A predominantly plant-based diet reduces the risk of developing several chronic diseases, including cancer and cardiovascular disease (CVD) coronary heart disease and stroke. It is often assumed that antioxidants, including vitamin C, vitamin E, the carotenoids (e.g., β-carotene, lycopene, and lutein), selenium, and the flavonoids (e.g., quercetin, kaempferol, myricetin, luteolin, and apigenin), contribute to this protection by interfering passively with oxidative damage to DNA, lipids, and proteins. This hypothesis is supported by numerous *in vitro* studies in animals and humans. A large number of descriptive, case–control, and cohort studies have also demonstrated an inverse association between high intakes and/or plasma levels of antioxidants and risk of CVD and cancer at numerous sites, as well as other conditions associated with oxidative damage, such as age-related macular degeneration, cataracts, and chronic obstructive pulmonary disease (COPD).

These findings provided a strong incentive for the initiation of intervention studies to investigate whether a lack of dietary antioxidants is causally related to chronic disease risk and if providing antioxidant supplements confers benefits for the prevention and treatment of these conditions. This article summarizes the findings of the largest primary and secondary trials published to date and considers their implications for future research and current dietary advice.

Cardiovascular Disease

Of all the diseases in which excess oxidative stress has been implicated, CVD has the strongest supporting evidence. Oxidation of low-density lipoprotein (LDL) cholesterol appears to be a key step in the development of atherosclerosis, a known risk factor in the development of CVD. Small studies have demonstrated reductions in LDL oxidation (mostly *in vitro*) following supplementation with dietary antioxidants (particularly vitamin E, which is primarily carried in LDL-cholesterol), suggesting that they may provide protection against the development of heart

disease. A number of large intervention trials using disease outcomes (rather than biomarkers such as LDL oxidation) have also been conducted to try to demonstrate a protective effect of vitamin E, β-carotene, and, to a lesser extent, vitamin C supplements on cardiovascular disease. Most have been carried out in high-risk groups (e.g., smokers) or those with established heart disease (i.e., people with angina or who have already suffered a heart attack).

Primary Prevention

The results of most primary prevention trials have not been encouraging (**Table 1**). For example, in the Finnish Alpha-Tocopherol Beta-Carotene Cancer Prevention (ATBC) study, approximately 30 000 male smokers received vitamin E (50 mg/day of α-tocopherol), β-carotene (20 mg/day), both, or an

Table 1 Summary of large intervention trials (>1000 subjects) investigating the role of antioxidants and CVD in primary prevention

Trial	Characteristics of subjects	Sex	Length of follow-up (years)	Treatment	Effect of antioxidant supplementation
ATBC	29 133 smokers, Finland	Male	6	50 mg α-tocopherol and/or 20 mg β-carotene	No significant effect on fatal or nonfatal-CHD or total strokes with either supplement Increase in deaths from hemorrhagic stroke in vitamin E group Increase in hemorrhagic stroke (+62%) and total mortality (+8%) in β-carotene group
CARET	14 254 smokers, 4 060 asbestos workers, United States	Male and Female	4	30 mg β-carotene and 25 000 IU retinol	Increase in deaths from CVD (+26%) (terminated early)
LCPS	29 584 poorly nourished, China	Male and Female	5	15 mg β-carotene, 30 mg α-tocopherol, and 50 µg selenium	Small decline in total mortality (+9%) Reduction in deaths from stroke in men (−55%) but not women
PHS	22 071 physicians, United States	Male	12	50 mg β-carotene and/or aspirin (alternate days)	No effect on fatal or nonfatal myocardial infarction or stroke
PPP	4 495 with one or more CVD risk factors, Italy	Male and Female	$3\frac{1}{2}$	Low-dose aspirin and/or 300 mg α-tocopherol	No effect on CVD deaths or events (but inadequate power due to premature interruption of trial)
SCPS	1720 with recent nonmelanoma skin cancer, Australia	Male and Female	8	50 mg β-carotene	No effect on CVD mortality
VACP II	1 204 former asbestos workers, Australia	Male and Female	5	30 mg β-carotene or 25 000 IU retinol (no placebo group)	No effect of β-carotene on CHD deaths
WHS	39 876, United States	Female	2	50 mg β-carotene (alternate days)	No effect on fatal or nonfatal CVD

ATBC, Alpha Tocopherol Beta Carotene Prevention Study; CARET, Beta Carotene and Retinol Efficacy Trial; LCPS, Linxian Cancer Prevention Study; PHS, Physicians Health Study; PPP, Primary Prevention Project; SCPS, Skin Cancer Prevention Study; VACP, Vitamin A and Cancer Prevention; WHS, Women's Health Study; CHD, Coronary Heart Disease; CVD, Cardiovascular disease.

inactive substance (placebo) for approximately 6 years. There was no reduction in risk of major coronary events with any of the treatments despite a 50% increase in blood vitamin E concentrations and a 17-fold increase in β-carotene levels. Moreover, with vitamin E supplementation, there was an unexpected increase in risk of death from hemorrhagic stroke and a small but significant increase in mortality from all causes with β-carotene supplementation (RR, 1.08; 95% confidence interval (CI), 1–16). An increase in CVD deaths was also observed in the Beta-Carotene and Retinol Efficacy Trial (CARET), which tested the effects of combined treatment with β-carotene (30 mg/day) and retinyl palmitate (25 000 IU/day) in 18 000 men and women with a history of cigarette smoking or occupational exposure to asbestos compared to the placebo group (RR, 1.26; 95% CI, 0.99–1.61).

Secondary Prevention

The most positive results from secondary prevention trials came from the Cambridge Heart Antioxidant Study (CHAOS), a controlled trial on 2002 heart disease patients with angiographically proven coronary atherosclerosis randomly assigned to receive a high dose of vitamin E (400 or 800 IU/day) or placebo (**Table 2**). Those receiving the supplements were 77% less likely to suffer from nonfatal heart disease over the $1\frac{1}{2}$-year trial period than those who did not receive vitamin E (RR, 0.23; 95% CI, 0.11–0.47), although there was no reduction in CVD deaths. However, other large secondary prevention trials with longer follow-up have been less encouraging. For example, in a further analysis of the ATBC study, the β-carotene supplementation was associated with an increased risk of coronary heart disease (CHD) deaths among men who had a previous heart attack and were thus at high risk of subsequent coronary events. There were significantly more deaths from fatal CHD in the β-carotene group (RR, 1.75; 95% CI, 1.16–2.64) and in the combined β-carotene and vitamin E group compared to the placebo group (RR, 1.58; 95% CI, 1.05–2.40). The Heart Outcomes Prevention Evaluation Study (HOPE) observed no benefit from vitamin E supplementation (400 IU/day) on CVD or all-cause mortality. The Heart Protection Study in the United Kingdom examined the effect of 5 years of

Table 2 Summary of large intervention trials (>1000 subjects) investigating the role of antioxidants and CVD in secondary prevention[a]

Trial	Characteristics of subjects	Sex	Length of follow-up (years)	Treatment	Effect of antioxidant supplementation
ATBC	1862 smokers with previous MI, Finland	Male	$5\frac{1}{2}$	50 mg α-tocopherol and/or 20 mg β-carotene	No effect on total coronary events (fatal and nonfatal) Increase in deaths from fatal CHD in β-carotene ($+75\%$) and combined β-carotene/vitamin E group ($+58\%$) vs placebo
	1795 heavy smokers with previous angina, Finland				No effect on symptoms or progression of angina or on total coronary events
CHAOS	2002 patients with coronary atherosclerosis, United Kingdom	Male and Female	$1\frac{1}{2}$	300 or 800 IU α-tocopherol	Reduction in nonfatal MI (-77%) but no effect on CVD mortality
GISSI	11324 patients with recent MI, Italy			300 mg α-tocopherol and/or 1 g n-3 PUFA	No benefit from vitamin E
HOPE	9541 known CVD or diabetes, Canada	Male and Female	4–6	400 IU α-tocopherol and/or ACE inhibitor	No effect on MI, stroke, or CVD death
HPS	20536 with known vascular disease or at high risk, United Kingdom	Male and Female	≥ 5	20 mg β-carotene, 600 mg α-tocopherol, and 250 mg vitamin C	No effect on fatal or nonfatal MI or stroke

[a]Secondary prevention is defined as including patients with known or documented vascular disease.
ACE, angiotensin converting enzyme; ATBC, Alpha Tocopherol Beta Carotene Prevention Study; CHAOS, Cambridge Heart Antioxidant Study; GISSI, GISSI Prevenzione Trial; HOPE, Heart Outcomes Prevention Evaluation Study; HPS, Heart Protection Study; CHD, Coronary Heart Disease; CVD, cardiovascular disease; MI, myocardial infarction; PUFA, polyunsatutated fatty acids.

supplementation with a cocktail of antioxidant vitamins (600 mg vitamin E, 250 mg vitamin C, and 20 mg β-carotene) alone or in combination with the lipid-lowering drug Simvastatin or placebo in more than 20 000 adults with CHD, other occlusive arterial disease, or diabetes mellitus. Although blood levels of antioxidant vitamins were substantially increased, no significant reduction in the 5-year mortality from vascular disease or any other major outcome was noted. In the Italian GISSI-Prevenzione Trial dietary fish oils reduced the risk of fatal or nonfatal CVD in men and women who had recently suffered from a heart attack but vitamin E supplementation (300 mg daily for $3\frac{1}{2}$ years) did not provide any benefit. In these three trials, no significant adverse effects of vitamin E were observed.

Systematic reviews and meta-analyses of the clinical trials to date have therefore concluded that despite evidence from observational studies, people with a high occurrence of CVD often have low intakes or plasma levels of antioxidant nutrients. Supplementation with any single antioxidant nutrient or combination of nutrients has not demonstrated any benefit for the treatment or prevention of CVD.

Cancer

The oxidative hypothesis of carcinogenesis asserts that carcinogens generate reactive oxygen species that damage RNA and DNA in cells, predisposing these cells to malignant changes and enhanced cancer risk. Most, but not all, damage is corrected by internal surveillance and repair systems involving dietary antioxidants, as well as endogenous antioxidant mechanisms. Antioxidants are therefore proposed to prevent cell damage by neutralizing free radicals and oxidants, thus preventing subsequent development of cancer.

β-Carotene

Many of the randomized controlled trials (RCTs) investigating a protective role for antioxidant nutrients in cancer prevention (**Table 3**) have focused on β-carotene. A study in Linxian, China, of a rural population with poor nutritional status found that supplementation with a combination of β-carotene, selenium, and vitamin E for 5 years provided a 21% reduction in stomach cancer mortality and a 13% reduction in all cancer deaths. Although interesting, the population studied was likely to have very low intakes of a number of micronutrients and this study does not contribute to knowledge about the effects of individual antioxidants or offer any insight into

their effects on populations with good nutritional status.

The findings of a number of large double-blind RCTs in well-fed subjects using high-dose β-carotene supplements (either alone or in combination with other agents) have generally been unsupportive of any protective effect, although most have only focused on high-risk groups (e.g., smokers, asbestos workers, and older age groups). In the ATBC Cancer Prevention Trial, in which 29 000 male smokers were randomly assigned to receive β-carotene and/ or α-tocopherol or placebo each day, β-carotene showed no protective effect on the incidence of any type of cancer after approximately 6 years. In fact, concern was raised following the publication of the findings of this trial because those randomized to receive this vitamin had an 18% higher risk of lung cancer (RR, 1.18; 95% CI, 3–36) as well as an 8% higher total mortality than nonrecipients. Subgroup analyses suggested that the adverse effect of β-carotene on lung cancer risk was restricted to heavy smokers and that the risk appeared to be transient, being lost at follow-up 4–6 years after cessation of supplementation.

The CARET was also terminated early because of similar findings; subjects receiving a combination of supplements (30 mg β-carotene and vitamin A daily) experienced a 28% increased risk of lung cancer incidence compared with the placebo group (RR, 1.28; 95% CI, 1.04–1.57). Subgroup analyses also suggested that the effect was found in current, but not former, smokers. In contrast, in the Physicians Health Study, supplementation of male physicians with 50 mg β-carotene on alternate days had no effect on cancer incidence (men who were smokers did not experience any benefit or harm). The Heart Protection Study also demonstrated no effect on 5-year cancer incidence or mortality from supplementation with 20 mg β-carotene in combination with vitamins E and C in individuals at high risk of CVD, despite increases in blood concentrations of these nutrients (plasma β-carotene concentrations increased 4-fold). They did not, however, find any harmful effects from these vitamins.

A number of trials have attempted to investigate the effect of β-carotene supplementation on nonmelanoma skin cancer, the most common forms of which are basal cell and squamous cell carcinomas (these types of cells are both found in the top layer of the skin). However, none have shown any significant effect on skin cancer prevention. For example, the Physicians Health Study found no effect after 12 years of β-carotene supplementation on the development of a first nonmelanoma skin cancer. The Nambour Skin Cancer Prevention Trial of 1621

Table 3 Summary of large intervention trials (>1000 subjects) investigating the role of antioxidants and cancer in primary prevention

Trial	Characteristics of subjects	Sex	Length of follow-up (years)	Treatment	Effect of antioxidant supplementation
ATBC	29 133 smokers, Finland	Male	5–8	50 mg α-tocopherol and/ or 20 mg β-carotene	18% increase in lung cancer in β-carotene group (no effect in vitamin E group) 34% reduction in incidence of prostate cancer in vitamin E group No effect of either vitamin on colorectal, pancreatic, or urinary tract cancer
CARET	14 254 smokers, 4060 asbestos workers, United States	Male and Female	4	30 mg β-carotene and 25 000 IU retinol	Lung cancer increased by 28%
HPS	20 536 at high CVD risk, United Kingdom	Male and Female	≥5	20 mg β-carotene, 600 mg α-tocopherol, and 250 mg vitamin C	No effect on cancer incidence or mortality
LCPS	29 584 poorly nourished, China	Male and Female	5	15 mg β-carotene, 30 mg α-tocopherol, and 50 μg selenium	Cancer deaths declined by 13% Stomach cancer declined by 21%
NSCPT	1621 (73% without skin cancer at baseline), Australia	Male and Female	$4\frac{1}{2}$	30 mg β-carotene with or without sunscreen application	No effect on basal cell or squamous cell carcinoma
PHS	22 071 physicians, United States	Male	12	50 mg β-carotene and/or aspirin (alternate days)	No effect on incidence of malignant neoplasms or nonmelanoma skin cancer
VACP II	1204 former asbestos workers, Australia	Male and Female	5	30 mg β-carotene or 25 000 IU retinol (no placebo group)	No effect of β-carotene on cancer mortality
WHS	39 876, United States	Female	2	50 mg β-carotene (alternate days)	No effect on cancer incidence

ATBC, Alpha Tocopherol Beta Carotene Prevention Study; CARET, Beta Carotene and Retinol Efficacy Trial; HPS, Heart Protection Study; LCPS, Linxian Cancer Prevention Study; NSCPT, Nambour Skin Cancer Prevention Trial; PHS, Physicians Health Study; VACP, Vitamin A and Cancer Prevention; WHS, Women's Health Study; CVD, Cardio Vascular disease.

men and women followed for nearly 5 years (most of whom had no history of skin cancer at baseline) showed that those supplemented with 30 mg β-carotene did not experience any reduction in risk of basal cell or squamous cell carcinoma or the occurrence of solar keratoses (precancerous skin growths that are a strong determinant of squamous cell carcinoma). A 5-year trial of 1805 men and women with recent nonmelanoma skin cancer (the Skin Cancer Prevention Study) also found that supplementation with 50 mg of β-carotene gave no protection against either type of skin cancer, although this may have been because these cancers have a long latency period of approximately 12 years (**Table 4**).

Together, these trials suggest that β-carotene supplements offer no protection against cancer at any site and, among smokers, may actually increase the risk of lung cancer. Investigators have sought to

explain these findings by proposing that components of cigarette smoke may promote oxidation of β-carotene in the lungs, causing it to exert a prooxidant (rather than antioxidant) effect and act as a tumor promoter.

Vitamin C

There are no published RCTs of vitamin C alone in primary prevention, but data from the small number of trials of vitamin C in combination with other nutrients have not provided any support for a role for high-dose vitamin C supplementation in cancer prevention (**Table 3**). The Linxian trial found no significant effect of supplementing Chinese men and women with 120 mg vitamin C and 30 μg molybdenum daily for 5 years on the risk of cancers of the oesophagus or stomach. The Polyp Prevention Study, a trial of 864 patients with previous

Table 4 Summary of large intervention trials (>1000 subjects) investigating the role of antioxidants and cancer in secondary prevention[a]

Trial	Characteristics of subjects	Sex	Length of follow-up (years)	Treatment	Effect of antioxidant supplementation
NPCT	1312 with history of basal or squamous cell carcinoma, United States	Male and Female	$4\frac{1}{2}$	200 µg selenium	No effect on incidence of skin cancer
					Reduce cancer mortality (50%), cancer incidence (37%), prostate cancer (63%), colorectal cancer (58%), and lung cancer (46%)
SCPS	1805 with recent nonmelanoma skin cancer, United States	Male and Female	5	50 mg β-carotene	No effect on occurrence of new nonmelanoma skin cancer

[a]Secondary prevention defined as subjects with documented cancer including nonmelanoma skin cancer (although some of the primary prevention trials did not exclude those with nonmelanoma skin cancer at baseline).
NPCT, Nutritional Prevention of Cancer Trial; SCPS: Skin Cancer Prevention Study.

adenoma, found no effect of either β-carotene or a combination of vitamins E and C (1000 mg) on the incidence of subsequent colorectal adenomas. The Heart Protection Study also found no beneficial effects of supplementation with these three vitamins on cancer mortality. However, trials have generally been carried out on those with diets containing sufficient amounts of vitamin C and there is a need for further studies in people with low intakes.

Vitamin E

The ATBC trial showed no significant effect of α-tocopherol supplementation (50 mg/day) on risk of lung, pancreatic, colorectal, or urinary tract cancers among heavy smokers (**Table 3**). However, in a post hoc subgroup analysis a 34% reduction in the risk of prostate cancer was seen in men who received this supplement. Although interesting, prostate cancer was not a primary endpoint of this study, and no other studies have supported a preventative effect of vitamin E for prostate cancer. The Heart Protection Study found no effect of vitamin E in combination with vitamin C and β-carotene on cancer incidence or mortality. Two smaller, short-term intervention studies found no effect of α-tocopherol supplementation on mammary dysplasia or benign breast disease. Several trials have also been unable to demonstrate a protective effect of vitamin E supplementation on the risk or recurrence of colorectal adenomatous polyps.

Selenium

A few trials have suggested that selenium supplementation may have a protective effect on liver cancer in high-risk groups living in low-selenium areas. The provision of selenium-fortified salt to a town in

Qidong, China, with high rates of primary liver cancer, reduced the incidence of this cancer by 35% compared with towns that did not receive this intervention (**Table 3**). Trials have also demonstrated the incidence of liver cancer to be significantly reduced in subjects with hepatitis B and among members of families with a history of liver cancer receiving a daily supplement of 200 µg of selenium for 4 and 2 years, respectively.

The Nutritional Prevention of Cancer Trial in the United States also supported a possible protective role of selenium (**Table 4**): 1312 patients (mostly men) with a previous history of skin cancer were supplemented with either placebo or 200 µg selenium per day for $4\frac{1}{2}$ years and those receiving selenium demonstrated significant reductions in the risk of cancer incidence (37%) and mortality (50%). Although selenium was not found to have a protective effect against recurrent skin cancer, the selenium-treated group had substantial reductions in the incidence of lung, colorectal, and prostate cancers of 46, 58, and 63%, respectively. Further analysis showed the protective effect on prostate cancer to be confined to those with lower baseline prostate-specific antigen and plasma selenium levels. Although these data need confirmation, they suggest that adequate selenium intake may be important for cancer prevention.

Other Diseases Associated with Oxidative Damage

Type 2 Diabetes

Type 2 diabetes is associated with elevated oxidative stress (especially lipid peroxidation) and declines in antioxidant defense. This is thought to be due in part to elevated blood glucose levels (hyperglycemia), but severe oxidative stress may also precede and accelerate the development of type 2 diabetes and then of diabetic complications (CVD and microvascular complications such as retinopathy, neuropathy, and nephropathy).

Small-scale human trials have shown administration of high doses of vitamin E to reduce oxidative stress and improve some CVD risk factors, such as blood glycated hemoglobin, insulin, and triglyceride levels, in people with diabetes. Such trials have also indicated benefit from vitamin E in improving endothelial function, retinal blood flow, and renal dysfunction. However, the findings of large clinical trials investigating the role of individual or a combination of antioxidant nutrients in reducing the risk of CVD and microvascular complications in people with diabetes have generally been disappointing. For example, the Heart Outcomes Prevention Evaluation Trial investigated the effects of vitamin E and the drug Ramipril in patients at high risk for CVD events and included a large number of middle-aged and elderly people with diabetes (more than 3600). An average of $4\frac{1}{2}$ years of supplementation with 400 IU of vitamin E per day was found to exert no beneficial or harmful effect on CVD outcomes or on nephropathy. The Primary Prevention Project trial found no effect of vitamin E (300 mg/day) supplementation for 3 or 4 years in diabetic subjects, and the Heart Protection Study, which included a number of people with diabetes, also reported no benefit of a combination of antioxidant vitamins on mortality or incidence of vascular disease.

Chronic Obstructive Pulmonary Disease (COPD)

The generation of oxygen free radicals by activated inflammatory cells produces many of the pathophysiological changes associated with COPD. Common examples of COPD are asthma and bronchitis, each of which affects large numbers of children and adults. Antioxidant nutrients have therefore been suggested to play a role in the prevention and treatment of these conditions. A number of studies have demonstrated a beneficial effect of fruit and vegetable intake on lung function. For example, regular consumption of fresh fruit rich in vitamin C (citrus fruits and kiwi) has been found to have a beneficial effect on reducing wheezing and coughs in children.

Vitamin C is the major antioxidant present in extracellular fluid lining the lung, and intake in the general population has been inversely correlated with the incidence of asthma, bronchitis, and wheezing and with pulmonary problems. Although some trials have shown high-dose supplementation (1–2 g/day) to improve symptoms of asthma in adults and protect against airway responsiveness to viral infections, allergens, and irritants, this effect has been attributed to the antihistaminic action of the vitamin rather than to any antioxidant effect. The results of these trials have also been inconsistent, and a Cochrane review of eight RCTs concluded that there is insufficient evidence to recommend a specific role for the vitamin in the treatment of asthma. However, a need for further trials to address the question of the effectiveness of vitamin C in asthmatic children was highlighted.

Other dietary antioxidants have been positively associated with lung function in cohort studies but the findings of clinical trials have been mixed. In a study of 158 children with moderate to severe asthma, supplementation with vitamin E (50 mg/day) and vitamin C (250 mg/day) led to some improvement in lung function following ozone exposure. However, the much larger ATBC trial found no benefit from supplementation with α-tocopherol (50 mg/day) and β-carotene (20 mg/day) on symptoms of COPD, despite the fact that those with high dietary intakes and blood levels of these vitamins at baseline had a lower prevalence of chronic bronchitis and dyspnea. A small trial investigating the effects of selenium supplementation in asthmatics found that those receiving the supplements experienced a significant increase in glutathione peroxidase levels and reported improvement in their asthma symptoms. However, this improvement could not be validated by significant changes in the separate clinical parameters of lung function and airway hyperresponsiveness. Therefore, there is little evidence to support the role of other nutrients in COPD treatment.

Macular Degeneration and Cataracts

The eye is at particular risk of oxidative damage due to high oxygen concentrations, large amounts of oxidizable fatty acids in the retina, and exposure to ultraviolet rays. In Western countries, age-related macular degeneration (AMD) is the leading cause of blindness among older people. Cataracts are also widespread among the elderly and occur when the lens is unable to function properly due to the formation of opacities within the lens. These develop when proteins in the eye are damaged by photooxidation; these damaged proteins build up, clump, and precipitate. It has been proposed that antioxidants may prevent cellular damage in the eye by reacting with free radicals produced during the process of light absorption.

The results of intervention trials in this area have also been mixed. The Age-Related Eye Disease Study in the United States investigating the effects of combined antioxidant vitamins C (500 mg), E (400 IU), and β-carotene (15 mg) with and without 80 mg zinc daily for 6 years showed some protective effect (a reduction in risk of approximately 25%) on the progression of moderately advanced AMD but no benefit on the incidence or progression or early AMD or cataracts. The Lutein Antioxidant Supplementation Trial, a 12-month study of 90 patients with AMD, found significant improvements in visual function with 10 mg/day lutein (one of the major carotenoids found in the pigment of a normal retina) alone or in combination with a number of other antioxidant nutrients. The Roche European Cataract Trial, providing a combined daily supplement of β-carotene, vitamin C, and vitamin E among adults with early signs of age-related cataract, showed a small deceleration in the progression of cataract after 3 years.

However, the Linxian trial found no influence of vitamin supplementation on risk of cataract; the ATBC trial found no reduction in the prevalence of cataracts with vitamin E, β-carotene, or both among male smokers; and the Health Physicians Study of more than 22 000 men showed no benefit from 12 years of supplementation with β-carotene (50 mg on alternate days) on cataract incidence. In fact, current smokers at the beginning of this trial who received the supplement experienced an increased risk of cataract (by approximately 25%) compared to the placebo group. The Vitamin E, Cataract and Age-Related Maculopathy Trial also reported no effect of supplementation with vitamin E for 4 years (500 IU/day) on the incidence or progression of cataracts or AMD.

Possible Explanations for the Disagreement between the Findings of Observational Studies and Clinical Trials

Various explanations have been given for the different findings of observational studies and intervention trials. Clearly, nonrandomized studies are unable to exclude the possibility that antioxidants are simply acting as a surrogate measure of a healthy diet or lifestyle and that the protective effect of certain dietary patterns, which has been presumed to be associated with dietary antioxidants, may in fact be due to other compounds in plant foods, substitution of these foods for others, or a reflection of other health behaviors common to people who have a high fruit and vegetable intake. However, although intervention studies provide a more rigorous source of evidence than observational studies, they are not without

weaknesses from a nutritional perspective and the trials have been criticized for a number of reasons:

- The nature of the supplements used: It has been suggested that the synthetic forms used in most trials may have different biological activity or potency from natural forms of these vitamins, although trials using the natural forms have not found different clinical effects. The type of isomer used has also been questioned (e.g., β-carotene versus other carotenoids such as lycopene or lutein or α-tocopherol versus γ-tocopherol). Trials have not investigated other potentially beneficial antioxidants in foods, such as flavonoids and lycopenes.

- The use of high doses of one or two antioxidants: Mechanistic and epidemiological data suggest that antioxidants act not only individually but also cooperatively and in some cases synergistically. Single supplements may interfere with the uptake, transport, distribution, and metabolism of other antioxidant nutrients. An optimal effect would therefore be expected to be seen with a combination of nutrients at levels similar to those contained in the diet (corresponding to higher levels of intake associated with reduced risk in the observational studies). The findings of clinical trials testing the effect of a cocktail of antioxidant nutrients at low doses are awaited, but the Heart Protection Study did not demonstrate a protective effect of multiple antioxidants and a small RCT of 160 patients with coronary disease, using a combination of antioxidant nutrients (800 IU α-tocopherol, 1000 mg vitamin C, 25 mg β-carotene, and 100 μg selenium twice daily) for 3 years, showed no benefit for secondary prevention of vascular disease.

- Insufficient duration of treatment and follow-up: Most of the intervention trials published to date (except the Physicians Health Study, which found no effect despite 12 years of follow-up) had durations of treatment and follow-up lasting only approximately 4–6 years. Diseases such as cancer and CVD develop over a long period of time and trials may have been too short to demonstrate any benefit.

- The use of high-risk groups: Many of the supplementation trials have not been undertaken on normal 'healthy' individuals but on those with preexisting oxidative stress, either through smoking or through preexisting disease, among whom increasing antioxidant intake may not have been able to repair the oxidative damage process sufficiently to affect cancer or CVD risk.

- Lack of information about the impact of genetic variability: Unknown genetic factors (interacting with nutrition) may explain some of the lack of effect in intervention studies. A greater understanding of the impact of factors such as genotype, age, and ill health on the interactions between antioxidants and reactive oxygen species would be helpful in designing future trials.

The Supplementation en Vitamines et Minéraux AntioXydants Study (SU.VI.MAX) has taken account of many of these issues in its design. This is a randomized, placebo-controlled trial testing the efficacy of supplementation among more than 12 000 healthy men and women over an 8-year period with a cocktail of antioxidant vitamins (120 mg vitamin C, 30 mg vitamin E, and 6 mg β-carotene) and minerals (100 µg selenium and 20 mg zinc) at doses achievable by diet (approximately one to three times the daily recommended dietary allowances) on premature death from CVD and cancer. Early reports suggest that this regime has not demonstrated an effect on CVD risk but has led to a 31% decrease in cancer incidence and a 37% reduction in total mortality among men but not women. This may reflect higher dietary intakes of these nutrients among the women in the trial compared to men, but publication of these results is still awaited. However, this is a good illustration of the type of nutritional approach that may be needed in the future.

Conclusion

Although there is a substantial body of evidence that diets rich in plant foods (particularly fruit and vegetables) convey health benefits, as do high plasma levels of several antioxidant nutrients found in these foods, a causal link between lack of antioxidants and disease occurrence or between antioxidant administration and disease prevention remains to be established. There is a lack of understanding of the mechanisms underpinning the apparent protective effect of plant foods and, as yet, no clear picture of which components are effective and hence no way of predicting whether all or just some plant foods are important in this respect.

If future trials do demonstrate a reduction in chronic disease risk with antioxidant supplementation, this cannot be definitively attributed to the antioxidant effect of these nutrients because other biological functions may also play a role. For example, in addition to retarding LDL oxidation, vitamin E may help to protect against CVD via its action on platelet aggregation and adhesion or by inhibition of the proliferation of smooth muscle cells. Furthermore, although vitamin C, vitamin E, and selenium have been shown to decrease the concentration of some of the biomarkers associated with oxidative stress, the relationship between many of these biomarkers and chronic disease remains to be elucidated.

The intervention studies highlight the lack of information on the safety of sustained intakes of moderate to high doses of micronutrient supplements and long-term harm cannot be ruled out, particularly in smokers. Further evidence is required regarding the efficacy, safety, and appropriate dosage of antioxidants in relation to chronic disease.

Currently, the most prudent public health advice continues to be to consume a variety of plant foods.

See also: **Antioxidants**: Diet and Antioxidant Defense; Observational Studies. **Ascorbic Acid**: Physiology, Dietary Sources and Requirements; Deficiency States. **Cancer**: Epidemiology and Associations Between Diet and Cancer; Effects on Nutritional Status. **Carotenoids**: Chemistry, Sources and Physiology; Epidemiology of Health Effects. **Coronary Heart Disease**: Hemostatic Factors; Lipid Theory. **Diabetes Mellitus**: Etiology and Epidemiology; Classification and Chemical Pathology; Dietary Management. **Lipoproteins**. **Lung Diseases**. **Selenium**. **Stroke, Nutritional Management**. **Vitamin E**: Metabolism and Requirements; Physiology and Health Effects.

Further Reading

Asplund K (2002) Antioxidant vitamins in the prevention of cardiovascular disease: A systematic review. *Journal of Internal Medicine* **251**: 372–392.

British Nutrition Foundation (2001) *Briefing Paper: Selenium and Health*. London: British Nutrition Foundation.

British Nutrition Foundation (2003) *Plants: Diet and Health. A Report of the British Nutrition Foundation Task Force* Goldberg G (ed.) Oxford: Blackwell Science.

Clarke R and Armitage J (2002) Antioxidant vitamins and risk of cardiovascular disease. Review of large-scale randomised trials. *Cardiovascular Drugs and Therapy* **16**: 411–415.

Evans J (2002) Antioxidant vitamin and mineral supplements for age-related macular degeneration. *Cochrane Database Systematic Review* **2**: CD000254.

Lawlor DA, Davey Smith G, Kundu D *et al.* (2004) Those confounded vitamins: What can we learn from the differences between observational versus randomised trial evidence? *Lancet* **363**: 1724–1727.

Lee I (1999) Antioxidant vitamins in the prevention of cancer. *Proceedings of the Association of American Physicians* **111**: 10–15.

Mares JA (2004) High-dose antioxidant supplementation and cataract risk. *Nutrition Review* **62**: 28–32.

Morris C and Carson S (2003) Routine vitamin supplementation to prevent cardiovascular disease: A summary of the evidence for the US Preventive Services Task Force. *Annals of Internal Medicine* **139**: 56–70.

National Academy of Sciences Food and Nutrition Board (2000) *Dietary Reference Intakes for Vitamin C, Vitamin E, Selenium and Carotenoids*. Washington, DC: National Academy Press.

Ram F, Rowe B, and Kaur B (2004) Vitamin C supplementation for asthma. *Cochrane Database Systematic Review* **3**: CD000993.

Stanner SA, Hughes J, Kelly CNM *et al.* (2004) A review of the epidemiological evidence for the 'antioxidant hypothesis.' *Public Health Nutrition* **7**: 407–422

Vivekananthan D, Penn MS, Sapp SK *et al.* (2003) Use of antioxidant vitamins for the prevention of cardiovascular disease: Meta-analysis of randomised trials. *Lancet* **361**: 2017–2023.

APPETITE

Contents

Physiological and Neurobiological Aspects

J C G Halford, University of Liverpool, Liverpool, UK
J E Blundell, University of Leeds, Leeds, UK

© 2005 Elsevier Ltd. All rights reserved.

Appetite Regulation and Expression

Traditionally it has been thought that appetite is influenced solely by body components or by metabolism. These influences are commonly referred to as the glucostatic, aminostatic, thermostatic, or lipostatic hypotheses. Each suggests that a single variable such as glucose, amino acids, heat generation, or adipose tissue stores plays the major role in modulating the expression of appetite. It can be accepted that all four variables can be monitored and each can exert some influences over food consumption. In the last few years research has given renewed support to the lipostatic hypothesis, specifically, the identification of the adipose signal leptin. The short-term consequences of food ingestion generated by a meal also produce a powerful inhibition on further intake (satiety). We can draw a distinction between short-term satiety signals generated by the physiological consequences of meal intake (episodic), and the long-term signals generated by the body's constant metabolic need for energy (tonic). This distinction may be a useful starting point in our examination of the integration of the CNS systems responsible for the expression of appetite.

Episodic Events: Hunger, Satiety and the Appetite Cascade

A good place to start is the psychological experiences of hunger and satiety that underpin the pattern of eating behavior. Hunger can be defined as the motivation to seek and consume food initiating a period of feeding behavior. The process that brings this period to an end is termed satiation. Satiation processes ultimately lead to the state of satiety in which the hunger drive, and consequently eating behavior, is inhibited. The processes of satiation determine the meal size and the state of satiety determines the length of the post meal interval. The net effect of these systems can be considered before (preprandial or cephalic phase), during (prandial), and after (postprandial) a meal (see **Figure 1**).

Preconsumption physiological signals are generated by the sight and smell of the food, preparing the body for ingestion. Such afferent sensory information, carried to the brainstem via cranial nerves, stimulates hunger before eating and during the initial stages of consumption (the prandial phase). During the prandial phase the CNS receives postingestive sensory afferent input from the gut reflecting both the amount of food eaten and earliest representations of its nutrient content. Mechanoreceptors in the gut detect the distension of gut lining caused by the presence of food aiding the estimation of the volume of food consumed. Gut chemoreceptors detect the chemical presence of various nutrients in the gastrointestinal tract providing information on the composition (and possible energy content) of the food consumed. Prandial and postprandial signals are generated by the detection of nutrients that

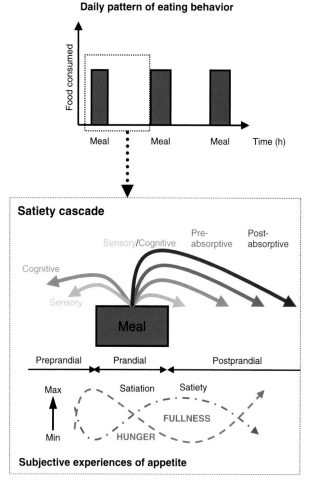

Figure 1 The satiety cascade. The signals generated prior to (preprandial), during (prandial), and after (postprandial) the consumption of a meal critical to short-term (episodic) meal-by-meal appetite regulation throughout the day.

have been absorbed from the gastrointestinal tract and have entered the circulation in the periphery (postabsorptive satiety signals). Circulating nutrients that are either metabolized in the periphery (e.g., liver) activate central nervous system (CNS) receptors (e.g., in brainstem), or they enter and affect the brain directly and act as postabsorptive metabolic satiety signals.

Neural Structures Critical to the Expression of Appetite

The CNS receives information generated by the sensory experience of eating, and from the periphery indicating the ingestion, absorption, metabolism, and storage of energy. To regulate appetite a variety of structures within the CNS integrate multiple signals, to assess the biological need for energy, to generate or inhibit conscious experiences of hunger, and subsequently to initiate the appropriate behavioral action. Information reaches the CNS via three main routes:

1. Signals from the periphery: peripheral receptors in the gut (distension and chemo-receptors) and metabolic changes in the liver (energy conversion and energy status) send afferent signals via the vagus nerve to the nucleus of the solitary tract/area postrema (NST/AP) complex in the brainstem.
2. Signals from specific receptors within the brain: receptors in the CNS, particularly in the brainstem detecting circulating levels of nutrients, their metabolites, and other factors within the periphery.
3. Substances crossing the blood–brain barrier entering the brain: factors such as neurotransmitter precursors, leptin or insulin cross the blood–brain barrier and directly alter CNS neurochemical activity, particularly in key hypothalamic nuclei and associated limbic areas.

Original theories of the neural control of appetite conceptualize food intake to be controlled by the opposing action of two hypothalamic centers (lateral hypothalamus, LH; and ventral medial hypothalamus, VMH). However, with later precision technologies numerous hypothalamic and nonhypothalamic nuclei have been implicated in the control of both hunger and satiety. For instance, infusions of various agents in or near the paraventricular nucleus (PVN), a key hypothalamic site, produce either marked increases or decreases in food intake and of specific macronutrients. Other key limbic sites identified as playing critical roles in appetite regulation include the arcuate nucleus (ARC), nucleus accumbens (NAc), the amygdala, posterior hypothalamus and the dorsal medial hypothalamus. Nonhypothalamic/limbic regions key to the expression of appetite include the NTS/AP adjacent areas in the hindbrain that relay vagal afferent satiety signals from the periphery (particularly receptors in the gastrointestinal tract and liver) to the hypothalamus. This area of the brainstem appears to possess receptors sensitive to levels of circulating nutrients and afferent sensory information from the mouth including taste (carried by cranial nerves).

Interrelated Levels of the System

Before we go on to consider the individual systems underpinning the expression of appetite it is useful to try and understand how neural, nutritional, and psychological events interact before, during, and after a meal. The biopsychological system underlying the expression of appetite can be conceptualized as having three domains (**Figure 2**):

1. Psychological events (e.g., subjective sensations of hunger, satiety, hedonics, and cravings) accompanying observable behavioral operations (meal intake, snacking behavior, food choice) and their measurable consequences (energy intake and macronutrient composition of food consumed).
2. Peripheral physiology and metabolic events related to the effect of absorbed nutrients and

their utilization or subsequent conversion for storage (i.e., the changes in the body due to either energy intake and/or energy deficit).
3. Neurochemical (classic neurotransmitters, neuropeptides, and hormones) and metabolic interactions within the CNS (i.e., how various signals of the body's energy status are detected in the brain).

The expression of appetite reflects the synchronous operation of events and processes in all three domains.

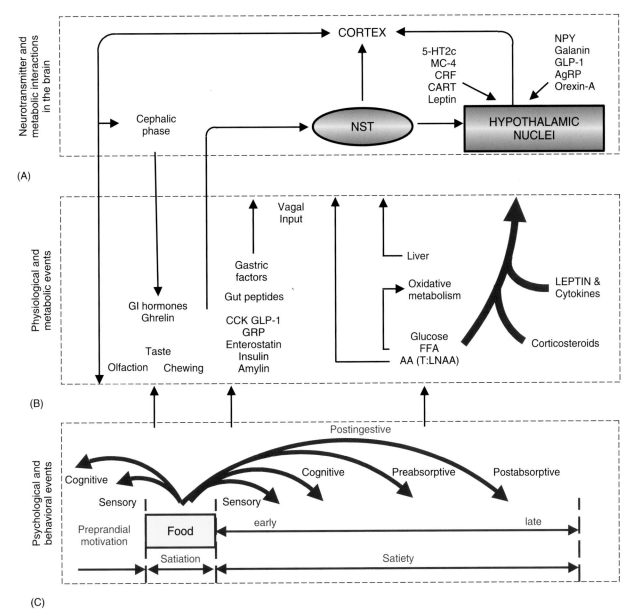

Figure 2   The psychobiological expression of appetite and the three levels of operation: (A) psychological and behavioral events; (B) physiological and metabolic operations; and (C) neurochemical and metabolic interactions within the CNS. *Abbreviations*: 5-HT, serotonin; AA, amino acids; AgRP, agouti-related peptide; CART, cocaine and amphetamine-regulated transcript; CCK, cholecystokinin; CRF, corticotropin releasing factor; FFA, free fatty acids; GI, gastrointestinal; GLP-1, glucagon-like peptide-1; GRP, gastric releasing peptide; MC, melanocortin; NPY, neuropeptide Y; T/LNAA, NTS, nucleus tractus solitarius; T/LNAA, tryptophan large neutral amino acids ratio.

Initiation and Stimulation of Eating: Mechanisms Underpinning Hunger

The intimate contact of mainly chemical, but also physical, stimuli with receptors in the mucosa of the nose and mouth set up orosensory effects of food stimuli. This is in turn transmitted to the brain by afferent fibers of primary olfactory, gustatory, and somatosensory neurons of cranial nerves 1, 5, 7, 9, and 10. These peripheral inputs appear to make contact with dopamine and opioid neurotransmitters in the brain. The cephalic phase of appetite control refers to physiological responses engendered by the sight or smell of food, which are anticipatory and serve to prepare the system for the imminent ingestion of food. Cephalic phase responses occur in the mouth (anticipatory secretion of saliva), stomach, and small intestine and represent preprandial changes that are precursors for the onset of a meal.

In addition it has been proposed that changes in blood glucose may serve as a signal for meal initiation. Recent evidence provides some support for a role for 'transient declines' in blood glucose in humans leading to increased expression of hunger and the initiation of eating. Potent feeding responses can also be obtained by microinjection of peptides to the brain of animals. A number of peptides, including β-endorphin, dynorphin, neuropeptide Y (NPY), orexins (OX-A and OX-B), galanin, agouti-related peptide (AgRP), and melanin-concentrating hormone (MCH) increase food intake.

Neuropeptide Y (NPY) is probably the most studied appetite stimulatory peptide. NPY is found throughout the CNS and in particular abundance in the PVN of the hypothalamus. Hypothalamic NPY neurons that are implicated in appetite regulation project from the ARC to the PVN. Infusing NPY directly into the CNS or increasing release of NPY within the PVN promotes meal initiation and produces an immediate and marked increase in food intake, delaying the onset of satiety. The hyperphagic effects of NPY appear to be mediated by both NPY Y1 and Y5 receptors. Endogenous NPY is sensitive to a variety of peripherally generated signals. It is stimulated by the gut factor ghrelin, but inhibited by the pancreatic hormone amylin, the adiposity signal leptin, and the satiety neurotransmitter serotonin (5-HT). Like NPY, galanin-induced hyperphagia has been well documented. Early studies demonstrated that direct infusion of galanin into the hypothalamus of rodents stimulated feeding behavior. Moreover, high concentrations of galanin and its receptors are found in the hypothalamus in areas associated with appetite regulation.

A more recently discovered CNS stimulatory system is that of the orexins. The endogenous orexin system is integrated with other critical hypothalamic energy regulatory systems. The system consists of two peptides, termed orexin-A and orexin-B, along with two orexin receptors, orexin-1 (OX1) and orexin-2 (OX2). The strongest and most reliable effect on food intake is produced by orexin-A. The endogenous orexin system responds to insulin-induced hypoglycemia and food restriction. Moreover, leptin reduces orexin-A concentration in the hypothalamus, and partially blocks orexin-A induced changes in feeding behavior.

Not all stimulatory peptide systems are within the brain. Ghrelin is a peripherally secreted hormone responsive to nutritional status. Human plasma ghrelin increases during fasting and decreases after food intake. Unlike the other gut-derived factors detailed in this review, ghrelin stimulates rather than inhibits feeding behavior. Both peripheral and central infusions of ghrelin have been shown to stimulate food intake in rats and mice, an effect in part mediated by central NPY. In lean humans, endogenous plasma ghrelin levels rise markedly before a meal and are suppressed by food intake. In lean healthy volunteers, ghrelin infusions increase food intake, premeal hunger, and prospective consumption.

Satiety: Peripheral Physiological Influences

Intake of energy can only be achieved (in mammals) through the gastrointestinal tract, and energy intake is limited by the capacity of the tract. Humans are periodic feeders and usually meals are separated by periods (intermeal intervals) of 3–5 h during which little food is eaten. It can be noted that the periodicity of meal eating is compatible with the time taken by the gastrointestinal tract to process a meal. After the ingestion of a meal the stomach mixes the meal with gastric secretions that aid its liquefaction and delivers the mixture at a steady rate into the small intestine for further chemical digestion and absorption. Four hours after ingestion most of the meal has left the stomach and the majority of nutrients have been absorbed. It seems obvious that the stomach must be involved in the termination of eating (satiation). Indeed stomach distension is regarded as being an important satiety signal. A good deal of experimental evidence indicates that gastric distension can arrest eating behavior, but the effect may be short lived. By itself, gastric distension does not appear to produce the sensation of satiety and cannot be the only factor controlling meal size. Indeed, chemicals released by gastric stimuli or by food processing in the gastrointestinal tract are critical to the episodic control of appetite. Many of these chemicals are peptide neurotransmitters, and many peripherally administered peptides cause changes in food consumption.

There is evidence for an endogenous role for cholecystokinin (CCK), pancreatic glucagon, gastrin releasing peptide (GRP), and somatostatin. Much recent research has confirmed the status of CCK as a hormone mediating meal termination (satiation) and possibly early phase satiety. Food consumption (mainly protein and fat) stimulates the release of CCK (from duodenal mucosal cells), which in turn activates CCK-A type receptors in the pyloric region of the stomach. This signal is transmitted via afferent fibers of the vagus nerve to the nucleus tractus solitarius (NTS) in the brainstem. From here the signal is relayed to the hypothalamic region where integration with other signals occurs. Direct infusions of CCK dose-dependently reduce food intake in mice, rats and monkeys, and in human volunteers the CCK octopeptide CCK-8 reduces food intake and enhances satiety. Peripheral CCK-8 administration has also been shown to increase the release of serotonin in the hypothalamus, a neurotransmitter that has been implicated in the integration of episodic satiety signals.

Other potential peripheral satiety signals include peptides such as enterostatin, neurotensin, and glucagon-like peptide (GLP-1). Researchers are continually searching for components of peripheral metabolism that could provide information to the brain concerning the pattern of eating behavior. There is considerable current interest in the peptide called enterostatin. It is formed by the cleavage of procolipase that produces colipase and this 5 amino acid activation peptide. The administration of enterostatin reduces food intake and, since it is increased after high-fat feeding, it has been suggested that enterostatin could be a specific fat-induced satiety signal. Another gut factor stimulated by the ingestion of dietary fat is intestinal glycoprotein apolipoprotein A-IV produced in the human small intestine and released into intestinal lymph in response to dietary lipids.

Glucagon-like peptide 1 (GLP-1) is a hormone that is released from the gut into the bloodstream in response to intestinal carbohydrate. Endogenous GLP-1 levels increase after meals with the largest increase in response to carbohydrate ingestion. In humans, infusions of glucose directly into the gut or the ingestion of carbohydrate produces a decrease in appetite and an increase in blood GLP-1. A series of studies by Meier and coworkers in both lean and obese human volunteers demonstrated that infusions of synthetic human GLP-1 enhanced ratings of fullness and satiety and reduced food intake and spontaneous eating behavior. Recent research has also focused on amylin, a pancreatic hormone, which also has a potent effect on both food intake and body weight. Peripheral administration of amylin reduces food intake in mice and rats, and meal size in rats.

One further source of biological information relevant to the control of appetite concerns fuel metabolism. The products of food digestion may be metabolized in peripheral tissues or organs, or may enter the brain directly. Most research has involved glucose metabolism and fatty acid oxidation in the hepatoportal area. The main hypothesis suggests that satiety is associated with an increase in fuel oxidation. Indirect evidence is provided by the use of antimetabolites that block oxidation pathways or impair fuel availability and lead to increases in food intake. It is argued that membranes or tissues sensitive to this metabolic activity modulate afferent discharges that are relayed to the brain via the vagus nerve. Pathways in the CNS that are sensitive to this metabolic signaling have begun to be mapped out. It is difficult to identify CNS mechanisms that specifically integrate short-term satiety signals alone into appetite regulation. Generally, the peripheral release and detection of various gut peptides could account for their satiety function. However, direct entry into, and action on receptors in the CNS, may also contribute to their satiety action. The one central factor clearly associated with episodic satiety, rather than tonic energy status, is serotonin (see below).

Tonic Signals: The Moderating Effects of Energy Status

Appetite is not only derived from the daily flux of physiology associated with meals and eating behavior but also must respond to the long-term (tonic) energy status of the organism. Factors derived from the processes of energy storage and the status of the body's energy stores must also contribute to appetite and its expression (e.g., indicators of glucose metabolism and fat storage). Blood carries various substances (other than nutrients) generated in organs implicated in nutrient metabolism and energy storage such as the liver, the pancreas and in adipose tissue depots that reflect the body's energy status and that have been shown to have potent effects on food intake (insulin, glucagons, and leptin). The number of potentially active metabolites and by-products produced by energy metabolism of differing nutrients is vast providing a wide range of potential indicator substances.

As noted earlier one of the classical theories of appetite control has involved the notion of a so-called long-term regulation involving a signal that informs the brain about the state of adipose tissue stores. This idea has given rise to the notion of a lipostatic or ponderostatic mechanism. Indeed, this is a specific example of a more general class of peripheral appetite (satiety) signals believed to circulate in the blood reflecting the state of depletion or repletion of energy reserves that directly modulate brain mechanisms. Levels of substances such as satietin and adipsin, or cytokine signals such as interleukin-6 (IL-6) tumor-necrosing factors (e.g., TNFα) may all be influenced by adipose tissue. Levels of other circulating hormones, for example, gonadal steroids (androgens, estrogens, and progesterone) also reflect the body fat mass, and so its energy status. Gonadal steroids have potent effects on (both increasing and reducing) food intake, meal size and frequency, body weight, and per cent body fat.

Leptin (ob Protein)

For 40 years, scientists searched for a mechanism by which the brain could monitor body fat deposition in order to keep an animal's body weight constant. In 1994, a gene that controlled the expression of a protein produced by adipose tissue was identified. Circulating levels of this protein (the ob protein) could be measured in normal weight mice. However, in obese ob/ob mice, which display marked overeating, this protein was absent due to a mutation of the ob gene. A series of studies demonstrated that the absence of this protein was responsible for overconsumption and obesity in the obese ob/ob. As the ob protein reduces food intake and also increases metabolic energy expenditure, both of which would result in weight loss, it was named leptin from the Greek 'leptos' meaning thin. In general, circulating levels of leptin appear to reflect the current status of body fat deposition and increase with the level of adiposity demonstrating the responsiveness of endogenous leptin to weight gain and energy status.

Since the identification of leptin and its receptor researchers have isolated numerous CNS hypothalamic neuropeptide systems, which mediate the hypophagic action of leptin. NPY, the melanocortins, corticotropin releasing factor (CRF), cocaine and amphetamine regulated transcript (CART), and the orexins may all be part of the circuit linking adipose tissue with central appetite regulatory mechanisms. Certainly the fact that leptin has multiple effects on complex hypothalamic appetite systems, consisting of wide ranging but integrated regulatory neuropeptides, would appear to support the view that leptin is a major factor in body weight regulation. There is evidence of synergy between leptin and the short-term meal-generated satiety factor CCK. Systemic administration of CCK enhances leptin-induced decreases in food intake and augments weight loss in rodents.

Integration of Episodic and Tonic Signals within the CNS

As stated previously, certain brainstem, hypothalamic, and other limbic sites appear critical in the regulation of food intake and feeding behavior. Within these sites numerous neurochemicals (first neurotransmitters and then neuropeptides) have been identified as potent inhibitors and stimulators of feeding behavior. 5-HT has been implicated as a critical CNS satiety factor in the short-term regulation of food intake. Specifically, the 5-HT system appears to be sensitive to meal-generated satiety factors such as CCK, enterostatin, and ingested macronutrients. Moreover, 5-HT drugs appear to enhance satiety, suppress CNS NPY release, and inhibit hunger. 5-HT appears to mediate the effects of episodic meal-generated satiety on appetite. The second CNS system to be involved is that of the melanocortins, which appear integral in the action of circulating leptin on intake and (like 5-HT) its agonists also inhibit NPY functioning. Thus, the melanocortins may mediate the effects of tonic energy status on appetite.

Of all the monoamines, 5-HT has been most closely linked with the episodic process of satiation and the state of satiety. Moreover, it has been known for a long time that serotoninergic drugs reliably reduce food intake and body weight, both in animals and humans. A number of researchers have identified the critical role of 5-HT_{1B} and 5-HT_{2C} in mediating the satiety effect of 5-HT. Direct agonists of 5-HT_{1B} and 5-HT_{2C} have been shown to reduce intake and to produce changes in feeding behavior consistent with the operation of satiety. Studies with selective 5-HT_{1B} and 5-HT_{2C} agonists in humans confirm their satiety-enhancing properties. Hypothalamic areas, including the PVN, have been implicated in 5-HT hypophagia. 5-HT activation suppresses the levels of the appetite stimulatory peptide NPY within the PVN. Conversely, blocking 5-HT synthesis or antagonizing 5-HT receptors increases NPY functioning in the PVN. This interaction between 5-HT and NPY may be one of the critical mechanisms in short-term (episodic) appetite, determining the generation of either hunger or satiety. As mentioned previously, 5-HT function has been linked to peripheral signals triggered by fat ingestion, such as CCK and enterostatin. Moreover, CNS levels of the 5-HT precursor tryptophan are directly affected by dietary carbohydrate, through its action on the tryptophan/large neutral amino acid competition to cross the blood–brain barrier. Thus, CNS 5-HT is sensitive to both fat and carbohydrate ingestion.

The melanocortins are one of the inhibitory systems through which the tonic adiposity signal leptin inhibits food intake. Like leptin, the role of CNS melanocortins was revealed through the investigation of a genetic mouse model of obesity (agouti (A y/a)) syndrome. These animals were obese, displayed marked hyperphagia, and produced excessive amounts of agouti, an endogenous antagonist of melanocortin receptors. The hyperphagia was linked specifically to blockade of the melanocortin MC4R receptor. Children who are unable to synthesize endogenous melanocortin receptor agonists also display abnormal eating patterns and obesity. It soon became apparent that the melanocortin receptor MC4R, and a number of its endogenous agonists (such as αMSH), and antagonists (such as AgRP) were part of the endogenous body weight regulation system. MC4R receptors are expressed widely throughout the CNS and in the hypothalamus and these systems appear to mediate the effects of a number of factors such as leptin and insulin. For instance, CNS administration of MC4R receptor agonists inhibits NPY-induced hyperphagia.

Even if tonic signals such as leptin are generated independently from episodic signals they must feedback to reduce intake by altering subjective experiences of hunger and satiety. Increases and decreases in endogenous circulating leptin do have an effect on the modulation of subjective experiences of hunger. Moreover, endogenous leptin levels may fluctuate

across the day, in part as a consequence of meal consumption and the effects this has on metabolism. Individuals with an inability to produce leptin experience constant hunger and without the tonic leptin signal the constant drive for energy is unleashed and leads to continuous and voracious food-seeking behavior. Similarly, specific deficits in a system that responds to circulating leptin, in this case the absence of functional melanocortin MC4R receptors, produces similar effects on appetite and intake. These extreme examples demonstrate the inability of short-term meal-generated episodic signals alone to block the override demand for energy (expressed as continuous hunger) generated by tonic basal metabolism.

Summary: Episodic and Tonic Factors in the Regulation of Appetite

Endogenous 5-HT and leptin represent two aspects of negative feedback integral to the appetite control

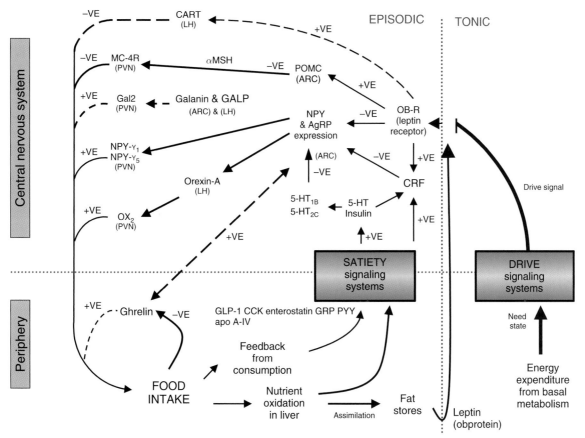

Figure 3 The integration of peripherally generated episodic and tonic signals critical to the expression of appetite. Signals generated by both meal consumption and fat deposition are integrated into a complex hypothalamic system of neuropeptides, which in turn either stimulate or inhibit subsequent food intake. Abbreviations: 5-HT, serotonin; αMSH, alpha melanocortin stimulating hormone; AgRP, agouti-related peptide; A-IV, apoliproprotein-IV; ARC, arcuate nucleus; CART, cocaine and amphetamine-regulated transcript; CCK, cholecystokinin; CRF, corticotropin releasing factor; GAL, galanin; GLP-1, glucagon-like peptide-1; GRP, gastric releasing peptide; LH, lateral hypothalamus; MC, melanocortin; NPY, neuropeptide Y; OX, orexin; PVN, paraventricular hypothalamus; POMC, pre-pro-opiomelanocortin; PYY, peptide YY.

system (see **Figure 3**). Both systems appear to inhibit NPY functioning, the effect of leptin being partly mediated by melanocortins and other excitatory and inhibitory neuropeptides. 5-HT mediates the effect of meal-derived satiety factors derived from pre- and postingestive processes (such as CCK and enterostatin relsease) and promotes meal termination, prolonging the intermeal interval. By such a mechanism the body deals with the daily physiological fluxes that result from meal intake ensuring an approximately appropriate daily energy intake. Circulating leptin accurately reflects the current status of the body's energy store. Leptin levels continually modify total daily and meal food intake to maintain a sufficient but not excessive level of energy deposition. Thus, 5-HT and leptin represent two classes of signals: short-term episodic and long-term tonic feedback, respectively. The net result of the action both episodic and tonic signals will be an adjustment in the expression of appetite, adjusting subsequent feeding behavior to compensate for previous intake and energy stored.

See also: **Appetite**: Psychobiological and Behavioral Aspects. **Brain and Nervous System**. **Hunger**. **Lipoproteins**.

Further Reading

Blundell JE (1991) Pharmacological approaches to appetite suppression. *Trends in Pharmacological Sciences* 12: 147–157.

Blundell JE and Halford JCG (1998) Serotonin and appetite regulation: Implications for the treatment of obesity. *CNS Drugs* 9(6): 473–495.

Gehlert DR (1999) Role of hypothalamic neuropeptide Y in feeding and obesity. *Neuropeptides* 33: 329–338.

Halford JCG, Cooper GD, Dovey TM, Ishii Y, Rodgers RJ, and Blundell JCG (2003) Pharmacological Approaches to Obesity treatment, Current Medical Chemistry. *Central Nervous System Agents* 3: 283–310.

MacNeil DJ, Howard AD, Guan XM, Fong TM, Nargaund RP, Bednarek MA, Goulet MT, Weinberg DH, Strack AM, Marsh DJ, Chen HY, Shen CP, Chen AS, Rosenblun Cl, Macneil T, Tota M, MacIntyre ED, and Van der Ploeg LHT (2002) The role of melanocortins in body weight regulation: opportunities for the treatment of obesity. *European Journal of Pharmacology* 440(2–3): 141–157.

Meier JJ, Gallwitz B, Schmidt WE, and Nauck MA (2002) Glucagon-like peptide 1 as a regulator of food intake and body weight: therapeutic perspectives. *Eur. J. Pharmacol.* 440: 267–279.

Moran TH (2000) Cholecystokinin and satiety: current perspectives. *Nutrition* 16: 858–865.

Morton GJ and Schwartz MW (2001) The NPY/AgRP neuron and energy homeostasis. *International Journal of Obesity* 25(supplement 5): s56–62.

Rodgers RJ, Ishii Y, Halford JCG, and Blundell JE (2002) Orexins and appetite regulation. *Neuropeptides* 36(5): 303–326.

Woods SC and Seeley RJ (2000) Adiposity signals and the control of energy homeostasis. *Nutrition* 16: 894–902.

Zhang Y, Proenca R, Maffei M, Barone M, Leopold L, and Friedman JM (1994) Positional cloning of the mouse obese gene and its human homologue. *Nature* 372: 425–432.

Psychobiological and Behavioral Aspects

R J Stubbs and S Whybrow, The Rowett Research Institute, Aberdeen, UK
J E Blundell, University of Leeds, Leeds, UK

© 2005 Elsevier Ltd. All rights reserved.

The Nature of Feeding Behavior and Appetite 'Regulation'

Mammalian feeding occurs regularly and intermittently and despite a general lack of conscious nutritional knowledge on the part of the animal, usually appears to match energy intake (EI) and nutrient intakes with requirements. How is this achieved? The common explanation is that appetite, EI, or feeding behavior are regulated to ensure that physiological requirements are met. However, there is a lack of direct evidence for this regulation. It may be that neither feeding behavior nor appetite are regulated in a strictly physiological sense since: (1) neither are held constant within certain narrow limits; and (2) feeding responses are not an inevitable response to an altered physiological signal or need. Feeding behavior is responsive to a number of induced states such as pregnancy, cold exposure, growth and development, and weight loss. These responses have often been cited as evidence of a system that is regulated. It is probable that aspects of body size and composition are regulated and that changes in feeding behavior are functionally coupled to those regulatory processes. Indeed, feeding behavior might be said to be adaptive rather than regulated since patterns of food intake are flexible, responsive, and anticipatory, enabling the animal to adapt to changes in the state of the internal and external environment.

Hunger and satiety often have a large learned, anticipatory component rather than being the direct consequences of unconditioned physiological signals *per se*, such as reduced gastrointestinal content. Such physiological events can act as important cues for feeding but they do not necessarily directly determine that behavior.

The mechanism by which feeding behavior is coupled to physiological (and other events) is the process of learning. To understand feeding behavior, hunger, and satiety processes, the mechanism by which learning links feeding behavior to physiological, sensory, nutritional, situational, and other learning cues must be appreciated. This is true for mice and men. This mechanism is termed 'associative conditioning' of preferences, appetites, and satieties.

Learned Appetites, Satieties, and Feeding Behavior

Animals and humans learn (or become conditioned) to associate a given food with the physiological consequences of having ingested it. They associate certain proximal stimuli such as the smell, color, taste, or texture of a food (the conditioning stimulus) with a set of sensations that are directly felt (sensory afferent inputs), in relation to the external stimulus and to the endogenous changes such as physiological and neuroendocrine responses to food. The physiological changes that occur as a result of ingesting the food are termed the 'unconditioned stimulus.' The subject forms a learned or 'conditioned association' between the conditioning stimulus and the unconditioned stimulus (the

detectable consequence of eating), which informs them of the sensory and physiological consequences of ingesting that food. This process is summarized in **Figure 1**. Conditioned or learned associations are most efficiently established if the food is sensorially distinct, if there is a significant detectable postingestive consequence of ingesting the food and if a training or learning schedule is encountered (e.g., by repeated exposure to the food under similar conditions). Learning is facilitated by social interaction.

As regards appetite 'regulation' a problem arises when foods are constructed to look and taste like foods with a different composition. For some time after the initial exposure to the food subjects will respond to it in a manner that is determined not by immediate exposure to the food but by what they have learned during the previous period of exposure to the similar foods upon which the learning was originally based. Only if the food produces a very large unconditioned stimulus will this previously learned response be instantly over-ridden. This raises the possibility that the use of food mimetics (e.g., artificial sweeteners) may disrupt stable patterns of learned feeding behavior in consumers at large.

The above view of the nature of feeding behavior has implications for the way the appetite system functions in lean and overweight people.

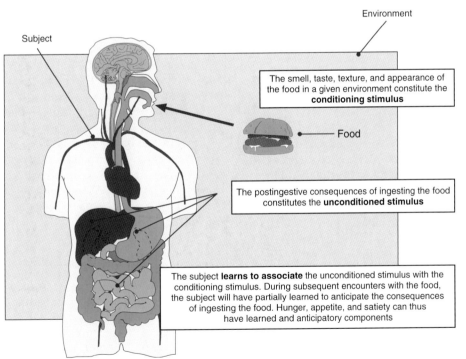

Figure 1 The process by which the subject learns to associate the postingestive consequences of eating with the food eaten and the environment in which it was eaten. Environmental influences can vary in strength from negligible effect to, in extremis, influences so strong that they can constitute the major factor determining a subject's subsequent response to that food.

Physiologists have expended considerable time and effort in attempting to understand how feeding behavior is geared to the regulation of a stable body weight. Obesity is therefore seen as a consequence of defects in this regulation. The evidence from behavioral studies suggests that feeding behavior is inherently more responsive to decreases rather than increases in body weight. Second, current secular trends in body weight suggest that, over time, it is relatively easy to increase body weight, which infers body weight is not tightly regulated, at least with reference to weight gain. For instance, according to the National Health and Nutrition Examination Survey (NHANES) ongoing dietary surveys of American adults, average weight change amounts to a gain of 0.2–$2.0\,\mathrm{kg\,year^{-1}}$. Third, while obese subjects exhibit differences in their feeding behavior and physiology, the literature is remarkably short of clear lean–obese differences in feeding behavior of a type that suggest defects in a regulatory system. For example, evidence suggests that the obese tend to select a diet rich in fat, which in itself facilitates over consumption. However, the tendency to select fat cannot be viewed as a defect in physiological regulation. It may be far more profitable to attempt to understand how feeding responds to environmental and endogenous stimuli, and which of these responses are functional and/or adaptive and which are not. This consideration influences the methodological approaches that attempt to investigate how feeding behavior responds to endogenous and environmental influences.

Methodological Issues

Measuring Hunger

Hunger is a subjectively expressed construct that people use to express a motivation to eat. The most appropriate measure of hunger is its subjective expression at a given time. This is achieved by asking subjects to mark a visual analog scale, which takes the form of a straight line with two extreme representations of hunger anchored at either end. It is most useful to track changes in subjective hunger over time and in relation to feeding events, diet composition, or physiological parameters. Hunger itself exhibits a large learned component (see above) as reflected by the fact that most of the variation in the subjectively expressed hunger of human subjects is accounted for by time. If hunger is plotted against time in Western subjects feeding ad libitum then it generally exhibits three peaks and troughs, which broadly correspond to the three main

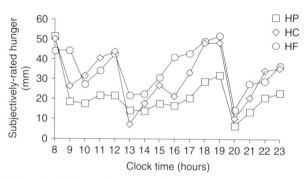

Figure 2 Subjective hunger tracked during waking hours in six subjects feeding on isoenergetically dense high-protein (HP), high-fat (HF), and high-carbohydrate (HC) diets. Subjects exhibit the three peaks and troughs of hunger that typify the Western feeding schedule.

meal times of a Western feeding schedule (**Figure 2**). While subjective hunger is a relatively poor proxy for the amount eaten it is a reasonably good predictor of when eating will occur. It is important to recognize that hunger can be influenced by a large number of factors and so a search for 'the hunger signal' is likely to prove fruitless. Thus, a large survey of over 600 men, women, boys, and girls could find no clear constellation of traits, sensations, or characteristics that typified hunger. Several laboratories have found inverse correlations between indices of postprandial carbohydrate utilization and hunger. While the postprandial utilization of carbohydrate is likely to influence hunger and indeed may act as a learned cue that conditions hunger it is not the exclusive physiological signal that determines hunger. A variety of hormones and drugs, the sight and smell of food, its perceived palatability, timing, and social situation can all influence hunger.

A number of proxy measures of hunger, such as salivation, have been made in an attempt to characterize hunger more objectively. These approaches have had relatively limited success and are difficult to compare across environmental circumstances. Satiety (or postingestive satiety (PI satiety)) is reciprocally related to hunger and can therefore be measured as such.

Measurement of Appetite

Appetite is specific to foods, exhibits wide intersubject variability, and tends to decline for a specific food as that food is eaten, leading to selection of other foods. Appetite is therefore said by Le Magnen to be sensory specific. The sensory specificity of appetite has been shown to relate *inter alia* to the postingestive consequences (satiation and satiety) of having ingested a food. The most objective measure of appetite for a given food in a specific experimental situation is therefore the amount of that food that a subject chooses to eat. Appetite is not rigidly determined by physiological signals *per se*, although they may greatly influence it. Both the palatability of a food and the appetite for it tend to co-vary and are often increased subsequent to a period of negative energy balance. Two examples are dieting and illness, both of which lead to lowered intake and a subsequent rebound in appetite. As discussed above the appetite for a food will be learned on the basis of the consequences of having ingested that food on previous eating occasions. Because of this it is possible to use covertly manipulated foods to deceive subjects into behaving in a manner largely determined by prior learned experience. If this were not so such deception would be impossible because the physiological signals produced by the sensorially similar yet nutritionally different food would immediately translate (through physiological signals) into behavioral compensation. This fact has implications for consumers since food technology can now dissociate the sensory and nutritional properties of foods, which may undermine the learned basis of food intake control in some people.

Measures of Feeding Behavior

There are many different techniques that can be used to measure feeding behavior in a number of different environmental situations (see 00000 and 00000). These techniques are used in real-life and/or laboratory studies of feeding. Generally, in the laboratory, specific aspects of the system are manipulated at the cognitive, sensory, gastrointestinal, or even the metabolic level by, for example, deceiving subjects about the energy content of foods, altering the sensory variety of the diet, and administering nasogastric or parenteral infusions, respectively. A number of other manipulations can be achieved. Because the environment can have such a large influence on feeding behavior it is important to consider a particular influence on feeding in several contexts. For instance, the effects of fat on energy intake have been considered in several laboratory and real-life contexts. Under most sets of circumstances dietary fat appears to be a risk for excess intake. The relationship between the experimental context and how it influences the investigations made is depicted in **Figure 3**.

Sensory Stimulation and Palatability

Palatability can be measured as the subjective preference for a food, its subjective pleasantness, or indeed the amount (in grams) of a food a subject eats. The relative palatability of a food can be determined by choice tests or taste tests relative to other standard ingestants (e.g., the 5% sugar solution). However, there has been much more controversy over the actual definition of palatability. In general the palatability of a food can be thought of as: (1) the momentary subjective orosensory pleasantness of a food; or (2) its sensory capacity to stimulate ingestion of that

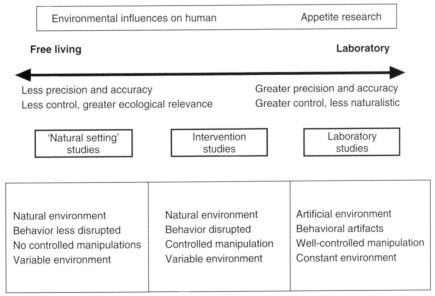

Figure 3 The constraints and limitations that the experimental environment places on studies of human feeding. In general the environment ranges from totally free living, which is realistic but very difficult to make measurements in, to the laboratory where measurements are easy but may be contaminated by artifacts due to the artificiality of the laboratory surroundings.

food. However, the second definition should not be taken to indicate that there is a direct correlation between the perceived palatability of a food and the amount of that food which is ingested. As with hunger, the coupling between the expressed sensation and the amount of food or energy ingested is loose. This definition takes account of the fact that the palatability of the food is jointly determined by the nature of the food (smell, taste, texture, and state), the sensory capabilities and metabolic state of the subject, and the environment in which the food and subject interact. Palatability is therefore not stable; indeed, the palatability of a food typically declines as its own ingestion proceeds. Work on military personnel suggests that the decline in preference for highly preferred foods (e.g., chocolate) is greater than that for staple foods such as bread, which exhibit more stable preference profiles. Palatability can be dissociated from sensory intensity since sensory intensity increases with the concentration of the compound or food being tasted; palatability generally shows a parabolic n-shaped curve with increasing sensory intensity of the food. Palatability can be conditioned, as can aversions. Palatability of a food generally increases with food deprivation.

Because of the mutable nature of palatability and sensory preference the role that they play in determining EI and degree of overweight are unclear. Short-term experiments suggest that more preferred foods stimulate hunger and food intake. Recent work in American and French consumers suggest that on a palatability scale of 1–7 subjects rarely select any food below a score of 3 and that palatability does increase the size of meals. But these works do not address energy balance. Indeed, virtually no published evidence supports the notion that altering dietary palatability or sensory variety *per se* will influence longer term energy balance of human subjects, despite the common perception that increasing dietary palatability will increase intake. This perception is so strong that the food industry feels unable to sacrifice the palatability of their products in developing healthier options, as the risk of decreased consumer acceptance is believed to be too high.

Certain combinations of the sensory and nutritional profiles of foods (e.g., sweet, high-fat foods) are conducive to overconsumption. This effect is often due to the combination of sensory stimuli and the postingestive effects of the food, which re-enforce each other. The individual sensory and nutritional stimuli in isolation are often less effective. Thus, cafeteria regimes, which can produce obesity in rats, typically alter the composition of the diet by increasing its fat content. When rats are given petroleum jelly in chow as a fat mimetic, they initially prefer this diet to normal chow. This preference soon becomes extinct, suggesting that sensory factors alone do not maintain preference.

Sensory Stimuli and Body Weight

It was originally proposed that obese subjects are more susceptible to external stimuli such as sensory stimuli than lean subjects who were more reliant upon internal physiological cues. This predicted that in a Western context the numerous external food stimuli would promote excess EI in susceptible individuals. As can be appreciated from the above, the interplay between 'external' and 'internal' signal is much more complex and interactive than was initially supposed. Nevertheless, given the multiplicity of afferent inputs that can influence feeding it is possible that some subjects have learned to base feeding predominantly on some cues rather than others. However, dividing these cues into simply internal and external sources is perhaps oversimplified. Current questionnaires that attempt to characterize a subject's responsiveness to food do so by dissociating 'externality,' 'restraint' and 'emotionality.'

Systematic differences have been found in sensory preference profiles, but not perceptions of intensity of various tastes between lean and obese subjects. Recent work has suggested that subjects with a history of weight fluctuation have an enhanced sensory preference for high-fat stimuli that are sweet. It has also recently been shown that sensory preference for fats is associated with degree of fatness in adults and children. This may be important. While there is little evidence that sensory stimuli alone promote positive energy balances, there is evidence that people select foods they prefer. Since high-fat foods are usually more energy dense than lower fat foods, preferential selection of these foods can lead to excess EIs without any apparent change in the amount of food eaten. Thus, sensory factors are likely to play a role in the selection of foods that are conducive to weight gain.

Sensory Versus Nutritional Determinants of Intake

The major problem with the concept of sensory preference or palatability as determinants of hyperphagia and obesity in humans is: (1) that there is little direct evidence for this effect *per se* (because the appropriate experiments are very difficult to carry out); and (2) both animals and humans appear to acquire sensory preferences for foods dense in readily available energy. Dissociation of the sensory characteristics and postingestive consequences of ingesting a food becomes difficult and perhaps artificial. It seems that at the present time the data from animal studies tends to suggest that maximal sensory preference for a food or diet is achieved when the sensory stimulus is reinforced by the metabolic consequences that form part of the satiety sequence. Indeed, there is controversial evidence that ingestion of one sensory stimulus (sweetness) without the associated nutrient (carbohydrate) promotes ingestion of energy shortly afterwards. The contribution of sensory and nutritional determinants of feeding is still poorly understood in humans.

Meal Patterns, Appetite, and Energy Balance

The effect of meal patterns on appetite and energy balance is also an unresolved issue. It has been noted that snacking and commercially available snack food are often believed to elevate EI. However, there is considerably less evidence that meal or snack patterns contribute to the development of obesity. It is important to note at this point that the relationship between a meal and a snack relates to timing and size of ingestive events in meal-feeding animals. In nonhuman species (and indeed humans) who engage in numerous small feeding bouts throughout their diurnal cycle there is little if any distinction between a meal and a snack. Meal-feeding animals are conditioned to ingest the majority of their EI in a few large ingestive events in their diurnal cycle, at approximately the same time points. Under these conditions, a snack can be defined as an energetically small, intermeal ingestive event (SIMIE). To avoid confusion with a common use of the word to describe a certain type of commercially available food, we use the phrase 'commercially available snack foods' to describe those specific foods. Commercially available snack foods tend to differ from the rest of the diet as they are more energy dense, high in fat and carbohydrate and low in protein, and usually contain a large fraction of their edible mass as dry matter. They are by no means the only food eaten as a SIMIE in many people at large.

There are two alternative hypotheses about how snacking may influence EI and body weight: (1) snacking helps 'fine tune' meal-time EI to match intake with requirements; or (2) habitual consumption of calorific drinks and snacks between meals is a major factor driving EI up and predisposing people to weight gain and obesity.

The evidence in relation to meal patterns, appetite, EI, and body weight is, however, indirect and fragmentary. On aggregate, cross-sectional studies tend to support no or a negative relationship between meal frequency and BMI. However, Bellisle et al. (1991) convincingly argue that examinations of the relationship between snacking and energy balance in free-living subjects are extensively flawed by misreporting, misclassification of meals and snacks, and potentially by reverse causality. Under these conditions it is difficult to draw clear conclusions about the effects of snacking in cross-sectional studies. It is therefore important to conduct controlled laboratory interventions over a number of days in humans. These studies suggest that in the short to medium term adding mandatory snacks to the diet leads to overconsumption. This effect is most pronounced in those who do not habitually snack and least pronounced in those who do. It is also of note that rats tend to be 'snackers' and Western humans tend to be meal feeders. The rat tends to adjust EI by varying meal frequency, the human by varying meal size. However, if rats are meal fed, they learn to adjust EI by varying meal size. Humans placed in time isolation begin to adjust intake by varying meal frequency. These comparisons illustrate the fact that adjustment of intake to energy or nutrient requirements occurs within a conditioned time framework, which itself is variable depending on the conditioning environment. Despite large changes in the pattern of feeding, EI can still be adjusted to satisfy requirements.

Social and Situational Influences on Feeding Behavior

There are a number of social and situational influences on food intake in humans. In general, the shorter the time period of measurement the greater the effect of situational and social influences. Thus, there are a large number of factors that can influence single meal size in humans. These factors are summarized in **Figure 4**.

Time of day appears to influence meal size in that the amount eaten and the EI increases on going from breakfast, to lunch to the evening meal. Meal size also increases across the feeding period in rats. It has been suggested that this occurs in learned anticipation of the energy requirements in the fasting period (night for humans, day for rats)[6]. Meal size and EI

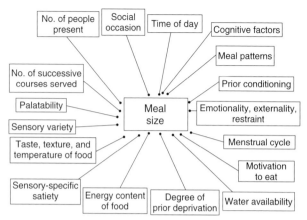

Figure 4 Major factors known to affect single meal size in humans. In general, the shorter the time interval of measurement the greater the influence of these factors on feeding behavior.

tend to be greater at weekends than on weekdays in Western adults. Meal size also varies as a power function of the number of people present at a meal. DeCastro has termed this effect 'social facilitation' of feeding. Social facilitation and daily routine account for much of this effect.

Seasonality can influence feeding. A number of studies suggest that EI, meal size, and eating rate are all elevated in the autumn. In one particular study hunger was associated with meal size in winter and spring, but not so clearly in the autumn.

Cognitive and Social Cues

Throughout the 1960s and 1970s a large number of behavioral studies examined the effect of cognitive and social cues (perceived energy content of foods, salience of cues, eating behavior of others present) on feeding in relation to the externality hypothesis. While a large number of studies found that so-called external cues do relate to short-term feeding behavior, a large number of others did not. However, the presence of external cues alone does not reliably predict how much food people will eat. Neither does the presence of external cues always relate to lean–obese differences in feeding patterns. Some of these differences in relation to cognitive and social cues are better explained in relation to dietary restraint. 'Restraint' is a term used to describe people who are attempting to limit or reduce their body weight by means of cognitive energy restriction (dieting). In doing so it is proposed that they are placing their motivation in relation to feeding at odds with physiological feeding stimuli. Placing

cognition at odds with physiological drives can result in pathologies of eating since the normal 'regulatory' processes are cognitively undermined. According to Herman and Polivy, these aberrations can extend into disturbances of emotion and cognition, which, *in extremis*, may partially underlie the increase in the prevalence of eating disorders. Furthermore, it is argued that restraint will increase the probability that a person will break a diet. It has been shown that an intervention (usually a preload) that breaks the rules of restraint, almost paradoxically induces a greater intake. This phenomenon has been termed 'counter-regulation.' This effect is cognitive, since it can be induced by deceiving a restrained eater into believing that a preload was high in calories. Because the concept of restraint has predictable behavioral outcomes it is a useful tool in characterizing different people with respect to their feeding behavior.

Macronutrients and Appetite

Food and nutrient ingestion influence human appetite through multiple feedbacks at several levels, which can be traced through the processes of food location, ingestion, digestion, absorption, and metabolism. Satiety is therefore maintained by a functional sequence or cascade of sequential physiological events that reinforce each other. Removing parts of a food or nutrient's effects from this sequence will therefore diminish its impact on satiety.

Protein

Protein suppresses EI to a greater extent than any of the other macronutrients. This effect is apparent in free-living subjects and in the laboratory. There may be a critical threshold in the amount of protein required to suppress subsequent EI since studies that have found little effect of protein relative to other macronutrient preloads have only used small amounts of energy in the preloads. Thus, protein appears to be particularly satiating when given in moderate and large amounts (**Figure 5**).

The mechanisms responsible for the apparent appetite-restraining effect of protein have not yet been determined. Essential amino acids when ingested in excess of requirement form a physiological stress that must be disposed of by oxidation. It is known that animals will alter feeding behavior in order to alleviate a physiological stress. Pigs, in particular, appear capable of learning to select a protein:energy ratio in the diet that is optimal for growth, as can rats.

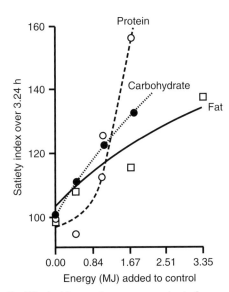

Figure 5 Effect of increasing energy content of macronutrient loads on satiety index subjectively expressed over 3.25 h. (Reproduced from Weststrate JL (1992) Effect of nutrients on the regulation of food intake. Unilever Research, Vlaardingen, The Netherlands.

Carbohydrates

By the mid 1990s it was generally accepted that carbohydrates are absorbed, metabolized, and stored with less energetic efficiency than dietary fat and were protective against weight gain. Indeed, a general perception was developing that because *de novo* lipogenesis appears limited when humans feed on Western diets, carbohydrate ingestion does not promote fat storage. At the same time the notion that carbohydrate metabolism or stores exert powerful negative feedback on EI became quite firmly established. By the same reasoning, diets high in carbohydrates were deemed to be more satiating, specifically because they were high in carbohydrates. High-fat diets were seen to promote overconsumption because they are relatively low in carbohydrate.

Recently, doubts have surfaced about the paramount role of carbohydrates as the central nutrient around which energy balance is regulated and body weight controlled. Several rigorous tests of carbohydrate-specific models of feeding have suggested that carbohydrate oxidation or stores do not exert powerful negative feedback on EI. Rather, as macronutrients come in the diet (where fat is disproportionately energy dense) there appears to be a hierarchy in the satiating efficiency of the macronutrients protein, carbohydrate, and fat. Per megajoule of energy ingested protein induces supercaloric compensation, carbohydrate generates approximately caloric compensation, and fat precipitates subcaloric compensation, and hence often excess EI. When energy density is controlled protein is

still far more satiating than carbohydrates or fats (at least when ingested in excess of 1–1.5 MJ loads). Under these conditions differences in the satiating efficiency of carbohydrates and fats become subtle. Some studies are now showing that it is possible to overeat when consuming a high-carbohydrate, energy-dense diet. Furthermore, in recent studies where both fats and sugars are added to the diet, there is no evidence that increasing sugar intake levers fat out of the diet and protects against weight gain.

The foods most capable of limiting EI (both voluntary and metabolizable) are those rich in unavailable complex carbohydrates. However, humans are not too fond of these foods. The average Western adult's fiber intake is spectacularly low.

It has recently been suggested that carbohydrates with a high glycemic index are especially conducive to weight gain. The evidence relating to the glycemic index of carbohydrates and appetite control is currently very inconclusive. It is likely several factors associated with readily absorbed carbohydrates can promote higher energy intakes. These include their sweetness, ready solubility, and ease with which they can be added to foods and absorbed across the gut wall. It may be a coincidence that these traits also determine the high glycemic load of these carbohydrates. Thus, while certain high-glycemic-index carbohydrates may promote higher energy intakes the effect may not be due to their glycemic index *per se*.

Fat

Numerous studies have now shown that when humans or animals are allowed to feed ad libitum on high-fat (HF) energy-dense diets, they consume similar amounts (weight) of food but more energy (which is usually accompanied by weight gain) than when they feed ad libitum on lower fat, less energy-dense diets. However, fat is not likely to be the only risk factor for over consumption and few analyses take account of how fat may interact with other nutrients. For instance, sweet high-fat foods have a potent effect on stimulating EI.

We are beginning to gain insights into the effects of types of fat on appetite control, due to the search for forms of fat that do not predispose the general population to weight gain. There is already some evidence that certain subtypes of fat limit the excess EI that occurs as a consequence of ingesting a high-fat diet. In the future specific nutrients could be tailored to exert quantitatively significant effects on appetite control, tissue deposition, and energy balance. In this context it is of note that certain isomers of conjugated linoleic acid (CLA) can be used to suppress appetite and fat deposition in animals and perhaps humans.

The Combined Effects of Macronutrients and Energy Density on Energy Intake

There has recently been considerable debate as to whether the effects of diet composition on EI can be simply explained in terms of dietary energy density. Here energy density is defined as the metabolizable energy per unit weight of ready to eat food. The major determinants of dietary energy density are water and fat, with water having the greatest effect. In general the energy density of ready to eat foods is largely determined by a fat–water seesaw, with energy density falling as the water content of food rises and as the fat content of foods falls. Protein and carbohydrate contribute relatively little to dietary energy density. There is considerable scope for technological developments that can alter the energy density of foods without compromising palatability.

Energy density exerts profound effects in constraining EI in short-to-medium term studies. Subjects behave differently in longer-term interventions because they learn to adjust their feeding behavior. Energy density is a factor, which at high levels can facilitate excess EI, and at low levels constrains EI. However, the effects that dietary energy density may exert on appetite and EI should be considered in the context of other nutritional and non-nutritional determinants of EI rather than as a substitute for those considerations.

Multifactor models appear more appropriate to explain nutritional determinants of feeding since they explain a far greater proportion of the variance in EI than single nutrient-based models (see **Figure 6**).

Micronutrients

There is currently very little data on the effect of micronutrients on feeding behavior and body weight under normal feeding conditions. There is evidence that rodents will learn to select a diet that alleviates a micronutrient deficiency. It may also be supposed that the administration of a micronutrient that will, for instance, improve a deficiency-related defect in nutrient metabolism will also improve appetite for that nutrient, and perhaps appetite in general. For instance, heat-stressed chickens will learn to consume more of a food rich in ascorbic acid, which apparently helps alleviate the stress.

See also: **Appetite**: Physiological and Neurobiological Aspects. **Dietary Intake Measurement**: Methodology; Validation. **Dietary Surveys**. **Energy**: Balance. **Hunger**. **Meal Size and Frequency**. **Obesity**: Definition, Etiology and Assessment.

Further Reading

Blundell JE (1979) Hunger, appetite and satiety – Constructs in search of identities. In: Turner M (ed.) *Nutrition and Lifestyles*, pp. 21–42. London: Applied Science Publishers.

Blundell JE and Stubbs RJ. Diet and food intake in humans. In: Bray GA, Bouchard C, and James WPT (eds.) *International Handbook of Obesity*, 2nd edn. Dekker Inc.(in press).

Booth DA, Lee M, and Macleavey C (1976) Acquired sensory control of satiation in man. *British Journal of Psychology* **67**: 137–147.

De Castro JM (1997) How can energy balance be achieved by free-living human subjects? *Proc Nutr Soc* **56**: 1–14.

Forbes JM (1995) *Diet, Voluntary Food Intake and Selection in Farm Animals*. Oxford: CAB International.

Friedman MI and Tordoff MG (1986) Fatty acid oxidation and glucose utilisation interact to control food intake in rats. *American Journal of Physiology* **251**: R840–R845.

Herman P and Polivy J (1991) Fat is a psychological issue. *New Scientist* 19th November: 41–45.

Hill AJ, Rogers PJ, and Blundell JE (1995) Techniques for the experimental measurement of human eating behaviour and food intake: a practical guide. *International Journal of Obesity* **19**: 361–375.

Langhans W and Scharrer E (1992) The metabolic control of food intake. *World Review of Nutrition and Diet* **70**: 1–68.

Le Magnen J (1992) *Neurobiology of Feeding and Nutrition*. California Academic Press, Millbrae, CA.

Mattes R (1990) Hunger ratings are not a valid proxy measure of food intake in humans. *Appetite* **15**: 103–113.

Mattes RD (1985) Gustation as a determinant of ingestion: methodological issues. *American Journal of Clinical Nutrition* **41**: 672–683.

Mayer J (1955) The regulation of energy intake and the body weight. *Annals of the New York Academy of Science* **63**: 15–43.

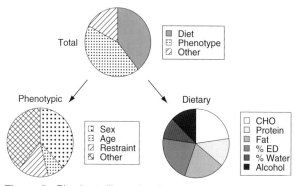

Figure 6 Pie charts illustrating the percentage of the variability in energy intake ascribable to different sources in 102 subjects self recording their food intake for 7 consecutive days. Approximately 39% of the variability was due to diet and ~40% was due to intersubject variability. These two major sources of variation are subdivided further. These charts clearly illustrate that the determinants of energy intake in human adults is multifactorial. ED, energy density.

Monello LF and Mayer J (1967) The Hunger and satiety sensations of men, women, boys and girls. *American Journal of Clinical Nutrition* 20: 253–261.

Ramirez I (1990) What do we mean when we say palatable food? *Appetite* 14: 159–161.

Schachter S and Rodin J (1974) *Obese Humans and Rats.* Washington DC: Erlbaum/Halsted.

Spitzer L and Rodin J (1981) Human eating behaviour: a critical review of studies in normal weight and overweight individuals. *Appetite* 2: 293–329.

Stubbs J, Ferres S, and Horgan G (2000) Energy density of foods: effects on energy intake. *Critical Reviews in Food Science and Nutrition* 40(6): 481–515.

ARTHRITIS

L A Coleman, Marshfield Clinic Research Foundation, Marshfield, WI, USA

R Roubenoff, Millennium Pharmaceuticals, Inc., Cambridge, MA, USA and Tufts University, Boston, MA, USA

© 2005 Elsevier Ltd. All rights reserved.

Introduction

There are many different types of arthritis, which, broadly defined, can be categorized into two major groups: degenerative and inflammatory. Osteoarthritis (OA) is the most common type of degenerative arthritis. In an inflammatory arthritis such as rheumatoid arthritis (RA) there is a systemic illness with inflammation of many joints. There is evidence of a systemic immune response; there is also activation of the acute-phase response. The systemic inflammation leads to altered energy and protein metabolism and wasting of body cell mass and muscle mass, described as 'rheumatoid cachexia.'

Dietary management of these two major types of arthritis differs substantially. In OA, the primary goal of dietary management is prevention via weight loss. Very little is known about the prevention of RA; the primary goal is treatment of inflammatory symptoms and prevention of joint damage and disability. We discuss dietary therapies including modification of dietary fatty acids and supplementation, in addition to vitamin and mineral supplementation and elimination diets; and make recommendations for optimizing dietary intake in order to attempt to alleviate disease symptoms.

Definitions and Etiology

Over a hundred types of arthritis are currently recognized. Among the degenerative arthritides, OA is the most common form, and the prototype of this group. In OA there is inflammation within the joint, but there is no evidence of whole-body inflammation, a key feature in distinguishing OA from the inflammatory arthritides. In general, OA affects a few joints, usually the large weight-bearing joints of the lower extremities, such as the knees and hips. Osteoarthritis can also affect the hands, especially in women, but without the systemic illness that characterizes inflammatory diseases such as RA. The etiology of OA is unknown, but the primary pathological problem is degradation of the cartilage leading to loss of joint space and bony overgrowth, causing pain first with weight-bearing, then with passive motion, and finally at rest.

In contrast, in an inflammatory arthritis such as RA there is a systemic illness with inflammation of many joints, usually the small joints of the hands, wrists and feet, often spreading to include the knees and hips. There is evidence of a systemic immune response, with activation of clones of autoreactive T cells and increased production of many cytokines, including interleukin (IL)-1β, tumor necrosis factor (TNF)-α, IL-6, and others. There is also activation of the acute-phase response, with reduced albumin synthesis and increased production of fibrinogen, C reactive protein, and other acute-phase reactants. The systemic inflammation leads to altered energy and protein metabolism and wasting of body cell mass and muscle mass, described as 'rheumatoid cachexia.'

Prevalence

Osteoarthritis is the most common joint affliction, and its prevalence increases dramatically with age. Radiographic evidence of OA is seen in 70% of people aged over 65 years, but symptoms do not necessarily correspond with X-ray changes. Osteoarthritis of the hip has been reported in 7–25% of adults aged 55 years and older, while knee OA is approximately twice as common, and OA of the hands three times as common. Rheumatoid arthritis, on the other hand, affects 1–2% of the population, but generally attacks many more joints than OA and is associated with a twofold or higher increased risk of death. Other inflammatory arthritides, such as the seronegative spondyloarthropathies, are much less common.

Clinical Features

The term 'arthritis' simply means the presence of pain and inflammation (heat, swelling, redness) in a joint. Joint pain without inflammation is 'arthralgia', and may be due to disease within the joint or in the surrounding soft tissues, ligaments, and tendons. Degenerative arthritis such as OA is generally a disease of the large weight-bearing joints of the lower extremities, such as the knees and hips. In addition, OA commonly strikes the distal interphalangeal (DIP) and first carpometacarpal joints of the hands, especially in women. The affected joints have pain on motion, mild swelling, and sometimes intra-articular effusions or swelling. As the disease progresses, bony overgrowth becomes clinically apparent, coinciding with the development of osteophytes on radiographic examination. These osteophytes, together with loss of joint space, are the radiographic hallmarks of OA, and reflect new bone formation at the joint margins. Over time, the range of motion in the joint is restricted, first by pain, later by loss of joint space, and finally by the osteophytes. Treatment of OA is essentially symptomatic, using analgesics and nonsteroidal anti-inflammatory drugs (NSAIDs) to reduce pain and limit the intra-articular inflammation. However, this treatment is seldom completely satisfactory, and progression of the disease is usually seen. Joint replacement surgery has revolutionized the care of end-stage OA, allowing return of function of joints that are otherwise immobile.

In inflammatory arthritis the situation is quite different. Rheumatoid arthritis is a symmetric, additive polyarthritis involving up to several dozen small joints of the hands, wrists, and feet, often with involvement of the knees, hips and ankles, and sometimes the elbows, shoulders and cervical spine. There is pain, swelling, and warmth in the affected joints and stiffness upon awakening or after prolonged immobility that can last for several hours. Unlike OA, in RA there is evidence of whole-body inflammation with activation of the acute-phase response. This leads to suppression of albumin gene expression and upregulation of the production of acute-phase proteins such as C reactive protein, transferrin, and fibrinogen. In addition, there is suppression of serum iron, increased zinc, and increased

Table 1 Examples of drug side effects on nutritional status

Effect	Drugs
Appetite increased	Alcohol, insulin, steroids, thyroid hormone, sulfonylureas, some psychoactive drugs, antihistamines
Appetite decreased	Bulk agents (methylcellulose, guar gum), glucagon, indometacin, morphine, cyclophosphamide, digitalis
Malabsorption	Neomycin, kanamycin, chlortetracycline, phenindione, p-aminosalicylic acid, indometacin, methotrexate
Hyperglycemia	Narcotic analgesics, phenothiazines, thiazide diuretics, probenecid, phenytoin, coumarin
Hypoglycemia	Sulfonamides, aspirin, phenacetin, β-blockers, monoamine oxidase inhibitors, phenylbutazone, barbiturates
Plasma lipids reduced	Aspirin and p-aminosalicylic acid, L-asparaginase, chlortetracycline, colchicine, dextrans, fenfluramine, glucagon, phenindione, sulfinpyrazone, trifluperidol
Plasma lipids increased	Oral contraceptives (estrogen-progestogen type), adrenal corticosteroids, chlorpromazine, ethanol, thiouracil, growth hormone, vitamin D
Protein metabolism decreased	Tetracycline, chloramphenicol

From The Merck Manual of Diagnosis and Therapy, Edition 17, p. 22, edited by Mark H. Beers and Robert Berkow. Copyright 1999 by Merck & Co., Inc., Whitehouse Station, NJ.

whole-body protein breakdown and resting metabolic rate. Treatment begins with rest, physical therapy, and use of NSAIDs to reduce pain. Low-dose oral corticosteroids, equivalent to 5–10 mg day^{-1} of prednisone, are often necessary to control symptoms. However, these therapies do not alter the natural history of the disease. The best chance of doing so rests with the so-called 'slow-acting anti-rheumatic drugs' (SAARDs), such as methotrexate, TNF-α inhibitors, and other medications that have been shown to prevent erosions. It should be noted that some of these medications may also affect the nutritional status of individuals with RA via either altered appetite, blood sugar, plasma lipids, absorption, or protein metabolism (**Table 1**).

Role of Diet in the Management of Inflammatory Arthritis

Nutritional Assessment in Rheumatoid Arthritis

It is important to recognize that patients with RA do not have normal nutritional status. Compared with healthy persons of the same weight, age, race, gender, and height, patients with RA have lower body cell mass (especially muscle mass) and increased fat mass. This condition has been termed 'rheumatoid cachexia,' and it occurs despite adequate and even excessive dietary intake. This cachexia is generally seen in the presence of hypermetabolism (elevated resting energy expenditure) and hypercatabolism (elevated protein breakdown), along with reduced physical activity. These metabolic abnormalities are linked to increased production of the catabolic cytokines IL-1β and TNF-α. The problems are further exacerbated by reduced physical activity, which reduces the anabolic stimulus to muscle, and disordered growth hormone kinetics. In addition, patients with RA have lower concentrations of serum albumin and other markers of visceral protein status, and often have anemia of chronic disease with disordered iron metabolism.

Although many foods or food components have been considered as possible treatments for RA, most studies have focused on either supplementation (particularly the use of fish oil) or the use of an elimination diet, especially fasting or a vegetarian regimen.

Supplementation with Dietary Fatty Acids

Various dietary fatty acids have been shown to have numerous immunomodulatory effects. Arachidonic acid (AA, 20:4 *n-6*) is synthesized in mammalian tissues from the essential fatty acid linoleic acid (18:2 n-6), found in many plant products. The release of AA from cell membrane phospholipids via the action of phospholipase A_2 results in the subsequent production of AA-derived eicosanoids, such as prostaglandin (PG) E_2 and leukotriene (LT) B_4, which have potent proinflammatory and chemotactic effects. Alternatively, when AA is replaced with an *n-3* fatty acid in the diet, such as eicosapentaenoic acid (EPA, 20:5 *n-3*) or docosahexaenoic acid (DHA, 22:6 *n-3*), there is competitive inhibition of the use of AA as a substrate, and eicosanoids with different biological activity (PGE$_3$ and LTB$_5$) are produced through the cyclooxygenase and 5-lipoxygenase cellular metabolic pathways (**Figure 1**). More specifically, EPA-derived eicosanoids result in decreased platelet aggregation, reduced neutrophil chemotaxis, and anti-inflammatory effects. Omega-3 fatty acids are derived primarily from marine sources, including fish and shellfish. Because modulation of dietary fatty acids can alter cellular eicosanoid production, it has been hypothesized that increased consumption of *n-3* fatty acids can affect the immunologic and inflammatory responses accompanying RA.

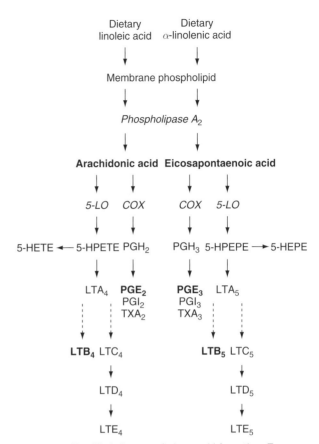

Figure 1 Simplified diagram of eicosanoid formation. Enzymes are italicized. Key intermediates are in bold. *COX*, cyclooxygenase; 5-HEPE, 5-hydroxyeicosapentaenoic acid; 5-HETE, 5-hydroxyeicosatetraenoic acid; 5-HPETE, 5-hydroperoxyeicosatetraenoic acid; 5-HPEPE, 5-hydroperoxyeicosapentaenoic acid; LT, leukotriene; PG, prostaglandin; TX, thromboxane.

Eicosapentaenoic acid supplementation causes modest improvement in the number of tender joints and fatigue among patients with RA although clinical benefits have generally been small, subjective, and transient. Possible mechanisms for this improvement in clinical symptoms of inflammation include decreased LTB$_4$ production, altered neutrophil membrane lipid composition, reduced interleukin-1 (IL-1) production, or a change in the α-tocopherol content of the diet. Overall, findings suggest that clinical benefits of dietary supplementation with *n-3* polyunsaturated fatty acids (PUFAs) are more commonly observed among patients consuming higher dosages of fish oil, for longer periods than those previously studied. Indeed, beneficial clinical effects have been observed for as long as 1 year among patients with RA ingesting 2.6 g daily of *n-3* PUFA supplements. In terms of optimal dosage of supplementation, however, a level of 130 mg kg^{-1} day^{-1} (9 g of *n-3* PUFAs in a person weighing 70 kg) has been shown to result in no additional improvement compared with patients receiving doses ranging from 3 to 6 g daily. Therefore, although the optimal level of fish oil supplementation is yet to be determined, there does appear to be an upper limit beyond which no additional benefit exists for patients.

Although some studies seem to suggest modest clinical improvements as a result of dietary fish oil supplementation in patients with RA, the question of the effects of a patient's medical regimen on the efficacy of fish oil supplementation remains. Nonsteroidal anti-inflammatory agents are known to inhibit the cyclooxygenase enzyme system, which is the same pathway that seems to be inhibited by EPA and DHA. It is therefore possible that in studies of fish oil supplementation where patients are simultaneously maintained on NSAIDs, the effect of EPA is diminished, since the cyclooxygenase pathway is already inhibited by concurrent treatment with NSAIDs. Several studies have attempted to address this issue and have demonstrated a modest effect of n-3 fatty acid supplementation in both patients who are treated with NSAIDs and those who are not, suggesting that concurrent treatment with NSAIDs does not seem to diminish the effect of n-3 fatty acids. On the other hand, a clinically important NSAID-sparing effect of fish oil among patients who discontinue NSAIDs has not been demonstrated, suggesting that the benefits of fish oil supplementation are modest at best, relative to the effects of medication.

Although the majority of studies regarding manipulation of dietary fatty acids have focused on fish oil supplementation, other fatty acids have also been studied. The use of α-linolenic acid, the precursor of EPA and DHA, has not been shown to be of any benefit in RA. However, γ-linolenic acid, found in blackcurrant seed, evening primrose, and borage seed oils, has resulted in clinically important reductions in the signs and symptoms of disease activity in patients with RA, perhaps via a reduction in PGE_2, IL-1, and IL-6. Because these oils do not cause an unpleasant fishy taste and odor in recipients, they may be preferred to fish oils for chronic treatment.

In summary, most studies of dietary supplementation with n-3 fatty acids suggest a modest improvement in clinical symptoms associated with RA, which are to some extent dose-and time-dependent. The most consistent clinical benefits have been reductions in tender joint counts and morning stiffness. Studies do not suggest that benefits are great enough to warrant discontinuing patients' other medications. However, the use of fish oil supplements, or diets rich in marine fish, may further improve clinical symptoms among patients with RA. Beyond the possible benefits in terms

of controlling inflammatory symptoms of RA, increases in n-3 PUFAs are also associated with reduced risk of cardiovascular disease and other health benefits. Thus, there is reason to promote fish consumption among patients with RA consistent with general healthy eating recommendations. Both the American Heart Association and World Health Organization suggest consuming a minimum of two servings of fish per week, with one or more of the servings as oily fish. Those individuals who do not consume fish regularly may consider supplementation with modest levels of fish oils; however, until more is known about optimal dosages, caution should be taken with the use of concentrated high-dose fish oil supplements. Of note, there has been concern raised over environmental contamination of some types of marine fish with methylmercury. Therefore, eating a variety of fish will help to reduce any potentially negative health effects due to environmental contaminants.

Vitamin and Mineral Supplementation

Most studies involving vitamin or mineral supplementation in RA have focused on either the antioxidant nutrients (vitamin C, vitamin E, beta carotene, selenium) or B vitamins. Various studies have examined the effects of vitamins C, E, and selenium supplementation on the management of RA. In general, results from randomized controlled trials of vitamin E supplementation have been of relatively short duration and have led to conflicting results so that there continues to be a lack of concrete evidence to support vitamin E supplementation at a particular dosage. Nonetheless, patients with RA could certainly be encouraged to increase their intake of vitamin E-rich foods, including edible vegetable oils (sunflower, safflower, canola, olive), unprocessed cereal grains, and nuts. Similarly, the effect of dietary sources of other antioxidant nutrients, such as selenium and vitamin C, on inflammatory symptoms in RA has also been ambiguous. It should be emphasized that providing individual nutrient supplements does not necessarily offer the same overall benefit as when nutrients are obtained from whole foods. It is possible that the combination of nutrients that are present in whole foods, or even some unidentified components of a food, are responsible for any observed beneficial effects, and that supplementing a typical diet with individual nutrients will not provide the same benefit.

We have studied vitamin B_6 levels in patients with RA and healthy controls, and found that plasma levels of pyridoxal-5-phosphate (PLP), the metabolically active form of vitamin B_6, were lower in patients with RA compared to control subjects. Furthermore, plasma levels of PLP were inversely associated with TNF-α production by peripheral blood mononuclear cells, suggesting that abnormal vitamin B_6 status may be contributing to inflammation in RA. However, there is no evidence to support the efficacy of oral vitamin B_6 supplements for treating the symptoms of RA at this time. Furthermore, large doses of vitamin B_6 can be toxic; therefore, as with the anti-oxidant nutrients, patients with RA would obtain the greatest benefit by increasing dietary sources of vitamin B_6, consistent with the dietary reference intake (DRI) for this nutrient. If supplementation is considered, it should not exceed twice the DRI level.

Fasting and Vegetarian Diets

An alternative approach to alleviating the symptoms associated with chronic inflammation is elimination of various foods or food components, most often by fasting or a vegetarian diet. Some studies have demonstrated a significant improvement in various objective and subjective measures of disease activity, including number of tender and swollen joints, Ritchie articular index, duration of morning stiffness, erythrocyte sedimentation rate (ESR), C reactive protein (CRP), grip strength and score on health assessment questionnaires, among patients with RA 6 weeks to 2 years after initiating a vegetarian diet. Furthermore, these clinical improvements were accompanied by changes in biochemical and immunological parameters consistent with a substantial reduction in inflammatory activity. Other studies, however, have demonstrated no clinical improvement among patients with RA following a vegetarian diet.

Several possible mechanisms have been proposed to explain the impact of elimination diets on clinical symptoms in RA. One possibility is that RA might be the result of hypersensitivity to environmental toxins or specifically to foods or food-related products, resulting in a food allergy of sorts that exacerbates symptoms of RA. However, true food intolerance, involving a systemic humoral immune response against food items, appears to be relatively uncommon among patients with RA. Another possible mechanism that has been proposed includes an alteration in the fatty acid content of the diet. Vegetarian diets contain more linoleic acid, but less AA, EPA, and DHA than omnivorous diets. Therefore, the eicosanoid precursors (AA, EPA, and DHA) must be produced endogenously from linoleic and α-linolenic acid (see **Figure 1**). It has been hypothesized that if this endogenous production cannot compensate for the absence of AA in the diet, then the precursor of the proinflammatory eicosanoids would be reduced, perhaps explaining the beneficial effect of vegetarian diets in patients with RA. Furthermore, it has also been demonstrated that fasting for 7 days resulted in decreased release of LTB_4 from neutrophils, in addition to reductions in morning stiffness, articular index, and ESR, but that this reduction in LTB_4 occurred despite an increased AA content of the serum, platelets, and neutrophils. These findings suggest that perhaps fasting may impair a metabolic step of AA conversion.

Other potential mechanisms include the possible effect of a vegetarian diet on antioxidant status, or on other dietary practices frequently associated with vegetarianism. Plant-based foods are naturally high in antioxidant nutrients (vitamin C, vitamin E, and beta-carotene) and low serum antioxidant levels have been associated with an increased risk of developing RA, although the specific mechanism involved remains unknown. Certainly, RA is associated with increased production of reactive oxygen species; these compounds seem to contribute to the inflammatory process, so a diet high in antioxidants could limit damage via their anti-inflammatory properties. While changes in fatty acid composition or antioxidant status seem to be the most plausible explanations for the potential benefit of adhering to a vegetarian diet, there are other possible mechanisms as well. Fasting, for example, suppresses inflammation and frequently a period of fasting is recommended prior to initiating an elimination or vegetarian diet; it is possible that this fasting period contributes to the reduction in inflammation among patients with RA following a vegetarian diet.

In summary, the notion that food sensitivity reactions contribute significantly to clinical symptoms associated with RA remains controversial. However, it seems that at least a small subgroup of patients with RA may benefit from individualized dietary manipulation involving elimination of specific foods or food components, in combination with other medical therapies. However, fasting and other elimination diets should be used with caution in light of the prevalence of rheumatoid cachexia in this population. Such patients are prone to further loss of cell mass during restrictive diets, and the net effect may be to do more harm than good.

Conclusions

Of the two primary approaches to the dietary management of inflammatory arthritis – supplementation and elimination diets – it appears that dietary supplementation with fish oil may result in the most consistent clinical benefits, although improvements still remain modest. Elimination diets, including fasting and vegetarian regimens, may provide some benefit for a limited number of patients with RA, but consistent alleviation of disease activity by objective clinical measures has not been demonstrated.

In neither case does the use of dietary management warrant discontinuing a patient's medical regimen; rather, diet may be useful as an adjunct to other more substantiated therapies. Perhaps the most prudent approach for patients with RA interested in attempting to control their disease activity through diet is to recommend a diet consistent with current recommendations for all individuals, including an intake high in fresh fruits, vegetables, and grains, with moderate amounts of lean meats and poultry, and an emphasis on fish, particularly marine fish high in *n*-3 fatty acid content. More definitive research demonstrating consistent, objective clinical benefits is needed before specific dietary manipulations for patients with RA can be recommended. In addition, there is growing evidence that exercise, both resistance and aerobic, has important beneficial effects on both inflammatory and degenerative arthritis.

Role of Diet in the Management and Prevention of Degenerative Arthritis

Much less is known about the role of diet in the treatment of OA and other degenerative arthritides. The above discussion regarding *n*-3 PUFAs in RA also may pertain to OA, although the strength of the effect has not been studied as thoroughly. However, the same eicosanoid metabolism occurs in OA as in RA, with the exception that the disorder is limited to the joint rather than involving the whole body. Thus, fish oils may well be of benefit in OA. Antioxidant intervention with vitamin E may also be effective in OA, with several studies showing an effect comparable with NSAIDs. Although not strictly nutrients, glucosamine and chondroitin sulfate, which are two of the constituents of normal cartilage that decline with arthritis, have been shown to be useful when given as an oral supplement, especially in patients with early OA.

In contrast to RA, where diet's main role is in the treatment and little is known about prevention, there is more known about dietary components that lead to OA than about nutritional management of OA. It is clear that OA of the lower extremities is largely a problem brought on by obesity, especially OA of the knee (and hip, to a much lesser extent),

suggesting that obesity seems to be a mechanical rather than systemic risk factor. Thus, maintaining body weight within the recommended ranges is probably the most important nutritional intervention to prevent OA. Weight loss leads to reduction in joint stress, and often reduces symptoms. In fact, recent studies have suggested that if all overweight and obese individuals reduced their body weight by 5 kg, or until their body mass index (BMI) was within the desirable range, 24% of surgeries for knee OA could be avoided. Furthermore, studies have demonstrated that exercise can improve OA symptoms even independently of weight loss, presumably by increasing muscle strength and thus improving the shock-absorbing power of the muscles, hence sparing the cartilage and joint. However, patients with OA have a great deal of difficulty with exercise, and their sedentary life style is reinforced by their joint pain, generally leading to weight gain after the onset of OA, which in turn exacerbates the disease, creating a vicious cycle. Exercise programs that increase physical activity and strengthen the muscles surrounding afflicted joints clearly improve symptoms in OA. Thus, OA can be thought of as a disease of overnutrition, while RA is generally a disease of undernutrition. Interestingly, recent twin studies have examined the role of genetic versus environmental factors as mediators of the obesity–OA relationship, and have suggested that shared genetic factors are not as important as environmental factors in mediating the obesity–OA relationship. Dietary modification leading to weight loss is a critical component of the management of OA.

See also: **Cytokines**. **Fatty Acids**: Omega-3 Polyunsaturated. **Obesity**: Complications. **Starvation and Fasting**. **Supplementation**: Dietary Supplements; Role of Micronutrient Supplementation. **Vegetarian Diets**.

Further Reading

Adam O, Beringer C, Kless T *et al.* (2003) Anti-inflammatory effects of a low arachidonic acid diet and fish oil in patients with rheumatoid arthritis. *Rheumatology International* **1**: 27–36.

Anderson RJ (2001) Rheumatoid arthritis: clinical and laboratory features. In: Klippel JH (ed.) *Primer on the Rheumatic Diseases*, 12th edn, pp. 218–225. Atlanta, GA: Arthritis Foundation.

Baker K, Nelson M, Felson DT *et al.* (2001) The efficacy of home-based progressive strength training in older adults with knee osteoarthritis: a randomized controlled trial. *Journal of Rheumatology* **28**: 1655–1665.

Belch JJF and Hill A (2000) Evening primrose oil and borage oil in rheumatologic conditions. *American Journal of Clinical Nutrition* **71**: 352S–356S.

Coggon D, Reading I, Croft P et al. (2001) Knee osteoarthritis and obesity. International Journal of Obesity and Related Metabolic Disorders 25: 622–627.

Goronzy JJ and Weyand CM (2001) Rheumatoid arthritis: epidemiology, pathology, and pathogenesis. In: Klippel JH (ed.) Primer on the Rheumatic Diseases, 12th edn, pp. 209–217. Atlanta, GA: Arthritis Foundation.

Hafstrom I, Ringertz B, Spangberg A et al. (2001) A vegan diet free of gluten improves the signs and symptoms of rheumatoid arthritis: the effects on arthritis correlate with a reduction in antibodies to food antigens. Rheumatology 40: 1175–1179.

McCabe BJ, Frankel EH, and Wolfe JJ (eds.) (2003) Handbook of Food-Drug Interactions. Boca Raton, FL: CRC Press.

Manek NJ, Hart D, Spector TD, and MacGregor AJ (2003) The association of body mass index and osteoarthritis of the knee joint: an examination of genetic and environmental influences. Arthritis and Rheumatism 48: 1024–1029.

Miller GD, Rejeski WJ, Williamson JD et al. and ADAPT Investigators (2003) The Arthritis Diet and Activity Promotion Trial (ADAPT): design, rationale, and baseline results. Controlled Clinical Trials 24: 462–480.

Nelson M, Baker K, Roubenoff R, and Lindner L (2002) Strong Women and Men Beat Arthritis. New York: Putnam.

Panush RS, Carter RL, Katz P, Kowsari B, Longley S, and Finnie S (1983) Diet therapy for rheumatoid arthritis. Arthritis and Rheumatism 26: 462–471.

Rall LC, Rosen CJ, Dolnikowski et al. (1996) Protein metabolism in rheumatoid arthritis and aging: effects of muscle strength training and tumor necrosis factor α. Arthritis and Rheumatism 39: 1115–1124.

Reginster JY, Deroisy R, Rovati LC et al. (2001) Long-term effects of glucosamine sulphate on osteoarthritis progression: a randomized, placebo-controlled clinical trial. Lancet 357: 251–256.

Rennie KL, Hughes J, Lang R, and Jebb SA (2003) Nutritional management of rheumatoid arthritis: a review of the evidence. Journal of Human Nutrition and Dietetics 16: 97–109.

Roubenoff R, Roubenoff RA, Selhub J et al. (1995) Abnormal vitamin B6 status in rheumatoid cachexia. Association with spontaneous tumor necrosis factor alpha production and markers of inflammation. Arthritis and Rheumatism 38: 105–109.

Roubenoff R, Walsmith J, Lundgren N et al. (2002) Low physical activity reduces total energy expenditure in women with rheumatoid arthritis: implications for dietary intake recommendations. American Journal of Clinical Nutrition 76: 774–779.

Sarzi-Puttini P, Comi D, Boccassini L et al. (2000) Diet therapy for rheumatoid arthritis: a controlled double-blind study of two different dietary regimens. Scandanavian Journal of Rheumatology 29: 302–307.

Skoldstam L, Hagfors L, and Johansson G (2003) An experimental study of a Mediterranean diet intervention for patients with rheumatoid arthritis. Annals of Rheumatic Disease 62: 208–214.

Walsmith J and Roubenoff R (2002) Cachexia in rheumatoid arthritis. International Journal of Cardiology 85: 89–99.

Relevant Website

http://www.euro.who.int/nutrition – World Health Organization website: CINDI (Countrywide Integrated Noncommunicable Disease Intervention) Dietary Guide. Provides a guide for healthy eating and healthy lifestyles, as suggested by the World Health Organization.

ASCORBIC ACID

Contents
Physiology, Dietary Sources and Requirements
Deficiency States

Physiology, Dietary Sources and Requirements

D A Bender, University College London, London, UK

© 2005 Elsevier Ltd. All rights reserved.

Ascorbic acid is a vitamin (vitamin C) for only a limited number of species: man and the other primates, bats, the guinea pig, and a number of birds and fishes.

In other species ascorbic acid is not a vitamin, but is an intermediate in glucuronic acid catabolism, and its rate of synthesis bears no relation to physiological requirements for ascorbate. Species for which ascorbate is a vitamin lack the enzyme gulonolactone oxidase (EC 1.11.3.8) and have an alternative pathway for glucuronic acid metabolism.

Ascorbic acid functions as a relatively nonspecific, radical-trapping antioxidant and also reduces the tocopheroxyl radical formed by oxidation of vitamin E. It has a specific metabolic function as the redox coenzyme for dopamine β-hydroxylase and peptidyl glycine hydroxylase, and it is required to maintain the iron of 2-oxoglutarate-dependent hydroxylases in the reduced state.

Absorption, Transport, and Storage

In species for which ascorbate is not a vitamin, intestinal absorption is passive, while in human beings and guinea pigs there is sodium-dependent active transport of the vitamin at the brush border membrane, with a sodium-independent mechanism at the basolateral membrane. Dehydroascorbate is absorbed passively in the intestinal mucosa and is reduced to ascorbate before transport across the basolateral membrane.

At intakes up to about 100 mg per day, 80–95% of dietary ascorbate is absorbed, falling from 50% of a 1 g dose to 25% of a 6 g and 16% of a 12 g dose. Unabsorbed ascorbate is a substrate for intestinal bacterial metabolism.

Ascorbate and dehydroascorbate circulate in the bloodstream both in free solution and bound to albumin. About 5% of plasma vitamin C is normally in the form of dehydroascorbate. Ascorbate enters cells by sodium-dependent active transport; dehydroascorbate is transported by the insulin-dependent glucose transporter and is accumulated intracellularly by reduction to ascorbate. In poorly controlled diabetes mellitus, tissue uptake of dehydroascorbate is impaired because of competition by glucose, and there may be functional deficiency of vitamin C despite an apparently adequate intake.

About 70% of blood-borne ascorbate is in plasma and erythrocytes (which do not concentrate the vitamin from plasma). The remainder is in white cells, which have a marked ability to concentrate ascorbate; mononuclear leukocytes achieve 80-fold concentration, platelets 40-fold, and granulocytes 25-fold, compared with the plasma concentration.

There is no specific storage organ for ascorbate; apart from leukocytes (which account for 10% of total blood ascorbate), the only tissues showing a significant concentration of the vitamin are the adrenal and pituitary glands. Although the concentration of ascorbate in muscle is relatively low, skeletal muscle contains much of the body pool of 5–8.5 mmol (900–1500 mg) of ascorbate.

Metabolism and Excretion

As shown in **Figure 1**, oxidation of ascorbic acid proceeds by a one-electron process, forming monodehydroascorbate, which disproportionates to ascorbate and dehydroascorbate. Most tissues also contain monodehydroascorbate reductase (EC 1.6.5.4), a flavoprotein that reduces the radical back to ascorbate. Dehydroascorbate is reduced to ascorbate by dehydroascorbate reductase (EC 1.8.5.1), a glutathione-dependent enzyme; little is oxidized to diketogulonic acid in human beings.

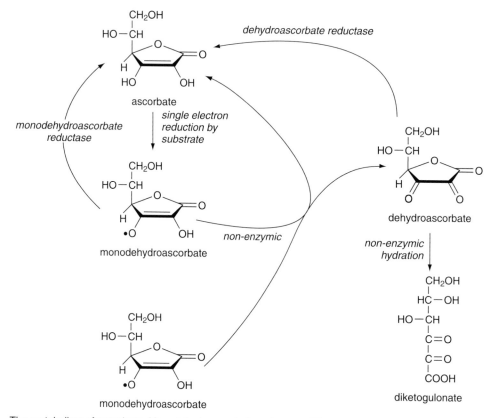

Figure 1 The metabolism of ascorbate. Monodehydroascorbate reductase, EC 1.6.5.4; dehydroascorbate reductase, EC 1.8.5.1.

Both ascorbate and dehydroascorbate are filtered at the glomerulus, then reabsorbed by facilitated diffusion. When glomerular filtration exceeds the capacity of the transport systems, at a plasma concentration of ascorbate above about $85\,\mu mol/l$, the vitamin is excreted in the urine in amounts proportional to intake.

It has been reported that approximately 25% of the dietary intake of ascorbate is excreted as oxalate; this would account for about 40% of the total urinary excretion of oxalate. However, there is no known metabolic pathway for the synthesis of oxalate from ascorbate, and it is likely that all or most of the oxalate found in urine after loading doses of ascorbate is formed nonenzymically, after the urine has been collected. Even in people at risk of forming oxalate renal stones it is unlikely that normal or high intakes of ascorbate pose any additional hazard.

Metabolic Functions of Ascorbic Acid

Ascorbic acid has specific and well-defined roles in two classes of enzymes: copper-containing hydroxylases and the 2-oxoglutarate-linked, iron-containing hydroxylases. It also increases the activity of a number of other enzymes *in vitro*—a nonspecific reducing action rather than reflecting a metabolic function of the vitamin. In addition, ascorbic acid has a number of less specific effects due to its action as a reducing agent and oxygen radical quencher. There is also evidence that ascorbate has a role in regulating the expression of connective tissue protein (and some other) genes; its mechanism of action is unknown.

Copper-Containing Hydroxylases

Dopamine β-hydroxylase (EC 1.14.17.1) is a copper-containing enzyme involved in the synthesis of the catecholamines noradrenaline and adrenaline from tyrosine in the adrenal medulla and central nervous system. The active enzyme contains Cu^+, which is oxidized to Cu^{2+} during the hydroxylation of the substrate; reduction back to Cu^+ specifically requires ascorbate, which is oxidized to monodehydroascorbate.

A number of peptide hormones have a terminal amide, and amidation is essential for biological activity. The amide group is derived from a glycine residue in the precursor peptide, by proteolysis to leave a carboxy terminal glycine. This is hydroxylated on the α-carbon; the hydroxyglycine decomposes nonenzymically to yield the amidated peptide and glyoxylate. This reaction is catalyzed by peptidyl glycine hydroxylase (peptidyl α-amidase, EC 1.14.17.3); like dopamine β-hydroxylase, it is a

copper-containing enzyme, and it requires ascorbate as the electron donor.

2-Oxoglutarate-Linked, Iron-Containing Hydroxylases

A number of iron-containing hydroxylases (**Table 1**) share a common reaction mechanism, in which hydroxylation of the substrate is linked to decarboxylation of 2-oxoglutarate. Ascorbate is required for the activity of all of these enzymes, but it does not function as either a stoichiometric substrate or a conventional coenzyme (which would not be consumed in the reaction).

Proline and lysine hydroxylases are required for the postsynthetic modification of collagen, and proline hydroxylase also for the postsynthetic modification of osteocalcin in bone and the Cl_q component of complement. Aspartate β-hydroxylase is required for the postsynthetic modification of protein C, the vitamin K-dependent protease which hydrolyzes activated factor V in the blood-clotting cascade. Trimethyllysine and γ-butyrobetaine hydroxylases are required for the synthesis of carnitine.

The best studied of this class of enzymes is procollagen proline hydroxylase; it is assumed that the others follow essentially the same mechanism. As shown in **Figure 2**, the first step is binding of oxygen to the enzyme-bound iron, followed by attack on the 2-oxoglutarate substrate, resulting in decarboxylation to succinate, leaving a ferryl radical at the active site of the enzyme. This catalyzes the hydroxylation of proline, restoring the free iron to undergo further reaction with oxygen.

It has long been known that ascorbate is oxidized during the reaction, but not stoichiometrically with hydroxylation of proline and decarboxylation of 2-oxoglutarate. The purified enzyme is active in the absence of ascorbate, but after about 5–10 s (about 15–30 cycles of enzyme action) the rate of reaction falls. The loss of activity is due a side reaction of the highly reactive ferryl radical in which the iron is oxidized to Fe^{3+}, which is catalytically inactive—so-called uncoupled decarboxylation of

Table 1 Vitamin C-dependent, 2-oxoglutarate-linked hydroxylases

Aspartate β-hydroxylase	EC 1.14.11.16
γ-Butyrobetaine hydroxylase	EC 1.14.11.1
p-Hydroxyphenylpyruvate hydroxylase	EC 1.14.11.27
Procollagen lysine hydroxylase	EC 1.14.11.4
Procollagen proline 3-hydroxylase	EC 1.14.11.7
Procollagen proline 4-hydroxylase	EC 1.14.11.2
Pyrimidine deoxynucleotide dioxygenase	EC 1.14.11.3
Thymidine dioxygenase	EC 1.14.11.10
Thymine dioxygenase	EC 1.14.11.6
Trimethyllysine hydroxylase	EC 1.14.11.8

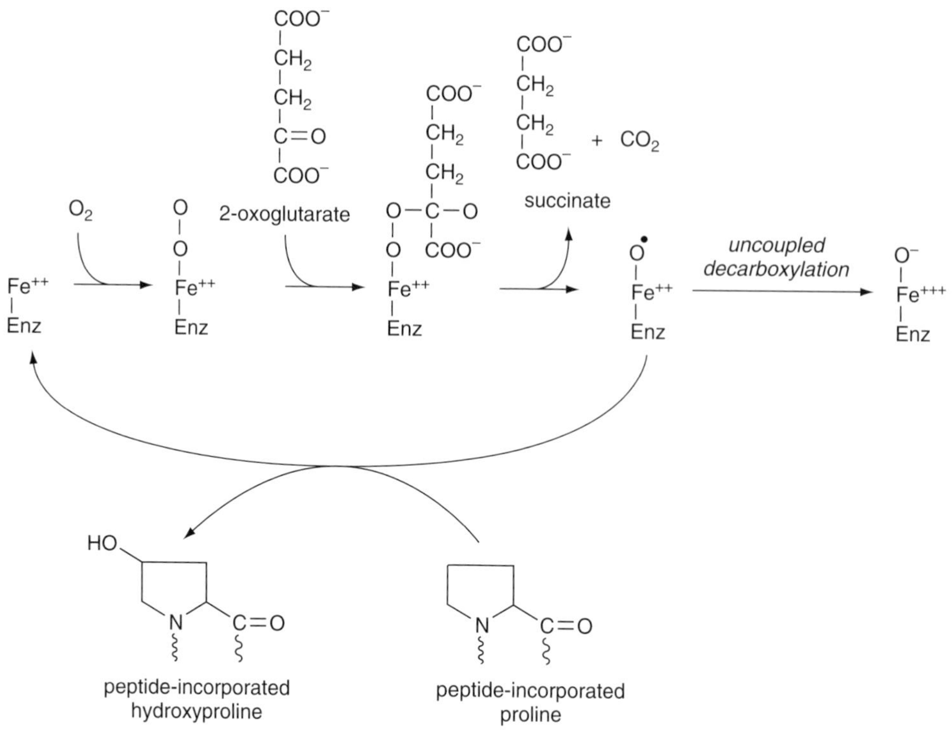

Figure 2 The reaction of procollagen proline hydroxylase.

2-oxoglutarate. Activity is only restored by ascorbate, which reduces the iron back to Fe^{2+}.

The Role of Ascorbate in Iron Absorption

Inorganic dietary iron is absorbed as Fe^{2+} and not as Fe^{3+}; ascorbic acid in the intestinal lumen not only maintains iron in the reduced state but also chelates it, increasing absorption considerably. A dose of 25 mg of vitamin C taken together with a meal increases the absorption of iron approximately 65%, while a 1 g dose gives a 9-fold increase. This is an effect of ascorbic acid present together with the test meal; neither intravenous administration of vitamin C nor supplements several hours before the test meal affects iron absorption, although the ascorbate secreted in gastric juice should be effective. This is not a specific effect of ascorbate; a variety of other reducing agents including alcohol and fructose also enhance the absorption of inorganic iron.

Inhibition of Nitrosamine Formation

Oral bacteria can reduce nitrate to nitrite which, under the acidic conditions of the stomach, can react with amines in foods to form carcinogenic N-nitrosamines. In addition to dietary sources, a significant amount of nitrate is formed endogenously by the metabolism of nitric oxide—1 mg/kg body weight/day (about the same as the average dietary intake), increasing 20-fold in response to inflammation and immune stimulation, and nitrate is secreted in saliva.

Ascorbate reacts with nitrite forming NO, NO_2, and N_2, so preventing the formation of nitrosamines. In addition to ascorbate in foods, there is considerable secretion of ascorbate in the gastric juice, and inhibition of gastric secretion for treatment of gastric ulcers, as well as reducing vitamin B_{12} absorption, also inhibits this presumably protective gastric secretion of ascorbate.

However, while ascorbate can deplete nitrosating compounds under anaerobic conditions, the situation may be reversed in the presence of oxygen. Nitric oxide reacts with oxygen to form N_2O_3 and N_2O_4, both of which are nitrosating reagents, and can also react with ascorbate to form NO and monodehydroascorbate. It is thus possible for ascorbate to be depleted, with no significant effect on the total concentration of nitrosating species. It remains to be determined whether or not ascorbate has any significant effect in reducing the risk of nitrosamine formation and carcinogenesis.

Antioxidant and Prooxidant Actions of Ascorbate

Chemically, ascorbate is a potent reducing agent, both reducing hydrogen peroxide and also acting as a radical trapping antioxidant, reacting with superoxide and a proton to yield hydrogen peroxide or with the hydroxy radical to yield water. In each case the product is monodehydroascorbate, which, as shown in **Figure 1**, undergoes dismutation to ascorbate and dehydroascorbate. In studies of ascorbate depletion in men there is a significant increase in abnormalities of sperm DNA, suggesting that vitamin C may have a general, nonspecific radical-trapping antioxidant function.

Ascorbate also acts to reduce the tocopheroxyl radical formed by oxidation of vitamin E in cell membranes and plasma lipoproteins. It thus has a vitamin E sparing antioxidant action, coupling lipophilic and hydrophilic antioxidant reactions.

The antioxidant efficiency of ascorbate is variable. From the chemistry involved, it would be expected that overall 2 mol of tocopheroxyl radical would be reduced per mole of ascorbate because of the reaction of 2 mol of monodehydroascorbate to yield ascorbate and dehydroascorbate. However, as the concentration of ascorbate increases, so the molar ratio decreases, and it is only at very low concentrations of ascorbate that it tends toward the theoretical ratio. This is because, as well as its antioxidant role, ascorbate can be a source of hydroxyl and superoxide radicals.

At high concentrations, ascorbate can reduce molecular oxygen to superoxide, being oxidized to monodehydroascorbate. Both Fe^{3+} and Cu^{2+} ions are reduced by ascorbate, again yielding monodehydroascorbate; the resultant Fe^{2+} and Cu^+ are reoxidized by reaction with hydrogen peroxide to yield hydroxide ions and hydroxyl radicals. Thus, as well as its antioxidant role, ascorbate has prooxidant action; the net result will depend on the relative rates of formation of superoxide and hydroxyl radicals by autooxidation and metal-catalyzed reactions of ascorbate, and the trapping of these radicals by ascorbate.

It seems likely that the prooxidant actions of ascorbate are of relatively little importance *in vivo*. Except in cases of iron overload there are almost no transition metal ions in free solution, they are all bound to proteins, and because the renal transport system is readily saturated, plasma and tissue concentrations of ascorbate are unlikely to rise to a sufficient extent to lead to significant radical formation.

Assessment of Vitamin C Status

The early method of assessing vitamin C nutritional status was by testing the extent of saturation of the body's reserves by giving a test dose of 500 mg (2.8 mmol) and measuring the amount excreted in the urine. In a subject with high status, more or less all of the test dose is recovered over a period of 5 or 6 h.

More sensitive assessment of status is achieved by measuring the concentration of the vitamin in whole blood, plasma, or leukocytes. Criteria of adequacy are shown in **Table 2**. The determination of ascorbate in whole blood is complicated by nonenzymic oxidation of the vitamin by hemoglobin, and most studies rely on plasma or leukocyte concentrations of ascorbate.

A problem arises in the interpretation of leukocyte ascorbate concentrations because of the different capacity of different classes of leukocytes to accumulate the vitamin. Granulocytes are saturated at a concentration of about 530 pmol/10^6 cells, while mononuclear leukocytes can accumulate 2.5 times more ascorbate. A considerable mythology has developed to the effect that vitamin C requirements are increased in response to infection, inflammation, and trauma, based on reduced leukocyte concentrations of ascorbate in these conditions. However, the fall in leukocyte ascorbate can be accounted for by an increase in the proportion of granulocytes in response to trauma and infection (and hence a fall in the proportion of mononuclear leukocytes). Total leukocyte ascorbate is not a useful index of vitamin C status without a differential white cell count.

There is increased formation of 8-hydroxyguanine (a marker of oxidative radical damage) in DNA during (short-term) vitamin C depletion, and the rate of removal of 8-hydroxyguanine from DNA by excision repair, and hence its urinary excretion, is affected by vitamin C status. This suggests that measurement of urinary excretion of

Table 2 Plasma and leukocyte ascorbate concentrations as criteria of vitamin C nutritional status

		Deficient	Marginal	Adequate
Whole blood	mmol/l	<17	17–28	>28
	mg/l	<3.0	3.0–5.0	>5.0
Plasma	mmol/l	<11	11–17	>17
	mg/l	<2.0	2.0–3.0	>3.0
Leukocytes	pmol/10^6 cells	<1.1	1.1–2.8	>2.8
	µg/10^6 cells	<0.2	0.2–0.5	>0.5

8-hydroxyguanine may provide a biomarker of optimum status, as a basis for estimating requirements.

Requirements

While the minimum requirement for ascorbate is firmly established, there are considerable differences between the reference intakes published by different national and international authorities. Depending on the chosen criteria of adequacy, and assumptions made in interpreting experimental results, it is possible to produce arguments in support of reference intakes ranging from 30 to 100 mg/day. Studies of intakes associated with reduced risks of cancer and cardiovascular disease suggest an average requirement of 90–100 mg/day and a reference intake of 120 mg/day.

Minimum Requirement

The minimum requirement for vitamin C was established in the 1940s in a depletion/repletion study, which showed that an intake of less than 10 mg per day was adequate to prevent the development of scurvy, or to cure the clinical signs. At this level of intake, wound healing is impaired, and optimum wound healing requires a mean intake of 20 mg per day. Allowing for individual variation, this gives reference intake of 30 mg/day, which was the UK figure until 1991 and the WHO/FAO figure until 2001.

Requirements Estimated from the Plasma and Leukocyte Concentrations of Ascorbate

The plasma concentration of ascorbate shows a sigmoidal relationship with intake. Below about 30 mg/day it is extremely low and does not reflect increasing intake to any significant extent. As the intake rises above 30 mg/day, so the plasma concentration begins to increase sharply, reaching a plateau of 70–85 µmol/l, at intakes between 70 and 100 mg/day, when the renal threshold is reached and the vitamin is excreted quantitatively with increasing intake.

The point at which the plasma concentration increases more or less linearly with increasing intake represents a state where reserves are adequate and ascorbate is available for transfer between tissues. This corresponds to an intake of 40 mg/day and is the basis of the UK, EU, and FAO figures. At this level of intake the total body pool is about 5.1 mmol (900 mg). It has been argued that setting requirements and reference intakes on the basis of the steep part of a sigmoidal curve is undesirable, and a more appropriate point would be the intake at which the plasma concentration reaches a plateau, at an intake of around 100–200 mg/day.

The US/Canadian reference intakes of 75 mg for women and 90 mg for men are based on studies of leukocyte saturation during depletion/repletion studies.

Requirements Estimated from Maintenance of the Body Pool of Ascorbate

An alternative approach to estimating requirements is to determine the fractional rate of catabolism of total body ascorbate; an appropriate intake would then be that required to replace losses and maintain the body pool.

Clinical signs of scurvy are seen when the total body pool of ascorbate is below 1.7 mmol (300 mg). The pool increases with intake, reaching a maximum of about 8.5 mmol (1500 mg) in adults— 114 µmol (20 mg)/kg body weight. The basis for the 1989 US RDA of 60 mg was the observed mean fractional turnover rate of 3.2% of a body pool of 20 mg/kg body weight/day, with allowances for incomplete absorption of dietary ascorbate and individual variation.

It has been argued that a total body pool of 5.1 mmol (900 mg) is adequate; it is threefold higher than the minimum required to prevent scurvy, and there is no evidence that there are any health benefits from a body pool greater than 600 mg. The observed body pool of 8.5 mmol in depletion/repletion studies was found in subjects previously consuming a self-selected diet, with a relatively high intake of vitamin C, and therefore might not represent any index of requirement. Assuming a total body pool of 5.1 mmol and catabolism of 2.7%/day, allowing for efficiency of absorption and individual variation gives a reference intake of 40 mg/day.

Because the fractional turnover rate was determined during a depletion study, and the rate of ascorbate catabolism varies with intake, it has been suggested that this implies a rate of 3.6%/day before depletion. On this basis, and allowing for incomplete absorption and individual variation, various national authorities arrive at a recommended intake of 80 mg.

The rate of ascorbate catabolism is affected by intake, and the requirement to maintain the body pool cannot be estimated as an absolute value. A habitual low intake, with a consequent low rate of catabolism, will maintain the same body pool as a habitual higher intake with a higher rate of catabolism.

Dietary Sources and High Intakes

It is apparent from the list of rich sources of vitamin C in **Table 3** that the major determinant of vitamin C intake is the consumption of fruit and

Table 3 Rich sources of vitamin C

	Portion (g)	mg/portion
Black currants	80	160
Oranges	250	125
Orange juice	200	100
Strawberries	100	60
Grapefruit	140	56
Melon	200	50
Green peppers	45	45
Sweet potato	150	38
Loganberries	85	34
Spinach	130	33
Red currants	80	32
White currants	80	32
Pineapple	125	31
Brussels sprouts	75	30
Mangoes	100	30
Satsumas	100	30
Tangerines	100	30
Turnips	120	30
Gooseberries	70	28
Potato chips	265	27
Broccoli	75	26
Swedes	120	24
Spring greens	75	23
Artichokes, globe	220	22
Potatoes	140	21
Avocados	130	20
Leeks	125	20
Lemons	25	20
Okra	80	20
Peas	75	20
Raspberries	80	20
Tomato juice	100	20
Plantain, green	85	17
Bilberries	80	16
Blackberries	80	16
Kidney	150	15
Tomatoes	75	15
Bananas	135	14
Cauliflower	65	13
Beans, broad	75	11
Cabbage	75	11
Nectarines	110	11
Parsnips	110	11
Rhubarb	100	10

vegetables; deficiency is likely in people whose habitual intake of fruit and vegetables is very low. However, clinical signs of deficiency are rarely seen in developed countries. The range of intakes by healthy adults in Britain reflects fruit and vegetable consumption: the 2.5 percentile intake is 19 mg per day (men) and 14 mg per day (women), while the 97.5 percentile intake from foods (excluding supplements) is 170 mg per day (men) and 160 mg per day (women). Smokers may be at increased risk of deficiency; there is some evidence that the rate of ascorbate catabolism is 2-fold higher in smokers than in nonsmokers.

There is a school of thought that human requirements for vitamin C are considerably higher than those discussed above. The evidence is largely based on observation of the vitamin C intake of gorillas in captivity, assuming that this is the same as their intake in the wild (where they eat considerably less fruit than under zoo conditions), and then assuming that because they have this intake, it is their requirement—an unjustified assumption. Scaling this to human beings suggests a requirement of 1–2 g per day.

Intakes in excess of about 80–100 mg per day lead to a quantitative increase in urinary excretion of unmetabolized ascorbate, suggesting saturation of tissue reserves. It is difficult to justify a requirement in excess of tissue storage capacity.

A number of studies have reported low ascorbate status in patients with advanced cancer—perhaps an unsurprising finding in seriously ill patients. One study has suggested, on the basis of an uncontrolled open trial, that 10 g daily doses of vitamin C resulted in increased survival. Controlled studies have not demonstrated any beneficial effects of high-dose ascorbic acid in the treatment of advanced cancer.

High doses of ascorbate are popularly recommended for the prevention and treatment of the common cold. The evidence from controlled trials is unconvincing, and meta-analysis shows no evidence of a protective effect against the incidence of colds. There is, however, consistent evidence of a beneficial effect in reducing the severity and duration of symptoms. This may be due to the antioxidant actions of ascorbate against the oxidizing agents produced by, and released from, activated phagocytes, and hence a decreased inflammatory response.

Scorbutic guinea pigs develop hypercholesterolemia. While there is no evidence that high intakes of vitamin C result in increased cholesterol catabolism, there is evidence that monodehydroascorbate inhibits hydroxymethylglutaryl CoA reductase, resulting in reduced synthesis of cholesterol, and high intakes of ascorbate may have some hypocholesterolaemic action. There is limited evidence of benefits of high intakes of vitamin C in reducing the incidence of stroke, but inconsistent evidence with respect to coronary heart disease.

Regardless of whether or not high intakes of ascorbate have any beneficial effects, large numbers of people habitually take between 1 and 5 g per day of vitamin C supplements. There is little evidence of any significant toxicity from these high intakes. Once the plasma concentration of ascorbate reaches the renal threshold, it is excreted more or less quantitatively with increasing intake.

Because the rate of ascorbate catabolism increases with increasing intake, it has been suggested that abrupt cessation of high intakes of ascorbate may result in rebound scurvy because of 'metabolic conditioning' and a greatly increased rate of catabolism. While there have been a number of anecdotal reports, there is no evidence that this occurs.

See also: **Antioxidants**: Diet and Antioxidant Defense. **Ascorbic Acid**: Deficiency States. **Cholesterol**: Factors Determining Blood Levels. **Diabetes Mellitus**: Dietary Management. **Fruits and Vegetables. Iron. Vitamin E**: Physiology and Health Effects.

Further Reading

Basu TK and Schorah CI (1981) *Vitamin C in Health and Disease.* p. 160. London: Croom Helm.

Bender DA (2003) Ascorbic acid (vitamin C). In: *Nutritional Biochemistry of the Vitamins*, 2nd edn., pp. 357–384. New York: Cambridge University Press.

Benzie IF (1999) Vitamin C: Prospective functional markers for defining optimal nutritional status. *Proceedings of the Nutrition Society* 58: 469–476.

Chatterjee IB (1978) Ascorbic acid metabolism. *World Review of Nutrition and Dietetics* 30: 69–87.

England S and Seifter S (1986) The biochemical functions of ascorbic acid. *Annual Review of Nutrition* 6: 365–406.

Ginter E (1978) Marginal vitamin C deficiency, lipid metabolism and atherogenesis. *Advances in Lipid Research* 16: 167–220.

Rivers JM (1987) Safety of high-level vitamin C ingestion. *Annals of the New York Academy of Sciences* 498: 445–451.

Sato P and Udenfriend S (1978) Studies on vitamin C related to the genetic basis of scurvy. *Vitamins and Hormones* 36: 33–52.

Sauberlich HE (1994) Pharmacology of vitamin C. *Annual Review of Nutrition* 14: 371–391.

Smirnoff N (2000) Ascorbic acid: Metabolism and functions of a multi-facetted molecule. *Current Opinion in Plant Biology* 3: 229–235.

Deficiency States

C J Bates, MRC Human Nutrition Research, Cambridge, UK

© 2005 Elsevier Ltd. All rights reserved.

Scurvy: The History, and Discovery of Vitamin C

Scurvy is traditionally associated with long sea voyages (**Table 1**), which typically lasted for several years; the seamen's diets were confined to whatever could be stored at room temperature for long periods. In the absence of refrigeration, their diets typically consisted of dried biscuits and other dry cereal foods (wheat flour and oatmeal), salted meat, dried peas, cheese, butter, and ale, i.e., whatever could be dried and preserved, often for long periods in adverse tropical climates. The signs and symptoms that were commonly described in classical accounts of scurvy, written long before its cause was understood, included lassitude, swollen joints, putrid and bleeding gums, failure of wound healing and the opening of old wounds and sores, intradermal bleeding due to capillary fragility, heart failure, and sudden death (**Table 2**). Although nowadays we carefully distinguish the symptoms of true scurvy (now known to be produced specifically by vitamin C deficiency) from conditions such as beriberi (thiamine deficiency, which is associated with oedema of the lower limbs), vitamin A deficiency (associated with night-blindness and corneal lesions), and rickets (caused mainly by a lack of exposure to sunlight in children), in the older literature these conditions were often not recognized as distinct. Signs and symptoms of scurvy occurred on land in times of siege or during prolonged military campaigns where dietary variety and access to fresh foods were severely restricted. While some medical practitioners and leaders became convinced that the cause of scurvy was dietary and that cure and prevention were possible by including fresh plant food such as scurvy grass, decoctions of evergreen needles etc. in the diet (**Table 1**), many remained convinced, right up to the beginning of the twentieth century, that other factors such as 'foul vapours' or infections were to blame. Indeed, before the recognition and discovery of essential micronutrients and experimental animal studies in the early years of the twentieth century, which confirmed that small amounts of certain complex organic molecules are needed in the diet to maintain health, the idea that food needed to supply anything other than energy, protein, certain minerals, and water was not generally accepted.

Although ad hoc treatments for scurvy had been successfully applied in many situations before the eighteenth century, the definitive proof of a dietary cure is attributed to James Lind, whose controlled trial of several different treatments of the disease on board HMS Salisbury, followed by his *Treatise of the Scurvy* published in 1753, provided the decisive evidence that persuaded the British Admiralty to insist on the inclusion of citrus fruit regularly in the naval diet (**Table 1**). Lind showed that a 'rob' or decoction of oranges could rapidly cure the disease, and the application of his discovery rapidly brought about dramatic reductions in the incidence of and mortality due to scurvy. However, the labile component in fruit that was responsible for protection against scurvy was not isolated until 1928. Its

Table 1 Scurvy and vitamin C; selected historical milestones, 1500–1950

1536	Jacques Cartier used a leaf extract of evergreen-tree needles to cure scurvy in explorers in Newfoundland
1593	Sir Richard Hawkins successfully used citrus fruit (amongst other cures and precautions) as a cure for scurvy in sailors
1753	James Lind's *Treatise of the Scurvy* described the first controlled nutrition experiment, in which oranges and lemons, but not other treatments, cured scurvy in sailors
Late eighteenth century	Successful public-health practices were introduced to reduce scurvy in the British navy based on citrus-fruit rations (Sir Gilbert Blane); Captain James Cook's long sea voyages used, and benefited from, this new knowledge
Late nineteenth century	Outbreaks of 'Barlow's disease' (infantile scurvy) in young children receiving mainly condensed cow's milk
Early twentieth century	Guinea-pig model of human scurvy developed by Holst and Frohlich in Norway; this enabled antiscorbutic foods and extracts to be studied in the laboratory
1928	Isolation of crystalline 'hexuronic acid' by Albert Szent-Gyorgyi in Cambridge, followed by its recognition as 'the antiscorbutic vitamin', alias vitamin C, by Charles King in Pittsburgh
1933	Norman Haworth (UK) and Tadeus Reichstein (Switzerland) separately synthesized vitamin C (L-ascorbic acid) and resolved its structure
Mid twentieth century	Human studies showed 10 mg vitamin C per day to be sufficient to prevent or cure scurvy; animal studies showed that vitamin C is essential for normal collagen and hence connective-tissue formation, thereby resolving the biochemical basis for many of the clinical signs of scurvy

chemical structure was proved by *de novo* synthesis from common sugars a few years later (**Table 1**). Paradoxically, crystalline ascorbic acid (vitamin C) was first isolated, not from a plant source such as fruit or green leaves, but from an animal source, namely adrenal glands, where high concentrations are also found. Indeed, the original motivation for the isolation of the crystalline material by Albert Szent-Gyorgyi in Hopkins' laboratory in Cambridge arose from his attempt to isolate a new adrenal hormone. The 'hexuronic acid' that he crystallized was not immediately equated with the antiscorbutic vitamin. Fortunately, studies by Charles Glen King in Pittsburgh led to the recognition of this unstable easily oxidized sugar derivative as the long-sought antiscorbutic principle, vitamin C or L-ascorbic acid.

Table 2 The signs and symptoms of scurvy, and evidence of inadequate tissue levels of vitamin C

Clinical signs and symptoms of scurvy in adults
Petechiae (small hemorrhagic spots), perifollicular hemorrhages, and larger sheet hemorrhages, especially of the skin of the limbs and trunk
Positive 'Hess test' (pressure or suction test) for increased capillary fragility
Hyperkeratosis of hair follicles; hairs abnormally coiled (ecchymoses)
Swollen and bleeding gums
Swollen painful joints, with effusions and arthralgia
Failure of wound healing and breakdown (reopening) of old wounds
Oedema, dyspnoea, dry eyes and mouth
Lassitude and impaired mental state
Sudden heart failure, often leading to sudden death, in severe cases

Clinical signs and symptoms in young infants
Painful joints leading to frog-like lying appearance; bleeding into the joints
Swelling ('beading') of rib cage and swelling of long-bone joints
Changes in x-ray appearance of the epiphyses of the long bones: 'ground glass' appearance, differing from that of rickets (with which infantile scurvy was often confused)
Intracranial hemorrhages, 'bulging eyes', and anemia in some cases; gums affected only if teeth already erupted

Biochemical evidence of inadequate vitamin C status
Serum or plasma vitamin C concentration $<0.2\,mg\,dl^{-1}$ ($<11\,\mu mol\,l^{-1}$)
Buffy-coat vitamin C concentration $<15\,\mu g$ ($<85\,nmol$) per 10^8 white cells
Untreated subjects with clinical scurvy invariably have very low biochemical vitamin C levels, but people may have very low biochemical levels without having clinical evidence of scurvy; very low intakes for periods of months to years, plus additional stresses, increase the likelihood of clinical scurvy

Degradation, Turnover, and Factors that Induce Increased Requirements for Vitamin C

The instability of vitamin C in air, and especially in neutral or alkaline aqueous solution, is attributable to the fact that in the presence of oxygen or other oxidizing agents it readily undergoes two successive one-electron oxidation steps to produce dehydro-ascorbate. Since the oxidation products are also unstable and undergo an irreversible lactone ring opening to diketogulonic acid, the vitamin is very easily destroyed, both in foods and (to a lesser extent because of efficient recycling mechanisms) in the body. Diketogulonic acid is one of several degradation products of vitamin C that cannot be reconverted to the vitamin and are further degraded to stable excretory products, such as oxalic acid, by oxidative metabolism. Of all the micronutrients that are essential for human health and survival, vitamin C is the most easily destroyed during drying and other traditional methods of preserving food. Citrus fruits contain other organic acids that inhibit this process of oxidation by lowering the pH of the fruit juice. This enables them, and extracts of them, to preserve at least some of their vitamin content for several weeks and even months of storage and thereby helps them to prevent and cure scurvy.

It remains largely a mystery why some people succumb to classical scurvy after a short period of virtually zero intake, whereas others survive for much longer. It has been speculated that some people may be able to produce all of the enzymes of the vitamin C synthetic pathway, including gulonolactone oxidase, which is normally absent from humans. However, this now seems unlikely, and it is more probable that the retention and recycling mechanisms for the vitamin are more efficient in some people than in others. We now know, for example, that smokers have a higher turnover of endogenous vitamin C than non-smokers, presumably because of the free-radical oxidant species in cigarette smoke. People with infections also have increased vitamin C turnover, which is associated with the liberation of pro-oxidant substances (such as hypochlorous acid) that are used by the body to kill bacteria. Some people have isoforms of certain blood proteins such as haptoglobins that are associated with relatively low levels of vitamin C in the blood. Very occasionally, there arise non-lethal mutations of vitamin C-dependent pathways whose abnormalities can be treated with high vitamin C intakes. A well-characterized example is Ehlers–Danlos syndrome, type VI, which is associated with impaired collagen lysyl hydroxylation and presents with a variety of clinical and biochemical connective-tissue (collagen-related) defects. However, much more research is needed to determine which of many possible genetic and environmental factors modulate the turnover of vitamin C in the body and to determine individual requirements and hence relative resistance to scurvy. Although 100–200 mg of the vitamin per day is needed to approach saturation of the tissues of humans, the amount needed to prevent or cure scurvy is less than $10 \, \text{mg day}^{-1}$, as was shown by experiments involving prolonged periods of feeding with depleted diets in the middle of the twentieth century (**Table 1**). Today, overt clinical scurvy is rare. It is occasionally seen in refugee camps or in elderly people with poor diets that are devoid of the usual sources of the vitamin. The latter high-risk group contains many individuals who are unable to chew fresh fruit and vegetables because of bad dentures or poor gastric tolerance of acidic or fibrous foods (see below).

An essential dietary requirement for vitamin C (L-ascorbic acid) is shared with humans by only a small number of other vertebrates, including primates, guinea pigs and agoutis, and some birds and fishes. Most mammals synthesize the vitamin in their livers from hexose sugars; birds synthesize it in their kidneys. The final enzyme in the pathway, L-gulono-lactone oxidase, has been lost in several unrelated species, suggesting a vulnerable and easily mutated locus on the genome. Presumably this mutation was neutral or advantageous during the natural selection of man's ancestors, when human and related-primate diets were rich in plant-derived sources of the vitamin.

Well-Established Metabolic Functions of Vitamin C that are Impaired in Deficiency

Studies of guinea pigs (and other species requiring a dietary source of vitamin C) have revealed that, when deprived of the vitamin, characteristic lesions of growing bones, failure of wound-healing of skin and bones, capillary defects, and other lesions arise, all of which point to a failure of the new synthesis of, or repair processes for, connective tissues and especially the protein collagen, which is the major extracellular protein and comprises a third of all the protein in the body (**Table 1**). As the biochemical pathway of collagen biosynthesis became better understood, during the middle years of the twentieth century, it became clear that certain unusual and characteristic hydroxylated amino-acids, comprising two different hydroxylated forms of proline and one of lysine, occurred uniquely in collagen. These were not coded for by the genome or inserted by the amino-acid-assembly machinery of the cell but instead were created by 'post-translational' amino-acid hydroxylation processes that took place after the nascent pro-collagen polypeptide chain had been synthesized on the polysomal messenger RNA. Some of the prolyl residues of the pro-collagen molecule were then hydroxylated to hydroxyprolyl residues, and some of the lysyl residues were hydroxylated to hydroxylysyl residues. The hydroxylated prolyl residues are essential for subsequent collagen triple-helix formation and hence for the secretion of nascent collagen; the hydroxylated lysyl residues form part of the essential pyridinoline-type crosslinks that stabilize the collagen fibers, especially those in bone. In the absence of sufficient vitamin C, these hydroxylation reactions rapidly fail, because the iron at the active center of the 'mixed function oxidase' enzymes that catalyze them is rapidly inactivated by oxidation. Vitamin C, specifically, is needed to keep the essential ferrous residues at the hydroxylase-enzyme active centers in the reduced, active, form. In the absence of the vitamin, these enzymes are inactivated after only a few cycles of hydroxylation.

The essential function of vitamin C in collagen maturation can go a long way towards explaining many of the clinical lesions of scurvy (**Table 2**). However, recent evidence indicates that the vitamin may also act directly on the transcription and translation of collagen mRNA and on the synthesis of other parts of the cell machinery that are needed for the formation of normal connective tissues. Parts of this process have yet to be clarified.

Vitamin C also plays a cofactor-like role in the reactions of several other enzymes that split molecular oxygen, notably members of the group of enzymes that are classified as 'mixed-function oxidases.' Two enzymes containing ferrous iron that are involved in carnitine biosynthesis (trimethyl lysine hydroxylase and γ-butyrobetaine hydroxylase) fall into this category. Aspartate β-hydroxylase, which is needed for the post-synthetic modification of protein kinase C, also requires vitamin C. Another enzyme that requires vitamin C is the copper enzyme dopamine β-hydroxylase, and, in this reaction, ascorbic acid is needed to reduce cupric copper to the cuprous form at the active site. Peptidyl glycine hydroxylase (peptidyl α-amidase) is also a copper enzyme that requires vitamin C as cosubstrate. Vitamin C can increase the activities of several other enzymes, by a non-specific reducing or protective action that is shared by other cellular reductants. This action is, however, distinct from

the functions described above, which are more specific to vitamin C.

In the course of its functional roles, ascorbic acid is oxidized in two successive one-electron reversible steps, and it is thought that most, if not all, of its essential biological actions are centred around this key redox cycle. The first oxidation product is the free-radical form of the vitamin, which is known variously as 'monodehydroascorbate,' 'semidehydroascorbate,' or 'ascorbate free radical' (AFR). Although this intermediate shares with most other free radicals the properties of having a relatively short half life and a high degree of chemical reactivity, it is, nevertheless, more stable than many other free radicals, contrasting with the highly reactive and damaging radicals such as hydroxyl or superoxide radical that are derived from molecular oxygen. By reacting with, and thus quenching, these damaging oxygen free radicals, ascorbate can act as a free-radical chain terminator and can thereby protect vulnerable macromolecules such as DNA, lipids, and proteins from oxidative damage by free-radical chain reactions. Such reactions would otherwise cause extensive damage, including genetic damage (to DNA), the formation of potentially atherogenic oxidized lipids, and oxidative inactivation of enzymes. For this reason, ascorbic acid is thought to possess important 'protective' antioxidant properties that are not directly connected with its other cofactor-like or cosubstrate-like roles in enzyme reactions. Ascorbate probably also protects host tissues against damage by oxidants such as hypochlorous acid that are produced in the normal course of bacterial killing by white cells.

The second one-electron oxidation step in ascorbate oxidation produces dehydroascorbate from the free-radical intermediate AFR. Both of these oxidized forms can be recycled to ascorbate either by non-enzymatic reactions with glutathione as the reductant (electron acceptor) or by pyridine nucleotide-dependent enzymatically catalyzed reactions. Thus, the two sequential one-electron oxidation steps from ascorbate to dehydroascorbate are fully reversible in vivo. However, the subsequent spontaneous non-enzymatic reaction comprising hydrolysis of the 1,4-lactone ring is not reversible, so that the product of this reaction, diketogulonic acid, has no provitamin activity. Normally, about 3% of the vitamin C in the body is degraded every day, and this loss must be replaced from the diet. Nevertheless, many weeks at or near zero intake are usually needed to reach scorbutic levels, if the tissues are reasonably well supplied to begin with.

Measurement of Vitamin C Status; Biochemical Tests for Adequacy and Deficiency

In species (such as humans) that cannot synthesize vitamin C in their bodies, the vitamin concentration in tissues and blood compartments (plasma, erythrocytes, and white blood cells) varies characteristically with the dietary intake of the vitamin. Since the blood-compartment concentrations mirror the concentrations in most other cells and tissue compartments, tissue vitamin C status can be monitored by measuring the concentration in plasma or blood, even though the blood concentrations are generally lower than those in most tissues. The concentration ratios between extracellular and various intracellular compartments are determined by active transport systems that concentrate the vitamin inside many cell types. At high intakes of the vitamin, the intestinal absorption process is overwhelmed, so that some of the ingested vitamin remains unabsorbed and is destroyed in the lower intestine by intestinal bacteria. The maximum steady-state level in plasma can be temporarily exceeded following a high bolus intake, but the excess vitamin is rapidly excreted in the urine once the renal threshold for filtration and reabsorption is exceeded. These safety mechanisms limit the maximum concentration of the vitamin to which the tissues are exposed.

For many years, the best biochemical measure of vitamin C status was considered to be the buffy coat, or total white-cell concentration of the vitamin (**Table 2**), expressed as micrograms per 10^8 white cells, the cell count in the assay sample usually being estimated by an electronic cell counter. This status index varied predictably with the magnitude of the total body vitamin C stores during controlled (animal) depletion studies. However, in practice it has proved to be a difficult test to use in human studies and especially in surveys, as it requires complex laboratory operations to be performed immediately after collecting the blood. It is also difficult to harmonize between laboratories, and, since it measures the average vitamin C content across several different white-cell types, whose individual proportions and relative vitamin C contents may vary considerably, its interpretation was not always straightforward. In addition, infection has rather unpredictable effects on the values obtained. For all of these reasons, this assay has fallen out of favor and is now rarely used. The concentration of the vitamin in erythrocytes or whole blood is not an ideal alternative, partly because hemoglobin can catalyze the oxidative destruction of the vitamin *in vitro* and partly because erythrocyte concentrations do not mirror other body compartments in a simple manner.

Serum or plasma vitamin C has therefore become the most commonly used status assay. In order to avoid short-term fluctuations caused by recent bolus intakes from food or supplements, it is preferable to collect an overnight-fasting blood sample. Since the vitamin is extremely easily oxidized, the sample must be carefully preserved unless the assay is to be performed immediately. The usual approach is to add freshly prepared metaphosphoric acid, usually at between 2 and 5% w/v, which precipitates plasma proteins, chelates transition-metal ions, and provides a protective acidic environment of a suitable pH. If stored, the samples must be kept at a low temperature, e.g., at $-25\,^{\circ}C$ for not more than a week or two or at $-80\,^{\circ}C$ for up to 1–2 years. There are many alternative physicochemical and chemical assay methods for measuring vitamin C in extracts of plasma or serum. These include (a) the measurement of its chemical reducing action on reducible dyes such as dichlorophenol indophenol and (b) the formation of either a colored osazone or a fluorescent derivative with orthophenylene diamine, after conversion to dehydroascorbate. Quantitation by absorbance or by electrochemical detection after separation by high-performance liquid chromatography is favored by many workers. This procedure has the advantage of being relatively specific (i.e., free from most forms of interference) and highly sensitive, but it is more time-consuming than the simpler nonchromatographic methods. Different methods may differ with respect to their specificity and their sensitivity to problems of interference as well as in the precautions that are needed to avoid oxidative destruction of the vitamin during the assay. Careful validation and robust quality-control procedures are essential.

Plasma or serum levels below $11\,\mu mol\,l^{-1}$ ($<0.2\,mg$ per $100\,ml$) are considered to be evidence of biochemical deficiency, and if this is severe and prolonged, the risk of clinical deficiency, i.e., scorbutic signs and symptoms, gradually increases. Intakes below around $20\,mg\,day^{-1}$ are likely to result in plasma levels in this range. Studies of human volunteers in the middle of the twentieth century showed clearly that an intake of $10\,mg$ vitamin C per day in a healthy adult is sufficient to prevent clinical scurvy, and this small amount is also sufficient to cure scorbutic signs and symptoms (**Table 1**).

Assay methods based on urinary excretion of vitamin C have been used to study status, but they are too cumbersome and difficult to interpret to be useful in population studies. There are no well-established functional assays available to define vitamin C status and requirements at present. An older method known as the 'Hess test,' which measures relative capillary fragility under pressure or suction (**Table 2**), is useful only if subclinical scurvy is present and is rarely attempted today. Studies of collagen crosslinks or oxidative damage to macro-molecules such as DNA or lipids may yield evidence about functional status in the future, but this remains a research challenge and is not yet an available option for routine studies or surveys.

Occurrence of Low Intakes and Poor Biochemical Status in Present-Day Societies

Although scurvy is rare, biochemical evidence of poor vitamin C status is not uncommon in certain high-risk groups in different human populations. Studies in The Gambia in West Africa, for instance, have shown that there is a regular seasonal cycle of availability of foods rich in vitamin C, with a good availability in the dry season alternating with a severe shortage during the rainy season. Plasma, buffy-coat, and breast-milk concentrations are all, on average, adequate in the dry season but are severely reduced during the rains. Functional and health-related parameters also deteriorate during the rains, but it has so far proved difficult to reverse this deterioration by vitamin C supplements alone. Therefore, robust evidence of health consequences of this seasonal availability cycle has not yet been obtained.

From recent surveys in the UK, **Table 3** shows the prevalence of low intakes of vitamin C (estimated from the proportion of participants receiving less than the lower reference nutrient intake (LRNI), which is the amount deemed to be sufficient for only a few people in a population group, namely the 2.5% with

the lowest requirements). Also shown in **Table 3** is the prevalence of plasma concentrations below the lower cut-off of normality, set at $0.2 \, \text{mg} \, \text{dl}^{-1}$ or $11 \, \mu\text{mol} \, \text{l}^{-1}$. This is shown for several subgroups of the British population of different ages, from data collected in three nationally representative population surveys during the decade 1990s. It is clear from these results that very few people were getting less than the LRNI for vitamin C over a 4 day or 7 day period of weighed-intake estimates of their diets. Low plasma levels were likewise relatively uncommon in the younger age groups; however, they were more common in older people and were especially prevalent, at almost 40%, in older people living in institutions such as nursing homes. These relatively low plasma levels seen in frail older people are likely to be caused by factors other than very low intakes of the vitamin. In the UK, unlike The Gambia, there was relatively little evidence of a major seasonal variation in vitamin C intake or status at the end of the twentieth century.

Other studies have shown that vitamin C absorption does not appear to be abnormally low in healthy older people. However, there is growing evidence that the multiple pathologies associated with old age (and with debility at any age) are associated with increased turnover of the vitamin. Older people with very low levels of vitamin C are at higher risk of dying sooner than those with high levels, although short-term vitamin supplements generally fail to reverse this increased risk. It thus appears that vitamin C status can act as a barometer of health as well as being a marker of adequacy of vitamin C intake. Further research is needed to determine the key mechanisms that affect the rate of vitamin C turnover and its control in different age

Table 3 Prevalence of low vitamin C intakes and low plasma vitamin C concentrations in Britain at the end of the twentieth century: data from the National Diet and Nutrition Surveys[a]

Age group	LRNI[b] (mg day^{-1})	Intake less than LRNI[b]	C Less than 11 μmol l^{-1} plasma vitamin
Pre-school 1.5–4.5 years	8	8/723 = 1.1%	24/723 = 3.3%
Young people 4–18 years			
4–10 years	8	1/423 = 0.2%	6/422 = 1.4%
11–14 years	9	0/307 = 0%	4/307 = 1.3%
15–18 years	10	1/271 = 0.4%	8/271 = 3.0%
Adults 65 years and over			
Free-living 65–79 years	10	8/606 = 1.3%	88/606 = 14.5%
Free-living 80+ years	10	7/274 = 2.5%	45/274 = 16.4%
Institution-living	10	2/248 = 0.8%	98/248 = 39.5%

[a]Confined to those participants who provided both a weighed-intake record for 4 or 7 days and a blood sample for the biochemical analysis. Source: National Diet and Nutrition Survey Series, commissioned jointly by the Department of Health and MAFF, whose responsibility has since been transferred to the Food Standards Agency. The National Diet and Nutrition Survey Reports are published by The Stationery Office.
[b]Lower reference nutrient intake, deemed to be sufficient for only 2.5% of the population who have the smallest requirements.

groups and different metabolic states. Since frail older people are at high risk of developing pressure sores and of needing surgery for a variety of ailments, there seems to be a potential public-health advantage in avoiding the development of very low vitamin C stores in this vulnerable age group, as a sensible precautionary measure.

See also: **Antioxidants**: Diet and Antioxidant Defense. **Ascorbic Acid**: Physiology, Dietary Sources and Requirements. **Fruits and Vegetables**. **Nutritional Assessment**: Biochemical Indices. **Older People**: Nutritional-Related Problems. **Supplementation**: Role of Micronutrient Supplementation.

Further Reading

Barnes MJ and Kodicek E (1972) Biological hydroxylations and ascorbic acid with special regard to collagen metabolism. *Vitamins and Hormones* 30: 1–43.

Bates CJ, Prentice AM, and Paul AA (1994) Seasonal variations in vitamins A, C, riboflavin and folate intakes and status of pregnant and lactating women in a rural Gambian community. *European Journal of Clinical Nutrition* 48: 660–668.

Carpenter KJ (1986) *The History of Scurvy and Vitamin C.* Cambridge: Cambridge University Press.

Institute of Medicine (2000) *Dietary Reference Intakes for Vitamin C, Vitamin E, Selenium and Carotenoids.* Washington, DC: National Academy Press.

Kivirikko KI and Myllyla R (1982) Posttranslational enzymes in the biosynthesis of collagen: intracellular enzymes. *Methods in Enzymology* 82: 245–304.

Langlois MR, Delanghe JR, de Buyzere ML, Bernard DR, and Ouyang J (1997) Effect of haptoglobin on the metabolism of vitamin C. *American Journal of Clinical Nutrition* 66: 606–610.

Packer L and Fuchs J eds. (1997) *Vitamin C in Health and Disease.* New York: Marcel Dekker Inc.

Pinnell SR, Krane SM, Kenzora JE, and Glimcher MJ (1972) A heritable disorder of connective tissue. Hydroxylysine-deficient collagen disease. *New England Journal of Medicine* 286: 1013–1020.

Sato P and Udenfriend S (1978) Studies on vitamin C related to the genetic basis of scurvy. *Vitamins and Hormones* 36: 33–52.

Atherosclerosis *see* **Cholesterol**: Sources, Absorption, Function and Metabolism. **Coronary Heart Disease**: Prevention

B

B Vitamins *see* **Cobalamins**. **Niacin**. **Pantothenic Acid**. **Riboflavin**. **Thiamin**: Physiology; Beriberi. **Vitamin B₆**

Bacteria *see* **Infection**: Nutritional Interactions; Nutritional Management in Adults

---

Bases *see* **Electrolytes**: Acid-Base Balance

Beer *see* **Alcohol**: Absorption, Metabolism and Physiological Effects; Disease Risk and Beneficial Effects; Effects of Consumption on Diet and Nutritional Status

---

BEHAVIOR

E L Gibson, University College London, London, UK
M W Green, Aston University, Birmingham, UK

© 2005 Elsevier Ltd. All rights reserved.

Introduction

The effects of diet on behavior have long been a topic of folklore, superstition, and popular mythology and more recently the subject of rigorous, and not so rigorous, scientific study. Most research into dietary effects on human behavior has assessed changes in mood or mental function after eating (or drinking) or after fasting. Typical measures of mental function include reaction time, attention, memory, problem solving, and intelligence. In addition, research has addressed the effects of diet on disturbed behavior, including attention-deficit–hyperactivity disorder (ADHD) in children, antisocial behavior and aggression, mental illness – for example depression – and dementia (**Table 1**).

Clearly, chronic malnutrition can seriously affect behavior by impairing brain development, and acute malnutrition may result in insufficient nutrients being available for optimal cognitive function. However, this article concentrates on dietary effects on behavior that are not the result of chronic malnutrition or of pharmacologically active ingredients of the diet such as alcohol or caffeine. Rather, the behaviors arise from more subtle effects of variation in nutrient intake within the normally nourished population.

Effects of Meals

The commonest way in which food can affect behavior is the change in mood and arousal that occurs after eating a meal. This might sound trite, but it is not trivial: this general meal effect is probably the most reliable example of an effect of diet on behavior. Many animals, including

Table 1 Examples of nutritional variables known or suspected to affect behavior, mood, and cognition

Food restriction
Early-life undernutrition
Chronic semi-starvation
Dieting to lose weight
Short-term fasting (e.g., missing a meal)

Meal effects
Pre- to post-meal changes
Meal timing (e.g., morning, afternoon, night)
Meal size
Macronutrient composition (acute and chronic effects)

Amino-acids
Neurotransmitter precursors (e.g., tryptophan, tyrosine, phenylalanine)
Phenylketonuria

Sugars
Sucrose (dietary intake)
Glucose (supplement, tolerance)

Micronutrients
Iodine
Iron
Selenium
B-vitamins: B_1, B_6, B_{12}, folate
Vitamin C
Vitamin E

Diabetes
Acute effects of hypoglycemia
Chronic effects

Pharmacological
Caffeine
Alcohol
Nutraceuticals (e.g., plant compounds)

humans, tend to be aroused, alert, and even irritable when hungry. This encourages their search for food. However, their mental processes become distracted by this task, to the detriment of other behaviors. After eating a satiating meal, we and other animals become calm, lethargic, and may even sleep.

Nevertheless, even this seemingly straightforward phenomenon can be distorted and can vary across individuals and situations. The impact of a food or drink will depend on the person's initial state. For example, thirsty people improved their vigilance when allowed to drink water, whereas when people were asked to drink when not thirsty, their performance deteriorated. Numerous experiments have shown that manipulation of the structure of meals results in variation in postprandial changes in mood and mental function. One obvious facet of meals that has been investigated is what is eaten, i.e., nutrient composition; the other two main aspects of meal structure that have been studied are meal timing and meal size. Of course, the effect of a meal on appetite also represents a behavioral effect, but this aspect is covered elsewhere in this encyclopedia.

Besides any nutritional effects, two other influences on behavior are known to interact with attempts to measure dietary effects on behavior. First, most people are very habitual in their choice of food and in the size and timing of their meals. As a result, they have learned a set of beliefs and expectations about the impact of their habitual dietary regime. Therefore, particularly in short-term tests, these expectations may override or mitigate physiological changes. Dietary experiences that differ from a person's habitual eating pattern could lead their behavior to change through cognitive rather than (or as well as) physiological influences.

Second, there are circadian rhythms and sleep–wake cycles in arousal and performance, which complicate the interpretation of meal effects, as we discuss in the next section.

Meal Timing

Does the timing of a meal in the day make a difference to any effects on behavior? In other words, do any behavioral effects differ between breakfast, midday, and evening meals or between mid-morning and afternoon snacks?

Breakfast The potential effects of breakfast on performance and well-being continue to attract much interest, not least from industry, especially concerning the performance of schoolchildren. Pollitt and colleagues have argued that children are likely to be more susceptible than adults to the effects of fasting, owing to their greater brain metabolic demands relative to their glycogenic and gluconeogenic capacity. The numerous studies in this area have produced inconsistent results, which is partly attributable to variation in the populations studied, their nutritional status, and the designs used. There is a consensus that breakfast is more likely than not to benefit schoolchildren's performance, particularly if the children are already nutritionally vulnerable and have mental abilities with room for improvement.

In all of us, there is a tendency for levels of arousal and alertness to rise during the morning, reaching a peak near midday. Some evidence suggests that breakfast may help to control this arousal, so that attention can be successfully focused on the task in hand. Conversely, omitting breakfast may increase autonomic reactivity, leading to less-focused attention. This effect could explain the finding that children without breakfast showed better recall of objects to which they had not been asked to attend; such attention to irrelevant stimuli is also known to occur with increased anxiety. Furthermore, increasing hunger is likely to be distracting.

Less attention has been paid to the effects of breakfast in adults. However, there are several studies of the effects of giving breakfast to students that show a benefit in spatial and verbal-recall tasks 1–2 h later, compared with missing breakfast. Interestingly, attention-based and reaction-time tasks were not improved by breakfast, and a logical-reasoning task was even slightly impaired. Perhaps performance in those tests benefits more from mild arousal, which could be acutely reduced by some breakfasts. These studies did not determine whether performance later in the morning is affected by breakfast. Differential effects of breakfast content and size will be discussed below.

Midday meal Several studies have demonstrated a drop in performance after the midday meal, particularly in vigilance tasks requiring sustained attention. However, this 'post-lunch dip' may not simply be an effect of eating, because vigilance has also been found to decline from late morning to early afternoon in subjects not eating lunch. That is, there is an underlying circadian rhythm in performance that is confounded by the effect of a midday meal. In fact, using noise stress to arouse subjects during a midday meal prevented any decline in performance due to the meal. It has also been shown that the more anxious one is feeling prior to lunch, the less one will experience a post-lunch dip in performance. In support of this, another study found that subjects scoring highly on a personality measure of extraversion and low on neuroticism were more likely to be affected by a post-lunch dip. These are examples of the importance of individual differences and context for meal effects.

Evening meal There are few studies of the effects of eating later in the day, although there has been some interest in the effects of meals during night shifts. Accuracy of performance declines with eating during a night shift, but, unlike the effects of lunch, pre-meal anxiety levels had no effect. One study in students on the effects of eating a large freely chosen evening meal found little evidence for consistent changes in performance relative to missing the meal. Despite this, the students who omitted the

meal reported feeling more feeble and incompetent and less outgoing than those who had eaten.

Snacks One study specifically addressed whether an afternoon snack (approximately 1–1.2 MJ (240–290 kcal) of yoghurt or confectionery) eaten 3 h after lunch (or no lunch) affected task performance. A beneficial effect of the snack was found on memory, arithmetic reasoning, and reaction time 15–60 min later. The comparison was with performance after a 'placebo' zero-energy drink (participants were unaware of the energy content). This rather different placebo does not preclude effects due to differences in sensory experience and expectations. Moreover, whether or not lunch had been eaten beforehand had little effect on the outcome, suggesting that any nutritional effects must be isolated to the acute impact of the snack. It is known that snacks of this size eaten after a meal have only a small effect on blood glucose, although insulin rises sufficiently to inhibit lipolysis and suppress the release of plasma free fatty acids later in the post-prandial period.

The authors reported that these performance benefits from an afternoon snack were not found with a snack eaten in the late morning. The most likely reason is that the beneficial effect depends on the decline in alertness that normally occurs during the afternoon.

Other studies have found differential effects of the macronutrient content of snacks; these are discussed below.

Meal Size

The effect of meal size on behavior has been little studied, perhaps because there are a number of methodological difficulties and an absence of theory. For example, what counts as a large or small meal? Should the difference be measured in terms of absorbed energy, or weight or volume eaten, or even consumption time? If absorbed energy is used as the measure, then behavioral outcomes would need to be measured with a sufficient delay for differences in energy absorption to be discriminable. Moreover, the influence of expectations and habit might confound experimental nutritional differences.

Two studies in adults found that eating large lunches (at least 4 MJ (1000 kcal)) impaired vigilance relative to eating small or medium-sized lunches. There was also evidence that this effect depended on the meal size being different from that habitually consumed. In adolescents, a larger breakfast (2.6 MJ (634 kcal), on average) resulted in poorer vigilance but better short-term memory 3 h later, compared with a smaller breakfast (1.6 MJ (389 kcal), on average). Thus, there is some evidence that vigilance is adversely affected by a large meal.

Meal Composition

Carbohydrate versus protein The effects of varying the nutrient composition of meals have been studied extensively, rather more for mood than performance. This is largely because of evidence that plasma and brain levels of precursor amino-acids for the synthesis of monoamine neurotransmitters (chemicals responsible for signalling between nerve cells), strongly implicated in mood disorders, can depend on the ratio between carbohydrate and protein in the diet. Synthesis of the neurotransmitter serotonin (or 5-hydroxytryptamine (5-HT)) depends on the dietary availability of the precursor essential amino-acid, tryptophan, owing to a lack of saturation of the rate-limiting enzyme, tryptophan hydroxylase, which converts tryptophan to 5-hydroxytryptophan (see **Figure 1**). An important complication is that

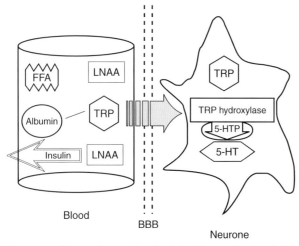

Figure 1 The pathways involved in the synthesis of the neurotransmitter 5-hydroxytryptamine (5-HT; serotonin) from the precursor essential amino-acid, tryptophan (TRP). Tryptophan is taken up by neurones from the blood, but its passage across the blood–brain barrier (BBB) is in competition with that of another group of essential amino-acids known as the large neutral amino-acids (LNAA). Thus, the ratio of tryptophan to total LNAA determines how much tryptophan enters the brain. Most tryptophan is normally bound to albumin in plasma, so it is not available for uptake into the brain. However, after a carbohydrate-rich low-protein meal, increased release of insulin raises levels of free fatty acids (FFA) in plasma, and these displace tryptophan from albumin. In addition, insulin promotes tissue uptake of the LNAA from plasma. Hence, the ratio of tryptophan to total LNAA increases and more tryptophan enters the brain. Increased availability of tryptophan in neurones drives greater synthesis of 5-HT because the rate-limiting enzyme, tryptophan hydroxylase, which converts tryptophan to the intermediate 5-hydroxytryptophan (5-HTP), is not fully saturated.

tryptophan competes with several other amino-acids, the large neutral, primarily branched-chain, amino-acids (LNAA), for the same transport system from blood to brain. If the protein content of a meal is sufficiently low, for example less than 5% of the total energy as protein, then relatively few amino-acids will be absorbed from the food in the gut. At the same time, insulin will stimulate tissue uptake of competing amino-acids from the circulation, and the plasma ratio of tryptophan to those amino-acids (tryptophan/LNAA) will rise, favoring more tryptophan entry to the brain. Conversely, a high-protein meal, which would be less insulinogenic, results in the absorption of large amounts of competing amino-acids into the blood, especially the branched-chain amino-acids (leucine, isoleucine, and valine). On the other hand, tryptophan is scarce in most protein sources and is readily metabolized on passage through the liver: thus, the plasma ratio of tryptophan to competing amino-acids falls after a protein-rich meal. Indeed, the protein-induced reduction in plasma tryptophan ratio often seems to be more marked than any carbohydrate-induced rise. Such effects also depend on the interval since, and nutrient content of, the last meal.

This evidence is particularly relevant to dietary effects on mood and arousal, because 5-HT has long been implicated in sleep and in affective disorders such as depression and anxiety. However, cognitive performance might also be affected, given the known role of 5-HT in responsiveness to environmental stimuli and stressors, impulsivity, and information processing. Importantly, there is evidence that the dietary availability of tryptophan can influence brain function in humans: for instance, feeding a tryptophan-free diet, which considerably reduced plasma tryptophan (and so could be expected to impair 5-HT function), induced depression in previously recovered depressives and in people with a genetic predisposition to depression. Furthermore, a tryptophan-free drink has been shown to impair performance in tests of visuospatial and visual-discrimination learning and memory.

There is evidence that people feel calmer and sleepier after snacks or meals rich in carbohydrate but virtually free of protein (an unusual situation) than after protein-rich meals containing little carbohydrate. This is compatible with changes in 5-HT function, but these studies did not determine whether this is due to an increase in 5-HT after the carbohydrate-rich meal or a decrease after the protein-rich meal, which could prevent the postprandial sleepiness. Furthermore, adding more than 5–6% protein (of total energy) to the carbohydrate meal has been shown to prevent the increased synthesis of central

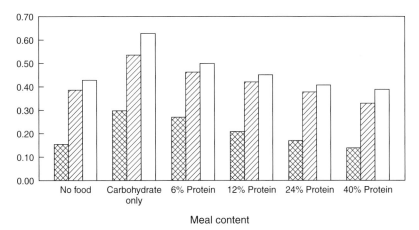

Figure 2 The effect in rats of no meal, a carbohydrate meal with no protein, and meals with increasing amounts of protein on the plasma ratio of tryptophan to the large neutral amino-acids with which tryptophan competes for entry across the blood–brain barrier (cross-hatched bars), levels of tryptophan in the hypothalamus of the rat brain (hatched bars, expressed in $\mu mol\,g^{-1}$), and levels of 5-hydroxytryptophan, an intermediate precursor of serotonin synthesis, in the hypothalamus (open bars, expressed in $0.1\,\mu g\,g^{-1}$). The rise in tryptophan entering the brain after a carbohydrate meal drives increased serotonin synthesis, but this effect is progressively inhibited by increasing protein content.

5-HT, relative to fasted levels, in both rats and people (see **Figure 2**). Also, even pure carbohydrate does not appear to induce sleepiness in everyone.

Another difficulty in comparing the effects of carbohydrate and protein intakes is that relative changes in mood and performance might be due to a protein-induced increase in plasma tyrosine, the precursor amino-acid for synthesis of the catecholamine neurotransmitters (adrenaline, noradrenaline, dopamine), which also competes with LNAA for entry into the brain. In catecholamine systems where the neurones are firing rapidly, acute physiological increases in brain tyrosine (e.g., by feeding a high-protein diet) can raise the tyrosine hydroxylation rate and catecholamine turnover. Such systems include dopaminergic neurones involved in arousal, attention, and motivation. Nevertheless, high-protein meals in humans do not always raise the plasma tyrosine–LNAA ratio; the effect depends on nutritional status and time of day, for example.

Differential effects on performance have been seen with less extreme variations in protein and carbohydrate intakes. For example, a lunch of 55% energy as protein and 15% as carbohydrate produced faster responses to peripheral stimuli, but greater susceptibility to distraction, than eating the reverse proportions of protein and carbohydrate. Sleepiness was not affected by macronutrient composition in that study. However, with these protein–carbohydrate ratios, the plasma tryptophan–LNAA ratio could still be lowered by the protein-rich meal relative to the ratio after the carbohydrate-rich meal, even if tryptophan/LNAA does not rise from pre-meal levels

after a carbohydrate-rich meal with much more than 5% protein (**Figure 2**).

A delay of at least 2 h after eating may be necessary for changes in neurotransmitter precursors to influence behavior. Earlier effects may be related to changes in glucose availability and levels of insulin and counter-regulatory hormones such as adrenaline, glucagon, and cortisol. These changes could underlie recent results after breakfasts of 20:80, 50:50, and 80:20 protein–carbohydrate ratios (1.67 MJ, 400 kcal). A measure of central attention initially improved after the carbohydrate-rich breakfast, but later improved after the protein-rich ones; the opposite was found for peripheral attention. This study also found that the 80% protein breakfast produced the best short-term memory performance about 1–2 h after eating, but not at 3.5 h.

Effects of dietary fat Most studies of the effects of fat have varied its level together with that of carbohydrate, while keeping protein constant and so allowing equicaloric meals. Comparisons have been made of low-fat (e.g., 11–29% of energy as fat), medium-fat (e.g., 45% of energy as fat), and high-fat (e.g., 56–74% of energy as fat) breakfasts, mid-morning and midday meals, and intraduodenal infusions of lipid or saline. On balance, high-fat meals appear to increase subsequent fatigue and reduce alertness and attention, relative to high-carbohydrate/low-fat meals. However, there are inconsistencies in changes in specific moods and the effects of meal timing: for instance, feelings of drowsiness, confusion, and uncertainty were found to increase after both low- and high-fat lunches but not after a medium-fat lunch. One possibility is that mood may be adversely affected by meals that differ substantially from habitual ones in macronutrient composition. An alternative is that similar mood effects could be induced (albeit by different mechanisms) by high carbohydrate in one meal and high fat in the other: for example, 1.67 MJ (400 kcal) drinks of pure fat or carbohydrate taken in the morning both increased an objective measure of fatigue relative to a mixed-macronutrient drink, although the two single-nutrient drinks had opposite effects on plasma tryptophan/LNAA ratios.

In many of these studies, the meals were designed to disguise variation in fat level from the participants. It is therefore possible that effects on mood may have resulted from discrepancies between subjects' expectations of certain post-ingestive effects and the actual effects that resulted from neurohormonal responses to the detection of specific nutrients in the duodenum and liver. A case in point may be the increase in tension, 90 min after lunch, with increasing fat intake reported by predominately female subjects: this might reflect an aversive reaction to (unexpected) fat-related post-ingestive sensations.

Postprandial declines in arousal can be quite noticeable 2.5–3 h after high-fat meals, but fat in mid-morning meals seems to be more sedating than fat ingested at lunchtime, which might relate to expectations. By comparison, when lipid was infused directly into the duodenum, a decline in alertness was apparent much sooner, by 30–90 min after the meal. These effects of fat may result from increased release of the gastric regulatory hormone cholecystokinin. However, in a study comparing ingestion of pure fat, carbohydrate, and protein (1.67 MJ (400 kcal) at breakfast), measures of memory, attention, and reaction time deteriorated more after carbohydrate and protein than after fat. This beneficial effect of fat was attributed to the demonstrated relative absence of glycemic and hormonal (insulin, glucagon, and cortisol) perturbations in the 3 h following fat ingestion.

Carbohydrates, Stress, Mood, and Mental Function

Susceptibility to Mood Enhancement by Diet

The possibility that a carbohydrate-rich low-protein meal could raise 5-HT function gave rise to the proposal that some depressed people may self-medicate by eating carbohydrate, so leading to increased 5-HT release in a manner reminiscent of the effects of antidepressant drugs, which enhance

aspects of 5-HT function by inhibiting the removal of 5-HT from the synaptic cleft between nerve cells. For the most part, however, early behavioral and pharmacological evidence for such a phenomenon was not very convincing.

Nevertheless, recent research provides some further support for beneficial effects of carbohydrate-rich protein-poor meals on mood and emotion in some people. When participants were divided into high and low stress-prone groups, as defined by a questionnaire, carbohydrate-rich protein-poor meals prior to a stressful task were found to block task-induced depressive feelings and the release of the glucocorticoid stress hormone cortisol, but only in the high stress-prone group. This finding was replicated using high- and low-tryptophan-containing proteins (α-lactalbumin and casein, respectively). It was argued that, because stress increases 5-HT activity, the poor response to stress of the sensitive group might indicate a deficit in 5-HT synthesis that is improved by this dietary intervention.

There is another link between macronutrient intake, stress, and mood. Chronic dysfunction of the stress-sensitive hormone cortisol and its controlling hypothalamic pituitary adrenal (HPA) axis is associated with depression and anxiety and with abdominal obesity. Moreover, protein-rich meals that prevent a meal-induced fall in arousal also stimulate the release of cortisol in unstressed people, and the degree of this effect is positively correlated with the probability of poor psychological well-being. Chronically, a carbohydrate-rich diet is associated with better overall mood state and lower average plasma cortisol than a high-protein diet. Acutely, a carbohydrate preload, but not protein or fat load, enhances cortisol release during stress. This may be related to findings from both human and animal research that suggest that eating carbohydrate-rich and perhaps high-fat foods can help restore normal HPA axis function and glucocorticoid stress responses. Raised levels of cortisol in stressed people contribute to insulin resistance, which in turn promotes abdominal obesity. However, insulin resistance may increase the likelihood of high-carbohydrate low-protein foods raising brain tryptophan and 5-HT levels, because of increased levels of plasma fatty acids, which result in more unbound tryptophan in plasma. Conversely, it has also been found that high baseline cortisol predicts induction of depression by dietary depletion of tryptophan. This might underlie recent findings that insulin-resistant people are less prone to suicide and depression, both of which are believed to be increased by low 5-HT function. Similarly, patients with seasonal affective disorder show increased insulin resistance in the winter, together with a greater predilection for sugar-rich foods. Unfortunately, despite this protective effect, insulin resistance is a substantial risk to health because of its association with cardiovascular disease.

Sugars and Opioids

Endogenous opioids are released during stress and are known to be important for adaptive effects such as resistance to pain. They are also involved in motivational and reward processes in eating behavior, such as the stimulation of appetite by palatable foods. Perhaps the best evidence for opioid involvement in an interaction between stress and eating is the finding that, in animals and human infants, the ingestion of sweet and fatty foods, including milk, alleviates crying and other behavioral signs of stress. Recently, this effect was shown to depend on sweet taste rather than calories, as non-nutritive sweeteners also reduce crying. This stress-reducing effect can be blocked by opioid antagonists. The conclusion that adults select sweet fatty foods for opioid-mediated relief of stress is tempting, but remains speculative. Also, such behavior would need to be explained in the context of stress itself enhancing endogenous opioid release.

Glucose, Mood, and Mental Function

The possibility that ingesting glucose can alter mood and improve mental function has generated considerable research interest. However, there is space here only to summarize and interpret the key findings and controversies. The interest in glucose arises from two observations: first, that the primary source of energy for brain function is glucose, and, second, that mental function and mood deteriorate when blood glucose concentration falls below basal physiological levels (hypoglycemia; $<3.6 \, \mathrm{mmol \, l^{-1}}$). The first observation must be qualified by recent evidence that, first, in times of metabolic demand, the brain can also use lactate very effectively as an energy source, and, second, the brain contains significant stores of glycogen in specialized cells called astrocytes, which can be metabolized for energy by neighboring neurones. Nevertheless, in rats, extracellular glucose levels in a specific region of the brain critical for memory, the hippocampus, decline to a greater extent during more demanding memory tasks, and this decline is prevented by a systemic glucose load.

Hypoglycemia is rarely induced by normal food, although large quantities of sugar-rich drinks taken on an empty stomach might do so in some people. Yet, many studies of the effects of glucose use a method similar to the oral glucose tolerance test (OGTT), in which fasted patients drink aqueous solutions containing 50–75 g of some form of glucose. This is meant to be not a normal nutritional manipulation but a test of glucoregulation. Associations have been reported between rapid and substantial declines in blood glucose after OGTTs and aggressive thoughts and behavior. However, this might be mediated by greater counter-regulatory hormone release.

In studies comparing sugar-rich drinks with zero-energy sweet placebos, many participants report no effect on mood, but some report a rise in subjective energy within an hour, followed by increased calmness. In children, controlled studies failed to support the popular myth that sugar is excitatory: again, it either had no effect or was calming. However, it is worth noting that some adults, and probably children, are especially sensitive to rapid drops in blood glucose, showing counter-regulatory hormone release and 'hypoglycemic symptoms' even though actual hypoglycemic levels of glucose are not reached.

It may be that beneficial effects of glucose ingestion become consistently apparent only when demands are placed on mental function. The findings on glucose and cognitive performance can be summarized as follows.

- The majority of studies that administered a glucose drink found subsequent improvements in performance compared with administration of a placebo, particularly in tests of short-term memory or vigilance tasks that require a large component of 'working memory'.
- Improvements in performance can be associated with rising or falling blood glucose levels, even independently of consuming a glucose load.
- Young healthy subjects require more demanding tasks than the elderly to detect a beneficial effect of glucose load.
- Associations between performance and glucose may be mediated by individual glucoregulatory efficiency.
- Both glucoregulation and performance are influenced by hormones, such as adrenaline and cortisol, that are sensitive to stressful or arousing cognitive tasks.
- Personality, stress-sensitivity, and task involvement can influence glucose uptake and disposal and, hence, the effects of glucose on cognition.

However, one important pattern does emerge: memory performance is worse in poorer than in better glucoregulators (**Figure 3**). This is true not just for elderly patients but also among a healthy student population, especially if the task is sufficiently demanding. High peak blood glucose predicts poor memory performance in elderly patients, whether or

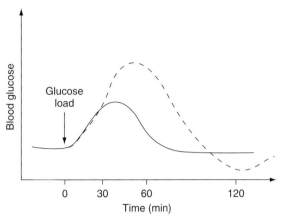

Figure 3 A model of changes in blood glucose levels after a glucose load in people who are either good regulators (solid line) or poor regulators (broken line) of blood glucose. The increased peak and delayed recovery of blood glucose levels in poor regulators suggests glucose intolerance and insulin resistance. In such people, there may be a brief period of mild hypoglycemia prior to a return to baseline levels. This difference in glucoregulation has been demonstrated in both young and elderly people without diabetes. Poor glucoregulation predicts poor cognitive performance in challenging tests, especially those involving memory.

not a glucose load has been given prior to testing. This relationship between raised glucose levels and poor memory performance could underlie a recent finding that a snack with a high glycemic index (greater plasma glucose rise) resulted in poorer memory performance 2–3 h later than a snack with a low glycemic index. Even so, it seems that a glucose load can lessen the memory deficit present in young and old poor glucoregulators (with little consistency or no effect in good glucoregulators).

One reason why poor glucoregulation predicts poor memory performance may be that glucose intolerance is associated with higher basal and stress-induced cortisol secretion. Cortisol is known to impair memory, probably by an action on hippocampal neurones that includes inhibition of glucose uptake. However, the substantial rise in insulin induced by a glucose load in poor glucoregulators may overcome the negative impact of cortisol in some cases: hyperinsulinemia induced independently of hyperglycemia has been shown to ameliorate memory deficits in patients with Alzheimer-type dementia.

Two other mechanisms might explain the ability of a glucose load to improve performance in subsequent challenging tasks. One is an increase in sympathetic activation by the glucose load: adrenaline is known to enhance memory. The other is increased synthesis and release of the neurotransmitter acetylcholine during challenging tasks: acetylcholine is known to be critically involved in learning and memory and is synthesized from dietary choline and from acetyl CoA, which is a by-product of glucose metabolism.

Hyperactivity and Antisocial Behavior

In children, there is an increasing frequency of the diagnosis of ADHD, a condition characterized by inattention, impulsive and disruptive behavior, learning difficulties, and increased levels of gross motor activity and fidgeting. Also, the prevalence of food allergies and intolerances has been increasing. Perhaps it is not surprising that dietary explanations and treatments for ADHD have been sought regularly for several decades, given theories of allergic reactions or intolerance to food additives, ingredients in chocolate, and even refined sugar (often grouped as the 'Feingold theory', after an early instigator of unproven dietary intervention). There has also been a long-standing interest in the possibility that antisocial behavior in children and adults might in part result from poor nutrition, although early studies were poorly designed. Behavioral effects of sugar and of many additives have by and large not been supported by controlled studies; however, determining unequivocally whether the behavior of young children is affected by specific dietary components is difficult. ADHD may be associated with disrupted eating behavior and poor nutrition, so that removal of a number of nutrient deficiencies might improve behavior. In addition, parents or unqualified health professionals may devise unsuitable dietary regimes that can increase the risk of undernutrition. As a result, there is little consensus as to what in the diet may or may not provoke disturbed behavior in children, other than that only a small minority of children are likely to be affected. Nevertheless, a recent British study, in which children were given a collection of food colorings and preservatives, or a placebo, in drinks, found a deterioration in the behavior reported by parents for both hyperactive and normal children given the additives, which seemed unrelated to allergic history. This effect was not detectable in a clinical setting. Clearly, a definitive answer will require more research.

Nevertheless, one promising line of research has involved supplementation with *n*-3 and *n*-6 highly unsaturated essential fatty acids: a recent study of ADHD children found improvement in the supplemented group on several behavioral measures after 3 months. Furthermore, a recent randomized placebo-controlled trial of dietary supplementation in young adult prisoners in the UK found a substantial reduction in antisocial behavior. The supplement used was a multivitamin and mineral preparation taken together with a combined *n*-3 and *n*-6 fatty-acid supplement, for a period varying from 2 weeks to 9 months. Other effects of essential fatty acids on cognition are discussed below.

Micronutrients and Mental Function

There has been, over the years, an increasing body of evidence suggesting that vitamin and mineral status is significantly related to both brain development in childhood and the degree of cognitive decline experienced as we age. Indeed, it is certainly the case that deficiencies of some vitamins are associated with negative neurological symptoms such as neural-tube defects. The work examining vitamin and mineral supplementation comprises both cohort studies and nutritional interventions and has generated much confusing and contradictory data. To a large degree, this confusion and contradiction result from variation in a number of factors such as the methodological rigour of each study, the measures of cognitive function used, and the precise nutrient being studied.

Early work in this area concentrated on the notion that supplementing the diet of schoolchildren with multivitamin supplements would improve both their IQ scores and their academic achievement. This work was controversial and marked by a number of deficiencies, such as any clear indication of whether the participants were nutritionally compromised prior to treatment, difficulties in determining which, if any, of the vitamins in the cocktail were producing effects, and the lack of any clear hypotheses regarding the mechanisms responsible. The consensus now is that supplementation will benefit cognitive development and IQ (especially non-verbal) in a minority of children who are not otherwise adequately nourished. In Britain and the USA at least, there is particular concern that a significant proportion of adolescents, especially girls, are deficient in iron. There is good evidence that iron deficiency contributes to poor cognitive ability, perhaps in association with low vitamin C status, which has also been linked to reduced cognitive function. Iron is known to be essential for the synthesis and function of neurotransmitters, such as dopamine, noradrenaline, and serotonin (5-HT). Selenium is another mineral that may be important for brain function, and low levels of selenium have been associated with cognitive decline and depressed mood in the European population.

Much recent work, however, has concentrated on the use of vitamins in the treatment of age-related cognitive decline and dementia and, to varying degrees, is more scientifically rigorous than the earlier work. The overwhelming majority of the experimental work has targeted the action of two groups of micronutrients: antioxidants and B-complex vitamins. Research into the effects of antioxidant vitamins, whilst showing some promise in that correlational studies show that levels of these vitamins (vitamin E most consistently) are associated with function in a range of cognitive domains, is more contradictory when one considers the clinical intervention trials. The work on B-complex vitamins is, however, more consistent and supported by a strong hypothetical basis. This relies on the roles of vitamins B_{12} and folate in methylation of membrane phospholipids (see below) and neurotransmitters and in breaking down the toxic sulfur amino-acid homocysteine. High levels of homocysteine are now considered by some to be a far greater risk factor for the development of coronary and vascular problems than are high levels of cholesterol. Elevated levels of homocysteine may be a cause of minor ischemic events, which, cumulatively, lead to a degradation of cognitive function due to either subclinical deficiencies of or problems with the absorption of B-complex vitamins. Indeed, a large number of studies have consistently demonstrated relationships between homocysteine levels, B-complex vitamin levels, and neuropsychological task performance. The number of direct intervention trials that have supplemented the diets of the elderly with B-complex vitamins is, however, small. Whilst some studies have shown no net benefit of supplementation on the cognitive function of the elderly, a larger number of studies have shown a stabilization of cognitive function and a reduction in homocysteine levels resulting from B-complex vitamin supplementation. As with the studies of antioxidant vitamins, however, these studies must be interpreted with a degree of caution since they use differing dosages, periods of supplementation, and measures of neuropsychological function.

Lipids

Lipids have attracted a good deal of research interest in terms of their possible effects on psychological function. The main nutrients studied fall into three groups: cholesterol, n-3 and n-6 essential fatty acids, and phospholipids. In general, the theoretical basis underpinning the effects (or lack of effects) of these nutrients on psychological function relates to how their relative concentrations affect cell-membrane fluidity. The rigidity of lipid bilayers of cell membranes is thought to be essential for neurotransmitter function because it maintains maximum exposure of receptors at the synaptic cleft between neurones.

Cholesterol

The interest in cholesterol as a substance that is related to psychological well-being stems back to the 1980s. During this period, a number of epidemiological studies found that individuals with low cholesterol levels were more prone to aggressive behavior and at greater risk of suicide and violent death. In addition, it was found that non-human primates increased their incidence of aggressive behavior when kept on a low-cholesterol diet. In terms of neuropsychological function, a number of studies have found associations between cholesterol levels and choice reaction time and/or memory function. Two of these studies sought actively to reduce cholesterol levels by pharmacological or dietary means: both found that lowering cholesterol produced small but statistically significant impairments in memory and attention. Conversely, however, a number of studies have demonstrated that high cholesterol levels are a significant risk factor for the development of Alzheimer's dementia. One mechanism for the negative effects of cholesterol lowering may be that neural cell walls lose their rigidity, thereby decreasing the relative exposure of serotonin (5-HT) membrane receptors at the synaptic cleft and impeding 5-HT signal transmission.

Essential Fatty Acids

There is a body of evidence suggesting that dietary supplementation with docosahexanoic acid (DHA; 22:6, *n*-3) and arachidonic acid (AA; 20:4, *n*-6) is effective in reducing the symptoms of clinical depression and schizophrenia. These fatty acids are also important for the development of the central nervous system in mammals. Recent work has demonstrated that maternal supplementation with these particular fatty acids during pregnancy significantly improves children's IQ at age 4 compared with children whose mothers took corn oil during pregnancy. There is no convincing evidence yet concerning the effects of essential-fatty-acid supplementation on the cognitive function of the elderly, although one study has found a correlational link between *n*-3 fatty-acid intake and the risk of developing Alzheimer's dementia. The proposed modes of action of these fatty acids involve their antithrombotic and anti-inflammatory properties in addition to their being a primary component of membrane phospholipids in the brain.

Phospholipids

The final group of lipids that has been investigated in terms of possible psychological benefits is the phospholipids and, in particular, phosphotidylserine. As with cholesterol, the proposed mode of action whereby this substance affects psychological function is via alterations in cell-membrane fluidity. A number of studies have claimed that dietary supplementation with phosphotidylserine can arrest the symptoms of both age-related decline and full dementia. In general, however, these studies have been poorly carried out and suffer from procedural difficulties such as a lack of appropriate control populations, alterations in dosage during the trial, and use of unvalidated or inappropriate neuropsychological assessment measures. Indeed, some of the more methodologically rigorous trials have specifically shown that phosphotidylserine supplementation exerts no significant effect on psychological function. The evidence for the efficacy of phosphotidylserine is, therefore, unclear.

Food Deprivation

There is evidence to suggest psychological effects of undernutrition. In severe cases, such as anorexia nervosa, neuropsychological function is impaired primarily as a result of structural changes in brain anatomy resulting from starvation. Evidence that undernutrition is associated with psychological problems in those not suffering from eating disorders was first hinted at in the Minnesota Study of Semi-Starvation in the 1950s. Volunteers who were kept on a half-calorie-intake diet for a period of months reported mood swings, increased irritability, poorer memory, and an inability to concentrate. These self-reported effects were not supported by objective testing, but the lack of a non-deprived control group means that there may have been an affect that could have been masked by a practice effect.

Dieting to lose weight is one of the most common food-choice-related behaviors in the Developed World, and it has been consistently associated with negative psychological consequences such as preoccupation with body shape and depression. In addition, a number of investigators have found that dieting to lose weight is associated with impairments in cognitive function, with dieters performing more poorly than non-dieters on measures of reaction time, immediate memory, and the ability to sustain attention. This is unlikely to be due to pre-existing differences between individuals who happen to be dieting and those who are not dieting at the time of testing since, within individuals, performance is poorer when dieting than when not dieting. It is unlikely that these effects are due to the gross physical effects of food deprivation since experimentally induced food deprivation of varying lengths fails to produce a comparable impairment in task performance; in addition, poorer task performance is found amongst dieters who claim not to have lost any weight over the course of the diet.

Rather than being a function of food deprivation per se, the poorer task performance amongst current dieters appears to be a function of the preoccupying concerns with hunger and body shape that are characteristic of dieters. Indeed, the impairments in task performance amongst dieters appear to be comparable in both structure and magnitude to those that result from the preoccupying concerns that are characteristic of clinical depression and anxiety disorders. Specifically, the primary deficit appears to be a reduction in the amount of available working-memory capacity, working memory being the primary cognitive system that allocates processing capacity to ongoing cognitive operations. A threshold hypothesis has been formulated to account for this phenomenon. Non-dieting highly restrained eaters are characterized by an enduring trait concern with body shape, which consumes a certain amount of working-memory capacity (explaining why non-dieting restrained eaters perform at a level intermediate between the levels of current dieters and unrestrained eaters). When they decide to diet, they then experience preoccupations with food and an increased desire to eat; this extra drain on working-memory capacity reaches a point where insufficient capacity is available to maintain task performance. Support for this hypothesis can be seen in the results of a study in which highly restrained non-dieters were instructed to imagine eating their favorite food or to imagine their favorite holiday whilst performing a reaction-time task. When imagining their favorite food, but not their favorite holiday, restrained non-dieters performed as poorly as current dieters on the reaction-time task.

Although evidence seems to be mounting that the poor cognitive function of current dieters is due to psychological and not biological factors, work continues to examine some of the more subtle possible biological mechanisms that may underlie the effects. One possible mechanism is that a low dietary intake of the amino-acid tryptophan (the precursor for 5-HT) leads dieters to have impaired serotonergic function. However, analysis of the urine of dieters for the 5-HT metabolite 5-hydroxyindoleacetic acid found no evidence for this. Another possibility (not yet investigated) is that, by avoiding red meat, dieters experience mild iron deficiency, with deleterious consequences for hemoglobin status, brain oxygen supply, and neurotransmitter function.

The types of dieter studied so far are those who attempt to lose weight in an unsupported and unsupervised manner. Comparisons between this type of dieter and those who attempt to lose weight in the context of an organized weight-loss group reveal dramatic differences. Those who diet as part of a group do not show the impairments in task performance typical of unsupported dieters. In addition, unsupervised dieters display an elevated stress response after 1 week of attempted weight loss (as measured by salivary cortisol levels), whereas supported dieters do not. It would appear, therefore, that the poor performance characteristic of unsupervised dieting is a result of the stress associated with this type of weight-loss attempt and that the psychological manifestation of this stress is the preoccupying thoughts outlined above.

Functional and Pharmacological Components of Foods and Drinks

There is growing interest, particularly in the food and beverage industry, in developing foods and drinks with functional properties (nutraceuticals) attractive to the consumer. These include effects on behavior, such as improvements in cognitive function, mood, and physical performance. Components of interest include caffeine, herbal extracts such as ginkgo biloba and panax ginseng, micronutrients, essential fatty acids, amino-acids, and carbohydrates. There is some support for beneficial effects of these components, but they are not reviewed further here.

Conclusion

The scientific understanding of dietary effects on behavior has moved in from the fringes of respectability sufficiently to attract substantial commercial interest. Advances in nutritional and neuropsychological knowledge, experimental design, and sensitivity of measures of behavior and brain function have produced replicable findings in some areas to mollify earlier scepticism. New understanding of the impact of nutrition on brain function and of predictors of individual susceptibility has allowed reinterpretation of old data. Promising areas with encouraging developments in understanding include the interactions between macronutrients, stress, and mood disorders, and the effects of vitamins, minerals, and lipids on cognition, dementia, and psychiatric disorders. Some findings, including recent discoveries of poorly nourished sectors of the population, suggest useful interventions. Nevertheless, research in this field is at an early stage, and the coming years should bring further revelations relating to the link between diet and behavior. With industrial backing, few may escape the consequences.

See also: **Appetite**: Psychobiological and Behavioral Aspects. **Brain and Nervous System. Caffeine. Children**: Nutritional Problems. **Diabetes Mellitus**: Etiology and Epidemiology. **Eating Disorders**: Anorexia Nervosa. **Exercise**: Diet and Exercise. **Fatty Acids**: Omega-3 Polyunsaturated; Omega-6 Polyunsaturated. **Food Choice, Influencing Factors. Food Folklore. Food Intolerance. Glucose**: Metabolism and Maintenance of Blood Glucose Level; Glucose Tolerance. **Glycemic Index. Homocysteine. Hunger. Hyperactivity. Hypoglycemia. Iodine**: Deficiency Disorders. **Iron. Lipids**: Composition and Role of Phospholipids. **Meal Size and Frequency. Older People**: Nutrition-Related Problems. **Premenstrual Syndrome. Sports Nutrition. Supplementation**: Dietary Supplements; Role of Micronutrient Supplementation. **Vitamin E**: Metabolism and Requirements.

Further Reading

Awad N, Gagnon M, Desrochers A, Tsiakas M, and Messier C (2002) Impact of peripheral glucoregulation on memory. *Behavioral Neuroscience* 116: 691–702.

Benton D (2002) Carbohydrate ingestion, blood glucose and mood. *Neuroscience and Biobehavioral Reviews* 26: 293–308.

Berr C (2002) Oxidative stress and cognitive impairment in the elderly. *Journal of Nutrition Health and Aging* 6: 261–266.

Bruinsma KA and Taren DL (2000) Dieting, essential fatty acid intake and depression. *Nutrition Reviews* 58: 98–108.

Dallman MF, Pecoraro N, Akana SF *et al.* (2003) Chronic stress and obesity: a new view of "comfort food". *Proceedings of the National Academy of Sciences of the United States of America* 100: 11696–11701.

Ernst E (1999) Diet and dementia: is there a link? A systematic review. *Nutritional Neuroscience* 2: 1–6.

Fernstrom JD (1994) Dietary amino acids and brain function. *Journal of the American Dietetic Association* 94: 71–77.

Gesch CB, Hammond SM, Hampson SE, Eves A, and Crowder MJ (2002) Influence of supplementary vitamins, minerals and essential fatty acids on the antisocial behavior of young adult prisoners: randomised, placebo controlled trial. *British Journal of Psychiatry* 181: 22–28.

Gibson EL and Green MW (2002) Nutritional influences on cognitive function: mechanisms of susceptibility. *Nutrition Research Reviews* 15: 169–206.

Green MW (2001) Dietary restraint and craving. In: Hetherington MM (ed.) *Food Cravings and Addiction.* pp. 521–548. Leatherhead: Leatherhead Food RA.

Hillbrand M and Spitz RT (1996) *Lipids, Health and Behavior.* Washington, DC: American Psychological Society.

Kalmijn S, Feskens EJM, Launer LJ, and Kromhout D (1997) Poly-unsaturated fatty acids, antioxidants and cognitive function in very old men. *American Journal of Epidemiology* 145: 33–41.

Krummel DA, Seligson FH, and Guthrie HA (1996) Hyperactivity: is candy causal? *Critical Reviews in Food Science and Nutrition* 36: 31–47.

Markus CR, Olivier B, Panhuysen GEM *et al.* (2000) The bovine protein alpha-lactalbumin increases the plasma ratio of tryptophan to the other large neutral amino acids, and in vulnerable subjects raises brain serotonin activity, reduces cortisol concentration, and improves mood under stress. *American Journal of Clinical Nutrition* 71: 1536–1544.

Pollitt E and Mathews R (1998) Breakfast and cognition: an integrative summary. *American Journal of Clinical Nutrition* 67: 804S–813S.

Reynolds EH (2002) Folic acid, ageing, depression, and dementia. *BMJ* 324: 1512–1515.

Riggs K, Spiro A, Tucker K, and Rush D (1996) Relations of vitamin B_{12}, vitamin B_6, folate, and homocysteine to cognitive performance in the Normative Aging Study. *American Journal of Clinical Nutrition* 63: 306–314.

Rogers PJ (2001) A healthy body, a healthy mind: long-term impact of diet on mood and cognitive function. *Proceedings of the Nutrition Society* 60: 135–143.

Sher L (2001) Role of thyroid hormones in the effects of selenium on mood, behavior, and cognitive function. *Medical Hypotheses* 57: 480–483.

Smith AP and Jones DM (eds.) (1992) *Handbook of Human Performance*, vol. 2, *Health and Performance.* London: Academic Press.

Story M and Neumark-Sztainer D (1998) Diet and adolescent behavior: is there a relationship? *Adolescent Medicine* 9: 283–298.

Tucker DM, Penland JG, Sandstead HH *et al.* (1990) Nutrition status and brain function in aging. *American Journal of Clinical Nutrition* 52: 93–102.

Wolraich ML, Wilson DB, and White W (1995) The effect of sugar on behavior or cognition in children: a meta-analysis. *JAMA,* 274: 1617–1621.

Beriberi *see* **Thiamin**: Beriberi

Beverages *see* **Alcohol**: Absorption, Metabolism and Physiological Effects; Disease Risk and Beneficial Effects; Effects of Consumption on Diet and Nutritional Status. **Tea**

BIOAVAILABILITY

R J Wood, Tufts University, Boston, MA, USA

© 2005 Elsevier Ltd. All rights reserved.

Introduction

Bioavailability is an important consideration in a number of areas of nutrition, including the derivation of Dietary Reference Intakes, estimation of potential impact of changes in dietary pattern, the selection of specific food fortificants, and the formulation of whole meal products, such as infant formulas or meal replacements. In this article, the role of food processing in nutrient bioavailability, specific determinants of nutrient bioavailability, methods for measuring bioavailability, and bioavailability of food fortificants are discussed.

Definition

Nutrient bioavailability is defined as the fraction of a nutrient in a food that is absorbed and utilized. In practice, however, measurements of bioavailability have focused on either direct measurement of absorption or determination of the change in some functional or biochemical endpoint reflecting absorption and utilization of the nutrient. In general, the bioavailability of all nutrients can be estimated by measuring absorption alone because, once absorbed, nutrients are freely available for biological utilization, irrespective of their original dietary source. For example, consider the case of iron bioavailability. Iron absorption can be measured directly from a food by a variety of methods (described in more detail later). In addition, absorbed iron enters the plasma iron pool carried on the protein transferrin. In turn, this absorbed iron will be used in large part (about 80%) immediately in the synthesis of hemoglobin by erythrocyte precursor cells in the bone marrow. The fraction of iron that is utilized for hemoglobin synthesis is not dependent in any way on the food source of that iron. Thus, food iron bioavailability can be conveniently measured and compared in relative terms among various sources by determining the change in blood hemoglobin after consumption of various forms of iron in iron-deficient subjects. Thus, nutrient bioavailability can be estimated by measuring these appropriate endpoints, such as hemoglobin incorporation for iron, hepatic tissue or mineral content of bone for various bone-seeking minerals, or more

generally as growth stimulation under nutrient limiting conditions, etc.

An exception to the 'absorption equals bioavailability' rule is selenium. One form of dietary selenium is selenomethionine. This selenium-containing compound is handled by the body exactly like the amino acid methionine and gets readily incorporated into methionine-containing proteins. However, the selenium found in selenium-dependent enzymes is in the form of a special amino acid called selenocysteine, which must be synthesized in the body during the process of incorporation of selenocysteine into these selenoproteins. Selenomethionine catabolism will result in the release of this selenium into an active endogenous selenium pool, which serves as the source of selenium for selenocysteine synthesis. Thus, selenium in selenomethionine is not immediately available to support selenium-dependent functions in the body.

Effects of Food Processing

Food processing can have positive or negative effects on nutrient bioavailability. For example, milling of grains removes all or part of the external covering of the grain (bran) that contains high amounts of phytic acid, an important inhibitor of bioavailability of divalent minerals, such as iron, zinc, and copper. One disadvantage of this form of food processing is that much of the mineral content of grains is in the bran fraction and is lost in the process of milling. To compensate for this loss of mineral (and some vitamins as well) grain products can be 'enriched' by fortifying the flour made from the milled grain with specific micronutrients. Simple food processing techniques, such as sprouting or fermentation, are also effective in lowering the phytate content and increasing mineral bioavailability of grains. Other techniques used in food manufacturing, such as browning, which produces the Maillard reaction, and extrusion, can have negative effects on bioavailability of certain nutrients. Processing practices that affect the polyphenol content of cereals and legumes can influence nutrient bioavailability. Polyphenols interact with plant proteins and form tannin–protein complexes that can inactivate enzymes or lead to protein insolubility adversely influencing amino acid and protein bioavailability. The antinutritional properties of polyphenols can be decreased by removing them from grain with chemical treatments (such as alkaline treatment and ammonia) or removing from grain the polyphenol-rich pericarp and testa by pearling.

Importance of Nutrient Bioavailability to Human Nutrition

Assessment of bioavailability of nutrients is an essential component of deriving dietary reference intakes (DRIs), guidelines for optimal intake of individual nutrients established for North American populations. Many DRIs are based on evaluation of available physiological data to determine the obligatory daily needs for a nutrient to replace losses, or the amount needed for optimal growth of tissues, and an estimate of overall dietary bioavailability of the nutrient in question. In many populations, the content of a nutrient in the diet (e.g., iron or zinc) may be sufficient to meet recommended intake, but bioavailability is suboptimal due to the presence of high levels of inhibitory substances (such as phytate) in the diet leading to a high risk of developing this nutrient deficiency.

Determinants of Nutrient Bioavailability

Speciation

Speciation refers to the form of the nutrient found in food, which may in turn influence the absorption of the nutrient in the gastrointestinal tract. For example, this term could be applied to *cis-* or *trans*-forms of unsaturated fatty acids found in partially hydrogenated oils; individual coenzyme forms of vitamins, such as free thiamin, thiamin pyrophosphate (TPP), thiamin monophosphate (TMP) and thiamin triphosphate (TTP), or the various coenzyme forms of riboflavin – flavin mononucleotide (FMN) and adenine dinucleotide (FAD), or for vitamin B_6 – pyridoxine, pyridoxamine, and pyridoxal; or minerals, such as ferrous or ferric forms of nonheme iron or heme iron; or the selenomethionine, selenite, or selenate form of selenium.

Digestion and Metabolism

During the transit of digested food material through the gastrointestinal tract many changes occur in the intestinal lumen that could influence nutrient bioavailability. Digestion of food constituents is an important aspect of nutrient bioavailability. The secretion of acid into the stomach following food ingestion activates certain digestive enzymes, as well as creating an acidic environment that influences mineral solubility and extraction from food. In this regard, the choice of a mineral to use for supplementation purposes might be influenced by certain physiological conditions, such as achlorhydria. Aging is associated with a decrease in gastric acid secretion in many elderly persons leading to either hypochlorhydria or achlorhydria,

characterized by either low or complete absence of acid secretion, respectively, leading to a neutral or slightly alkaline gastric pH. This raised pH condition in the stomach can have detrimental effects on micronutrient bioavailability. For example, elderly persons with achlorhydria are at risk of vitamin B_{12} deficiency because of an inability to remove properly protein-bound vitamin B_{12} from food when it enters the stomach. In these subjects, the capacity to absorb vitamin B_{12} is normal, however, because they can readily absorb crystalline (nonprotein-bound) vitamin B_{12} from a supplemental vitamin B_{12} dose. Lowering the gastric pH towards normal by administering hydrochloric acid restores vitamin B_{12} absorption from food.

In achlorhydric elderly persons the absorption of calcium carbonate from a dietary supplement after an overnight fast is very poor, presumably because calcium carbonate is a relatively insoluble calcium salt and needs gastric acid to be solubilized. Again, these subjects have normal calcium absorption if the calcium is delivered in a more soluble form, such as calcium citrate. In addition to elderly persons who develop achlorhydria, a large number of people regularly use gastric acid-lowering medications, such as the gastric proton pump inhibitor omeprazole, for antiulcer therapy. These medications can reduce zinc absorption and presumably may affect the absorption of other divalent minerals. Acidification of the gastric contents and solubilization of minerals in the gastric juice is important because many mineral nutrients are preferentially absorbed in the duodenum (upper small intestine) and need to be available in free or low-molecular-weight complexes when they leave the stomach to facilitate contact with intestinal nutrient transporters on the apical (luminal) surface of the absorptive enterocytes.

The lower gastrointestinal tract can also be a potentially important site affecting the bioavailability of bioactive substances found in food. In this regard, intestinal bacteria found in the large intestine can influence bioavailability. Bacteria are instrumental in the metabolic conversion of certain phytonutrients into forms that are more readily absorbed. In addition, bacteria likely play an important role in the enhancing effects of prebiotics on mineral bioavailability. Consumption of nonabsorbable carbohydrates, such as inulin, can have a positive effect on mineral absorption. A possible mechanism of this effect is that the nonabsorbable carbohydrates pass the small intestine and enter into the large intestine where they serve as a food substrate for bacteria. The metabolism of these prebiotic substances by intestinal bacteria lowers the pH of the lumen of the large intestine and may thereby serve to solubilize some insoluble mineral complexes that have passed through the small intestine. The freed mineral would then be available for absorption from the large intestine, thereby increasing overall mineral bioavailability. Other scenarios are possible as well, such as the release of short-chain fatty acids by the bacteria, that may facilitate mineral absorption.

Chelation

Chelation is the process whereby an organic moiety acts as a ligand to bind a metal ion through two or more coordination bonds. Some low-molecular-weight compounds that may be released during the digestion of food can act as metal chelators and increase metal solubility in the intestinal lumen. In some circumstances, chelated forms of metals are naturally present in food, such as heme iron (part of hemoglobin or myoglobin protein) found in meat. Heme is a stable protoporphyrin ring-containing compound that protects a central iron atom from interacting with other potentially deleterious compounds, such as phytic acid, that would reduce its availability and inhibit iron absorption. Nonheme iron bioavailability is affected by various enhancing and inhibitory substances found in food. In contrast, heme iron bioavailability is not. The heme moiety is absorbed intact by the enterocyte. Inside the enterocyte a cytosolic enzyme heme oxygenase breaks apart the protoporphyrin ring and releases the caged iron atom, which can then be transferred out into the blood.

Bioavailability Enhancers and Inhibitors

Various food substances have been identified that act as enhancers or inhibitors of divalent mineral absorption. In general, these food factors influence nutrient bioavailability by either forming relatively insoluble complexes with nutrients or preventing them from interacting with their respective nutrient transporter, or by protecting the nutrient from such untoward interaction maintaining it in a state that can be absorbed or as an absorbable chelated complex (e.g., heme iron).

A list of factors known to influence mineral bioavailability is given in **Table 1**.

Table 1 Dietary enhancers and inhibitors of mineral bioavailability

Enhancers	Inhibitors
Ascorbic acid	Polyphenols (especially galloyl groups)
Organic acids	Phytic acid
Meat factor	Myricetin
Alcohol	Chlorogenic acid (coffee)
Inulin	Insoluble dietary fiber

General Physiology of Nutrient Absorption

Nutrients enter the blood by passing through the intestinal mucosa. Intestinal nutrient transport can occur via two distinct pathways. One is termed the paracellular pathway and represents the movement of a nutrient between the absorptive enterocytes on the intestinal villi. This transport pathway is an energy-independent diffusional process and depends on the electrochemical gradient across the mucosa and its permeability characteristics to the nutrient in question. The characteristics of the diffusional pathway are not regulated in response to nutrient deficiency or excess. A second transport pathway represents the transcellular movement of a nutrient across the intestine. The transcellular transport rate of the nutrient is composed of both diffusional and carrier-mediated transport pathways. Often in response to changes in nutrient status the number of nutrient carriers will be changed to facilitate appropriate increases or decreases in intestinal absorption to help maintain nutrient homeostasis. Within a class of nutrients there can be substantial differences in absorption rates. For example, in the case of minerals, monovalent minerals (such as sodium, potassium, and iodine) are absorbed at very high efficiency approximating complete absorption, while multivalent elements (such as chromium, heavy metals, and iron) are relatively poorly absorbed (1–20%). In addition, because some nutrient transporters, e.g., the divalent metal transporter DMT-1 that is responsible for intestinal iron transport, can also transport more than one type of mineral, unintended alterations in the absorption rate of one mineral may occur by a process of co-adaptation in response to changes in the status or physiologic need for another mineral. For example, in iron deficiency, iron absorption is increased, but the absorption of cadmium and lead are also inadvertently increased. However, these effects (homeostatic regulation and co-adaptation) are responses to a change in physiological state and should not be confused with alterations in nutrient 'bioavailability' *per se*, a characteristic of an individual food, a complex mixed meal, or a longer term characteristic of a particular dietary pattern.

Methods for Measuring Nutrient Bioavailability

In Vitro Bioavailability Technique

Nutrient bioavailability, estimated as absorbability alone, can be measured by various *in vitro* methods. *In vitro* methods have obvious distinct advantages in that they are less expensive, rapid, and amenable to high throughput analyses. Often, experimental *in vitro* methods involve an initial 'digestion phase' where the food is treated with acid and digestive enzymes to simulate the initial steps of food breakdown. The digestion phase is then followed by a second phase wherein the goal is to estimate the potential relative availability of a nutrient. This usually involves the measurement of the concentration of the soluble nutrient of interest in a supernatant of the digested food following centrifugation or after dialysis of the digested food products across a semi-permeable membrane designed to select only low-molecular-weight complexes. Variations on this theme include the addition of radioactive isotopes following the digestion phase and the *in vitro* measurement of cellular uptake of the nutrient in a cell culture preparation or some appropriate index of nutrient uptake. In the case of iron, for example, cellular synthesis of ferritin, an iron storage protein, has been used. Similar applications of this *in vitro* technique are now appearing in the scientific literature for the measurement of phytochemical bioavailability, such as beta-carotene, lycopene, lutein, etc. However, although promising at the moment, there is little confidence that these methods can adequately replace *in vivo* methods of measuring nutrient bioavailability.

In Vivo Bioavailability Techniques

Various animal models and techniques have been used to estimate nutrient bioavailability. A primary concern that must be initially addressed in using animal models to estimate nutrient bioavailability is whether these various model systems accurately reflect nutrient bioavailability in humans. For example, usual experimental animal models, such as rats and mice, cannot be used to assess beta-carotene bioavailability because the absorptive mechanism in these rodents for this nutrient is quite different from that in humans. In contrast, the ferret appears to be a suitable animal model to at least mimic this carotenoid's intestinal absorptive pathway. Similarly, poor correlation of iron bioavailability between chicks and humans for elemental iron powders has raised questions about the suitability of that species for estimating nutrient bioavailability of iron.

Measuring Nutrient Bioavailability in Humans

The first consideration is often whether it is necessary to have an accurate quantitative estimate of nutrient bioavailability, or whether an estimate of relative bioavailability compared to a known standard nutrient source will suffice. An accurate quantitative measure of bioavailability might be necessary when the intention is to provide data to derive a recommendation for dietary intake to meet a nutrient requirement. In this case, it is important to have a reasonably good estimate of the true fraction of a given dose of the ingested nutrient that could be absorbed and utilized, for example, to replace endogenous losses of the nutrient.

A common application of bioavailability measurements is to compare relative bioavailability between two or more sources of a nutrient. For example, one might be concerned with determining the calcium bioavailability from milk compared to calcium derived from a vegetable source such as broccoli or calcium-fortified orange juice. There are many techniques available to measure relative nutrient bioavailability under *in vivo* conditions based on a comparison of the rise in plasma level (or urinary excretion) of the nutrient or rate of appearance in plasma of a radioactively labeled nutrient after an oral test dose. An important technical advance in measuring food mineral bioavailability in humans was the validation of an extrinsic tag method. Extrinsic tag studies were validated by measuring the extent of absorption of a mineral isotope mixed exogenously (the 'extrinsic tag') with a food compared to that of an intrinsic tag where the absorption of the isotope is determined from an intrinsically labeled food source. The intrinsic tag is often achieved by growing plants hydroponically in a solution enriched in a radioactive or stable mineral isotope to label the plant food of interest during growth, or by supplying the mineral isotope tag to a growing animal used for meat, or one that was used for milk production, for example. These studies have shown that in most cases the ratio of absorption of the extrinsic to the intrinsic isotope was approximately one, indicating that the extrinsically added isotope tag became homogenously incorporated into the pool of absorbed mineral found endogenously in the food of interest. The use of the extrinsic tag method has greatly facilitated the study of relative bioavailability of minerals from food in human subjects.

A large and growing number of people are consuming dietary supplements. However, due to the relative difficulty of labeling these supplements, in most cases, little information on the bioavailability of the nutrients in the supplements is available. A study of vitamin and mineral bioavailability from a popular multinutrient supplement found good absorption of the water-soluble vitamins (B vitamins and vitamin C) from the tablet but relatively poor absorption of copper and zinc.

Food Fortification

In the summer of 1941 a National Nutrition Conference for Defense was held that led to the recommendation that there should be improvement of the nutritive value of certain low-cost stable food products (e.g., flour and bread) by nutrient enrichment to replace nutrients lost during the milling and refining process. This led to recommendations to fortify milk with vitamin D, margarine with vitamin A, and salt with iodine using the new recommended dietary allowances (RDAs) established by the Committee on Food and Nutrition of the National Research Council (currently the Food and Nutrition Board) as a yardstick to judge the appropriate levels of fortification. Standards of identity for 'enriched' flour' were initially established that allowed for the addition of the 'basic four': iron, thiamin, niacin, and riboflavin (with optional calcium). In subsequent years, the standard of identity concept was expanded to include some other enriched foods. As of 1998, the Food and Drug Administration mandated that folate be added to the standards of identity for enriched breads, flours, corn meals, pastas, rice, and other grain products.

Micronutrient Fortification in the UK

In the UK, fortification of foods is subject to the Food Safety Act 1990. Fortification of certain micronutrients to margarine and most types of flour is mandatory. Calcium, iron, thiamin, and niacin are required to be added to both white and brown flours, but not to wholemeal flours. The level of required fortification is shown in **Table 2**.

Margarine is required to be fortified with vitamin A and D to levels comparable with or exceeding those found in butter. Additional mandatory fortification requirements determine the nutrient content of infant formulas and follow-on formulas, weaning foods, and foods intended to be used in energy-restricted diets. In the UK, voluntary fortification is allowed for certain products, such as breakfast cereal, soft drinks, and milks. In most cases the level of fortification per serving is between 15% and 33% of the relevant RDA.

Table 2 Nutrients required to be added to white and brown flours in the United Kingdom

Nutrient	Amount of nutrient (mg) per 100 g flour
Calcium	235–390
Iron	Not less than 1.65
Thiamin	Not less than 0.24
Niacin	Not less than 1.6

Bioavailability of Food Fortificants

The bioavailability of nutrients added to food can be determined by a number of factors. For example, in some cases the reactivity of added nutrients can cause untoward reactions that adversely affect the organoleptic properties of food. In these cases, there must be a trade-off of some kind and it may be necessary to intentionally select a somewhat less bioavailable form of a nutrient to provide an acceptable consumer product or to provide an acceptable shelf life to the product under given field conditions. Moreover, once added to a food, the bioavailability of a fortificant can be altered by various food manufacturing processes, such as those that demand high heat and pressure. Normal home food preparation techniques can also affect nutrient bioavailability. In addition, plant breeding and horticultural practices can contribute to the development and use of superior plant varieties supplying additional or more bioavailable micronutrients. For example, genetic engineering of plants has led to the development of rice and other grain products that have lower phytate content and higher mineral bioavailability. The development of 'Golden Rice,' which is rich in β-carotene, a dietary precursor of vitamin A, represents a well-known example of genetic plant engineering to enhance nutrient intakes. There is increasing interest in genetic manipulation of plant stocks to achieve higher content of potentially healthful phytonutrients, such as lycopene and lutein. Internationally, the traditional focus of fortification has been directed at the 'Big 3' – deficiencies of vitamin A, iodine, and iron – due to the widespread prevalence of deficiencies of these particular micronutrients and well-known adverse health effects of these nutrient deficiencies.

Bioavailability of Fortified Iron

A list of iron sources that are generally recognized as safe (GRAS) by the US Food and Drug Administration (FDA) is given in **Table 3**. However, as shown in **Table 4**, the bioavailability of different iron sources varies widely. Moreover, even within a given source of iron, such as the elemental iron powders commonly used to fortify various ready-to-eat breakfast cereals and other products, a significant disparity (5–148%) in relative bioavailability (compared to ferrous sulfate) can be observed. To some extent, these differing bioavailability estimates reflect the influence of the characteristics of the fortified product in terms of its contribution of various enhancers or inhibitors (**Table 1**) on iron bioavailability. In addition, other factors also can affect the bioavailability of elemental iron powders, such as the particle size of the fortificant

Table 3 Iron and zinc compounds listed as generally recognized as safe by the US Food and Drug Administration

Iron compounds	Zinc compounds
Elemental iron	Zinc sulfate
Ferrous ascorbate	Zinc chloride
Ferrous carbonate	Zinc gluconate
Ferrous citrate	Zinc oxide
Ferrous fumarate	Zinc stearate
Ferrous gluconate	
Ferrous lactate	
Ferrous sulfate	
Ferric ammonium citrate	
Ferric chloride	
Ferric citrate	
Ferric pyrophosphate	
Ferric sulfate	

compound – a finer particle size is associated with greater iron bioavailability.

There is very limited information available concerning the bioavailability of calcium or other nutrients added as a fortificant to various products. One study in elderly women found that calcium citrate malate used to fortify orange juice had equivalent bioavailability to calcium from milk or calcium from a calcium carbonate supplement. In a study with adult subjects, the

Table 4 Average relative bioavailability in humans of various iron sources used as iron fortification compounds

Average relative bioavailability	Iron compound	Approximate iron content (%)
>90% group		
106[a]	Ferrous lactate	19
100	Ferrous sulfate 7H$_2$O	20
100	Ferrous fumarate	33
92	Ferrous succinate	35
>60–<90% group		
89	Ferrous gluconate	12
75	Electrolytic elemental Fe powders	97
74	Ferric saccharate	10
74	Ferrous citrate	24
62	Ferrous tartrate	22
Variable (%)		
21–74	Ferric pyrophosphate	25
25–32	Ferric orthophosphate	28
13–148	H-reduced elemental Fe powder	97
5–20	Carbonyl elemental Fe powder	99

[a]Relative to absorption of iron from ferrous sulfate = 100%
Adapted from Lynch S (2002) Food iron absorption and its importance for the design of food fortification strategies. *Nutrition Reviews* **60**: S3–S15.

bioavailability of a single 25 000 IU dose of vitamin D$_2$ was assessed from whole milk, skim milk, and vitamin D-fortified oil given with toast. No difference in peak serum vitamin D$_2$ was found following these three treatments, suggesting that the fat content of whole milk does not influence vitamin D bioavailability. It has also been shown that consumption of vitamin D-fortified orange juice (1000 IU/240 ml) for 12 weeks significantly increased serum 25-hydroxyvitamin D concentrations.

Fat content of a meal may have an important effect on carotenoid bioavailability. The absorption of carotenoids (α-carotene, β-carotene, and lycopene) from salad vegetables was found to be undetectable if a fat-free salad dressing was used, but substantially greater absorption occurred with a full-fat salad dressing. The amount of fat needed to promote optimal absorption of vitamin E and carotenoids may be rather limited. No difference in absorption of vitamin E and α- or β-carotene was observed when supplements were administered with either 3 g or 36 g of dietary fat. In contrast, lutein ester absorption was more than twice as great when consumed with the higher fat level.

Bioavailability of food sources of folate are usually only about 50% of synthetic folic acid. This systematic difference may be due to the occurrence of polyglutamyl folic acid in foods that reduce folate absorption.

See also: **Calcium**. **Carotenoids**: Chemistry, Sources and Physiology. **Cobalamins**. **Copper**. **Food Fortification**: Developed Countries; Developing Countries. **Iodine**: Physiology, Dietary Sources and Requirements. **Microbiota of the Intestine**: Prebiotics. **Osteoporosis**. **Selenium**. **Vitamin A**: Biochemistry and Physiological Role. **Zinc**: Physiology.

Further Reading

Backstrand J (2002) The history and future of food fortification in the United States: a public health perspective. *Nutrition Reviews* **60**: 15–26.

Bouis HE (2003) Micronutrient fortification of plants through plant breeding: can it improve nutrition in man at low cost? *Proceedings of the Nutrition Society* **62**(2): 403–411.

Calvo MS and Whiting SJ (2003) Prevalence of vitamin D insufficiency in Canada and the United States: importance to health status and efficacy of current food fortification and dietary supplement use. *Nutrition Reviews* **61**(3): 107–113.

Chavasit V and Nopburabutr P (2003) Combating iodine and iron deficiencies through the double fortification of fish sauce, mixed fish sauce, and salt brine. *Food and Nutrition Bulletin* **24**(2): 200–207.

Dary O and Mora JO (2002) Food fortification to reduce vitamin A deficiency: International Vitamin A Consultative Group recommendations. *Journal of Nutrition* **132**(supplement 9): 2927S–2933S.

Delange FM (2003) Control of iodine deficiency in Western and Central Europe. *Central Europe Journal of Public Health* **11**(3): 120–123.

Fairweather-Tait SJ and Teucher B (2002) Iron and calcium bioavailability of fortified foods and dietary supplements. *Nutrition Review* **60**(11): 360–367.

Johnson-Down L, L'Abbe MR, Lee NS, and Gray-Donald K (2003) Appropriate calcium fortification of the food supply presents a challenge. *Journal of Nutrition* **133**(7): 2232–2238.

Lutter CK and Dewey KG (2003) Proposed nutrient composition for fortified complementary foods. *Journal of Nutrition* **133**(9): 3011S–3020S.

Lynch S (2002) Food iron absorption and its importance for the design of food fortification strategies. *Nutrition Reviews* **60**: S3–S6.

Meltzer HM, Aro A, Andersen NL, Koch B, and Alexander J (2003) Risk analysis applied to food fortification. *Public Health and Nutrition* **6**(3): 281–291.

Penniston KL and Tanumihardjo SA (2003) Vitamin A in dietary supplements and fortified food: too much of a good thing? *Journal of the American Dietetic Association* **103**(9): 1185–1187.

Quinlivan EP and Gregory JK 3rd (2003) Effect of food fortification on folic acid intake in the United States. *American Journal of Clinical Nutrition* **77**(1): 8–9.

Rosado JL (2003) Zinc and copper: proposed fortification levels and recommended zinc compounds. *Journal of Nutrition* **133**(9): 2985S–2989S.

BIOTIN

D M Mock, University of Arkansas for Medical Sciences, Little Rock, AR, USA

© 2005 Elsevier Ltd. All rights reserved.

Biotin is a water-soluble vitamin that is generally classified in the B complex group. Biotin was discovered in nutritional experiments that demonstrated a factor in many foodstuffs capable of curing the scaly dermatitis, hair loss, and neurologic signs induced in rats fed dried egg white. Avidin, a glycoprotein found in egg white, binds biotin very specifically and tightly. From an evolutionary standpoint, avidin probably serves as a bacteriostat in egg white; consistent with this hypothesis is the observation that avidin is resistant to a broad range of bacterial proteases in both the free and biotin-bound form. Because avidin is also resistant to pancreatic proteases, dietary avidin binds to dietary biotin (and probably any biotin from intestinal microbes) and prevents absorption, carrying the biotin through the gastrointestinal tract. Biotin is synthesized by many intestinal microbes; however, the contribution of microbial biotin to absorbed biotin, if any, remains unknown. Cooking denatures avidin, rendering this protein susceptible to digestion and unable to interfere with absorption of biotin.

Absorption and Transport

Digestion of Protein-Bound Biotin

The content of free biotin and protein-bound biotin in foods is variable, but the majority of biotin in meats and cereals appears to be protein-bound via an amide bond between biotin and lysine. Neither the mechanisms of intestinal hydrolysis of protein-bound biotin nor the determinants of bioavailability have been clearly delineated. Because this bond is not hydrolyzed by cellular proteases, release is likely mediated by a specific biotin—amide hydrolase (biotinidase, EC 3.5.1.12). Biotinidase mRNA is present in pancreas and, in lesser amounts, in intestinal mucosa. Biotinidase is also present in many other tissues, including heart, brain, liver, lung, skeletal muscle, kidney, plasma, and placenta. Biotinidase also likely plays a critical role in intracellular recycling of biotin by releasing biotin from intracellular proteins such as carboxylases during protein turnover.

Intestinal Absorption and Transport into Somatic Cells

At physiologic pH, the carboxylate group of biotin is negatively charged. Thus, biotin is at least modestly water-soluble and requires a transporter to cross cell membranes such as enterocytes for intestinal absorption, somatic cells for utilization, and renal tubule cells for reclamation from the glomerular filtrate. In intact intestinal preparations such as loops and everted gut sacks, biotin transport exhibits two components. One component is saturable at a k_m of approximately 10 μM biotin; the other is not saturable even at very large concentrations of biotin. This observation is consistent with passive diffusion. Absorption of biocytin, the biotinyl-lysine product of intraluminal protein digestion, is inefficient relative to biotin, suggesting that biotinidase releases biotin from dietary protein. The transporter is present in the intestinal brush border membrane. Transport is highly structurally specific, temperature dependent, Na^+ coupled, and electroneutral. In the presence of a sodium ion gradient, biotin transport occurs against a concentration gradient.

In rats, biotin transport is upregulated with maturation and by biotin deficiency. Although carrier-mediated transport of biotin is most active in the proximal small bowel of the rat, the absorption of biotin from the proximal colon is still significant, supporting the potential nutritional significance of biotin synthesized and released by enteric flora. Clinical studies have provided evidence that biotin is absorbed from the human colon, but studies in swine indicate that absorption of biotin from the hindgut is much less efficient than from the upper intestine; furthermore, biotin synthesized by enteric flora is probably not present at a location or in a form in which bacterial biotin contributes importantly to absorbed biotin. Exit of biotin from the enterocyte (i.e., transport across the basolateral membrane) is also carrier mediated. However, basolateral transport is independent of Na^+, electrogenic, and does not accumulate biotin against a concentration gradient.

Based on a study in which biotin was administered orally in pharmacologic amounts, the bioavailability of biotin is approximately 100%. Thus, the pharmacologic doses of biotin given to treat biotin-dependent inborn errors of metabolism are likely to be well absorbed. Moreover, the finding of high bioavailability of biotin at pharmacologic doses provides at least some basis for predicting that bioavailability will also be high at the physiologic doses at which the biotin transporter mediates uptake.

Studies of a variety of hepatic cell lines indicate that uptake of free biotin is similar to intestinal uptake; transport is mediated by a specialized carrier system that is Na^+ dependent, electroneutral, and structurally specific for a free carboxyl group. At large concentrations, transport is mediated by diffusion. Metabolic trapping (e.g., biotin bound covalently to intracellular proteins) is also important. After entering the hepatocyte, biotin diffuses into the mitochondria via a pH-dependent process.

Two biotin transporters have been described: a multivitamin transporter present in many tissues and a biotin transporter identified in human lymphocytes. In 1997, Prasad and coworkers discovered a Na^+-coupled, saturable, structurally specific transporter present in human placental choriocarcinoma cells that can transport pantothenic acid, lipoic acid, and biotin. This sodium-dependent multivitamin transporter has been named SMVT and is widely expressed in human tissues. Studies by Said and

coworkers using RNA interference specific for SMVT provide strong evidence that biotin uptake by Caco-2 and HepG2 cells occurs via SMVT; thus, intestinal absorption and hepatic uptake are likely mediated by SMVT. The biotin transporter identified in lymphocytes is also Na^+ coupled, saturable, and structurally specific. Studies by Zempleni and coworkers provide evidence in favor of monocarboxylate transporter-1 as the lymphocyte biotin transporter.

A child with biotin dependence due to a defect in the lymphocyte biotin transporter has been reported. The SMVT gene sequence was normal. The investigators speculate that lymphocyte biotin transporter is expressed in other tissues and mediates some critical aspect of biotin homeostasis.

Ozand and collaborators described several patients in Saudi Arabia with biotin-responsive basal ganglia disease. Symptoms include confusion, lethargy, vomiting, seizures, dystonia, dysarthria, dysphagia, seventh nerve paralysis, quadriparesis, ataxia, hypertension, chorea, and coma. A defect in the biotin transporter system across the blood–brain barrier was postulated. Additional work by Gusella and coworkers has suggested that SLC19A3 may be responsible for the reported defect.

The relationship of these putative biotin transporters to each other and their relative roles in intestinal absorption, transport into various organs, and renal reclamation remain to be elucidated.

Transport of Biotin from the Intestine to Peripheral Tissues

Biotin concentrations in plasma are small relative those of other water-soluble vitamins. Most biotin in plasma is free, dissolved in the aqueous phase of plasma. However, small amounts are reversibly bound and covalently bound to plasma protein (approximately 7 and 12%, respectively); binding to human serum albumin likely accounts for the reversible binding. Biotinidase has been proposed as a biotin binding protein or biotin carrier protein for the transport into cells. A biotin binding plasma glycoprotein has been observed in pregnant rats. Although the importance of protein binding in the transport of biotin from the intestine to the peripheral tissues is not clear, the immunoneutralization of this protein led to decreased transport of biotin to the fetus and early death of the embryo.

Transport of Biotin into the Central Nervous System

Biotin is transported across the blood–brain barrier. The transporter is saturable and structurally specific for the free carboxylate group on the valeric acid side chain. Transport into the neuron also appears to involve a specific transport system with subsequent trapping of biotin by covalent binding to brain proteins, presumably carboxylases.

Placental Transport of Biotin

Biotin concentrations are 3- to 17-fold greater in plasma from human fetuses compared to those in their mothers in the second trimester, consistent with active placental transport. The microvillus membrane of the placenta contains a saturable transport system for biotin that is Na^+ dependent and actively accumulates biotin within the placenta, consistent with SMVT.

Transport of Biotin into Human Milk

More than 95% of the biotin in human milk is free in the skim fraction. The concentration of biotin varies substantially in some women and exceeds the concentration in serum by one or two orders of magnitude, suggesting that there is a system for transport into milk. Metabolites account for more than half of the total biotin plus metabolites in early and transitional human milk. With postpartum maturation, the biotin concentration increases, but inactive metabolites still account for approximately one-third of the total biotin plus metabolites at 5 weeks postpartum. Studies have not detected a soluble biotin binding protein.

Metabolism and Urinary Excretion of Biotin and Metabolites

Biotin is a bicyclic compound (**Figure 1**). One of the rings contains an ureido group (—N—CO—N—). The tetrahydrothiophene ring contains sulfur and has a valeric acid side chain. A significant proportion of biotin undergoes catabolism before excretion (**Figure 1**). Two principal pathways of biotin catabolism have been identified in mammals. In the first pathway, the valeric acid side chain of biotin is degraded by β-oxidation. β-Oxidation of biotin leads to the formation of bisnorbiotin, tetranorbiotin, and related intermediates that are known to result from β-oxidation of fatty acids. The cellular site of this β-oxidation of biotin is uncertain. Spontaneous (nonenzymatic) decarboxylation of the unstable β-keto acids (β-keto-biotin and β-keto-bisnorbiotin) leads to formation of bisnorbiotin methylketone and tetranorbiotin methylketone; these catabolites appear in urine.

In the second pathway, the sulfur in the thiophane ring of biotin is oxidized, leading to the formation of biotin-L-sulfoxide, biotin-D-sulfoxide, and biotin

sulfone. Sulfur oxidation may be catalyzed by a NADPH-dependent process in the smooth endoplasmic reticulum. Combined oxidation of the ring sulfur and β-oxidation of the side chain lead to metabolites such as bisnorbiotin sulfone. In mammals, degradation of the biotin ring to release carbon dioxide and urea is quantitatively minor. Biotin metabolism is accelerated in some individuals by anticonvulsants and during pregnancy, thereby increasing in urine the ratio of biotin metabolites to biotin.

Animal studies and studies using brush border membrane vesicles from human kidney cortex indicate that biotin is reclaimed from the glomerular filtrate against a concentration gradient by a saturable, Na^+-dependent, structurally specific system, but biocytin does not inhibit tubular reabsorption of biotin. Subsequent egress of biotin from the tubular cells occurs via a basolateral membrane transport system that is not dependent on Na^+. Studies of patients with biotinidase deficiency suggest that there may be a role for biotinidase in the renal handling of biotin.

On a molar basis, biotin accounts for approximately half of the total avidin-binding substances in human serum and urine (**Table 1**). Biocytin, bisnorbiotin, bisnorbiotin methylketone, biotin-D,L-sulfoxide, and biotin sulfone account for most of the balance.

Biliary Excretion of Biotin and Metabolites

Biliary excretion of biotin and metabolites is quantitatively negligible based on animal studies. When [^{14}C]biotin was injected intravenously into rats, biotin, bisnorbiotin, biotin-D,L-sulfoxide, and bisnorbiotin methylketone accounted for less than 2% of the administered ^{14}C, but urinary excretion accounted for 60%. Although the concentrations of biotin, bisnorbiotin, and biotin-D,L-sulfoxide were approximately 10-fold greater in bile than in serum of pigs, the bile-to-serum ratios of biotin and metabolites were more than 10-fold less than those of bilirubin, which is actively excreted in bile.

Metabolic Functions

In mammals, biotin serves as an essential cofactor for five carboxylases, each of which catalyses a critical step in intermediary metabolism. All five of the mammalian carboxylases catalyze the incorporation of bicarbonate as a carboxyl group into a substrate and employ a similar catalytic mechanism.

Biotin is attached to the apocarboxylase by a condensation reaction catalyzed by holocarboxylase synthetase (**Figure 1**). An amide bond is formed

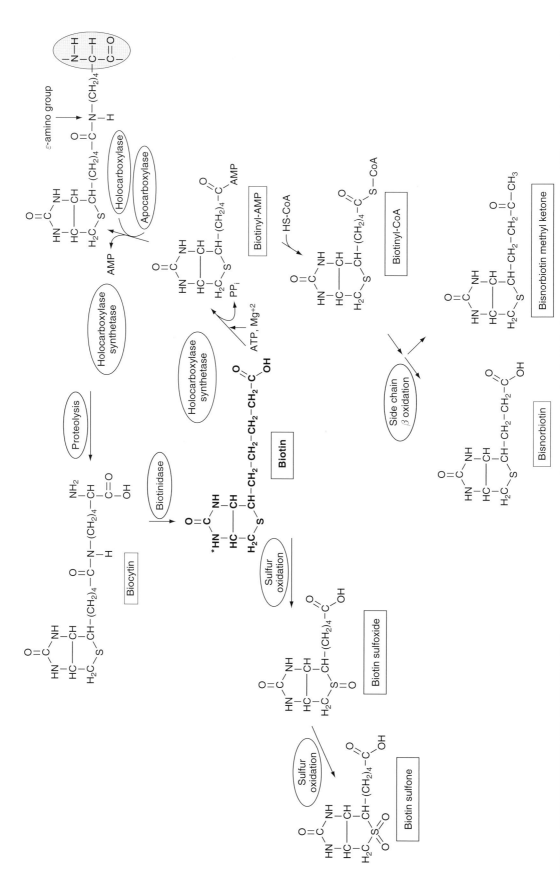

Figure 1 Biotin metabolism and degradation. Ovals denote enzymes or enzyme systems; rectangles denote biotin, intermediates, and metabolites. AMP, adenosine monophosphae; ATP, adenosine triphosphate; CoA, coenzyme A; Pp, pyrophosphate; *, site of attachment of carboxyl moiety.

Table 1 Normal range for biotin and metabolites in human serum and urine[a]

Compound	Serum (pmol/l)	Urine (nmol/24 h)
Biotin	133–329	18–127
Bisnorbiotin	21–563	6–39
Biotin-D,L-sulfoxide	0–120	5–19
Bisnorbiotin methylketone	0–120	2–13
Biotin sulfone	ND	1–8
Biocytin	0–26	1–13
Total biotinyl compounds	294–1021[b]	46–128

[a]Normal ranges are reported ($n = 15$ for serum; $n = 16$ for urine, except biocytin, $n = 10$).
[b]Including unidentified biotin metabolites.
ND, not determined.

between the carboxyl group of the valeric acid side chain of biotin and the ε-amino group of a specific lysyl residue in the apocarboxylase; these regions contain sequences of amino acids that are highly conserved for the individual carboxylases both within and between species.

In the carboxylase reaction, the carboxyl moiety is first attached to biotin at the ureido nitrogen opposite the side chain; then the carboxyl group is transferred to the substrate. The reaction is driven by the hydrolysis of ATP to ADP and inorganic phosphate. Subsequent reactions in the pathways of the mammalian carboxylases release carbon dioxide from the product of the carboxylase reaction. Thus, these reaction sequences rearrange the substrates into more useful intermediates but do not violate the classic observation that mammalian metabolism does not result in the net fixation of carbon dioxide.

Regulation of intracellular mammalian carboxylase activity by biotin remains to be elucidated. However, the interaction of biotin synthesis and production of holoacetyl-CoA carboxylase in

Escherichia coli has been extensively studied. In the bacterial system, the apocarboxylase protein and biotin (as the intermediate biotinyl-AMP) act together to control the rate of biotin synthesis by direct interaction with promoter regions of the biotin operon, which in turn controls a cluster of genes that encode enzymes that catalyze the synthesis of biotin.

The five biotin-dependent mammalian carboxylases are acetyl-CoA carboxylase isoforms I and II (also known as α-ACC (EC 6.4.1.2) and β-ACC (EC 6.4.1.2)), pyruvate carboxylase (EC 6.4.1.1), methylcrotonyl-CoA carboxylase (EC 6.4.1.4), and propionyl-CoA carboxylase (EC 6.4.1.3). ACC catalyzes the incorporation of bicarbonate into acetyl-CoA to form malonyl-CoA (**Figure 2**). There are two isoforms of ACC. Isoform I is located in the cytosol and produces malonyl-CoA, which is rate limiting in fatty acid synthesis (elongation). Isoform II is located on the outer mitochondrial membrane and controls fatty acid oxidation in mitochondria through the inhibitory effect of malonyl-CoA on fatty acid transport into mitochondria. An inactive mitochondrial form of ACC may serve as storage for biotin.

The three remaining carboxylases are mitochondrial. Pyruvate carboxylase (PC) catalyzes the incorporation of bicarbonate into pyruvate to form oxaloacetate, an intermediate in the Krebs tricarboxylic acid cycle (**Figure 2**). Thus, PC catalyzes an anaplerotic reaction. In gluconeogenic tissues (i.e., liver and kidney), the oxaloacetate can be converted to glucose. Deficiency of PC is probably the cause of the lactic acidemia, central nervous system lactic acidosis, and abnormalities in glucose regulation observed in biotin deficiency and biotinidase deficiency. β-Methylcrotonyl-CoA carboxylase (MCC) catalyzes an essential step in the degradation of the branched-chain amino acid leucine (**Figure 2**). Deficient activity of MCC leads to metabolism of

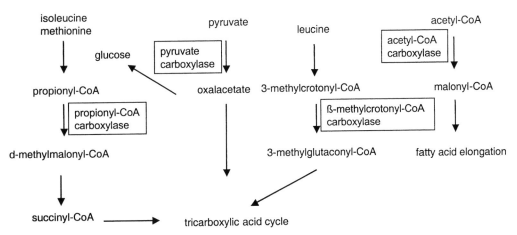

Figure 2 Interrelationship of pathways catalyzed by biotin-dependent enzymes (shown in boxes).

3-methylcrotonyl-CoA to 3-hydroxyisovaleric acid and 3-methylcrotonylglycine by an alternate pathway. Thus, increased urinary excretion of these abnormal metabolites reflects deficient activity of MCC.

Propionyl-CoA carboxylase (PCC) catalyzes the incorporation of bicarbonate into propionyl-CoA to form methylmalonyl-CoA; methylmalonyl-CoA undergoes isomerization to succinyl-CoA and enters the tricarboxylic acid cycle (**Figure 2**). In a manner analogous to MCC deficiency, deficiency of PCC leads to increased urinary excretion of 3-hydroxy-propionic acid and 3-methylcitric acid.

In the normal turnover of cellular proteins, holo-carboxylases are degraded to biocytin or biotin linked to an oligopeptide containing at most a few amino acid residues (**Figure 1**). Biotinidase releases biotin for recycling. Genetic deficiencies of holocarboxylase synthetase and biotinidase cause the two types of multiple carboxylase deficiency that were previously designated the neonatal and juvenile forms.

A Potential Role for Biotin in Gene Expression

In 1995, Hymes and Wolf discovered that biotini-dase can act as a biotinyl-transferase; biocytin serves as the source of biotin, and histones are specifically biotinylated. Approximately 25% of total cellular biotinidase activity occurs in the nucleus. Zempleni and coworkers demonstrated that the abundance of biotinylated histones varies with the cell cycle, that biotinylated histones are increased approximately twofold compared to quiescent lymphocytes, and that histones are debiotinylated enzymatically in a process that is at least partially catalyzed by biotini-dase. These observations suggest that biotin plays a role in regulating DNA transcription and regulation.

Although the mechanisms remain to be elucidated, biotin status has been shown to clearly effect gene expression. Cell culture studies suggest that cell pro-liferation generates an increased demand for biotin, perhaps mediated by increased synthesis of biotin-dependent carboxylases. Solozano-Vargas and cowor-kers reported that biotin deficiency reduces messenger RNA levels of holocarboxylase synthetase, α-ACC, and PCC and postulated that a cyclic GMP-dependent signaling pathway is involved in the pathogenesis.

Studies have been conducted on diabetic humans and rats that support an effect of biotin status on carbohydrate metabolism. Genes studied include glu-cokinase, phosphoenolpyruvate carboxykinase (PEPCK), and expression of the asialoglycoprotein receptor on the surface of hepatocytes. The effect of biotin status on PEPCK expression was particularly striking when diabetic rats were compared to nondia-betic rats. However, most studies have been per-formed on rats in which metabolic pathways have been perturbed prior to administration of biotin. Thus, the role of biotin in regulation of these genes during normal biotin status remains to be elucidated.

Hyperammonemia is a finding in biotin defi-ciency. Maeda and colleges have reported that ornithine transcarbamoylase (an enzyme in the urea cycle) is significantly reduced in biotin-deficient rats.

Assessment of Biotin Status

Measurement of Biotin

For measuring biotin at physiological concentrations (i.e., $100 \, \mathrm{pmol \, l^{-1}}$ to $100 \, \mathrm{nmol \, l^{-1}}$), a variety of assays have been proposed, and a limited number have been used to study biotin nutritional status. Most published studies of biotin nutritional status have used one of two basic types of biotin assays: bioassays (most studies) or avidin-binding assays (several recent studies).

Bioassays are generally sensitive enough to mea-sure biotin in blood and urine. However, the bacter-ial bioassays (and perhaps the eukaryotic bioassays as well) suffer interference from unrelated sub-stances and variable growth response to biotin ana-logues. Bioassays give conflicting results if biotin is bound to protein.

Avidin-binding assays generally measure the abil-ity of biotin (i) to compete with radiolabeled biotin for binding to avidin (isotope dilution assays), (ii) to bind to avidin coupled to a reporter and thus pre-vent the avidin from binding to a biotin linked to solid phase, or (iii) to prevent inhibition of a bioti-nylated enzyme by avidin. Avidin-binding assays generally detect all avidin-binding substances, although the relative detectabilities of biotin and analogues vary between analogues and between assays, depending on how the assay is conducted. Chromatographic separation of biotin analogues with subsequent avidin-binding assay of the chroma-tographic fractions appears to be both sensitive and chemically specific.

Laboratory Findings of Biotin Deficiency

Although various indices have been used to assess biotin status, these have been validated in humans only twice during progressive biotin deficiency. In both studies, marginal biotin deficiency was induced in normal adults by feeding egg white. The urinary excretion of biotin declined dramatically with time on the egg-white diet, reaching frankly abnormal values in 17 of 21 subjects by day 20 of egg-white feeding. Bisnorbiotin excretion declined in parallel, providing evidence for regulated catabolism of biotin. In most subjects, urinary excretion of 3-hydroxyisovaleric acid increased steadily. By day 14 of egg-white feeding, 3-hydroxyisovaleric acid excretion was abnormally increased in 18 of 21 subjects, providing evidence that biotin depletion decreases the activity of MCC and alters leucine metabolism early in progressive biotin deficiency. Based on a study of only 5 subjects, 3-hydroxyisovaleric acid excretion in response to a leucine challenge may be even more sensitive than 3-hydroxyisovaleric acid excretion. Urinary excretions of 3-methylcrotonyl-glycine, 3-hydroxypropionic acid, and 3-methylcitric acid are not sensitive indicators of biotin deficiency compared to 3-hydroxyisovaleric acid excretion.

In a single study, plasma concentrations of free biotin decreased to abnormal values in only half of the subjects. This observation provides confirmation of the impression that blood biotin concentration is not an early or sensitive indicator of marginal biotin deficiency.

Lymphocyte PCC activity is an early and sensitive indicator of marginal biotin deficiency. In 11 of 11 subjects, lymphocyte PCC activity decreased to abnormal values by day 28 of egg-white feeding and returned to normal in 8 of 11 within 3 weeks of resuming a general diet with or without biotin supplement.

Odd-chain fatty acid accumulation is also a marker of biotin deficiency. The accumulation of odd-chain fatty acid is thought to result from PCC deficiency (**Figure 3**); the accumulation of propionyl-CoA likely leads to the substitution of a propionyl-CoA moiety for acetyl-CoA in the ACC reaction and to the incorporation of a three- (rather than two-) carbon moiety during fatty acid elongation. However, in comparison to lymphocyte PCC activity and urinary excretion of 3-hydroxyisovaleric acid, odd-chain fatty acids accumulate in blood lipids more slowly during biotin deficiency and return to normal more gradually after biotin repletion.

Requirements and Allowances

Data providing an accurate estimate of the dietary and parenteral biotin requirements for infants, children, and adults are lacking. However, recommendations for biotin supplementation have been formulated for oral and parenteral intake for preterm infants, term infants, children, and adults (**Table 2**).

Table 2 Adequate intake of biotin

Life-stage group	Adequate intake (μg/day)
Infants (months)	
0–6	5
7–12	6
Children (years)	
1–3	8
4–8	12
Males and females (years)	
9–13	20
14–18	25
≥19	30
Pregnancy	30
Lactation	35

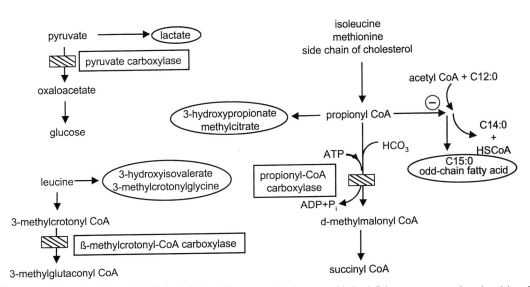

Figure 3 Organic acids and odd-chain fatty acids accumulate because biotin deficiency causes reduced activity of biotin-dependent enzymes. Hatched bars denote metabolic blocks at deficient carboxylases; ovals denote accumulation of products from alternative pathways.

Dietary Sources, Deficiency, and High Intakes

Dietary Sources

There is no published evidence that biotin can be synthesized by mammals; thus, the higher animals must derive biotin from other sources. The ultimate source of biotin appears to be de novo synthesis by bacteria, primitive eukaryotic organisms such as yeast, moulds, and algae, and some plant species.

The great majority of measurements of biotin content of foods have used bioassays. Recent publications provide evidence that the values are likely to contain substantial errors. However, some worthwhile generalizations can be made. Biotin is widely distributed in natural foodstuffs, but the absolute content of even the richest sources is low compared to the content of most other water-soluble vitamins. Foods relatively rich in biotin are listed in **Table 3**. The average daily dietary biotin intake has been estimated to be approximately 35–70 μg.

Circumstances Leading to Deficiency

The fact that normal humans have a requirement for biotin has been clearly documented in two situations: prolonged consumption of raw egg white and parenteral nutrition without biotin supplementation in patients with short bowel syndrome and other causes of malabsorption. Based on lymphocyte carboxylase activities and plasma biotin levels, some children with severe protein–energy malnutrition are biotin deficient. Investigators have speculated that the effects of biotin deficiency may be responsible for part of the clinical syndrome of protein–energy malnutrition.

Biotin deficiency has also been reported or inferred in several other clinical circumstances, including long-term anticonvulsant therapy, Leiner's disease, sudden infant death syndrome, renal dialysis, gastrointestinal diseases, and alcoholism. Studies of biotin status during pregnancy and of biotin supplementation during pregnancy provide evidence that a marginal degree of biotin deficiency develops in at least one-third of women during normal pregnancy. Although the degree of biotin deficiency is not severe enough to produce overt manifestations of biotin deficiency, the deficiency is sufficiently severe to produce metabolic derangements. A similar marginal degree of biotin deficiency causes high rates of fetal malformations in some mammals. Moreover, data from a multivitamin supplementation study provide significant albeit indirect evidence that the marginal degree of biotin deficiency that occurs spontaneously in normal human gestation is teratogenic.

Clinical Findings of Frank Deficiency

The clinical findings of frank biotin deficiency in adults, older children, and infants are similar. Typically, the findings appear gradually after weeks to several years of egg-white feeding or parenteral nutrition. Thinning of hair and progression to loss of all hair, including eyebrows and lashes, has been reported. A scaly (seborrheic), red (eczematous) skin rash was present in the majority; in several, the rash was distributed around the eyes, nose, mouth, and perineal orifices. These cutaneous manifestations, in conjunction with an unusual distribution of facial fat, have been termed 'biotin deficiency facies.' Depression, lethargy, hallucinations, and paraesthesia of the extremities were prominent neurologic symptoms in the majority of adults. The most striking neurologic findings in infants were hypotonia, lethargy, and developmental delay.

The clinical response to administration of biotin has been dramatic in all well-documented cases of

Table 3 Foods relatively rich in biotin

Food	ng biotin/g food	serving size (g)	μg biotin/serving
Chicken liver, cooked	1872.00	74	138.00
Beef liver, cooked	416.00	74	30.80
Egg, whole, cooked	214.00	47	10.00
Peanuts, roasted, salted	175.00	28	4.91
Egg, yolk, cooked	272.00	15	4.08
Salmon, pink, canned in water	59.00	63	3.69
Pork chop, cooked	45.00	80	3.57
Mushrooms, canned	21.60	120	2.59
Sunflower seeds, roasted, salted	78.00	31	2.42
Chili	5.20	441	2.29
Hot dog, chicken and pork, cooked	37.00	56	2.06
Egg, white, cooked	58.00	35	2.02
Banana pudding	10.20	170	1.73
Strawberries, fresh	15.00	111	1.67

biotin deficiency. Healing of the rash was striking within a few weeks, and growth of healthy hair was generally present by 1 or 2 months. Hypotonia, lethargy, and depression generally resolved within 1 or 2 weeks, followed by accelerated mental and motor development in infants. Pharmacological doses of biotin (e.g., 1–10 mg) have been used to treat most patients.

High Intakes

Daily doses up to 200 mg orally and up to 20 mg intravenously have been given to treat biotin-responsive inborn errors of metabolism and acquired biotin deficiency. Toxicity has not been reported.

See also: **Brain and Nervous System**. **Breast Feeding**. **Cofactors**: Organic. **Meat, Poultry and Meat Products**. **Microbiota of the Intestine**: Prebiotics. **Pregnancy**: Role of Placenta in Nutrient Transfer.

Further Reading

Bender DA (1999) Optimum nutrition: Thiamin, biotin, and pantothenate. *Proceedings of the Nutritional Society* **58**: 427–433.

Cronan JE Jr (2002) Interchangeable enzyme modules. Functional replacement of the essential linker of the biotinylated subunit of acetyl-CoA carboxylase with a linker from the lipoylated subunit of pyruvate dehydrogenase. *Journal of Biological Chemistry* **277**: 22520–22527.

Flume MZ (2001) Final report on the safety assessment of biotin. *International Journal of Toxicology* **20**(supplement 4): 1–12.

McCormick DB (2001) Bioorganic mechanisms important to coenzyme functions. In: Rucker RB, Suttie JW, McCormick DB, and Machlin LJ (eds.) *Handbook of Vitamins*, 3rd edn, pp. 199–212. New York: Marcel Dekker.

McMahon RJ (2002) Biotin in metabolism and molecular biology. *Annual Reviews in Nutrition* **22**: 221–239.

Mock DM (1992) Biotin in human milk: When, where, and in what form? In: Picciano MF and Lonnerdal B (eds.) *Mechanisms Regulating Lactation and Infant Nutrient Utilization*. New York: John Wiley.

National Research Council, Food and Nutrition Board, and Institute of Medicine (1998) Dietary reference intakes for thiamin, riboflavin, niacin, vitamin B-6, folate, vitamin B-12, pantothenic acid, biotin, and choline. In *Recommended Dietary Allowances.*, pp. 374–389. Washington, DC. National Academy Press.

Pacheco-Alvarez D, Solorzano-Vargas RS, and Del Rio AL (2002) Biotin in metabolism and its relationship to human disease. *Archives of Medical Research* **33**: 439–447.

Solbiati J, Chapman-Smith A, and Cronan JE Jr (2002) Stabilization of the biotinoyl domain of *Escherichia coli* acetyl-CoA carboxylase by interactions between the attached biotin and the protruding "thumb" structure. *Journal of Biological Chemistry* **277**: 21604–21609.

Wolf B (2001) Disorders of biotin metabolism. In: Scriver CR, Beaudet AL, Sly WS, and Valle D (eds.) *The Metabolic and Molecular Basis of Inherited Disease*, vol. 3, pp. 3151–3177. New York: McGraw-Hill.

Zempleni J and Mock DM (2001) Biotin. In: Song WO and Beecher GR (eds.) *Modern Analytical Methodologies in Fat and Water-Soluble Vitamins*, pp. 459–466. Baltimore: John Wiley.

Blood Lipids/Fats *see* **Hyperlipidemia**: Overview. **Lipoproteins**

Blood Pressure *see* **Hypertension**: Etiology

BODY COMPOSITION

D Gallagher and S Chung, Columbia University, New York, NY, USA

© 2005 Elsevier Ltd. All rights reserved.

Introduction

Historically, the measurement of the body and its components centered around cadaver analyses where specific tissues and organs were extracted from the body for inspection. The extraction of tissue samples from the living body was a step forward in allowing for the analyses of tissue morphology in a state more closely resembling the *in vivo* state. However, both cadaver and *in vitro* tissue analyses are subject to inaccuracies when extrapolations are being made to the living body. Nevertheless, much of our understanding of human body composition in both children and adults has roots in these approaches. During the twentieth century, significant advances were made in the development of *in vivo* methods of body composition analysis thanks to the disciplines of physics, engineering, and medicine. Methodologies with minimal or no risk to the participant have allowed for the assessment of body composition in growth and development, aging, and disease.

The physiological significance of knowing the composition of the body greatly depends on the question of interest. Common applications involving medical/clinical diagnoses include osteopenia/osteoporosis; muscle wasting; sarcopenia; lipodystrophy; altered states of hydration; malnutrition; and obesity. There are also metabolic consequences (e.g., insulin resistance) associated with high and low levels of body fat and where the fat is distributed. From a nutritional perspective, the interest in body composition has increased multifold with the global increase in the prevalence of obesity and its complications. This chapter will focus on our current state of body composition knowledge and how this knowledge was determined with the available most advanced methodologies.

Body Composition Determination

There is no single gold standard for body composition measurements *in vivo*. All methods incorporate assumptions that do not apply in all individuals and the more accurate models are derived by using a combination of measurements, thereby reducing the importance of each assumption. The most commonly used technique today with good reproducibility in children and adults is dual-energy X-ray absorptiometry.

Dual-Energy X-Ray Absorptiometry (DXA)

The DXA method evolved from earlier single and dual photon absorptiometry methods for evaluating bone mineral. DXA systems share in common an x-ray source that, after appropriate filtration, emits two photon energy peaks. The attenuation of the two energy peaks relative to each other depends on the elemental content of tissues through which the photons pass. Bone, fat, and lean soft tissues are relatively rich in calcium/phosphorus, carbon, and oxygen, respectively. DXA systems are designed to separate pixels, based on appropriate models and relative attenuation, into these three components. There are no known factors, including hydration effects that significantly influence the validity of DXA fat and bone mineral estimates. Excessive or reduced fluid volume would be interpreted as changes in lean soft tissue. The radiation exposure is minimal and can be used in children and adults of all ages. DXA measures in persons who fit within the DXA field-of-view have good reproducibility for total body and regional components.

Hydrodensitometry/Air Plethysmography

One of the oldest methods of measuring body composition, the determination of body volume by water displacement (Archimedes principle) allows for the estimation of fat-free mass (FFM) density (where an assumption is made that densities of fat and FFM are constant) from which percent body fat is calculated using a two-compartment body composition model. Today there are a number of additional methods for measuring body volume, including air displacement plethysmography. Limitations with this approach include the assumptions of stable densities of fat and FFM across the age range where this may not be true in older individuals and across race/ethnic groups where it is now known that the density of FFM in Blacks is higher.

Dilution Techniques

Since fat is relatively anhydrous, the body's water is found primarily in the body's FFM compartment where approximately 73% of a healthy non-obese adults FFM compartment is water. The body's water pool can be measured using tracers which after administration, dilute throughout the body.

Basic assumptions involved with tracer dilution for body composition determination include equal distribution though out the pool of interest and dilution is complete within a specific period of time without any loss. Examples of commonly used tracers include deuterium oxide for total body water and sodium bromide for extracellular water.

Whole-Body Counting

A small constant percentage of total body potassium (TBK) is radioactive (^{40}K) and emits a γ-ray. With appropriate shielding from background, this γ-ray can be counted using scintillation detectors. As the ratio of ^{40}K to ^{39}K is known and constant, ^{39}K or "total body potassium" can be estimated accordingly. All of the body's potassium is within the FFM compartment and the proportion of the body FFM compartment TBK/FFM ratio is relatively stable in the same subject over time and between different subjects. However, with increasing age or when comparing young versus elderly, the TBK to FFM ratio decreases.

Magnetic Resonance Imaging/Computed Tomography

The use of computed tomography (CT) has had limited application in body composition research due primarily to radiation exposure. Its use has primarily been limited to single slice acquisitions in the abdomen and mid-thigh whereby information on adipose tissue distribution and muscle cross-sectional area have been derived. The use of magnetic resonance imaging (MRI) has resulted in important advances in body composition phenotyping. MRI studies are safe and instruments are available in most hospital or related facilities. Expense is a limiting factor. The importance of both CT and MRI is that both methods acquire cross-sectional images of the body at pre-defined anatomic locations. Image analysis software then allows estimation of the adipose tissue, skeletal muscle, and organs based on pixel intensity. Acquiring images at predefined intervals and integrating the area between slices allows reconstruction of an entire organ of interest such as skeletal muscle mass. A significant advancement made possible by these imaging methods has been the characterization of a tissue distribution, such as adipose tissue where it is now possible to quantify visceral, subcutaneous, and intermuscular depots at the regional and whole-body level.

Bioimpedance Analysis (BIA)

BIA is a simple, low-expense, noninvasive body composition measurement method. BIA is based on the electrical conductive properties of the human body. Measures of bioelectrical conductivity are proportional to total body water and the body compartments with high water concentrations such as fat free and skeletal muscle mass. BIA assumes that the body consists of two compartments, fat and FFM (Body weight = Fat + FFM). BIA is best known as a technique for the measurement of percent body fat although it has more recently been used for estimating skeletal muscle mass too.

Anthropometry

For routine clinical use, anthropometric measurements (circumference measures and skinfold thickness) have been preferred due to ease of measurement and low cost. Waist circumference and the waist-hip ratio measurements are commonly used surrogates of fat distribution, especially in epidemiology studies. Waist circumference is highly correlated with visceral fat and was recently included as a clinical risk factor in the definition of the metabolic syndrome. Specifically, waist circumferences greater than 102 cm (40 in) in men and greater than 88 cm (35 in) in women are suggestive of elevated risk.

Skinfold thicknesses which estimate the thickness of the subcutaneous fat layer are highly correlated with percent body fat. Since the subcutaneous fat layer varies in thickness throughout the body, a combination of site measures is recommended, reflecting upper and lower body distribution. Predictive percent body fat equations based on skinfold measures are age and sex specific in adults and children.

Body Mass Index (BMI)

The body mass index (BMI = weight kg/height m^2) continues to be the most commonly used index of weight status, where normal weight is a BMI $18.5-25.9$ kg/m^2; overweight is a BMI $25.0-29.9$ kg/m^2; and obese a BMI >30.0 kg/m^2. BMI is a commonly used index of fatness due to the high correlation between BMI and percent body fat in children and adults. The prediction of percent body is dependent on age (higher in older persons), sex (higher in males), and race (higher in Asian compared to African American and Caucasian).

In Vivo Neutron Activation

Nitrogen, carbon, hydrogen, phosphorus, sodium, chlorine, calcium, and oxygen are all measurable *in vivo* by methods known as neutron activation analysis. A source emits a neutron stream that interacts with body tissues. The resulting decay products of activated elements can be counted by detectors and elemental mass established. Carbon, nitrogen, and calcium can be used to estimate total body fat, protein, and bone mineral mass using established equations. Neutron activation analysis is uniquely valuable in body composition research as there are no known age or sex effects of currently applied equations, however, facilities that provide these techniques are limited.

Models in Body Composition

The use of models in the assessment of body composition allows for the indirect assessment of compartments in the body. Typically, a compartment is homogenous in composition (e.g., fat), however, the simpler the model the greater the assumptions made and the greater the likelihood of error. The sum of components in each model is equivalent to body weight (**Figure 1**). These models make assessments at the whole-body level and do not provide for regional or specific organ/tissue assessments.

The basic two-compartment (2C) model (**Table 1**) is derived from measuring the density of fat-free mass (FFM) by hydrodensitometry and subtracting FFM from total body weight thereby deriving fat mass (body weight – FFM = fat mass). FFM is a heterogeneous compartment consisting of numerous tissues and organs. A 2C approach becomes inadequate when the tissue of interest in included within the FFM compartment. Nevertheless, the 2C model is routinely and regularly used to calculate fat mass from hydrodensitometry, total body water, and total body potassium.

A three-compartment (3C) model consists of fat, fat-free solids, and water. The water content of FFM is assumed to be between 70% and 76% for most species and results from cross-sectional studies in adult humans show no evidence of differences in the hydration of FFM with age. The fat-free solids component of FFM refers to minerals (including bone) and proteins. The 3C approach involves the measurement of body density (usually by hydrodensitometry) and total body water by an isotope dilution technique. Assumptions

Table 1 Multicompartment body composition models

Model	Equations for % fat	Reference
2C	$100 \times (4.971/D_b - 4.519)$	a
3C	$100 \times (2.118/D_b - 0.78 \times (TBW/W) - 1.354)$	b
4C	$100 \times (2.747/D_b - 0.727 \times (TBW/W) + 1.146 \times (BMC/W) - 2.0503)$	c
6C	$100 \times (2.513/D_b - 0.739 \times (TBW/W) + 0.947 \times (TBBM/W) - 1.79)$	d

[a]Behnke AR Jr, Feen BG, and Welham WC (1942) The specific gravity of healthy men. *Journal of the American Medical Association* **118**: 495–498.
[b]Siri WE (1961) Body composition from fluid spaces and density: analysis of methods. In: Brozek J and Hensch el A (eds.) *Techniques for Measuring Body Composition*, pp. 223–224. Washington, DC: National Academy of Science.
[c]Boileau RA, Lohman TG, and Slaughter MH (1985) Exercise and body composition of children and youth. *Scandinavian Journal of Sports Sciences* **7**: 17–27.
[d]Heymsfield SB, Wang ZM, and Withers RT (1996) Multicomponent molecular level models of body composition analysis. In: Roche AF, Heymsfield SB, and Lohman TG (eds.) *Human Body Composition*, pp. 129–147. Champaign: Human Kinetics.
D_b, body density; TBW, total body water; W, body weight; BMC, bone mineral content; TBBM, total body bone mineral.

are made that both the hydration of FFM and the solids portion of FFM are constant. Since bone mineral content is known to decrease with age, the 3C approach is limited in its accuracy in persons or populations where these assumptions are incorrect.

A four-compartment (4C) model involves the measurement of body density (for fat), total body water, bone mineral content by dual-energy X-ray absorptiometry (DXA), and residual (residual = body weight – (fat + water + bone)). This model allows for the assessment of several assumptions that are central to the 2C model. The 4C approach is frequently used as the criterion method against which new body composition methods are compared in both children and adults.

The more complex 4C model involves neutron activation methods for the measurement of total body nitrogen and total body calcium, where total body fat = body weight – total body protein (from total body nitrogen) + total body water (dilution volume) + total body ash (from total body calcium). A six-compartment model is calculated as follows: fat mass (measured from total body carbon) = body weight – (total body protein + total body water + bone mineral + soft tissue mineral (from a combination of total body potassium, total body nitrogen, total body chloride, total body calcium) + glycogen (total body nitrogen) + unmeasured residuals). However, the availability of neutron activation facilities is limited and therefore the latter models are not readily obtainable by most researchers.

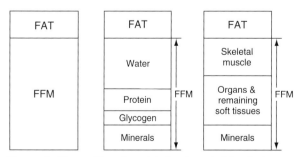

Figure 1 Three different models for characterizing body composition compartments. Components are as labeled: FFM, fat-free body mass.

At the organizational level, a five-level model was developed where the body can be characterized at five levels. The following are the levels and their constituents: atomic = oxygen, carbon, hydrogen, and other (level 1); molecular = water, lipid, protein, and other (level 2); cellular = cell mass, extracellular fluid, and extracellular solids (level 3); tissue-system level = skeletal muscle, adipose tissue, bone, blood, and other (level 4); and whole body (level 5).

Tissues and Organs

The aforementioned models do not allow for subregion and/or specific organ and tissue measurements. For example, skeletal muscle mass (SM) is contained within the FFM compartment. SM represents the single largest tissue in the adult body and is equivalent to ~40% of body weight in young adults, decreasing to ~30% of young values at elderly ages. SM is one of the more difficult components to quantify. Estimates of SM are commonly derived from anthropometry, total body potassium, and DXA using modeling approaches previously described. The use of magnetic resonance imaging (MRI) in body composition research has allowed for a good estimation of SM, adipose tissue (AT), and select organs *in vivo*, in all age groups with no risk to the participant (**Figure 2**). Moreover, AT distribution, including subcutaneous adipose tissue (SAT), visceral adipose tissue (VAT), and intermuscular adipose tissue (IMAT) is also measurable using a whole-body multislice MRI protocol (**Figure 3**). In studies relating body composition to energy expenditure, high metabolic rate organs including liver, kidneys, heart, spleen, and brain are also measurable using MRI.

Bone mineral content and bone mineral density of specific body sites (e.g., radius, hip, lumbar spine) are most commonly measured using DXA. Bone mass and microarchitecture are important determinants of bone strength, with microarchitectural deterioration being one of the specific changes associated with

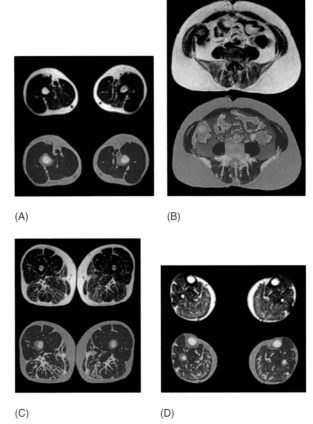

(A)　　　　　　　　　　　　(B)

(C)　　　　　　　　　　　　(D)

Figure 3 Cross-sectional images from (A) upper arm, (B) trunk (L4-L5 level), (C) mid-thigh, and (D) mid-calf in an elderly female volunteer. IMAT, intermuscular adipose tissue (pink); SM, skeletal muscle (red); SAT, subcutaneous adipose tissue (green); VAT, visceral adipose tissue (blue).

osteoporosis. Using high-resolution microcomputed tomography (micro-CT) and computer software, detailed analysis of three-dimensional (3D) architecture is feasible and allows microstructural 3D bone information to be collected.

Body Composition Applications During Growth

Skeletal muscle mass has a central role in intermediary metabolism, aerobic power, and strength. Its mass increases as a portion of body weight during growth, accounting for 21% at birth and 36% at adolescence. The essential role of skeletal muscle in many physiologic processes throughout the lifespan makes understanding of factors affecting it significant. The greater incidence of type 2 diabetes mellitus in adolescents in the US (particularly in girls from minority populations) and in Japan makes evaluation of race and sex differences in pediatric skeletal muscle mass (and adipose tissue or fat mass) especially important. Identification and

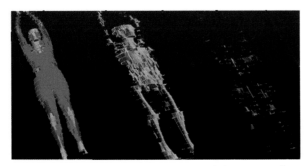

Figure 2 3D reconstructed image of whole-body scan (from MRI). Skeletal muscle (red); adipose tissue (green); bone, organs, and residual (yellow); intermuscular adipose tissue (pink).

characterization of differences could form the basis for further investigation of the associated metabolic implications.

Race differences in SM are known to exist as early as prepuberty. African-Americans have greater limb lean tissue mass compared to Asian and Caucasian children, while Caucasian children have greater amounts than Asians throughout Tanner stages 1 to 5. Race differences in total body bone mineral content adjusted for total body bone area, age, height, and weight have been reported in prepubertal African-American, Asian, and Caucasian females and males. African-American children had greater total body bone mineral content than Asian and Caucasian children, while differences between Asian and Caucasian children are less clear. Collectively, these findings suggest that the proportions of specific FFM subcomponents may differ by race. Although mechanisms leading to bone and skeletal muscle differences between races are not well understood, endocrine factors may be involved.

Sex differences in FFM have been reported from birth throughout childhood with females having smaller amounts than males. Total body bone mineral content is less in Tanner 1 females compared to males in African-Americans, Asians, and Caucasians. The mechanism for this sex difference in unclear. Gonadal steroids are significant mediators of adult sexual dimorphism of body composition, including fat-free soft tissues. Prepubertal females have higher concentrations of circulating estradiol than prepubertal males, and gonadotropin and gonadal steroids increase gradually in both males and females from the age of 5 years. Thus, prepuberty is a period with sex differences in circulating concentrations of sex steroids and of changes in these concentrations with advancing age. The earlier skeletal maturation of females, for example, has been attributed to the greater estradiol level in females compared to males. However, non-hormonal (possibly genetic) mechanisms may also play a role.

Fat or adipose tissue distribution is recognized as a risk factor for cardiovascular disease in both adults and children. An android or male fat pattern, with relatively greater fat in the upper body region, is associated with negative metabolic predictors whereas a gynoid or female fat pattern, with relatively greater fat in the hip and thigh areas, is associated with less metabolic risk. More and more studies are showing that the syndrome develops during childhood and is highly prevalent among overweight children and adolescents. While the concept of the metabolic syndrome referred initially to the presence of combined risk factors including VAT, dyslipidemia, hypertension, and insulin resistance in adults, it is now known to exist in children, especially where obesity and/or higher levels of VAT are present. Although sex-specific patterns of fat distribution had previously been thought to emerge during puberty, sex and race differences in fat distribution are now known to exist in prepubertal children. The implications are that a specific body composition pattern may differ by sex and race. An example is the relationship of blood pressure to central fat distribution in boys compared to girls where a significant positive relationship between trunk fat and blood pressure was reported in boys but not girls, and was independent of race, height, weight, and total body fat. Understanding the predictors of blood pressure in children is important since childhood blood pressure has been shown to track into adulthood in longitudinal studies. Children whose blood pressure levels were in the highest quintile, were two times more likely to be in the highest quintile 15 years later. Identification of clinically useful body composition measures would allow for the identification of children at increased risk for hypertension, who could benefit from monitoring.

Race differences in fat distribution among prepubertal Asians, African-Americans, and Caucasians also exist. Previous reports in adolescents have suggested significantly smaller hip circumferences in Asian females at all pubertal stages compared to Caucasians and Hispanics and greater trunk subcutaneous fat in Asian females compared to Caucasians. Differences in subcutaneous fat mass and fat distribution in Asian compared to Caucasian adults have also been described. Understanding the sex- and race-specific effects of puberty on regional body composition may help delineate the developmental timing of specific health risk associations.

Race difference in blood pressure has been reported in many studies of adults, where a higher prevalence of hypertension has been found among African-American women, placing this group at a higher risk for cardiovascular-related morbidities and mortality. Previous studies attempting to determine whether this race difference appears in childhood or early in adulthood have produced inconclusive findings.

Body Composition Applications During Aging

During the adult life span, body weight generally increases slowly and progressively until about the seventh decade of life, and thereafter, declines into old age. An increased incidence of physical disabilities and comorbidities is likely linked to aging-associated body composition changes. Characterization of the aging processes has identified losses in muscle mass, force, and strength, which collectively are defined as 'sarcopenia.' Little is known about the overall rate at which sarcopenia develops in otherwise healthy elderly subjects, if this rate of progression differs between women and men, and the underlying mechanisms responsible for age-related sarcopenia. Peak SM mass is attained in the young adulthood years and slowly declines thereafter. During the latter adult years, SM decreases more rapidly as body fat becomes more centralized. Anthropometric equations have been developed for predicting appendicular skeletal muscle (ASM = SM of the limbs) in the elderly where sarcopenia was defined as ASM (kg)/height^2 (m^2) less than two standard deviations below the mean of the young reference group. In the elderly men, the mean ASM/height^2 was approximately 87% of the young group. The corresponding value in women was approximately 80%. **Table 2** shows the estimated prevalence's of sarcopenia in the same survey sample for each ethnic group, by age and sex. The same authors have reported that obese and sarcopenic persons have worse outcomes than those who are nonobese and sarcopenic.

Even in healthy, weight-stable elderly persons, changes in body composition over a 2-year period can include decreases in SM mass and bone mineral content with corresponding increases in IMAT and VAT, after adjusting for their baseline values, despite no detectable changes in physical function or food intake.

In adults, excess abdominal or VAT is recognized as an important risk factor in the development of coronary heart disease and non-insulin dependent diabetes mellitus. Waist circumference and the waist:hip ratio are commonly used to predict visceral fat accumulation in epidemiological studies. However, waist circumference is unable to differentiate VAT from SAT. As a result, persons with similar waist circumferences could have markedly different quantities of VAT and abdominal SAT. Skinfold thickness has been used as a continuous

variable grading adiposity or adipose tissue distribution within study populations.

The most accurate measurement of VAT requires imaging techniques (MRI and computed tomography (CT)), which are expensive and not readily available in many clinical settings. **Figure 3B** shows an MRI-derived cross-sectional image at the L4-L5 level with adipose tissue depots identified. The AT located between muscle bundles (IMAT; **Figure 3**) and visible by MRI and CT may be negatively associated with insulin sensitivity. In the elderly, greater IMAT (as suggested by lower skeletal muscle attenuation by CT) is associated with lower specific force production. Currently, there is no simple or clinic-based method to measure adipose tissue located between the muscle groups, defined in our laboratory as intermuscular adipose tissue (IMAT). IMAT has been reported to be significantly negatively correlated with insulin sensitivity and higher in type 2 diabetic women compared to nondiabetic women.

Sex and race differences in body composition are well established in adults. Men acquire higher peak SM mass than women and some evidence exists suggesting that men may lose SM faster than women with age. Moreover, it is well established that women have a larger amount of total body fat or total adipose tissue than men. Among races, African-American adult men and women have larger amounts of SM than Asian and Caucasians even after adjusting for differences in body weight, height, age, and skeletal limb lengths.

Efforts are ongoing to better understand variations in IMAT as a function of age, race, and level of fatness. IMAT deposits appear comparable in size in adult African-Americans, Asians, and Caucasians at low levels of adiposity but accumulate as a greater proportion of TAT in African-Americans compared to Caucasians and Asians subjects (58 g IMAT/kg TAT in African-Americans; 46 g IMAT/kg TAT in

Table 2 Prevalance (%) of sarcopenia[a] in the New Mexico Elder Health Survey, by age, sex, and ethnicity, 1993–1995

Age group (years)	Men		Women	
	Hispanic (n = 221)	Non-Hispanic whites (n = 205)	Hispanics (n = 209)	Non-Hispanic whites (n = 173)
<70	16.9	13.5	24.1	23.1
70–74	18.3	19.8	35.1	33.3
75–80	36.4	26.7	35.3	35.9
>80	57.5	52.6	60.0	43.2

[a]Appendicular skeletal muscle mass/height^2 (kg/m^2) less than two standard deviations below the mean value for the young adults from Gallagher D, Visser M, De Meersman RE *et al.* (1997) Appendicular skeletal muscle mass: effects of age, gender, and ethnicity. *Journal of Applied Physiology* **83**: 229–239.
Adapted from Baumgartner RN, Koehler KM, Gallagher D *et al.* (1998) Epidemiology of sarcopenia among the elderly in New Mexico. *American Journal of Epidemiology* **147**: 755–763.

Caucasians; 44 g IMAT/kg TAT in Asians). Across race groups, VAT deposits also appear comparable in size at low levels of adiposity but with increasing adiposity VAT accumulates more in Asians and Caucasians compared to IMAT, although accumulation rates for IMAT and VAT do not differ in African-Americans. While the association between greater amounts of abdominal or VAT and increased insulin resistance and the metabolic syndrome is well established compared to the peripherally located SAT, the role of the IMAT compartment in the metabolic alterations leading to the development of insulin resistance warrants further investigation, especially as it may influence race/ethnicity differences in dysglycemia. Collectively, sex and race differences exist in body composition in children and adults.

Physiological Application: Two Examples

Example 1

Expressing heat production relative to body mass is required when comparing energy expenditure rates between individuals that differ in size. Age and gender-specific resting energy expenditure (REE) norms based on body weight and stature-derived were developed in the early 1900s by Kleiber and showed that adult mammals differing widely in body size had similar metabolic rates relative to body weight raised to the 0.75 power. Two components are usually considered as representative of whole-body metabolically active tissue, body cell mass (BCM), and FFM. BCM is typically estimated as the exchangeable potassium space that can be measured by total body potassium. The FFM component can be measured using two-component body composition methods.

In studies assessing REE, FFM is considered the principal contributor to energy requirements, and is commonly used as a surrogate for metabolically active tissue. However, this practice is inherently flawed as it pools together numerous organs and tissues that differ significantly in metabolic rate. The brain, liver, heart, and kidneys alone account for approximately 60% of REE in adults while their combined weight is less than 6% of total body weight or 7% of FFM. The skeletal muscle component of FFM comprises 40–50% of total body weight (or 51% of FFM) and accounts for only 18–25% of REE. REE varies in relation to body size across mammalian species. Within humans, REE per kg of body weight or FFM is highest in newborns ($\sim$56 kcal kg^{-1} day^{-1}), declines sharply until 4 years, and slowly thereafter reaching adult values ($\sim$25 kcal kg^{-1} day^{-1}). Among adults,

REE is lower in the later adult years, to an extent beyond that explained by changes in body composition. That is, the loss of FFM cannot fully explain the decrease (5–25%) in REE in healthy elderly persons.

Recent attention has been given to modeling REE based on available information on organ- and tissue-specific metabolic rates combined (**Table 3**) with the mass of these tissues as determined by MRI. Whole-body REE can be calculated from organ- tissue mass (REE$_c$) and then compared to REE measured using indirect calorimetry (REE$_m$) for individuals or groups. REE (in kJ day^{-1}) of each organ- tissue component (subscript i) can be calculated using the following equation:

$$REE_i = OMR_i \times M_i \qquad [1]$$

where OMR (organ metabolic rate) is the metabolic rate constant (in kJ per kg per day) for each organ-tissue component (**Table 3**) and M is the mass of the corresponding organ/tissue (in kg). Whole-body REE (in kJ per day) is calculated as the sum of the seven individual organ-tissue REE

$$REE_c = \sum_{i=1}^{7} (REE_i) \qquad [2]$$

The whole-body REE equation is:

$$REE_C = 1008 \times M_{brain} + 840 \times M_{liver} + 1848$$
$$\times M_{heart} + 1848 \times M_{kidneys} + 55$$
$$\times M_{SM} + 19 \times M_{AT} + 50 \times M_{residual} \qquad [3]$$

This approach has allowed for the hypothesis to be tested that the proportion of FFM as certain

Table 3 Organ and tissue coefficients used in developing models

	Weight (kg)[a]	Density (kg l^{-1})[a]	Metabolic rate (kJ kg^{-1} day^{-1})[b]
Skeletal muscle	28.0	1.04	55
Adipose tissue	15.0	0.92	19
Liver	1.8	1.05	840
Brain	1.4	1.03	1008
Heart	0.3	1.03	1848
Kidneys	0.3	1.05	1848
Residual	23.2	*	50

[a]Adapted from Snyder WS, Cook MJ, Nasset ES *et al.* (1975) Report of the task group on reference men. *International Commission on Radiological Protection* 23. Oxford: Pergamon.
[b]Adapted from Elia M (1992) Organ and tissue contribution to metabolic rate. In: Kinney JM and Tucker HN (eds.) *Energy Metabolism. Tissue Determinants and Cellular Corollaries*, pp. 61–77. New York: Raven Press.
*Residual mass was not assigned a density but was calculated as body mass minus sum of other measured mass components.

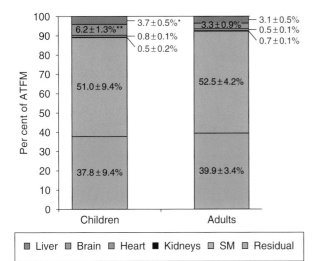

Figure 4 Proportional contribution of each organ/tissue to Adipose Tissue Free Mass (ATFM). Liver (▣), brain (▣), heart (▣), kidneys (■), skeletal muscle mass (▣), residual mass (▣), * $p < 0.01$ and ** $p < 0.001$ for children vs. adults. Reproduced with permission from Hsu A, Heshka S, Janumala I, Song MY, Horlick M, Krasnow N, and Gallagher D (2003) Larger mass of high-metabolic-rate organs does not explain higher resting energy expenditure in children. *American Journal of Clinical Nutrition* **77**: 1506–11.

high metabolic rate organs, specifically liver and brain, is greater in children compared to young adults (**Figure 4**). Findings thus far have shown that after accounting for this disproportion, the specific organ/tissue metabolic constants available in the literature (**Table 3**) are not adequate to account for REE in children. These results therefore imply that the decline in REE per kilogram body weight (or per kilogram FFM) during the growth years is likely due to both changes in body composition and changes in the metabolic rate of individual organs/tissues. When this approach was applied to young adults (31.2 ± 7.2 years), REE_c and REE_m were highly correlated, with no significant differences between them. When this approach was applied to persons over 70 years, both older men and women had significantly lower REE_m compared to REE_c, and the magnitude of the differences were 13% and 9.5%, respectively, for men and women. These findings suggest that even after adjustment for age-related organ and tissue atrophy in the elderly, whole body REE by indirect calorimetry continues to be lower than expected. The latter suggests that the metabolic rate constants used (**Table 3**) for specific organs and tissues may not be appropriate in the elderly.

At the individual or clinic level, the measurement of REE by indirect calorimetry is frequently unavailable. An alternate approach has been to estimate REE based on body weight, height, age, and sex. Many studies have examined the association between these basic and easily acquired measures and REE. A small number of studies have included FFM in their REE prediction equations. **Table 4** lists published equations for the prediction of REE in healthy individuals.

Example 2

The global increase in the prevalence of childhood overweight and obesity and their associations with disease during childhood and adulthood is now alarming public health officials. One approach to understanding the pathways between overweight/obesity and disease is identifying the factors that cause excess weight gain. The time *in utero* is considered a critical period. During the growth and development years, the periods known as 'adiposity rebound' and adolescence are considered critical periods in the development and persistence of overweight in the pediatric age group. Children born small or large for gestational age appear to be at increased risk for cardiovascular disease and diabetes in adulthood. To what extent the growth trajectory between birth and adulthood influences the risk of disease burden is unclear. Important questions that need to be answered include the role that adiposity or fat accretion and adipose tissue distribution has on the development of disease. To answer such questions, the measurement of body composition needs to occur at the organ/tissue level beginning as early as birth, if not earlier. The current MRI methodology allows for such measurements after birth although no data exists thus far where infants have been followed longitudinally into adolescence or adulthood.

Conclusion

The measurement of body composition allows for the estimation of body tissues, organs, and their distributions in living persons without inflicting harm. It is important to recognize that there is no single measurement method in existence that allows for the measurement of all tissues and organs and no method is error free. Furthermore, bias can be introduced if a measurement method makes assumptions related to body composition proportions and characteristics that are inaccurate across different populations. The clinical significance of the body compartment to be measured should first be determined before a measurement method is selected since the more advanced techniques are less accessible and more costly.

Table 4 REE prediction equations based on anthropometrics or body composition

Authors	Subjects/gender/nation	Weight status	Age (years)	Equation
Harris & Benedict (1919)	239/M-F/USA	NW	29 ± 14 (X ± SD)	F: **BMR** = 9.5 wt (kg) + 1.9 ht (cm) − 4.7 age (years) + 655 M: **BMR** = 13.8 wt (kg) + 5.0 ht (cm) − 6.8 age (years) + 66
Robertson & Reid (1952)	2310/M-F/UK	NS	Range (3–80)	**RMR** = BSA (m²) × 24 × age-specific value
Altman & Dittmer (1968)	>200/M-F/USA	NW	Range (3–16)	F: **REE** = 0.778 wt (kg) + 24.11 M: **REE** = 0.815 wt (kg) + 21.09
Dore et al. (1982)	140/F/UK	NW, OW, OB	Variable	**REE** = 8.24 wt (kg) + 0.02 FFM (kg) − 3.25 age (years) + 712
Bernstein (1983)	202/M(154)/USA	OW, OB	40 ± 12 (X ± SD)	**RMR** = 7.48 wt (kg) − 0.42 ht (cm) − 3.0 age (years) + 844 **REE** = 22 FFM (kg) + 6.4 FM (kg) − 2.1 age (years) + 251
Garrow & Webster (1985)	104/F/UK	NW, OW, OB	Variable	**REE** = 24.2 FFM (kg) + 5.8 (% fat) + 310
Joint FAO/WHO/UN (1985)	11 000/M-F/Multi	NW, OW, OB	Variable	3–10 years F: **REE** = 22.5 wt (kg) + 499 3–10 years M: **REE** = 22.7 wt (kg) + 495 10–18 years F: **REE** = 17.5 wt (kg) + 651 10–18 years M: **REE** = 12.2 wt (kg) + 746 18–30 years F: **BMR** = 55.6 wt (kg) + 1397.4 ht (m) + 146 30–60 years F: **BMR** = 36.4 wt (kg) − 104.6 ht (m) + 3619 18–30 years M: **BMR** = 64.4 wt (kg) − 113.0 ht (m) + 3000 30–60 years M: **BMR** = 47.2 wt (kg) + 66.9 ht (m) + 3769
Schofield (1985)	7549/M-F/UK	NW, OW, OB	Range (<3 to >60)	Under 3 years F: **BMR** = 0.068 wt (kg) + 4.281 ht (m) − 1.730 Under 3 years M: **BMR** = 0.0007 wt (kg) + 6.349 ht (m) − 2.584 3–10 years F: **BMR** = 0.071 wt (kg) + 0.677 ht (m) + 1.553 3–10 years M: **BMR** = 0.082 wt (kg) + 0.545 ht (m) + 1.736 10–18 years F: **BMR** = 0.035 wt (kg) + 1.948 ht (m) + 0.837 10–18 years M: **BMR** = 0.068 wt (kg) + 0.574 ht (m) + 2.157 18–30 years F: **BMR** = 0.057 wt (kg) + 1.184 ht (m) + 0.411 18–30 years M: **BMR** = 0.063 wt (kg) − 0.042 ht (m) + 2.953 30–60 years F: **BMR** = 0.034 wt (kg) + 0.006 ht (m) + 3.530 30–60 years M: **BMR** = 0.048 wt (kg) − 0.011 ht (m) + 3.670 Over 60 years F: **BMR** = 0.033 wt (kg) + 1.917 ht (m) + 0.074 Over 60 years M: **BMR** = 0.038 wt (kg) + 4.068 ht (m) − 3.491
Owen (1986)	44/F/USA	NW, OW, OB	29 ± 14 (X ± SD)	F: **RMR** = 7.18 wt (kg) + 795
Owen (1987)	60/M/USA	NW, OW, OB	29 ± 14 (X ± SD)	M: **RMR** = 10.2 wt (kg) + 879
Owen (1988)	104/M-F/USA	NW, OW, OB	29 ± 14 (X ± SD)	**REE** = 23.6 FFM (kg) + 186
Ravussin & Bogardus(1989)	249/M-F/USA	NW, OW, OB	Variable	**REE** = 21.8 FFM (kg) + 392
Maffeis et al. (1990)	130/M-F/Italy	NW, OW, OB	Range (6–10)	F: **REE** = (35.8 wt (kg) + 15.6 ht (cm) − 36.3 age (years) + 1552)/4.18 M: **REE** = (28.6 wt (kg) + 23.6 ht (cm) − 69.1 age (years) + 1287)/4.18
Mifflin et al. (1990)	498/M-F/USA	NW, OW, OB	Range (19–78)	F: **RMR** = 9.99 wt (kg) + 6.25 ht (cm) − 4.92 age (years) − 161 M: **RMR** = 9.99 wt (kg) + 6.25 ht (cm) − 4.92 age (years) + 5 **REE** = 19.7 FFM (kg) + 413

Continued

Table 4 Continued

Cunningham (1991)	Meta-analysis	NW, OW, OB		REE = 21.6 FFM (kg) + 370
Hayter & Henry (1994)	2999/M/UK	NW, OW, OB	Range (18–30)	M: RMR = 51.0 wt (kg) + 3500
Piers et al. (1997)	39/M/Australia	NW, OW	Range (18–30)	M: RMR = 51.0 wt (kg) + 3415
van der Ploeg et al. (2001)	38/M/Australia	NW, OW	24.3 ± 3.3 (X ± SD)	18–30 years M: RMR = 48.2 wt (kg) + 25.8 ht (cm) − 49.6 age (years) + 113 18–30 years M: RMR = 21.0 wt (kg) − 56.2 age (years) + 76.1 FFM 4C (kg) + 2202
van der Ploeg et al. (2002)	41/M/Australia	NW, OW	44.8 ± 8.6 (X ± SD)	30–60 years M: RMR = 41.92 wt (kg) + 13.79 ht (cm) − 14.89 age (years) + 1939 30–60 years M: RMR = 91.85 FFM 4C (kg) + 1463
Siervo et al. (2003)	157/F/Italy	NW, OW, OB	23.8 ± 3.8 (X ± SD)	F: RMR = 11.5 wt (kg) + 542.2

M, male; F, female; NS, not specific; NW, normal weight; OW, overweight; OB, obesity; X, mean; SD, standard deviation; BSA, body surface area; wt, weight; ht, height; BMR, basal metabolic rate; RMR, resting metabolic rate; REE, resting energy expenditure; FFM, fat-free mass; FFM 4C, fat-free mass via the four-compartment body composition model; FM, fat mass.

Adapted from the following references: Altman P and Dittmer D (1968) *Metabolism*. Bethesda: Federation of American Societies for Experimental Biology; Bernstein RS, Thornton JC, Yang MU *et al.* (1983) Prediction of the resting metabolic rate in obese patients. *American Journal of Clinical Nutrition* **37**: 595–602; Cunningham JJ (1991) Body composition as a determinant of energy expenditure: a synthetic review and a proposed general prediction equation. *American Journal of Clinical Nutrition* **54**: 963–969; Dore C, Hesp R, Wilkins D, and Garrow JS (1982) Prediction of requirements of obese patients after massive weight loss. *Human Nutrition Clinical Nutrition* **36C**: 41–48; Garrow JS and Webster J (1985) Are pre-obese people energy thrift? *Lancet* **1**: 670–671; Harris JA and FG Benedict (1919) *A Biometric Study of Basal Metabolism in Man*, pp. 1–266. Washington DC: Carnegie Institution; Hayter JE and Henry CJK (1994) A re-examination of basal metabolic rate predictive equations: the importance of geographic origin of subjects in sample selection. *European Journal of Clinical Nutrition* **48**: 702–707; Joint FAO/WHO/UN Expert Consultation (1985) *Energy and Protein Requirements*. Technical Reports Series 724. Geneva: World Health Organization; Maffeis C, Schutz Y, Micciolo R Zoccante L, and Pinelli L (1993) Resting metabolic rate in six- to ten-year-old obese and non-obese children. *Journal of Pediatrics* **122**: 556–562; Mifflin MD, St Jeor TS, Hill LA *et al.* (1990) A new predictive equation for resting energy expenditure in healthy individuals. *American Journal of Clinical Nutrition* **51**: 241–247; Owen OE (1988) Resting metabolic requirements of men and women. *Mayo Clinic Proceedings* **63**: 503–510; Owen OE, Holup JL, D'Allessio DA *et al.* (1987) A reappraisal of the caloric requirements of men. *American Journal of Clinical Nutrition* **46**: 875–885; Owen OE, Kavle E, Owen RS *et al.* (1986) A reappraisal of caloric requirements in healthy women. *American Journal of Clinical Nutrition* **44**: 1–19; Piers LS, Diffey B, Soares MJ *et al.* (1997) The validity of predicting the basal metabolic rate of young Australian men and women. *European Journal of Clinical Nutrition* **51**: 333–337; Ravussin E and Bogardus C (1989) Relationship of genetics, age, and physical fitness to daily energy expenditure and fuel utilization. *American Journal of Clinical Nutrition* **49**: 968–975; Robertson JD and Reid DD (1952) Standards for the basal metabolism in normal people in Britain. *Lancet* **1**: 940–943; Schofield WN (1985) Predicting basal metabolic rate, new standards and review of previous work. *Human Nutrition Clinical Nutrition* **39C**: 5–41; Siervo M, Boschi V, and Falconi C (2003) Which REE prediction equation should we use in normal-weight, overweight and obese women? *Clinical Nutrition* **22**: 193–204; van der Ploeg GE and Withers RT (2002) Predicting the metabolic rate of 30–60-year-old Australian males. *European Journal of Clinical Nutrition* **56**: 701–708; van der Ploeg GE, Gunn SM, Withers RT, Modra AC, Keeves JP, and Chatterton BE (2001) Predicting the resting metabolic rate of young Australian males. *European Journal of Clinical Nutrition* **55**: 145–152.

Acknowledgments

This work was supported by Grants HL70298, DK42618 (Project 4), and HD42187 from the National Institutes of Health.

See also: **Bone. Obesity**: Definition, Etiology and Assessment; Childhood Obesity. **Older People**: Physiological Changes.

Further Reading

Baumgartner RN, Koehler K, Gallagher D *et al.* (1998) Epidemiology of sarcopenia among the elderly in New Mexico. *American Journal of Epidemiology* **147**: 755–763.

Ding M, Odgaard A, Linde F, and Hvid I (2002) Age-related variations in the microstructure of human tibial cancellous bone. *Journal of Orthopedic Research* **20**: 615–621.

Elia M (1992) Organ and tissue contribution to metabolic rate. In: Kinney JM and Tucker HN (eds.) *Energy Metabolism. Tissue Determinants and Cellular Corollaries*, pp. 61–77. New York: Raven Press.

Ellis KJ (2000) Human body composition: *in vivo* methods. *Physiological Reviews* **80**: 649–680.

Forbes GB (1987) *Human Body Composition: Growth, Aging, Nutrition, and Activity*. New York: Springer-Verlag.

Gallagher D, Belmonte D, Deurenberg P *et al.* (1998) Organ-tissue mass measurement allows modeling of REE and metabolically active tissue mass. *American Journal of Physiology* **275**: E249–E258.

Goran MI (2001) Metabolic precursors and effects of obesity in children: a decade of progress, 1990–1999. *American Journal of Clinical Nutrition* **73**: 158–171.

He Q, Horlick M, Fedun B, Wang J, Pierson RN Jr, Heshka S, and Gallagher D (2002) Trunk fat and blood pressure in children through puberty. *Circulation* **105**: 1093–1098.

Kleiber M (1961) *The Fire of Life, and Introduction to Animal Energetics*. New York: Wiley.

Roche AF, Heymsfield SB, and Lohman TG (eds.) (1996) *Human Body Composition*. Champaign: Human Kinetics.

Snyder WS, Cook MJ, Nasset ES *et al.* (1975) Reports of the task group on reference men. *International Commission on Radiological Protection* 23. Oxford: Pergamon.

Wang Z, Pierson RN Jr, and Heymsfield SB (1992) The five level model: a new approach to organizing body composition research. *American Journal of Clinical Nutrition* **56**: 19–28.

BONE

B M Thomson, Rowett Research Institute, Aberdeen, UK

© 1999 Elsevier Ltd. All rights reserved.

This article is reproduced from the previous edition, pp. 185–190, © 1999, Elsevier Ltd.

Introduction

Bone serves as a framework for the body and as a metabolic reserve of calcium and phosphate at times of mineral deficiency. It consists of cells from two distinct lineages, bone-forming osteoblasts and bone-resorbing osteoclasts, and the calcified extracellular matrix that these cells secrete and remodel.

Bone formation begins in the embryo, either via a cartilaginous intermediate, as in the case of the long bones, or via a membranous intermediate, as in the case of the flat bones of the skull. Continued production of cartilage at specialized sites on the long bones, termed growth plates, and the subsequent conversion of this cartilage into bone results in longitudinal postnatal growth. Skeletal growth and development is regulated by genetic, mechanical and hormonal mechanisms. In general, genetic influences dictate the basic structure of the skeleton, while responses to mechanical loading adjust the strength of particular bones to their functional environment.

Simultaneously, hormonal mechanisms coordinate the movement of calcium and phosphate to and from the skeleton, thereby enabling bone to act as a reservoir of these minerals at times of calcium stress (e.g., pregnancy and lactation). At the cellular level, bone growth is coordinated by an array of interacting cytokines and growth factors, which control bone cell division, maturation and activity.

Failure of the mechanisms controlling bone cell function, especially during bone turnover in adults, leads to bone loss, and this can produce clinical osteoporosis. Other skeletal disease states result from nutritional deficiency, e.g., rickets, or from genetic defects, e.g., osteopetrosis or osteogenesis imperfecta.

Bone Types, Composition and Structure

There are two types of bone in the skeleton – flat bones, e.g., the skull, and long bones, e.g., the femur. The principal anatomical features of a long bone are shown in **Figure 1**.

Bone matrix

Bone matrix is a composite material that derives its strength from a compression-resistant mineral phase and a tension-resistant network of collagen fibers. Bone's mineral phase – calcium hydroxyapatite,

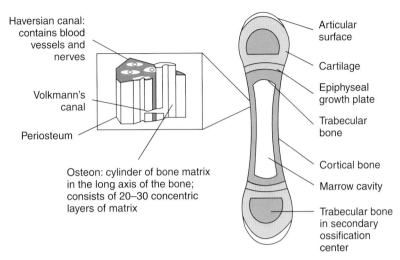

Figure 1 The anatomy of a long bone, e.g., the femur. Inset shows an enlarged section of cortical bone.

$Ca_{10}(PO_4)_6(OH)_2$ – is subdivided into a mosaic of tiny microcrystallites, thereby creating a large surface area for ion exchange and limiting the spread of cracks. Bone matrix also contains a number of specialized noncollagenous proteins, such as osteocalcin, osteonectin and osteopontin.

Macroscopic architecture

Two types of internal bone architecture are visible to the naked eye. Cortical bone, the stronger but heavier of the two forms, comprises the outer wall of all bones and fulfils a mainly mechanical function (see insert, **Figure 1**). It consists of parallel cylinders of matrix (osteons) arranged along the load-bearing axis of the bone.

Within each osteon the matrix is deposited in concentric layers, each 2–3 μm thick, with a predominant fiber direction (like multilayer plywood). The central canal of each osteon contains bone cells, blood vessels and nerves.

Trabecular bone, the second architectural form, is found at the ends of long bones and in the middle of the vertebrae. It consists of a latticework of bony struts, each 100–500 μm thick. Although weaker than cortical bone, it is more cellular and hence more metabolically active.

Bone Cells

Osteoblasts

Bone-forming cells are called osteoblasts. They are characterized by high levels of alkaline phosphatase, an enzyme required for matrix mineralization, and display structural features reflecting their intense secretory activity (e.g., prominent endoplasmic reticulum).

Osteoblasts are arranged as a closely packed layer of cells on growing bone surfaces, with each cell producing around three times its own volume of bone in about 3 days. Newly synthesized bone matrix is produced in an unmineralized form (termed osteoid) and consists of highly crosslinked collagen I fibers (which give the tissue its tensile strength) and a number of noncollagenous proteins such as osteocalcin. Osteoid is also rich in osteoblast-derived growth factors – insulin-like growth factor II (IGF-II) and transforming growth factor β – and these may regulate local bone turnover. Once formed, osteoid is mineralized. In cortical bone, crystal growth begins at sites along the collagen fibrils and is regulated by inhibitory molecules released by the osteoblasts.

Approximately 10–20% of osteoblasts become entombed in the matrix that they have produced and are termed osteocytes. They remain linked to the bone surface via long cell processes and appear to respond to mechanical loading. Osteocytes may therefore be responsible for coupling of mechanical stimulation to bone growth.

Osteoblasts contribute to the control of bone resorption, responding to bone-resorbing signals by producing degradative enzymes and by releasing molecules that increase osteoclast activity and recruitment. Osteoblasts may therefore coordinate bone turnover by switching from bone formation to the control of bone resorption.

Origin of the osteoblast Osteoblasts are derived from stem cells located near bone surfaces. These stem cells can give rise to cartilage, fat and fibrous tissues in experimental systems, suggesting that osteoblasts form part of a superfamily of connective-tissue cells.

The stem cells divide and mature into preosteoblasts, an intermediate cell type, which displays some osteoblast-like features, e.g., type I collagen production, alkaline phosphatase and osteonectin mRNA, but which lacks the intense alkaline phosphatase activity and highly developed endoplasmic reticulum of the mature cells.

Terminal differentiation into mature osteoblasts is associated with the cessation of cell division, the production of osteopontin and osteocalcin, and changes in both oncogene expression and nuclear protein–DNA interactions. Further changes in regulatory nuclear proteins accompany the onset of mineralization.

Osteoclasts

Osteoclasts are large $(3000–250000\,\mu m^3)$ highly mobile multinucleate cells (10–20 nuclei), which contribute to bone remodeling and calcium homeostasis by resorbing bone. The osteoclast's resorptive apparatus consists of a central 'ruffled border', a highly folded region of cell membrane across which acid and degradative enzymes are extruded, and a peripheral 'clear zone', which seals the osteoclasts onto the bone.

Osteoclasts dissolve bone mineral by secreting acid across their ruffled borders using proton-pumping ATPases. Acid production also requires carbonic anhydrase – an enzyme used for acid production by the stomach, which is absent in some forms of the lethal bone disease osteopetrosis. The organic components of bone are degraded by lysosomal enzymes; one of these, acid phosphatase, is used as a marker for osteoclast activity.

Origin of the osteoclast Osteoclasts are descended from blood-cell-forming interleukin-3-dependent stem cells located in the bone marrow and are therefore part of the same superfamily of cells as macrophages, lymphocytes and red blood cells. Partially differentiated mononuclear preosteoclasts migrate via the circulation to resorption sites, where they proliferate and acquire differentiated features (e.g., acid phosphatase and calcitonin receptors), before fusing into multinucleate osteoclasts and beginning to resorb.

Regulation of Bone Cell Activity

Genetic and mechanical

While genetic influences dictate the basic structure of the skeleton, responses to mechanical loading adapt bone to its functional environment. In general, physical strain stimulates bone formation, while disuse (e.g., paralysis) results in bone loss. As a consequence, the cortical width of a professional tennis player's serving arm may be increased by 35% relative to the other arm. Such adaptation optimizes the balance between skeletal strength and weight.

Systemic regulation of serum calcium: the calciotropic hormones, parathyroid hormone, calcitonin, and dihydroxyvitamin D₃

Serum calcium is maintained within tight limits $(2.2–2.6\,mmol\,l^{-1})$, a process necessary for the maintenance of many cellular activities including neuromuscular function.

Parathyroid hormone (PTH) releases calcium into the blood by mobilizing bone mineral at times of calcium shortage. It binds to receptors on preosteoblastic cells and signals the release of osteoclast activating factors. It also promotes calcium retention by the kidney and uptake from the gut.

Calcitonin is produced in response to a rise in serum calcium. It acts directly on osteoclasts and inhibits bone resorption.

Vitamin D metabolites regulate serum calcium and are essential for skeletal growth and development. The parent compound, vitamin D, is essentially inactive and requires two hydroxylation steps before gaining biological activity. The second of these hydroxylation steps is tightly regulated by PTH. Once formed, the most potent vitamin D metabolite, 1,25-dihydroxyvitamin D₃ $(1,25(OH)_2D_3)$, increases intestinal calcium absorption and promotes bone matrix mineralization. It also alters cell differentiation, influencing chondrocyte maturation within the growth plate and regulating gene expression in osteoblastic cells.

Systemic hormones that regulate skeletal growth or function: growth hormone, oestradiol, and vitamin A

Growth hormone stimulates bone growth by prompting cell division amongst the chondrocytes of the growth plate. It acts in part by stimulating IGF-I production.

While there is no doubt that the decreased levels of oestradiol that follow normal or artificially induced menopause lead to increased bone loss, oestradiol's role in skeletal biology remains obscure. The recent discovery of oestradiol receptors in osteoblasts suggests it may have a direct effect on osteoblastic cells.

Vitamin A is important for the maintenance of normal bone remodeling. It may also participate in the control of three-dimensional pattern formation during limb bud development.

Local regulation of bone cell proliferation, maturation, and function by polypeptide growth factors

A variety of growth factors (e.g., fibroblast growth factor and IGF-I) stimulate the division of preosteoblastic cells. Other signal molecules (e.g., transforming growth factor β) are associated with developmental events such as the formation of the vertebrae, jaws, and palate. Osteoblasts produce many of these growth factors themselves and deposit them in their extracellular matrix, suggesting that they coordinate small groups of cells at specific locations. Osteoclast recruitment is regulated by a variety of blood cell growth factors, termed 'colony stimulating factors'. Several of these are produced by osteoblastic cells. Osteoblasts have also been shown to produce factors that stimulate mature osteoclasts to resorb.

Mechanisms of Bone Growth

Flat bones and long bones arise by two distinct mechanisms.

Growth of long bones (e.g., femur): endochondral ossification

The principal stages of long-bone growth are shown in **Figure 2**. Long bones begin as cartilaginous regions in the early embryo. They grow as rapidly dividing peripheral cells add new chondrocytes to the outside of the structure and as older cells in the body of the cartilage divide, enlarge, and secrete matrix (**Figure 2A**).

The oldest chondrocytes (located in the middle) expand, calcify their matrix, and are termed 'hypertrophic' (**Figure 2B**). Osteoblasts then secrete a bony layer around the midshaft of the cartilage, forming the 'primary bone collar'. This structure is extended and thickened by successive generations of osteoblasts.

Once established, the primary bone collar is penetrated at several points by osteoclasts (**Figure 2C**). These rapidly erode the calcified cartilage of the interior to leave only a supportive framework inside the bone collar. As the peripheral bone gains in strength, osteoclasts remove this framework to leave the marrow cavity.

Continued growth of long bones: the growth plate Long-bone growth continues at specialized 'epiphyseal growth plates' (**Figure 3**). Proliferating chondrocytes at the top of the growth plate add new cells, while their more mature descendants secrete matrix and enlarge, thereby producing longitudinal growth. Ultimately, the chondrocytes hypertrophy and calcify their matrix. Osteoclasts present in the marrow cavity invade this calcified cartilage, destroying the horizontal septa separating the chondrocytes. This leaves vertical bars of calcified cartilage projecting into the marrow cavity, and these act as a framework for subsequent bone deposition.

Complete calcification of the growth plate at the end of puberty marks the end of longitudinal growth.

Intramembranous ossification (e.g., the bones of the cranium)

The flat bones of the skull begin as highly vascularized sheets of embryonic tissue. Undifferentiated cells within these sheets differentiate directly into osteoblasts and form a radiating network of bony spicules lying parallel to the surface of the brain. During growth, successive generations of osteoblasts add new bone to the outside and periphery of this structure, while osteoclasts resorb from the inner surface to maintain proportional thickness and shape.

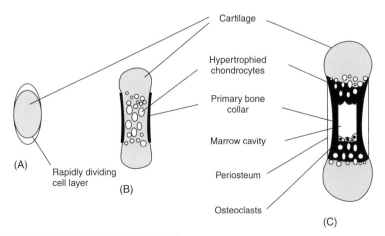

Figure 2 The principal stages of embryonic long-bone growth.

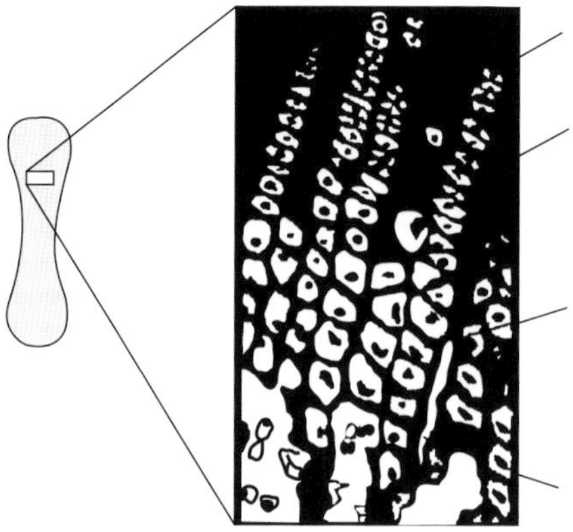

Rapidly dividing chondrocytes add new cells to growth plate

Maturing chondrocytes expand and synthesize matrix

Hypertrophic chondrocytes calcify their matrix

Osteoclasts invade calcified cartilage, leaving vertical bars of material as a framework for subsequent bone formation

Figure 3   Continued longitudinal growth at the growth plate.

Bone Atrophy: Hormonal Influences and the Effect of Age

Bones grow in size and strength until peak bone mass is attained around the age of 35 years. Peak mass varies between demographic subgroups (25–30% higher in males than females 10% higher in blacks than whites), although there is a large variation within each group (1 woman in 40 has a peak mass less than the average for women aged 65 years). Bone mass subsequently declines with age and as a result of a variety of factors that predispose an individual to bone loss. The observed bone mass of an individual over 35 years therefore represents their peak bone mass minus both the cumulative age-related bone loss and any losses resulting from disease or specific risk factors.

Bone turnover and age-related bone loss

Bone is continuously broken down and replaced throughout life, thereby mobilizing calcium for systemic needs and preventing the accumulation of old fatigue-fractured material. Typically, 4% of cortical bone and 25% of trabecular bone are replaced each year.

Turnover begins with the recruitment of osteoclast precursors. These mature, fuse into multinucleate osteoclasts, and resorb a depression 60 μg deep in the bone surface over a period of about 10 days. Osteoblasts derived from undifferentiated cells located in the vicinity of the resorption site then replace the resorbed material. The entire process lasts approximately 4 months.

After the fourth decade of life, bone reformation fails to replace completely the resorbed bone, so that bone turnover produces a net bone loss. This so-called 'age-related bone loss' (0.3% and 1% of peak bone mass per year in males and females,

respectively) occurs regardless of sex, physical activity, nutrition, or socioeconomic status. Its rate depends upon the frequency of remodeling cycles and the imbalance between the amount of bone resorbed and replaced at each remodeling event.

Age-related bone loss therefore occurs more rapidly in trabecular bone (which turns over more rapidly) and is increased by factors that promote bone turnover (transient calcium deficiency). Risk factors or disease states associated with either low peak bone mass or increased rates of loss include small body size, nulliparity, inactivity, early natural menopause, anorexia, thyrotoxicosis, and Cushing's syndrome.

Ultimately, the combination of reduced bone mass and disrupted trabecular architecture (as individual bony struts are severed or removed from the lattice) leads to reduced bone strength and increased fracture risk.

Other causes of bone loss: hyperparathyroidism and malignant disease

Hyperparathyroidism is an endocrine disorder characterized by raised serum calcium levels and increased cortical bone loss. It is usually caused by a benign adenoma, which secretes excessive PTH, thereby increasing both bone resorption and calcium retention by the kidney. Pathological bone loss is also a feature of many malignant disease states. Bone destruction may result from osteoclast activation in the immediate vicinity of invading tumors or from the systemic effects of circulating factors released by the tumor cells.

Oestrogen

Sex-hormone status and the pubertal growth spurt are important in determining bone mass at maturity. Conversely, bone loss accelerates in the first years after the menopause as the skeleton adapts to declining oestrogen levels. In general, postmenopausal women who lose bone fastest have the lowest endogenous sex-hormone levels. Although the skeletal role of oestrogens at the cellular level remains unclear, recent findings suggest that oestrogens may have a direct effect on osteoblastic cells.

Osteopetrosis

Osteopetroses are a class of rare genetic disorders characterized by defective osteoclast function and a consequent failure of bone remodeling. Symptoms vary with severity but may include skeletal malformation with dense but fragile bones. Recurrent infection and spontaneous bleeding may result from the crowding out of the marrow cavity by unresorbed bone and mineralized cartilage.

See also: **Body Composition. Calcium.**
Carbohydrates: Regulation of Metabolism. **Glucose**: Metabolism and Maintenance of Blood Glucose Level.

Growth and Development, Physiological Aspects. **Osteoporosis**. **Vitamin A**: Physiology. **Vitamin D**: Physiology, Dietary Sources and Requirements; Rickets and Osteomalacia.

Further Reading

Favus MJ (1990) *Primer on the Metabolic Bone Diseases and Disorders of Mineral Metabolism* California: American Society for Bone and Mineral Research.

Goss RJ (1978) *The Physiology of Growth* New York: Academic Press.

Ham AW (1969) *Histology*, 6th edn. Philadelphia: Lippincott.

Riggs BL (1988) *Osteoporosis: Etiology, Diagnosis and Management* New York: Raven Press.

Thomson BM and Loveridge N (1992) Bone growth. In: *The Control of Fat and Lean Deposition*, 51st University of Nottingham Easter School in Agricultural Science. Oxford: Butterworth Heinemann.

Vaughan JM (1970) *The Physiology of Bone*. Oxford: Clarendon Press.

BRAIN AND NERVOUS SYSTEM

J D Fernstrom and M H Fernstrom, University of Pittsburgh, Pittsburgh, PA, USA

© 2005 Elsevier Ltd. All rights reserved.

Design of the Nervous System

The nervous system has two principal cell types: neurons and glia. Neurons (like wires) conduct electrical signals and are organized into circuits to perform specific functions. They have a unique cellular architecture: small cellular extensions (dendrites) receive chemical and electrical signals from other neurons; a longer extension (the axon, which can be up to a meter in length) sends electrical signals down its length to one or more nerve terminals. Nerve terminals contain neurotransmitters, molecules released by arriving electrical signals that modify the electrical activity of adjacent neurons. Neurons have considerable energy needs; indeed the brain, which is 2% of body weight, consumes 15–20% of the body's daily energy intake. Glial cells, which constitute about 60% of the brain's cell mass, provide physical and metabolic support for neurons, and insulate axons and nerve terminals, to ensure privacy in electrical signaling. The glial

cells found in peripheral nerves serve the same functions.

The nervous system is broadly divided into two parts: the central and peripheral nervous systems. The central nervous system (CNS) consists of the brain, retina, and spinal cord, and contains complex neuronal circuits that control body functions (e.g., blood pressure, breathing, hunger, movement). The peripheral nervous system consists of groups of neurons that mostly lie outside of the CNS, and either supply sensory information to the CNS, or send CNS commands to effector cells, such as muscle and gland cells.

The Blood–Brain Barrier

Each portion of the nervous system is separated from the blood (and thus the rest of the body) by a metabolic 'barrier,' which modulates the access of nutrients to and the removal of metabolites from the neurons and glia within it. For the brain and spinal cord, this barrier is termed the 'blood–brain barrier' (BBB; there is also a blood–cerebrospinal fluid (CSF) barrier; CSF is made from blood); for the retina, it is called the 'blood–retinal barrier,' and for peripheral neurons, the 'blood–nerve barrier.' The functions of these barriers are very similar. The focus of the following discussion will be the BBB, because it has been studied the most.

The BBB is located in the endothelial cells that make up the brain's capillaries. Unlike capillaries elsewhere in the body, the endothelial cells of brain capillaries are tightly joined, such that nothing passes into (or out of) brain without passing through these cells. The BBB thus presents a continuous lipid barrier to molecules. One implication is that the ease with which molecules in blood gain access to brain should depend on their lipid solubility: the more lipid soluble, the greater the accessibility to brain by diffusion. However, most molecules of biologic importance to brain are not lipid soluble, and thus do not easily diffuse across lipid membranes into brain. Examples include glucose, amino acids, and water-soluble vitamins. Consequently, endothelial cell membranes must be more than just lipid barriers; indeed, embedded in them are specific transport carriers that mediate the brain uptake of most nutrients.

Energy Substrates

The brain uses glucose as its primary energy substrate. Glucose is not lipid-soluble, and thus requires a BBB transporter. The glucose transporter has a maximal transport capacity for glucose of $1.4\,\mu mol$ per min per gram brain, or about $1200\,g\,day^{-1}$ for the entire brain (a human brain weighs $1400\,g$). The human brain consumes 15–20% of the body's oxygen; brain glucose utilization is therefore about $100\,g\,day^{-1}$. The BBB transporter thus has a maximal capacity for transporting glucose well in excess of that demanded daily by the brain.

Inside the brain, glucose is rapidly taken up into neurons by a cellular glucose transporter. Within the neuron, glucose enters the glycolytic pathway. The initial enzyme, hexokinase, has a very high affinity for glucose, and is fully saturated at normal brain glucose concentrations. Hence, overall, each step in the glucose pipeline from blood to brain neurons is designed to maximize glucose supply for neuronal energy production. It only fails when the blood glucose supply is abruptly curtailed, such as when a diabetic patient injects too much insulin and blood glucose levels rapidly fall (the transporter cannot compensate for such abrupt drops in blood glucose). The effect is dramatic: confusion, delirium, seizures, coma, and finally death occur as blood glucose drops to very low levels. Such effects are most rapidly reversed by the infusion of glucose, suggesting that no other compound in blood readily substitutes for glucose as the brain's primary energy substrate.

Normally, the body carefully maintains blood glucose concentrations. During starvation, however, blood glucose falls enough to cause the brain to recruit an additional energy source, i.e., ketone bodies. Ketone bodies are liver-produced by-products of the breakdown of stored fat (fatty acids), and provide an extended supply of energy when the input of food-derived energy is low. The brain uses ketone bodies whenever their blood levels rise; blood ketone body concentrations rise in starvation. The BBB ketone body transporter (ketone bodies are not lipid soluble) is induced in starvation, enhancing the flow of ketone bodies into brain. During prolonged starvation, more than half of the energy used by the brain is derived from ketone bodies. Continued use of some glucose appears obligatory, however, and is supplied via liver gluconeogenesis.

The chronic ingestion of high-fat diets also elevates blood ketone body concentrations, promoting their use by the brain for energy production. However, extremely high levels of fat must be consumed, and such diets are unpalatable. Hence, diet is not thought normally to influence cerebral energy production via dietary fat manipulation of ketone body supply to brain. Very high-fat diets are occasionally used clinically to treat intractable seizures. Though the beneficial effect is linked to levels of circulating ketone bodies, the mechanism is presently unknown.

Amino Acids and Protein

Neurons and glial cells in brain use amino acids to produce proteins. In addition, certain amino acids are used to produce small functional molecules such as neurotransmitters. Does diet influence amino acid flow into brain, and their use in generating proteins and transmitters? The path from diet to brain proceeds from amino acid absorption from the gastrointestinal tract, insertion into the circulation, and extraction by brain. This extraction process involves the BBB, which contains a number of transporters for amino acids. The properties of these transporters dictate how much of each amino acid enters (and exits) the brain. Currently, six carriers have been identified. Of special interest are two carriers: (1) the large neutral amino acid (LNAA) carrier, which is shared by several amino acids (some are precursors for neurotransmitters: phenylalanine, tyrosine, tryptophan, histidine). The carrier is competitive, allowing changes in the plasma concentration of any one LNAA to affect not only that amino acid's BBB transport, but also that of each of its transport competitors. Glutamine, an LNAA present in brain in high concentrations, drives the brain uptake of the other LNAA, by serving as the principal amino acid counter-transported from brain to blood each time an LNAA is taken up into brain; and (2) the acidic amino acid carrier, which transports glutamic and aspartic acids. This carrier primarily transports glutamate and aspartate from the brain to the circulation. The other transporters include one selective for basic amino acids, two selective for subgroups of the small, neutral amino acids, and one selective for taurine.

The carriers that move amino acids into brain are those that transport primarily essential amino acids (the large, neutral, and basic amino acids), while those that move amino acids out of brain are those transporting nonessential amino acids (the acidic and small neutral amino acids). A small, net influx into brain of the essential amino acids no doubt reflects their consumption in brain by biosynthetic and metabolic pathways. The net efflux of the nonessential amino acids, notably aspartate, glutamate, glycine and cysteine may serve to remove from brain amino acids that act directly as excitatory transmitters or cotransmitters. The brain carefully compartmentalizes these amino acids metabolically, because they excite neurons, and a mechanism to remove them from brain may be a component of this compartmentalization design.

Changes in dietary protein intake have no effect on brain protein synthesis in adults. Indeed, the chronic ingestion of very low levels of dietary protein does not depress brain protein synthesis; brain cells may thus be efficient in retaining and reusing amino acids released during intracellular protein breakdown. In neonatal and infant animals, however, low levels of protein intake are associated with below normal rates of protein synthesis in brain. But, the presumed mechanism of this association, reduced uptake of essential amino acids into brain and abnormally low brain concentrations of these amino acids, has not been proven. Hence, at present, there is no convincing evidence linking dietary protein intake and brain protein synthesis via a limitation of amino acid availability to brain. For neurotransmitters, the evidence of this diet–brain link is more certain, and provides interesting examples of the fundamentally different manner in which the brain uses transport carriers to handle amino acids that are neurotransmitter precursors, and those that are neurotransmitters themselves. Good examples are tryptophan (an LNAA) and glutamate (an acidic amino acid), which have been most extensively studied.

Tryptophan (TRP) is the precursor for the neurotransmitter serotonin (5HT). The TRP concentration in brain rapidly influences the rate of 5HT synthesis: raising brain TRP concentrations increases synthesis, while lowering brain TRP decreases synthesis. Brain TRP uptake and concentrations are directly influenced by the plasma concentrations of TRP and its BBB LNAA transport competitors. The plasma concentrations of TRP and the other LNAA are readily modified by food intake, thereby linking diet to brain 5HT synthesis. Dietary proteins and carbohydrates are the food components that change brain TRP and 5HT: carbohydrate ingestion increases plasma TRP, while lowering the plasma concentrations of its LNAA competitors, causing BBB TRP uptake, brain TRP concentrations, and 5HT synthesis all to increase. The ingestion of a meal containing protein raises plasma concentrations of both TRP and its LNAA competitors. As a consequence, TRP experiences no change in competition for BBB transport (and sometimes a reduction, at high-protein intakes), and brain TRP concentrations and 5HT production do not change (or may decline). Hence, a key feature of the LNAA transporter, its competitive nature, explains the impact of meals containing or lacking protein on the production of a molecule important to normal brain function (5HT).

Chronic dietary effects are also observed. For example, chronic ingestion by rats of diets containing proteins with high ratios of one or more LNAA to TRP cause brain TRP and 5HT concentrations to decline. And, the chronic ingestion of diets low in protein causes the plasma concentrations of all LNAAs to decline (including TRP), and brain TRP and 5HT. In this case, brain TRP falls not because of a change in BBB competition, but simply because the BBB uptake of all LNAA declines with falling plasma concentrations (the transporter becomes unsaturated, eliminating competition).

Other LNAA are neurotransmitter precursors in substrate driven pathways in brain. Phenylalanine and tyrosine are substrates for catecholamine synthesis, and histidine is the precursor of histamine. Like TRP, the brain concentrations of these amino acids are influenced by their competitive BBB uptakes from the circulation, and thus the diet.

The nonessential amino acid glutamate (GLU) is an excitatory neurotransmitter, causing neurons that express GLU receptors to depolarize. Because GLU is excitatory, responsive neurons can become overexcited, when subjected to prolonged GLU exposure, and die. The term "excitotoxicity" was coined to describe this effect, and led to the concern that GLU ingested in food (as a constituent of dietary proteins; as a flavoring agent) might cause the brain to become flooded with GLU, causing widespread neurotoxicity. The BBB acidic amino acid transporter prevents this from occurring: it primarily transports GLU out of, not into the brain. Consequently, the BBB functions as a 'barrier' to GLU penetration from the blood.

Another mechanism also protects brain neurons from excessive exposure to GLU. Glial cells rapidly remove GLU from brain extracellular fluid and convert it to an electrically inert amino acid, glutamine. While glial cells efficiently absorb neuronal GLU, they can just as readily clear any GLU that strays into the brain from the circulation.

Fatty Acids and Choline

Fatty Acids

The brain uses fatty acids to synthesize the complex fat molecules that form neuronal and glial cell membranes. This process is more active in growing animals than in adults. The brain synthesizes some fatty acids from smaller molecules, but their uptake from the circulation is also an important source, and is the only source for certain fatty acids (the essential fatty acids, which cannot be manufactured in the body). The details of the uptake process are not well understood.

From the nutritional perspective, diet influences essential fatty acid availability to brain, with potentially important functional consequences. In almost all mammals, there are two essential fatty acids: linoleic acid and α-linolenic acid (termed polyunsaturated fatty acids; PUFAs). In the nervous system (as elsewhere), linoleic and α-linolenic acids are incorporated into phospholipid molecules, and inserted into cellular membranes, where they influence membrane fluidity and membrane-associated functions (e.g., the functionality of receptors and transporters). In addition, the linoleic acid in membrane lipids can be released and converted into arachidonic acid, a key precursor in the synthesis of prostaglandins and leukotrienes, families of important signaling molecules. α-Linolenic acid can be converted into docosahexanoic acid, a molecule found in very large amounts in the rods and cones of the retina, and in nerve terminal membranes in brain. Docosahexanoic acid is thought to be a key component of phototransduction, and has been demonstrated to have important effects on vision. Dietary modifications in essential fatty acid intake might therefore be expected to influence membrane functions in brain, leading to alterations in brain function (as has been demonstrated for vision).

Choline

Choline occurs in the body as a constituent of lipid molecules in cell membranes, as a source of methyl groups, and as a precursor for the neurotransmitter acetylcholine. Choline is not an essential nutrient in humans, and deficiencies are rarely seen, since it is ubiquitous in the diet. However, in recent decades, dietary choline has been a focus of interest, because of the possibility that changes in choline intake could influence neuronal acetylcholine synthesis. Acetylcholine (ACh) is a neurotransmitter; its synthesis in and release by brain neurons is influenced by choline availability, which in turn can be altered by dietary choline intake, either in the form of free or fat-bound choline (phosphatidylcholine). In this context, oral choline and phosphatidylcholine have found some application in human diseases thought to involve ACh. For example, they have been used successfully to treat movement disorders such as tardive dyskinesia, a drug-induced muscular disorder in schizophrenic patients linked to low ACh function. However, they proved to be of little value in controlling abnormal muscle movements associated with Huntington's disease (also linked to low ACh function). Dietary choline and phosphatidylcholine supplements have also been studied as potential memory enhancers, since CNS ACh neurons play an important role in memory. Patients with Alzheimer's disease have been most studied but, in general, the disappointing outcome has been that neither choline nor phosphatidylcholine has afforded much improvement in memory.

Vitamins

Neurons and glia have the same functional demands for vitamins as do other cells in the body. Their access to brain is thus an important consideration, particularly given the existence of the BBB. Water-soluble vitamins are transported across the BBB and, in some cases, the blood-CSF barrier, most often by nonenergy requiring carriers. After they are taken up into neurons and glial cells, most are rapidly converted into their biologically active derivatives, namely cofactors in enzyme-mediated reactions. Since cofactors are recycled, dietary deficiencies in one or another vitamin do not immediately lead to brain dysfunction, inasmuch as cofactor pools may take extended periods of time to become depleted. Although fat-soluble vitamins are lipid soluble, their passage through the BBB most likely involves more than simply diffusion.

Water-Soluble Vitamins

Folic acid is transported into brain as methylenetetrahydrofolic acid, the major form of folic acid in the circulation. It is then transported rapidly into neurons and glia from the CSF/extracellular fluid. Once inside cells, folates are polyglutamated. Methylenetetrahydrofolate is used by neurons and glia in reactions involving single carbon groups, such as in the conversion of serine to glycine or homocysteine to methionine. Once methylenetetrahydrofolate is consumed in these reactions, folic acid is transported out of the brain into the circulation. Folate has become an issue of neurologic concern because of a link between folate deficiency and abnormal CNS development. The incidence of spina bifida, a serious spinal cord abnormality, rises above the population mean in the children of women who are folate-deficient during pregnancy. Moreover, the incidence of spina bifida can be reduced by folic acid supplementation during pregnancy, beginning prior to conception. Initiating supplementation before conception is essential, since the basic design of the CNS is laid down during the first trimester. At present, the mechanism(s) by which folic acid deficiency leads to the improper formation of the spinal cord is unknown. Folate deficiency may also be linked to depression in adults, and occasional studies suggest that folate supplementation can improve mood in depressed patients. The mechanism(s) by which folate modifies mood is presently unknown.

Ascorbic acid (vitamin C) is actively transported into the brain extracellular fluid through the blood–CSF barrier, from which it is actively transported into cells. Brain ascorbate pools show minimal fluctuations over a wide range of plasma ascorbate concentrations, which presumably explains the absence of CNS signs in ascorbate deficiency. To date, the only defined biochemical function of ascorbic acid in brain is as a cofactor for the enzyme that converts dopamine to noradrenaline (norepinephrine) (though ascorbate is thought by some to function as an antioxidant).

Thiamine (vitamin B_1) is taken up into brain by a BBB transporter; small amounts also gain entry via transport from blood into CSF. It is then transported into neurons and glia; conversion to thiamine pyrophosphate effectively traps the molecule within the cell. In nervous tissue, thiamine functions as a cofactor in important enzymes of energy metabolism. Severe thiamine deficiency in animals reduces thiamine pyrophosphate levels, and the activities of thiamine-dependent reactions. It causes loss of the coordinated control of muscle movement; the exact biochemical mechanism is not clear. The functional deficits are rapidly corrected with thiamine treatment, suggesting that neurons have not been damaged or destroyed. Thiamine deficiency in humans (beriberi; Wernicke's disease) produces similar deficits in the control of muscle movements, and also mental confusion. Korsakoff's syndrome, which occurs in almost all patients with Wernicke's disease, involves a loss of short-term memory and mental confusion. Severe thiamine deficiency in humans appears to produce neuronal degeneration in certain brain regions. The motor abnormalities can be corrected with thiamine treatment, but the memory dysfunction is not improved.

Riboflavin enters brain via a saturable BBB transport carrier. It is then transported into neurons and glia, and trapped intracellularly by phosphorylation and conversion to flavin adenine dinucleotide. Flavin adenine dinucleotide functions as a cofactor in carboxylation reactions. The brain contents of riboflavin and its derivatives are not notably altered in states of riboflavin deficiency or excess.

Pantothenic acid is transported into brain by a BBB transport carrier. Neurons and glial cells take up pantothenic acid slowly by a mechanism of facilitated diffusion. Inside the cell, the vitamin becomes a component of coenzyme A, the coenzyme of acyl group transfer reactions. Relative to other tissues, the brain contains a high concentration of pantothenate, mostly in the form of coenzyme A. Brain coenzyme A concentrations are not depleted in pantothenate deficiency states.

Niacin (vitamin B_3) is transported into brain as niacinamide, primarily via the BBB. Most niacin in brain is derived from the circulation, though brain may be able to synthesize small amounts. Niacin is taken up into neurons and glia and rapidly converted to nicotinamide adenine dinucleotide. The half-life of nicotinamide adenine dinucleotide in brain is considerably longer than in other tissues. Nicotinamide adenine dinucleotide and nicotinamide adenine dinucleotide phosphate are involved in numerous oxidation-reduction reactions. Dietary niacin deficiency in the presence of a low intake of TRP causes pellagra in humans, a deficiency disease that includes mental depression and dementia, loss of motor coordination, and tremor. The mechanism(s) for these effects have not been identified.

Pyridoxine (vitamin B_6) is taken up into brain via a transport carrier that has not been well described. The vitamin can be transported in any of its nonphosphorylated forms (pyridoxine, pyridoxal, pyridoxamine). Once within the brain extracellular fluid, the vitamin is readily transported into neurons and glia and phosphorylated (primarily to pyridoxal phosphate or pyridoxine phosphate). Pyridoxal phosphate is a cofactor in a variety of neurotransmitter reactions, such as aromatic-L-amino acid decarboxylase (an enzyme of monoamine biosynthesis), glutamic acid decarboxylase (the enzyme of γ-amino butyric acid [GABA] synthesis), and GABA transaminase (the enzyme that catabolizes GABA). In humans, pyridoxine deficiency is rare, because of its widespread occurrence in foodstuffs. However, when identified, it has been associated with increased seizure activity, an effect dissipated by pyridoxine treatment. This effect may be linked to the production of GABA, an inhibitory neurotransmitter.

Biotin is transported into brain by a BBB carrier. It is a coenzyme for a variety of key carboxylation reactions in gluconeogenesis, fatty acid synthesis, and amino acid metabolism. Normally, biotin is recycled in cells during protein (enzyme) turnover, but not in brain; brain cells are thus more immediately dependent than other cells on circulating biotin availability. Biotin deficiency is rare; when it occurs, it can involve CNS symptoms (depression, sleepiness). The underlying basis for these effects is presently unknown.

Cobalamin (vitamin B_{12}) is thought to be transported into brain by a carrier-mediated mechanism. Little is known about this process, or about the function of vitamin B_{12} in the nervous system. Vitamin B_{12} deficiency is associated with neurologic abnormalities, which are presumed to derive from the demyelinization of CNS axons seen in advanced deficiency cases. These effects are reversed if vitamin B_{12} treatment is provided early enough; left untreated, axonal degeneration occurs. Vitamin B_{12} may be important in neuronal repair mechanisms, which may become compromised in deficiency states. Nervous system damage associated with vitamin B_{12} deficiency can occur at any age.

Fat-Soluble Vitamins

Of the fat-soluble vitamins, vitamin A (retinol) has been the most studied in relation to the CNS. The others have been much less well examined, though vitamin E is currently of some interest, because of its function as an antioxidant. The CNS is not thought to be a major focus of action for vitamins D and K, and thus little information is available regarding their roles in brain function.

The principal role of vitamin A in the CNS is as a component of the photoreceptive pigment of the eye, rhodopsin. In the blood, vitamin A circulates bound to retinol-binding protein and transthyretin (prealbumin). Its transport into retinal cells occurs at the blood–retinal barrier (the retinal pigmented epithelial (RPE) cells), after the retinol–protein complex binds to retinol-binding protein receptors. Once bound, retinol is released into the RPE cell. The retinol-binding protein and transthyretin molecules are released back into the circulation. Inside the RPE cell, retinol binds to a specific protein, and ultimately is esterified to a fatty acid. This molecule serves as the substrate for the conversion of retinol into the visually active form of the molecule, 11-*cis*-retinaldehyde, which then finds its way into the photoreceptor cell to be bound to opsin to form rhodopsin, the light-responsive pigment of the eye. When light strikes rhodopsin, phototransduction occurs and 11-*cis*-retinaldehyde is isomerized to all-*trans*-retinaldehyde, hydrolyzed from opsin, and released by the photoreceptor into the extracellular space (the opsin is retained and reused). The all-*trans*-retinaldehyde is shuttled into the RPE cell, where it is reconverted into 11-*cis*-retinaldehyde, and then recycled to the photoreceptor cells again to form rhodopsin.

From the nutritional perspective, retinal cells have an efficient system for managing and maintaining vitamin A pools. Hence, depletion of retinal vitamin A pools secondary to dietary deficiency only occurs over an extended time period. Deficiency appears functionally as 'night-blindness,' as rhodopsin levels decline. Extended vitamin A deficiency leads to a loss of photoreceptor elements, and eventually of the photoreceptor cells themselves. The cause of this cellular degeneration is not well understood.

Vitamin E is an antioxidant and free radical scavenger that protects fatty acids in cellular membranes. It is transported in blood associated with lipoproteins. The mechanism of its transfer into nervous tissue is unknown. Dietary vitamin E deficiency is extremely rare in humans. It occurs in association with certain abnormalities of vitamin E transport and fat absorption, and sometimes in individuals with protein-calorie malnutrition. The neurological manifestations are peripheral nerve degeneration, spinocerebellar ataxia, and retinopathy. Vitamin E has been proposed to play a role in a number of CNS diseases linked to oxidative damage. One example is Parkinson's disease, a movement disorder caused by the degeneration of certain groups of brain neurons. Evidence of oxidative damage is present in the brains of Parkinsonian patients, though controlled clinical trials of vitamin E supplementation have proved to be of no benefit. Such negative findings question the likelihood of a vitamin E link to the etiology of the degenerative changes. A second example is Alzheimer's dementia, which is associated with a progressive, ultimately catastrophic degeneration of the brain. Several types of oxidative damage have been found in the brains of Alzheimer's patients, though it is presently unclear if this damage is cause or effect. Vitamin E supplementation can slow the progression of Alzheimer's disease. However, such findings do not indicate if vagaries in vitamin E intake over an extended period of time are a cause of the disease.

Minerals

All of the essential minerals are important for cellular functions in brain, as they are elsewhere in the body. These are sodium, potassium, calcium, magnesium, iron, copper, zinc, manganese, cobalt, and molybdenum. While most function as cofactors in enzymatic reactions, sodium and potassium are key ions in electrical conduction in neuronal membranes, calcium functions as a second messenger within neurons, and magnesium is an important component of certain neurotransmitter receptors. The diet normally provides more than adequate amounts of almost all minerals, except possibly for calcium, iron, magnesium, and zinc. The BBB permeability to most metals is quite low. For example, although the brain extracts 20–30% of the glucose in blood in a single capillary transit, it extracts <0.3% of any metal. The mechanisms of transport into brain for most metals are unknown. However, some details regarding the transport and/or functions of iron, calcium, and copper are available.

Iron circulates bound to the protein transferrin. Iron uptake into brain occurs primarily at the BBB, and involves a transferrin receptor-mediated endocytosis of the iron–transferrin complex by capillary endothelial cells. Iron dissociates from transferrin inside the cell, and is delivered into the brain interstitial fluid; the transferrin is returned to the circulation. Brain iron associates with ferretin, and is stored intracellularly. The bulk of the iron-ferretin stored in brain resides in glial cells and is laid down early in postnatal life. Marked regional differences in iron and ferretin concentrations occur in brain; levels in some areas are as high as those in liver. This distribution, however, does not correlate with the density of transferrin receptors in brain capillaries; it is presently unknown how or why the unequal distribution of iron develops. Numerous enzymes in brain are iron requiring, including several hydroxylases involved in neurotransmitter production, and a key metabolic enzyme, monoamine oxidase.

Iron deficiency can cause impairments in attention and cognition in children. Similar effects are seen in animals. In iron-deficient rats, brain iron concentrations decline, with newborn and infant animals showing more rapid declines than older animals. Iron repletion in brain occurs in infant and adult rats with iron supplementation, but not in animals depleted at birth. While outside of the brain, the activities of many iron-dependent enzymes are depressed by iron deficiency, their activities are unaffected inside the brain. However, a reduction in certain dopamine receptors occurs, along with aberrations in dopamine-dependent behaviors (dopamine is a CNS neurotransmitter). The inability of brain iron stores to recover in rats made iron deficient as newborns coincides with a persistence of dopamine-linked behavioral deficits, despite normal repletion of iron stores elsewhere in the body. Restoration of normal behavior with iron supplementation, along with brain iron stores, is seen in animals made iron deficient at other ages.

Iron deficiency also interferes with myelinization. Since marked glial proliferation and myelin formation occur early in infancy, iron deficiency during this period could prevent the optimal development of neuronal communications (glial cells provide insulation for axons and synapses). This effect could account for some of the behavioral deficits associated with neonatal iron deficiency.

Calcium is actively transported into the CNS, primarily via the blood–CSF barrier, and is not vitamin D sensitive. Since calcium concentrations in the circulation are regulated, under most circumstances, this process should also help to maintain brain calcium uptake and levels in the face of vagaries in calcium intake. Deficiencies in brain calcium should thus be a relatively rare occurrence.

Copper functions as a cofactor for numerous enzymes, including dopamine β-hydroxylase (DBH), which converts dopamine to noradrenaline. Dietary copper deficiency in humans is fairly rare. When produced in animals, it leads to reduced DBH activity in neurons and cells anywhere in the nervous system that synthesize noradrenaline. The mechanism of copper transport into the brain is presently unknown. Copper deficiency occurs as an X-linked genetic disease of copper transport in Menkes' syndrome, in which tissue and brain copper levels become extremely low, and produce neurodegeneration. Children with Menkes' syndrome die at a very young age.

See also: **Amino Acids**: Chemistry and Classification; Metabolism; Specific Functions. **Ascorbic Acid**: Physiology, Dietary Sources and Requirements. **Biotin**. **Calcium**. **Choline and Phosphatidylcholine**.

Cobalamins. Copper. Fatty Acids: Metabolism. **Folic Acid. Glucose**: Metabolism and Maintenance of Blood Glucose Level. **Niacin. Pantothenic Acid. Protein**: Synthesis and Turnover. **Riboflavin. Thiamin**: Physiology. **Vitamin A**: Physiology; Biochemistry and Physiological Role. **Vitamin E**: Metabolism and Requirements.

Further Reading

Davson H, Zlokovic B, Rakic L, and Segal MB (1993) *An Introduction to the Blood-Brain Barrier.* Boca Raton, CRC Press.

Fernstrom JD and Fernstrom MH (2001) Diet, monoamine neurotransmitters and appetite control. In: Fernstrom JD, Uauy R, and Arroyo P (eds.) *Nutrition and Brain, Nestlé Nutrition Workshop Series Clinical and Performance Program,* vol. 5, pp. 117–134. Basel: Karger.

Fernstrom JD and Garattini S (eds.) (2000) International Symposium on Glutamate. *Journal of Nutrition* 130(4S): 891S–1079S.

Innis SM (1994) The 1993 Borden Award Lecture: Fatty acid requirements of the newborn. *Canadian Journal of Physiology and Pharmacology* 72: 1483–1492.

Spector R (1989) Micronutrient homeostasis in mammalian brain and cerebrospinal fluid. *Journal of Neurochemistry* 53: 1667–1774.

Zigmond MJ, Bloom FE, Landis SC, Roberts JL, and Squire LR (eds.) (1999) *Fundamental Neuroscience.* New York: Academic Press.

BREAST FEEDING

C K Lutter, Pan American Health Organization, Washington, DC, USA

© 2005 Elsevier Ltd. All rights reserved.

Nutritional demands during the first year of life are greater than at any other time. During this period, a healthy newborn triples its birth weight and doubles its length and the size of its brain. The benefits of breast feeding during this critical period of development, even in the most privileged environments, are undisputable. Consequently, there are also measurable risks for those infants not breast fed, which include increases in diarrhea, acute respiratory infections, and otitis media and short- and long-term deficits in intellectual development. Not breast feeding may also be associated with increased risk of some chronic diseases and obesity, although the evidence for these relationships is still accumulating. Not breast feeding may also be associated with increased risk of some chronic diseases. In developing countries, the risks of not breast-feeding are magnified many times over and also include increased mortality. Because of these benefits, breast feeding should be promoted as a cultural and behavioral norm rather than as interchangeable with formula feeding.

Breast feeding also benefits women's health. Breast feeding reduces the risk of ovarian and premenopausal breast cancer and also promotes postpartum weight loss. Because it delays the return of menses, it reduces fertility and, in the absence of modern contraceptives, increases birth intervals. This article provides a broad overview of the physiological and nutritional aspects of breast milk and behavioral aspects of breast feeding, followed by a summary of global and national initiatives to improve breast feeding practices and data on breast feeding trends in Latin America.

Breast Feeding Recommendations

Both the World Health Organization (WHO) and the United Nations Children's Fund (UNICEF) recommend exclusive breast feeding for 6 months and continued breast feeding together with provision of safe, appropriate, and hygienically prepared complementary foods until 2 years of age or beyond. The American Academy of Pediatrics Section on Breastfeeding also recommends exclusive breast feeding for 6 months. Breast feeding is defined as exclusive if breast milk is the sole source of infant nutrition with no other liquids (including water) or food given, although medicinal and/or vitamin drops are permitted. Partial or mixed breast-feeding is used to describe infants who are not exclusively breast-fed. In a comprehensive review, WHO provided the scientific underpinnings of the recommended duration of exclusive breast feeding and noted that infants who were exclusively breast fed for 6 months experienced less morbidity from gastrointestinal infection than those who were exclusively breast fed for only 3 or 4 months. Also, exclusive breast feeding for 6 months, as opposed to only 3 or 4 months, resulted in no measurable deficits in growth among infants from either developing or developed countries.

The public health challenge is to support women to follow global breast feeding recommendations so as to ensure the healthiest start in life for all the world's children. Adherence to the recommended

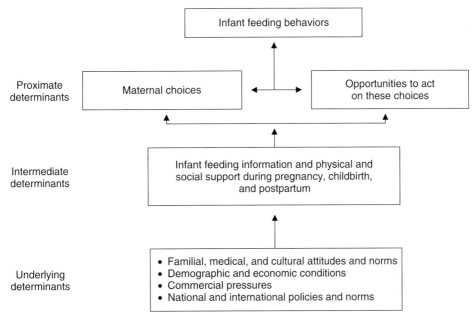

Figure 1 Determinants of infant feeding behaviors.

breast feeding behaviors or lack thereof results from a complex series of physiological and behavioral interactions between a mother and her infant—interactions that take place within a larger familial, community, and global setting (**Figure 1**). Although breast feeding occurs when a mother puts her child to the breast or allows her toddler to suckle, a woman's decision to breast feed and to act on this decision are dependent on a number of determinants, not all of which favor breast-feeding or are within her control. These determinants include infant feeding attitudes and norms among family members, the medical profession, peers, and employers; the availability of information and access to skilled assistance to prevent and/or address breast-feeding (BF) problems; and, during the period of BF initiation and exclusive breast feeding, nearly unrestricted access between mother and infant.

Breast Milk

Breast milk is a unique bioactive substance that changes composition, within and between feedings and over time, to suit the needs of the growing infant. More than 200 different constituents of breast milk have been identified, many of which have dual roles, and more continue to be discovered as analytic techniques improve. Breast milk includes true solutions, colloids, membranes, membrane-bound globules, and living cells. Its three distinct stages occur when colostrum, transitional, and mature milk are secreted; each aids newborns in their physiologic adaptation to extrauterine life.

Compared to mature milk, colostrum, produced during the first week of life, has a higher protein and lower fat content and is rich in immunoglobulins, antibodies, and antioxidants. Compared to colostrum, transitional milk, produced from 7 days to between 10 days and 2 weeks postpartum, has lower immunoglobulins and total protein content and higher lactose, fat, and total caloric content.

Women experience the shift to transitional milk as a feeling of fullness in the breasts, which occurs between 40 and 72 h after birth. This occurs sooner for multiparas than primiparas. Milk volume increases dramatically after birth from less than 100 ml/day to approximately 500 ml/day by day 5 and approximately 650 ml/day by month 1 and 750 ml/day by month 3 (**Figure 2**). Exclusively breast fed infants consume 714, 784, and 776 ml/day between 0 and 2, 3 and 5, and 6 and 8 months, respectively. Mature milk has an energy density of approximately 75 kcal/ml, which translates into a

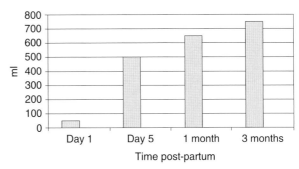

Figure 2 Average volume of breast milk production.

daily caloric intake of 450–550 kcal/day. This is entirely sufficient to satisfy current energy recommendations for infants for the first 6 months of life.

Once breast milk supply has been established, the volume produced depends on infant demand; frequent exclusive breast feeding is critical for stimulating optimal milk production. This is why it is so important that infants be breast fed on demand, day and night: The more often milk is removed from the breasts, the more milk a woman produces. The process of lactation requires both milk synthesis and its release into the alveoli and the lactiferous sinuses for removal by the suckling infant. Milk production is mediated by prolactin and its release by oxytocin. The decrease in plasma progesterone after birth initiates the process of lactogenesis. For several days following birth, lactogenesis does not depend on suckling; however, by day 3 or 4, milk secretion declines if milk is not removed from the breast. Therefore, any practices, such as the use of prelacteal feeds, supplemental bottles, or feeding on a schedule, that interfere with the infant's desire or ability to nurse effectively are likely to undermine the successful establishment of lactation. Also, because infant demand is the primary determinant of milk production, the early introduction of other liquids or complementary foods will displace the energy and nutrients provided by breast milk rather than provide an additional source of nutrition.

Lipids comprise the primary source of energy and are the most variable constituent of breast milk and vary in concentration during a feeding, between breasts, during the day, and over time. They also vary in concentration among women by as much as 50%. Research on the lipid component of breast milk has focused on its association with improved cognitive development and possible role in the prevention of obesity and other chronic degenerative diseases in breast fed children compared to formula-fed children. Particular attention has been paid to the dietary omega-3 polyunsaturated fatty acid, docosahexaenoic acid (DHA), which has been shown to enhance retinal development and visual acuity and may provide a physiologic explanation for the superior cognitive development that is documented in breast fed children. Following the lead of Japan and numerous European countries, the US Food and Drug Administration has permitted the addition of DHA to infant formula.

Proteins in breast milk include casein, serum, albumin, α-lactabumin, β-lactoglobulins, immunoglobulins, and other glycoproteins. Lactoferrin, an iron binding protein, inhibits the growth of certain iron-dependent bacteria in the gastrointestinal track and may protect against certain gastrointestinal infections. Lactose is the predominant carbohydrate of breast milk. It has been shown to enhance calcium absorption as well as provide a readily available source of galactose, which is essential to central nervous system development. Although concerns have been raised about the adequacy of breast milk to satisfy protein requirements for 6 months, a number of well-controlled studies have shown that protein needs can met through exclusive breast feeding.

The nutrients in breast milk most affected by maternal nutritional status are the water-soluble vitamins and the fat-soluble vitamins. With few exceptions, maternal stores and intake do not affect the mineral content of breast milk. Micronutrients affected by maternal intake and nutritional status include thiamin, riboflavin, vitamin B_6, vitamin B_{12}, vitamin A, iodine, and selenium. Those not affected include folate, vitamin D, calcium, iron, copper, and zinc. Particular attention has been paid to iron content of breast milk because of the relatively low breast milk content compared to theoretical needs. Breast milk iron, however, is highly bioavailable and exclusively breast fed term infants of normal birth weight are not at risk for iron deficiency anemia or depletion of iron stores. Iron supplements, beginning at 2 months, are recommended for preterm or low-birth-weight infants. Zinc, another mineral essential to human development, is also highly bioavailable in breast milk. Breast milk volume does not appear to be influenced by maternal nutritional status, except in situations of extreme food deprivation and famine.

Benefits of Breast Feeding

Breast feeding contributes to both maternal and infant nutrition and health through a number of important mechanisms. It provides a complete source of nutrition for the first 6 months of life for normal, full-term infants and provides one-half and one-third of energy needs for the second half of the first year and the second year of life, respectively. It also contributes significantly to protein and micronutrient requirements. Numerous studies have shown that during illness, whereas intake of complementary foods declines significantly, breast milk intake does not decrease. Because of the well-established superiority of breast milk over other infant feeding modes, women cannot ethically be randomized in infant feeding studies and as a result most data on the benefits of breast-feeding and the risks of not breast feeding are observational. However, the dose–response effect observed in such studies, even when donor breast milk is provided through a nasogastric tube to premature newborns, provides evidence of causality.

A large-scale study involving more than 17 000 infants in which breast feeding promotion was randomized and morbidity results analyzed on an 'intention to treat' basis, with breast feeding promotion as the treatment, also provides evidence of causality. Infants born in hospitals and provided care in clinics randomized to breast feeding promotion were 40% less likely to have more than one case of gastrointestinal infection and 50% less likely to have atopic eczema than infants not randomized to this intervention (**Figure** 3). The intervention significantly increased the duration of exclusive breast feeding at 3 months from 6 to 43% and the duration of partial breast-feeding at 1 year from 11 to 20%. Therefore, this study proved through a causal design that better breast feeding practices reduce risk of diarrhea and eczema, and that hospital and clinic-based interventions can result in large-scale shifts in behavior.

A pooled analysis of longitudinal data from Brazil, Pakistan, and the Philippines showed that during infancy breast feeding resulted in a 6-fold reduction in mortality during the first month of life, a 4-fold reduction in the second month, and a 2-fold reduction thereafter (**Figure** 4). In none of the studies was exclusive breast feeding sufficiently prevalent to examine the additional preventive effect of exclusive breast feeding over partial breast feeding. However, case–control studies that have examined breast feeding and mortality show that infants who are exclusively breast fed for the first 2 months of life have a 24-fold reduced risk of diarrhea compared to those exclusively bottle fed (**Figure** 5).

It is well established that breast-fed infants have a different pattern of growth. The fact that the nutrient composition of breast milk is qualitatively and

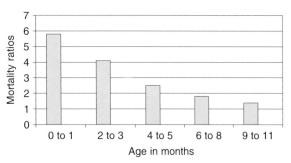

Figure 4 Increased risk of mortality associated with not breast feeding. (From World Health Organization (2000) WHO Collaborative Study Team on the role of breastfeeding on the prevention of infant mortality: Effect of breastfeeding on infant and child mortality due to infectious diseases in less developed countries: A pooled analysis. *Lancet* **355**: 451–455.)

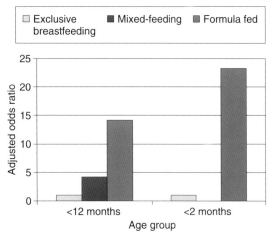

Figure 5 Exclusive breast feeding and risk of mortality from diarrhea in Brazil. (From Victora CG, Vaughan JP, Lombardi *et al.* (1987) Evidence for protection by breast-feeding against infant deaths from infectious diseases in Brazil. *Lancet* **2**(8554): 319–321.)

quantitatively different than formula, coupled with the epidemic of obesity among children in developed countries, has led a number of investigators to examine its association with infant feeding mode. In one of the largest studies to date of more than 9000 German schoolchildren, a dose–response between the duration of breast feeding and risk of obesity at age 5 or 6 years was reported (**Figure** 6). However, not all studies have found a relationship. Because most of the research to date has been carried out in developed countries, where breast feeding is more common among the better educated and affluent who are also more likely to practice other healthful behaviors, the possibility of bias persists.

More than 11 studies have documented an association between breast feeding and cognitive development. In the longest follow-up to date, a study

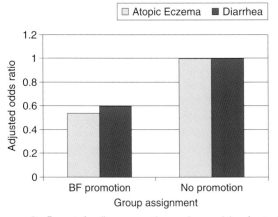

Figure 3 Breast feeding promotion reduces risk of atopic eczema and diarrhea. (Source: Kramer MS, Chalmers B, Hodnett E *et al.* (2001) Promotion of breastfeeding intervention trial (PROBIT): A randomized trial in the Republic of Belarus. *Journal of the American Medical Association* **285**(4):413–420.)

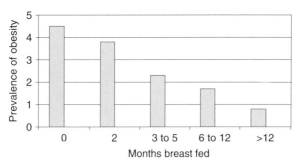

Figure 6 Months of breast feeding and prevalence of obesity in German schoolchildren. (From Von Kries R, Koletzko B, Sauerwald T *et al.* (1999) Breast feeding and obesity: Cross sectional study. *British Medical Journal* **319**: 147.)

also showed that adults who as infants had been breast fed for at least 9 months grew up to be significantly more intelligent than those breast-fed 1 month or less. After adjusting for a variety of factors, a dose–response relationship between the length of breast feeding and a number of different intelligence quotient measures was found in Danish adults who had been breast fed as infants. The total difference for those breast fed between 7 and 9 months versus less than 1 month was 6.6 points.

The longer women breast feed, the more they are protected against breast cancer. A reanalysis of data from 47 studies in 30 countries included more than 50 000 women with breast cancer and nearly 97 000 without it. Women who developed breast cancer were less likely to have breast fed, or if they had, the length of time they had breast fed was significantly shorter than that of women who were free of breast cancer. The effect of breast feeding on risk of breast cancer did not differ between women in developed and developing countries, and it did not vary significantly by age, menopausal status, ethnic origin, the number of births a woman had, her age when her first child was born, or any of a number of other personal characteristics examined. Based on the size of the effect, it is estimated that the cumulative incidence of breast cancer in developed countries would be reduced by more than half, from 6.3 to 2.7 per 100 women by age 70, if women had the average number of births and lifetime duration of breast feeding that has until recently been prevalent in developing countries.

Not surprisingly, not breast feeding results in significantly greater health care expenditures. Among middle-class children from the United States and Scotland, the excess cost of health care services for diarrhea, lower respiratory tract illness, and otitis media during the first year of life was estimated to be between $331 and $475 per never-breast fed infant in 1995. These costs were calculated on the basis of

2033 excess office visits, 212 excess days of hospitalization, and 609 excess prescriptions for each 1000 never-breast fed infants compared to 1000 infants breast fed exclusively for at least 3 months.

Breast Feeding Initiatives

In response to concerns about the use of infant formula in environments where lack of breast feeding resulted in large numbers of infant who became severely ill or died, a grassroots global initiative took hold in the 1970s to promote international and national efforts to protect, promote, and support breast feeding. These efforts culminated in 1981 with the nearly unanimous adoption by the World Health Assembly (WHA) of the International Code of Marketing of Breast-Milk Substitutes. This document and subsequent relevant WHA resolutions, collectively known as the Code, provide guidelines for the marketing of breast milk substitutes, bottles, and teats. To ensure infant feeding decisions free from the influence of marketing pressures, the Code provides guidelines on a number of issues associated with increases in formula feeding, including direct promotion to the public, donations to health care institutions, free supplies to mothers, and the use of baby images on labels that glorify bottle feeding. Its implementation is monitored by a 2-year reporting cycle by countries to the WHA and by the International Code Documentation Centre in Penang, Malaysia. Despite continued violations by infant food companies and the lack of enforcement in many developed countries, the Code has provided an important tool for regulating and monitoring the infant food industry to ensure that its marketing practices do not undermine breast feeding.

The 1990 Innocenti Declaration, which set four operational targets that all governments should achieve by 1995, was endorsed by the 45th WHA. These targets included appointment of a national breast feeding coordinator and establishment of a multisectoral national breast feeding committee; ensuring that all health facilities providing maternity services fully practice the 10 steps to successful breast feeding (**Table 1**) set out in the WHO/UNICEF statement; taking action to give effect to the Code; and enacting imaginative legislation to protect the breast feeding rights of working women. This declaration provided the basis for the WHO/UNICEF Baby Friendly Hospital Initiative (BFHI), which was developed in 1991, piloted in 12 countries, and inaugurated as a global initiative in 1992. BFHI promotes hospital practices consistent with early initiation, an environment conducive to BF, appropriate clinical management of BF, and compliance

Table 1 WHO/UNICEF 10 steps to successful breast feeding

Step 1. Have a written breast-feeding policy that is routinely communicated to all health care staff.

Step 2. Train all health care staff in skills necessary to implement this policy.

Step 3. Inform all pregnant women about the benefits and management of breast feeding.

Step 4. Help mothers initiate breast feeding within a half-hour of birth.

Step 5. Show mothers how to breast feed and how to maintain lactation even if they should be separated from their infants.

Step 6. Give newborn infants no food or drink other than breast milk, unless medically indicated.

Step 7. Practice rooming-in—allow mothers and infants to remain together—24 h a day.

Step 8. Encourage breast feeding on demand.

Step 9. Give no artificial teats or pacifiers (also called dummies or smoothers) to breast feeding infants.

Step 10. Foster the establishment of breast feeding support groups and refer mothers to them on discharge from the hospital or clinic.

Table 2 Trends in breast feeding practices

Country	Year	Initiation (%)	Median duration BF (months)	
			Exclusive BF	Any BF
Bolivia	1989	96.4	NA	16.9
	1994	96.3	3.3	17.5
	1998	96.6	3.9	18.0
Colombia	1986	NA	NA	11.6
	1990	93.4	0.6	12.7
	1995	94.5	0.5	11.3
	2000	95.5	0.7	13.1
Costa Rica	1981	NA	NA	7.2
	1986	NA	NA	9.3
	1993	NA	NA	9.1
Dominican Republic	1986	92.7	NA	8.1
	1991	92.0	0.4	9.0
	1996	93.2	0.6	7.6
Ecuador	1994	95.0	2.0	15.7
	1999	97.0	2.2	15.5
El Salvador	1988	93.1	NA	15.2
	1993	91.2	0.8	15.5
	1998	94.0	0.9	17.7
Guatemala	1987	NA	NA	19.9
	1995	95.6	1.7	19.8
	1998	96.5	0.9	19.9
Haiti	1977	NA	NA	15.6
	1994	96.3	0.4	17.5
	2000	97.4	0.4	18.5
Honduras	1986	NA	NA	17.3
	1991	NA	NA	17.2
	1996	96.0	2.1	17.3
Jamaica	1989	96.0	NA	12.4
	1993	94.0	NA	12.4
Nicaragua	1992–1993	91.9	0.6	12.3
	1998	92.4	0.7	12.2
Paraguay	1990	92.8	0.4	10.5
	1995/6	93.6	0.3	11.4
	1998	94.2	NA	11.5
Peru	1991–1992	96.0	0.8	17.3
	1996	96.8	2.7	19.5
	2000	97.8	4.2	21.6

BF, breast feeding; NA, not available.

with certain key provision of the Code, such as no donations of free or subsidized infant formula. Certification is awarded to hospitals that comply with a set of standardized Baby Friendly criteria developed by WHO and UNICEF. Worldwide, nearly 20 000 hospitals are certified as Baby Friendly.

At the same time that the Code and BHFI were being implemented, numerous projects worked to develop training materials in lactation management and counseling skills and provided funding for widespread dissemination of training courses. National governments also actively implemented campaigns to promote breast feeding. In Latin America, these efforts are likely responsible for a resurgence of breast feeding.

Global Breast Feeding Practices

The most comprehensive data on breast feeding come from the Demographic and Health Surveys conducted with support from the US Agency for International Development. These surveys are nationally representative and conducted throughout the developing world. In a number of countries, multiple surveys permit the analysis of trends. Overall, the data show that although the vast majority of women—more than 90% in all countries—initiate breast feeding, the duration of exclusive breast feeding is far less than the recommended 6 months (**Table 2**). In most countries, the duration of breast feeding is unchanged. Several countries are showing increases and in only one does there appear to be a decrease. However, concurrent with

the time period during which the surveys took place, numerous demographic changes occurred that are negatively associated with breast-feeding, such as increased female employment and education and increased urbanization. When adjusted for these changes, highly significant improvements in breast feeding are seen in many countries, particularly those in which breast feeding promotion efforts have been most active.

See also: **Infants**: Nutritional Requirements; Feeding Problems. **Lactation**: Physiology; Dietary Requirements. **United Nations Children's Fund**. **World Health Organization**.

Further Reading

Aguayo VM, Ross JS, Kanon S et al. (2003) Monitoring and compliance with the Code of Marketing of Breast-Milk Substitutes in West Africa: Multisiet cross sectional survey in Togo and Burkina Faso. British Medical Journal 326: 1–6.

Ball TM and Wright AL (1999) Health care costs of formula-feeding in the first year of life. Pediatrics 103: 870–876.

Butte NF (2001) The role of breastfeeding in obesity. Pediatric Clinics of North America 48(1): 189–198.

Collaborative Group on Hormonal Factors in Breast Cancer (2002) Breast cancer and breastfeeding: Collaborative reanalysis of individual data from 47 epidemiological studies in 30 countries, including 50 302 women with breast cancer and 96 973 women without the disease. Lancet 360: 187–195.

Kramer MS, Chalmers B, Hodnett E et al. (2001) Promotion of breastfeeding intervention trial (PROBIT): A randomized trial in the Republic of Belarus. Journal of the American Medical Association 285(4): 413–420.

Kramer MS and Kakuma R (2001) The Optimal Duration of Exclusive Breastfeeding: A Systematic Review, WHO/NHD/01.08, WHO/FCH/CAH/01.23. Geneva: World Health Organization.

Lawrence RA and Lawrence RM (1999) Breastfeeding: A Guide for the Medical Profession. St. Louis: Mosby.

Mortensen EL, Michaelsen KF, Sanders SA et al. (2002) The association between duration of breastfeeding and adult intelligence. Journal of the American Medical Association 287: 2365–2371.

Victora CG, Vaughan JP, Lombardi et al. (1987) Evidence for protection by breast-feeding against infant deaths from infectious diseases in Brazil. Lancet 2(8554): 319–321.

Von Kries R, Koletzko B, Sauerwald T et al. (1999) Breast feeding and obesity: Cross sectional study. British Medical Journal 319: 147.

World Health Organization (1981) The International Code of Marketing of Breast-Milk Substitutes. Geneva: World Health Organization.

World Health Organization (1989) Protecting, Promoting, and Supporting Breastfeeding: The Special Role of Maternity Services. Geneva: World Health Organization.

World Health Organization (2000) WHO Collaborative Study Team on the role of breastfeeding on the prevention of infant mortality: Effect of breastfeeding on infant and child mortality due to infectious diseases in less developed countries: A pooled analysis. Lancet 355: 451–455.

BURNS PATIENTS

S A Hill, Southampton General Hospital, Southampton, UK

© 2005 Elsevier Ltd. All rights reserved.

Of all insults to the body, burns elicit the most profound stress response. This response encompasses hormonal, metabolic, and immunologic changes, which are complicated by the loss of the many protective functions of an intact skin. The initial hypermetabolic state induces intense protein catabolism, which must be checked by aggressive nutritional support in order to limit morbidity and mortality. Following this intense period of catabolism, which lasts 10–14 days, there is a gradual reduction in the metabolic rate, catabolic processes decrease, the wound heals, and anabolic processes predominate. Nutritional support must also continue throughout these latter stages, which may take many weeks, so that anabolism can be supported and fuel reserves replenished. A diet high in carbohydrate (CHO) and protein but low in fat will not only suppress catabolism and favor anabolism but also support an appropriate immunological response.

Hypermetabolism and Hypercatabolism

The burn wound is the focal point of all the circulatory, metabolic, and inflammatory responses associated with injury (**Figure 1**).

Metabolic Response

Increased glucose demand is initially met by glycogenolysis. When glycogen stores are exhausted, lipolysis and protein catabolism increase to supply gluconeogenic substrates. This hypermetabolic response is accompanied by increased cardiac output, increased oxygen consumption, and increased thermogenesis. The physical loss of skin cover has other major effects, including fluid loss, increased heat loss by evaporation, and loss of local immune function. Skin grafting will provide some cover for burned areas but the use of allografts increases the total area of damaged skin. Early excision and grafting is associated with increased survival in patients with more than 70% burns compared with conservative management. Donor split-skin graft sites heal within 7–14 days, unlike the burned area, which continues to make increased metabolic demands for weeks after the initial insult. Measurements of energy requirements take into account whole body metabolism and include any demands made by donor sites. Recent work suggests that early coverage with artificial 'skin' may reduce the hypercaloric requirements of the patient.

The sympathoadrenal axis is stimulated as a result of thermal injury, with increased plasma levels of epinephrine, norepinephrine, and cortisol. In addition, levels of both glucagon and insulin

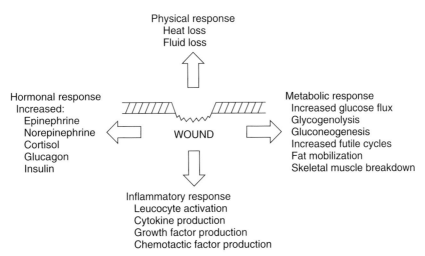

Figure 1 Schematic representation of the central nature of the burn wound in triggering physical, hormonal, metabolic, and inflammatory responses.

increase, although an apparent insulin resistance develops in peripheral tissues. There is an increase in core temperature, which appears to be mediated centrally by the hypothalamus in response to cytokine release, possibly interleukin-1 (IL-1). Plasma levels of glucose are maintained and may even increase, although glucose flux is greatly increased. Metabolic demands for glucose and amino acids increase and the body responds to meet these demands (**Table 1**). The degree of hypermetabolism and oxygen consumption are closely related to the extent and depth of burn injury. As a result, basal energy expenditure increases and is doubled for a 60% burn (**Figure 2**). Catecholamines augment

cardiac and circulatory performance, which increases blood flow to the wound. Liver and kidney blood flow also increase, with increased delivery of gluconeogenic precursors, increased glucose release into the circulation, and increased nitrogen clearance. The release of fat from adipose tissue is stimulated by catecholamines. In the liver, fat metabolism to glycerol and free fatty acids produces energy as long as an adequate glucose supply replenishes oxaloacetic acid for oxidation of acetyl CoA, the product of triacylglycerol oxidation.

Table 1 Metabolic and circulatory responses to burn injury

Wound	Whole body
Damage	Increase in catecholamines, cortisol, glucagon, insulin
	Hepatic switch to synthesis of acute phase proteins
Increased blood flow to the wound	Increased cardiac output
Increased metabolism of glucose	Increased gluconeogenesis
	Increased free fatty acid flux
	Increased oxygen consumption
	Futile substrate cycling of carbohydrate intermediates and fatty acids
Increased heat loss	Increased core temperature: hypothalamic mediated
Attempted repair	Increased amino acid flux
	Release of arginine and glutamine from skeletal muscle
	Increased nitrogen loss
Inflammatory response	Inhibition of maximum inflammatory response by cortisol
	Cytokine and eicosanoids increase inflammation

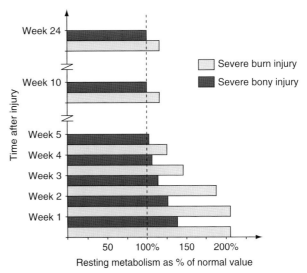

Figure 2 The stress response to thermal injury is greater than that to any other insult. The resting energy requirements in burns patients are greater for longer than for any other injury. (Adapted with permission from Long CL, Schaffel N, Geiger JW *et al.* (1979) Metabolic response to injury and illness: Estimation of energy and protein needs from indirect calorimetry and nitrogen balance. *Journal of Parenteral and Enteral Nutrition* **3**(6): 452–456.)

Thus, both continued oxygen and glucose must be supplied to prevent ketoacidosis. Heat production and energy wastage occur as a result of a 2- or 3-fold increase in futile cycling of substrates; glucose, pyruvate, and fructose-6-phosphate are all involved in these reactions.

Gluconeogenesis can occur only in the liver and is increased by catecholamines and glucagon. The plasma levels of gluconeogenic amino acids (alanine and glutamine) initially increase during the first 2 days, when glycogen is preferentially metabolized, but subsequently decrease. Days 4–7 are associated with a maximal decrease in plasma levels of gluconeogenic amino acids, whereas muscle production and hepatic consumption are both increased.

Catabolic Response

Release of gluconeogenic amino acids from skeletal muscle results in loss of muscle mass. Deamination of these amino acids, during the generation of carbon skeletons for glucose synthesis, increases nitrogen production with subsequent conversion to urea, which is excreted by the kidneys. Urinary nitrogen loss following thermal injury is largely from skeletal muscle breakdown, but a significant contribution of approximately 25–30% comes from the burn exudate. The rate of nitrogen loss is related to total burn area (TBA) and can be as much as 3 or 4 g/kg/day at its peak (**Figure 3**). These high rates of nitrogen loss persist for the first 7–10 days and then gradually decline until the burn area is healed and

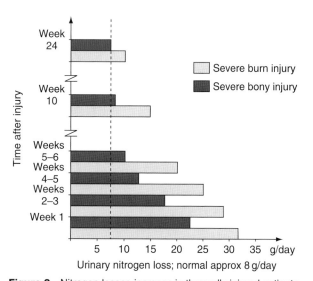

Figure 3 Nitrogen losses increase in thermally injured patients and remain high for a longer period than for any other injury. (Adapted with permission from Long CL, Schaffel N, Geiger JW *et al.* (1979) Metabolic response to injury and illness: Estimation of energy and protein needs from indirect calorimetry and nitrogen balance. *Journal of Parenteral and Enteral Nutrition* **3**(6): 452–456.)

body stores of nitrogen are replenished; this may take many months. Nutritional support provides an exogenous source of calories and protein, which limits autocanabalism of skeletal muscle with a reduction in infective complications, increased survival rates, and reduced hospital stay.

Inflammatory Response

Local and systemic factors lead to an increase in inflammatory cell infiltration of the burn wound with removal of damaged tissue in preparation for epithelialization and wound healing. The cytokine cascade precipitated by stress hormones in response to injury involves tumor necrosis factor-α (TNF-α), which subsequently activates leucocyte production of IL-1, IL-6, platelet-derived growth factor, and eicosanoids (prostaglandins, thromboxanes, and leukotrienes). These in turn amplify the cellular and cytokine responses by release of chemotactic factors. TNF-α and the cytokines are also mediators of the increased metabolic and catabolic response seen in burns patients. TNF-α will increase acute-phase protein synthesis and increase loss of amino acids from skeletal muscle. However, it is also associated with the healing process in that wound healing is stimulated as a result of vascular proliferation and collagen synthesis. Excessive release of TNF-α can be harmful and is associated with muscle wasting, excessive weight loss, increased nitrogen loss, systemic inflammatory response syndrome, and debility.

These early immune reactions give way, in the second and third week postburn, to injury immunosuppression. This takes the form of reduced responsiveness of lymphocytes, impaired production of IL-2, and changes in immune cell phenotypes. Burn injury inhibits the T-helper 1 response but promotes a T-helper 2 response. As a result, IL-2 and interferon-γ (IFN-γ) production is reduced, which increases the risk of infection. Membrane lipid composition also influences lymphocyte and macrophage functions in terms of signaling and eicosaniod production. There is a reduction in *n*-6 (mainly arachidonic) fatty acids and an increase in PGE$_2$, which can lead to immunosuppression. Dietary replacement of *n*-6 by *n*-3 polyunsaturated fatty acids (PUFAs) reduces immunosuppression by altering membrane composition and eicosanoid series production. Nutritional studies have focused on the influence that enteral feed composition has on immune function—so-called immune-enhancing diets. The theoretical elements of interest are *n*-3 PUFAs and the amino acids arginine and glutamine. The evidence base for a clinically measurable advantage of such immune-enhancing preparations is yet to be fully established. Small studies have shown a reduction in wound infection rate and a possible reduction in length of stay per percentage total body surface area burned.

Nutritional Requirements

In the absence of an exogenous nutrient supply, autocanabalism would result in major morbidity and mortality. Nutritional supply of energy and protein in excess of normal requirements prevents such complications.

Calories

Adults Much work has focused on developing an easy-to-apply formula for predicting the number of calories required to maintain weight in the severely burned patient. Many of these formulas are simply based on percentage burn area and body surface area, but others are complex—arrived at by regression analysis. Recent evaluations of these formulas, compared to indirect calorimetry, suggest that none perfectly predict a patient's true requirements. The most reliable are summarized in **Table 2**. Requirements vary considerably depending on multiple factors including time after burn injury, not all of which can be taken into consideration in the formulas used (**Table 3**). Because of major within- as well as between-patient variation, it is agreed that

Table 2 Formulas for predicting calorie requirements in adults that compare favorably with indirect calorimetric measurements ($1.3 \times$ REE)

Xie formula[a]
$1000 + (25 \times BSAB)$ kcal/m²/day *or* $4184 + (105 \times BSAB)$ kJ/ m²/day

Zawacki formula[b]
1440 kcal/m²/day *or* 6025 kJ/ m²/day

Milner formula[c]
$(BMR \times 24 \times BSA) + (0.274 + (0.0079 \times BSAB) - (0.004 \times DPB))$ kcal/m²/day *or*
$(BMR \times 24 \times BSA) + (1.146 + (0.0331 \times BSAB) - (0.017 \times DPB))$ kJ/m²/day

[a]Xie WG *et al.* Estimation of the calorie requirements of burned Chinese adults. *Burns.* 1993, **19**: 146–9.
[b]Zawacki BE *et al.* Does increased evaporative water loss cause hypermetabolism in burned patients? *Annals of Surgery.* 1970, **171**: 236–40.
[c]Milner EA, Cioffi WG, Mason AD, McManus WF, and Pruitt BA Jr. A longitudinal study of resting energy expenditure in thermally injured patients. [Journal Article] *Journal of Trauma-Injury Infection & Critical Care.* **37**(2): 167–70.
BSAB, body surface area burned; BMR, basal metabolic rate; DPB, days postburn.

Table 3 Factors that may alter total energy requirements in burns patients

Number of days after burn injury
Changes in environmental temperature and humidity
Changes in core body temperature, including sepsis, infection
Inhalation injury
Activity level
Surgical interventions; grafting
Dressing changes
Pain and anxiety
Sedative drugs

indirect calorimetry should be used to predict resting energy requirements (REEs) throughout the recovery period.

By measuring oxygen uptake and carbon dioxide production, the REE of the patient can be derived. Recent work has established that although body weight can be maintained on a regimen of a caloric intake of 1.3–1.5 times the REE, this reflects increasing fat accumulation despite persistent catabolism of skeletal protein. The catabolism appears to persist despite nutritional manipulation. It has been suggested that lean mass can only be maintained by pharmacological means with the use of insulin, insulin-like growth factor-1 (IGF-1), or anabolic steroids such as oxandrone.

Children Pediatric patients, who account for at least 35% of all burn injuries, are a challenge to nutritional support teams. Compared to adults, they have lower lean body mass and fat reserves and have a higher basal metabolic rate. Extra allowances are needed for growth and development, particularly during the infant and adolescent growth spurts. Many different pediatric formulas are used (**Table 4**). Indirect calorimetry indicates that those predicting lower calorie requirements may be more accurate.

For pediatric patients, for whom requirements have been particularly difficult to predict using formulas, indirect calorimetry has been of great importance in determining adequate calorie intake and measured energy expenditure should be multiplied by a factor of 1.5 to provide adequate calories for weight maintenance in children with burns.

Balance of Energy-Producing Substrates

Energy requirements may be met by glucose, fat, and protein. There has been much interest in the relative proportions of these three sources, and it now seems that 20–25% should be supplied as protein but only 15% as fat.

Table 4 Examples of formulas used to predict energy requirements in children

Wolfe[a]

BMR × 2 kcal/24 h

Males	BMR equation	Females	BMR equation
0–3	$(60.9 \times W) - 54$	0–3	$(61 \times W) - 51$
3–10	$(22.7 \times W) + 459$	3–10	$(22.5 \times W) + 499$
10–18	$(17.5 \times W) + 651$	10–18	$(12.2 \times W) + 746$

Modified Galveston formulas[b]

Less than 1 year old: 2100 kcal/m² BSA + 1000 kcal/m² BSA burned

Less than 12 years old: 1800 kcal/m² BSA + 1300 kcal/m² BSA burned

12–18 years old: 1500 kcal/m² BSA + 1500 kcal/m² BSA burned

Curreri junior formulas[c]

Daily calorie needs[d]

 Birth–1 year: basal RDA in kcal + (15 kcal/% burn)

 1–3 years: basal RDA in kcal + (25 kcal/% burn)

 4–15 years: basal RDA in kcal + (40 kcal/% burn)

[a]O'Neil CE, Hutsler D, and Hildreth MA. Basic nutritional guidelines for pediatric burn patients. *Journal of Burn Care & Rehabilitation.* 1989, **10**(3): 278–84.
[b]Hildreth MA, Herndon DN, Desai MH, and Duke MA. Reassessing caloric requirements in pediatric burn patients. *Journal of Burn Care Rehabilitation* 1988, **9**(6): 616–8.
[c]Day T, Dean P, Adams MC, Luterman A, Ramenofsky ML, and Curreri PW. Nutritional requirements of the burned child: the Curreri junior formula. *Proceedings of the American Burn Association* 1986, **18**: 86.
[d]RDA (kcal) varies with age: 0–0.5 years, 320; 0.5–1 years, 500; 1–3 years, 740; 4–6 years, 950; 7–10 years, 1130; 11–14 years, 1440 (male) and 1310 (female); 15–18 years, 1760 (male) and 1370 (female).
BMR, basal metabolic rate; BSA, body surface area; RDA, recommended daily allowance; W, weight in kilograms.

Carbohydrate

Adults A high carbohydrate:fat ratio is associated with better maintenance of body weight. However, this may reflect increased fat accumulation rather than an increase in protein synthesis. Hyperglycemia alone can increase alanine efflux from skeletal muscle, without stimulating protein synthesis. Euglycemia, using exogenous insulin with high glucose delivery, can inhibit amino acid oxidation and favor amino acid synthesis. This may reflect an effect of IGF-1, which is released in response to insulin. In addition, hyperglycemia stimulates hepatic lipogenesis and increased CO_2 production, which may prevent weaning from ventilatory support. Hyperglycemia must therefore be prevented.

Children In children, carbohydrate is more effective than fat in promoting nitrogen retention by reducing the need for protein catabolism and subsequent gluconeogenesis. In infants, 5% dextrose in water parenterally can be used at 5 mg/kg/min initially and increased to a maximum of 15 mg/kg/min over the course of the first few days postinjury to provide 40–50% of calorie requirements. In older children, as in adults, glucose administration at a maximum rate of 5–7 mg/kg/min is recommended. These are parenteral recommendations; enteral feeding guidelines have not been established, although in general, carbohydrate should be limited to 50% of calorie intake.

Fat

Adults Feeding regimens that simply overfeed with a normal diet lead to problems in the recovery phase; muscle wasting persists together with central obesity. Reduction in fat administration largely prevents these problems if protein calories replace lipid calories (**Figure 4**). Fat cannot be excluded from the diet; a minimum fat content of 4% of total calories will ensure a supply of essential fatty acids. A diet containing 15% fat will meet such requirements as well as provide a delivery medium for fat-soluble vitamins. Dietary fat is largely composed of long-chain triacylglycerols (LCTs), and excess LCTs are associated with hepatic steatosis, reticuloendothelial system blockage, and immunosuppression. Varying the composition of the fats supplied to burns patients may alleviate some of these problems. Medium-chain fatty acids, particularly *n*-3 PUFA found in fish oil, appear beneficial in maximizing whole body protein synthesis in an animal model of burn injury. There is a decrease in plasma *n*-6 fatty acids after burn injury, so replacement with *n*-3 PUFA results in the production of prostanoid and eicosanoid series associated with less immunosuppression than those arising from *n*-6 PUFA metabolism. The use of low-fat feed, supplemented with *n*-3 PUFAs, reduces protein catabolism and increases IGF-1, particularly 2 or 3 weeks

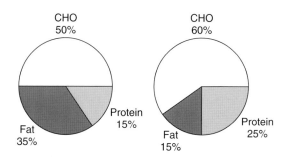

Figure 4 Pie charts demonstrating the difference in proportion of carbohydrate, fat, and protein calories required by burns patients (right) compared to normal patients (left).

postburn. Limiting fat to 15% total calorie intake reduces wound infection rate, improves healing rate, reduces the incidence of pneumonia, improves nutritional markers, and reduces hospital stay. Such benefits have been seen both with and without the addition of *n*-3 PUFAs.

Children A fat intake of 2 or 3% of total calories is the minimum recommended for the prevention of essential fatty acid deficiency in pediatric patients. For intravenous fat administration in infants, a maximum of 4 g/kg lean body weight is suggested.

Protein

Adults Protein calories comprise a significant proportion of the energy requirement of a severely burned patient. Intact protein, rather than amino acids, is associated with better weight maintenance and improved survival. Nitrogen loss must be estimated regularly in a burn patient in order to ensure adequate nitrogen replacement. Total nitrogen loss (TNL) is impossible to measure accurately since 20–30% of nitrogen loss occurs in the exudate from wounds. There is some doubt regarding the use of urinary urea nitrogen (UUN) to estimate total urinary nitrogen (TUN), from which TNL is usually calculated. In healthy, unstressed subjects, urea comprises 80% of the TUN, but ureagenesis is inconsistent after burn injury and varies widely depending on the extent and course of illness. If measurement of TUN is available this will reflect nitrogen loss more accurately:

$$TNL = TUN + 4\,g/day \text{ or } (UUN \times 1.25) + 4\,g/day$$

Total nitrogen loss must then be compared with nitrogen supply (NS) to calculate the nitrogen balance (NB):

$$NB = TNL - NS$$

The aim is to keep a positive balance, and a suitable starting point would be 2 or 3 g protein/kg lean body weight/day; 6.25 g protein is equivalent to 1 g nitrogen. Urinary excretion of 3-methyl histidine has been used as a measure of skeletal protein catabolism. Nitrogen input from blood products is appreciable, accounting for 15% of total nitrogen intake, but is often ignored when calculating nitrogen balance, which therefore underestimates protein intake.

Amino acids play an important role in adaption to burn injury both as gluconeogenic substrates and as substrates for acute phase protein synthesis and wound repair. Arginine flux appears to be increased in burns patients, but plasma levels of arginine and glutamine appear to be greatly reduced following burn injury. These changes have prompted supplementary feeding with particular amino acids. Interest has focused on ornithine α-ketoglutarate (OAK) and its metabolites arginine and glutamine. OAK is also a precursor for proline, the incorporation of which into collagen is a rate-limiting step in collagen synthesis. Arginine also increases collagen deposition, and in animal models of burn injury increased arginine provision has been associated with increased wound healing and improved immune function. There is evidence of a clinically important reduction in healing time and infectious episodes following OAK-, arginine-, or glutamine-supplemented feeding in human studies. Glutamine is the most abundant amino acid in the body and is the major fuel source for the intestine. Its presence prevents villous atrophy and maintains mucosal integrity as well as stimulates blood flow to the gut. Glutamine supplementation of feed reduces the incidence of gram-negative bacteremia in patients with severe burns. The proposed mechanism is the reduction in bacterial translocation across the gut wall; glutamine has been shown to reduce bacterial translocation in a rat model. However, the evidence for a significant clinical effect of arginine- or glutamine-supplemented enteral feed is still equivocal.

Children Protein needs are often estimated by formulas based on lean body weight. To estimate preburn weight, the 50th centile weight for height should be used. For children younger than 1 year old, 3 or 4 g protein/kg lean body weight is suggested to provide adequate nutritional support for graft coverage and healing; this should be reduced to 2.5–3 g protein/kg lean body weight for children 1–3 years of age. In older children, protein requirements are further reduced to 1.5–2.5 g/kg lean body weight. When nitrogen balance is calculated for children, the following formulas have been suggested:

$$\text{Age } 0-4 \text{ years: } TNL = UUN + 2$$

$$\text{Age } 4-10 \text{ years: } TNL = UUN + 3$$

$$\text{Age } >10 \text{ years: } TNL = UUN + 4$$

Protein-enriched diets, containing 25% calories as protein compared to 16% in normal diets, have been associated with improved nitrogen balance, improved immune function, and fewer infective episodes in children with severe burns. Until recently, albumin was a mainstay of fluid requirements in children with severe burns, which contributes to protein provision. However, studies have shown increased morbidity and mortality in critically ill patients given albumin. It seems that the outcome for children with severe burns is no worse if they receive albumin supplementation only when albumin levels decline below 10 g/l (or 15 g/l in the presence of intolerance of enteral feed). Use of albumin should be reviewed regularly.

Vitamins

Specific vitamin requirements in burns patients have not been established, but levels may decline in the hypermetabolic state. As a minimum, the recommended daily allowance should be given following injury. For minor burns of 10–20% body surface area, supplementation with a single multivitamin tablet orally should replace vitamin losses sustained during injury. For larger burns, additional supplementation is advised, especially vitamin C (ascorbic acid), which is of benefit in wound healing and has experimentally been shown to possess free radical scavenging properties that may help to limit tissue damage. A recommended dose is 1 g daily in two divided doses for all patients with major burns; children younger than age 3 years should receive half this dose daily. The essential, fat-soluble, vitamin A may also confer some advantages in wound healing and immunomodulation. A dose of 10 000 IU daily is recommended for all patients with major burns who are older than the age of 3 years; younger children should receive half this amount daily. Wherever possible, both vitamin and micronutrients should be administered by the enteral route. If such supplements are added to total parenteral nutrition (TPN), dosing schedules should take into account the increased bioavailablity via this route and a dose reduction may be advisable. Monitoring of levels of micronutrients should guide replacement by the parenteral route.

Trace Elements

Trace elements are present in the body in amounts less than one part per million by weight; many are essential components of metalloenzymes. Following burn injury, significant amounts of these trace elements may be lost. The acute phase reaction is characterized by a decrease in plasma levels of copper, iron, selenium, and zinc and an increase in the plasma levels of the carrier proteins ferritin and caeruloplasmin. Although iron levels decline following burn trauma, it has been shown that excessive administration of iron is harmful and that low plasma levels of iron appear to be of

benefit in reducing microbial replication. In contrast, increased intravenous administration of copper, zinc, and selenium during the first week following burn injury resulted in fewer complications, an improved leucocyte response, a rapid return of the plasma levels of these trace minerals, as well as a shorter hospital stay. Zinc, copper, and manganese are essential for wound healing; serum zinc levels decrease following stress and burn injury largely due to increased urinary loss. Zinc supplementation, 220 mg daily, should be considered for all patients with major burns. Inclusion of trace elements in both enteral and parenteral nutrition is essential.

Adjunctive Treatments

There is great interest in a pharmacological role for growth hormone (GH) and/or IGF-1 in reversal of the catabolic state and stimulation of anabolic processes. GH stimulates production of IGF-1, which improves amino acid transport and enhances gluconeogenesis from exogenously supplied amino acids. Blood levels of IGF-1 are markedly reduced in burn patients following injury and remain so for the first week, after which levels increase; these changes correlate with IGF binding protein-3 levels. This binding protein prevents plasma proteolysis of IGF-1. GH and IGF-1 have both been used in experimental models of burn injury, and their effectiveness at limiting catabolism and enhancing mucosal proliferation is encouraging. In children GH treatment accelerates donor site healing and increases protein synthesis. GH has also been shown to exert immunomodulatory effects, which may contribute to a reduced incidence of infection. Other growth factors have also been used experimentally and in animal models improve the rate of healing and strength of burn wounds (**Table 5**). However, the role for such hormonal therapies has yet to be firmly established in clinical management plans.

Table 5 Growth factors identified as potential adjunctive therapy in wound healing

Growth hormone
Insulin-like growth factor-1
Epidermal growth factor
Transforming growth factors (α and β)
Platelet-derived growth factor
Fibroblast growth factors (1–7)
Erythropoeitin
Granulocyte macrophage colony-stimulating factor

Nutritional Management

Nutritional management of the burn patient is an important facet of overall management. It is important to involve a multidisciplinary feeding team to manage nutrient intake and organize nutritional assessment. A warm, ambient temperature is essential for reducing fluid and heat loss and keeping the patient comfortable. Metabolic rate increases with discomfort and dressing changes can be a continual source of stress. Thus, analgesic requirements must be adequate or anesthesia administered. There has been a move toward continuing enteral feed in the immediate perioperative period. The risk of aspiration seems to be very low, particularly if jejunal feeding is used. Even when nasogastric feeding is used, starvation times can be minimized without

apparent increased risk. As a result, 60% rather than 6% of caloric requirements can be met on days of surgery/dressing changes.

Route of Feeding

Wherever possible, the enteral route should be used. The American Gastroenterological Association has strongly endorsed this view and stated that routine parenteral nutrition is contraindicated if the enteral route is available. Nasogastric, nasojejunal, and percutaneous enteral access tubes have all been used successfully when feeding is introduced as soon after burn injury as possible. Jejunal feeding is associated with a higher success rate than gastric feeding and may be continued even in the presence of gastric stasis. Increased mortality has been associated with

Table 6 Scheme for nutritional monitoring in a patient with a burn injury

Day 0	Record:
	a. Age
	b. Height
	c. Urine output
	d. Oral fluid/food intake
	
	Investigate:
	a. Plasma prealbumin
	b. Electrolytes and urea
	c. Hemoglobin and hematocrit
	
	Intervention:
	a. If burn area >20%, place nasoenteral feeding tube, nasojejunal if possible,
	   start feeding according to calculated values
	b. Intravenous crystalloid, blood, and colloid according to center protocol
		Estimate:
		a. Ideal body weight
		b. % TBA
		c. Need for dressings/
		   surgery/activity
		d. Fluid loss

Day 2/3	Investigate: a. Indirect calorimetry, energy requirement, calorie balance b. 24-h UUN c. Urinary myoglobin d. Hematocrit Intervention: a. Adjust calorie intake to match calculated need b. If intolerant of enteral feeding, reduce to 10–30 ml/h and start TPN to supplement calorie and nitrogen delivery	
Day 4/5 and twice weekly	Investigate: a. Plasma prealbumin b. Hematocrit c. Indirect calorimetry, as above Intervention: a. Calculate nitrogen balance; adjust nitrogen intake b. Adjust calorie intake	
Day 6/7 and weekly	Investigate: a. Weight b. Trace elements c. Weekly need for dressing changes and/or surgery d. Is enteral absorption improving? Stop/reduce TPN e. Is oral intake increasing? Is enteral supplementation still needed? Intervention: a. Adjust calorie intake to account for (c) above b. Add trace elements if indicated c. Review route(s) of feeding	

the use of central venous catheters and TPN in patients with severe burn injury. This is related to both catheter-associated morbidity and depression of gut function. Glutamine is relatively unstable and has not been included in parenteral formulations. New preparations containing the dipeptide or acetylated form of glutamine will be available in the future that may be of benefit to patients who are dependent on TPN.

Patients with burn injuries greater than 10% are often unable or unwilling to increase their oral intake to meet calorie needs, which are higher by a factor of 1.3 compared to normal. For patients with <20% burns, calorie intake can often be met by supplemental nocturnal feeding through a fine-bore feeding tube. For burns >20%, nasoenteral supplementation is essential. Evidence suggests that the earlier nutrition is started, the greater the attenuation of the hypermetabolic and catabolic response. Early feeding, within 6 h of injury, is optimal. Enteral delivery of glucose and glutamine maintains mucosal integrity and reduces gut ischaemia, as shown by a reduction in arterial-to-intraluminal CO_2 gap. This latter measure can identify an imbalance between calories presented and oxygen delivered to the gut and may be used to adjust enteral feeding levels to prevent excessive delivery.

Some patients are intolerant of enteral feeding, especially those needing mechanical ventilation, who require high levels of opiate analgesia and exogenous norepinephrine support. In these patients, TPN is needed. Wherever possible, a slow, continuous presentation of enteral feed should also be provided to prevent intestinal mucosal atrophy and preserve immune function. Whichever routes are required, calorie provision should be guided by nutritional monitoring of energy expenditure and nitrogen balance.

Nutritional Monitoring

There are a variety of ways to monitor nutritional status in the burn patient; body weight, nutritional intake, nitrogen balance, and laboratory indices all play a role in nutritional assessment. A scheme for continuing nutritional assessment is given in **Table 6**.

Success of the chosen nutrition plan must be monitored and the plan adjusted accordingly. Energy expenditure and nitrogen losses should be measured once or twice weekly for calorie and nitrogen balance calculations. The choice of additional biochemical markers to assess overall nutritional state is difficult and no one marker adequately predicts actual nutritional state at all times during the course of injury. The constitutively produced prealbumin, with its short half-life and independence from exogenous albumin administration, is often used.

Pediatric patients often exhibit growth delays and special attention must be paid to younger children who are less than their ideal body weight at the time of injury. Nutritional support is often required for many weeks after discharge from hospital, and outpatient follow-up of growth in children is essential.

See also: **Amino Acids**: Metabolism. **Cytokines**. **Nutritional Support**: Adults, Enteral.

Further Reading

ASPEN board of directors (2002) Guidelines for the use of parenteral and enteral nutrition in adult and pediatric patients. *Journal of Parenteral and Enteral Nutrition* 26(1, supplement): 88SA–90SA.

Bessey PQ and Wilmore DW (1988) The burned patient. In: Kinney JM, Jeejeebhoy KN, Hill GL *et al.* (eds.) *Nutrition and Metabolism in Patient Care*, pp. 672–700. Philadelphia: WB Saunders.

Cynober L (1989) Amino acid metabolism in thermal burns. *Journal of Parenteral and Enteral Nutrition* 13(2): 196–205.

Dickerson RN, Gervasio JM, Riley ML *et al.* (2002) Accuracy of predictive methods to estimate resting energy expenditure of thermally-injured patients. *Journal of Parenteral and Enteral Nutrition* 26(1): 17–29.

Gamliel Z, DeBiasse MA, and Demling RH (1996) Essential microminerals and their response to burn injury. *Journal of Burn Care and Rehabilitation* 17: 264–272.

Herndon DN, Nguyen TT, and Gilpin DA (1993) Growth factors: Local and systemic. *Archives of Surgery* 128: 1227–1234.

Martindale RG and Cresci GA (2001) Use of immune-enhancing diets in burns. *Journal of Parenteral and Enteral Nutrition* 25(2): S24–S26.

Peck M (2001) American Burn Association Clinical Guidelines. Initial nutrition support of burn patients. *Journal of Burn Care and Rehabilitation* 22: 595–665.

Pratt VC, Tredget EE, Clandin T *et al.* (2002) Alterations in lymphocyte function and relation to phospholipid composition after burn injury in humans. *Critical Care Medicine* 30(8): 1753–1761.

Rettmer RL, Williamson JC, Labbé RF *et al.* (1992) Laboratory monitoring of nutritional status in burn patients. *Clinical Chemistry* 38(3): 334–337.

Rodriguez DJ (1996) Nutrition in patients with severe burns: State of the art. *Journal of Burn Care and Rehabilitation* 17: 62–70.

CAFFEINE

M J Arnaud, Nestle S.A., Vevey, Switzerland

© 2005 Elsevier Ltd. All rights reserved.

During the period 1820–1827, three white crystalline substances called 'caffein' or 'coffein,' 'guaranin,' and 'thein' were isolated from green coffee beans, guarana, and tea, respectively. These substances were shown in 1838–1840 to be identical. Later, caffeine was also discovered in maté prepared from *Ilex paraguariensis* and kola nuts. Since then, caffeine has been shown to be a natural constituent of more than 60 plant species.

Two other related compounds, theophylline and theobromine, have also been isolated from tea and cocoa beans, respectively while a third, paraxanthine, was isolated from human urine (**Figure 1**). By the end of the nineteenth century, all of these methylated xanthines had been synthesized. Caffeine, both natural and synthetic, has been used as a flavoring agent in food and beverages and as an active component of a variety of over-the-counter pharmaceutical products and drugs. A regulation adopted by the European Commission requires the compulsory labeling 'high caffeine content' when soft drinks contain more than 150 mg caffeine per liter.

In addition to natural caffeine obtained by the industrial decaffeination process, caffeine can also be obtained by the methylation of theobromine and also by total chemical synthesis using dimethylcarbamide and malonic acid.

Chemistry

Caffeine (M_r 194.19) is also called, more systematically, 1,3,7-trimethylxanthine, 1,3,7-trimethyl-2,6-dioxopurine, or 3,7-dihydro-1,3,7-trimethyl-l*H*-purine-2,6-dione and has been referred to as a purine alkaloid.

Caffeine is odourless and has a characteristic bitter taste. It is a white powder (density ($d^{18/4}$) 1.23) moderately soluble in organic solvents and water. However, its solubility in water is considerably increased at higher temperatures (1% (w/v) at 15 °C and 10% at 60 °C). Its melting point is 234–239 °C and the temperature of sublimation at atmospheric pressure is 178 °C. Caffeine is a very weak base, reacting with acids to yield readily hydrolyzed salts, and relatively stable in dilute acids and alkali. Caffeine forms unstable salts with acids and is decomposed by strong solutions of caustic alkali.

In aqueous solution, caffeine is nonionized at physiological pH. Dimers as well as polymers have been described. The solubility of caffeine in water is increased by the formation of benzoate, cinnamate, citrate, and salicylate complexes. In plants, chlorogenic acid, coumarin, isoeugenol, indolacetic acid, and anthocyanidin have been shown to complex with caffeine.

Caffeine exhibits an ultraviolet absorption spectrum with a maximum at 274 nm and an absorption coefficient of 9700 in aqueous solution. Upon crystallization from water, silky needles are obtained containing 6.9% water (a 4/5 hydrate).

Determination

Caffeine has traditionally been identified in foods by ultraviolet spectrophotometry of an organic solvent extract after suitable cleanup by column chromatography. Such methods tend to be laborious and may be subject to interference from other ultraviolet-absorbing compounds. Recently, high-performance liquid chromatography has been more extensively used. This technique, often in conjunction with solid phase extraction, can provide accurate data for the determination of caffeine in foods and physiological samples.

Absorption, Distribution, and Elimination

Following oral ingestion, caffeine is rapidly and virtually completely absorbed from the gastrointestinal tract into the bloodstream. Mean plasma

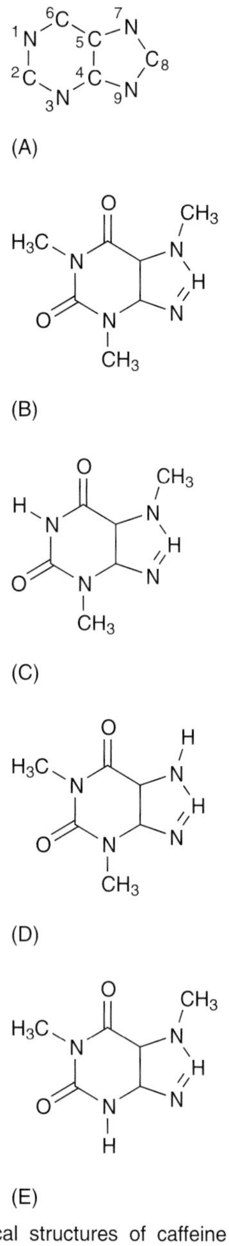

(A)

(B)

(C)

(D)

(E)

Figure 1 Chemical structures of caffeine and the dimethyl-xanthines. (A) Purine ring nomenclature according to E. Fischer; (B) caffeine; (C) theobromine; (D) theophylline; (E) paraxanthine. From Dews (1984).

concentrations of 8–10 mg l^{-1} are observed following oral or intravenous doses of 5–8 mg kg^{-1}. The plasma kinetics of caffeine can be influenced by a number of factors, including the total dose of caffeine, the presence of food in the stomach, and low pH values of drinks, which can modify gastric emptying. Caffeine enters the intracellular tissue water and is found in all body fluids: cerebrospinal fluid, saliva, bile, semen, breast milk, and umbilical cord blood. A higher fraction of the ingested dose of

caffeine is recovered in sweat compared to urine. The fraction of caffeine bound to plasma protein varies from 10 to 30%.

There is no blood–brain barrier and no placental barrier limiting the passage of caffeine through tissues. Therefore, from mother to fetus and to the embryo, an equilibrium can be continuously maintained.

The elimination of caffeine is impaired in neonates because of their immature metabolizing hepatic enzyme systems. For example, plasma half-lives of 65–103 h in neonates have been reported compared to 3–6 h in adults and the elderly.

Gender, exercise, and thermal stress have no effect on caffeine pharmacokinetics in men and women. Cigarette smoking increases the elimination of caffeine, whereas decreases have been observed during late pregnancy or with the use of oral contraceptives and in patients with liver diseases. Drug interactions leading to impaired caffeine elimination are frequently reported.

There is no accumulation of caffeine or its metabolites in the body and less than 2% of caffeine is excreted unchanged in the urine. Some rate-limiting steps in caffeine metabolism, particularly demethylation into paraxanthine that is selectively catalyzed by *CYP1A2*, determine the rate of caffeine clearance and the dose-dependent pharmacokinetics in humans.

Important kinetic differences and variations in the quantitative as well as qualitative metabolic profiles have been shown between species, thus making extrapolation from one species to another very difficult. All of the metabolic transformations include multiple and separate pathways with demethylation to dimethyl- and monomethylxanthines, formation of dimethyl- and monomethylurates, and ring opening yielding substituted diaminouracils (**Figure 2**). The reverse biotransformation of theophylline to caffeine is demonstrated not only in infants but also in adults.

From metabolic studies, an isotopic caffeine breath test has been developed that detects impaired liver function using the quantitative formation of labeled carbon dioxide as an index. From the urinary excretion of an acetylated uracil metabolite, human acetylator phenotype can be easily identified and the analysis of the ratio of the urinary concentrations of other metabolites represents a sensitive test to determine the hepatic enzymatic activities of xanthine oxidase and microsomal 3-methyl demethylation, 7-methyl demethylation, and 8-hydroxylation. Quantitative analyses of paraxanthine urinary metabolites may be used as a biomarker of caffeine intake. Fecal excretion is a minor elimination route, with recovery of only 2–5% of the ingested dose.

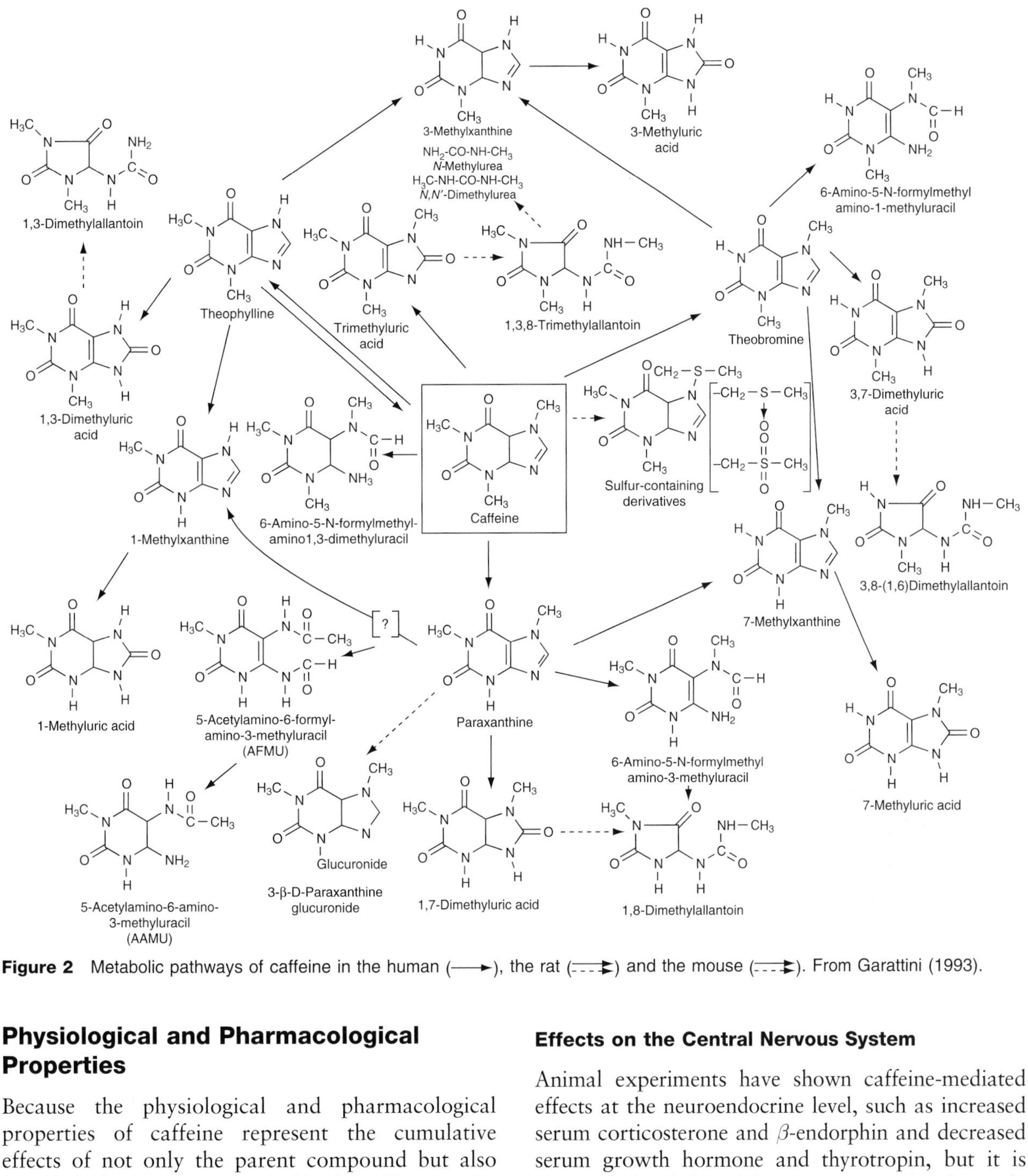

Figure 2 Metabolic pathways of caffeine in the human (———▶), the rat (===▶) and the mouse (---▶). From Garattini (1993).

Physiological and Pharmacological Properties

Because the physiological and pharmacological properties of caffeine represent the cumulative effects of not only the parent compound but also its metabolites, it is quite possible that effects attributed to caffeine *per se* are in fact mediated by one or more of its metabolites. It must also be noted that most of the knowledge about caffeine's effects has been derived from acute administration to fasted subjects submitted to a period of caffeine abstinence in order to ensure low plasma caffeine concentrations. It is thus difficult to extrapolate the results to the usual pattern of caffeine consumption in which most people consume it at different intervals throughout the day and over periods of years.

Effects on the Central Nervous System

Animal experiments have shown caffeine-mediated effects at the neuroendocrine level, such as increased serum corticosterone and β-endorphin and decreased serum growth hormone and thyrotropin, but it is expected that habitual human consumption has only marginal or inconsistent neuroendocrine effects. Caffeine is described as a central nervous system (CNS) stimulant, and the increased formation and release of neurotransmitters such as catecholamines, serotonin, γ-aminobutyric acid, norepinephrine, and acetyl-choline have been reported.

Behavioral effects can be observed in humans after acute and moderate doses of $1–5\ mg\ kg^{-1}$ of caffeine. In these studies, the subjects felt more alert and active with improved cognitive function, including vigilance, learning, memory, and mood state. It was claimed that they would be better able to cope with their jobs when bored or fatigued and after night work and sleep deprivation. Population-based studies of the effect of caffeine intake on cognition showed a positive trend, especially among elderly women. Comparative studies on regular and deprived caffeine consumers suggest that reversal of caffeine withdrawal is a major component of the effects of caffeine on mood and performance.

A dose-dependent delay in sleep onset is found as well as a decrease in total sleep time and an impairment of sleep quality characterized by an increased number of spontaneous awakenings and body movements. In premature infants, sleep organization appears to be unaffected by treatment with 5 mg/kg/day caffeine to prevent apnoea.

The observation that sensitive subjects are more likely to have trembling hands is considered to be a CNS effect and not a direct effect on muscle. Caffeine doses higher than $15 \, mg \, kg^{-1}$ induce headaches, jitteriness, nervousness, restlessness, irritability, tinnitus, muscle twitchings, and palpitations. These symptoms of chronic excessive caffeine intake are part of the criteria used to make the diagnosis of caffeinism. The same symptoms have been reported in adults on abrupt cessation of caffeine use.

With $100–200 \, mg \, kg^{-1}$ doses, mild delirium appears, followed by seizures and death. Although tolerance with low doses led to a pleasant stimulation, alertness, and performance benefits, on withdrawal, headache, drowsiness, fatigue, and anxiety were reported.

Epidemiology and laboratory studies suggest beneficial effects of caffeine consumption in the development of Parkinson's disease and the mechanisms involved may be mediated through adenosine A_{2A} receptors. The role of these receptors in neuronal injury and degeneration, as well as in other diseases such as Alzheimer's disease, has important therapeutic potential but needs further investigation.

Effects on the Cardiovascular System

Caffeine produces a direct stimulation of myocardial tissue leading to an increase in the rate and force of contraction. This direct cardiac effect can be inhibited by a depressant effect on the heart via medullary vagal stimulation. These opposing effects may explain why bradycardia, tachycardia, or no change can be observed in individuals receiving similar doses of caffeine. The traditional clinical view that caffeine induces arrhythmias in humans has not been confirmed by controlled experimental studies.

Caffeine decreases peripheral resistance by direct vasodilatation and increases blood flow to a small extent. This effect results from the relaxation of smooth muscle of blood vessels. For coronary arteries, vasodilatation is also observed in vitro, but the effects of caffeine in human coronary arteries in vivo are unknown. Different effects of caffeine on circulation can be observed in different vascular beds and, for example, the treatment of migraine headaches by caffeine is mediated through the vasoconstriction of cerebral arteries. It has also been shown that caffeine is capable of attenuating postprandial hypotension in patients with autonomic failure.

The observed cardiovascular effects consist of a 5–10% increase in both mean systolic and diastolic blood pressure for 1–3 h. A significant association was found between caffeine-related increase in systolic blood pressure and caffeine-related increase in pain tolerance. However, in contrast to the acute pressor effect reported, several epidemiological studies showed that habitual caffeine intake lowers blood pressure. Heart rate is decreased by 5–10% during the first hour, followed by an increase above baseline during the next 2 h. These effects are not detectable in regular coffee drinkers, suggesting that a complete tolerance can be developed. The tolerance to chronic caffeine intake can explain contradictory results reported in the literature. A few studies suggest that caffeine is partly responsible for the homocysteine-raising effect of coffee. This effect is associated with increased risk of cardiovascular disease, but it is uncertain whether this relation is causal.

Epidemiological studies designed to establish a relationship between caffeine intake and the incidences of myocardial infarction, mortality from ischaemic heart disease, or cerebrovascular accidents have provided conflicting results and have failed to establish a significant correlation.

Effects on Renal Functions

In humans, the administration of a single dose of $4 \, mg \, kg^{-1}$ caffeine increases the urinary excretion of sodium, calcium, magnesium, potassium, chloride, and urine volume. The mechanism of this mild diuresis has been attributed to an increase in renal blood flow, an increased glomerular filtration, and a decrease in tubular reabsorption of sodium ions and other ions. Although these effects appeared more pronounced for a higher acute dose of $10 \, mg \, kg^{-1}$, a review concluded that caffeine consumption stimulates a mild diuresis similar to water. There was no evidence of a fluid–electrolyte imbalance as well as disturbed thermoregulation, and caffeine was not detrimental to exercise performance or health.

Tolerance to the diuretic action of caffeine was demonstrated more than 50 years ago and was shown to develop on chronic caffeine intake so that the clinical significance of hypokalemia and calciuria is difficult to evaluate. Although controversial, some epidemiological studies have implicated caffeine in the increased risk for poor calcium retention. For calcium intakes lower than 750 mg per day, increased rate of bone loss and lower bone density were reported. However, it has been suggested that the effect on bone of high caffeine intake requires a genetic predisposition toward osteoporosis. In individuals who ingest calcium recommended daily allowances, there is no evidence of any effect of caffeine on bone status and calcium economy.

Effects on the Respiratory System

In caffeine-naive subjects, a dose of $4 \, \text{mg kg}^{-1}$ increases the mean respiratory rate. This effect is not found in chronic caffeine ingestion. Several mechanisms have been suggested, such as an increase in pulmonary blood flow, an increased supply of air to the lungs due to the relaxation of bronchiolar and alveolar smooth muscle, an increase in sensitivity of the medullary respiratory center to carbon dioxide, stimulation of the central respiratory drive, an improved skeletal muscle contraction, and an increase in cardiac output.

At higher doses ($7 \, \text{mg kg}^{-1}$), caffeine ingested by trained volunteers alters ventilatory and gas exchange kinetics during exercise, leading to a transient reduction in body carbon dioxide stores.

Effects on Muscles

Caffeine has been shown to have a bronchial and smooth muscle relaxant effect and to improve skeletal muscle contractility. Significant increases in hand tremor and forearm extensor electromyogram were observed in human subjects after the ingestion of $6 \, \text{mg kg}^{-1}$ of caffeine. This effect is more likely due to a CNS stimulatory effect than to direct action on the muscle fibers. Skeletal muscle fatigue can be reversed by high concentrations of caffeine obtained only *in vitro* but not *in vivo*.

Effects on the Gastrointestinal System

Caffeine relaxes smooth muscle of the biliary and gastrointestinal tracts and has a weak effect on peristalsis. However, high doses can produce biphasic responses, with an initial contraction followed by relaxation. Caffeine seems to have no effect on the

lower oesophageal sphincter. The increase in both gastric and pepsin secretions is linearly related to the plasma levels obtained after the administration of a dose of $4–8 \, \text{mg kg}^{-1}$. In the small intestine, caffeine modifies the fluid exchange from a net absorption to a net excretion of water and sodium.

The role of caffeine in the pathogenesis of peptic ulcer and gastrointestinal complaints remains unclear, and no association has been found in clinical and epidemiological studies.

Effects on Energy Metabolism

Acute administration of caffeine produces a 5–25% increase in the basal metabolic rate. Inactive subjects exhibit a greater increase in resting metabolic rate than do exercise-trained subjects. It is concluded that endurance training seems to result in a reduced thermogenic response to a caffeine challenge.

These modifications of energy metabolism were associated with significant increases in serum free fatty acids, glycerol, and lactate concentrations, whereas inconsistent findings were reported for blood glucose levels. Acute administration of caffeine was shown to decrease insulin sensitivity and to impair glucose tolerance, possibly as a result of elevated plasma epinephrine. However, it is not understood why a large and long-term epidemiological study associated significant lower risks for type 2 diabetes in both men and women with total caffeine intake. The lipolytic effect is generally explained by the inhibition of phosphodiesterase, the release of catecholamine, or adenosine receptor antagonism. The increased availability of free fatty acids and their oxidation may have a glycogen-sparing effect. However, increasingly more results do not support the hypothesis that caffeine improves endurance performance by stimulating lipolysis, and some of the ergogenic effects in endurance exercise performance may occur directly at the skeletal muscle and CNS levels. In addition, this effect may be suppressed by the simultaneous ingestion of a high-carbohydrate meal, which is a common practice prior to competition.

Despite the controversy among scientists concerning the ergogenic potential of caffeine on sport performance, it is accepted that caffeine will not improve performance during short-term, high-intensity work, whereas an increase in both work output and endurance in long-term exercise is expected. Most studies also show that the duration and the magnitude of the ergogenic effect of caffeine are greater in nonusers than in users.

Based on the assumption that caffeine may enhance athletic performance, the International

Olympic Committee defined an upper concentration limit of 12 µg/ml in urine samples, above which an athlete was disqualified. However, in the World Anti-Doping Agency Executive Committee Meeting (September 2003), it was observed that the stimulant effect of caffeine is obtained at levels lower than 12. As a consequence, caffeine was removed from the 2004 list of prohibited substances because athletes must be allowed to behave like other people in society and may thus be allowed to drink coffee.

Safety and Toxicology

The acute oral LD_{50} (dose sufficient to kill one-half of the population of tested subjects) of caffeine is more than $200 \, mg \, kg^{-1}$ in rats, $230 \, mg \, kg^{-1}$ in hamsters and guinea pigs, $246 \, mg \, kg^{-1}$ in rabbits, and $127 \, mg \, kg^{-1}$ in mice. The sensitivity of rats to the lethal effects of caffeine increases with age, and higher toxicity is observed in male than in female rats.

Vomiting, abdominal pain, photophobia, palpitations, muscle twitching, convulsions, miosis, and unconsciousness were described in several reports of nonfatal caffeine poisonings in children who ingested $80 \, mg \, kg^{-1}$ caffeine. In several fatal accidental caffeine poisonings, cold chills, stomach cramps, tetanic spasms, and cyanosis were reported. The likely lethal dose in adult humans has been estimated to be approximately 10 g, which corresponds roughly to $150–200 \, mg \, kg^{-1}$. With daily doses of $110 \, mg \, kg^{-1}$ given via intragastric cannula to female rats over 100 days, hypertrophy of organs such as the salivary gland, liver, heart, and kidneys was reported. Caffeine also induced thymic and testicular atrophy. Developmental and reproductive toxicity was associated with high, single daily doses of caffeine. The no-effect level for teratogenicity is $40 \, mg \, kg^{-1}$ caffeine per day in the rat, although delayed sternebral ossification can be observed at lower doses. This effect has been shown to be reversed in the postnatal period. Available epidemiological evidence suggests that maternal caffeine consumption does not cause morphological malformation in the fetus. Caffeine intake has been linked with reduced fetal size in some studies, particularly when intake was more than 600 mg per day, whereas others have not shown an impact on growth. High daily levels given as divided doses in rats were less toxic than when given as a single dose, in which case reduced fetal body weight was the only effect observed.

Caffeine at high concentration levels has mutagenic effects in bacteria and fungi and causes chromosomal damage in vitro. However, there is consensus that caffeine is not mutagenic in higher animals.

An epidemiological study showed no chromosomal aberrations in lymphocytes of normal, caffeine-exposed people, and other studies reported an increased frequency of micronucleated blood cells and the absence of mutagenic compounds in urine. In long-term studies, caffeine was shown to have no carcinogenic potential in rodents. Caffeine has not been classified as carcinogenic in animals or humans by the International Agency for Research on Cancer.

Therapeutic Uses

The most extensively investigated and most firmly established clinical application of caffeine is the control of neonatal apnoea in premature infants. The respirogenic properties of theophylline were first reported, and caffeine is increasingly being used as a substitute for theophylline because of its wider therapeutic index. For infants with a body weight of 2.5 kg, the therapeutic loading doses varied from 5 to $30 \, mg \, kg^{-1}$, followed by a maintenance dose of $3 \, mg \, kg^{-1}$ per day. Plasma caffeine levels must be controlled carefully to reach $10–20 \, mg \, l^{-1}$.

Because of the bronchial muscle relaxant effect, caffeine is used in chronic obstructive pulmonary disease and for the treatment of asthma. The use of caffeine in the treatment of children with minimal brain dysfunction, to increase the duration of electroconvulsive therapy-induced seizure, for allergic rhinitis, as well as for atopic dermatitis has also been described. Recently, caffeine has been used as a diagnostic test for malignant hyperthermia and in the diagnosis of neuroleptic malignant syndrome, a complication of neuroleptic therapy.

Caffeine is found in many drug preparations, both prescription and over-the-counter. Caffeine is present in drugs used as stimulants, pain relievers, diuretics, and cold remedies. When used as an analgesic adjuvant, the potency of the analgesic drug is significantly enhanced by the addition of caffeine.

Although caffeine has been shown to promote thermogenesis in humans, it is no longer allowed as an ingredient in weight-control products in the US market because long-term clinical studies demonstrate that it does not help those wishing to lose weight.

Biochemical Mechanisms of Action

The physiological and pharmacological properties of caffeine cannot be explained by a single biochemical mechanism. Three principal hypotheses have been investigated to explain the diverse actions of caffeine.

The first biochemical effect described was the inhibition of phosphodiesterase, the enzyme that catalyzes the breakdown of cyclic adenosine 3′,5′-phosphate (cAMP). Caffeine was shown to increase cAMP concentrations in various tissues. This inhibition occurs at large concentrations (millimolar range) and is of limited importance with regard to the physiological effects of caffeine at levels at which it is normally consumed.

Calcium translocation is the second mechanism frequently suggested from experiments using skeletal muscles. However, high concentrations of caffeine are also necessary to modify intracellular calcium ion storage.

In the plasma, increased levels of β-endorphin, epinephrine, norepinephrine, corticosterone, ACTH, renin, and angiotensin I and decreased levels of growth hormone, thyroxine, triiodothyronine, and thyrotropin were reported with high caffeine doses. The mechanisms responsible for these various effects are largely unknown, and the mediation of adenosine receptors is suggested. The antagonism of benzodiazepine at the receptor level is observed at lower caffeine concentrations (0.5–0.7 mM) than those required for phosphodiesterase inhibition.

The third mechanism, antagonism of the endogenous adenosine, is the most plausible mode of action because caffeine exerts its antagonism at micromolar levels. Its main metabolite, paraxanthine, is as potent as caffeine in blocking adenosine receptors. Caffeine is more potent at A_{2A} receptors and less potent at A_3 receptors compared to A_1 and A_{2B} receptors. An upregulation of adenosine receptor is the postulated biochemical mechanism of caffeine tolerance.

Adenosine receptor antagonism appears to be the mechanism that explains most of the effects of caffeine on CNS activity, intestinal peristalsis, respiration, blood pressure, lipolysis, catecholamine release, and renin release. However, some effects, such as opiate antagonism or effects that are similar to those of adenosine, must be mediated by other mechanisms, such as the potentiation by caffeine of inhibitors of prostaglandin synthesis.

See also: **Brain and Nervous System**. **Diabetes Mellitus**: Etiology and Epidemiology. **Energy**: Balance; Requirements. **Exercise**: Beneficial Effects; Diet and Exercise. **Sports Nutrition**. **Tea**.

Further Reading

Armstrong LE (2002) Caffeine, body fluid–electrolyte balance and exercise performance. *International Journal of Sport Nutrition and Exercise Metabolism* 12: 205–222.

Arnaud MJ (1987) The pharmacology of caffeine. *Progress in Drug Research* 31: 273–313.

Clarke RJ and Macrae R (eds.) (1988) Physiology. In *Coffee*, vol. 3. London: Elsevier.

Clarke RJ and Vitzhum OG (eds.) (2001) *Coffee. Recent Developments*. London: Blackwell Science.

Debry G (1994) *Coffee and Health*. Paris: John Libbey Eurotext.

Dews PB (ed.) (1984) *Caffeine*. Berlin: Springer-Verlag.

Dews PB, O'Brien CP, and Bergman J (2002) Caffeine: Behavioural effects of withdrawal and related issues. *Food and Chemical Toxicology* 40: 1257–1261.

Garattini S (ed.) (1993) *Caffeine, Coffee and Health*. New York: Raven Press.

Graham TE (2001) Caffeine and exercise, metabolism, endurance and performance. *Sports Medicine* 31: 785–807.

James JE (1991) *Caffeine and Health*. London: Academic Press.

Lorist MM and Tops M (2003) Caffeine, fatigue, and cognition. *Brain and Cognition* 53: 82–94.

Nawrot P, Jordan S, Eastwood J *et al.* (2003) Effects of caffeine on human health. *Food Additives and Contaminants* 20: 1–30.

Schmitt JAJ (2001) *Serotonin, Caffeine and Cognition. Psychopharmacological Studies in Human Cognitive Functioning*. Maastricht, The Netherlands: Neuropsych.

Snel J and Lorist MM (eds.) (1998) *Nicotine, Caffeine and Social Drink, Behaviour and Brain Function*. Amsterdam: Harwood Academic.

World Health Organization–International Agency for Research on Cancer (1991) *IARC Monographs on the Evaluation of Carcinogenic Risks to Humans: Coffee, Tea, Mate, Methylxanthines and Methylglyoxal*, vol. 51. Lyon, France: WHO–IARC.

CALCIUM

L H Allen, University of California at Davis, Davis, CA, USA
J E Kerstetter, University of Connecticut, Storrs, CT, USA

© 2005 Elsevier Ltd. All rights reserved.

Calcium is an essential nutrient. Although most of the calcium in the body is found in bones and teeth, the other 1% has critical, life-sustaining functions.

Most people in the world, including those in industrialized countries, fail to consume the recommended amounts of calcium, which will ultimately result in poor bone health and increase the risk of osteoporosis. Adequate calcium intake is critical to the achievement of peak bone mass in the first several decades of life, the retention of bone during middle adulthood, and the minimization of bone loss during the last several decades. Without adequate intake, the intestine, bone, and renal systems have intricate ways of retaining more calcium and normalizing serum calcium levels. These three primary tissues of calcium homeostasis (intestine, bone, and kidneys) are dynamic in their handling of calcium, reacting to dietary intake, physiological need, or disease processes. This article discusses calcium absorption, regulation, function, metabolism, and excretion as well as the changes in calcium physiology during the lifespan.

Absorption and Transport

Intake and Distribution

The dietary intake of calcium in the United States is approximately 20 mmol (600–1200 mg) per day unless supplements are consumed. Approximately 73% of dietary calcium is supplied from milk products, 9% from fruits and vegetables, 5% from grains, and the remaining 12% from all other sources. Approximately 25% of women take a nutritional supplement that contains calcium, but supplement use by men and children is much lower.

Approximately 25–50% of dietary calcium is absorbed and delivered to the exchangeable calcium pool. Of the 25–30 mol (1000–1200 g) of calcium in the body, 99% is found in the skeleton and teeth. The remaining 1% is in the blood, extracellular fluid, muscle, and other tissues. The extracellular pool of calcium turns over 20–30 times per day in adults, whereas bone calcium turns over every 5 or 6 years. A remarkably large amount is filtered through the kidneys, approximately 250 mmol (10 000 mg) per day, of which approximately 98% is reabsorbed, so that urinary excretion of the mineral is only 2.5–5 mmol (100–200 mg) per day (**Figure 1**).

Intestinal Calcium Absorption

The efficiency of dietary calcium absorption depends on two major factors: its interaction with other dietary constituents and physiological/pathological factors. Dietary factors that reduce the total amount of

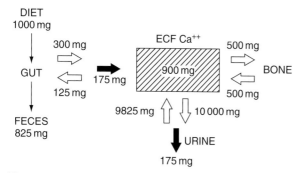

Figure 1 Daily calcium turnover.

calcium absorbed by the intestine include phosphate, oxalate, phytate, fiber, and very low calcium intakes, whereas those that increase absorption include protein (or specific amino acids, lysine and arginine) and lactose in infants. The physiological/pathological factors that decrease intestinal calcium absorption include low serum $1,25(OH)_2$ vitamin D (the form of the vitamin that effects calcium absorption), chronic renal insufficiency, hypoparathyroidism, aging, and vitamin D deficiency, whereas increased absorption is observed during growth, pregnancy, primary hyperparathyroidism, sarcoidosis, and estrogen and growth hormone administration. The interindividual variability in intestinal calcium absorption is very high for reasons that are not entirely clear. On tightly controlled diets, a homogenous group of subjects can have intestinal calcium absorptions ranging from 10 to 50%.

Dietary calcium is complexed to food constituents such as proteins, phosphate, and oxalate, from which it needs to be released prior to absorption. The role of gastric acid (or the lack thereof induced by commonly used proton pump inhibiting drugs) in intestinal calcium absorption is not well established, although achlorhydria can impair absorption in the fasted state.

Calcium crosses the intestinal mucosa by both active and passive transport. The active process is saturable, transcellular, and occurs throughout the small intestine. The transcellular pathway is a multistep process, starting with the entry of luminal calcium into the enterocyte (possibly via a calcium channel) and translocation of calcium from the microvillus border of the apical plasma membrane to the basolateral membrane followed by extrusion out of the enterocyte. Calbindin, a calcium binding protein that is regulated by the hormonal form of vitamin D, $1,25(OH)_2D_3$, affects every step in the movement of calcium through the enterocyte, including entry into the cell, movement in the cell interior, and transfer into the lamina propria. Although details of the movement of calcium through intestinal cells are still under investigation, it appears that the vitamin D-dependent calcium binding protein calbindin-D_{9k} and the plasma membrane calcium-pumping ATPase 1b (PMCA1b) are critical transport molecules in the cytoplasm and basolateral membrane, respectively. The active transport pathway is predominant at lower levels of calcium intake, and it becomes more efficient in calcium deficiency or when intakes are low and also when calcium requirements are high during infancy, adolescence, and pregnancy. It becomes less efficient in vitamin D-deficient individuals and in elderly women after menopause.

The passive transport pathway is nonsaturable and paracellular. It occurs throughout the small intestine and is unaffected by calcium status or parathyroid hormone (PTH). It is relatively independent of $1,25(OH)_2D_3$, although this metabolite has been found by some investigators to increase the permeability of the paracellular pathway. A substantial amount of calcium is absorbed by passive transport in the ileum due to the relatively slow passage of food through this section of the intestine. The amount of calcium absorbed by passive transport will be proportional to the intake and bioavailability of calcium consumed.

Fractional calcium absorption increases in response to low intake but varies throughout life. It is highest during infancy (60%) and puberty (25–35%), stable at approximately 25% in adults, and then declines with age (by approximately 2% per decade after menopause). There is little difference in calcium absorption efficiency between Caucasians and African Americans. The lower urinary calcium and better calcium conservation in African Americans probably contributes to their higher bone mineral density.

Storage

The skeleton acts as the storage site for calcium. Bone calcium exists primarily in the form of hydroxyapatite $(Ca_{10}(PO_4)_6(OH)_2)$, and this mineral comprises 40% of bone weight. In the short term, the release of calcium from bone serves to maintain serum calcium concentrations. In the longer term, however, persistent use of skeletal calcium for this purpose without adequate replenishment will result in loss of bone density. The storage of very small amounts of calcium in intracellular organelles and its subsequent release into cytosol acts as an intracellular signal for a variety of functions.

Between 60 and 80% of the variance in peak bone mass is explained by genetics, including polymorphisms in the vitamin D–receptor gene and in genes responsible for insulin-like growth factor-1 (IGF-1) and collagen production.

Metabolism and Excretion

Regulation by Hormones

The concentration of ionized calcium in serum is closely regulated because it has profound effects on the function of nerves and muscles, blood clotting, and hormone secretion. The principal regulators of calcium homeostasis in humans and most terrestrial vertebrates are PTH and the active form of vitamin D, $1,25(OH)_2$ vitamin D_3 (**Figure 2**).

PTH is a single-chain polypeptide that is released from the parathyroid when there is a decrease in the calcium concentration in extracellular fluid. The calcium-sensing

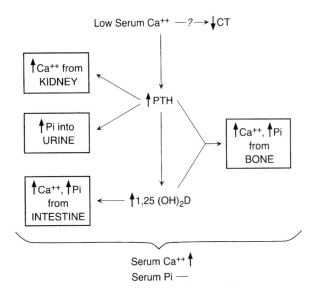

Figure 2 Hormonal regulation of calcium metabolism.

receptor (acting as the thermostat for calcium) is found on the parathyroid gland, where it detects small perturbations in serum ionized calcium. The decline in serum calcium induces an increase in PTH secretion. PTH has the effect of restoring extracellular calcium concentrations by stimulating the resorption of bone to release calcium, by increasing the renal reabsorption of calcium, and by enhancing the renal conversion of $25(OH)D_3$ to the active, hormonal form of the vitamin, $1,25(OH)_2$ vitamin D_3. The active form of vitamin D then increases the synthesis of intestinal calcium binding protein (CaBP), leading to more efficient intestinal calcium absorption. PTH release is inhibited when serum calcium and $1,25(OH)_2$ vitamin D_3 increase or when serum phosphate is decreased. The highly regulated interactions among PTH, calcium, $1,25(OH)_2$ vitamin D_3, and phosphate maintain blood calcium levels remarkably constant despite significant changes in calcium intake or absorption, bone metabolism, or renal functions. The extracellular calcium concentration is the most important regulator of PTH secretion and occurs on a minute-by-minute basis. Acute PTH administration leads to release of the rapidly turning over pool of calcium near the bone surface. Chronic administration of PTH increases osteoclast cell number and activity. Interestingly and paradoxically, intermittent PTH administration is anabolic, increasing formation of trabecular bone. In the kidney, PTH has three major functions: It increases calcium reabsorption, inhibits phosphate reabsorption, and enhances the synthesis of the active form of vitamin D. All of these actions are designed to defend against hypocalcemia.

There are two sources of vitamin D: the diet (where it is found as the fortificant vitamin D_2 or natural D_3) or synthesis in skin during exposure to ultraviolet radiation (sunlight). The vitamin enters the circulation and is transported on a vitamin D binding protein to the liver, where it is hydroxylated to 25(OH) cholecalciferol, which leaves the liver, is bound again to the binding protein in the circulation, and enters the kidney where it is hydroxylated again to $1,25(OH)_2D_3$, the most active metabolite of the vitamin. The primary biological effect of $1,25(OH)_2D_3$ is to defend against hypocalcemia by increasing the efficiency of intestinal calcium absorption and by stimulating bone resorption. $1,25(OH)_2D_3$ interacts with the vitamin D receptor on the osteoblasts, and via RANKL/RANK it stimulates the maturation of osteoclasts that function to dissolve bone, releasing calcium into the extracellular space. The recently discovered RANK ligand, a member of the tumor necrosis factor superfamily, and its two receptors (RANK and osteoprotegerin) are pivotal regulators of osteoclastic bone resorption, both *in vivo* and *in vitro*. More of the active metabolite is produced during calcium deficiency or after a low calcium intake in order to restore serum calcium by increasing intestinal calcium absorption, renal calcium reabsorption, and bone turnover.

Serum vitamin D concentrations decline in winter and are generally related to vitamin D intake and sunlight exposure. When serum $25(OH)D_3$ concentrations decline below 110 nmol/l, PTH levels increase, contributing to the bone loss that occurs in vitamin D deficiency and that is evident in northern Europe, the United States, Japan, and Canada during winter months. Rickets is becoming a more recognized health problem, particularly in infants of African American mothers who are not taking vitamin D supplements or consuming adequate amounts of vitamin D-fortified milk and who are exclusively breast-feeding their infants. In the US national nutrition survey conducted in the 1990s, 42% of African American women had low 25(OH) vitamin D concentrations in plasma. Thus, vitamin D deficiency is more prevalent than once believed, and it is particularly a risk for the elderly due to their reduced capacity for synthesizing vitamin D precursors in their skin, in those who are infirm and/or in nursing homes or living at more northern or southern latitudes, or in other situations in which the skin is not exposed to sunlight. The result of vitamin D deficiency is normal serum calcium and elevated PTH and alkaline phosphatase. The secondary hyperparathyroidism causes increased osteoclastic activity, calcium loss from bone, and ultimately bone loss.

Several other hormones also affect calcium metabolism. Notably, estrogens are necessary for the maintenance of balance between bone resorption and accretion.

The decrease in serum estrogen concentrations at approximately the time of menopause is the primary factor contributing to the elevated rate of bone resorption that occurs at this stage of life and that is the primary contributory factor to osteoporosis. Estrogen treatment will reduce bone resorption within a few weeks and subsequently lead to higher serum concentrations of PTH and $1,25(OH)_2D_3$ and improved intestinal absorption and renal reabsorption of calcium. Testosterone also inhibits bone resorption, and lack of this hormone can cause osteoporosis in men. Glucocorticoids, sometimes used to treat conditions such as osteoid arthritis, inflammatory bowel disease, and asthma, inhibit both osteoclastic and osteoblastic activity, impair collagen and cartilage synthesis, and reduce calcium absorption. Consequently, excessive bone loss often results from glucocorticoid treatment or occurs when excessive amounts of the hormone are secreted, such as in Cushing's disease. Oral calcium supplements should be considered for patients receiving exogenous glucocorticoids. Thyroid hormones stimulate bone resorption so that bone abnormalities occur in both hyper- and hypothyroidism. Growth hormone stimulates cartilage formation, the formation of $1,25(OH)_2D$, and intestinal calcium absorption. Insulin stimulates collagen production by osteoblasts and impairs the renal reabsorption of calcium.

Excretion

Ionized calcium in the plasma is freely filtered by the kidney so that very large amounts enter the kidney each day, but 99.8% of this calcium is reabsorbed throughout the nephron. Regulated active transport occurs in the distal convoluted tubule and involves vitamin D, CaBP, and PTH. Typically, approximately 2.5–6 mmol (100–240 mg) of calcium is excreted in urine daily.

Dietary calcium has a relatively small impact on urinary calcium (e.g., only 6–8% of an increase in dietary calcium intake will appear in the urine). The major food components that affect urinary calcium are protein, phosphorus, caffeine, and sodium. For each 50-g increment in dietary protein, approximately 1.5 mmol (60 mg) of additional calcium is lost in urine. The higher amounts of phosphorus consumed concurrently with a high-protein diet can blunt, but not eliminate, this phenomenon. Dietary phosphorus (as well as intravenously administered phosphorus) increases PTH synthesis and subsequently stimulates renal calcium reabsorption and reduces the urinary excretion of calcium. Caffeine causes a reduction in renal reabsorption of calcium and a subsequently increased loss of urinary calcium soon after it is consumed. It has been shown repeatedly in animals and humans that dietary sodium, in the form of salt (NaCl), increases urinary calcium excretion. On average, for every 100 mmol (2300 mg) of sodium excreted in urine, there is an approximately 0.6–1 mmol (24–40 mg) loss of calcium in free-living healthy populations of various ages. Because most of the urinary calcium is of bone origin, it is commonly hypothesized that those nutrients or food components that are hypercalciuretic are also detrimental to the skeleton. On the other hand, thiazide medications are hypocalciuric and, as such, may have modest positive effects on bone.

Metabolic Functions

The most obvious role of calcium is to provide structural integrity and strength in bones and teeth. Approximately 99% of the total body calcium content is used for this purpose. Bone also serves as a reservoir of calcium that can be drawn upon when serum calcium concentrations decline. The remaining 1% of the body's calcium is contained in blood, extracellular space, muscle, and other tissues, in which calcium concentrations are kept relatively constant. The maintenance of constant serum calcium concentrations at approximately 2.5 mmol/l is critical for a number of cellular functions.

The extracellular concentration of calcium is in the 10^{-3} M range, whereas in the cytosol it is approximately 10^{-6} M. Almost all of the intracellular calcium is bound within organelles such as the nucleus, endoplasmic reticulum, and vesicles. Cytosolic calcium concentrations are very low and influenced greatly by release of some calcium from cellular organelles. Therefore, a small change in the release of calcium from intracellular sites or transport across the cell membrane results in a relatively large change in cytosolic calcium concentration. Binding of a hormone or a growth factor to a plasma membrane receptor increases inositol triphosphate release, which in turn increases the free intracellular calcium concentration. The ionized calcium then binds to calmodulin, followed by a conformation change in the protein to trigger cellular events such as muscle contraction, nerve conduction, cell movement and differentiation, cell division, cell-to-cell communication, and secretion of hormones such as insulin. In these roles, calcium acts as an intracellular messenger.

Calcium may play a role in energy regulation and risk of obesity. Dietary calcium regulation of circulating $1,25(OH)_2D_3$ in turn regulates the concentration of calcium in adipocytes. When adipocyte intracellular calcium concentration increases, this promotes the expression of lipogenic genes, and fat breakdown is reduced leading to accumulation of lipid in adipocytes. Through this pathway, low-calcium diets appear to promote fat deposition, whereas high-calcium intakes afford some protection from obesity.

Changes in Calcium Metabolism during the Life Span

The total body calcium content of the newborn infant is approximately 0.75 mol (30 g), which increases during growth to approximately 1000 g in adult women and 1200 g in adult men. This represents an average daily accumulation of approximately 2.5–3.7 mmol (100–150 mg) from infancy to adulthood.

The efficiency of calcium absorption is highest during infancy (approximately 60%), and the amount absorbed from breast milk does not appear to be affected by calcium consumed in solid foods. During the growth spurt of adolescence, calcium retention and accretion increase to peak at approximately 200–300 mg per day in girls and boys, respectively. It involves the action of growth hormone, IGF-1, and sex steroids. The onset of menstruation in girls is associated with a rapid decline in bone formation and resorption. Intestinal calcium absorption is predictably more efficient during the growth spurt and also decreases subsequently. Importantly, it is thought that calcium intakes during the period of growth can affect the peak bone mass achieved and therefore influence the amount of bone mineral remaining when osteoporosis begins in later life. Bone mass may continue to accumulate up to approximately age 30 years, although the amount gained is relatively small after age 18 years.

During pregnancy, a relatively small amount of calcium, approximately 625–750 mmol, is transported to the fetus. Most of this calcium is thought to be obtained through greater efficiency of maternal intestinal calcium absorption, possibly induced by increases in $1,25(OH)_2D_3$ production. For this reason, a higher calcium intake during pregnancy is probably not required.

Most studies have reported that there is no increase in intestinal calcium absorption during lactation even when dietary intake of the mineral is relatively low. Changes in biochemical markers and kinetic studies using isotopes indicate that the source of much of the calcium secreted in breast milk is the maternal skeleton, as well as more efficient renal reabsorption and subsequently lower urinary excretion of the mineral. Bone calcium is restored at the end of lactation as the infant is weaned, when ovarian function returns and menstruation resumes. At this time, intestinal calcium absorption increases, urinary calcium remains low, and bone turnover rates decline to normal levels. There is no strong evidence that lactation per se or maternal calcium intake during lactation affect later risk of osteoporosis in women. Thus, there is no strong rationale for increasing maternal calcium intake during lactation. Breast milk calcium concentration is relatively unaffected by maternal intake, and it remains stable throughout lactation.

Menopause begins a period of bone loss that extends until the end of life. It is the major contributor to higher rates of osteoporotic fractures in older women. The decrease in serum estrogen concentrations at menopause is associated with accelerated bone loss, especially from the spine, for the next 5 years, during which approximately 15% of skeletal calcium is lost. The calcium loss by women in early menopause cannot be prevented unless estrogen therapy is provided. Calcium supplements alone are not very helpful in preventing postmenopausal bone loss. Upon estrogen treatment, bone resorption is reduced and the intestinal calcium absorption and renal reabsorption of calcium are both increased. Similarly, amenorrheic women have reduced intestinal calcium absorption, high urinary calcium excretion, and lower rates of bone formation (compared to eumenorrheic women). In both men and women, there is a substantial decline in intestinal absorption of calcium in later life.

Calcium Deficiency

When calcium absorption is chronically low, because of low intakes, poor bioavailability, or conditions that impair intestinal absorption, there is a decrease in the serum ionized calcium concentration. This in turn stimulates the release of PTH, which returns serum calcium to normal by increasing renal calcium reabsorption, stimulating the renal production of $1,25(OH)_2D_3$, and inducing bone reabsorption. The result of long-term calcium deficiency is accelerated bone loss in older individuals or the inability to fully achieve peak bone mass in younger individuals.

Dietary Sources

Food Sources

The majority of dietary calcium in industrialized countries comes from milk products; one serving (i.e., 250 ml milk or yogurt or 40 g cheese) contains approximately 7.5 mmol (300 mg). Nondairy sources (fruits, vegetables, and grain products) supply approximately 25% of total calcium. When substantial amounts of grains are consumed, for example, in breads or as maize products, these can be important sources, although the calcium in cereals tends to be less bioavailable than that in dairy products. Other foods high in calcium include tofu set with a calcium salt, kale, broccoli, and, increasingly, calcium-fortified juices and cereals. No matter what the source, a high percentage of people in both industrialized and less wealthy countries fail to meet recommended guidelines for optimal calcium intake.

Bioavailability

Several dietary constituents decrease the bioavailability of calcium in food. Increasing fiber intake by, for example, replacing white flour by whole wheat flour in a typical Western diet has long been associated with negative calcium balance even when calcium intakes meet recommended levels. Likewise, the fiber in fruits and vegetables can cause negative calcium balance. In cereals, phytic acid is the main constituent of fiber that binds calcium, making it unavailable for absorption. The fermentation of bread during leavening reduces phytate content substantially, making calcium more bioavailable. In fruits and vegetables, the uronic acids in hemicellulose are strong calcium binders, as is the oxalic acid present in high concentrations in foods such as spinach. Calcium bioavailability from beans is approximately half and that from spinach approximately one-tenth of the bioavailability from milk. In contrast, calcium absorption from low-oxalate vegetables, such as kale, broccoli, and collard greens, is as good as that from milk. The difference in calcium absorption between the various forms of supplements is not large.

Dietary fat does not affect calcium absorption except in individuals with diseases that impair fat malabsorption (e.g., short bowel syndrome, celiac disease, and pancreatitis). In these conditions, the calcium forms an insoluble and unabsorbable 'soap' with the unabsorbed fat in the alkaline lumen of the small intestine, potentially resulting in impaired bone mineralization. In addition, the luminal calcium is not available to precipitate the oxalates, meaning that the free oxalates will be hyperabsorbed leading to increased risk for renal oxalate stones. Neither dietary phosphorus nor a wide range of phosphorus-to-calcium ratios affect intestinal calcium absorption in very low-birth-weight infants and adults.

Lactose improves calcium absorption in young infants, in whom absorption of calcium is predominantly by passive transport. In adults, the presence of lactose in the diet has little effect on the efficiency of calcium absorption.

Effects of High Calcium Intakes

Calcium can inhibit the absorption of both heme iron (found in meat, fish, and poultry) and non-heme iron. The mechanism by which this occurs remains controversial, but the inhibition probably occurs within the mucosal cells rather than in the intestinal lumen. This interaction is of concern because calcium supplements are taken by many women who may have difficulty maintaining adequate iron stores. Approximately 300–600 mg of calcium, as a supplement or in foods, reduces the absorption of both heme and non-heme iron by approximately 30–50% when consumed in the same meal. The inhibitory effect on iron absorption is inversely related to iron status so that it is relatively unimportant above a serum ferritin concentration of approximately 50–60 µg/l. Thus, consideration should be given to monitoring the iron status of menstruating women with low iron stores who take calcium supplements. There is no inhibitory effect when calcium and iron supplements are consumed together in the absence of food, and inhibition may be less with calcium citrate.

In the past, it was common to restrict dietary calcium in patients with a history of calcium oxalate stones. However, recent data suggest that a severe calcium restriction in patients with oxalate stones is not only ineffective but also can lead to bone demineralization. For the prevention of recurrent stone formation, a diet restricted in oxalate, sodium, and animal protein is probably most effective. Only if absorptive hypercalciuria is present should a moderate calcium restriction be imposed.

Long-term consumption of approximately 1500–2000 mg calcium per day is safe for most individuals, although there will be some reduction in the efficiency of iron absorption. However, higher intakes from supplements (62.5 mmol or 2.5 g per day) can result in milk–alkali syndrome (MAS), with symptoms of hypercalcemia, renal insufficiency, metabolic alkalosis, and severe alterations in metabolism. Based on risk of developing MAS, the upper limit for calcium intake is 2500 mg per day for adults and children.

See also: **Bioavailability**. **Bone**. **Dairy Products**. **Lactation**: Dietary Requirements. **Pregnancy**: Nutrient Requirements; Safe Diet for Pregnancy. **Vitamin D**: Physiology, Dietary Sources and Requirements; Rickets and Osteomalacia.

Further Reading

Bronner F (1992) Symposium: Current concepts of calcium absorption. *Journal of Nutrition* 122: 641–686.

Heaney RP (2003) How does bone support calcium homeostasis? *Bone* 33: 264–268.

Institute of Medicine (1997) *Dietary Reference Intakes for Calcium, Phosphorus, Magnesium, Vitamin D and Fluoride*. Washington, DC: National Academy Press.

Prentice A (2000) Calcium in pregnancy and lactation. *Annual Reviews in Nutrition* 20: 249–272.

Prentice A (2004) Diet, nutrition and the prevention of osteoporosis. *Public Health Nutrition* 7: 227–243.

Specker BL (2004) Nutrition influences bone development from infancy through toddler years. *Journal of Nutrition* 134: 691S–695S.

Wasserman RH and Fullmer CS (1995) Vitamin D and intestinal calcium transport: Facts, speculations and hypotheses. *Journal of Nutrition* 125: 1971S–1979S.

Weaver CM and Heaney RP (1999) Calcium. In: Shils ME, Olson JA, Shike M *et al.* (eds.) *Modern Nutrition in Health and Disease*. Philadelphia: Lea & Febiger.

Zemel MB and Miller SL (2003) Dietary calcium and dairy modulation of adiposity and obesity risk. In *Primer on the Metabolic Bone Diseases and Disorders of Mineral Metabolism*, 5th edn. Washington, DC: American Society for Bone and Mineral Research.

Calories *see* **Energy**: Balance; Requirements. **Energy Expenditure**: Indirect Calorimetry; Doubly Labeled Water

CANCER

Contents

Epidemiology and Associations Between Diet and Cancer

G A Colditz, Harvard Medical School, Boston, MA, USA

© 2005 Elsevier Ltd. All rights reserved.

Sources of Evidence Linking Diet and Cancer

Laboratory scientists have known since the early twentieth century that various nutritional manipulations can influence the occurrence of tumors in animals. Despite this discovery of the relationship between diet and cancer in animals, widespread interest in the study of diet and cancer in humans did not develop until more recently when the large international differences in cancer rates were correlated with variations in dietary factors. In fact, investigators have found strong correlations between estimated per capita fat consumption and breast cancer rates internationally, raising the possibility that dietary fat may have an important role in the etiology of breast cancer. Other observations such as those demonstrating that migrating populations adopted, sooner or later, the cancer rates of their new host population strengthened the evidence that international differences were the result not of genes, but of noninherited factors, including diet. The study designs used to investigate diet and cancer in humans are discussed below.

Descriptive Studies

Rates of cancer show large differences between countries for many malignancies. International correlations compare disease rates with lifestyle factors such as per capita consumption of specific dietary factors.

Age-adjusted rates of colon and breast cancer are up to five times higher in some countries than others. Dakar in Senegal (0.6) and Poona (3.1) and Bombay (3.5) in India, have the lowest incidence rates of colon cancer per 100 000 males; in contrast, the USA has the highest recorded rates of 32.2 in Connecticut and 31.4 in New York.

Strong nutritional correlates exist for specific cancers. These studies, also known as ecological studies use the country or other geographic area as the unit of measure rather than the individual. For example, Armstrong and Doll in 1975 compared per capita total fat intake and national breast cancer mortality rates among women and found a correlation of 0.89: Countries with higher fat intake had higher breast cancer mortality. They also compared per capita fat intake and mortality from colon cancer and observed a correlation of 0.85 for men and 0.81 for women.

The most important of the existing strengths of correlation studies is that the contrasts in dietary intake are very large. For example, the range of fat intake within a population tends to be small compared with the range of far intake among different populations.

Although correlation studies have opened the door to new leads in the study of diet and cancer, certain limitations have prevented these investigations from advancing past the level of hypothesis generation. First and foremost, there are many factors other than dietary differences that distinguish countries with a high incidence from those with a low incidence. This makes it difficult to identify dietary factors as the primary explanation for the differences in the etiology of cancers. For example, besides consuming a diet with a higher proportion of energy from fat, populations of countries that are more industrialized will also have shifted from an agrarian to an urbanized, sedentary society with lower total energy expenditure. Therefore, with increasing industrialization exposure to many aspects of life will decrease exercise and increase fat intake. Consider the example of colon cancer. The international correlation between fat and colon cancer mortality in men is 0.85, and for meat it is 0.85. There is also a correlation between gross national product and colon cancer mortality (0.77 for men); more industrialized countries have higher economic production and higher rates of cancer. Owing to the many factors that are associated with industrialization it is not possible to separate our which factor is important in the etiology of colon cancer, lack of physical activity or increased consumption of fat or meat. Studies with data on lifestyle factors at the individual level are needed to clarify which of these variables is important (see below).

Special-Exposure Groups

Within populations there are groups that have atypical dietary patterns which may provide valuable information in the probe for further information on the relationship of diet and cancer. These groups are called special-exposure groups and are often defined by ethnic or religious characteristics. In addition to offering many of the advantages of correlation studies, the number of alternative explanations for any observations may be reduced if the special-exposure group lives in the same area as the comparison group.

As a largely vegetarian group, the Seventh-Day Adventists have been used in studies of meat earing and cancer. Studies of these groups, however, are limited in the same ways that other ecological studies are limited. For example, although lower rates of colon cancer have been observed among Seventh-Day Adventists—supporting the hypothesis that meat is related to colon cancer—there are other lifestyle choices that characterize the group, such as low rates of tobacco use and alcohol intake, which could also modify their rates of colon cancer.

Evidence from Descriptive Studies

In 1981, Doll and Peto made an estimate based largely on descriptive studies that 35% of cancers in the USA may be attributable to dietary factors; but reflecting uncertainty in the sources of data used for this estimate, they noted that the range of possible dietary contribution was from as low as 10% to as high as 70%. The marked variation in the rates of most cancers among countries is evidence that dietary factors may influence the development of cancer. The potential range of dietary factors that may influence cancer risk are presented in **Table 1**. Despite the fact that descriptive studies provide an excellent source of hypotheses, it is necessary to conduct analytical studies to collect data that will provide more definitive evidence.

Table 1 Examples of suspected dietary factors influencing cancer risk

Dietary factor	Site of cancer
Increased risk	
Overnutrition/Obesity	Endometrium, gallbladder, breast, colon
Alcohol	Liver, oesophagus, larynx, pharynx, breast, colon
Beer	Rectum
Fat (especially saturated)	Colorectum, breast, prostate
Red meat	Colorectum
Salt	Stomach, nasopharynx
Heterocyclic amines (from cooked meat)	Colorectum
Decreased risk	
Fiber	Colorectum, breast
Vitamins A, C, E	Many sites
Protease inhibitors	Colorectum
Calcium, vitamin D	Colorectum
Folate	Colorectum
Lycopene	Prostate
Carotenoids	Lung
Phytooestrogens	Breast

Time Trends within Countries

The analysis of cancer trends over time can lead to useful findings in the study of diet and cancer. By looking at the change in cancer rates in a specific population over time and comparing these rates with changes in specific factors over the same period (e.g., changes in dietary habits), investigators can uncover possible associations supporting the dietary factors hypotheses. For example, researchers have examined vital statistics for Japanese natives and US whites to unveil changes in cancer mortality and related antecedent patterns of lifestyle in the two populations. These investigations have uncovered that animal fat consumption in Japan steadily increased from a daily level of 6.5 g per person in 1955 to 27.6 g in 1987; at the same time the Japanese rate of colon cancer in men rose at a rapid pace; in fact, the mortality rates owing to colon cancer in men almost trebled over this time. This evidence lends more support to the hypothesis that mortality from colon cancer in men is influenced by high dietary fat consumption.

Similar data were collected in Singapore to determine trends in the incidence of breast cancer: in 1996 an average annual increase in breast cancer incidence of 3.6% over a 25-year period for all women was reported. The most convincing evidence that the observed trend was real was that it was clearly cohort-related rather than period-related. The risk was observed to increase in successive birth cohorts from the 1890s to the 1960s. Changes in dietary consumption patterns (e.g., the adoption of a more 'Western' diet) fall among other factors cited as having a possible effect on the continuing increase in rates of breast cancer among women in Singapore. Like descriptive studies, time-trend studies are a valuable source for hypotheses generation, but more definitive evidence is required from analytical epidemiology to uncover any real associations between dietary factors and cancer rates.

Migrant Studies

Migrant studies examine the rates of specific diseases in migrating populations. These studies are important in addressing the possibility that observed correlations in ecological studies are owing to genetic factors. Generally, results from migrant studies have so far found that the migrating group takes on the rate of cancer of the new country. Hence genetic factors are excluded as the dominant cause for varying rates of cancer between countries. A good example of this is seen in the Japanese migrant population to the USA. Japan has low rates of cancers of the breast, colon, and prostate, while the rates of these cancers among Japanese migrants to the USA move toward the higher US rates. The increased risk of breast cancer among migrants occurs primarily in later generations, leading investigators to believe that the causal factors operate early in life. Investigators also consider major changes in the rate of disease that occur within a population over time as evidence that nongenetic factors play an integral role in the etiology of cancer. The limitations of migrant studies are similar to those of ecological studies.

Analytical Studies

Cohort studies Cohort studies involve the collection of information from healthy participants who are followed over time and observed for the occurrence of new cases of disease (incident cases). During or at the end of follow-up, the disease frequency within a cohort may be measured as either a cumulative incidence rate (the number of cases divided by the entire base population) or an incidence density rate (the number of cases divided by the total follow-up time accumulated by all members of the population, or 'person-time' follow-up). The relative risk is the rate of disease (cumulative incidence rate or incidence density rate) in the exposed (e.g., those with a high intake of dietary fat) divided by the rate of disease in the unexposed (e.g., those on a low-fat diet). A relative risk of 2 implies that the exposed group has twice the rate of disease compared with the unexposed group.

For illustration, in a study of 121 700 women, a group of participants who completed dietary questionnaires and had no previous diagnosis of cancer in 1980, were followed through 1988 to address the hypothesis that dietary fat increases and fiber intake decreases the risk of breast cancer. This outcome was defined by histologically confirmed cases of breast cancer. In one analysis, the primary exposure of interest was energy-adjusted intake of total dietary fiber. Among the women in the highest quintile of energy-adjusted dietary fiber intake there were 299 cases of breast cancer compared with 305 cases among the women in the lowest quintile. This gave a relative risk (with adjustment for established breast cancer risk factors as well as alcohol intake) of 1.02 for those in the highest quintile of energy-adjusted dietary fiber intake compared with those in the lowest quintile.

There is also a growing body of evidence available from cohort studies for the assessment of dietary fat intake and breast cancer in developed countries. The average relative risk was 1.03. This observation was based on the results from nine prospective studies with at least 50 incident breast cancer cases each ($n = 2742$) and a large comparison series (i.e., noncases). At the same time, as these results suggest no overall association for total fat intake, emerging evidence suggests that monounsaturated fat may be protective against breast cancer.

The use of cohort studies can be advantageous in many ways when studying the relationship between diet and cancer. A cohort study allows the assessment of multiple effects of a given dietary exposure. Dietary data can be updated during follow-up and the temporal relation between diet and cancer can be addressed. For example, the beneficial effects of alcohol in reducing the risk of gallstone formation and coronary heart disease, and the potentially deleterious effects of alcohol on cancer and hemorrhagic stroke, can be weighed against each other in a cohort study. It is also possible to measure the absolute rates of disease according to the level of food or nutrient intake.

Among the limitations of cohort studies is the concern that current practice, usage, or exposure may change over the duration of the follow-up, limiting the ability to come to any relevant conclusions in studies of diet and cancer that have measured exposure just once at the beginning of the study. Controlling for extraneous variables such as smoking, which are related both to risk of cancer and to dietary intake, and separating the effects of specific dietary factors from those that exist together, also limit the range of knowledge that can be extracted from cohort studies.

Some investigators believe that the large number of subjects required to study rare disease and the high expense of management and maintenance also limit the usefulness of cohort studies. Others believe that the larger overall monetary investment most cohort studies require can be advantageous: More variables can be studied and in the long run further hypotheses can be generated and more conclusions produced than in a single case–control study that relies on recall of past habits.

Case–control studies In case–control studies information is obtained from diseased participants and compared with information provided by disease-free controls with respect to a possible risk factor (e.g., level of a dietary factor). Data collected from these studies can be used to evaluate the hypothesis that the risk factor is a cause of the disease. The cases are selected from a defined population, such as a country population. The population represents those at risk of developing the disease under study. Each time someone in the defined population is diagnosed with the disease during the duration of the study, this individual joins the case series. As each case arises from the population, one or more controls should be sampled to estimate the prevalence of the exposures among those remaining free from disease. The controls may be chosen from any population of individuals that provides valid information about those at risk for the disease. It is important to choose controls so that their probability of selection is unrelated to the exposure being studied.

In the study of the relationship of diet and cancer, case–control studies may be used to evaluate the hypotheses that individual or multiple dietary factors are the cause of the cancer under investigation. For example, a study in 1977 identified all cases of lung cancer diagnosed during an 18-month period from 1972 in three Singapore hospitals. Controls were chosen from other hospital patients free of any smoking-related diseases. There were a total of 233 cases and 300 controls interviewed regarding their frequency of consumption of dark-green leafy vegetables and food preparation habits. The investigation found a substantially increased risk of lung cancer among those reporting a low consumption of dark-green leafy vegetables.

Case–control studies are better suited to the study of rare diseases because in cohort studies tens of thousands of individuals must be followed in order to study the most common cancers. It is also thought that case–control studies may be quicker and less expensive to conduct because they require fewer subjects, and they are therefore often employed as an alternate mode of investigation to cohort studies.

Among the limitations of case–control studies is the comparability of information between the cases and the controls. While in a cohort study the exposure of interest is measured before the onset of disease, in case–control studies the exposure is assessed in individuals who (in most cases) already know their own disease status. Often the person collecting the data will also know the disease status of the patient. This may influence the accuracy of the data collected, either through differential recall by cases and controls, or by an interviewer being more persistent in questioning cases than controls. In cohort studies neither the participant nor the investigator knows whether or not the subject will be a case or noncase by the end of the follow-up period.

Intervention studies In principle, the most powerful means of determining the effects of dietary factors on cancer risk is an intervention study (i.e., a randomized trial). In randomized trials bias is removed because of the equal distribution of risk factors in each group. For example, it has been proposed that a randomized trial of fat reduction could help uncover the mystery of the relationship between dietary fat intake and breast cancer. The Women's Health Initiative was started by the US National Institutes of Health with the goal of enrolling and randomizing several tens of thousands of women, half of whom will be trained to follow a diet deriving less than 20% of energy from fat. Unfortunately, such a trial would not be able to address the most promising modification of the dietary fat hypothesis—that dietary fat reduction at an early age may reduce breast cancer risk several decades later. Other problems with such a randomized trial include the difficulty of maintaining compliance with a diet incompatible with prevailing food consumption habits, and the gradual secular decline in total fat consumption already under way which may reduce the size of the comparison of fat intake between the intervention group and the control groups. The Women's Health Initiative Trial will also counsel the women in the intervention group to adopt a diet that is high in fruits, vegetables, and grain products as well as low in total and saturated fat, therefore making it more difficult to distinguish between the effect of the fat reduction and that of increasing intake of fruits, vegetables, and grain products. All in all, intervention studies may in principle have a great chance of determining effects of dietary factors on cancer risk, but trials of sufficient duration and size may not be feasible because of long-term compliance and cost.

Epidemiological Issues in the Study of Diet and Cancer

Resolved and Unresolved Issues

Some of the issues that researchers have encountered in their attempt to uncover the mystery of the dietary factors linked to cancer include the difficulty of distinguishing the importance of parts of dietary factors from the overall effect of each dietary factor (e.g., total dietary fat intake compared with type of dietary fat intake). In a meta-analysis in 1990 of 12 case–control studies of dietary fat intake and cancer, 4 studies observed a significant positive association, 6 uncovered nonsignificant positive associations, and 2 saw inverse associations. When the data were analyzed together there was a positive association observed for both total fat intake and saturated fat intake. Investigators must ask themselves which factor has larger implications in the study of diet and cancer, as not all studies have included analyses of the individual types of fats along with their data on overall fat consumption. In the study of the influence of dietary fiber intake (which includes crude fiber and many soluble fiber fractions) on cancer rates, there is debate about the most appropriate method of biochemical analysis for determining fiber content of individual foods. This same issue arises with the study of most dietary factors and could affect any important advances in the study of diet and cancer.

Biochemical indicators of food and nutrient intake have two fundamental uses in epidemiological studies. Most often they serve as a 'surrogate' for actual dietary intake in studies of disease occurrence. For nutrients that vary widely in concentration within foods and for which food composition tables are inaccurate, biochemical indicators may be the most feasible way of measuring intake. Within-food variation may occur owing to differences in food storage, processing, or preparation, or may be owing to geographical differences in soil nutrient content. For example, it has been found that selenium content in US soil can vary by as much as 100-fold, which in turn causes the selenium content of swine muscle to vary more than 15-fold. Another example is that of fat. When the composition of fats in commercial food products is not known to study participants, it is possible to assess the fat components of the diet by subcutaneous fat aspirates which reflect long-term dietary patterns.

Like most exposures in chronic disease, nutrient exposures relevant to disease are usually long-term. As the promotion period for cancers may be years or decades, it is usually desirable that a biomarker indicates the cumulative effect of diet over an extended period of time. There are a couple of methods to surpass the barrier of an indicator that is only sensitive to short-term intake, and to overcome the day-to-day intake fluctuations that occur with most nutrients: (1) experimental studies, in which nutrient levels are manipulated; and (2) sampling levels in individuals longitudinally. Biomarkers of nutrient levels in blood or other tissues can provide a useful assessment of intake of certain nutrients, although the above considerations must be acknowledged, and careful attention must be given to specimen collection, storage, and analysis in order to avoid misclassification or bias. With an expanding array of biochemical indicators that have been validated as measures of dietary intake, their use in nutritional epidemiology will continue to grow.

The limited range of diet within most populations adds its own set of complexities to the epidemiological study of nutrition and cancer. For example, in the majority of populations where foods high in fat are readily available, very few individuals consume less than 30% of their energy from fat. This makes it difficult to study the impact of reducing fat intake to less than 30% of total energy intake. At the same time, some individuals of a relatively homogeneous population may have very different dietary patterns: For example, a range of dietary fat intake from 25% to 40% of total energy was seen within a cohort of 52 000 male health professionals in the USA.

Given that most neoplasms have a long induction period (the time from an exposure to a carcinogen to the development of cancer), often spanning several decades, accurate measure of long-term dietary intake is of utmost importance in the study of the implications of diet on cancer. Therefore, short-term methods of dietary assessment such as 24-h recalls are usually insufficient. In the context of case–control studies these short-term methods are inappropriate because they measure current diet, and it has been found that individuals alter their diet after the diagnosis of cancer. The most feasible method of measuring long-term intakes in large numbers of individuals is the food frequency questionnaire: These questionnaires measure the usual frequency of a selected list of foods.

Food frequency questionnaires to assess dietary intake need to be carefully designed. First of all, the food items on the questionnaire must represent the major source of nutrients of interest within the study population. Depending on the consistency of the concentration of a nutrient in a given food, the precision of dietary questionnaires varies. Food frequency questionnaires may provide rankings by level of intake but they do not quantify actual intake. A dietary questionnaire may efficiently distinguish between participants with low-fiber and high-fiber intakes in a given population, but it will not necessarily provide a precise assessment of the absolute fiber intake. In the case of larger studies, it is possible for a random sample of participants to provide a more comprehensive assessment of intake by keeping several weeks of dietary records. This additional information will provide a more precise quantification of dietary intake by helping estimate true dose–response relationships between a nutrient and diet expressed in absolute intake.

Summary of Known Relations between Diet and Cancer

A wealth of studies since the 1970s have clearly documented the relations between diet and a growing number of cancers (**Table 2**). Convincing evidence based on consistent findings from epidemiological studies conducted in diverse populations now shows that diet is an established cause of prostate, breast, digestive tract, airway, and urinary tract cancers. With these rich epidemiological data we can more confidently conclude that some 30% of cancer is attributable to diet. Public health officials have taken the accumulated evidence and developed strategies for minimizing cancer risk. Among these recommendations is a diet high in vegetables, fruits, and legumes and low in red meat, saturated fat, salt, and sugar. They suggest that carbohydrates be consumed as whole grains such as whole meal bread and brown rice rather than as white bread and rice. Any added fats should come from plant sources and should be unhydrogenated, an example being olive oil, which may potentially be beneficial. Given the evergrowing knowledge of the association between diet and cancer, and the subsequent recommended prevention strategies, it is time that researchers and public health officials combined their efforts

Table 2 Levels of evidence for major forms of cancer by foods, energy-generating nutrients, dietary exposure to selected nonnutrients, and nutrition-related indicators

	Suggestive evidence	*Strong evidence*	*Convincing evidence*
Increased risk			
Major food groups			
– Cereals	Stomach		
– Meat	Pancreas	Large bowel	
– Eggs and egg products	Stomach		
– Sugars	Large bowel		
Macronutrients			
– Proteins (animal)	Large bowel, pancreas, endometrium		
– Carbohydrates (total)	Stomach, pancreas		
– Saturated fat (animal)	Large bowel, lung, endometrium		Prostate
Nonnutrients			
– Alcohol		Oesophagus, pancreas	Oral cavity, large bowel, cervix uteri, breast
– Salt (NaCl)		Stomach	Nasopharynx
Nutritional covariates			
– Height	Ovary, prostate	Breast, large bowel	Large bowel, premenopausal breast = inverse association postmenopausal breast = positive association, endometrium, kidney, oesophagus
– Obesity			
– Hot drinks		Oesophagus	
Decreased risk			
Major food groups			
– Vegetables	Liver, pancreas, breast, endometrium, cervix uteri, ovary, prostate	Oesophagus, stomach, larynx, lung, urinary bladder	Oral cavity, large bowel, kidney
– Fruits	Liver, pancreas, breast, endometrium, cervix uteri, ovary, kidney	Oral cavity, oesophagus, stomach, larynx	Large bowel, lung, urinary bladder
Macronutrients			
– Fiber	Large bowel, pancreas		
– Monounsaturated fat	Breast		
Nutritional covariates			
– Physical activity	Endometrium, prostate	Breast	Large bowel, breast
– Folate			Colon, breast

not only to uncover the mysteries of diet and cancer but also to balance the 'war on cancer' treatment with more extensive efforts in prevention.

See also: **Alcohol**: Disease Risk and Beneficial Effects. **Cancer**: Epidemiology of Gastrointestinal Cancers Other Than Colorectal Cancers; Epidemiology of Lung Cancer; Effects on Nutritional Status. **Dietary Fiber**: Potential Role in Etiology of Disease. **Dietary Surveys**. **Vegetarian Diets**.

Further Reading

Ames BN, Gold LS, and Willett WC (1995) The causes and prevention of cancer. *Proceedings of the National Academy of-Sciences USA* **92**: 5258–5265.

Armstrong B and Doll R (1975) Environmental factors and cancer incidence and mortality in different countries, with special reference to dietary practices. *International Journal of Cancer* **15**: 617–631.

Colditz GA and Willett W (1991) Epidemiologic approaches to the study of diet and cancer. In: Alfin-Slater RB and Kritchevsky D (eds.) *Cancer and Nutrition*. New York: Plenum.

Doll R and Peto R (1981) The causes of cancer: Quantitative estimates of avoidable risks in the United States today. *Journal of the National Cancer Institute* **66**: 1191–1308.

Giovannucci E, Stampher MJ, Colditz GA *et al.* (1993) A comparison of prospective and retrospective assessments of diet in the study of breast cancer. *American Journal of Epidemiology* **137**: 502–511.

Seow A, Duffy SW, McGee MA *et al.* (1996) Breast cancer in Singapore: Trends in incidence 1968–1992. *International Journal of Epidemiology* **25**: 40–45.

Trichopoulos D, Li FP, and Hunter DJ (1996) What causes cancer? *Scientific American* **275**: 80–87.

Trichopoulos D and Willett WC (eds.) (1996) Nutrition and cancer. *Cancer Causes and Control* 7: 3–180.

Willett WC (1989) *Nutritional Epidemiology*. Oxford: Oxford University Press.

Willett WC, Colditz GA, and Mueller NE (1996) Strategies for minimizing cancer risk. *Scientific American* **275**: 88–95.

Wydner EL, Yasuyuki F, Harris RE *et al.* (1991) Comparative epidemiology of cancer between the United States and Japan. *Cancer* **67**: 746–763.

Epidemiology of Gastrointestinal Cancers Other Than Colorectal Cancers

H-Y Huang, Johns Hopkins University, Baltimore, MD, USA

© 2005 Elsevier Ltd. All rights reserved.

This article addresses the epidemiology of esophageal cancer, stomach cancer, pancreatic cancer, and small intestine cancer. People with any of these cancers are often diagnosed at 60–80 years of age. The incidences are higher among men than among women and vary widely with geographic location and population, suggesting that environmental factors are important in the development of these cancers.

Esophageal Cancer

The esophagus is a hollow tube, approximately 10 in long in adults. It conveys food from the pharynx to the stomach. Mucous glands in the lining of the esophagus secret mucus to aid in lubrication. Absorption in the esophagus is nil.

Descriptive Epidemiology

Worldwide, esophageal cancer is the eighth most common cancer and the sixth most common cause of cancer death, accounting for approximately 450 000 new cases and a similar number of deaths in 2002. More than 70% of esophageal cancer is squamous cell carcinoma, and approximately 20% is adenocarcinoma. Squamous cell carcinoma arises from dysplasia in the middle and lower third of the esophagus epithelial lining, whereas adenocarcinoma usually develops in the glandular tissue in the distal esophagus. The incidence of esophageal cancer varies tremendously with geographic location and populations throughout the world, with a maximum ratio of 500 to 1. In central and Southeast Asia, the Far East, and the Middle East, squamous cell carcinoma is the predominant form of esophageal cancer, whereas in the United States and Europe, adenocarcinoma of the esophagus has been rapidly increasing since 1970s, particularly in Caucasian men, to approach or surpass the rate of squamous cell carcinoma. In the United States, African Americans have an approximately 2-fold increased risk for esophageal cancer compared to Caucasians, possibly because of an unhealthy lifestyle.

Disease Process

There may be no symptoms of esophagus cancer during the early stages. As the cancer develops, nonspecific symptoms occur, including dysphagia, weight loss, chronic cough, and pain in the retrosternal, back, or right upper abdomen. In more than 50% of esophagus cancer cases, the cancer is either unresectable or has metastasized at the time of diagnosis. The prognosis of esophagus cancer depends on disease stages and tumor sizes. For resectable esophagus cancer, the 5-year survival rate ranges from 15 to 24%. For metastasized esophagus cancer, the 5-year survival rate is less than 5%.

Although both squamous cell carcinoma and adenocarcinoma of the esophagus are responsive to chemotherapy, the treatment effect rarely lasts more than 1 year. Radiotherapy may reduce the chance of perioperative morbidity and mortality, but it may increase the risk for local and regional complications such as esophagotracheal fistulas. Research is under way to determine whether an improved treatment efficacy can be achieved by combined chemotherapy, radiotherapy, and surgery.

Risk Factors

Squamous cell carcinoma Factors that cause chronic irritation and esophageal mucosa inflammation may increase the risk for esophageal squamous cell carcinoma. These factors include moderate to heavy alcohol drinking, smoking, achalasia, diverticuli, and consumption of extremely hot beverages, coarse grains or seeds, lye, and caustic spices.

The importance of alcohol consumption in the carcinogenesis of esophageal squamous cell carcinoma is well recognized. However, the mechanisms by which alcohol increases cancer risk have not been elucidated. Alcohol may cause chronic irritation to the esophagus, and it may increase cell proliferation and enhance the permeability of carcinogens to cells. An alcohol metabolite, acetaldehyde, is known to be a carcinogen. Risk for esophageal squamous cell carcinoma is higher for spirits drinkers, followed by wine and beer drinkers.

Cigarette smoke is a rich source of carcinogens, such as benzo(a)pyrene and volatile nitrosamines. It also contains free radicals, reactive oxygen species, and reactive nitrogen species that are capable of initiating and propagating oxidative damage to lipids, proteins, and DNA, leading to several degenerative diseases including cancer. Alcohol drinking may account for approximately 80% of squamous cell esophageal cancer cases, whereas tobacco use may account for approximately 60%. Simultaneous use of alcohol and tobacco further increases esophageal cancer risk.

Achalasia is a swallowing disorder caused by degeneration of the intrinsic autonomic nerves in the esophagus wall and lower esophageal sphincter, leading to decreased or absent peristalsis in the esophageal smooth muscle or impaired relaxation of the lower esophageal sphincter. Approximately 20–29% of achalasia patients may develop esophageal cancer within 15–20 years, predominantly squamous cell carcinoma, possibly because of increased inflammation, bacterial growth, and chemical irritation caused by prolonged contact of food ingredients with esophageal mucosa. In contrast, the likelihood of malignant transformation from diverticuli is less than 1%, although the mechanisms of carcinogenesis are speculated to be the same as those for achalasia.

Low income is associated with squamous cell carcinoma of the esophagus, independent of alcohol and tobacco use, suggesting that other factors associated with poverty may play a role. In Africa and Far East countries, incidences of esophageal cancer are high in regions where starchy food is the predominant food in the diet, and this may have been an indication of poor nutritional status. Several studies have reported that very low intake of fresh fruits and vegetables is associated with higher risk of esophagus cancer. Conversely, high intake of fruits and vegetables, particularly citrus fruits, may confer preventive benefits. Frequent consumption of highly salted meat, pickled vegetables, cured meat, and smoked meat was found to be associated with esophageal cancer risk; these foods contain carcinogenic compounds such as heterocyclic amines and N-nitroso compounds.

Familial aggregation of esophageal squamous cell carcinoma has been reported, but it may reflect genetic predisposition as well as common environmental exposures. Hereditary squamous cell carcinoma of the esophagus develops in approximately 95% of people with a genetic abnormality at chromosome 17q25 that causes a rare autosomal dominant disorder, nonepidermolytic palmoplantar keratoderma.

Adenocarcinoma The risk factor profile of esophageal adenocarcinoma is quite different from that of squamous cell carcinoma. Tobacco use is associated with adenocarcinoma of the esophagus, but the association is less strong than that with squamous cell carcinoma. High intakes of fiber, vitamin C, vitamin B_6, folate, and β-carotene were found to be associated with a lower risk. However, unlike squamous cell carcinoma, esophageal adenocarcinoma does not consistently develop more often in people with frequent alcohol consumption or low income.

Gastroesophageal reflux disease (GERD) is strongly associated with adenocarcinoma of the esophagus. In the process of gastroesophageal reflux, acid fluid regurgitates into the gastroesophageal junction and causes a sensation of heartburn. GERD can be caused by hiatal hernia, esophageal ulcer, and use of drugs that relax the lower gastroesophageal sphincter and increase reflux. Alcohol, tobacco, obesity, and pregnancy may also contribute to GERD.

Barrett's esophagus represents intestinal metaplasia of the squamous epithelium in the distal esophagus. Barrett's esophagus develops in approximately

5–10% of people with GERD and is associated with a 30- to 125-fold increased risk for esophageal adenocarcinoma.

In the United States, the incidence of adenocarcinoma of the esophagus has increased more than 350% since the 1970s. Obesity has been hypothesized to be one of the factors responsible for this increase by augmenting abdominal pressure and gastroesophageal reflux frequency. However, evidence has not been consistent to support this hypothesis.

Prevention

For primary prevention, smoking cessation and avoidance of heavy alcohol intake may significantly reduce the risk for squamous cell carcinoma. A healthful diet with fresh fruits and vegetables but no highly salted, preserved, or smoked food should lead to a reduction in the risk for both of the major forms esophageal cancer. For secondary prevention, routine screenings by endoscopes may confer benefits to individuals with Barrette's esophagus. Treatment with endoscopic ablation combined with proton pump inhibitors may retard Barrett's esophagus to normal squamous mucosa.

Research has been under way to determine the chemopreventive effects of 13-cis-retinoic acid, nonsteroidal antiinflammatory drugs (e.g., aspirin and sulindac), selenium, and ornithine decarboxylase inhibitor, α-difluoromethylornithine, in patents with Barrett's esophagus. These agents also hold promise for preventing squamous cell carcinoma. Other chemopreventive agents that may be useful for reducing both types of esophageal cancer include ascorbic acid, polyphenols (e.g., ellagic acid and epigallocatechin-3-gallate), and sulfhydryl compounds. These agents have been shown in animal models to inhibit nitrosamine formation and enhance the activities of detoxifying enzymes such as glutathione-S-transferase and glutathione peroxidase, but evidence from humans is sparse.

Stomach Cancer

The stomach is located between the esophagus and the duodenum on the left side of the abdominal cavity. It serves as a short-term reservoir of foodstuff and provides digestive functions. Gastric epithelium secrets mucus, hydrochloric acid, hormones (e.g., gastrin), protease, lipase, gelatinase, and other enzymes. The movement of the stomach is controlled by the autonomic nervous system and several hormones in the digestive system.

Descriptive Epidemiology

Worldwide, stomach cancer is the fourth most common cancer and the second most common cause of cancer deaths, accounting for approximately 989 000 new cases and 850 000 deaths in 2001 and 2002, respectively. Stomach cancer can be classified as diffuse or intestinal. The former has an earlier onset with similar occurrences by sex and by geographic areas, whereas the latter has a later onset and develops more often in men than women. There is a wide variation (more than 10-fold) in the incidence of the intestinal type, suggesting that environmental factors are important determinants. Japan, Korea, China, Eastern Europe, Central America, and South America have higher incidences, whereas southern Asia, India, North America, and Africa have lower incidences. A wide range of incidence also occurs within countries.

The incidence and mortality rates of stomach cancer have been declining for several decades because of a reduction in childhood *Helicobacter pylori* infection, improved nutritional status, and reductions in exposures to carcinogens in preserved food. However, because of increases in life expectancy, the absolute number of stomach cancer cases has been increasing.

Disease Process

Approximately 90% of stomach cancer is adenocarcinoma. Other forms of stomach cancer include lymphomas and sarcomas. Symptoms such as excessive belching, heartburn, stomachache, and back pain may occur. Internal bleeding may appear as blood in the vomit or as black, tar-like feces, or it may be so slight that it is undetected. The prognosis of stomach cancer is poor and dependents on disease stages; 5-year survival rate is approximately 20% in the United States.

Risk Factors

Helicobacter pylori infection *Helicobacter pylori* infection can cause inflammatory responses that induce atrophic gastritis and intestinal metaplasia of gastric mucosa, resulting in reduced gastric acidity, which in turn facilitates in vivo formation of carcinogenic N-nitroso compounds and leads to the intestinal type of stomach cancer. In addition, *H. pylori* infection can trigger a cascade of inflammatory responses and oxidative damage to induce cell proliferation and malignant transformation, leading to the diffuse type of stomach cancer. It was estimated that *H. pylori* infection accounted for approximately 50–60% of stomach cancer cases and was associated with an approximately sixfold increased risk at least 10 years prior to diagnosis. These may have been underestimated because of the possibility of loss of the infection or antibody due to extensive replacement of gastric mucosa with intestinal metaplasia in people with stomach cancer.

Infection of *H. pylori* is common—50% worldwide and 90% in developing countries. However, only a small percentage develops into stomach cancer, suggesting that factors such as diet and genetic susceptibility modify risk.

Dietary factors Pickled vegetables and smoked, cured, salted, or dried fish or meat contain nitrite or *N*-nitroso compounds. These preserved foods, as well as grilled or charcoal flame-broiled food that contains polycyclic aromatic hydrocarbons, have been shown to be associated with increased risk of stomach cancer in most studies. Despite the fact that vegetables are a major source of nitrate, evidence suggests an inverse association between fresh fruits and vegetables and stomach cancer risk; the associations for yellow- or green-colored vegetables and citrus fruits are particularly strong. A few studies have reported a lower risk for stomach cancer among people consuming more allium vegetables, onions, and garlic. Some, but not all, studies have found a positive association between starchy food consumption and stomach cancer risk.

Vitamin C intake is consistently found to be inversely associated with stomach cancer risk in observational studies. Vitamin C can act as a powerful water-soluble antioxidant as well as an effective scavenger of nitrite. Protective roles of α-tocopherol and β-carotene are suggestive but less strong. These micronutrients may also be surrogate markers of healthy dietary pattern or lifestyle.

Evidence is inconsistent regarding the role of alcohol, coffee, or black tea consumption in the development of stomach cancer. However, green tea consumption was associated with a lower risk in several studies, presumably because of its polyphenol content.

High intake of salt is associated with a higher risk of stomach cancer. Animal studies have demonstrated that salt per se can damage gastric mucosa and induce gastritis. However, in humans, high salt intake correlates positively with intake of processed meat or fish that contains nitrosamines. Hence, it is unclear whether salt evokes stomach cancer or is merely a marker of other exposures.

Cigarette smoking Tobacco use is associated with a 1.5- to 2.0-fold increased risk for stomach cancer, and it has been estimated to account for 10–17% of stomach cancer cases. These estimates may have been confounded by other factors such as poor diet.

Familial factors Familial aggregation of stomach cancer derives mostly from common environmental exposures and lifestyle factors. Hereditary stomach cancer is rare. Germline mutations in the gene coding for cell adhesion protein E-cadherin (CDH1) were found to be associated with stomach cancer of the diffuse type. Germline mutation of *p53* has also been reported. People with hereditary nonpolyposis colorectal cancer are also at higher risk for stomach cancer.

Prevention

Evidence points to the importance of improving diet and eradicating *H. pylori* infection. A diet rich in fresh fruits and vegetables without highly salted, preserved, or smoked food will theoretically offer benefits in primary prevention. In countries where the incidence of stomach cancer is high, screening for *H. pylori* may be effective for secondary prevention. To this end, programs of mass screening and eradication of *H. pylori* by antibiotics are being performed in Japan. However, because only a small proportion of individuals with *H. pylori* colonization develop stomach cancer, concerns have been raised regarding the possibility of antibiotic resistance by a mass *H. pylori* eradiation program. Use of vaccines against *H. pylori* may be an alternative approach.

Pancreatic Cancer

The pancreas is an elongated organ locating in close proximity to the duodenum. It consists of three parts—head, body, and tail—and is partitioned into lobules by connective tissue. Approximately 85% of the pancreas is composed of exocrine cells called acini that secret digestive enzymes such as proteases, lipase and amylase, ribonuclease, gelatinase, deoxyribonuclease, and elastase. These digestive enzymes, together with bicarbonate secreted from the epithelial cells lining small pancreatic ducts, enter into pancreatic ducts and subsequently to the lumen of the duodenum. Embedded in the exocrine tissue are endocrine tissues called Islets of Langerhans that secret endocrine enzymes, such as insulin and glucagon.

Descriptive Epidemiology

Worldwide, there were approximately 230 000 pancreatic cancer cases and a similar number of deaths due to pancreatic cancer in 2002. Pancreatic cancer is the fifth and sixth most common cause of cancer death in men and women, respectively, in most Western countries. The incidence of pancreatic cancer has declined slightly, with an average annual change of −0.04%, from 1975 to 1998 in the United States, presumably as a result of smoking cessation. In contrast, the incidences in Japan and European countries are increasing.

Disease Process

Adenocarcinoma in the head of the pancreas accounts for 80–90% of pancreatic cancer. Pancreatic cancer is a devastating disease because it is rapidly fatal; the case fatality ratio is 0.99, median survival is 6 months or less, 1-year survival is approximately 20–30%, and 5-year survival is less than 5%. There is no effective screening modality for pancreatic cancer. The disease is difficult to diagnose and detect because the disease process is either silent or present with nonspecific symptoms, such as unexplained weight loss, back pain, nausea, jaundice, and altered intestine habits. In approximately 80–90% of cases, the cancer is diagnosed at a nonresectable stage when even small tumors have metastasized to other organs, most commonly the liver. Patients undergo cachexia, a complex metabolic syndrome clinically presenting with progressive weight loss and depletion of reserves of adipose tissue and skeletal muscle. Pancreatic cancer cells are particularly resistant to radiotherapy and chemotherapy, rendering the treatment unsuccessful. The lack of a useful screening tool and the poor prognosis of this disease highlight the importance of primary prevention.

Risk Factors

The etiology of pancreatic cancer is largely unknown. Prospective follow-up epidemiologic studies are the better study designs for determining a temporal relationship between exposures and disease outcomes. However, the rarity of pancreatic cancer makes it difficult to examine an association with sufficient statistical power. Most studies are case–control designs in which information of lifestyle and environmental exposures is collected from pancreatic cancer cases or proxies after cancer diagnoses and from selected controls with no pancreatic cancer. Such study design is prone to recall biases and information biases, and a temporal relationship cannot be determined. Once nonspecific symptoms occur, the aggressive disease processes make it difficult to complete data collection before a patient dies of the disease.

To date, the only risk factors of pancreatic cancer that have been well accepted are oldage and cigarette smoking. Pancreatic cancer is more common in men than women, possibly because of differences in

lifestyle factors and environmental exposures. African Americans, New Zealand Maoris, native Hawaiians, and Jews have higher incidences, whereas individuals in India or Nigeria and Seventh-Day Adventists have lower incidences. Hereditary pancreatitis and germline mutations may account for 10–15% of pancreatic cancer cases. Purported but unproven risk factors include diet, obesity, diabetes mellitus, chronic pancreatitis, *H. pylori* colonization, gastric or duodenal acidity, and occupational exposures to carcinogens. Socioeconomic status is not associated with pancreatic cancer risk.

Cigarette smoking Cigarette smoking has been consistently shown to be associated with a 2- or 3-fold increased risk and accounts for 25–30% of pancreatic cancer cases. Higher risk has been associated with increased numbers of cigarettes smoked. Cigarette smoking may interact with hereditary factors to increase pancreatic cancer risk. It was estimated that smokers who had a family history of pancreatic cancer had a sixfold increased risk compared to nonsmokers who did not have a family history, whereas a three- or fourfold increased risk was found in nonsmokers who had a family history or smokers who did not have a family history compared to nonsmokers with no family history.

Inherited gene mutations Inherited mutations of genes account for approximately 10% of pancreatic cancer cases. *BRCA2* mutations are the most common, accounting for approximately 7%. Pancreatic cancer caused by these mutations often presents as 'apparently sporadic' because of the low penetrance of *BRCA2* mutations. High-penetrance germline mutations in the *CDKN2A (p16)* gene that cause the familial atypical multiple mole and melanoma syndrome are also associated with higher risk for pancreatic cancer. Inherited mutations of *LKB/STK11* gene cause the Peutz–Jeghers syndrome, characterized by hamartomatous gastrointestinal polyps, mucocutaneous melanotic spots, and, in 30% of patients, pancreatic cancer. Inherited defects in a DNA mismatched repair gene causing hereditary nonpolyposis colorectal cancer and inherited mutations of the cationic trypsinogen gene causing acute pancreatitis at young age may also cause pancreatic cancer.

Dietary factors Higher intakes of fat, carbohydrate, animal protein, fried food, cured meat, or smoked meat have been associated with a higher risk for pancreatic cancer. In contrast, higher intakes of vitamin C, fiber, or, more generally, fresh fruits and vegetables and higher serum concentrations of folate and pyridoxine are associated with lower risk for pancreatic cancer. Alcohol, tea, or coffee consumption is not associated with pancreatic cancer.

Diabetes mellitus The temporal relationship between diabetes and pancreatic cancer is uncertain. A twofold increased risk of pancreatic cancer has been reported for people diagnosed with diabetes at least 5 years prior to pancreatic cancer diagnosis. The latency period of pancreatic cancer is unknown, but an estimate of at least 10 years has been reported. Hence, diabetes may be a consequence rather than a cause of pancreatic cancer. Interestingly, familial pancreatic cancer was not found to be associated with diabetes. In addition, approximately 50% of individuals who have non-insulin-dependent diabetes mellitus are not aware of the disease, and many pancreatic cancer patients are diagnosed with diabetes at the time of the cancer diagnosis.

Chronic pancreatitis Both hereditary and sporadic forms of chronic pancreatitis have been found to increase pancreatic cancer risk. In the inflammatory processes of chronic pancreatitis, cytokines, reactive oxygen species, and mediators of the inflammatory pathway (e.g., NF-κB and COX-2) may increase cell turnover, cause loss of tumor suppressor genes, stimulate oncogene expression, and lead to pancreatic malignancy. Heavy alcohol consumption may increase the risk of chronic pancreatitis.

Prevention

Smoking cessation may be the first choice for the primary prevention of pancreatic cancer. However, evidence to support this rationale is lacking. An effective screening modality for pancreatic cancer has not been developed.

Small Intestine Cancer

The small intestine is approximately 20 feet long and consists of three sections: the duodenum, jejunum, and ileum. The small intestine performs extensive digestion and absorption functions. It also secrets secretin, which stimulates the pancreas to produce digestive enzymes.

Descriptive Epidemiology

Cancer of the small intestine is very rare; the age-adjusted incidence is approximately 1.4 per 100 000—less than 2% of all gastrointestinal malignancies. The incidence of small intestine cancer is higher in Maori of New Zealand and Hawaiians, and it is lower in India, Romania, and other areas of Eastern Europe. In the United States, the incidences of adenocarcinoma, lymphoma, and carcinoid have only slightly increased since 1980s; even for lymphoma, which has had the largest increase, the annual rate of increase has been no more than 1 per 1 million.

Disease Process

There are four types of small intestine cancer, each with unique characteristics: adenocarcinoma, carcinoid, lymphoma, and sarcoma. In Western developed countries, approximately 30–40% of small intestine cancer is adenocarcinoma, predominantly in the duodenum, and carcinoid and lymphoma occur more often in the jejunum or ileum, whereas sarcoma may develop anywhere in the small intestine. In developed countries, lymphoma is very rare and occurs more often in older people with relatively good survival. In contrast, in developing countries, lymphoma is the main type of small intestine cancer, and it occurs more often in younger individuals, anywhere in the small intestine, with poor survival. Hence, prognosis of small intestine cancer depends on the type, geographic location (which may be an indication of etiology and/or the advancement of treatment), and disease stages. Clinical presentation may include abdominal pain, weight loss, abdominal mass, anemia, nausea/vomiting, bleeding, obstruction, jaundice, and anorexia before diagnosis. Overall, the 5-year survival rate is approximately 80% for carcinoid, 60% for lymphoma, 45% for sarcoma, and 20% for adenocarcinoma.

Risk Factors

Due to the rarity of small intestine cancer, etiologic investigation has relied on only a few small case–control studies. A lack of histology data has further undermined the strength of the evidence.

Tobacco use, alcohol consumption, and dietary factors such as high animal protein, high animal fat, sugar, and salted, cured, or smoked food were associated with small intestine cancer in some but not all studies. Small intestine adenoma, familial adenomatous polyposis, hereditary nonpolyposis colorectal cancer, peptic ulcer, celiac sprue, and cholescystectomy have been found to be associated with increased risk for small intestine adenocarcinoma. In people with Crohn's disease, a 16- to more than 100-fold increased risk for small intestine adenocarcinoma has been reported, but unlike most adenocarcinomas that occur in the duodenum, these patients tend to have adenocarcinomas in the elium. The reasons for the increased risk are uncertain, but it has been hypothesized to be due to the medication for treating Crohn's disease.

Prevention

Because very little is known about the etiology of small intestine cancer, no preventive strategy has been proposed.

Conclusion

The wide variation in the incidences of cancers of the esophagus, stomach, pancreas, and small intestine by geographic location and by population suggest that environmental factors play an important role in the etiology. Indeed, several risk factors are commonly shared by these cancer sites, including tobacco use, a diet low in fresh fruits and vegetables, and a diet high in salted, cured, or smoked food. Strategies for gastrointestinal cancer prevention should aim to counteract these risk factors. In addition, avoidance of heavy alcohol consumption and eradication of *H. pylori* may significantly reduce the incidence of esophageal cancer and stomach cancer, respectively. Studies are under way to test the efficacy of chemoprevention agents in the prevention of esophageal cancer and stomach cancer in high-risk populations. The development of noninvasive screening tests, such as molecular or imaging technology, is needed for early detection and better prognosis.

See also: **Alcohol**: Disease Risk and Beneficial Effects. **Ascorbic Acid**: Physiology, Dietary Sources and Requirements. **Diabetes Mellitus**: Etiology and Epidemiology. **Fruits and Vegetables**. **Small Intestine**: Disorders. **Stomach**: Disorders.

Further Reading

Enzinger PC and Mayer RJ (2003) Esophageal cancer. *New England Journal of Medicine* 349(23): 2241–2252.

Ghadirian P, Ekoe JM, and Thouez JP (1992) Food habits and esophageal cancer: An overview. *Cancer Detection and Prevention* 16(3): 163–168.

Heath EI, Limburg PJ, Hawk ET, and Forastiere AA (2000) Adenocarcinoma of the esophagus: Risk factors and prevention. *Oncology (Huntington)* 14(4): 507–514.

Lange J and Siewert JR (eds.) (2000) *Esophageal Carcinoma: State of the Art.* New York: Springer.

Levin B (1999) An overview of preventive strategies for pancreatic cancer. *Annals of Oncology* 10(supplement 4): 193–196.

Lowenfels AB and Maisonneuve P (1999) Pancreatic cancer: Development of a unifying etiologic concept. *Annals of the New York Academy of Sciences* 880: 191–200.

Neugut AI, Jacobson JS, Suh S, Mukherjee R, and Arber N (1998) The epidemiology of cancer of the small bowel. *Cancer Epidemiology Biomarkers & Prevention* 7(3): 243–251.

Palli D (2000) Epidemiology of gastric cancer: An evaluation of available evidence. *Journal of Gastroenterology* 35(supplement 12): 84–89.

Plummer M, Franceschi S, and Munoz N (2004) Epidemiology of gastric cancer. *IARC Scientific Publications* 2004(157): 311–326.

National Cancer Institute (2001, February) Report of the Pancreatic Cancer Progress Review Group. Available at http://prg.nci.nih.gov/pancreatic/default.html.

National Cancer Institute (2002, December) Report of the Stomach/Esophageal Cancers Progress Review Group. Available at http://prg.nci.nih.gov/stomach/finalreport.html.

Sharma P and Sampliner RE (eds.) (2001) *Barrett's Esophagus and Esophageal Adenocarcinoma.* Malden, MA: Blackwell Science.

Epidemiology of Lung Cancer

A J Alberg and J M Samet, Johns Hopkins Bloomberg School of Public Health, Baltimore, MD, USA

© 2005 Elsevier Ltd. All rights reserved.

At the start of the twentieth century, lung cancer was a rare disease, whereas by its end it had become a leading cause of death and the most common cause of cancer death in the United States. The occurrence of most cases can be explained by environmental agents; cigarette smoking was identified as its predominant cause in the 1950s. With the role of smoking well established, research on lung cancer has focused on environmental and genetic factors that may determine lung cancer risk in smokers. Genetic factors have been the subject of increased scrutiny because the risk of cancer may be determined in part by interindividual variation in the metabolism and detoxification of environmental agents, such as cigarette smoke, as well as variation in susceptibility to DNA damage and in DNA repair capability.

The role of diet as an environmental factor that may determine lung cancer risk in smokers remains a topic of considerable interest. Studies on diet and lung cancer in humans began in the 1970s as part of a broader search for factors determining susceptibility to the carcinogenic effects of tobacco smoke. Early animal studies showed that vitamin A depletion caused loss of differentiation of the respiratory epithelium, a histopathological state analogous to the dysplasia found in cigarette smokers at risk for lung cancer. In animal studies, these changes reverted with nutrient repletion, raising the prospect that dietary interventions could reduce lung cancer risk in cigarette smokers. Early epidemiological studies indicated that indices of vitamin A consumption were associated, in the expected protective direction, with lung cancer risk. An influential 1981 publication by Buckley and colleagues shifted emphasis to β-carotene rather than retinol, and by the early 1980s clinical trials of β-carotene as a chemopreventive agent had been initiated. Observational evidence continued to show that measures of vitamin A and carotene intake were inversely associated with lung cancer risk; the weight of evidence favored fruits and vegetables as the carriers of the chemopreventive agents. In the mid-1990s, the hypothesis that β-carotene and retinol were protective was disproved in large clinical trials that unexpectedly showed increased risk in smokers randomized to the active agents. Hypotheses concerning specific carotenoids and other dietary components have since been advanced along with more general theories involving dietary antioxidants and oxidant stress from smoking and other factors.

Lung Cancer

Respiratory Carcinogenesis

The term 'lung cancer' refers to a histologically and clinically diverse group of malignancies arising in the respiratory tract, primarily but not exclusively from cells lining the airways of the lung. Beginning with the trachea, the airways branch dichotomously through 20 or more generations. Most cancers arise in the larger airways of the lung, typically at the fourth through the eighth generations. There, the airways are lined by a ciliated epithelium that includes secretory cells and glands and also neuroepithelial cells. The specific cells of origin of lung cancer are unknown; candidates include the secretory cells, pluripotential basal cells, and neuroepithelial cells. Only a small proportion of lung cancers in smokers have been considered as originating in the lung's periphery, but with the current trend of increasing adenocarcinoma this proportion may be increasing.

Lung cancer is thought to arise from a sequence of genetic changes that move a cell from a normal to a malignant state. Diverse genetic changes in oncogenes and tumor suppressor genes have been found in lung cancers, although the specific longitudinal sequence of these changes has not been characterized. Nonetheless, our evolving understanding of respiratory carcinogenesis, as a sequential progression from normal cell to clinical cancer, implies that there may be multiple points for interrupting the sequence and thereby preventing cancer.

Risk Factors for Lung Cancer

The increase in the incidence of lung cancer during the first half of the twentieth century prompted intensive epidemiological investigation of the disease, with the identification of a number of causal agents. Cigarette smoking is by far the most prominent cause of lung cancer, and the worldwide epidemic of lung cancer is largely attributable to smoking. However, occupational exposures have placed a number of worker groups at high risk and there is evidence that indoor and outdoor air pollution also increases lung cancer risk generally. The observed familial aggregation of lung cancer suggests that genetic factors may also determine risk. Extensive research is in progress on the specific genes that may determine risk in smokers; experience to date has supplied some leads but the evidence has been mixed for most of the genes studied.

In smokers, the risk of lung cancer depends largely on the duration of smoking and the amount smoked; risk increases exponentially with both, but more steeply with duration than amount. A safe level of smoking has not been shown, and even the secondhand tobacco smoke involuntarily inhaled by nonsmokers increases lung cancer risk. Fortunately, lung cancer risk declines in those who stop smoking, although not to the level of those who have never smoked; risk is present even after 30 years of abstention and currently in the United States approximately half the lung cancer cases occur in former smokers.

A number of occupational exposures increase lung cancer risk; the substances involved include radon (found in underground mines), arsenic, asbestos, chromium, chloromethyl ethers, nickel, and polycyclic aromatic hydrocarbons. For these agents, risk increases with the level of exposure, and synergism with smoking has been shown for several, such as asbestos and radon. Many other agents are suspected occupational carcinogens.

Indoor and outdoor air also contains respiratory carcinogens. Combustion sources contaminate outdoor air with polycyclic aromatic hydrocarbons and radionuclides, and outdoor air pollution is thought to contribute to a few percent of lung cancers in general. Carcinogens in indoor air vary with the setting but may include radon, tobacco smoke, smoke from wood or coal burning, and cooking fumes. In the United States, radon is estimated to cause approximately 14 000 lung cancer deaths annually.

Lung Cancer Histopathology

As assessed by the clinical approach of light microscopy, primary cancer of the lung occurs as multiple histological types, the most common being squamous cell carcinoma (epidermoid carcinoma), adenocarcinoma, large cell carcinoma, and small cell carcinoma. The other malignancies include adeno-squamous carcinomas, carcinoid tumors, and bronchial gland carcinomas. The pathogenetic bases of the four principal histological types are uncertain, and various cells of origin and pathways of differentiation have been hypothesized. In addition, a careful examination of multiple sections from the same case shows tumors to be frequently heterogeneous, with elements of several histological types. Observer variation in classifying histological types of lung cancer is well documented and should be considered when interpreting research findings on a histological basis.

Few links have been made between specific histological types and particular etiological agents. Cigarette smoking increases risk for squamous cell carcinoma, adenocarcinoma, large cell carcinoma, and small cell carcinoma, although the risks tend to increase less steeply with extent of smoking for adenocarcinoma, the most common type in never-smokers. Most occupational carcinomas are not associated with risk for a particular histological type of lung cancer. The evidence for specific links is strongest for chloromethyl ether and radon progeny. Some studies of diet and lung cancer risk have provided analyses stratified by histological type, but these histology-specific analyses provide no specific biological insights.

Although knowledge of the etiological and pathological bases of the different types of lung cancer remains limited, trends of lung cancer histology have been monitored in the general population. A trend of increasing proportion of adenocarcinoma has been documented in many regions throughout the world. For example, in the United States during the past three decades adenocarcinoma remained the most common type of lung cancer in women and increased in men so that it is now also the most common histologic type of lung cancer in men. The hypothesis has been advanced that this shift reflects temporal changes in the carcinogens delivered by smoking as well as a changing topography of smoking.

Diet

Dietary Hypotheses and Mechanisms

Epidemiological research on diet and lung cancer has been both hypothesis driven and descriptive, exploring associations between foods or nutrient indexes and lung cancer risk. Interest in macronutrients has emphasized indices of dietary fat, which was long ago noted to have the capacity to act as a tumor promoter. Micronutrients have been extensively studied, spurred initially by the pioneering epidemiological work of Bjelke and the original

vitamin A and β-carotene hypotheses. Bjelke and subsequent researchers originally focused on vitamin A because of its role in cellular differentiation and the promise of the initial observational findings, but this line of inquiry was subsequently expanded to include antioxidant micronutrients, with an emphasis on β-carotene. The more general hypothesis has been advanced that antioxidant micronutrients may protect against oxidative damage to DNA and thereby protect against cancer. Hypotheses concerning specific beverages have also been proposed; for example, animal studies have shown alcohol consumption to be associated with changes in lung lipids, including surfactant, and in levels of enzymes that can activate procarcinogens and mutagens. Another epidemiologic approach, empirical rather than hypothesis driven, has been to explore the intakes of several specific foods or food groups for associations with lung cancer risk. The identification of protective associations between fruit and vegetable consumption and lung cancer resulted from the use of this more empirical approach.

Certain methodological issues are relevant to a discussion of diet and lung cancer. When investigating a potential link between diet and lung cancer, the potent role of cigarette smoking in the etiology of lung cancer, along with the current differences in the diets of smokers compared with nonsmokers, makes the potential confounding effects of cigarette smoking an acute concern. Even when there is an attempt to control for smoking, residual confounding of diet–lung cancer associations may still occur. Cigarette smoke can directly affect circulating concentrations of dietary factors (**Figure 1**); for example, smokers tend to have lower levels of circulating antioxidant micronutrients even after accounting for differences in dietary intake.

Aspects of the design and conduct of epidemiological studies in general further limit interpretation of

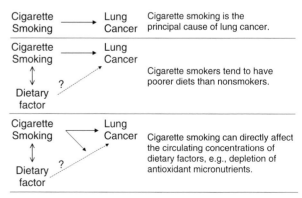

Figure 1 Cigarette smoking complicates the study of diet and lung cancer.

specific dietary studies. Approaches to dietary assessment are not fully standardized, and there may be differences between studies in the number of foods queried, the measurement of serving sizes, and the interview approach employed. There is also uncertainty regarding the biologically relevant exposure window or windows for lung cancer, and dietary agents may plausibly act in early and/or later stages of carcinogenesis. Clinically diagnosed lung cancer reflects a series of complex molecular genetic events that occur over a long period, and the relevant windows for dietary exposures are uncertain. Case–control studies usually measure past diet during some reference period, whereas cohort studies tend to focus on current diet. Most of the epidemiologic research has taken the form of case–control studies, many of which focus on diet during the 5 years preceding diagnosis. These studies provide direct information concerning dietary factors in the later stages of carcinogenesis. To the extent that such measures reflect usual adult (or lifetime) diet, the results of these studies may also be relevant to the role of diet in earlier stages of carcinogenesis. However, because lung cancer tends to be rapidly fatal, many case–control studies include data collected from deceased subjects' next-of-kin. Data from surrogate respondents are probably less accurate than self-reported data, and using such information is certain to introduce substantial misclassification.

Evidence concerning relationships between lung cancer and fruits, vegetables, micronutrients, phytochemicals, fat, body mass index, beverages, and meat intake is reviewed here. For these agents, there is no basis for anticipating that some threshold of intake is relevant to protection (or risk). Rather, a dietary factor that protects against lung cancer would theoretically be expected to confer greater protection when present in greater amounts, and vice versa. Consequently, this review emphasizes dose–response trends, with a monotonic dose–response relationship considered to provide the strongest evidence favoring an association. To focus on the most relevant evidence, the summary tables include only studies that controlled for age and cigarette smoking and case–control studies with more than 200 lung cancer cases. Smaller studies would not be expected to have sufficiently precise estimates to be informative.

Dietary Associations with Lung Cancer

Fruit In total, the evidence favors a protective association between greater fruit consumption and lower lung cancer risk, with associations in the protective direction in 18 of 31 studies (**Table 1**). When stratified by gender, the overall protective association holds more often than not for both males and females. No clear pattern emerges when studies have examined specific fruits or classes of fruits. For example, apples and citrus fruits are associated with reduced risk of lung cancer in some studies but not in others.

Vegetables Evidence for a protective association for vegetable consumption parallels the evidence for fruit consumption, with 18 of 33 studies showing associations at least weakly in the protective direction (**Table 1**). The overall evidence thus points strongly toward a protective association, which has been observed in both males and females. In addition to vegetable intake as a whole, the results for a number of specific vegetables, such as carrots and cruciferous vegetables, have been consistently associated with a reduced risk of lung cancer, at least for the highest versus the lowest categories of consumption.

Micronutrients Two different strategies have been used to evaluate the relationship of micronutrients to lung cancer. One approach has been to use data summarized from food-frequency questionnaires to estimate micronutrient intake. A second approach has been to draw blood samples from study participants and assay the concentrations of micronutrients in circulation. The former approach provides a better average measure of micronutrient 'exposure,' whereas the latter approach has the advantage of measuring micronutrient concentrations closer to the level of cells, where the biologic effect is postulated to occur. However, a single assay of circulating micronutrient concentrations may not reflect the biologically appropriate window of exposure. The evidence is most abundant for vitamins A, C, and E and for total carotenoids and β-carotene. A body of evidence is also accumulating for α-carotene, β-cryptoxanthin, lutein, and lycopene.

The majority of studies on dietary retinol show no association with lung cancer risk (**Table 2**). On the other hand, studies of dietary intake of β-carotene, total carotenoids, and vitamin C point more consistently toward an inverse association, with results at least equally divided between showing some evidence of protective association and showing no association (**Table 2**). As with β-carotene, studies of additional provitamin A carotenoids α-carotene and β-cryptoxanthin have also been evenly divided between showing no association and showing a protective association with lung cancer. Conversely, only a minority of studies of the non-provitamin A carotenoids lycopene and lutein have suggested that higher intakes are associated with decreased risk of lung cancer.

Studies based on micronutrients measured from blood samples drawn after an individual is diagnosed with lung cancer showed that lung cancer

Table 1   Estimated relative risk of lung cancer according to frequency of fruit and vegetable consumption[a]

First author (year)	Sex	Fruits					Vegetables					Also adjusted for
		1	2	3	4	5	1	2	3	4	5	
Case–control studies												
Alavanja (1993)	F	1.0	1.1	0.8	1.1	—	1.0	0.8	0.9	0.8	1.0	Previous lung disease, daily energy intake
Axelsson (1996)	M	1.0	0.8	0.7	—	—	1.0	0.7	0.4	—	—	Marital status, occupation
Brennan (2000)	M/F	1.0	0.9	1.0	—	—	1.0	0.9	0.7	—	—	Sex, center (all nonsmokers)
Darby (2000)	M/F	—	—	—	—	—	1.0	0.8	0.9	0.9	—	Sex
De Stefani (1999)	M	1.0	0.6	0.5	—	—	1.0	0.7	0.5	—	—	Residence, education, family history, body mass index, total energy and fat intake
Dorgan (1993)	M/F	1.0	1.0	0.9	—	—	1.0	0.9	0.7	—	—	Passive smoking, education, occupation
Fontham (1988)	M/F	1.0	0.8	0.7	—	—	1.0	0.8	0.7	—	—	Race, sex
Gao (1993)	M	1.0	0.8	0.5	—	—	1.0	0.7	0.6	—	—	
Hu (1997)	M/F	—	—	—	—	—	1.0	1.1	0.8	—	—	Sex, area of residence, income
Jain (1990)	M/F	1.0	0.9	1.0	1.1	—	1.0	0.7	0.7	0.6	—	
Kreuzer (2002)	F	1.0	0.6	0.7	—	—	1.0	0.6	0.5	—	—	Region (all nonsmokers)
Kubik (2002)	F	1.0	0.7	—	—	—	1.0	0.8	—	—	—	Residence, education
Le Marchand (1989)	M	—	—	—	—	—	1.0	0.9	0.7	0.4	—	Ethnicity, cholesterol intake
Mayne (1994)	M	1.0	0.4	0.7	0.7	—	1.0	1.1	1.3	0.6	—	
	F	1.0	0.6	0.5	0.6	—	1.0	1.0	0.8	0.5	—	
Mohr (1999)	M/F	1.0	1.0	1.2	0.8	—	1.0	1.0	1.0	1.0	—	Sex, race, education
Swanson (1992)	M	1.0	0.7	1.5	0.9	—	—	—	—	—	—	Income, education
Swanson (1997)	F	1.0	1.0	1.0	0.9	0.8	1.0	0.9	0.7	0.8	0.6	
Takezaki (2001)	M	1.0	1.2	1.0	1.0	— (AC)	1.0	1.1	1.1	1.0	— (AC)	Season and year of visit, prior lung disease, green vegetable and meat intake
		1.0	0.9	0.8	0.6	— (SCC)	1.0	1.3	0.7	0.8	— (SCC)	
	F	1.0	0.7	0.8	0.7	— (AC)	1.0	0.7	0.9	0.8	— (AC)	
Wu-Williams (1990)	F	1.0	1.0	1.4	1.5	—	1.0	1.1	1.0	0.9	—	Education
Prospective studies												
Breslow (2000)	M/F	1.0	1.2	0.8	0.9	—	1.0	1.0	1.3	0.9	—	Sex
Chow (1992)	M	1.0	0.8	0.8	0.7	—	1.0	1.1	1.1	1.2	—	Occupation
Feskanich (2000)	M/F	1.0	1.1	1.0	1.1	0.9	1.0	0.9	0.8	0.9	0.8	Energy intake
Fraser (1991)	M/F	1.0	0.3	0.3	—	—	1.0	1.4	1.1	—	—	Sex
Hirvonen (2001)	M	1.0	0.9	0.9	0.7	—	1.0	1.0	0.9	0.7	—	Group
Jansen (2001)	M	1.0	0.6	0.7	—	—	1.0	0.7	0.9	—	—	Country, energy and fruit/vegetable intake
Knekt (1999)	M	1.0	0.9	0.6	—	—	1.0	0.9	0.8	—	—	
Kromhout (1987)	M	1.0	1.1	1.0	—	—	—	—	—	—	—	
Neuhouser (2003)	M/F	1.0	0.8	0.7	0.7	0.6	1.0	0.6	0.8	0.6	0.8	Sex, asbestos exposure, ethnicity, enrollment center
Ocke (1997)	M	1.0	0.5	0.5	—	—	1.0	0.8	0.9	—	—	Energy intake
Shibata (1992)	M	1.0	1.1	1.0	—	—	1.0	1.1	1.0	—	—	
	F	1.0	0.8	0.7	—	—	1.0	0.7	0.6	—	—	
Steinmetz (1983)	F	1.0	0.8	0.5	0.8	—	1.0	0.7	0.5	0.5	—	
Voorips (2000)	M/F	1.0	0.7	0.6	0.6	0.8	1.0	1.1	1.0	1.0	0.7	Sex, family history, education

[a]1 = lowest consumption category. The exposure categories of low to high are for summary purposes only and do not correspond to identical categories across studies.
AC, adenocarcinoma; F, female; M, male; SCC, squamous cell carcinoma.

cases had circulating concentrations of retinol, β-carotene, total carotenoids, vitamin E, and vitamin C that were 20% or more lower than those of noncases. However, the possibility that preclinical and clinically diagnosed lung cancer and concomitant changes in diet can lead to decreases in circulating micronutrient levels limits the inferences that may be drawn from studies based on blood samples taken after the diagnosis of lung cancer.

Data from prospective cohort studies are not subject to the previous limitation. In these studies, blood is collected from a population that is initially cancer-free and the population is then followed for the occurrence of lung cancer. The results of such

Table 2 Estimated relative risk of lung cancer according to intake of selected micronutrients[a]

First author (year)	Sex	Retinol 1	2	3	4	5	β-Carotene 1	2	3	4	5	Total carotenoids 1	2	3	4	5	Vitamin C 1	2	3	4	5
Case-control studies																					
Alavanja (1993)	F	1.0	1.4	0.8	0.9	1.3	1.0	0.9	0.9	1.0	1.0	1.0	0.9	0.9	0.9	1.3	1.0	1.5	1.1	1.3	1.5
Bond (1987)	M	1.0	0.9	0.9	—	—	—	—	—	—	—	1.0	1.0	0.9	—	—	—	—	—	—	—
Byers (1984)	M	1.0	0.8	0.5	—	—	—	—	—	—	—	1.0	0.7	0.4	—	—	—	—	—	—	—
	(SCC)	1.0	0.8	0.7	—	—(SM) —(AD)	—	—	—	—	—	—	—	—	—	—	—	—	—	—	—
Byers (1987)	M	1.0	0.9	0.6	—	—	—	—	—	—	—	1.0	1.0	0.9	0.8	—	1.0	1.0	0.9	0.8	—
	F	1.0	1.0	1.2	—	—	—	—	—	—	—	1.0	0.7	1.1	0.9	—	1.0	0.9	0.7	0.9	—
De Stefani (1999)	M/F	—	—	—	—	—	1.0	0.8	0.6	0.4	—	1.0	0.8	0.6	0.4	—	1.0	0.9	1.0	1.0	—
Fontham (1988)	M/F	1.0	0.9	0.9	—	—	—	—	—	—	—	1.0	1.0	0.9	—	—	1.0	0.9	0.7	—	—
Hinds (1984)	M/F	1.0	0.8	0.9	0.7	—	—	—	—	—	—	1.0	0.8	0.7	0.6	—	1.0	0.8	0.8	0.8	—
Jain (1990)	M/F	1.0	1.0	0.1	1.2	—	1.0	0.9	0.8	1.1	—	1.0	0.9	0.8	1.1	—	—	—	—	—	—
Le Marchand (1989)	M	1.0	1.0	1.1	1.1	—	1.0	1.3	0.8	0.5	—	1.0	1.0	0.5	0.4	—	1.0	1.0	0.5	0.4	—
Mayne (1994)	M	1.0	0.9	—	—	—	1.0	0.6	—	—	—	—	—	—	—	—	—	—	—	—	—
	F	1.0	1.0	—	—	—	1.0	0.8	—	—	—	—	—	—	—	—	—	—	—	—	—
Mettlin (1979)	M	1.0	1.0	—	—	—	—	—	—	—	—	—	—	—	—	—	—	—	—	—	—
Mettlin (1989)	M/F	—	0.9	0.6	—	—	1.0	0.9	0.8	0.6	0.5	—	—	—	—	—	—	—	—	—	—
Samet (1985)	M/F	1.0	0.8	0.7	—	—	—	—	—	—	—	1.0	0.9	0.8	—	—	—	—	—	—	—
Ziegler (1986)	M	1.0	1.2	1.2	—	—	—	—	—	—	—	1.0	0.2	1.5	—	—	—	—	—	—	—
Prospective studies																					
Chow (1992)	M	1.0	1.1	1.2	0.8	0.9	1.0	0.8	1.0	1.0	0.8	1.0	1.0	0.8	1.1	0.8	1.0	0.7	0.9	0.7	0.8
Holick (2002)	M	1.0	1.0	1.0	1.0	1.0	1.0	0.9	0.9	0.8	0.9	1.0	1.0	0.9	0.8	0.8	—	—	—	—	—
Knekt (1999)	M	—	—	—	—	—	1.0	1.1	0.8	—	—	1.0	1.2	0.9	—	—	—	—	—	—	—
Kromhout (1987)	M	—	—	—	—	—	1.0	0.5	0.7	—	—	1.0	0.4	0.4	—	—	—	—	—	—	—
Michaud (2000)	M/F	—	—	—	—	—	1.0	1.1	1.0	1.0	0.8	1.0	1.0	1.0	0.8	0.7	1.0	0.7	0.8	0.8	0.7
Neuhouser (2003)	M/F	—	—	—	—	—	1.0	0.9	0.9	1.0	1.0	1.0	1.0	0.9	1.0	0.9	1.0	0.8	0.4	—	—
Ocke (1997)	M	—	—	—	—	—	1.0	0.7	0.7	—	—	—	—	—	—	—	—	—	—	—	—
Paganini-Hill (1987)	M	1.0	1.2	1.0	—	—	1.0	1.3	0.7	—	—	—	—	—	—	—	—	—	—	—	—
	F	1.0	0.7	0.9	—	—	1.0	0.3	0.7	—	—	—	—	—	—	—	—	—	—	—	—
Rohan (2002)	F	—	—	—	—	—	1.0	1.8	1.8	1.4	—	—	—	—	—	—	—	—	—	—	—
Shekelle (1981)	M	1.0	2.2	1.4	2.0	—	—	0.9	1.1	—	—	1.0	0.8	0.4	0.1	—	—	—	—	—	—
Shibata (1992)	M	—	—	—	—	—	1.0	0.9	0.6	—	—	1.0	0.9	1.1	—	—	—	—	—	—	—
	F	—	—	—	—	—	1.0	0.7	0.6	—	—	1.0	0.8	0.6	—	—	—	—	—	—	—
Speizer (1999)	F	—	—	—	—	—	1.0	1.1	0.8	1.0	0.8	1.0	1.2	1.0	1.0	0.9	1.0	0.9	1.2	0.6	1.4
Steinmetz (1993)	F	—	—	—	—	—	1.0	0.8	0.7	0.8	—	1.0	1.1	0.7	1.4	—	—	—	—	—	—
Voorrips (2000)	M	—	—	—	—	—	1.0	0.8	0.9	1.0	1.0	—	—	—	—	—	1.0	0.8	0.8	—	—
Yong (1997)	M/F	—	—	—	—	—	1.0	0.8	0.9	1.0	1.0	1.0	0.7	0.8	0.7	—	1.0	0.9	0.7	0.7	—

[a]1 = lowest consumption category. The exposure categories of low to high are for summary purposes only and do not correspond to identical categories across studies. AD, adenocarcinoma; F, female; M, male; SCC, squamous cell carcinoma; SM, small cell carcinoma.

prospective studies bolster the evidence supporting the premise that in general, the higher the circulating concentrations of carotenoids (α-carotene, β-carotene, β-cryptoxanthin, lutein, lycopene, and total carotenoids), the lower the risk of lung cancer. Circulating concentrations of retinol, tocopherol, and selenium have not been associated with a reduced risk of lung cancer in most studies.

Studies of both dietary intake and prediagnostic blood concentrations favor a protective association between provitamin A carotenoids (specifically β-carotene, α-carotene, and β-cryptoxanthin) and lung cancer. It is not known, however, if a generally protective association is specific to these carotenoids or whether carotenoid intake merely serves as a marker of the intake of other protective substances or healthier dietary habits in general. The evidence for vitamin C is scant but suggestive of a protective association, whereas the data on vitamin A, vitamin E, and selenium have yielded null findings.

Phytochemicals Phytochemicals are low-molecular-weight molecules produced by plants. Of the many classes of phytochemicals, those studied in relation to lung cancer include phytoestrogens, flavonoids, and glucosinoids.

The tumor-promoting effects of steroid hormones can be blocked by phytoestrogens. Soybeans are a primary source of a specific class of phytoestrogens known as isoflavonoids. The relatively few studies on isoflavonoids in relation to lung cancer have not provided evidence of a link.

Flavonoids exhibit potent antioxidant activity. Flavonoid intake has been at least weakly associated with reduced risk of lung cancer in three out of four studies to date.

Isothiocyanates are metabolites of the class of phytochemcials known as glucosinolates. Isothiocyanates could exert anticancer effects by blocking carcinogens via induction of phase II detoxification enzymes, such as glutathione S-tranferase. Cruciferous vegetables contain high concentrations of glucosinolates, and hence consumption leads to higher endogenous isothiocyanate levels. As with cruciferous vegetables, lung cancer risk is also consistently lower with higher intakes or urinary levels of isothiocyanates.

A postulated link between isothiocyanates and a common polymorphism in the *GSTM1* gene provides an example of a potential gene–diet interaction relevant to lung carcinogenesis. A growing focus in cancer epidemiology is to characterize interindividual susceptibility to cancer by studying polymorphisms in genes involved in DNA repair and in the metabolism and detoxification of potential carcinogens. Of further interest is how such genetic traits interact with environmental exposures to contribute to cancer risk. The role of glutathione S-transferase as a phase II detoxification enzyme has made a common polymorphism in the glutathione S-transferase M1 (*GSTM1*) gene of interest in relation to lung cancer. Results combined across studies show that compared to people with the *GSTM1* present genotype, those with the *GSTM1* null genotype had an increased risk of lung cancer.

When isothiocyanates have been studied in combination with *GSTM1*, the decreased risk of lung cancer associated with isothiocyanates has been especially pronounced in people with the *GSTM1* null genotype. This association may represent either the cancer-blocking activity of isothiocyanates playing an enhanced role in *GSTM1* null individuals or more efficient metabolism of isothiocyanates in those with the *GSTM1* present genotype. Regardless, this is one example of the potential interactions between genetic and dietary factors, an approach that may eventually advance our understanding of the nutritional epidemiology of lung cancer.

Fat and cholesterol Evidence that dietary fat may facilitate tumor growth was reported as early as 1940. Correlation exists between international or regional dietary fat consumption and lung cancer mortality. In case–control studies, total fat intake is consistently associated with lung cancer risk among men and women, but saturated fat, unsaturated fat, and cholesterol intake tend to be associated with lung cancer risk only among men (**Table 3**). The prospective evidence shows a slightly different picture, with both total fat and saturated fat intake strongly associated with lung cancer in men but not women, and unsaturated fat and cholesterol not consistently associated with lung cancer risk in men or women (**Table 3**). The equivocal nature of the evidence is reflected in the lack of consistent findings between the sexes and the results of a large, pooled cohort study of both sexes that found lung cancer risk was not strongly associated with fat (total, saturated, or unsaturated) or cholesterol intake.

Regarding cholesterol, there is inconsistency between the dietary data presented previously and serologic data. A review of 33 prospective cohort studies indicated that lower circulating cholesterol levels were predictive of greater lung cancer risk. Similar results were obtained after accounting for the possible preclinical effects of cancer on cholesterol levels by limiting analyses to cases of lung cancer that were diagnosed 5 or more years after the initial cholesterol measurement. This association may be due to a direct effect of cigarette smoking on lipid profiles or to differences in dietary patterns between smokers and nonsmokers. The lack of consistency between the serologic

Table 3 Estimated relative risk of lung cancer according to fat intake or cholesterol intake[a]

First author (Year)	Sex	Total fat 1	2	3	4	5	Unsaturated fat 1	2	3	4	5	Saturated fat 1	2	3	4	5	Cholesterol 1	2	3	4	5
Case–control studies																					
Alavanja (1993)	F	1.0	1.4	1.4	2.2	2.8	—	—	—	—	—	1.0	1.5	1.6	2.3	4.9	1.0	0.6	0.7	1.1	1.1
Byers (1984)	M	1.0	0.9	1.1	—	—(SCC)	—	—	—	—	—	—	—	—	—	—	—	—	—	—	—
		1.0	0.8	0.8	—	—(SM)	—	—	—	—	—	—	—	—	—	—	—	—	—	—	—
		1.0	1.2	1.0	—	—(AD)	—	—	—	—	—	—	—	—	—	—	—	—	—	—	—
Byers (1987)	M	1.0	1.6	1.8	2.0	—	—	—	—	—	—	—	—	—	—	—	1.0	1.3	1.7	1.4	—
Byers (1987)	F	1.0	1.9	1.0	1.4	—	—	—	—	—	—	—	—	—	—	—	1.0	1.5	1.1	0.9	—
De Stefani (1997)	M	1.0	1.2	1.4	2.9	—	1.0	1.3	1.7	1.8 (monounsaturated)	—	1.0	0.9	2.3	2.1	—	1.0	1.4	1.3	2.3	—
							1.0	1.2	2.2	1.8 (polyunsaturated)	—										
Goodman (1988)	M	1.0	2.3	2.0	2.2	—	1.0	3.5	2.1	2.5 (monounsaturated)	—	1.0	1.8	2.3	2.1	—	1.0	2.3	1.8	2.2	—
Goodman (1988)	F	1.0	0.4	0.8	0.9	—	1.0	0.5	0.6	0.9 (polyunsaturated)	—	1.0	0.6	1.0	1.4	—	1.0	0.6	1.5	0.9	—
Hinds (1983)	M/F	—	—	—	—	—	—	—	—	—	—	—	—	—	—	—	1.0	1.3	1.4	2.0	—
	M	—	—	—	—	—	—	—	—	—	—	—	—	—	—	—	1.0	1.2	1.4	2.3	—
	F	—	—	—	—	—	—	—	—	—	—	—	—	—	—	—	1.0	1.7	1.3	1.2	—
Jain (1990)	M/F	—	—	—	—	—	—	—	—	—	—	—	—	—	—	—	1.0	0.9	1.0	1.6	—
Swanson (1997)	F	1.0	1.4	1.3	2.3	—	—	—	—	—	—	—	—	—	—	—	1.0	1.2	0.9	1.0	1.2
Prospective studies																					
Bandera (1997)	M	1.0	1.3	1.4	—	—	1.0	1.2	1.4 (monounsaturated)	—	—	1.0	1.3	1.4	—	—	1.0	1.1	1.1	—	—
							1.0	1.1	1.0 (polyunsaturated)	—	—										
Bandera (1997)	F	1.0	0.9	1.1	—	—	1.0	0.9	1.0 (monounsaturated)	—	—	1.0	0.7	0.8	—	—	1.0	0.8	1.0	—	—
							1.0	0.9	0.9 (polyunsaturated)	—	—										
Heilbrun (1994)	M	—	—	—	—	—	—	—	—	—	—	—	—	—	—	—	1.0	0.7	1.0	1.0	—
Knekt (1991)	M	1.0	1.3	1.6	—	—	1.0	0.9	1.1 (monounsaturated)	—	—	1.0	1.4	1.6	—	—	1.0	0.8	1.1	—	—
							1.0	0.6	0.9 (polyunsaturated)	—	—										
Shekelle (1991)	M	—	—	—	—	—	—	—	—	—	—	—	—	—	—	—	1.0	1.3	1.9	—	—
Smith-Warner (2002)	M/F	1.0	1.0	1.0	1.0	—	1.0	1.0	1.0	1.0 (monounsaturated)	—	1.0	1.0	1.0	1.0	—	1.0	1.0	1.0	1.0	—
							1.0	1.0	1.0	1.0 (polyunsaturated)	—										
Speizer (1999)	F	1.0	1.0	0.9	0.9	1.1	—	—	—	—	—	1.0	1.0	1.1	1.1	1.1	1.0	1.0	1.3	1.3	1.3
Wu (1994)	F	1.0	0.9	0.9	0.8	—	—	—	—	—	—	—	—	—	—	—	1.0	0.6	0.9	0.9	—
		1.0	0.7	0.6	0.9	—	—	—	—	—	—	—	—	—	—	—	—	—	—	—	—
		1.0 (animal)	0.6	0.7	0.7	—(plant)	—	—	—	—	—	—	—	—	—	—	—	—	—	—	—

[a] 1 = lowest consumption category. The exposure categories of low to high are for summary purposes only and do not correspond to identical categories across studies.
AD, adenocarcinoma; F, female; M, male; SCC, squamous cell carcinoma; SM, small cell carcinoma.

and dietary cholesterol data is not unreasonable given that dietary cholesterol intake is not strongly associated with serum cholesterol levels. The results of a trial of 846 men living at a veteran's home in Los Angeles showed that compared to men randomized to receive a conventional US diet, those randomized to receive a diet that reduced cholesterol intake by half and reduced serum cholesterol by 13% had a 20% increased risk of lung cancer after 8 years of dietary intervention and 2 additional years of follow-up.

Body mass index Prospective studies consistently show low body mass index (BMI) and relative weight to be associated with an increased risk of lung cancer (**Table 4**). This association is observed in some case–control studies, which rely on retrospective ascertainment of BMI, but not in others. Confounding by cigarette smoking should be considered as an explanation for these findings because cigarette smoking is strongly associated both with the risk of lung cancer and with leanness. The need to further test the hypothesis that leanness is a susceptibility factor for lung cancer is indicated by the results of studies in which this association is still observed even after potential confounding by cigarette smoking has been carefully addressed by stratifying by smoking status and by the number of cigarettes smoked per day for smokers.

Beverages Confounding by cigarette smoking is ubiquitous to the study of diet and lung cancer, but perhaps no topic better epitomizes the challenges of controlling confounding by smoking than does beverage consumption. Several beverages, including alcohol, coffee, tea, and milk, have been studied for a possible link to lung cancer. The majority of studies that have adjusted for age and cigarette smoking have observed either null or weak associations between alcohol drinking and the risk of lung cancer (**Table 5**).

Three prospective cohort studies have shown heavy coffee consumption to be associated with an elevated risk of lung cancer after adjustment for cigarette smoking, whereas seven case–control studies have yielded findings that tend to fluctuate around the null (**Table 6**). The issue of confounding between coffee

Table 4 Relative risk of lung cancer according to body mass index[a]

First author (year)	Sex	Average follow-up (years)	Body mass index							Subgroup	Adjusted for
			1	2	3	4	5	6	7		
Chyou (1994)	M	25	1.0	0.9	0.9	0.7	—	—	—		Age, smoking
Drinkard (1995)	F	6	1.0	0.5	0.5	0.5	—	—	—	Total	Age, smoking, physical activity
			1.0	0.6	0.7	—	—	—	—	Never smokers	
			1.0	1.2	0.6	—	—	—	—	Former smokers	
			1.0	0.8	1.0	—	—	—	—	Current smokers	
Henley (2002)	M	14	0.9	1.0	—	—	—	—	—	Nonsmokers	Age, race, former smoker, marital status, education, asbestos exposure, socioeconomic status, intake of alcohol, fat, fruits, and vegetables
	F		1.2	1.0	—	—	—	—	—	Nonsmokers	
Kark (1995)	M	23	2.3	1.3	1.1	1.1	1.0	—	—	Total	Age, smoking, area of residence
			3.7	2.1	1.7	2.0	1.0	—	—	Smokers	
Knekt (1991)	M	15	1.8	1.5	1.4	1.0	—	—	—	Total	Age, smoking, social class, health status, stress
Lee (1992)	M	22/26	1.8	1.5	1.0	—	—	—	—	Follow-up 11–15 years	Age, cigarettes per day, physical activity
			1.0	1.1	1.0	—	—	—	—	Follow-up >15 years	
Olson (2002)	F	12	1.0	0.9	0.7	0.5	0.4	—	—	Total	Age, pack years smoking, smoking status, physical activity, education, beer consumption, height, BMI at age 18, waist circumference

[a]1 = lowest BMI. The exposure categories of low to high are for summary purposes only and do not correspond to identical categories across studies.
BMI, body mass index; F, female; M, male.

Table 5 Estimated relative risk of lung cancer according to alcohol intake[a]

First author (year)	Sex	Total alcohol						Beer						Wine						Hard liquor					
		1	2	3	4	5	6	1	2	3	4	5	6	1	2	3	4	5	6	1	2	3	4	5	6
Case–control studies																									
Mettlin (1989)	M/F	—	—	—	—	—	—	1.0	0.5	0.7	1.3	—	—	1.0	0.5	0.8	0.9	—	—	1.0	0.7	0.6	0.6	—	—
Wu-Williams (1990)	F	1.0	1.3	1.0	1.3	—	—	—	—	—	—	—	—	—	—	—	—	—	—	—	—	—	—	—	—
Bandera (1992)	M	1.0	—	—	—	1.6	—	1.0	—	—	—	1.9	—	1.0	—	—	—	0.7	—	1.0	—	—	—	1.1	—
De Stefani (1993)	M	1.0	1.4	1.6	2.2	—	—	1.0	0.7	1.4	3.4	—	—	1.0	1.2	1.3	1.5	—	—	1.0	0.9	1.3	1.1	—	—
Mayne (1994)	M/F	—	—	—	—	—	—	1.0	1.1	0.9	1.2	—	—	—	—	—	—	—	—	—	—	—	—	—	—
Carpenter (1998)	M/F	1.0	0.5	0.9	1.1	—	—	1.0	0.4	0.9	—	—	—	1.0	0.7	0.8	—	—	—	1.0	1.2	1.9	—	—	—
Korte (2002)	M/F	1.0	0.6	1.3	1.1	1.9	—	—	—	—	—	—	—	—	—	—	—	—	—	—	—	—	—	—	—
Dosemeci (1997)	M	1.0	1.6	1.7	1.7	—	1.4	—	—	—	—	—	—	—	—	—	—	—	—	1.0	1.7	1.9	1.6	—	—
Swanson (1997)	M	1.0	0.6	1.1	1.0	—	—	—	—	—	—	—	—	—	—	—	—	—	—	—	—	—	—	—	—
Murata (1996)	M	1.0	1.0	2.4	1.8	—	—	—	—	—	—	—	—	—	—	—	—	—	—	—	—	—	—	—	—
Zang (2001)	M	1.0	1.1	1.2	1.1	—	—	—	—	—	—	—	—	—	—	—	—	—	—	—	—	—	—	—	—
Prospective studies																									
Pollack (1984)	M	1.0	0.7	1.3	1.7	1.9	—	—	—	—	—	—	—	1.0	2.2	—	—	—	—	1.0	2.6	—	—	—	—
Chow (1992)	M	—	—	—	—	—	—	1.0	1.2	1.4	1.7	1.1	1.8	—	—	—	—	—	—	1.0	1.3	1.3	1.3	1.0	1.9
Potter (1992)	F	—	—	—	—	—	—	1.0	0.6	1.9	—	—	—	—	—	—	—	—	—	1.0	1.1	—	—	—	—
Kvale (1983)	M	1.0	—	1.3	—	—	—	—	—	—	—	—	—	—	—	—	—	—	—	—	—	—	—	—	—
Gordon (1984)	M	1.0 (continuous variable)						—	—	—	—	—	—	—	—	—	—	—	—	—	—	—	—	—	—
	F	0.7 (continuous variable)						—	—	—	—	—	—	—	—	—	—	—	—	—	—	—	—	—	—
Kono (1986/87)	M	1.0	0.6	0.4	0.8	0.9	—	—	—	—	—	—	—	—	—	—	—	—	—	—	—	—	—	—	—
Stemmermann (1990)	M	1.0	0.7	0.9	1.4	1.1	—	—	—	—	—	—	—	—	—	—	—	—	—	—	—	—	—	—	—
Breslow (2000)	M/F	1.0	0.9	1.2	2.1	—	—	—	—	—	—	—	—	—	—	—	—	—	—	—	—	—	—	—	—
(nonsmokers)		1.0	—	—	2.3	—	—	—	—	—	—	—	—	—	—	—	—	—	—	—	—	—	—	—	—
Bandera (1997)	M	1.0	0.8	1.1	—	—	—	—	—	—	—	—	—	—	—	—	—	—	—	—	—	—	—	—	—
	F	1.0	1.2	1.0	—	—	—	—	—	—	—	—	—	—	—	—	—	—	—	—	—	—	—	—	—
Prescott (1999)	M	1.0	0.8	1.0	0.9	1.2	1.6	1.0	1.1	1.4	—	—	—	1.0	0.8	0.4	—	—	—	1.0	1.2	1.5	—	—	—
	F	1.0	0.9	1.0	1.0	1.0	0.8	1.0	0.9	1.5	—	—	—	1.0	0.9	0.2	—	—	—	1.0	0.8	0.7	—	—	—
Woodson (1999)	M	1.0	1.0	1.0	0.9	1.0	—	1.0	1.0	0.8	0.9	0.9	—	1.1	1.0	0.8	—	—	—	1.1	1.0	1.0	1.1	1.1	—
Hirvonen (2001)	M	—	—	—	—	—	—	—	—	—	—	—	—	1.0	0.7	—	—	—	—	—	—	—	—	—	—
Djousse (2002)	M/F	1.0	1.2	1.1	1.3	—	1.2	—	—	—	—	—	—	—	—	—	—	—	—	—	—	—	—	—	—
Korte (2002)	M/F	1.0	1.0	0.9	1.0	1.5	—	—	—	—	—	—	—	—	—	—	—	—	—	—	—	—	—	—	—
CPS I and II, from Korte (2002)	M/F	1.0	1.0	1.0	1.2	1.4	—	—	—	—	—	—	—	—	—	—	—	—	—	—	—	—	—	—	—
Omenn (1996)	M/F	1.2	2.0	0.8	2.0	2.0	1.7	—	—	—	—	—	—	—	—	—	—	—	—	—	—	—	—	—	—

[a] 1 = lowest consumption category. The exposure categories of low to high are for summary purposes only and do not correspond to identical categories across studies.
F, female; M, male.

Table 6 Estimated relative risk of lung cancer according to frequency of tea, coffee, or milk consumption[a]

First author (year)	Sex	Tea						Coffee						Milk					
		1	2	3	4	5	6	1	2	3	4	5	6	1	2	3	4	5	6
								Case–control studies											
Brennan (2000)	M/F	—	—	—	—	—	—	—	—	—	—	—	—	1.0	1.0	0.8	—	—	—
Darby (2001)	M/F	—	—	—	—	—	—	—	—	—	—	—	—	1.0	0.9	1.1	2.1	—	—
Mendilaharsu (1998)	M smokers	1.0	0.7	0.7	0.9	0.5	0.3	1.0	1.1	1.3	0.8	1.2	1.2	—	—	—	—	—	—
Kreuzer (2002)	F nonsmokers	—	—	—	—	—	—	1.0	0.6	—	—	—	—	1.0	1.0	0.7	—	—	—
Kubik (2002)	F	1.0	1.0	—	—	—	(black)	—	—	—	—	—	—	1.0	0.8	—	—	—	—
		1.0	0.9	—	—	—	(green)												
		1.0	1.3	—	—	—	(herbal)												
Zhong (2001)	F nonsmokers	1.0	0.8	0.6	0.5	—	(green)	—	—	—	—	—	—	—	—	—	—	—	—
	F smokers	1.0	1.4	0.6	—	—	(green)												
Mohr (1999)	M/F	1.0	1.0	1.4	1.6	—	(green)	1.0	1.0	1.2	1.3	—	—	1.0	1.6	1.8	—	—	(whole)
														1.0	0.8	—	—	—	(2%)
														1.0	0.6	0.7	—	—	(skim)
Swanson (1997)	F													1.0	1.3	1.2	1.0	1.2	—
Takezaki (2001)	M, AC	1.0	1.1	1.1	1.3	—	(black)	1.0	0.9	1.2	—	—	—	1.0	1.0	0.9	0.8	—	—
	F, AC	1.0	1.0	1.1	1.1	—	(green)	1.0	0.8	0.8	1.3	—	—	1.0	0.8	1.0	0.7	—	—
	M, SCC	1.0	1.0	1.2	1.1	—	—	1.0	1.0	1.2	1.6	—	—	1.0	0.9	0.8	0.7	—	—
Tewes (1990)	F	1.0	1.4	—	—	—	(black)	—	—	—	—	—	—	—	—	—	—	—	—
		1.0	2.7	—	—	—	(green)												
Yoshiyuki (1995)	M	1.0	0.7	0.9	0.9	0.6	(Okinawan)	—	—	—	—	—	—	—	—	—	—	—	—
	F	1.0	0.7	0.8	0.8	0.4	(Okinawan)												
Mayne (1994)	M/F													1.0	0.9	3.3	1.6	—	(whole)
														1.0	1.3	0.8	0.8	—	(skim)
Mettlin (1989)	M/F	1.0	0.9	0.9	1.1	—	—	1.0	1.0	0.9	1.3	—	—	1.0	1.6	1.6	2.1	—	(whole)
														1.0	0.5	0.7	0.5	—	(2%)
														1.0	0.8	0.5	0.7	—	(skim)
Axelsson (1996)	M	1.0	0.9	1.2	0.7	—	—	1.0	0.9	1.2	1.6	—	—	1.0	0.9	1.4	1.7	—	—
								Prospective studies											
Goldbohm (1996)	M/F	1.0	0.9	1.0	0.8	0.9	1.1 (black)	—	—	—	—	—	—	—	—	—	—	—	—
Zheng (1996)	F	1.0	0.9	1.2	1.1	—	—	—	—	—	—	—	—	—	—	—	—	—	—
Breslow (2000)	M/F													1.0	1.4	1.0	—	—	(whole)
														1.0	0.9	0.5	—	—	(2%)
														1.0	1.0	0.6	—	—	(skim)
Hirvonen (2001)	M smokers	1.0	0.7	—	—	—	—	—	—	—	—	—	—	—	—	—	—	—	—
Fraser (1991)	M/F	1.0	—	—	—	—	—	—	—	—	—	—	—	1.0	1.0	0.9	—	—	—

[a] 1 = lowest consumption category. The exposure categories of low to high are for summary purposes only and do not correspond to identical categories across studies.
AC, adenocarcinoma; F, female; M, male; SCC, squamous cell carcinoma.

drinking and other health behaviors, particularly cigarette smoking, has not been addressed adequately, indicating that much stronger evidence is needed for coffee drinking to be considered a risk factor for lung cancer. Despite numerous in vitro and in vivo studies that have observed potential tumor-inhibitory effects of tea, the epidemiologic evidence does not provide support for a link between tea drinking and the risk of lung cancer (**Table 6**).

The associations observed between milk drinking and lung cancer depend on milk fat content. Milk drinking is not strongly associated with lung cancer risk when milk fat content is ignored. The associations between whole milk and lung cancer tend to be either null or in the direction of increased risk, whereas the associations for reduced fat or nonfat milk tend to be either null or in the protective direction (**Table 6**). Perhaps milk consumption, including the type of milk, is merely serving as a marker of fat intake.

Meat and fish Associations have been observed between red meat intake and increased lung cancer risk, but this evidence is counterbalanced by an equal number of null studies. The cooking method may play a role because heterocyclic amines from cooked meat may contribute to an increased lung cancer risk. The evidence does not support a strong link between fish consumption and lung cancer.

Diet and Prevention

Chemoprevention trials Three randomized, double-blind, placebo-controlled trials were undertaken in the 1980s and 1990s to test whether β-carotene supplementation protects against lung cancer. All three studies indicated that β-carotene supplementation in later adulthood does not protect against lung cancer (**Table 7**). To the contrary, β-carotene supplementation was associated with an increased risk of lung cancer among the high-risk populations of heavy smokers in the ATBC Cancer Prevention Study and smokers and asbestos-exposed workers in the CARET Study. No beneficial effect was observed for α-tocopherol supplementation in the ATBC Cancer Prevention Study.

These experimental results fail to corroborate the evidence from observational studies that favors a protective association between β-carotene and lung cancer. In fact, it is possible that β-carotene may exhibit prooxidant properties. Consistent with the results of observational studies, a protective association was noted when the data from the placebo controls in the ATBC Cancer Prevention Study were analyzed according to baseline serum and dietary β-carotene.

In interpreting the results of the ATBC and CARET studies, it is important to recognize that the studies enrolled older, high-risk individuals who had high cumulative exposure to tobacco smoke and/or asbestos. The results therefore presumably apply mainly to the latter stages of carcinogenesis. The doses administered were far higher than the normal dietary range, and the dose–response relationship for preventive effects, anticipated from the observational evidence, may not be applicable. Because antioxidant nutrients may exert their protective effect in the earlier stages of carcinogenesis, β-carotene may have been administered too late to halt the evolution of cellular changes that lead to lung cancer. Alternatively, compounds present in fruits and vegetables other than the micronutrients studied in the trials may protect against lung cancer. The protective associations for fruit and vegetable consumption were allied to the micronutrient

Table 7 Summary of randomized chemoprevention trials of micronutrients and lung cancer

Study (year)	Location	N	Number of cases	Study population	Years of follow-up	Regimen	Relative risk Incidence	Relative risk Mortality
ATBC (1994)	Finland	29 133	876	Male smokers, age 50–69 years	6 (median)	1. Placebo 2. AT (50 mg per day) 3. BC (20 mg per day) 4. AT + BC	0.98 (AT) 1.19 (BC)	1.02 (AT) 1.16 (BC)
CARET (1996)	United States	18 314	388	Asbestos-exposed smokers and heavy smokers Males and females, age 45–69 years	4 (average)	1. Placebo 2. BC (15 mg per day) + retinol (25 000 IU per day)	1.28	1.17 (all causes)
PHS (1996)	United States	22 071	170	Male physicians, age 40–84 years	12 (average)	1. Placebo 2. BC (50 mg on alternate days)	0.93	Not reported

AT, α-tocopherol; BC, β-carotene.

hypothesis, but the results of the chemoprevention trials raise questions about the potential payoff from large trials designed to test single micronutrients, unless there is a strong mechanistic basis or substantial observational evidence pointing to an individual micronutrient as the primary protective agent. Indeed, fruits and vegetables contain an abundance of antioxidants and phytochemicals with diverse anticarcinogenic activities. However, perhaps fruit and vegetable intake is acting as a marker of a healthier lifestyle that is associated with a low risk of cancer.

Conclusions

The past three decades have witnessed a tremendous increase in the information on diet and lung cancer. People who eat more fruits and vegetables in general have a lower risk of lung cancer than people who consume less of these foods. In observational studies, the same holds true for specific micronutrients, such as provitamin A carotenoids and vitamin C. The specific constituents of fruits and vegetables that confer protection are not known, and the results of the chemoprevention trials suggest a more complex role than researchers had previously thought. An important unanswered question is whether fruits and vegetables directly confer protection against cancer or whether estimates of fruit and vegetable consumption are indicators of differences between individuals who eat healthy and unhealthy diets that are leading to uncontrolled confounding. Nevertheless, the protective association noted for fruit and vegetable consumption has the potential to contribute to prevention. A diet adequate in fruit and vegetables is prudent for preventing chronic diseases in general.

Even for a dietary factor such as fruit or vegetable consumption that is generally associated with a reduced risk of lung cancer, the highest exposure category is usually associated with at most a halving of the risk of lung cancer. An association of this magnitude may result from residual confounding by cigarette smoking. Studies that control for cigarette smoking in the design are best suited to address the persistent concern about residual confounding by cigarette smoking. Examples are case–control studies in which cases and controls are closely matched on cigarette smoking history and studies limited to never-smokers.

Advances in the understanding of the role of diet in the etiology of lung cancer should not obscure the irrefutable fact that cigarette smoking is the predominant cause of lung cancer. Many important questions about the complex relationship between dietary habits and the development of lung cancer remain, but the path to permanently ending the epidemic of lung cancer is known: Prevent children from starting cigarette smoking and effectively assist addicted smokers to stop smoking cigarettes.

Acknowledgments

The authors thank Brant W. Hager for assistance in the preparation of the manuscript. This work was supported by funding from grants from the US National Cancer Institute (CA73790 and 5U01CA086308), the National Institute of Environmental Health Sciences (P30 ES03819), and the National Institute of Aging (5UO1AG018033).

See also: **Alcohol**: Disease Risk and Beneficial Effects. **Ascorbic Acid**: Physiology, Dietary Sources and Requirements. **Body Composition**. **Cancer**: Carcinogenic Substances in Food. **Carotenoids**: Chemistry, Sources and Physiology. **Cholesterol**: Sources, Absorption, Function and Metabolism; Factors Determining Blood Levels. **Fruits and Vegetables**. **Phytochemicals**: Classification and Occurrence; Epidemiological Factors. **Vitamin A**: Physiology.

Further Reading

Alberg AJ and Samet JM (2003) Epidemiology of lung cancer. *Chest* **123**: 21S–49S.
Samet JM (ed.) (1995) *Epidemiology of Lung Cancer*. New York: Marcel Dekker.
Schottenfeld D and Fraumeni JF (eds.) (1996) *Cancer Epidemiology and Prevention*, 2nd edn. Oxford: Oxford University Press.
Willett WC (1998) *Nutritional Epidemiology*, 2nd edn. Oxford: Oxford University Press.
World Cancer Research Fund (1997) *Food, Nutrition, and the Prevention of Cancer: A Global Perspective*. Washington, DC: American Institute for Cancer Research.

Dietary Management

C Shaw, Royal Marsden NHS Foundation Trust, London, UK

© 2005 Elsevier Ltd. All rights reserved.

Patients with cancer suffer from numerous eating difficulties due to the disease or treatments. However, if attention is paid to these problems and dietary intervention is early, patients can be relived from some of the symptoms and need not lose a great deal of weight. Many dietary problems may be anticipated if there is a known diagnosis and treatment plan, and a prompt referral to a dietician is beneficial. All patients should undergo a nutritional screening and assessment, and high-risk patients or those experiencing problems should be referred for advice and appropriate support.

Weight loss and poor nutritional status may lead to poor wound healing, increased risk of local and systemic infection, reduced tolerance to treatment, poor postoperative recovery, and reduced quality of life. Maintenance of good nutritional status is important to enable patients to complete their course of anticancer treatment.

Nutritional Support

Many cancer patients will require some form of nutritional support during the course of their illness (**Table 1**). When patients have an eating difficulty, the first course of action is to assess their oral intake. If patients are able to eat, then they should be given appropriate advice to maximize their oral intake. If patients are unable to swallow enough nourishment to maintain their weight, an enteral tube feed should be considered. The type of tube placed will depend on the following:

1. The anticipated length of time the feed will be required.
2. The physical state of the patient; for example, a nasogastric tube or percutaneous endoscopically placed gastrostomy tube may not be suitable for patients with complete oesophageal obstruction. A jejunostomy tube may be preferred following upper gastrointestinal tract surgery.
3. The wishes of the patient concerning the physical appearance of different tubes and the invasiveness of the procedure required to place them.

Table 1 Methods of nutritional support

Method	Route
Oral feeding	Oral feeding can be facilitated by
	Altering the consistency or timing of food or drink
	Fortifying food and drinks with protein and energy
	Altering the flavoring added to food
	Using sip feeds and dietary supplements
Enteral tube feeding	Nasogastric or nasojejunal tube Gastrostomy
	Percutaneous endoscopically guided Gastrostomy
	Radiologically inserted gastrostomy
	Percutaneous gastrostomy with a jejunal extension
	Jejunostomy
Parenteral nutrition	Central line
	Peripheral line

Numerous brands of enteral feeds are available. Most cancer patients will require complete, whole protein feeds providing $4–6\,kJ\,ml^{-1}$ ($1–1.5\,kcal\,ml^{-1}$). Only in cases of severe malabsorption, gastrointestinal fistula, or pancreatic insufficiency may elemental, peptide, or low-fat feeds be necessary.

The choice of feeding regimen will depend on the patient's mobility and activity during the day and on the volume of feed tolerated. It may be administered in the following ways: pump feeding overnight and/ or during the day; gravity feeding, which is usually provides a faster rate of feeding that does not require the precision of a pump; and bolus feeding.

Parenteral nutrition is required where the gastrointestinal tract cannot be used, such as in patients with complete bowel obstruction or severe malabsorption.

Practical Management of Eating Difficulties

Anorexia

Anorexia (loss of appetite) is often associated with other eating difficulties, such as nausea, taste changes, and constipation, and addressing these problems may improve the patient's appetite. Pain may also contribute to anorexia, and regular analgesia for pain may in turn help improve appetite, as may dietary alterations (**Table 2**). For patients who have severe anorexia, an appetite stimulant should be considered, such as dexamethasone, medroxyprogesterone acetate, or megestrol acetate.

Taste Changes

Cancer patients may suffer from lack of taste or 'taste blindness,' they may find that foods taste metallic or excessively salty or sweet, or they may find that foods taste abnormal. Depending on the taste change experienced, it is often worth excluding certain foods from the diet or using certain flavorings to try to stimulate the taste buds (**Table 3**).

Table 2 Dietary management of anorexia

Give small, frequent meals and snacks in preference to three meals daily.
Serve food on a small plate.
Ensure food looks appetizing.
Encourage any food the person prefers, even if it is all of one type (e.g., puddings).
Distract from eating (e.g., by conversation, watching television, or listening to music).
Give an alcoholic drink to be sipped before meals or with food.

Table 3 Suggestions for overcoming taste changes

Taste change	Suggestions
Excessively sweet	Reduce sugar content of food and drink. Add a pinch of salt to drinks and puddings.
Excessively salty	Avoid packet soups, gravy, and sauces. Avoid salted snacks (e.g., crisps and nuts) or try unsalted varieties. Avoid bacon and other cured or tinned meat. Add a pinch of sugar to sauces or soups.
Metallic taste	Soak red meat in acidic marinate (e.g., vinegar and wine). Eat white meat, fish, eggs, and cheese in preference to red meat. Avoid tea, coffee, and chocolate.
Taste blindness	Use extra flavorings: salt, pepper, pickles, mustard, herbs, and spices. Eat highly flavored food (e.g., curry).

Nausea and Vomiting

Nausea and vomiting must be controlled with antiemetic drugs. Some dietary suggestions may help patients with food choice when they are feeling nauseous (**Table 4**).

Dysphagia

Dysphagia (difficulty swallowing) may occur with solid food, semisolid foods such as porridge, or liquids. For the person who cannot manage solid food but is able to eat semisolids, altering the consistency of the food may be the only dietary change needed, encouraging food with extra sauce, soft puddings, and nourishing drinks.

For the patient who is only able to swallow fluids, close attention must be paid to their intake and dietary supplements are likely to be necessary. Some people who can only manage liquids choose to liquidize their food; this dilutes the nutrients, so meals should be fortified with butter, cream, glucose, cheese, etc. to add protein and energy.

If there is complete dysphagia to both solids and liquids, feeding by an enteral tube should be considered.

Table 4 Suggestions for food and fluids when person has nausea

Have cold food and drink in preference to hot because these have less odor.
Sip fizzy drinks.
Drink through a straw.
Try ginger flavors (e.g., ginger ale and ginger biscuits).
Eat small, frequent snacks to avoid the stomach from becoming completely empty.

In some instances, people can swallow solid food but aspirate liquids. Patients should undergo a complete assessment from a speech and language therapist to ascertain which textures are safe to swallow. It may be that thickened liquids such as milk shakes or those thickened with a commercial thickener are suitable, whereas thin liquids, such as tea and water, are aspirated. If thick fluids are also aspirated, it is usually safer to give nothing by mouth and to maintain hydration and nutrition through an enteral tube.

Mucositis and Stomatitis

If the mouth or throat is sore, eating can become very difficult. An analgesic taken before meals can help ease the pain and enable the person to eat a little more. Modifying the diet is also helpful (**Table 5**).

Xerostomia

Xerostomia (dry mouth) may be a long-term side effect of cancer treatment, and patients may need to use extra sauce with their foods or have soft food, and they usually need to sip a drink while eating. Chewing gum, preferably sugar-free, can stimulate saliva, although it should be avoided by those with no saliva because it will stick to their teeth. Pineapple can also stimulate saliva and eating it between meals may make the mouth more comfortable.

Good dental hygiene is particularly important because saliva protects the mouth against infection. If people with xerostomia also get mouth infections, the resulting mucositis makes it increasingly difficult for them to eat.

Trismus and Difficulty Chewing

Trismus (difficulty opening the mouth) and difficulty chewing may be overcome with soft food or, failing that, with nourishing drinks and dietary supplements. If the person loses weight and can manage very little orally, an enteral tube feed should be considered.

Table 5 Suggestions to relieve mucositis and stomatitis

Avoid citrus fruits and drinks.
Avoid salty, spicy food, vinegar, pickles, and other strong flavors.
Avoid carbonated drinks.
Have tepid food and drinks.
Iced drinks may be soothing (or may increase the pain).
Avoid dry foods that need extra chewing (e.g., toast).
Eat soft food and use extra sauce.

Gastrointestinal Fistulas

A fistula may develop anywhere in the gastrointestinal tract. The site of the fistula will determine the dietary management (**Table 6**).

Constipation

The cause of constipation must be considered initially. If it is due to a tumor pressing on the bowel (e.g., cancer of the ovary or colon), a low-fiber diet may be helpful. Low-fiber food is less bulky and may pass through the bowel more easily, particularly if accompanied by appropriate laxatives (e.g., stool softener).

If constipation is due to lack of fiber in the diet, then an increased fiber and fluid intake may be helpful. If constipation is due to analgesia, then appropriate laxatives need to be used in conjunction with any changes in the diet. In addition to fiber, a good fluid intake must be maintained to avoid constipation; approximately 2 litres per day is recommended.

Diarrhea

Diarrhea may be due to overflow from constipation, in which case the advice for constipation should be followed. Diarrhea due to intestinal hurry caused by bowel disease or drugs may be controlled with drugs and by avoiding excessive intake of high-fiber foods, which naturally pass through the bowel quickly. When malabsorption is suspected, a low-fat, elemental enteral tube feed should be considered. When diarrhoea is severe, it is important to replace the fluid lost to prevent dehydration. Oral rehydration solution is useful to replace fluid loses. Diarrhea caused by radiotherapy needs to be controlled with drugs, and a low-fiber diet is not thought to be helpful in this instance.

Intestinal Failure

A long-term side effect of pelvic radiotherapy may be enteritis resulting in intestinal failure. Extensive gastrointestinal surgery leaving less than 100 cm of small bowel, or a fistula in the small bowel causing high stoma losses, may also cause intestinal failure. Previous chemotherapy that may affect the function of the bowel can contribute to this condition. Intestinal failure is more likely to occur when the patient does not have a functioning colon (e.g., in the case of ileostomists or when the ileo-caecal valve is absent).

Dietary manipulation can greatly alleviate the symptoms of intestinal failure, such as thirst, dehydration, and high stoma losses or large volumes of diarrhea (**Table 7**).

An oral rehydration solution consisting of 20 g glucose, 3.5 g sodium chloride, 2.5 g sodium bicarbonate, and 1000 ml water provides 90 mmol of sodium per liter. It may be used chilled and to dilute weak fruit squashes. If the patient remains dehydrated despite following the advice detailed in **Table 7**, intravenous fluid replacement is necessary.

Drugs may be given to increase gut transit time or reduce fluid losses. If medication is in the form of capsules, these should be opened and the drugs given 60 min before meals. Suitable drugs include codeine phosphate, loperamide, rantidine, and octreotide. In the longer term, the following should be monitored:

Plasma electrolytes, ferritin, and vitamin D levels
Serum albumin, magnesium, zinc, calcium, phosphate, and alkaline phosphate
Folate and vitamin B_{12} concentrations
Prothrombin time
Body weight
Urinary sodium concentration

Bowel Obstruction

Bowel obstruction may be subacute or complete. In cases of complete bowel obstruction, the clinical condition of the patient must be considered. If it is

Table 6 Sites of fistulas and their management

Site	Management
Neck, salivary fistula	'Nil by mouth' and enteral tube feed until healed
Chyle leak (e.g., in neck)	Low-fat diet initially; if unsuccessful, a low-fat, medium-chain triglyceride enteral tube feed
	If unsuccessful, consider parenteral nutrition
Large bowel	Low-residue diet or elemental enteral tube feed
Small bowel	See **Table 7**

Table 7 Dietary management to reduce gut losses in intestinal failure

Restrict fluids to 500–1000 ml daily, increasing to 1500 ml.
Avoid drinks for 30 min before and 45 min after meals.
Avoid foods that are particularly high in fiber.
Sprinkle salt liberally on food.
Consider fat restriction if patient has a colon and there is evidence of steatorrhea.
Take salt and carbohydrate foods together to help sodium absorption.
If gut losses are 1000 ml or more, part or all of fluid intake should consist of an oral rehydration solution.

anticipated that the obstruction will resolve, or if aggressive treatment such as surgery is planned, parenteral nutritional support should be considered. Total parenteral nutrition may be inappropriate and is unlikely to be useful in cases in which the prognosis is poor and no treatment is possible.

Depending on the degree of obstruction, in cases of subacute obstruction the following action may be taken under medical supervision:

First day: sips of clear fluid, approximately $10 \, \text{ml} \, \text{h}^{-1}$
Second day: $30 \, \text{ml} \, \text{h}^{-1}$ clear fluid
Third day: $60 \, \text{ml} \, \text{h}^{-1}$ clear fluid
Fourth day: free clear fluids
Fifth day: free fluids, including milk, low-fiber soup, custard, and jelly
Sixth day: low-fiber diet, avoiding all fruit and vegetables, nuts, pulses, and whole grain cereals, whole meal bread, etc.

A patient who starts to vomit should return to the diet prescribed for the preceding day. If symptoms of bowel obstruction, such as abdominal pain and indigestion, remain controlled, fruit and vegetables may be introduced as tolerated, starting with small amounts.

Weight loss

Weight loss is often the consequence of the dietary problems described previously. The measures in **Table 8** should be considered to help prevent weight loss or encourage weight gain. It must be remembered that energy requirements may be elevated due to the physiological effects of malignancy. Much interest has focused on attempts to influence the metabolic alterations in cachexia via nutrients. Research has examined the possible role of eicosapentaenoic acid (EPA), an n-3 fatty acid, in reducing the inflammatory response in cachexia. A randomized trial in pancreatic cancer patients compared a high-energy drink fortified with EPA to a standard high-energy drink to examine whether this was more effective at promoting weight gain. The study failed

Table 8 Dietary advice to help prevent weight loss

Fortify food with cream, butter, cheese, oil, sugar, honey, glucose, jam, etc.
Have small, frequent snacks.
Use full-fat and full-sugar products.
Avoid large amounts of lower energy foods (e.g., fruit and vegetables).
Try dietary supplements, such as milky drinks and glucose polymer power.
Consider an overnight enteral tube feed to supplement the diet if weight loss continues despite following the previous advice.

to show any additional benefit of EPA in terms of weight gain.

Palliative Care

In some people, cancer will not be cured. Palliative care focuses on the relief of symptoms rather than aggressive curative treatment. The majority of people receiving palliative care will suffer from at least one eating difficulty. Much of the advice detailed previously for overcoming dietary problems is relevant, but it is often upsetting for these patients to have to pay close attention to their dietary intake. If patients are unconcerned about their poor dietary intake, it may be appropriate not to offer any advice; conversely, for those who are very concerned, the problem should be addressed seriously.

Alternative and Complementary Diets

The alternative and complementary diets considered here are modifications of a normal diet that are claimed to cure or treat cancer. Such diets are often followed for their anticipated antitumor effect. Often, they have not been tested or demonstrated to be effective in scientifically acceptable clinical trials. Patients may use other complementary therapies, such as healing, relaxation, visualization, homeopathy, and herbalism, in addition to making dietary changes. Dietary regimens may share common features:

Mainly vegetarian or vegan—alternatively, diets may limit red meat and allow limited free-range chicken and deep-sea fish
No manufactured or processed foods
Low in salt
Low in sugar
Low in fat
High in fiber, including raw fruit and vegetables and whole grains (these may be organic)
May include fruit and vegetable juices
High-dose vitamins and minerals

Nutritional inadequacies may arise in the patient who has a poor appetite. The diets may cause weight loss and are restrictive and time-consuming to prepare. Some ingredients may be difficult to obtain and are often costly. Studies appear to show no difference in survival rates between patients following complementary therapies and patients receiving conventional treatment alone. Patients who use complementary therapies, however, do report psychological benefits, such as feelings of hope and optimism. Patients should have enough information about the possible advantages and disadvantages before embarking on strict complementary or alternative diets.

The Potential Therapeutic Role of Vitamins

Much interest has been expressed in the therapeutic role of vitamins in cancer patients. This has led a number of alternative and complementary practitioners to advocate the use of high-dose vitamins for cancer patients. It has been know for some time that some vitamin-deficiency states may predispose some individuals to develop cancer. In a study of 29 000 vegetarian Chinese with a high frequency of oesophageal cancer, subjects were given supplements of β-carotene and vitamin E. Raising their daily intake above the minimum requirement reduced the incidence of deficiencies and reduced the number of oesophageal cancers. This type of study on vitamins and the etiology of cancer has led many practitioners and laypeople to extrapolate he role of vitamins into cancer treatment.

Although vitamins in food, especially vegetables and fruits, have been shown to be beneficial in reducing the incidence of particular types of cancer when included in the diet, the beneficial effects have not always been shown with vitamin and mineral supplements. Some supplements may promote tumor growth, as was seen in a study using β-carotene supplementation in patients with lung cancer. Supplementation increased the rate of tumor recurrence in such patients.

The potential therapeutic role of vitamins, such as vitamins D, K, B_6, B_{12}, and folate, has been investigated. However, additional studies are required to determine the role, if any, of such vitamins. It may be that some vitamins help protect against the side effects of tumor therapy, whereas some may modify tumor growth. Excessive dietary supplementation in cancer patients should be avoided until further evidence is available on the effects of vitamins on tumor growth.

See also: **Cancer**: Epidemiology and Associations Between Diet and Cancer; Epidemiology of Gastrointestinal Cancers Other Than Colorectal Cancers; Epidemiology of Lung Cancer; Effects on Nutritional Status. **Cobalamins**. **Colon**: Nutritional Management of Disorders. **Diarrheal Diseases**. **Eating Disorders**: Anorexia Nervosa. **Folic Acid**. **Nutritional Support**: Adults, Enteral; Adults, Parenteral; Infants and Children, Parenteral. **Supplementation**: Dietary Supplements. **Vitamin B$_6$**. **Vitamin D**: Physiology, Dietary Sources and Requirements. **Vitamin E**:

Metabolism and Requirements; Physiology and Health Effects. **Vitamin K**.

Further Reading

Bozzetti F (2001) Nutrition support in patients with cancer. In: Payne-James J, Grimble G, and Silk D (eds.) *Artificial Nutrition Support in Clinical Practice*, pp. 639–680. London: Greenwich Medical Media.

Cerhan JR, Potter JD, Gilmore JME *et al.* (2004) Adherence to the AICR cancer prevention recommendations and subsequent morbidity and mortality in the Iowa Women's Health Study Cohort. *Cancer Epidemiology, Biomarkers and Prevention* **13**(7): 1114–1120.

Downder SM, Cody MM, McCluskey P *et al.* (1994) Pursuit and practice of complementary therapies by cancer patients receiving conventional treatment. *British Medical Journal* **309**: 86–89.

Fearon KCH, von Meyenfeldt MF, Moses AGW *et al.* (2003) Effect of a protein and energy dense n-3 fatty acid enriched oral supplement on loss of weight and lean tissue in cancer cachexia: A randomised double blind trial. *Gut* **52**: 1479–1486.

Food Standards Agency Expert Group on Vitamins and Minerals (2003) *Safe Upper Limits of Vitamins and Minerals*. London: Food Standards Agency.

Gianotti L, Braga M, Nespoli L *et al.* (2002) A randomised controlled trail of preoperative oral supplementation with specialised diet in patients with gastrointestinal cancer. *Gastroenterology* **122**: 1763–1770.

Effects on Nutritional Status

C Shaw, Royal Marsden NHS Foundation Trust, London, UK

© 2005 Elsevier Ltd. All rights reserved.

Many patients with cancer experience nutritional problems during their treatment. The physiological effects of malignancy can cause increased nutritional requirements and a reduced nutritional intake. Anticancer treatment can produce side effects, including anorexia, mucositis, nausea, and vomiting, that can further reduce nutritional intake.

Weight loss and nutritional depletion of the cancer patient may interfere with anticancer treatment. Patients with cancer who lose weight may have a reduced tolerance to treatment due to poor wound healing and an increased susceptibility to infection. Weight loss may also contribute to a poor quality of life. Nutritional support of patients with cancer should be an integral part of treatment. Modification of oral intake may be sufficient to maintain nutritional status. There is also interest in nutrients that may modify cachexia in patients for whom altered metabolism is also contributing to weight loss. If the patient is unable to take sufficient nutrition orally, then food may be given through an enteral tube. Parenteral nutrition may be required when the gastrointestinal tract cannot be used.

Physiological Effects of Malignancy

Cancer cachexia is a syndrome suffered by many, but not all, patients with cancer. It is most prevalent in patients with tumors of the lung, head and neck, or gastrointestinal tract. Features of cachexia include weight loss, muscle wasting, lethargy, anorexia, early satiety, anemia of a nonspecific type, and altered host metabolism.

Weight loss is the most obvious feature of cachexia. In patients with cancer, an unintentional weight loss of 10% is deemed to be a significant change. Cachexia may be masked in people who were previously overweight or who have oedema. These people may be especially at risk of suffering from the consequences of cachexia, such as poor wound healing and increased risk of infection because their nutritional problems may not be addressed as promptly as those of patients who are obviously underweight. The causes of cancer cachexia are multifactorial (**Figure 1**).

Physiological Causes of Cancer Cachexia

Weight-losing patients with cancer may have a reduced energy intake, increased energy expenditure, or a combination of both. It has been estimated that 50–60% of cancer patients in hospital have abnormal resting energy expenditures, although this may be restricted to certain diagnoses, such as pancreatic, lung, and gastrointestinal cancers. Cachexia differs from uncomplicated starvation in that the usual adaptation to a reduced food intake, such as a reduction in energy expenditure and conservation of body protein stores, does not appear to take place. In the starving state, metabolic rate is decreased, weight loss occurs mostly from fat stores, and nitrogen losses are reduced; however, the reverse occurs in many patients with cancer.

Carbohydrate Metabolism

Some patients with cancer have been demonstrated to have a high rate of glucose turnover in both the fasting and the fed states and one cause may be increased Cori cycle activity. In the Cori cycle, glucose is metabolized anaerobically by the tumor, producing lactate (**Figure 2**). The tumor cannot utilize lactate and so it is returned to the liver where it is converted back into glucose. This utilizes energy, and the process is thus an energy-wasting cycle: Only 2 mol of ATP is produced by anaerobic glycolysis, and gluconeogenesis requires 6 mol of ATP. Had the lactate been metabolized aerobically via the Krebs cycle, 30 mol of ATP would have been synthesized. It has been estimated that Cori cycle activity may account for increased energy requirements of 1260 kJ (300 kcal) per day. Lactate has been shown to cause nausea, so it is possible that another side effect of the Cori cycle is reduced food intake.

Insulin resistance has been established as a common hormonal alteration, and raised levels of growth hormone seen in some patients with cancer may contribute to insulin resistance. Glucose intolerance is associated with sepsis, bed rest, starvation, and malnutrition, all of which may occur in cancer patients, making it difficult to establish how much the tumor contributes to glucose intolerance.

Protein Metabolism

Muscle wasting or loss is common in patients with cancer. It has been estimated that protein–energy malnutrition may be present in 50–80% of patients with cancer. Data from human studies indicate increased whole-body protein turnover, synthesis, and catabolism, increased hepatic protein synthesis, and reduced rates of albumin and skeletal muscle protein synthesis. It has been estimated that whole-body protein turnover in cancer patients is 32%

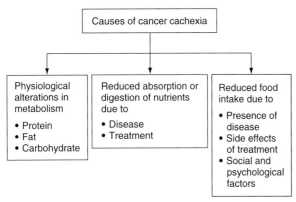

Figure 1 Causes of cancer cachexia.

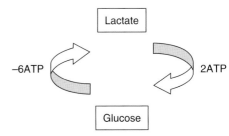

Figure 2 The Cori cycle.

higher than in noncancer patients and 35% higher than in starved normal subjects.

Glucose required by the tumor may be supplied from dietary glucose or by the conversion of amino acids into glucose. Weight-losing patients with cancer may have reduced plasma levels of amino acids alanine, glycine, and glutamine, possibly because these compounds are used for gluconeogenesis, and this may be a cause of increased protein catabolism.

Fat Metabolism

Loss of fat or adipose tissue is common in patients with cancer and is one of the most obvious signs of cachexia. Adipose tissue consists of triglycerides, which can be metabolized to yield free fatty acids and glycerol. In patients without cancer, glycerol concentrations are decreased postprandially because the body does not need to break down adipose tissue; however, patients with cancer have been shown to have raised glycerol concentrations in the fed state, which suggests they are in a hypermetabolic condition.

Alterations in carbohydrate and protein metabolism are greater than those for fat, and it is likely that loss of body fat is mostly due to raised energy expenditure as a consequence of glucose intolerance and cycling.

Differences between Malnourished Patients with and without Cancer

During starvation, the metabolism of people without cancer adapts in order to conserve body tissue. Patients with cancer, however, do not exhibit these mechanisms and therefore lose weight (**Table 1**).

The Role of Cytokines in Patients with Cancer

Cytokines are a range of polypeptides produced by cells of the immune system in response to an inflammatory action. Cytokines, including tumor necrosis factor, interleukins-1 and -6, and interferon-gamma, have been shown to induce some of the features of cancer cachexia when administered to humans. The tumors of patients with cancer may induce an inflammatory reaction resulting in raised levels of cytokines, or it may be that the cytokines produce proinflammatory cytokines. There may be amplification of the effect of cytokines by interaction between two or more.

There is much interest in the possible modulation of cytokine activity by fish oils that contain eicosapentenoic acid. Fish oil supplements rich in n-3 fatty acids may reduce production of cytokines and have been shown to inhibit fat and protein breakdown in animal models of cancer cachexia. Small studies of humans have demonstrated a reduction of proinflammatory cytokines in pancreatic cancer patients when given a supplement equivalent to 2 g of eicosapentaenoic acid (EPA) per day. However, in a clinical trial EPA-supplemented high-energy drinks and standard high-energy drinks slowed weight loss to the same extent.

Mechanisms of Cancer-Related Anorexia

Anorexia is the term given to loss of appetite, and it is thought that varying levels of neurotransmitters within the hypothalamus influence appetite. The neurotransmitter serotonin reduces appetite and neuropeptide Y stimulates appetite. Levels of neurotransmitters in the brain may be altered by plasma nutrients, hormones, and nerve impulses arriving from the gastrointestinal tract.

Although not all mechanisms controlling appetite are known, several theories have been suggested to account for anorexia in cancer patients. The amino acid tryptophan is usually bound to albumin. In cancer patients, because albumin synthesis may be reduced, there may be more free tryptophan circulating in the plasma. Tryptophan is a precursor of serotonin, which is known to inhibit appetite. This model has been used to examine appetite in animal models of cachexia but there is still debate as to whether this is the main cause of the anorexia of cachexia. Cytokines are also known to cause anorexia and, as discussed previously, cancer patients have raised levels of cytokines.

Effects of Treatment on Nutritional Status

Various treatments may be used for cancer with the goal of curing it or palliating symptoms (**Table 2**). All may potentially affect nutritional status.

The treatment chosen depends on the position of the tumor, its extent, and its sensitivity to radiotherapy or chemotherapy. Often, different treatments will be used in succession (e.g., surgery followed by chemotherapy, or radiotherapy followed by surgery).

Table 1 Metabolic differences between cancer patients and noncancer patients during starvation

Noncancer patients	Cancer patients
Reduced glucose tolerance	Increased glucose turnover
Reduced total body protein turnover, including reduced hepatic protein synthesis	Total body protein turnover maintained or increased
Slow weight loss, preferentially of stored fat	Rapid weight loss of fat and protein

Table 2 Treatment for cancer

Treatment	Examples
Surgery	Removal of tumor
	Removal of organ (e.g., gastrectomy, nephrectomy, colectomy)
	Palliation of symptoms (e.g., intestinal bypass, colostomy formation)
Chemotherapy	Single agent
	Combination of agents
	Drugs given as single dose or continuous infusion (e.g., methotrexate, epirubicin, mytoycin, fluorouracil)
Radiotherapy	External bean
	Single fractions daily
	Hyperfractionated
	Intensity modulated radiation therapy
	Brachytherapy—interstitial (e.g., iridium wires)
	Radioisotopes (e.g., iodine 131)
Biological therapies	Interferon
	Interleukin
Endocrine therapies	Tamoxifen
	Aminoglutethimide
	Goserelin
	Medroxyprogesterone acetate
	Megestrol acetate

Table 3 Side effects of chemotherapy that may affect nutritional status

Agent	Side effects
Methotrexate	Severe mucositis
	Nausea (dose dependent)
	Vomiting
Vincristine	Paralytic ileus
Fluorouracil	Diarrhea
	Occasional nausea
Cisplatin	Anorexia
	Severe prolonged nausea
	Nausea and vomiting
	Taste changes (particularly a metallic taste)
	Diarrhea (high doses)
Doxorubicin	Nausea
	Some vomiting
	Mucositis throughout gastrointestinal tract
Docetaxol	Diarrhea

Alternatively, treatments may be used concurrently (e.g., chemoradiation). The effect of treatment on nutritional status depends on the site of the tumor and the treatment given.

Surgery is used to remove all or part of the tumor or to bypass the tumor, thereby allowing organs to continue to function. There are often periods of starvation before and after surgery that may contribute to malnutrition in the cancer patient.

The trauma of surgery causes an increase in the production of catecholamines such as adrenaline, which results in the obligatory loss of nitrogen from the body. Repeated or extensive surgery contributes to an increase in metabolic rate and therefore contributes to nutritional depletion.

Chemotherapy is based on the use of drugs that interrupt the cell cycle and prevent cell multiplication. The drugs act on rapidly proliferating cells and also damage healthy cells, particularly those in the gastrointestinal tract and hair follicles. They may also cause nausea and vomiting, altered taste, nerve damage, and infertility. Drugs may be given orally, intravenously (bolus or continuous infusion), or intrathecally. High-dose chemotherapy may be used with a stem cell rescue. **Table 3** lists commonly used chemotherapeutic agents and their side effects that affect nutritional status.

Radiotherapy is the use of ionizing radiation to destroy malignant cells. External beam radiation is most commonly used. It may be used in combination with chemotherapy to enhance the effects of both treatments.

Biological therapies are based on the use of cytokines derived from cells in the immune system. Cytokines are administered to stimulate the body's immune response to reduce or prevent tumour growth and often cause anorexia.

Endocrine therapies are primarily used to control the growth of hormone-dependent cancers, such as cancer of the breast or prostate. Drugs may be used to block production of hormones or to block hormone receptors.

Head and Neck Cancer

Surgical resection is often used for cancers of the oropharynx. Removal of the tumor and reconstruction may lead to periods when the patient is not allowed to eat or drink in order to allow healing to take place. Resection of the mandible, tongue, maxilla, or pharynx may lead to difficulties with chewing or swallowing. There may be an increased risk of aspiration because of a poor ability to control food or fluids in the mouth or because of an alteration in the anatomy or cranial nerves required for swallowing.

Radiotherapy to the head and neck can have a significant impact on nutritional status with both early side effects, during or immediately after treatment, and late side effects, which may occur years after treatment (**Table 4**). Reduced food intake and weight loss due to soreness and dysphagia are particularly common and occur in up to approximately 90% of patients. A dry mouth (xerostomia) occurs when the salivary glands are irradiated and leave the teeth increasingly prone to tooth decay.

Table 4 Side effects of radiotherapy to the head and neck

Early	Late
Mucositis (inflammation of the mucosa)	Mucosal ulceration
	Xerostomia
Stomatitis (inflammation of the mouth)	Increased viscosity of saliva
Xerostomia (dry mouth)	Dysphagia
Increased viscosity of saliva	Altered taste
Dysphagia (difficulty swallowing)	Mouth blindness
Altered taste	Dental caries
Mouth blindness	Trismus (inability to open mouth)
Nausea	Fibrosis (formation of excessive fibrous tissue)
Anorexia	Stenosis (narrowing)
Loss of smell	Fistula
	Poor wound healing
	Osteoradionecrosis (degeneration of bone)

Chemotherapy may be used in combination with surgery and occasionally given concurrently with radiotherapy. Reduced food intake results from nausea, vomiting, learned food aversions, anorexia, and mucositis. Artificial nutritional support may be required during treatment if oral intake is significantly reduced.

Gastrointestinal Cancer

Surgery, chemotherapy, and radiotherapy treatments may be used for cancers of the gastrointestinal tract, depending on the site and type of disease. The impact of both disease and treatment on nutritional status is often great, particularly in upper gastrointestinal cancers.

Surgical resection of the upper gastrointestinal tract often affects the capacity to ingest food and fluids. Surgery that changes the length or motility of the small intestine affects the ability to digest and absorb food and fluids (**Table 5**). Tumors of the small intestine are rare, but small intestinal resection may be necessary because of strictures caused by previous abdominal or pelvic radiotherapy or because of adhesions from previous surgery.

Radiotherapy is often used to treat tumors of the gastrointestinal tract. It can severely affect the ingestion, digestion, and absorption of food and fluids (**Table 6**). Chronic malabsorption of bile salts contributes to fat malabsorption. Bile salts entering the colon inhibit water absorption and stimulate colonic peristalsis, causing fluid and electrolyte deficiencies.

Chemotherapy for gastrointestinal tumors is often associated with side effects such as anorexia, nausea, vomiting, and mucositis (inflammation of the

Table 5 Nutritional consequences of surgery to the gastrointestinal tract

Area of gastrointestinal tract resected	Impact on nutritional status
Oesophagus	Intestinal hurry (due to vagotomy and pyloroplasty)
	Reduced gastric capacity (due to stomach pull up)
	Stricture at anastomosis (surgical junction)
	Dumping syndrome
Stomach	Reduced capacity for food and fluids
	Early satiety
	Dumping syndrome
	Intestinal hurry (due to vagotomy and pyloroplasty)
	Fat malabsorption
	Anemia (lack of intrinsic factor)
Small intestine	General malabsorption
	Diarrhea
Terminal ileum	Malabsorption of vitamin B_{12}
	Fat malabsorption
	Decreased absorption of bile salts, fat-soluble vitamins, and minerals
	Short bowel syndrome

gastrointestinal mucosa). Learned food aversions, which arise through the association of particular foods with vomiting induced by chemotherapy, may also have an impact on nutritional intake.

Leukemias and Lymphomas

Systemic diseases such as leukemias and lymphomas are usually treated with chemotherapy. Chemotherapy is generally given intermittently to allow the bone marrow to recover. Patients experience anorexia, severe mucositis, nausea, vomiting, taste changes, food aversions, tiredness, and lethargy. Some drugs, such as doxorubicin, may reduce gut motility and increase the risk of gastrointestinal obstruction.

Table 6 Effects of radiotherapy on the gastrointestinal tract

Area irradiated	Side effects
Oesophagus	Dysphagia
	Mucositis
	Fibrosis
Stomach	Anorexia
	Nausea
	Vomiting
Abdomen and pelvis	Anorexia
	Nausea
	Vomiting
	Diarrhea
	Malabsorption
	Early enteritis
	Chronic enteritis

Radiotherapy may be used to treat isolated lymph nodes, as in the case of lymphoma, or it may be used to abolate the immune system prior to a bone marrow transplant or peripheral stem cell rescue. Profound neutropenia may results in bouts of sepsis and increased nutritional requirements due to pyrexia.

Bone Marrow Transplant

Bone marrow transplantation (BMT) carries a high risk of patients developing malnutrition due to the severe side effects of high-dose chemotherapy and whole-body irradiation. BMT may be used to treat acute myeloid leukemia, acute lymphoblastic leukemia, chronic myeloid leukemia, and lymphoma. Side effects that alter nutritional status are more likely to occur in allografts, in which the bone marrow from a matched or mismatched donor is used rather than the patient's own bone marrow. Graft versus host disease may occur in allogenic BMT. It is characterized by inflammation of the skin, which may cause increased nutritional requirements. Other symptoms include gastrointestinal involvement with severe diarrhoea; loss of blood, mucus, and tissue via the gastrointestinal tract; and increased fluid losses. There may also be liver involvement and altered liver function (**Table 7**).

Gynecological Cancer

Treatment for cancer of the ovary, uterus, or cervix can have a major impact on nutritional status (**Table 8**). Malignant disease, surgery, or radiotherapy in the pelvis can lead to adhesions, strictures of the bowel, malabsorption, and bowel obstruction. Irreversible damage may necessitate a gastrointestinal resection or the formation of an ileostomy or colostomy. Malignant ascites can impinge on the gastrointestinal tract due to pressure exerted by fluid within the abdomen, causing anorexia and early satiety. Chemotherapeutic drugs (e.g., cisplatin) used to treat gynecological cancers cause severe

Table 7 Side effects of bone marrow transplantation affecting nutritional status

Early	Late
Anorexia	Anorexia
Weight loss	Weight loss
Vomiting	Xerostomia
Stomatitis	Taste changes
Xerostomia	Chronic graft versus host disease
Diarrhea	
Malabsorption	Somnolence
Taste changes	
Acute graft versus host disease	

Table 8 Nutritional problems in gynecological cancer

Anorexia
Early satiety
Nausea
Vomiting
Taste changes
Radiation enteritis, early or late
Short bowel syndrome
Subacute bowel obstruction
Complete bowel obstruction

nausea and vomiting and therefore greatly reduce food intake.

Brain Tumors

Brain tumors are generally treated with surgery followed by radiotherapy or chemotherapy. A small percentage of patients may develop dysphagia as a result of the tumor, the treatment, or both, particularly in tumors of the brain stem. Patients may also experience taste changes, which can be severe and permanent, and somnolence following brain radiotherapy. High-dose steroids, such as prednisolone or dexamethasone, may cause increased appetite, steroid-induced diabetes mellitus, and weight gain.

Breast Cancer

Breast cancer patients are often treated with surgery, radiotherapy, and chemotherapy. Because surgery and radiotherapy are performed away from the gastrointestinal tract, these treatment modalities rarely have a major impact on nutritional status. Chemotherapy with drugs such as epirubicin may cause nausea, vomiting, and stomatitis (inflammation of the mouth), and docetaxol may cause diarrhea. In advanced disease, mediastinal nodes may cause dysphagia, and secondary liver disease may cause anorexia and nausea. Chemotherapy may cause general anorexia, lethargy, and nausea in some patients, although there is evidence that many breast cancer patients may gain weight during chemotherapy or when taking hormone treatments.

Cancer in Children

Malnutrition is common in children undergoing treatment for cancer because treatment is often aggressive and multimodal. Malnurition may occur in approximately one-third of all pediatric patients but is more common in certain diagnostic groups. High-risk diagnoses include Ewing's sarcoma, Wilms' tumor, head and neck tumors, advanced lymphomas, and neuroblastoma. Malnutrition and anticancer treatment in children may affect their future growth. The possible causes of malnutrition are listed in **Table 9**.

Table 9 Causes of malnutrition in children with cancer

Increased metabolic rate
Mechanical gastrointestinal problems (e.g., tumor pressing on stomach or gastrointestinal tract)
Malabsorption
Nausea
Vomiting
Taste abnormalities
Mucositis
Stomatitis
Dysphagia
Diarrhea
Somnolence
Behavioral and environmental factors
Poor eating habits
Learned food aversions
Noncompliance with dietary regimens

See also: **Ascorbic Acid**: Physiology, Dietary Sources and Requirements; Deficiency States. **Cancer**: Effects on Nutritional Status; Epidemiology and Associations Between Diet and Cancer. **Diabetes Mellitus**: Etiology and Epidemiology; Classification and Chemical Pathology. **Small Intestine**: Disorders; Structure and Function. **Stomach**: Disorders; Structure and Function.

Further Reading

Bozzetti F (2001) Nutrition support in patients with cancer. In: Payne-James J, Grimble G, and Silk D (eds.) *Artificial Nutrition Support in Clinical Practice*, pp. 639–680. London: Greenwich Medical Media.

Gibney E, Elia M, Jebb SA, Murgatroyd P, and Jennings G (1997) Total energy expenditure in patients with small-cell lung cancer: Results of a validated study using the bicarbonate–urea method. *Metabolism* **46**(12): 1412–1417.

Tisdale MJ (2003) The 'cancer cachectic factor.' *Supportive Care in Cancer* **11**(2): 73–78

Carcinogenic Substances in Food

D Anderson, University of Bradford, Bradford, UK
J C Phillips, BIBRA International Ltd, Carshalton, UK

© 2005 Elsevier Ltd. All rights reserved.

Introduction

Chemicals that are known or suspected to be carcinogenic to experimental animals and man are widespread throughout the environment. They occur naturally in the physical environment and are found in a very large number of higher plants, fungi and micro-organisms, many of which are part of the human diet. Some carcinogens have also been introduced into the human diet as a result of traditional cooking and preserving practices. Although carcinogens act through a wide variety of mechanisms, a substantial number have a common mechanism of action in that they react with the genetic material of the body, DNA. These so-called genotoxic carcinogens generally require metabolic activation to express their carcinogenicity. Although substantial efforts are being made to develop short-term, non-animal tests to predict the carcinogenicity of chemicals, animal bioassays remain the only reliable method for establishing the potential of a chemical to be a carcinogen, and form the basis of current approaches for the control of potentially carcinogenic chemicals in the human diet.

Naturally Occurring Carcinogens

It has been estimated that the total number of known chemicals exceeds 7 million, and that the great majority are naturally occurring. Although only a very small proportion (perhaps less than 0.01%) of these chemicals have been tested for carcinogenic potential in laboratory studies, a high proportion (as high as 50% in some evaluations) have been found to be positive. Therefore, even allowing for the imperfect selection and testing process, it is likely that there are a very large number of naturally occurring carcinogenic chemicals in the universe of chemicals, and therefore in the food we eat.

Naturally occurring substances identified as carcinogens in animals and humans by the range of approaches available for this purpose include inorganic compounds, organometallic compounds, and both simple and complex organic chemicals (see **Table 1**). These materials are present in the environment either as naturally occurring minerals or as a result of natural processes acting in the environment such as combustion, radioactive decay, or biodegradation of plant materials to oils. They are also widespread throughout the plant kingdom in both edible and nonedible plants and in many fungi and in unicellular organisms.

Inorganic Chemical Carcinogens

Many metallic elements are present as contaminants in food, being derived from a range of sources including the water used in food processing, soil residues, packaging, and cooking equipment. A number of metals and some of their salts have been shown to be carcinogenic in animals and humans, particularly to the lungs. These include arsenic,

Table 1 Examples of naturally occurring carcinogens

Inorganic chemicals
Arsenic; beryllium; chromium; cobalt; cadmium; lead; manganese; nickel
Polonium; radium; uranium; radon (gas)
Asbestos; silica (glassfiber); talc

Organic chemicals – complex mixtures
Mineral oils; shale oil; soot; wood shaving/dust

Organic chemicals in higher plants
Cycasin (betel nuts); saffrole (sassafras); pyrrolizidine alkaloids (Borginaceaea, Compositae); ptaquilosides (bracken); nitrosoalkaloids (tobacco)

Organic chemicals in lower order plants and microorganisms
Agaratine (mushrooms); aflatoxin, ochratoxin, sterigmatocystin (*Aspergillus* spp. and others); mitomycin, streptozotocin, daunomycin, actinomycin (*Streptomyces* spp.)

beryllium, cadmium, chromium, and nickel. Little is known about the mechanism by which metals cause cancer, although evidence is emerging that some metal ions affect the fidelity of an enzyme involved in the biosynthesis of DNA resulting in abnormal DNA being produced. A number of naturally occurring radioactive elements are also carcinogenic, particularly to the lungs. These include uranium, radium, and radon gas and may act by damaging DNA directly or by increasing oxidative damage as a result of an increase in reactive radical species. In addition, some naturally occurring minerals such as asbestos, silica, and talc are known to be carcinogenic to animals and humans under some circumstances.

Organic Chemicals – Complex Natural Mixtures

The earliest association made between the development of cancer in humans and exposure to an essentially natural rather than man-made chemical was that between scrotal (skin) cancer and soot by Percival Pott in 1775. However, the specific chemical(s) responsible (polycyclic aromatic hydrocarbons such as benzo(a)pyrene and 7,12-dimethylbenzanthracene) were not identified until more than a century later. Since then, a number of other naturally occurring materials have been shown to be carcinogenic. These have included mineral oils, shale oils, and wood dust/shavings, the oils being carcinogenic to the skin and wood dust to the nasal cavity. Inadvertent ingestion of small amounts of such materials with food may be difficult to avoid.

Organic Chemicals in Higher Plants

Although the acute toxicity of many plant species has been known since written records first appeared, only comparatively recently has the carcinogenicity

of plant-derived products been recognized. The list of confirmed animal carcinogens present in plants is still relatively small, and few, if any, are confirmed or suspected human carcinogens. However, developments in analytical chemistry will allow an increasingly detailed inventory to be made of chemicals in plants, which will undoubtedly result in the discovery of many more carcinogens in our foodstuffs. The recent identification of over 1000 chemicals in coffee beans, and the observation that whereas only 3% of the chemicals had been tested for carcinogenicity, nearly 70% of these tested positive, is a clear pointer to future directions. Although it can be argued that the majority of these compounds are present at very low levels in plants, and so the hazard to man from any individual compound may be small, reliable methods for assessing both hazard and risk of low-level exposure are not well developed. In addition, methods for assessing the hazard from complex mixtures of chemicals are also poorly developed, resulting in additional uncertainty in evaluating the hazard posed by natural materials. The identified chemical carcinogens in plants tend to be secondary metabolites, often present as part of the plants natural defense mechanism against predation (i.e., natural pesticides), and as such are widespread in fruit, vegetables, herbs, and spices (see **Table 2**).

Table 2 Some naturally occurring carcinogenic plant pesticides (a) and their sources (b)

(a)

Chemical class	Examples
Aldehyde	Crotonaldehyde; benzaldehyde; hexanal
Hydrazine/hydrazone	*N*-methyl-*N*-formylhydrazine; methylhydrazine; pentanal methylformylhydrazone
Alcohol	Methylbenzyl alcohol; catechol
Ester	Ethyl acrylate; benzyl acetate
Simple heterocycles	Coumarin; hydroquinone; saffrole; sesamol; 8-methoxypsoralen
Polyphenols	Quercetin

(b)

Generic source	Examples
Fruit	Apple; apricot; cherry; grapefruit; lemon; melon; peach pear; pineapple
Root vegetables	Carrot; onion; parsnip; radish; turnip
Brassica	Broccoli; Brussel sprout; cabbage
Herbs	Coriander; dill; fennel; mint; sage; tarragon
Spices	Allspice; carroway; cardamom; nutmeg; paprika; turmeric

One of the first classes of toxic compounds in plants to be identified were the pyrrolizidine alkaloids from the genus *Senecio*. Subsequently, more than 200 related compounds have been isolated from numerous families and species, many of which are potent liver toxins and liver carcinogens. Other classes of alkaloids found in the plant kingdom include derivatives of the nicotine alkaloids, such as N-nitrosonornicotine, which are present in tobacco leaves and are known to be carcinogenic to animals. Tobacco leaves also contain a range of compounds that have been shown to potentiate the carcinogenic effect of the alkaloids present.

Many other classes of carcinogenic plant products have been identified. These include glycosides of azoxy alcohols such as cycasin from betel nuts, a colon carcinogen; isoprene glycosides such as ptaquiloside found in bracken, a liver carcinogen; and phenolic alkylbenzenes such as safrole present in many herbs and vegetables, which are also principally liver carcinogens. Other phenolic compounds including flavanoids such as quercetin, rutin and kaemferol, and tannins such as trapain and brevifolin are potent mutagens but evidence for their carcinogenicity is lacking. In fact many of these compounds have been shown to exert anticarcinogenic effects.

Organic Chemical Carcinogens in other Edible Plants and in Microorganisms

Chemical carcinogens are also found in a wide range of lower plants, such as fungi, and in microorganisms. Simple and complex hydrazines are found in many species of mushroom and have been shown to produce tumors in many tissues of experimental animals. Mycotoxins such as aflatoxin B_1 and the related polynuclear compound produced by *Aspergillus* species are some of the most potent carcinogens known, being active at dose levels in the nanogram per kilogram range. Human exposure to such compounds occurs when cereal crops and nuts are stored in humid conditions, as they are in many parts of equatorial Africa and China. Aflatoxin B_1 is one of the few established human carcinogens found in the plant kingdom. Other carcinogenic compounds produced as natural products include the antibiotics adriamycin and daunomycin and the antineoplastic agent streptozotocin isolated from microorganisms of the genus *Streptomyces*.

Carcinogens Produced by Food Processing

Despite the widespread occurrence of potentially carcinogenic chemicals in the plant kingdom, most foodstuffs contain only low levels of these chemicals. However, it has now been recognized that a number of processes used in food preparation/processing can introduce significant amounts of carcinogens into the food or the local environment. The most widely studied of these processes are preservation of meats and fish by salting or smoking; grilling or broiling of meats, and cooking in vegetable oils.

Traditional methods for preserving meat and fish involve either salting or smoking. Epidemiological evidence has been found for an association between an increased incidence of cancer of the mouth and pharynx and intake of salted meat. It seems likely that a reaction between sodium nitrate and/or nitrite used for preserving the meat and alkylamides present in the meat results in the formation of N-nitrosamines and nitrosamides. These compounds have been shown to be potent carcinogens in animal experiments to the mouth, pharynx and other sites. Levels of nitrosamines in cured meats and fish can be as high as 100–200 ppb (parts per billion) for the simple alkylnitrosamines and between 10 and 100 ppb for volatile heterocyclic nitrosamines. Although dose levels required to induce tumor formation in animal studies are substantially higher than those likely to be ingested by man, there is a concern that the presence of nitrosamines in food presents a significant hazard to man.

Preservation of meats and fish by smoking has also been shown to introduce chemicals known to be carcinogenic to animals, particularly polycyclic aromatic hydrocarbons (PAHs), although direct evidence for an association between an increased incidence of human cancers and consumption of smoked meat and fish is lacking.

The frying or grilling of meats and fish has been found to generate significant quantities of heterocyclic nitrogenous compounds derived from amino acids present in foods. These so-called cooked food mutagens include 2-amino-3-methylimidazo[4,5-f]quinoline (IQ), 2-amino-3,8-dimethylimidazo[4,5-f]quinoxaline (methyl-IQ_x), 2-amino-1-methyl-6-phenylimidazo[4,5-b]pyridine (PhIP), 3-amino-1,4-dimethyl-5H-pyrido[4,3-b]indole (Trp-P-1), and 2-aminodipyrido[1,2-a:3′,2-d]imidazole (Glu-P-2). They are some of the most potent bacterial mutagens known and have been shown to induce a wide range of tumors in animals. Levels as high as 500 ppb have been found in grilled chicken and it has been suggested that they may be implicated in the induction of colon and breast cancer in humans. PAHs can also be generated by the grilling of meat and fish and both carcinogenic and noncarcinogenic compounds have been identified. Levels of one particular PAH in foods, the carcinogen benzo(a)pyrene, have been reported to vary from <1 ppb in grain to more than 30 ppb in singed meat.

Cooking foods in hot oils has also been found to generate a range of carcinogenic chemicals. Many of these are volatile and may therefore represent more of a hazard to the cook than to the food consumer. Thus, cooking with unrefined rapeseed or soya bean oil, which contain significant levels of the polyunsaturated fatty acid linolenic acid, has been shown to result in the release of aldehydes including formaldehyde, acetaldehyde and acrolein, hydrocarbons including 1,3-butadiene and benzene, and other chemicals. Many of these compounds are mutagenic to bacteria and carcinogenic in animals, and in areas of the world where such cooking practices are common (e.g., China), the incidence of lung cancer in the exposed population is high.

Mechanisms of Carcinogenicity

Chemical carcinogens induce neoplasia by a wide range of mechanisms involving either interaction with the hereditary material of the organism or interference with one of the many cellular control systems. The former compounds, known as genotoxic carcinogens, interact directly with DNA, resulting in a permanent heritable change to a cell following replication (i.e., an altered genotype). In contrast, nongenotoxic (epigenetic) carcinogens do not interact directly with DNA but cause cancer by other mechanisms.

Chemicals that react with DNA are invariably electrophiles (i.e., they possess one or more electron-deficient centers in the molecule) that target the nucleophilic (electron-rich) sites in the DNA. The electrophilic center may be present in the molecule itself (activation independent) as in β-propiolactone, dimethyl sulfate, and a,β-unsaturated aldehydes or be generated following metabolism (activation dependent) in the target species.

Examples of classes of compounds that are converted to reactive electrophiles by oxidative metabolism include nitrosamines, chlorinated alkanes, hydrazines, and polycyclic aromatic hydrocarbons. Because of the inherent reactivity of these species, they react not only with DNA, but also with other cellular macromolecules such as RNA and proteins. These reactions protect the cell against the carcinogenicity of the chemical by reducing the amount of electrophile available to react with DNA, but may lead to other forms of damage and ultimately cell death.

The enzyme system considered to be mainly involved in the activation of chemicals to carcinogenic species is the so-called mixed function oxidase system. This enzyme complex is centered on cytochrome P450 and is present in most, if not all, of the organs of the body. The enzyme system consists of a very large family of related isoenzymes of differing substrate specificity and has a widespread distribution in the animal kingdom. Early work with this enzyme system suggested that only certain isoenzymes were responsible for the activation of carcinogens, although it is now clear that different isoenzymes may activate the same compound in different species.

Most chemical carcinogens appear to be substrates of one particular isoenzyme called CYP1A1. Molecular modeling has shown that only relatively flat (planar) molecules are oxygenated by this cytochrome. Common carcinogens activated by this isoenzyme include PAHs, aflatoxin, and 9-hydroxyellipticine, whereas the related isoenzyme CYP1A2 activates arylamines and amides such as 2-acetylaminofluorene and the cooked food mutagens. Other subfamilies of cytochromes involved in activating carcinogens include CYP2E1, which is known to act on a wide range of small molecules such as dialkylnitrosamines, urethane, vinyl monomers and haloalkanes, and CYP3A, which also activates PAHs, aflatoxins, and cooked food mutagens.

The chemistry of the activation process varies with the type of carcinogen. The oxidation of aflatoxin B_1, for example, results in the formation of the 8,9-epoxide in a single step whereas the activation of PAHs, such as benzo(a)pyrene, is a multistep process involving an epoxide that is converted to a diol by epoxide hydrolase, which is then converted to the proximate carcinogenic species, a diolepoxide. Activation of arylamines and amides to DNA reactive species, in contrast, frequently involves an initial oxidation step to an N-hydroxy derivative, which is then further metabolized to a highly reactive N-O-ester. This latter reaction is catalyzed by a transferase enzyme, usually sulfotransferase or acetyltransferase for arylamines and glucuronotransferase for arylamides. Other oxidative reactions result in the formation of unstable compounds that decompose spontaneously to the ultimate carcinogenic species. Thus, simple nitrosamines are oxidized by CYP2E1 to an α-hydroxy intermediate, which breaks down to the electrophilic alkyldiazonium ion.

Enzyme systems other than the mixed function oxidase system may also be involved in the metabolic activation of carcinogens. Thus, for aflatoxins, there is evidence that prostaglandin H synthetase can activate this group of compounds and for arylamines, oxidation may be carried out by prostaglandin peroxidase, myeloperoxidase, or by flavin-containing monooxygenases.

The direct metabolic activation of compounds to carcinogenic species by phase II metabolism, a process normally associated with detoxification, can also occur. Thus safrole and related compounds are converted to their sulfate esters, the ultimate carcinogenic species by the phase II enzyme, sulfotransferase.

Metabolic Activation of Epigenetic Carcinogens

Since there is no common mechanism describing the action of epigenetic carcinogens, generalizations concerning the effect of metabolism on the activity of chemicals acting by a nongenotoxic mechanism are not possible. The activity of a number of epigenetic carcinogens is reduced as a result of metabolic activation, although in the case of one group of epigenetic carcinogens that produce renal tumors in the rat by binding to and preventing the degradation of a specific kidney protein, alpha-2-microglobulin, metabolic activation is required for carcinogenic activity. Compounds acting by this mechanism include isophorone and D-limonene, which are present naturally in many fruits.

Similarly, a wide range of structurally diverse chemicals induce liver tumors in rodents due to their ability to induce the proliferation of hepatic peroxisomes. Food contaminants such as phthalate diesters, which leach out of packaging materials, fall into this category, although no naturally occurring food chemical has yet been found to be a peroxisome proliferator. Some examples of nongenotoxic mechanisms of carcinogenesis are shown in Table 3.

Table 3 Some examples of nongenotoxic mechanisms of carcinogenesis

Mechanism	Examples of chemical classes
Promotion	Phorbol esters; barbiturates; chlorinated hydrocarbons
Peroxisome proliferation	Phthalate diesters; hypolipidemic drugs; chlorinated herbicides
Endocrine modulation	Androgens and estrogens; antithyroid agents
Cytotoxicity	Metal chelators; branched chain hydrocarbons

Carcinogenicity Tests

Animal Bioassays

As the mechanism of carcinogenesis in both humans and animals is not well understood, the only acceptable procedure for determining whether a chemical is likely to be a carcinogen is the examination of experimental animals exposed to the suspect material under carefully controlled conditions. This procedure relies on the assumption that animals will behave in essentially the same way as humans to carcinogen exposure, i.e., the mechanism of tumor induction will be similar in both animals and humans. Mechanistically based, short-term tests for carcinogenicity prediction not involving experimental animals are still a distant and elusive goal.

The basic approach for carcinogenicity testing involves administering the test material to two suitable animal species for a considerable proportion of their natural lifespan. Because of their small size and relatively short life expectancy, the rat and mouse are the species of choice, although the hamster is occasionally used. In the US, inbred strains of animals are widely used (the F344 rat and the B6C3F$_1$ hybrid mouse), although out-bred strains are commonly used in Europe. To examine the carcinogenic potential of food components, the test substance is usually given in the diet, although in some circumstances administration may be in the drinking water or by gavage. The study continues until a certain proportion in one or other of the treatment groups has died or has been killed in a moribund state. As a minimum, 50 animals are allocated at random to each of the experimental groups, allowing a statistically significant carcinogenic effect to be detected if five animals in a test group develop tumors and no animals in the control group do.

During the study, the animal's clinical state is regularly monitored and at the end of the study a complete necropsy is performed on all surviving animals. Any tumors found are classified as either neoplastic or non-neoplastic and some attempt is made to determine whether any tumors seen were the cause of the (early) death of the animal (fatal tumors) or were unrelated to the death (incidental tumors). The procedures of these bioassays are conducted under rigorous conditions defined by the Code of Good Laboratory Practice (GLP).

Tests are essentially of two types: the first, used widely under the National Toxicology Program (NTP) in the US, is designed to examine the ability of the test material to induce cancer in the species used; the second, is aimed at determining the cancer incidence in respect of dose – a classical dose–response study. The former requires a few treatment groups, including a relatively high-dose group in order to maximize the chance of detecting a carcinogenic effect, whereas the latter requires a wide range of dose groups to define accurately the dose–response relationship.

The analysis of a carcinogenicity bioassay is aimed at determining whether the administration of the test chemical has resulted in an increase in the incidence of tumors at one or more sites. In order to accomplish this analysis, two major confounding factors may have to be taken into consideration. The first is the effect of differences in mortality rates between the control and treated groups and the second is the effect of differences in food intake and its consequence on body weight. Both factors can substantially alter the tumor pattern observed in different groups. Early deaths may prevent the animals reaching tumor-bearing age, and reduced food intake and the associated reduction in body weight may result in a considerable reduction in tumor incidence.

The interpretation of the results of a bioassay are complex but most authorities work to the 'weight of evidence' principle. This evidence is taken in the light of the 'adequacy' of the bioassay, which is dependent on some of the factors previously discussed. Strong evidence for the compound being a genotoxic carcinogen would be increased malignant tumor incidence in two species, with tumors at multiple sites showing a clear dose–response relationship. Rare or unusual tumors at a site would be given added weight. Equivocal evidence may result from a statistically marginal result or only an increase in commonly occurring benign tumors. Tumor development in only one species and in association with species-specific toxicity is characteristic of nongenotoxic (or epigenetic) carcinogens. Sometimes, problems associated with such findings may be clarified by

further mechanistic studies or by reference to historical data. When the data from bioassays are considered in human risk assessment, other factors must clearly also be taken into consideration. These may include evidence of genotoxicity in short-term tests and data on metabolism and potential human exposure. Furthermore, a measure of risk at doses substantially below the bioassay dose may be needed. This may require an extrapolation using mathematical models. As yet no general agreement has been reached as to the most appropriate method, and so the calculated risk given by different methods may vary considerably. Thus, the final assessment may be made on quite pragmatic grounds, in which the experience and expertise of a number of individuals are drawn on to reach a consensus opinion.

Short-Term Predictive Tests

A large number of short-term tests have been developed in an attempt to predict carcinogenic potential and thereby reduce the reliance on animal tests. These include assays for detecting gene mutation, damage to chromosomes, or damage to the whole genome.

Gene mutation can be assessed in bacteria, yeasts, or mammalian cells in culture (see **Table 4**). Since many of the cell systems used are unable to activate metabolically the majority of test chemicals, an exogenous mammalian metabolizing system, the so-called S-9 mix, is incorporated into the assay. Chromosome damage can be measured in cell lines *in vitro* or by using animals exposed for a short time to the chemical. Structural damage produced can include chromosome and chromatid gaps and breaks, rings, fragments, dicentrics, translocations, and inversions. A short-term *in vivo* assay measuring

Table 4 Short-term test systems for predicting carcinogenic potential

Test system	Cell used	End point
Bacterial mutation	*Salmonella typhimurium* TA strains *Escherichia coli* WP2	Reversion to histidine independence
Mammalian gene mutation	Chinese hamster lung (V79) Chinese hamster ovary (CHO) Mouse lymphoma (L5178Y) Human transformed lymphoblastoid (TK6)	Loss of HPRT, TK, or Na^+/K^+ ATPase expression
Chromosome aberration *in vitro*	Chinese hamster fibroblast (CHL) Chinese hamster ovary (CHO) Human peripheral blood lymphocytes(PBL)	Chromosome/chromatid aberration (gaps, breaks, deletions)
Chromosome damage *in vivo*	Bone marrow erythrocytes (mouse)	Micronuclei induction
Heritable damage *in vivo*	Rodent germ cells	Dominant/lethal mutations; heritable translocations, etc.

HPRT, hypoxanthine phosphoribosyl transferase; TK, thymidine kinase.

unscheduled DNA synthesis (UDS) in rat liver or gut is recommended by most regulatory authorities if there is a positive response in any *in vitro* assay and a negative response in an *in vivo* cytogenetics assay. Other test methods and end points are under consideration by regulatory authorities as indicators of genotoxic potential including the COMET assay for assessing DNA damage, and aneuploidy, the change in chromosome number resulting from damage to the cellular architecture (spindle) controlling chromosome replication.

The last two decades have seen extensive efforts to determine whether short-term tests are suitable for predicting carcinogenic potential. The early validation studies suggested good predictability, with correct identification of over 90% of carcinogens (high sensitivity) and over 90% of noncarcinogens (high specificity). In later evaluations, a much lower figure (60%) was obtained. However, when carcinogens known to react by nongenotoxic mechanisms (e.g., hormones or peroxisome proliferators) were excluded, the predictability was improved suggesting that short-term tests are suitable for detecting those carcinogens that act by a genotoxic mechanism.

Although many regulatory authorities have guidelines for carcinogenicity evaluation, which include short-term tests, they all still require animal studies as the ultimate test for carcinogenicity. However, the use made of short-term tests varies. In the US, the Food and Drugs Administration (FDA) recommends a battery of short-term tests for all 'additives' for which cumulative dietary intake is expected to exceed 1.5 μg per person per day in order to assist in the interpretation of animal feeding studies. Some expert bodies, such as The International Agency for Research in Cancer, use short-term tests as an adjunct to animal carcinogenicity studies in their evaluation process, giving added weighting in their assessment of likely human hazard to an animal carcinogen that is also positive in short-term tests.

However, until a consensus can be reached as to what a positive or negative result in an animal feeding study means in terms of whether the compound may or may not be a human carcinogen, the further development of better (faster/cheaper) short-term tests may be a futile exercise.

Monitoring and Control of Hazards

The complex mixture of chemicals that constitute food, together with the uncertainty of the specific role of the various components in the diet, has made the control of potential carcinogens in food difficult. In particular, the realization that animal carcinogens, as identified by standard animal bioassays, are widely distributed in the general environment, including food, has made control by total elimination impossible.

Control of toxic agents in food particularly contaminants and additives has been achieved by examining their hazard in animal studies. Thus, the establishment of a no-observable-adverse-effect-levels (NOAEL) is followed by the setting of an allowable daily intake (ADI) through extrapolation based on the relative sensitivity of animals and humans to toxic events. This extrapolation may also take into consideration other properties of the chemical concerned, such as genotoxic potential. For genotoxic carcinogens, however, it is generally considered that there is no no-effect-level and therefore acceptable intake is based on estimation of likely risk. A maximum risk of 10^{-6} cancers in a lifetime is considered as an acceptable risk by some authorities, particularly those in the US, and acceptable exposure estimates extrapolated from animal data. For nongenotoxic carcinogens (and for some genotoxic carcinogens, particularly those that act as aneugens), no-effect levels are accepted, since the carcinogenic response is the result of a prior toxic event for which a no-effect-level can be determined. For additional safety, an arbitrary factor of 100 was applied to the NOAEL, to allow for interspecies variation ($\times 10$) and interindividual variability ($\times 10$). More recently, the two factors have been subdivided into variable factors (pharmacokinetic and pharmacodynamic) to reflect increased understanding of the mechanisms underlying the development of cancer and allow for factors associated with special groups such as infants and children. It must be said that the scientific basis to support either of these approaches (acceptable risk or no-effect-levels) is quite limited as even for the best-documented cases, the mechanism of the carcinogenic effect is poorly understood.

The unequivocal identification of human carcinogens is difficult since direct experimental approaches are precluded. Thus, epidemiological data involving both prospective and retrospective studies, and using case controls in certain investigations, has to be employed. These techniques have limited applications to diet-associated carcinogenesis and have proved most useful in identifying specific carcinogens in the work place or those used as therapeutic agents. The specific problem in identifying dietary carcinogens relate to the complexity of diet, the difficulty in identifying specific components, and the sensitivity of the epidemiological methods themselves. It would seem likely that epidemiological data will only be able to link specific chemical carcinogens in food with a carcinogenic effect in a few favorable circumstances, since such chemicals are likely to be present at low levels and induce only a small increase in tumor incidence over background levels. One such example was the identification of a carcinogenic hydrazone in the mushroom *Gyromitra esculenta,* as a result of an epidemiological study in Finland. Such methods have also indicated the relative importance of 'life style' factors in carcinogenesis: in particular, associations have been made between lack of dietary fiber and colon cancer, between a low intake of fresh fruit and vegetables and stomach cancer, and between excess dietary fat and colon and breast cancer, although the specific chemicals responsible have not been identified with any certainty.

Most of the activity aimed at controlling carcinogens in food has been directed at preventing addition of potentially carcinogenic substances to the existing background level of natural carcinogens. This has been tackled through the application of laws governing the adulteration of food, the first of which were enacted in the mid-nineteenth century in the UK. The current UK legislation is the 1990 Food Safety Act, governing the nature and quality of food and its nutritive value. This Act, like its forerunner, the 1955 Food and Drug Act, requires that the constituents of food should not be injurious to health. Thus, while there is no specific requirement for carcinogenicity testing in the current act, consideration is given to all available data, including the result of mutagenicity tests and long-term tests in animals.

The position in the US up to 1958 was similar to that in the UK. Food was considered adulterated if injury could arise from its use. Legislation was based on traditional food, added substances, and unavoidable added substances (contaminants). For added substances, listed in an inventory of over 3000 chemicals and often referred to as 'Everything Added to Food in the United States' (EAFUS), the food was considered adulterated if the added substance could render the food injurious to health; for unavoidably added substances, a balance was applied between the essential nature of the food material and the degree of contamination. These strictures applied to both carcinogenic and noncarcinogenic toxicants. In 1958 a change in emphasis was introduced through the Food Additives Amendment. This established a licensing scheme for substances deliberately added to foods or for substances that could migrate into food, but excluded materials that were generally, through usage, regarded as safe (GRAS). For licensing purposes, the material has to be shown to be 'safe' for its intended use, although in theory at least the GRAS substance could be a carcinogen.

In 1958 the Delaney Clause was enacted; this required that if there was evidence of carcinogenicity in any test system, the material should be prohibited from food usage. Improved analytical techniques have shown that many foods contain both unintentionally added and natural carcinogens, such as polynuclear aromatic hydrocarbons, nitrosamines, mycotoxins and arylamines, and no form of regulation could control these materials. Furthermore, bulk components of food may themselves play an important role in the development of carcinogenesis. The recognition that the exclusion of all potentially carcinogenic additives (under the Delaney Clause) is a practical impossibility has given way to the concept of 'safe' tolerance, and that 'safe levels' may be set by appropriate, conservative risk assessment in which an 'insignificant life time risk' of developing tumors of, for example, 10^{-6} is considered acceptable.

See also: **Cancer**: Epidemiology and Associations Between Diet and Cancer. **Fish**. **Food Safety**: Mycotoxins. **Meat, Poultry and Meat Products**. **Sodium**: Salt Intake and Health.

Further Reading

Arcos JC, Woo YT, Argus MF, and Lai D (1968–1985) *Chemical Induction of Cancer*, vols 1, 2A, 2B, 3A, 3B. New York: Academic Press.

Anderson D and Conning DM (1993) *Experimental Toxicology, The Basic Issues*, 2nd edn. London: Royal Society of Chemistry.

Ashby J and Tennant RW (1991) Definitive relationships among chemical structures, carcinogenicity and mutagenicity for 301 chemicals tested by the US NCI/NTP. *Mutation Research* **257**: 229–306.

Committee on Mutagenicity of Chemicals in Food, Consumer Products and the Environment (COM) (2000) *Guidance on a Strategy for Testing Chemicals for Mutagenicity*. London, UK: Department of Health.

Conning DM and Lansdown ABG (1983) *Toxic Hazards in Food*. London, UK: Croom Helm Ltd.

Hirono I (1987) *Naturally Occurring Carcinogens of Plant Origin. Toxicology, Pathology and Biochemistry* B.V. Amsterdam: Elsevier Science Publishers.

International Agency for Research on Cancer (1994) In: Hemminki K, Dipple A, Shuker DEG, Kadlubar FF, Segerback D, and Bartsch H (eds.) *DNA Adducts; Identification and Biological Significance*, IARC Scientific Publication No. 125. Lyon: IARC.

International Agency for Research on Cancer (1972–2002) *Evaluation of the Carcinogenic Risk of Chemicals to Humans*, Monograph Series No. 1–82. Lyon: IARC.

Lewis DFW, Bird MG, and Jacobs MN (2002) Human carcinogens: an evaluation study via the COMPACT and HazardExpert procedures. *Human and Experimental Toxicology* **21**: 115–122.

Nagao M and Sugimura T (1999) *Food Borne Carcinogens: Heterocyclic Amines*. Chichester, UK: Wiley.

Renwick AG (2000) The use of safety or uncertainty factors in the setting of acute reference doses. *Food Additives and Contaminants* 17: 627–635.

Scheuplein RJ (1990) Perspectives on toxicological risk – an example; food borne carcinogenic risk. In: Clayson DB, Munroe IC, Shubik P, and Swenberg JA (eds.) Progress in Predictive Toxicology, pp. 351–371. Amsterdam: Elsevier Science Publishers.

Williams GM and Weisburger JH (1991) Chemical carcinogenesis. In: Amdur MO, Doull J, and Klassen CD (eds.) *Casarett and Doull's Toxicology. The Basic Science of Poisons*, 4th edn., pp. 127–200. New York: Pergamon Press.

World Health Organisation (1999) Principles for the assessment of risks to human health of exposure to chemicals. *Environmental Health Perspectives*, No. 210.

CARBOHYDRATES

Contents

Chemistry and Classification

C L Stylianopoulos, Johns Hopkins University, Baltimore, MD, USA

© 2005 Elsevier Ltd. All rights reserved.

Introduction

Carbohydrates are the most abundant constituents of cereals, fruits, vegetables, and legumes. They are the major energy source in human nutrition and contribute to the texture and flavor of processed foods. They comprise a group of substances with different structures and varying physical, chemical, and physiological properties. Carbohydrates are polyhydroxy aldehyde or ketone molecules and their derivatives with the general formula $(CH_2O)_n$. Dietary carbohydrates are important in maintaining glycaemic homeostasis and gastrointestinal health. Furthermore, they contain necessary micronutrients, phytochemicals, and antioxidants.

Classification and Chemical Structure

Carbohydrates are classified into four categories according to their chemical structure and degree of polymerization: monosaccharides, disaccharides, oligosaccharides, and polysaccharides.

Monosaccharides

Monosaccharides are the simplest form of carbohydrate and cannot be further hydrolyzed into smaller subunits. According to their chain length, the monosaccharides can be divided into several categories, the more nutritionally important being the pentoses, with skeletons containing five carbon atoms (e.g., ribose), and the hexoses, with skeletons containing six carbon atoms (e.g., glucose).

The presence of asymmetrical carbon atoms in monosaccharides with different functional groups attached gives rise to optical activity, meaning that if polarized light is passed through a solution of these compounds, the plane of light will be rotated to the left (levorotatory or L form) or to the right (dextrorotatory or D form). As a result, mirror-imaged structures of the same compound exist and are called stereoisomers. Monosaccharides of the D form are more nutritionally important because the metabolic and digestive enzymes are specific for the D stereoisomers.

Monosaccharides demonstrate another type of stereoisomerism due to their formation of cyclic structures. The pentoses form furanose (five-membered rings), and the hexoses form pyranose (six-membered rings). Cyclization can produce two stereoisomers (the α and β configurations), and generally monosaccharide solutions contain an equilibrium mixture of these two forms. **Figure 1** illustrates D-glucose in its pyranose form in the α and β configurations. The isomerization produces compounds with different properties and has major metabolic importance, because of enzyme specificity for particular stereoisomers.

Glucose is the most abundant monosaccharide, and is a major cell fuel in the human body, and can be found unbound in body tissues and fluids. Glucose is the building block of several polysaccharides. Galactose and fructose are also used as cell

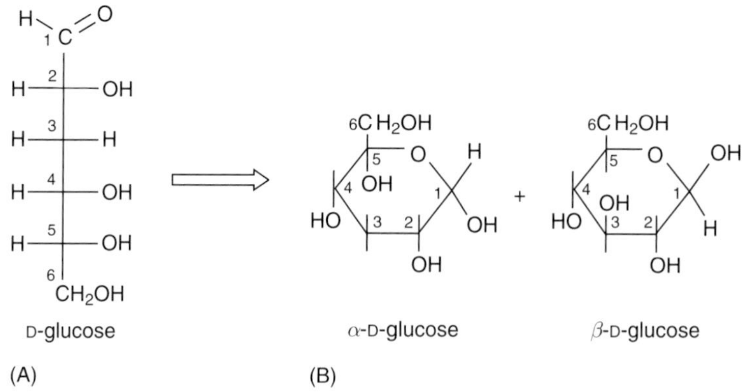

Figure 1 D-glucose molecule shown as (A) open chain and (B) a cyclic pyranose ring in the α and β configurations.

fuel. The most important monosaccharides and their significance are outlined in **Table 1**.

Several monosaccharide derivatives are constituents of polysaccharides, as well as food ingredients. Some nutritionally important monosaccharide derivatives and their significance are outlined in **Table 1**.

Table 1 Some nutritionally important monosaccharides

Class	Species	Significance
Hexoses	D-glucose	Major cell fuel, unbound in body fluids and tissues, building block of several polysaccharides
	D-fructose	Cell fuel, constituent of sucrose
	D-galactose	Cell fuel, constituent of lactose
	D-mannose	Constituent of plant cell wall polysaccharides and gums
Pentoses	L-arabinose, D-xylose	Constituent of plant cell wall polysaccharides
	D-ribulose, D-xylulose	Metabolite in pentose pathway
	D-ribose	RNA constituent
Uronic acids	D-glucuronic, D-galacturonic	Constituent of plant cell wall polysaccharides
	D-mannuronic, D-guluronic	Constituent of algal polysaccharides
Sugar alcohols	D-glucitol, D-xylitol	Food ingredient
	D-galactitol	Metabolite of galactose
Deoxysugars	D-deoxyribose	DNA constituent
	D-deoxygalactose	Constituent of algal polysaccharides
	L-fucose	Constituent of bacterial polysaccharides
	L-rhamnose	Constituent of pectic plant polysaccharides
Aminosugars	D-glucosamine, D-galactosamine	Constituent of aminosaminoglycans, cartilage

Disaccharides

Disaccharides consist of two monosaccharide units, linked by glycosidic bonds in the α or β orientation. The most important disaccharides are sucrose, lactose, and maltose. Sucrose consists of a molecule of α-glucose and a molecule of β-fructose linked together (**Figure 2A**). Lactose is found in milk and dairy products and consists of a molecule of galactose linked to a glucose molecule by a β-1,4glycosidic bond

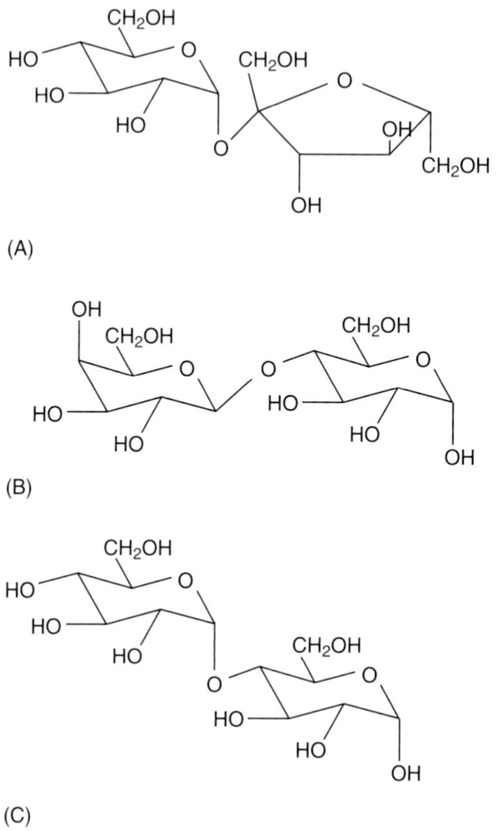

Figure 2 The molecular structures of (A) sucrose, (B) lactose, and (C) maltose.

Table 2 Some nutritionally important disaccharides

Class	Species	Significance
Disaccharide	Sucrose	Constituent of fruits, vegetables, and sweetener
	Lactose	Constituent of milk and dairy products
	Maltose, Isomaltose	Constituent of starch
	Trehalose	Food additive, constituent of mushrooms
	Lactulose	Lactose derivative, laxative
Disaccharide alcohols	Maltitol	Constituent of starch, sweetner
	Lactitol	Constituent of lactose, sweetener

(**Figure 2B**). Maltose is mainly produced by partial hydrolysis of starch and consists of two glucose units linked through an α-1,4glycosidic bond (**Figure 2C**). Some nutritionally important disaccharides and their significance are outlined in **Table 2**.

Oligosaccharides

Oligosaccharides consist of a chain of between three and nine monosaccharide units covalently linked to form large units and are named trioses, tetroses, etc, depending on the number of carbon atoms in their molecules. Oligosaccharides are distributed widely in plants and when digested yield their constituent monosaccharides. The major oligosaccharides are the raffinose series, formed by the linkage of galactose, sucrose, and glucose units, and the maltose series, formed by the linkage of glucose units. Some nutritionally important oligosaccharides and their significance are outlined in **Table 3**.

Polysaccharides

Polysaccharides consist of long chains of monosaccharide residues (more than nine) linked with glycosidic bonds. Polysaccharides found in nature usually have high molecular weights and are named after the component monosaccharide. These

Table 3 Some nutritionally important oligosaccharides

Class	Species	Significance
Maltoses	Maltotriose, Maltotetraose	Constituent of starch
Raffinoses	Raffinose, Stachyose, Verbascose	Constituent of vegetables and legumes
Fructoses	Fructotriose	Constituent of cereals and tubers
Lactoses	Fucosyl lactoses	Constituent of human breast milk

compounds consist of several hundred or even thousands of monosaccharide units. The properties of polysaccharides are determined by the species of monosaccharides in the polymer backbone, the types of linkages between residues, and the extent and type of chain branching.

Glucans are polymers of glucose and the major polysaccharides in the diet. The most important glucans are starch, glycogen, and cellulose. Glycogen is the short-term storage form of glucose in animal tissues. Starch is the most common digestible storage polysaccharide in plants, and cellulose is a major structural component of plant cell walls (**Figure 3**). Some nutritionally important polysaccharides and their significance are outlined in **Table 4**.

Polysaccharides with α linkages have a helical shape (e.g., the amylose starch molecule), while those with β linkages generally have a linear or flat ribbon-like molecule (e.g., the cellulose molecule) (**Figure 3**).

Polysaccharide molecules can be linear or branched. Branches can be formed through any unlinked hydroxyl group and vary from alternating and consecutive single-unit branches to multiple-unit branches (ramified structure). Polysaccharides that are highly branched tend to be soluble in water, because the chain structure prevents hydrogen bonding. Linear polysaccharides tend to be insoluble in water, unless they possess structural irregularities.

Nutritional Importance

Some carbohydrate types of specific importance in human nutrition are sugars and sugar alcohols, starch, and dietary fiber.

Sugars

The Food and Agriculture Organization (FAO) and the World Health Organization (WHO) expert consultation on carbohydrates use the term 'sugar' to describe monosaccharides and disaccharides. Sugars can be separated analytically from the food matrix by gas–liquid chromatography (GLC), high performance liquid chromatography, and enzymatic methods. Sugars are widely used in the food industry as sweeteners and preservatives. They improve the texture, body, palatability, and viscosity of foods and beverages.

The UK Department of Health distinguishes between 'intrinsic' and 'extrinsic' sugars. Intrinsic sugars are defined as those that occur naturally as part of the plant cell walls. Extrinsic sugars were defined as added sugars or those present when the

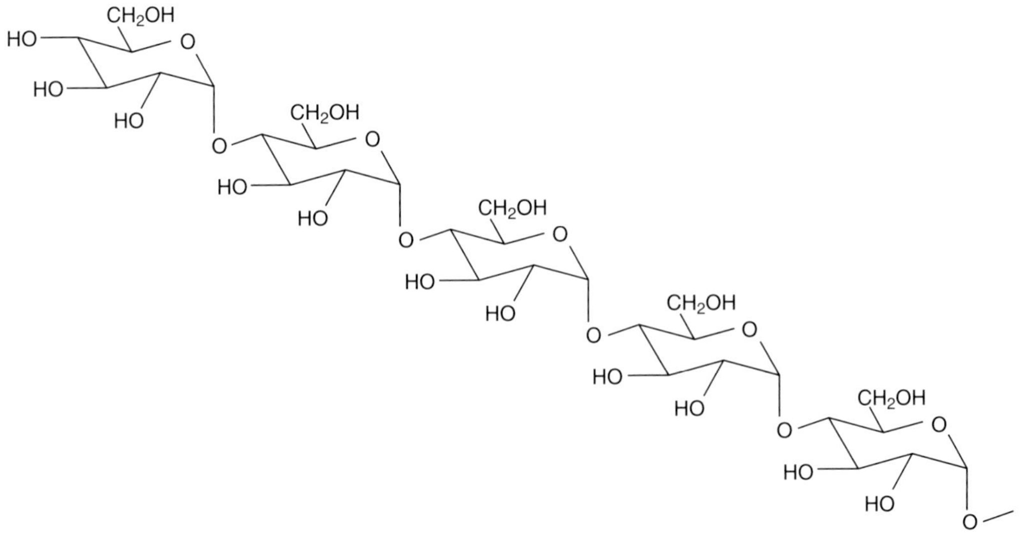

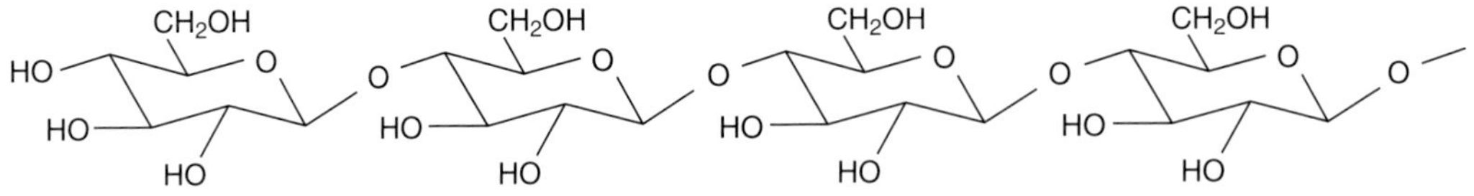

(A)

(B)

Figure 3 (A) Five units of an α-1,4-D-glucopyranose chain from a starch molecule (amylose). (B) Four units of a β-1,4-D-glucopyranose chain from a cellulose molecule.

food matrix has been disrupted. An additional term, 'non-milk' extrinsic sugar, is used to distinguish between milk and other extrinsic sugars. However, these terms have not been widely accepted.

Sugar Alcohols

Sugar alcohols are monosaccharide and disaccharide derivatives, such as sorbitol and xylitol, which are extensively used as sweeteners in the food industry. They have received increased attention because of their desirable properties of relative sweetness and limited digestion and absorption.

Starch

The most important, abundant, and digestible polysaccharide in human nutrition is starch. Starch comprises large chains of α-linked glucose residues, in the form of amylose or amylopectin. Amylose is a linear unbranched form of starch, which consists of α-1,4-linked glucose units (**Figure 3A**). Amylopectin is a branched-chain polymer, which consists of α-1,6-linked glucose units. Both forms of starch

can be found in cereals, potatoes, legumes, and other vegetables, with amylopectin comprising 80–85% and amylose 15–20% of total starch.

Dietary Fiber

There are several definitions of fiber, and no consensus exists among international organizations. The Association of Official Analytical Chemists International defines fiber as nondigestible animal and plant carbohydrates, based on the analytical methods for fiber separation using an enzymatic–gravimetric method (**Table 5**).

According to the new definition of the expert panel on macronutrients appointed by the Institute of Medicine of the National Academies of Science (**Table 5**), dietary fiber comprises intact nondigestible carbohydrates and lignin derived from plant sources. Functional fiber consists of nondigestible carbohydrates, derived from either plant or animal sources, that have shown favorable health outcomes for humans. Total fiber consists of both dietary and functional fiber. With this new definition of dietary and functional

Table 4 Some nutritionally important polysaccharides

Class	Species	Significance
Glucans	Starch	Storage polysaccharide in plants
	Glycogen	Short-term storage form of glucose in animal tissues
	Cellulose	Major structural component of plant cell walls
Galactans		Major constituents of noncellulosic matrix of plant cell wall
Xylans		Constituents of mature plant tissues
Mannans		Storage forms in several plants
Uronans	Galacturonans	Major components of water-soluble pectic fraction of plants
	Mannuronans	Components of algal polysaccharides
	Guluronans	Components of algal polysaccharides
Starch	Amylose, amylopectin	Most common digestible plant polysaccharides
Nonstarch	Cellulose	Major component of plant cell wall
	Pectin	Constituent of plant cell wall, food additive
	Hemicellulose	Constituent of plant cell wall
	Gums, mucilages	Plant hydrocolloids, food additives
	Algal polysaccharides	Constituents of algae and seaweed, food additives

fiber, new analytical methods should be developed and implemented to quantify accurately the total fiber component of foods.

Dietary and functional fiber cannot be digested by mammalian enzymes, and therefore they pass almost intact through the small intestine. Fiber consumption has potential health benefits, including the promotion of general gastrointestinal health and the prevention of several noncommunicable diseases.

Table 5 Current definitions of dietary fiber

Source	Definitions
AOAC[a]	Fiber: nondigestible animal and plant carbohydrates
IOM[b]	Dietary fiber: intact nondigestible carbohydrates and lignin, derived from plant sources
	Functional fiber: nondigestible carbohydrates derived from either plant or animal sources that have shown favourable health outcomes for humans
	Total fiber: dietary and functional fiber

[a]AOAC: Association of Official Analytical Chemists
[b]IOM: Institute of Medicine

Chemistry

Monosaccharides share the same functional groups, but their isomeric forms often exhibit differences in chemical reactions. Disaccharides exhibit a similar range of reactions to monosaccharides owing to the presence of similar functional groups. Oligosaccharides generally exhibit properties similar to those of monosaccharides and disaccharides with similar functional groups, but some oligosaccharides with nine monosaccharide units may exhibit similar properties to polysaccharides. In general, polysaccharides show slower reaction rates because of steric effects.

Solubility

Monosaccharides, disaccharides, and oligosaccharides have similar solubilities. Overall, they are very soluble in water. Sucrose is extremely soluble in water, while lactose is soluble to a lesser extent. Furthermore, they are insoluble in nonpolar organic solvents. They exhibit limited solubility in pure alcohols but are very soluble in aqueous alcohol solutions (70–80% v/v), and therefore these solutions are widely used for extraction and analysis. Oligosaccharides are less soluble than monosaccharides in aqueous alcohol solutions, and their solubility decreases as the number of monosaccharide units increases.

In general, polysaccharides form colloidal solutions in water, while some other polymers are extremely insoluble in water and require prior treatment with acid, alkali, or organic solvents to get them to dissolve. For example, β-1,4-mannans and glucans (e.g., cellulose) are very insoluble owing to hydrogen bonding between parallel chains. On the other hand, arabinoxylans are readily soluble in water, because the arabinosyl chains inhibit hydrogen bonding. Galactomannans are also readily soluble in water, producing viscous solutions, and are used as food additive gums. The α-linked glucans (e.g., amylose and amylopectin) have completely different solubilities. The glucan α-1,4-amylose is very soluble in warm water and forms colloidal solutions. When the amylose chains cool down, they form an amylose gel, which subsequently forms an insoluble crystalline material. Amylopectins are also very soluble in hot water but do not form an insoluble crystalline material to the same degree as amylose.

Reducing Properties

Monosaccharides are powerful reducing agents to a range of metals in alkaline solution, owing to the presence of aldo and keto groups. The extent of reduction varies among different monosaccharides. Disaccharides and oligosaccharides have the same reducing properties, except for sucrose, in which both hemi-acetal groups are combined. Polysaccharides usually contain one reducing group at the terminal end of the polymer chain and, as a result, have lower reducing properties.

Reactions in Acidic Solutions

When heated in strong acidic solutions, monosaccharides dehydrate and condense into a range of furans. The resulting furans condense with several reagents to generate colored products; hence the presence of monosaccharides and their derivatives can be verified. Under weaker acidic conditions, fructose is labile.

Reactions in Alkaline Solutions

In weak alkaline solutions, monosaccharides undergo isomerization of the aldose-keto group (enolization). In stronger alkaline solutions, they produce a series of degradation compounds, namely saccharinic acids. In the presence of ammonia, amino acids, and proteins, they condense repeatedly to generate a series of highly colored products (Maillard reaction); this reaction is used in the food industry to produce caramel colors.

Hydrolysis

Acid Disaccharides and oligosaccharides in mild acidic conditions are hydrolyzed to their constituent monosaccharides. The fructofuranosyl linkages of the fructooligosaccharides are quite susceptible to acid hydrolysis. Polysaccharides are also hydrolyzed to their constituent monosaccharides by acid hydrolysis, but the conditions necessary for complete hydrolysis depend on the solubilities of the polymers. The majority of polysaccharides (e.g., starch) are completely hydrolyzed under weak acidic conditions. However, cellulose requires treatment with strong acid for several hours prior to hydrolysis and subsequent heating under weak acidic conditions for the completion of the reaction. The uronans are very resistant to complete acid hydrolysis, and disaccharides of aldobiuronic acids are generally produced. Acid hydrolysis of polysaccharides results in extensive losses of their monosaccharide constituents.

Enzymatic Disaccharides are hydrolyzed in specific enzymatic solutions, and, therefore, this is a useful method for the analysis of sugar mixtures. Oligosaccharides are also susceptible to enzymatic hydrolysis. The maltooligosaccharides can be rapidly hydrolyzed by glucosidase enzymes.

Polysaccharides are more efficiently hydrolyzed to their monosaccharide constituents using specific enzymes. Fungal enzymes act specifically to hydrolyze different polysaccharides. The α-1,4 glycosidic linkages in starch can be hydrolyzed by various α amylases (e.g., salivary and pancreatic), producing maltose and isomaltose. The β-1,6 glycosidic linkages in amylopectin are not as easily hydrolyzed and require the presence of pullulanase – a fungal enzyme – to complete the hydrolysis.

Ester Formation

Monosaccharides contain hydroxyl groups and react with acids to form a variety of esters. The phosphate esters play a main role in carbohydrate metabolism. For example, the first step of glycolysis involves the production of the glucose-6-phosphate ester in a reaction catalyzed by the enzyme glucokinase in the presence of adenosine triphosphate. The uronic acids react with alcohols to form esters. The methyl esters of uronic acids are the most important in determining the physical properties of the uronans.

The presence of additional hydroxyl groups in disaccharides and oligosaccharides increases the number of sites for esterification reactions. Sucrose reacts with fatty acids to produce nondigestible esters, which have similar properties to the triacylglycerols.

The polysaccharide galacturonans, which are composed of an α-1,4 galacturonic acid chain with integrated rhamnose units, form salts with cations and may be esterified with methoxyl groups.

Substitution

Monosaccharides undergo substitution reactions with methyl iodide to produce methyl ether derivatives. These compounds have been used to identify the structure of polymers, because the sites of nonmethyl substituted groups are indicative of the branch points after hydrolysis. Monosaccharides undergo acetylation, which occurs on the free or the reduced molecule to produce acetylated alditols. These volatile compounds have been used to identify sugar mixtures by GLC. The presence of additional hydroxyl groups in disaccharides and oligosaccharides increases the number of sites for substitution reactions.

Abbreviations

D	dextrorotatory
FAO	Food and Agriculture Organization
GLC	gas–liquid chromatography
L	levorotatory
v/v	volume/volume
WHO	World Health Organization

Further Reading

Brody T (1999) *Nutritional Biochemistry*, 2nd edn, pp. 1–56. San Diego: Academic Press.

Eastwood M (2003) *Principles of Human Nutrition*, 2nd edn, pp. 195–122, 418–426, 486–509. Oxford: Blackwell.

FAO/WHO (1998) Carbohydrates in human nutrition. Report of a Joint FAO/WHO Expert Consultation. FAO. *Food and Nutrition Paper* **66**: 1–140.

Gray GM (2000) Digestion and absorption of carbohydrate. In: In: *Biochemical and Physiological Aspects of Human Nutrition*, 1st edn, pp. 91–106. Philadelphia: WB Saunders Company.

Groff JL and Gropper SS (2000) *Advanced Nutrition and Human Metabolism*, 3rd edn, pp. 70–105. Belmont: Wadsworth.

Institute of Medicine of the National Academies (2002) *Dietary Reference Intakes for Energy, Carbohydrate, Fiber, Fat, Fatty Acids, Cholesterol, Protein, Amino Acids*. Washington, DC: The National Academies Press.

Lewis BA (2000) Structure and properties of carbohydrates. In: In: *Biochemical and Physiological Aspects of Human Nutrition*, 1st edn, pp. 3–22. Philadelphia: WB Saunders Company.

Nantel G (2003) Glycemic carbohydrate: an international approach. *Nutrition Reviews* **61**: S34–S39.

Sanchez-Castillo CP, Hudson GJ, Englyst HN, Dewey P, and James WPT (2002) The importance of dietary carbohydrates. *Archivos Latinoamericanos de Nutricion* **52**: 321–335.

Sullivan DM and Carpenter DM (eds.) (1993) *Methods of Analysis for Nutritional Labeling*. Arlington: Association of Official Analytical Chemists.

Williams SR and Schlenker ED (2003) *Essentials of Nutrition and Diet Therapy*, 8th edn, pp. 47–65. St Louis: Mosby.

Regulation of Metabolism

C L Stylianopoulos, Johns Hopkins University, Baltimore, MD, USA

© 2005 Elsevier Ltd. All rights reserved.

Introduction

The three basic monosaccharides important in human nutrition are glucose, fructose, and galactose. Glucose is the product of the digestion of starch. In human metabolism, all simple sugars are converted into glucose. Glucose is the circulating form of carbohydrate in the bloodstream. Fructose is the sweetest of the simple sugars, and it is found in fruits and naturally occurring substances such as honey. Fructose consumption has increased greatly in the USA since the 1970s, when high-fructose corn syrup started to be widely used in food processing. High-fructose corn syrup is the major sweetening agent used by the food industry. Galactose is produced by the digestion of lactose, the major carbohydrate in milk.

Digestion

Most carbohydrates have to be converted to glucose in order to be used for energy production. The digestion of carbohydrates starts in the mouth, with mastication and the enzymatic action of salivary amylase, which converts starch to dextrins and maltose. Successive contractions of the stomach (peristalsis) move the food to the lower part of the stomach, while 20–30% of the carbohydrate is already converted to maltose. Peristalsis facilitates digestion in the small intestine, while the chemical digestion of carbohydrates is completed by pancreatic amylase (which continues the breakdown of starch to maltose) and intestinal disaccharidases (sucrase, lactase, and maltase for the breakdown of fructose, lactose, and maltose, respectively). The monosaccharide products of carbohydrate digestion are then absorbed into the portal circulation.

Absorption

Glucose accounts for the largest quantity of absorbed carbohydrate (80%), and galactose and fructose account for only a small amount (20%). The body quickly absorbs and transports the simple sugars, which enter the portal circulation via the capillaries of the intestinal villi and are transported to the liver. In the liver, fructose and galactose are converted to glucose, which is either used immediately for energy or stored in the form of glycogen. The liver can store approximately 5% of its mass in the form of glycogen, which can be readily converted to glucose for the production of energy.

Transport

Monosaccharides traverse the epithelial lining of the intestine by simple or facilitated diffusion or by active transport. The transport system for the passage of glucose and galactose through the apical membrane of the intestinal villi is called the Na^+-dependent glucose transporter (Na^+-dependent GLUT). Fructose uses a different transporter, called GLUT5, for the same passage. All monosaccharides are then transported from the enterocyte to the bloodstream by another sugar transporter known as GLUT2. The passage of glucose and galactose across both membranes of the intestine requires the presence of Na^+, while the passage of fructose is dependent on fructose concentration not Na^+ concentration.

Carbohydrates and Energy Metabolism

Glucose

The breakdown of glucose can be divided into two major parts: the anaerobic conversion of glucose to pyruvate, known as glycolysis, and the aerobic breakdown of pyruvate to carbon dioxide and water, which involves the tricarboxylic acid cycle and the electron transport chain.

Glycolysis is the series of enzymatic steps leading to the breakdown of one molecule of glucose to produce two molecules of pyruvate (**Figure 1**). Glycolysis occurs in the cytosol of different cells, and all human cells are capable of carrying out this process.

However, most glycolysis occurs in the liver, muscle, and adipose tissue.

The fate of pyruvate is determined by the cell type and the availability of oxygen. In the absence of oxygen, pyruvate is reduced to lactate in the cytosol. This occurs in the muscles during strenuous exercise, when the demands for energy are high. In cells that do not contain mitochondria, such as the erythrocytes, the glycolysis pathway is the only mechanism of energy production.

In the presence of oxygen, pyruvate is converted to acetyl coenzyme A (acetyl CoA) in the mitochondria and thus enters the tricarboxylic acid cycle and subsequently the electron transport chain. As a result, pyruvate is fully oxidized to carbon dioxide and water, and large amounts of energy are produced.

Fructose and Galactose

Fructose and galactose enter the glycolytic pathway through their conversion to intermediate compounds

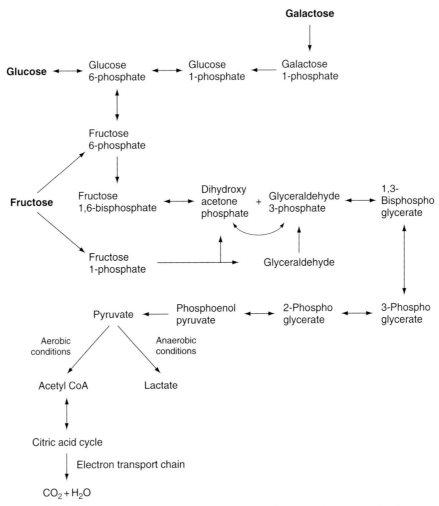

Figure 1 Outline of carbohydrate metabolism, including the points of entry of glucose, fructose, and galactose.

(**Figure 1**). This occurs primarily in the liver, and, as a result, these two monosaccharides are not generally available for uptake by other tissues. The end products of the catalysis of these monosaccharides are similar to glucose; however, when they are absorbed, they do not elicit the same hormonal response as glucose.

In the liver, breakdown of fructose, known as fructolysis, is initiated by the conversion of fructose to fructose 1-phosphate and subsequent hydrolysis to glyceraldehyde and dihydroxyacetone phosphate, a reaction catalyzed by fructose 1-phosphate aldolase. These products of hydrolysis can be used for further glycolytic conversion. Fructolysis in the liver bypasses the highly regulated step of phosphofructokinase and can produce a large amount of glycolytic metabolites. In the muscle and kidney cells, fructose can enter the glycolysis pathway through its conversion to fructose 6-phosphate, prior to the highly regulated phosphofructokinase step.

In the liver, galactose enters the glycolytic pathway through its phosphorylation to galactose 1-phosphate and subsequent epimerization to glucose 1-phosphate. This metabolic intermediate can either enter glycolysis by its conversion to glucose 6-phosphate or be used in glycogen synthesis, depending on the nutritional state of the organism.

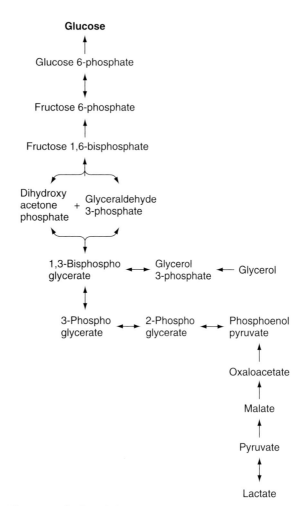

Figure 2   Outline of gluconeogenesis.

Glucose Production by the Liver and Kidneys

Gluconeogenesis

The biosynthesis of glucose from pyruvate, lactate, or other precursors is known as gluconeogenesis. It is not a direct reversal of glycolysis, since several steps of glycolysis are irreversible. Gluconeogenesis occurs mainly in the liver and less so in the kidney. These tissues contain all the necessary enzymes for gluconeogenesis and, furthermore, for the enzymatic activity of glycerol kinase, which allows glycerol to enter the gluconeogenic pathway at the level of glyceraldehyde 3-phosphate (**Figure 2**).

It is vital that the organism synthesizes glucose for those tissues that are unable to synthesize glucose. In humans, liver glycogen stores can sustain the body for 18 h without the ingestion of dietary carbohydrates. After this period, the liver must produce glucose for transport to other organs. The liver is the main gluconeogenic contributor (90%), while the kidney contributes gluconeogenically produced glucose to a lesser extent (10%).

Glycogenolysis

Glycogen is a branched polymer of glucose, which contains as many as 100 000 glucose units. The breakdown of glycogen for the production of glucose is known as glycogenolysis. Glycogen breakdown is initiated at the nonreducing ends of its branches. It consists of phosphorolysis of single glucose units by the cooperating enzymatic action of glycogen phosphorylase and the debranching enzyme. The product of phosphorolysis, glucose 1-phosphate, needs the additional action of phosphoglucomutase to convert it to glucose 6-phosphate. The liver contains the enzyme glucose 6-phosphatase for the hydrolysis of glucose 6-phosphate to free glucose, which can then be exported to the target tissues. However, the muscle and brain do not contain this enzyme, and the glucose 6-phosphate they produce enters the glycolytic pathway for energy production. Glycogen is a very efficient storage from of glucose, having an overall efficiency of storage of approximately 97%.

Control of Carbohydrate Metabolism

Hormonal Regulation

Hormones regulate (activate or inhibit) specific enzymes that catalyze the reactions of metabolic pathways. This is achieved mainly by covalent regulation or by conversion of the enzymes into their active or inactive form. Furthermore, hormones can control enzymes by induction or regulation of their transcription. Regulation of the expression of specific genes controls the concentrations of the enzymes and transport proteins necessary for carbohydrate metabolism.

Insulin When a meal is ingested, glucose is liberated as a result of the hydrolysis of dietary carbohydrate in the small intestine, and it is then absorbed into the blood. Increased glucose concentrations stimulate the production and secretion of insulin by the β cells of the pancreas. Insulin promotes the transfer of glucose into the target cells (i.e., skeletal muscle, liver, and adipose tissue) for use as energy and for storage in the form of glycogen, primarily in the liver.

Insulin also stimulates glycolysis by increasing the activity of glycogen synthase (**Figure 3**) and the transcription of glycolytic enzymes (**Figure 4**). Insulin inhibits gluconeogenesis by decreasing the transcription of several gluconeogenic enzymes (**Figure 4**) and by moderating the peripheral release of gluconeogenic precursors.

Fasting results in a decrease in insulin concentration and a reduction in glucose uptake by the muscle and adipose tissue, which use alternate forms of energy (e.g., free fatty acids). Glucose then becomes available for uptake by the brain, red blood cells, and renal medulla, which are strongly dependent on glucose for energy.

Glucagon Glucagon is a hormone secreted in the bloodstream by the α cells of the pancreas in response to low glucose levels. Glucagon counteracts the action of insulin, and its main role is to stimulate hepatic glucose output and to maintain glucose homeostasis. Glucagon stimulates glycogenolysis by activating glycogen phosphorylase and inhibits glycogen synthesis by inactivating glycogen synthase (**Figure 3**). Furthermore, glucagon stimulates gluconeogenesis by increasing the gene expression of gluconeogenic enzymes and by blocking glycolysis. In the liver, glucagon enhances the rate of gluconeogenesis by lipolysis, resulting in increased concentrations of free fatty acids and glycerol.

Catecholamines Epinephrine and norepinephrine are catecholamines that have a regulatory effect on

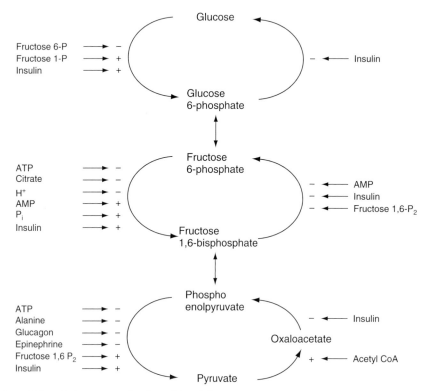

Figure 3 Points of regulation of glycogen synthesis and breakdown.

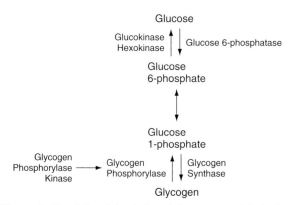

Figure 4 Regulation of glycolysis and gluconeogenesis in the liver.

carbohydrate metabolism. This effect is mainly dependent on the type of receptor present on each cell. Catecholamine receptors are divided into two types: two α receptors and three β receptors. The β and α-1 receptors stimulate catabolic reactions, while the α-2 receptor inhibits them. The presence of different catecholamine receptors on different cell types explains the selective breakdown of stores from certain tissues.

During fasting, catecholamines stimulate gluconeogenesis and glycogenolysis in the liver, as a result of increased secretion of glucagon by epinephrine. Catecholamines normally do not play a central role in maintaining glucose homeostasis during fasting, but they prevent hypoglycaemia when glucagon secretion is low.

Glucocorticoids Cortisol, the principal glucocorticoid, stimulates hepatic glucose output and the expression of genes encoding for gluconeogenic enzymes, thus stimulating gluconeogenesis. Cortisol is essential for the action of several hormones and has a much slower effect on hepatic glucose production than either glucagon or the catecholamines, taking several hours to take place.

Growth hormone Growth hormone, like cortisol, increases hepatic glucose production by changing substrate availability and promoting the expression of gluconeogenic enzymes. Growth hormone secretion is enhanced by starvation. Like cortisol, growth hormone affects hepatic glucose production much more slowly than glucagon or the catecholamines, taking several hours to occur.

Allosteric Enzyme Regulation

Allosteric enzymes are activated or inhibited by substances produced in the pathway in which the enzymes function. These substances are called

modulators and can alter the activity of allosteric enzymes by changing their conformation. Adenosine monophosphate (AMP), adenosine diphosphate (ADP), and adenosine triphosphate (ATP) are important modulators of allosteric enzymes in carbohydrate metabolism. The effects of ATP are opposed by those of AMP and ADP. When energy supply is adequate, ATP accumulates and negatively modulates enzymes that catalyze energy-producing or catabolic pathways, e.g., glycolysis. When energy is depleted and ATP concentration is decreased, AMP and ADP accumulate. As a result, allosteric enzymes in catabolic pathways are positively modulated and energy is produced. An increase in ATP inhibits further energy production and blocks glycolytic enzymes, while an increase in AMP or ADP stimulates glycolytic enzymes for energy production (**Figure 3**).

Directional Shifts

The majority of enzymes catalyze reversible reactions, and their action is highly dependent on the concentration of the reactants involved. An increase in the concentration of one reactant will drive the reaction in the direction that results in the breakdown of that reactant so as to achieve homeostasis. An example of a directional shift is the interconversion of glucose 1-phosphate and glucose 6-phosphate. During glucogenolysis, the concentration of glucose 1-phosphate increases and the reaction is driven towards the production of glucose 6-phosphate. During glycogen synthesis and gluconeogenesis, the concentration of glucose 6-phosphate increases and the reaction is driven towards the production of glucose 1-phosphate and, subsequently, towards the formation of glycogen.

Regulation of Gene Expression

Regulation of gene expression enables the human body to respond to changes in nutrient concentration. During increased availability of a specific nutrient, there is no need to express the genes encoding for enzymes involved in the metabolism of that nutrient. Gene expression is highly regulated by hormones, which respond to the concentration of nutrients in the blood. Selective expression of specific genes plays a major role in the regulation of carbohydrate metabolism.

Hormonal and nutrient concentrations affect several regulatory domains of genes that encode for enzymes involved in anabolic and catabolic pathways. High insulin and glucose concentrations increase mRNA levels and the transcription rates of the glycolytic enzymes and decrease those of the gluconeogenic enzymes. Glucagon has the opposite effect to insulin.

Glycogen Synthesis and Breakdown

The regulatory mechanism of glycogen synthesis and breakdown involves two counteracting enzymes: glycogen synthase and glycogen phosphorylase (**Figure 4**). Insulin activates glycogen synthase and therefore increases glycogen synthesis in the liver and muscle. When blood glucose levels decrease, glucagon inhibits glycogen synthase and activates glycogen phosphorylase in order to break down glycogen in the liver. Epinephrine also activates glycogen breakdown both in the liver and in skeletal muscle.

Peripheral Uptake of Glucose by Skeletal Muscle and Adipose Tissue

Glucose enters the target tissues by facilitated diffusion through a family of transporters known as glucose transporters (GLUTs). Five different isoforms of GLUTs have been isolated and characterized, GLUT1 to GLUT5. GLUT4 is mainly present in skeletal and cardiac muscle and in brown adipose tissue and differs significantly from the other isoforms in that it is stimulated by insulin. The other GLUTs do not require the action of insulin for glucose transport. GLUT1 and GLUT3 are responsible for glucose transport in most body tissues and are found in the brain, kidney, placenta, red blood cells, and fetal tissue. GLUT2 exists mainly in the liver and pancreas, and GLUT5 is responsible for glucose and fructose transport in the small intestine.

The GLUTs are encoded by different genes, and the regulation of their expression is highly tissue specific. GLUT4 is highly regulated by insulin, and its concentration is significantly increased in the presence of this hormone. As a result of the increase in GLUT4 concentration, there is increased glucose uptake by the adipose tissue and skeletal muscle.

Diseases of Carbohydrate Metabolism

Carbohydrate Malabsorption

Fructose intolerance and essential fructosuria   Fruc-Fructose intolerance and essential fructosuria are genetic defects of fructose metabolism. Fructose intolerance is an autosomal recessive disease, caused by a genetic defect in fructose 1-phosphate aldolase (aldolase B) in the liver. The symptoms of aldolase B deficiency occur when the infant is exposed to fructose. Aldolase B deficiency results in phosphate depletion and fructose 1-phosphate accumulation

in the liver. Consequently, gluconeogenesis and glycogenolysis are blocked, resulting in the inhibition of protein synthesis and subsequent liver failure.

Essential fructosuria is caused by a defect in the fructokinase gene. This disorder is asymptomatic and results in the excretion of fructose in the urine and in the conversion of fructose to fructose 6-phosphate in the muscle and adipose tissue.

Glucose and galactose malabsorption   Carbohydrate intolerance is a hereditary disorder that occurs infrequently and poses serious health risks. This disorder is caused by a deficiency in a digestive enzyme (e.g., sucrase-α-dextrinase) and defective glucose-galactose transport. Carbohydrate intolerance presents as the development of profuse infant diarrhoea immediately after birth.

Glycogen Storage Diseases

A lack of the enzyme glucose 6-phosphatase in the liver, kidney, and intestinal mucosa causes a disease known as Von Gierke's disease. This disease results in fasting hypoglycaemia, hepatomegaly, and recurrent acidosis. Genetic defects in glucose 6-phosphatase, glucose 6-phosphatase translocase, or pyrophosphate transporter result in a metabolic imbalance and an inability of the liver to maintain glucose homeostasis by either glycogenolysis or gluconeogenesis.

Gene mutations in the liver and muscle glycogen phosphorylases result in rare autosomal recessive disorders. In the liver, the disease results in glycogen accumulation and is known as Hers' disease. It is characterized by hypoglycaemia, hepatomegaly, and growth delay. In the muscle, the disease results in progressive muscle weakness and glycogen accumulation in the liver, and is known as McArdle's disease. It is characterized by exercise intolerance. A mutation in the debranching enzyme also results in glycogen accumulation in the liver and/or muscle and is known as Cori's disease. It is characterized by fasting hypoglycaemic convulsions, hepatomelagy, and myopathy.

Diabetes Mellitus

Diabetes mellitus is a group of metabolic disorders characterized by high levels of blood glucose (impaired glucose tolerance) and results from defects in insulin secretion, insulin action, or both. Diabetes mellitus is the seventh leading cause of death in the USA and is a major cause of premature mortality, stroke, cardiovascular disease, peripheral vascular disease, congenital malformations, perinatal mortality, and long-term and short-term disability. There are four principal types of diabetes mellitus: type 1 (formerly known as insulin-dependent diabetes mellitus), type 2 (formerly known as noninsulin-dependent diabetes mellitus), gestational diabetes (GDM), and maturity-onset diabetes of the young (MODY).

Type 1 diabetes   Type 1 diabetes is caused by autoimmune pancreatic β cell exhaustion and loss of insulin secretion. Onset of the disease occurs when most of the pancreatic β cells have been destroyed by the immune system. This form of diabetes is generally diagnosed in children and young adults and accounts for between 5% and 10% of all cases of diabetes mellitus.

Type 2 diabetes   Type 2 diabetes is a complex heterogenous disorder caused by interactions of various genetic and environmental factors. It is characterized by insulin resistance, obesity, a sedentary lifestyle, and occasionally by decreased insulin secretion. Because obesity and physical inactivity are increasing in children, the prevalence of paediatric type 2 diabetes has increased dramatically over the past 20 years to reach epidemic proportions. More than 85% of the cases of diabetes mellitus are type 2.

Gestational diabetes   GDM is a form of glucose intolerance that is diagnosed in some pregnant women. It is usually ameliorated after childbirth, but it increases the risk of developing type 2 diabetes in the future.

Maturity-onset diabetes of the young   MODY is an autosomal dominant trait that primarily affects insulin secretion and accounts for between 2% and 5% of the cases of diabetes. MODY can be caused by mutations in the glucokinase genes, leading to a reduced rate of glycolysis in the pancreas, reduced glycogen synthesis, and increased gluconeogenesis in the liver. It is diagnosed mostly in France and in the UK.

Abbreviations

ADP	Adenosine diphosphate
AMP	Adenosine monophosphate
ATP	Adenosine triphosphate
GDM	Gestational diabetes
GLUT1	Glucose transporter 1
GLUT2	Glucose transporter 2
GLUT3	Glucose transporter 3
GLUT4	Glucose transporter 4
GLUT5	Glucose transporter 5
MODY	Maturity-onset diabetes of the young

See also: **Diabetes Mellitus**: Etiology and Epidemiology; Classification and Chemical Pathology; Dietary Management. **Energy**: Metabolism. **Fructose**. **Galactose**. **Glucose**: Chemistry and Dietary Sources; Metabolism and Maintenance of Blood Glucose Level; Glucose Tolerance. **Glycemic Index**.

Further Reading

Brody T (1999) *Nutritional Biochemistry*, 2nd edn, pp. 57–132 and 157–271. San Diego: Academic Press.

Corssmit EPM, Romijn JA, and Sauerwein HP (2001) Regulation of glucose production with special attention to nonclassical regulatory mechanisms: a review. *Metabolism* 50: 742–755.

Eastwood M (2003) *Principles of Human Nutrition*, 2nd edn, pp. 195–212, 418–426 and 486–509. Oxford: Blackwell.

Gray GM (2000) Digestion and absorption of carbohydrate. In: *Biochemical and Physiological Aspects of Human Nutrition*, 1st edn, pp. 91–106. Philadelphia: WB Saunders Company.

Groff JL and Gropper SS (eds.) (2000) *Advanced Nutrition and Human Metabolism*, 3rd edn, pp. 70–105. Belmont: Wadsworth.

Jiang G and Zhang BB (2003) Glucagon and regulation of glucose metabolism. *American Journal of Physiology. Endocrinology and Metabolism* 284: E671–E678.

Levin RJ (1999) Carbohydrates. In: Shils ME, Olson JA, Shike M, and Ross AC (eds.) *Modern Nutrition in Health and Disease*, 9th edn, pp. 49–65. Media: Lippincott Williams & Wilkins.

McGrane MM (2000) Carbohydrate metabolism – synthesis and oxidation. In: *Biochemical and Physiological Aspects of Human Nutrition*, 1st edn, pp. 158–210. Philadelphia: WB Saunders Company.

Schlenker ED (2003) Carbohydrates. In: Williams SR and Schlenker ED (eds.) *Essentials of Nutrition & Diet Therapy*, 8th edn, pp. 47–65. St. Louis: Mosby.

Schlenker ED (2003) Digestion, Absorption, and Metabolism. In: Williams SR and Schlenker ED (eds.) *Essentials of Nutrition & Diet Therapy*, 8th edn, pp. 23–45. St. Louis: Mosby.

Stryer L (1995) *Biochemistry*, 4th edn, pp. 463–602. New York: WH Freeman and Company.

Tirone TA and Brunicardi FC (2001) Overview of glucose regulation. *World Journal of Surgery* 25: 461–467.

Tso P and Crissinger K (2000) Overview of digestion and absorption. In: *Biochemical and Physiological Aspects of Human Nutrition*, 1st edn, pp. 75–90. Philadelphia: WB Saunders Company.

Requirements and Dietary Importance

C L Stylianopoulos, Johns Hopkins University, Baltimore, MD, USA

© 2005 Elsevier Ltd. All rights reserved.

Introduction

Carbohydrates are an important energy source in the human diet. They generally supply about 45% of the energy requirement in developed countries and up to 85% in developing countries. Carbohydrates have been considered a fundamental source of nourishment and inexpensive and versatile staple of the diet.

The type and composition of dietary carbohydrates varies greatly among different food products. Dietary carbohydrates can be predominantly found in the form of sugar (monosaccharides and disaccharides) and starch or nonstarch polysaccharides. Furthermore, in the food industry they can be used in the form of hydrolyzed cornstarch, high-fructose corn syrups, modified starches, gums, mucilages, and sugar alcohols.

The current global emphasis for healthy eating focuses on increasing carbohydrate consumption, particularly in the form of whole grains, fruit, and vegetables. Epidemiological and clinical studies have shown a positive association between carbohydrate consumption and reduced risk of chronic disease and certain types of cancer.

Dietary Sources and Intakes

The major sources of carbohydrates are cereals, accounting for over 50% of carbohydrate consumed in both developed and developing countries, followed by sweeteners, root crops, pulses, vegetables, fruit, and milk products. Carbohydrate and nutrient intake in general can be estimated using data from food production and balance sheets, household surveys, and individual assessments (**Table 1**). **Figure 1** shows the trends in carbohydrate consumption by food group as a percentage of total carbohydrate in developed and developing countries, obtained from food balance data in 1994.

Sugars

The term 'sugar' includes monosaccharides and disaccharides. The most common monosaccharides are glucose (or dextrose), fructose, and galactose. Glucose is found in fruit, honey, maple syrup, and vegetables. Glucose is also formed from sucrose hydrolysis in honey, maple syrup and invert sugar, and from starch hydrolysis in corn syrups. The properties of glucose are important for improving food texture, flavor, and palatability. Glucose is the major cell fuel and the principal energy source for the brain. Fructose is found in honey, maple sugar, fruit, and vegetables. Fructose is also formed from sucrose hydrolysis in honey, maple syrup, and invert sugar. It is commonly used as a sweetener in soft drinks, bakery products, and candy in the form of high-fructose corn syrups. Galactose is found primarily in milk and dairy products.

The most common disaccharides are sucrose, lactose, and maltose. Sucrose is mostly found in sugar cane and beet, and in lesser amounts in honey, maple sugar, fruit, and vegetables. The properties of sucrose are important in improving viscosity, sweetness, and flavor of baked foods, ice cream, and desserts. Maltose is formed from starch digestion. It is also produced from the germination of grain for malt liquors. Lactose is found in milk and dairy products, and is not as sweet as glucose or sucrose.

In the second part of the twentieth century, sugar intake increased markedly in the US, because of increased consumption of added sugars in beverages and foods. According to the US Food Supply Data, consumption of added sugars has increased from 27 teaspoons/person/day in 1970 to 32 teaspoons/person/day in 1996, which represents a 23% increase. Soft drinks are the most frequently used form of added sugars, and account for one-third of total sugar intake. In Europe the trend of sugar consumption has been a steady one.

Table 1 Approaches for determination of trends in nutrient consumption worldwide

Approach	Advantages	Disadvantages
Food production	Figures available for every crop	Affected by agricultural practices, weather conditions, external forces
Food balance sheets	Figures available for every food item	Inadequate to determine food waste and spoilage
Household surveys	Figures close to actual food consumption	Inadequate to determine food consumption outside the home, food waste, and spoilage
Individual assessments	Figures close to actual food consumption	Data not available for all countries Diverse methods of assessment

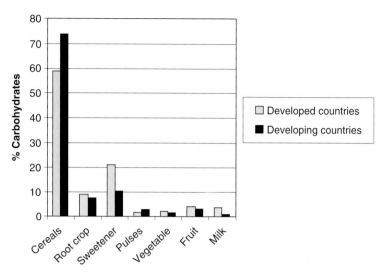

Figure 1 Trends in energy consumption by carbohydrate food group as a percentage of total carbohydrate in developed and developing countries, obtained from food balance data in 1994. Data obtained from FAO/WHO (1998). Carbohydrates in human nutrition. Report of a joint FAO/WHO expert consultation. *FAO Food and Nutrition Papers* 19 **66**: 1–140.

Polysaccharides

Starch   Starch is the most important and abundant food polysaccharide. Starch is predominantly derived from plant seed, such as wheat, maize, rice, oats, and rye, and from plant roots, such as potatoes. Legumes and vegetables also contribute to the starch content of the diet. Bread and pasta are popular forms of starch, while tropical starchy foods, such as plantains, cassava, sweet potatoes, and yams are increasingly contributing to carbohydrate intake. Starch accounts for 20–50% of total energy intake, depending on the total carbohydrate consumption.

Nonstarch   Nonstarch polysaccharides (NSP), formerly referred to as 'dietary fiber,' can either be soluble or insoluble and are mainly derived from cereals, especially wholegrain. Wheat, rice, and maize contain predominantly insoluble NSP, while oats, rye, and barley contain predominantly soluble NSP. Vegetables are also a source of NSP and contain equal amounts of insoluble and soluble NSP. Intakes of NSP range from about 19 g day^{-1} in Europe and North American countries to 30 g day^{-1} in rural Africa.

Health Effects of Carbohydrates

Carbohydrates are stored in the human body as glycogen mainly in the liver and muscle. The human body has a limited storage capacity for carbohydrates compared to fat. The total amount of carbohydrates stored in tissues and circulating in the blood as glucose is approximately 7.56 MJ (1800 kcal). Diets high in carbohydrate ensure adequate glycogen storage available for immediate energy utilization. Carbohydrates are the preferred energy source for the human brain and have an important role in reducing protein breakdown when energy intake is inadequate.

Dietary carbohydrates are absorbed in their hexose form (glucose, fructose, galactose) and provide 15.6 kJ g^{-1} (3.75 kcal g^{-1}) of energy. Although sugars and polysaccharides provide similar amounts of energy, they differ in their physiological and metabolic properties. The effects of carbohydrate-containing foods on blood glucose levels during digestion and absorption are variable, depending on the type of dietary carbohydrate. Postprandial glucose response is reduced when glucose absorption is slow. Glycemic index (GI) is used for the quantification of blood glucose response after carbohydrate consumption. GI is the area under the curve of the blood glucose increase 2 h after carbohydrate ingestion of a set amount of a particular food (e.g., 50 g) compared to the blood glucose increase 2 h after ingestion of the same amount of a reference food (white bread or glucose). GI is influenced significantly by the carbohydrate types and physical determinants of digestion rate (intact versus ground grains, cooked versus uncooked food, and soluble fiber content). Carbohydrate ingestion in the presence of fat and protein reduces the GI of a meal. The GI of carbohydrate-containing meals has been linked to several health outcomes. The role of carbohydrates in health is a growing area of research and has received a great amount of interest in the past decade.

Carbohydrates and Nutrient Density

Increased sugar consumption has generated concern in recent years because of the potential to displace the micronutrient content of the diet by increasing 'empty calories' and energy intake. There is some evidence that essential nutrient intake decreases with increasing total sugar intake. However, sugar intake has not been shown to accurately predict micronutrient ingestion. Moderate intakes of sugar coincide with sufficient nutrient intake. The risk of low micronutrient status is increased for individuals with a diet high in sugars and low in total energy intake, as in the case of children or people on restrictive diets. Data analysis on food intake of preschool children suggests that the intake of some micronutrients (calcium, zinc, thiamin, riboflavin, and niacin) is inversely related to sugar intake. However, the dilutional effects of sugars may be somewhat distorted by the fact that some rich sources of added sugars are also fortified with micronutrients, as in the case of breakfast cereals. The Dietary Reference Intake (DRI) Panel on Macronutrients, using national food intake data, reported that a clear dilutional effect on micronutrient intake starts when sugar intake approaches 25% of total calories. The American Heart Association dietary guidelines stress the consumption of fruit, vegetables, grains, and complex carbohydrates so that micronutrient requirements are met by whole rather than supplemented foods.

Several human studies have demonstrated that diets rich in NSP may reduce the bioavailability of minerals, such as iron, calcium, and zinc. Nevertheless, this effect is more likely due to the presence of phytate, which inhibits the absorption of those minerals, than the NSP content of the diet.

Carbohydrates and Obesity

Several studies have been conducted to establish an association between sugar ingestion and total energy intake. There have been consistent reports of a negative association between sugar intake and body mass index in adults and children. However, this observation could be confounded by the correlation of dietary fat and obesity, since high-fat diets are usually low in carbohydrates. Some ad libitum dietary studies have shown that diets low in sugar are associated with weight loss, maybe as a result of reduced calorie intake. Nevertheless, in human metabolic studies, no effect on weight or energy expenditure

was observed when carbohydrate was replaced by fat or protein in isocaloric diets.

Foods high in sugars or GI are highly palatable and it has been suggested that they create a potential risk for energy overconsumption and weight gain. However, there is no evidence to support this claim or confirm the role of GI in body weight regulation. Foods high in sugar have high energy density and thus decreasing their consumption can assist in weight reduction. On the contrary, foods rich in NSP are bulky and have less energy density and as a result induce greater satiety when ingested. It follows that diets rich in NSP may be useful for obesity prevention, since they prevent energy overconsumption. However, there is no evidence to indicate that increasing the carbohydrate content of a low-energy diet facilitates weight loss.

The consumption of sugar-sweetened soft drinks may contribute to weight gain because of the low satiety of liquid foods. Short-term human studies have shown that sugar-sweetened soft drink consumption does not result in a decrease of total energy intake. Thus, sugar-sweetened soft drinks can significantly increase the total caloric intake and result in weight gain. Consumption of these drinks has been associated with childhood obesity.

Carbohydrate and Cardiovascular Disease

Dietary factors influence the risk factors, such as obesity, diabetes, and hyperlipidemia, that lead to the development of cardiovascular disease (CVD). A diet rich in carbohydrates in the form of whole grain cereals, fruit, and vegetables may assist in the reduction of saturated fat and may increase the antioxidant content of the diet, thus reducing the risk of heart disease. On the contrary, a high intake of carbohydrates (>65% of total calories), especially in the form of refined sugars and starch, may increase serum triacylglycerol levels and adversely affect plasma lipoprotein profile. Short-term studies show a consistent relationship between sugar consumption and elevation of triacylglycerol levels as well as a decrease in plasma high-density lipoprotein (HDL) levels, which could result in increased atherosclerosis and heart disease risk. However, longitudinal cohort studies have failed to show a consistent association of sugar consumption with CVD, mainly because of the confounding factors associated with increased heart disease risk.

Certain NSP (for example β glycans) have been shown to reduce low-density lipoprotein (LDL) and total cholesterol levels on a short-term basis. Therefore, a protective effect for CVD has been shown with consumption of foods high in NSP. This protective effect has not been duplicated with NSP supplements. Furthermore, no long-term effect has been established.

High-GI diets have been shown to slightly increase hemoglobin A1c, total serum cholesterol and triacylglycerols, and decrease HDL cholesterol and urinary C-peptide in diabetic and hyperlipidemic individuals. In addition, low-GI diets have been shown to decrease cholesterol and triacylglycerol levels in dyslipidemic individuals. There are insufficient studies performed on healthy individuals and further research on the role of GI in lipid profile and CVD risk factors is warranted.

Carbohydrates and Type 2 Diabetes

There is little evidence from prospective studies to support a positive association between total dietary carbohydrate consumption and risk of type 2 diabetes. Some recent evidence suggests that rapidly digested refined sugars, which have a high GI, may increase the risk of type 2 diabetes. Short-term studies have shown that decreasing the GI of a meal can improve glucose tolerance and insulin sensitivity in healthy people. Furthermore, the substitution of high-GI with low-GI carbohydrates can decrease postprandial glucose and insulin levels. Some epidemiological studies have demonstrated a protective effect of NSP consumption against type 2 diabetes.

Carbohydrates and Dental Caries

The quantity and frequency of sugars in the diet play a significant role in the development of dental caries. Their digestion by salivary amylase provides an acid environment for the growth of bacteria in the mouth, thus increasing the rate of plaque formation. Sucrose is the most cariogenic of the sugars, followed by glucose, fructose, and maltose. The milk sugars (lactose and galactose) are considerably less cariogenic. There is no epidemiological evidence to support a cariogenic role of polysaccharide foods with no added sugars.

Dental caries is a multifaceted disease, affected not only by the frequency and type of sugar consumed, but also by oral hygiene and fluoride supplementation and use. Despite the increase in sugar consumption, the incidence of dental caries has decreased worldwide because of the increased use of fluoride and improvement in oral hygiene.

Carbohydrate and Cancer

Case-control studies have shown that colorectal cancer risk increases with high intakes of sugar-rich foods, while other studies have failed to prove such a relationship. Thus, there is insufficient evidence to support the role of sugar in the risk for colorectal cancer. On the contrary, carbohydrate consumption in the form of fruit, vegetables, and cereals has been shown to be protective against colorectal cancer.

Carbohydrate foods are a good source of phytoestrogens, which may protect against breast cancer. However, studies related to carbohydrate intake and breast cancer have been inconsistent and are insufficient to establish an association between carbohydrates and breast cancer risk.

The Health Professionals Follow-up Study showed a negative association of prostate cancer risk with high fructose intake. Additional data on the role of sugar consumption on prostate cancer risk is lacking. Some evidence suggests that increased fiber intakes are related to decreased prostate cancer risk.

Carbohydrates and Gastrointestinal Health

High intakes of NSP, in the range of $4-32\,g\,day^{-1}$, have been shown to contribute to the prevention and treatment of constipation. Population studies have linked the prevalence of hemorrhoids, diverticular disease, and appendicitis to NSP intakes, although there are several dietary and lifestyle confounding factors that could directly affect these relationships. High-carbohydrate diets may be related to bacterial growth in the gut and subsequent reduction of acute infective gastrointestinal disease risk.

Low-Carbohydrate Diets

The recent trend of weight loss diets promotes some level of carbohydrate restriction and increased protein consumption. Some examples are Dr Atkins New Diet Revolution, The South Beach Diet, and The Carbohydrate Addict's Diet. This dietary advice is contrary to that proposed by governmental agencies (US Department of Agriculture/Department of Health Services, National Institutes of Health) and nongovernmental organizations (American Dietetic Association, American Heart Association, American Diabetes Association, and American Cancer Society).

There is consistent evidence that weight loss in low-carbohydrate diets is triggered by negative energy balance resulting from low caloric intake, and that it is not a function of macronutrient composition. There is no scientific evidence to suggest that low-carbohydrate diets are more metabolically efficient than restricted calorie conventional diets. Several studies have shown that low-carbohydrate diets result in weight loss because of reduced caloric intake.

Low-carbohydrate diets promote the lipolysis of stored triacylglycerols known as ketosis, reduce glucose and insulin levels, and suppress appetite. As a result, there is an increase in blood uric acid concentration. Some studies have shown that the consumption of high amounts of nondairy protein results in a decline in kidney functions in individuals with mildly compromised kidney function. However, no such effect has been shown in individuals with normal kidney functions. Furthermore, low-carbohydrate diets can have side effects such as bad taste, constipation, diarrhea, dizziness, headache, nausea, thirst, and fatigue.

Low-carbohydrate diets lack essential vitamins and minerals because of inadequate consumption of fruit, vegetables, and grains, and require supplementation to achieve nutritional adequacy. Controlled trials of low-carbohydrate diets are necessary to establish long-term effectiveness and adverse health effects or benefits.

Requirements and Recommendations

According to the new definition of the expert panel appointed by the Institute of Medicine of the National Academies of Science (IOM), dietary reference intakes (DRIs) are defined as a set of reference values for nutrient intake, and include the estimated average requirement (EAR), recommended dietary allowance (RDA), adequate intake (AI), and tolerable upper intake level (UL). EAR refers to the average daily intake value of a nutrient that is estimated to fulfill the needs of healthy people in a particular lifestage or group. RDA refers to the minimum daily intake that fulfills the need of almost all healthy people in a particular lifestage or group. AI refers to the observed intake of a particular group of healthy people, and is used when there is lack of scientific experimentation for the determination of the EAR or the RDA. UL refers to the maximum daily intake level of a nutrient that is not likely to pose an adverse health effect for almost all people.

The DRIs for carbohydrate consumption of individual groups and lifestages are outlined in **Table 2**. These values are based on the average minimum amount of glucose needed for brain function. A UL for carbohydrates was not set because no studies have shown that excessive consumption of carbohydrates has a detrimental effect on health. Based on the dilutional effect of added sugars on micronutrients, the expert panel suggests a maximal intake of less than 25% of energy from added sugars. Total sugar intake can be decreased by limiting foods high in added sugars and consuming naturally occurring sugar products, like milk, dairy products, and fruit.

The IOM does not specify dietary requirements or recommendations for NSP consumption, but has provided recommended intakes for fiber, which includes NSP. The DRIs for total fiber consumption of individual groups and lifestages are outlined in **Table 3**. It has not been shown that a high fiber intake has a harmful effect in healthy individuals. Therefore, a UL for fiber has not been set.

There is insufficient evidence to support a recommendation by the IOM for the consumption of low-GI foods or the replacement of high-GI foods, like bread and potatoes. Although several studies propose adverse effects of high-GI carbohydrates and beneficial effects of low-GI foods, a recommendation on consumption of low-GI foods is a major dietary change that requires substantial scientific evidence. Therefore, a UL based on GI is not set.

The 1998 report of the Food and Agriculture Organization (FAO) and the World Health Organization (WHO) regarding the role of carbohydrates in human nutrition recommends the consumption of at least 55% of total energy in the form of carbohydrates from a variety of sources. The committee proposes that the majority of carbohydrates consumed should originate from NSP, principally from

Table 2 Carbohydrate requirements and recommendations (DRIs)

Age group/Life stage	EAR (g day^{-1})		RDA (g day^{-1})		AI (g day^{-1})
	Males	Females	Males	Females	
Infants (0–6 months)					60
Infants (6–12 months)					95
Children (1–18 years)	100	100	130	130	
Adults (>18 years)	100	100	130	130	
Pregnancy		135		175	
Lactation		160		210	

DRIs, dietary reference intakes; EAR, estimated average requirement; RDA, recommended dietary allowance; AI, adequate intake.- Data from Institute of Medicine of the National Academies (2002) *Dietary Reference Intakes for Energy, Carbohydrate, Fiber, Fat, Fatty Acids, Cholesterol, Protein, Amino Acids*. Washington, DC: The National Academies Press.

Table 3 Total fiber recommendations (DRIs)

Age group/Lifestage	AI (g day⁻¹)	
	Males	Females
Children (1–3 years)	19	19
Children (4–8 years)	25	25
Children (9–13 years)	31	26
Children (14–18 years)	38	26
Adults (19–50 years)	38	25
Adults (>51 years)	30	21
Pregnancy		28
Lactation		29

DRIs, dietary reference intakes; AI, adequate intake. Data from Institute of Medicine of the National Academies (2001) *Dietary Reference Intakes for Energy, Carbohydrate, Fiber, Fat, Fatty Acids, Cholesterol, Protein, Amino Acids.* Washington, DC: The National Academies Press.

cereals, vegetables, legumes, and fruit. Furthermore, it suggests that free sugars should be restricted to less than 10% of total energy. This report recognizes that there is no direct causal link between sugar consumption and chronic disease. However, sugars significantly increase the energy density of the human diet and high-sugar drinks have been associated with childhood obesity.

A 2002 report of the American Heart Association suggests the restriction of sugar consumption. This report recognizes that there are no beneficial effects of increased sugar consumption. On the contrary, some studies suggest that it may have adverse health effects. In order to enhance the nutrient density and reduce the energy density of the diet, increased consumption of high-sugar foods should be avoided.

See also: **Cancer**: Epidemiology and Associations Between Diet and Cancer; Effects on Nutritional Status. **Carbohydrates**: Chemistry and Classification; Regulation of Metabolism; Resistant Starch and Oligosaccharides. **Cereal Grains**. **Dental Disease**. **Diabetes Mellitus**: Etiology and Epidemiology. **Dietary Fiber**: Role in Nutritional Management of Disease. **Energy**: Metabolism. **Fructose**. **Fruits and Vegetables**. **Galactose**. **Glucose**: Chemistry and Dietary Sources. **Glycemic Index**. **Hypertension**: Etiology. **Lipids**: Chemistry and Classification. **Obesity**: Definition, Etiology and Assessment. **Sucrose**: Nutritional Role, Absorption and Metabolism; Dietary Sucrose and Disease. **World Health Organization**.

Further Reading

Anderson GH and Woodend D (2003) Consumption of sugars and the regulation of short-term satiety and food intake. *American Journal of Clinical Nutrition* 78(supplement): 843S–849S.

Brody T (1999) *Nutritional Biochemistry*, 2nd edn, pp. 57–192 and 457–475. San Diego: Academic Press.

Eastwood M (2003) *Principles of Human Nutrition*, 2nd edn pp. 195–212, 418–426 and 456–509. Oxford: Blackwell.

FAO/WHO (1998) Carbohydrates in human nutrition. Report of a joint FAO/WHO expert consultation. *FAO Food and Nutrition Papers 19* 66: 1–140.

Groff JL and Gropper SS (2000) *Advanced Nutrition and Human Metabolism*, 3rd edn, pp. 70–115. ch. 4. Belmont: Wadsworth.

Howard BV and Wylie-Rosett J (2002) Sugar and cardiovascular disease. A statement for healthcare professionals from the Committee on Nutrition of the Council on Nutrition, Physical Activity, and Metabolism of the American Heath Association. *Circulation* 106: 523–527.

Institute of Medicine of the National Academies (2002) *Dietary Reference Intakes for Energy, Carbohydrate, Fiber, Fat, Fatty Acids, Cholesterol, Protein, Amino Acids.* Washington, DC: The National Academies Press.

James WPT (2001) European diet and public health: the continuing challenge. *Public Health and Nutrition* 4: 275–292.

Johnson RK and Frary C (2001) Choose beverages and foods to moderate your intake of sugars: the 200 dietary guidelines for Americans – what's all the fuss about? *Journal of Nutrition* 131: 2766S–2771S.

Levin RJ (1999) Carbohydrates. In: Shils ME, Olson JA, Shike M, and Ross AC (eds.) *Modern Nutrition in Health and Disease*, 9th edn, pp. 49–65 ch. 3. Media: Lippincott Williams & Wilkins.

Ruxton CHS, Garceau FJS, and Cottrell RC (1999) Guidelines for sugar consumption in Europe: is a quantitative approach justified? *European Journal of Clinical Nutrition* 53: 503–513.

Saris WHM (2003) Sugars, energy metabolism, and body weight control. *American Journal of Clinical Nutrition* 78(supplement): 850S–857S.

Schlenker ED (2003) Carbohydrates. In: Williams SR and Schlenker ED (eds.) *Essentials of Nutrition and Diet Therapy*, 8th edn, pp. 47–65. St. Louis: Mosby.

Schlenker ED (2003) Digestion, Absorption, and Metabolism. In: Williams SR and Schlenker ED (eds.) *Essentials of Nutrition and Diet Therapy*, 8th edn, pp. 23–45. St. Louis: Mosby.

Touger-Decker R and van Loveren C (2003) Sugars and dental caries. *American Journal of Clinical Nutrition* 78(supplement): 881S–92S.

Relevant Websites

http://www.usda.gov – US Department of Agriculture and US Department of Health and Human Services (2000) Nutrition and your health: dietary guidelines for Americans, 5th edn.

Resistant Starch and Oligosaccharides

A Laurentin, Universidad Central de Venezuela, Caracas, Venezuela
C A Edwards, University of Glasgow, Glasgow, UK

© 2005 Elsevier Ltd. All rights reserved.

Introduction

In recent years, there has been increasing interest in those carbohydrates that escape absorption in the small intestine and enter the colon, where they may have specific health benefits due to their fermentation by the colonic microflora and their effect on gut physiology. This entry considers the definition, classification, dietary sources, methods of analysis, colonic fermentation, and health benefits of both resistant starch and oligosaccharides, and compares them with those of dietary fiber.

Resistant Starch

Definition

In 1992, a concerted action of European researchers defined resistant starch as "the sum of starch and the products of starch degradation not absorbed in the small intestine of healthy individuals." This concept completely changed our understanding of the action of carbohydrates in the diet because up until the early 1980s, it was thought that starches were completely digested and absorbed in the human small intestine. Three important considerations are attached to this physiological definition. First, resistant starch is made up not only of high-molecular weight polymers but also can include dextrins, small oligosaccharides, and even glucose, all derived from digested starch that escapes absorption. Second, resistant starches reach the human large intestine where they are metabolized by the complex colonic microflora. Finally, the actual amount of resistant starch in a food (i.e., the amount reaching the colon) depends on the physiology of the individual and it may be affected by age.

Classification and Dietary Sources

Food starches can be classified according to the way they are metabolized by the human small intestine into those that are rapidly digested, those that are slowly digested, and those that are resistant to digestion. Similarly, resistant starch has been classified into three types: physically inaccessible starch,

Table 1 Classification of resistant starch

Food source	Type[a]	Content in food (g per 100 g)	Contribution to total RS intake
Cereal products containing whole grains or grain fragments	RS_1	1–9	Minor
Brown breads			
Legumes			
Pastas			
Unripe bananas	RS_2	17–75	Very little
Uncooked potatoes			
High amylose starches			
Bread	RS_3	1–10	Major
Cornflakes			
Cooked cooled potatoes			
Legumes			
Amylose–lipid complex	Others	Not known	Unknown
Modified starches			

[a]RS_1, physically inaccessible starch; RS_2, resistant granules; RS_3, retrograded starch.

resistant starch granules, and retrograded starch (Table 1).

Physically inaccessible starch (RS$_1$) Type I resistant starch is physically inaccessible and is protected from the action of α-amylase, the enzyme that hydrolyzes the breakdown of starch in the human small intestine. This inaccessibility is due to the presence of plant cell walls that entrap the starch, for example, in legume seeds and partially milled and whole grains. RS_1 can also be found in highly compact processed food like pasta. The RS_1 content is affected by disruption of the food structure during processing (e.g., milling) and, to some extent, by chewing.

Resistant granules (RS$_2$) Starch granules are plant organelles where starch is produced and stored. Each plant has characteristic starch granules that differ in size, shape, amylose to amylopectin ratio, crystalline to amorphous material ratio, starch supramolecular architecture, and amylose–lipid complexes, amongst other features. It is believed that combinations of these factors make some granules more resistant to the attack of digestive enzymes than other granules. Type II resistant starch is found in unripe bananas, uncooked potatoes, and high amylose starches. RS_2 disappears during cooking, especially in water, because a combination of water and heat make the starch gelatinize, giving more access to amylases.

Retrograded starch (RS₃) Type III resistant starch is the most abundant of the resistant starches present in food. It is formed during usual food processing by cooking and then cooling. When starch is cooked in an excess of water, it gelatinizes, i.e., the granular structure is disrupted, the granule swells, and amylose leaks out of the amylopectin matrix. Then, when the food is cooled down, amylose (and more slowly amylopectin) recrystallizes to a new ordered and more compact structure (process known as retrogradation), which decreases access for digestive enzymes. RS₃ production can be affected by the amylose to amylopectin ratio, amount of water, and temperature during cooking, and the number of repeated cooking and cooling cycles. Retrograded starch can be found in bread, some brands of corn flakes, cooked-cooled potatoes, and legumes.

Others sources of resistant starch In recent years, amylose–lipid complex and modified starches have also been recognized as other sources of resistant starches (**Table 1**). Amylose–lipid complexes occur when fatty acids (12–18 carbons) are held within the helical structure of amylose. They are formed naturally during starch biosynthesis, but may also be produced during cooking. Lipids may interfere with amylose retrogradation, impairing the production of retrograded starch during processing. However, these complexes themselves have lower digestibility than cooked starch.

As well as naturally resistant starch complexes, there are different types of modified starches that are manufactured by the food industry for a variety of reasons. They can be defined as native starches that have been submitted to one or more physical, chemical, or enzymatic treatments promoting granular disorganization, polymer degradation, molecular rearrangements, oxidation, or chemical group addition. Modified starches can be classified into four main categories accordingly to their main physicochemical characteristic: pregelatinized, derivatized, cross-linked, and dextrinized starches (**Table 2**). However, they usually are known as physically, chemically, or enzymatically modified starch because of the way they are produced (**Table 3**). The digestibility of these modified starches is variable and depends on the type and extent of the treatment. Some authors have proposed a new category, type IV resistant starch, to include chemically modified starches. Indeed, it has been shown that cross-linked starches have a 15–19% decrease in *in vitro* digestibility when compared with their native starches, and hydroxypropylated starch is only 50% digestible. However, pregelatinized starches produced by drum drying and extrusion have a 3–6% and 5–11% decrease in digestibility, respectively. Part but not all of this reduction in digestibility is due to the formation of retrograded starch; therefore, physically modified starches should also be considered as a category of resistant starch.

In addition to the starch properties already described, several starchy foods (for instance, cereals and legumes) have antinutritional factors, such as lectins, tannins, phytates, and enzyme inhibitors (both protease and amylase inhibitors). Amylase inhibitors present in raw pulses may reduce the activity of amylase in the human small intestine. However, most of these factors, especially enzyme inhibitors, are inactivated during food processing and cooking.

Analysis

The definition of resistant starch is based on its physiological behavior in the human small intestine, i.e., resistant starch is a heterogeneous group of molecules from small monosaccharides to large polymers with different molecular weight, degree of polymerization, and supramolecular architecture.

Table 2 Classification of modified starches

Starch	Modifying agent	Physicochemical characteristic	Use in food
Pregelatinized	Extrusion Drum drying	Soluble in cold water	Cake and instant products
Derivatized	Acetyl Hydroxypropyl Phosphate	Stable at freeze-thawing cycles	Canned and frozen food
Cross-linked	Epiclorhydrine Trimetaphosphate	Stable at higher temperatures, extreme pH, and higher shear forces	Meat sauce thickeners Instant soup Weaning infant food Dressings
Dextrinized	Acid hydrolysis Oxidizing agents Irradiation Heat (pyrodextrins) Amylolytic enzymes	Soluble in cold water Lower or nil viscosity	Chewing gums Jelly Syrups

Table 3 Methods of modified starch production

Treatment	Modification	Description
Physically modified	Pregelatinization	Starch paste is precooked and dried by extrusion or drum drying
	Dextrinization	Starch polymers are hydrolyzed to smaller molecules by irradiation
Chemically modified	Derivatization[a]	Lateral groups are added to starch lateral chains
	Cross-linking[a]	Multifunctional groups are used to link two different starch molecules together
	Dextrinization	Starch polymers are hydrolyzed by oxidizing agents, acid hydrolysis, pyrodextrinization
Enzymatically modified	Dextrinization	Starch polymers are hydrolyzed to smaller molecules by incubation with amylases

[a]Double-derived starches are produced by combination of these two processes.

This complexity makes it difficult to quantify accurately. All *in vitro* methods therefore need to be corroborated against *in vivo* models; however, *in vivo* models are also very difficult to validate.

In general, *in vitro* methods try to imitate human small intestine digestion using different sample preparation (i.e., milling, chewing, etc.), sample pretreatment (i.e., simulation of oral or stomach digestion), sample treatment (i.e., different enzymes mixtures), sample post-treatment (i.e., different resistant starch solubilizing agents and enzyme mixtures), and incubation conditions (i.e., shaking/stirring, pH, temperature, time) (**Table 4**). The choice of each of these multiple factors represents a huge analytical problem because not only a compromise between physiological conditions and analytical handling has to be achieved, but also because the resistant starch content values must be in agreement with *in vivo* data.

On the other hand, in human *in vivo* methods, samples of digested food that reach the end of the small intestine are taken for analysis, either from ileostomy patients (i.e., where the large intestine has been removed) or from healthy volunteers using special cannulas in the ileum. Animals can also be employed for *in vivo* experiments, such as gnotobiotic (i.e., germ-free) and pseudognotobiotic (i.e., antibiotic treated) rats. In these cases, colonic bacterial fermentation is absent or suppressed by antibiotics and it is assumed that what reaches the end of the small intestine appears in feces. The main difficulty with these methods is that *in vivo* starch digestion may occur

during the whole transit through the small intestine, which varies between individuals and the type of meal consumed. Moreover, these studies are difficult to perform in healthy volunteers and the physiological significance of using ileostomy patients is debatable, for example, it may not relate to infants and children who have decreased digestive capacity.

The initial *in vitro* assays were adapted from the enzymatic-gravimetric method used for dietary fiber assessment, but could only measure RS_3. Soon new approaches to assess other types of resistant starch were developed. The Berry method, for instance, measures both RS_3 and RS_2 using an exhaustive incubation (16 h) of milled sample with α-amylase and pullulanase, following by centrifugation to separate the insoluble residue, which contains the resistant starch. This residue is treated with KOH to disperse retrograded and native starches, which are then hydrolyzed to glucose with amyloglucosidase. Finally, released glucose is quantified by a colorimetric assay. The Berry method has been subsequently modified by Faisant *et al.* and Goñi *et al.*: the pullulanase was eliminated from the enzyme mixture and a pretreatment with pepsin added to decrease starch-protein interactions (**Table 4**).

Other methods have been developed to assess all types of resistant starch. Indeed, the Englyst method was developed to assess all nutritionally important starch fractions, such as rapidly digestible and slowly digestible starches, along with the three types of resistant starches described above. In this method, resistant starch fractions are estimated altogether by difference between total and digestible starches. Sample preparation is kept to a minimum in an attempt to mimic the way food is consumed. After pretreatment with pepsin, the sample is incubated with a mixture of amyloglucosidase, invertase, and pancreatic enzymes for 2 h. Glucose released is then used to estimate the digestible starch. Next, total starch is measured as glucose released after solubilization of the nondigestible fractions with KOH, followed by amyloglucosidase hydrolysis. The Englyst method also allows evaluation of RS_1, RS_2, and RS_3. The main problem with this method is its low reproducibility, especially between laboratories, because of the technical difficulties involved. Two other methods include chewing by volunteer subjects as sample preparation. In the Muir method, for instance, the chewed sample is sequentially treated with pepsin and an amyloglucosidase–pancreatic amylase mixture to obtain the nondigestible fraction, which is then boiled with Termamyl (a thermostable α-amylase) and solubilized with dimethyl sulfoxide followed by another amyloglucosidase–pancreatic amylase mixture step to yield finally glucose. The Akerberg method is similar to the Muir method, but it includes other

Table 4 Comparison between different methods to measure resistant starch *in vitro*

Method	Sample				Treatment incubation	Types of RS measured[a]
	Preparation	Pretreatment	Treatment	Post-treatment		
Berry (1986)	Milling	None	Pancreatic α-amylase and pullulanase	KOH[b] Amyloglucosidase	Shaking for 16 h at 37 °C, pH 5.2	Sum of RS$_2$ and RS$_3$
Faisant *et al.* (1995)	Same as above	Same as above	Same as above, but without pullulanase	Same as above	Same as above, but pH 6.9	Same as above
Goñi *et al.* (1996)	Same as above	Pepsin	Same as above	Same as above	Same as above	Same as above
Englyst *et al.* (1992)	Minced or as eaten	Pepsin	Pancreatic α-amylase, amyloglucosidase, and invertase	Same as above	Shaking for 2 h at 37 °C, pH 5.2	RS$_1$, RS$_2$, RS$_3$, and total RS
Muir & O'Dea (1992)	Chewing	Salivary α-amylase then pepsin	Pancreatic α-amylase and amyloglucosidase	Thermostable α-amylase Dimethyl sulfoxide[b] Amyloglucosidase and pancreatic α-amylase	Stirring for 15 h at 37 °C, pH 5.0	Total RS
Akerberg *et al.* (1998)	Same as above	Same as above	Same as above	KOH[b] Thermostable α-amylase Amyloglucosidase	Stirring for 16 h at 40 °C, pH 5.0	Same as above
McCleary & Monaghan (2002)	Milling	None	Same as above	KOH[b] Amyloglucosidase	Shaking for 16 h at 37 °C, pH 6.0	Sum of RS$_2$ and RS$_3$

[a]RS, resistant starch; RS$_1$, physically inaccessible starch; RS$_2$, resistant granules; RS$_3$, retrograded starch.
[b]KOH and dimethyl sulfoxide are used as resistant starch solubilizing agents.

steps that permit the estimation of available starch and dietary fiber along with resistant starch (**Table 4**).

Recently, the most commonly used *in vitro* methods were extensively evaluated and a simplified version was proposed (McCleary method). Here, samples are treated with an amyloglucosidase–pancreatic amylase mixture only and the insoluble residue, after washing with ethanol, is dispersed with KOH, followed by the amyloglucosidase step to yield glucose. This protocol has been accepted by AOAC International (AOAC method 2002.02) and the American Association of Cereal Chemists (AACC method 32-40) (**Table 4**).

Regarding the quantification of the resistant fractions in modified starches, care must be taken because some nondigestible fractions are soluble in water and they can be lost during washing steps. This is particularly important with pregelatinized starches and pyrodextrins. One suitable way to look at the impact of the modification on the starch availability is measure total starch before and after the modification.

Dietary Intake

It is very difficult to assess resistant starch intake at present, because there are not enough data on the resistant starch content of foods. In addition, as the resistance of the starch to digestion depends on the method of cooking and the temperature of the food as eaten, the values gained from looking at old dietary intake data may be misleading. Despite this, an average value for resistant starch intake across Europe has been estimated as $4.1\,g\,day^{-1}$. Figures comparable with this estimation have been made in other countries, for instance, Venezuela ($4.3\,g\,day^{-1}$). It is very difficult to separate the benefits of slowly, but completely, digestible starches from those that are resistant. In some groups like small children, whose small intestinal digestive capacity is reduced, the very same food may provide more starch that is resistant to digestion than it would in normal adults.

Quantification of modified starch intake is even more difficult. First, food labels do not usually provide information about the nature of the modification used. Second, the commonly used method to estimate resistant starch can underestimate any nondigestible fractions that became soluble in water because of the modification. At present, there is no data available on how much modified starch is eaten.

Fermentation in the Colon

The main nutritional properties of resistant starch arise from its potential fermentation in the colon. The diverse and numerous colonic microflora ferments unabsorbed carbohydrates to short-chain fatty acids (SCFA), mainly acetate, propionate and butyrate, and gases (H_2, CO_2, and CH_4). Acetate is the main SCFA produced (50–70%) and is the only one to reach peripheral circulation in significant amounts, providing energy for muscle and other tissues. Propionate is the second most abundant SCFA and is mainly metabolized by the liver, where its carbons are used to produce glucose (via gluconeogenesis). Propionate has also been associated with reduced cholesterol and lipid synthesis. Finally, butyrate is mainly used as fuel by the colonic enterocytes, but has been shown *in vitro* to have many potential anticancer actions, such as stimulating apoptosis (i.e., programed cell death) and cancer cell differentiation (i.e., increasing expression of normal cell function), and inhibiting histone deacetylation (this protects the DNA). Resistant starch fermentation has been shown to increase the molar proportion of butyrate in the colon.

The main physiological effects of digestion and fermentation of resistant starch are summarized in **Table 5**. However, most of these effects have

Table 5 Physiological effects of resistant starch intake

Energy	$8{-}13\,kJ\,g^{-1}$; cf. $17\,kJ\,g^{-1}$ for digestible starches
Glycemic and insulinemic response	Depends on food, e.g., legumes (high in RS_1) and amylose-rich starchy foods (which tend to produce RS_3 on cooking) increase glucose tolerance, but cornflakes and cooked potatoes, both with high and similar glycemic indexes, have different resistant starch content
Lipid metabolism	Decreases plasma cholesterol and triacylglyceride levels in rat, but not in humans
Fermentability	Complete, although some RS_3 are more resistant
SCFA production	Increased production, especially butyrate
CO_2 and H_2 production	Occurs
Colonic pH	Decreased, especially by lactate production
Bile salts	Deoxycholate, a secondary bile salt with cytotoxic activity, precipitated due to the low pH
Colon cell proliferation	Stimulated in proximal colon, but repressed in distal colon; may be mediated by butyrate
Fecal excretion	At high dose, fecal bulk increases due to an increase in bacteria mass and water retention
Transit time	Increased intestinal transit at high dose
Nitrogen metabolism	Increased bacterial nitrogen and biomass
Minerals	May increase calcium and magnesium absorption in large intestine
Disease prevention	Epidemiological studies suggest prevention against colorectal cancer and constipation

been observed with a resistant starch intake of around $20–30 \,\mathrm{g\,day^{-1}}$, which represents from 5 to 7 times the estimated intake for the European population.

Oligosaccharides

Definition and Classification

Oligosaccharides are carbohydrate chains containing 3–10 sugar units. However, some authors also include carbohydrates with up to 20 residues or even disaccharides. Oligosaccharides can be made of any sugar monomers, but most research has been carried out on fructooligosaccharides (e.g., oligofructose) and galactooligosaccharides (e.g., raffinose, human milk oligosaccharides). Few oligosaccharides are hydrolyzed and absorbed in the small intestine (e.g., maltotriose), but nearly all enter the colon intact (nondigestible oligosaccharides). **Table 6** shows several examples of oligosaccharides (and disaccharides, for comparison purposes), their chemical structure, and source.

Dietary Sources and Intake

The first source of oligosaccharides in the human diet is mother's milk, which contains approximately $12 \,\mathrm{g\,l^{-1}}$. In human breast milk, there are over 100 different oligosaccharides with both simple and complex structures. They are composed of galactose, fucose, sialic acid, glucose, and N-acetylglucosamine. Most are of low molecular weight, but a small proportion are of high molecular weight. Ninety per cent of breast milk oligosaccharides are neutral; the remainder are acidic. Interestingly, the nature of these oligosaccharide structures is determined by the mother's blood group. These oligosaccharides may have

Table 6 Chemical structure and source of sugars and oligosaccharides

Common name	Simplified structure[a]	Source	NDO[b]
Sugars (disaccharides)			
Lactose	Galβ1 → 4Glc	Milk, milk products	No
Maltose	Glcα1 → 4Glc	Glucose syrups, hydrolysis of starch	No
Sucrose	Fruβ2 → 1Glc	Table sugar	No
Cellobiose	Glcβ1 → 4Glc	Hydrolysis of cellulose	Yes
Trehalose	Glcα1 → 1Glc	Mushrooms, yeast	No
Melibiose	Galα1 → 6Glc	Hydrolysis of raffinose	Yes
Gentiobiose	Glcβ1 → 6Glcβ	Plant pigments, like saffron	Yes
Trisaccharides			
Maltotriose	Glcα1 → 4Glcα1 → 4Glc	Glucose syrups, hydrolysis of starch	No
Umbelliferose	Galα1 → 2Glcα1 → 2Fruβ	Plant tissues	Yes
Raffinose	Galα1 → 6Glcα1 → 2Fruβ	Legume seeds	Yes
Planteose	Galα1 → 6Fruβ2 → 1Glc	Plant tissues	Yes
Sialylα(2–3)lactose	NeuAcα2 → 3Galβ1 → 4Glc	Human milk	Yes
Tetrasaccharides			
Stachyose	Galα1 → 6Galα1 → 6Glcα1 → 2Fruβ	Legume seeds	Yes
Lychnose	Galα1 → 6Glcα1 → 2Fruβ1 → 1Gal	Plant tissues	Yes
Isolychnose	Galα1 → 6Glcα1 → 2Fruβ3 → 1Gal	Plant tissues	Yes
Sesamose	Galα1 → 6Galα1 → 6Fruβ2 → 1Glc	Plant tissues	Yes
Pentasaccharides			
Verbacose	Galα1 → 6Galα1 → 6Galα1 → 6Glcα1 → 2Fruβ	Plant tissues	Yes
Lacto-N-fucopentaose I	Fucα1 → 2Galβ1 → 3GlcNAcβ1 → 3Galβ1 → 4Glc	Human milk	Yes
Lacto-N-fucopentaose II	Galβ1 → 3[Fucα1 → 4]GlcNAcβ1 → 3Galβ1 → 4Glc	Human milk	Yes
Fructans			
Oligofructose	[Fruβ2 → 1]Fruβ2 → 1Glc with 1–9 [Fruβ2 → 1] residues	Hydrolysis of inulin or synthesis from sucrose	Yes
Inulin (polysaccharide)	[Fruβ2 → 1]Fruβ2 → 1Glc with 10–64 [Fruβ2 → 1] residues	Artichokes	Yes

[a]Fru, D-fructose; Fuc, L-fucose; Gal, D-galactose; Glc, D-glucose; GlcNAc, N-acetylglucosamine; NeuAc, N-acetylneuraminic acid (or sialic acid).
[b]NDO, nondigestible oligosaccharides.

important function in the small intestine, where they can bind to the mucosa or to bacteria, interfering with pathogenic bacterial attachment and thus acting as anti-infective agents. As they are nondigestible, they enter the colon and may act as a major energy for the colonic microflora and promote the growth of typical lactic acid bacteria that are characteristic of the normal breast-fed infant. More recently, oligosaccharides have been added to some infant formulas to mimic the actions of those in human milk. Recently, several studies have shown that these promote the growth of bifidobacteria in feces and make the stools more like those of breast-fed infants in terms of consistency, frequency, and pH.

In adults, the main dietary sources of oligosaccharides are chicory, artichokes, onions, garlic, leeks, bananas, and wheat. However, much research has been carried out on purified or synthetic oligosaccharide mixtures, mostly fructooligosaccharides derived from inulin. The normal dietary intake of oligosaccharides is difficult to estimate, as they are not a major dietary component. Around $3 \, \mathrm{g \, day}^{-1}$ has been suggested in the European diet. However, with the increasing information on the health benefits of isolated oligosaccharide sources (see below) they are being incorporated into functional foods.

Analysis

In general, oligosaccharides are a less heterogeneous group of compounds than resistant starches. Almost all nondigestible oligosaccharides (some fructooligosaccharides are an exception) are soluble in 80% (v/v) ethanol solution, which makes them relatively easy to isolate from insoluble components. Liquid chromatography, more specifically high-performance anion exchange chromatography (HPAEC), has been extensively employed not only to separate mixtures of different oligosaccharides, but also to separate, identify, and quantify individual carbohydrate moieties after appropriate hydrolysis of the oligosaccharide to its individual monomers. A more comprehensive study of the oligosaccharide structure can be achieved using more sophisticated techniques, like nuclear magnetic resonance and mass spectrometry. However, from a nutritional viewpoint, where simpler methods are needed for quality control and labeling purposes, HPAEC is usually applied to quantify the monomers (and dimers) present before and after hydrolysis of the studied oligosaccharide with appropriate enzymes and then the oligosaccharide level is worked out by difference.

Fermentation in the Colon and Health Benefits

Most oligosaccharides escape digestion in the small intestine and are fermented by the colonic bacteria. They are rapidly fermented resulting in a low pH and have been shown to increase the survival of so-called probiotic organisms, i.e., lactobacilli and bifidobacteria. Probiotic bacteria have been show to have strain-specific effects, including reduction in duration of rotavirus and other infective diarrhea and reduction in symptoms of atopic eczema. They may also have some anticarcinogenic effects, but these have not been demonstrated in human *in vivo* studies. This action of oligosaccharides to promote the growth of bifidobacteria and lactobacilli defines them as prebiotics. Some studies are now investigating the synergistic effects of probiotics mixed with prebiotics. These mixtures are termed synbiotics. In addition to these actions, some oligosaccharides have similar health benefits to fermentable dietary fiber and resistant starch by increasing colonic fermentation, production of SCFA (especially butyrate), and reduction in colonic pH.

Resistant Starch, Oligosaccharides, or Just Dietary Fiber?

There has been much debate of the definition of dietary fiber and in particular whether it should include carbohydrates other than nonstarch polysaccharides. Recently, the American Association of Cereal Chemists (AACC) proposed a new definition of dietary fiber, which would include both oligosaccharides and resistant starch as well as associated plant substances. This new definition would also require complete or partial fermentation and demonstration of physiological effects such as laxation, and reduction in blood glucose or blood cholesterol. A similar approach to include beneficial physiological effects is also proposed by the Food and Nutrition Board of the US Institute of Medicine.

Thus, it is being increasingly recognized that oligosaccharides, resistant starch, and nonstarch polysaccharides are very similar especially in their effects on gut physiology and colonic fermentation. A comparison of their actions is summarized in **Table 7**. This inclusion of resistant starch and oligosaccharides in the definition of dietary fiber could have major implications for food labeling.

Table 7 The physiological effects of resistant starch, oligosaccharides, and dietary fiber

Physiological effect	Resistant starch	Oligosaccharides	Dietary fiber
Energy supply	$8-13\,kJ\,g^{-1}$	$8-13\,kJ\,g^{-1}$	$8-13\,kJ\,g^{-1}$
Increased glucose tolerance	Some foods	No	Some NSP[a]
Decreased plasma cholesterol and triacylglyceride levels	No	Not known	Some NSP
Fermentability	Complete	Complete	Variable
Production of SCFA	Yes	Yes	Yes
Increased butyrate production	High	High	Variable
CO_2 and H_2 production	Yes	Yes	Variable
Decreased fecal pH	Yes	Yes	Some NSP
Decreased production of deoxycholate	Yes	Yes	Some NSP
Increased colonocyte proliferation	Yes	Yes	Yes
Increased fecal bulk	At high dose	No	Variable
Faster whole gut transit time	At high dose	No	Yes
Increased bacterial nitrogen and biomass	Yes	Yes	Yes
Reduced mineral absorption in small intestine	No	No	Some NSP
Increased mineral absorption in large intestine	Yes	Yes	Some NSP
Possible prevention of colorectal cancer	Yes	Not known	Yes

[a]NSP, nonstarch polysaccharide.

See also: **Breast Feeding. Cereal Grains. Colon**: Structure and Function. **Dietary Fiber**: Physiological Effects and Effects on Absorption; Potential Role in Etiology of Disease; Role in Nutritional Management of Disease. **Legumes. Microbiota of the Intestine**: Prebiotics.

Further Reading

Blaut M (2002) Relationship of prebiotics and food to intestinal microflora. *European Journal of Nutrition* **41**(supplement 1): i11–i16.

Bornet FRJ, Brouns F, Tashiro Y, and Duvillier V (2002) Nutritional aspects of short-chain fructooligosaccharides: natural occurrence, chemistry, physiology and health implications. *Digestive and Liver Disease* **34**(supplement 2): S111–S120.

Champ M, Langkilde A-M, Brouns F, Kettlitz B, and Collet YL (2003) Advances in dietary fibre characterisation. 1. Definition of dietary fibre, physiological relevance, health benefits and analytical aspects. *Nutrition Research Reviews* **16**: 71–82.

Delzenne NM (2003) Oligosaccharides: state of the art. *Proceedings of the Nutrition Society* **62**: 177–182.

DeVries JW (2003) On defining dietary fibre. *Proceedings of the Nutrition Society* **62**: 37–43.

Ghisolfi J (2003) Dietary fibre and prebiotics in infant formula. *Proceedings of the Nutrition Society* **62**: 183–185.

Greger JL (1999) Non-digestible carbohydrates and mineral bioavailability. *Journal of Nutrition* **129**(supplement S): 1434S–1435S.

Kunz C, Rudloff S, Baier W, Klein N, and Strobel S (2000) Oligosaccharides in human milk: Structural, functional, and metabolic aspects. *Annual Review of Nutrition* **20**: 699–722.

McCleary BV (2003) Dietary fibre analysis. *Proceedings of the Nutrition Society* **62**: 3–9.

Roberfroid M (2002) Functional food concept and its application to prebiotics. *Digestive and Liver Disease* **34**(supplement 2): S105–S110.

Roberfroid MB (2003) Inulin and oligofructose are dietary fibres and functional food ingredients. In: Kritchevsky D, Bonfield CT, and Edwards CA (eds.) *Dietary Fiber in Health and Disease: 6th Vahouny Symposium*, pp. 161–163. Delray Beach, FL: Vahouny Symposium.

Topping DL, Fukushima M, and Bird AR (2003) Resistant starch as a prebiotic and synbiotic: state of the art. *Proceedings of the Nutrition Society* **62**: 171–176.

Carcinogens *see* **Cancer**: Carcinogenic Substances in Food

CAROTENOIDS

Contents

Chemistry, Sources and Physiology

B K Ishida and G E Bartley, Agricultural Research Service, Albany, CA, USA

Published by Elsevier Ltd.

Chemistry

Structure

Most carotenoids are 40-carbon isoprenoid compounds called tetraterpenes. Isoprenoids are formed from the basic five-carbon building block, isoprene (**Figure 1**). In nature, carotenoids are synthesized through the stepwise addition of isopentenyl diphosphate (IPP) units to dimethylallyl diphosphate (DMAPP) to form the 20-carbon precursor geranylgeranyl diphosphate (GGPP). Two molecules of GGPP are combined to form the first carotenoid in the biosynthetic pathway, phytoene, which is then desaturated, producing 11 conjugated double bonds to form lycopene, the red pigment in ripe tomato fruit (**Figure 1**). Nearly all other carotenoids can be derived from lycopene. Lycopene can be cyclized on either or both ends to form α- or β-carotene, and these in turn can be oxygenated to form xanthophylls such as β-cryptoxanthin, zeaxanthin, or lutein (**Figure 1** and **Figure 2**). Carotenoids having fewer than 40 carbons can result from loss of carbons within the chain (norcarotenoids) or loss of carbons from the end of the molecule (apocarotenoids). Longer carotenoids, homocarotenoids (C45–C50), are found in some bacterial species. The alternating double bonds along the backbone of carotenoid molecules form a polyene chain, which imparts unique qualities to this group of compounds. This alternation of single and double bonds also allows a number of geometrical isomers to exist for each carotenoid (**Figure 1**). For lycopene, the theoretical number of steric forms is 1056; however, when steric hindrance is considered, that number is reduced to 72. In nature most carotenoids are found in the all-*trans* form although mutants are known in plants, e.g., *Lycopersicon esculentum* (Mill.) var. Tangerine tomato, and eukaryotic algae that produce poly-*cis* forms of carotenoids. The mutant plant is missing an enzyme, carotenoid isomerase (CRTISO), which catalyzes the isomerization of the *cis* isomers of lycopene and its precursors to the all-*trans* form during biosynthesis. Light can also cause *cis* to *trans* isomerization of these carotenoids depending upon the surrounding environment. The isomeric form determines the shape of the molecule and can thus change the properties of the carotenoid affecting solubility and absorbability. *Trans* forms of carotenoids are more rigid and have a greater tendency to crystallize or aggregate than the *cis* forms. Therefore, *Cis* forms may be more easily absorbed and transported. End groups such as the β or ε rings of α-carotene and β-carotene and the amount of oxygenation will also affect carotenoid properties.

Chemical Properties

In general, carotenoids are hydrophobic molecules and thus are soluble only in organic solvents, having only limited solubility in water. Addition of hydroxyl groups to the end groups causes the carotenoid to become more polar, affecting its solubility in various organic solvents. Alternatively, carotenoids can solubilize in aqueous environments by prior integration into liposomes or into cyclic oligosaccharides such as cyclodextrins.

In general, carotenoid molecules are very sensitive to elevated temperatures and the presence of acid, oxygen, and light when in solution, and are subject to oxidative degradation.

Electronic Properties

What sets carotenoids apart from other molecules and gives them their electrochemical properties is the conjugated double bond system. In this alternating double and single bond system, the π-electrons are delocalized over the length of the polyene chain. This polyene chain or chromophore imparts the characteristic electronic spectra and photophysical and photochemical properties to this group of molecules. The highly delocalized π-electrons require little energy to reach an excited state so that light energy can cause a transition. The length of the conjugated polyene or

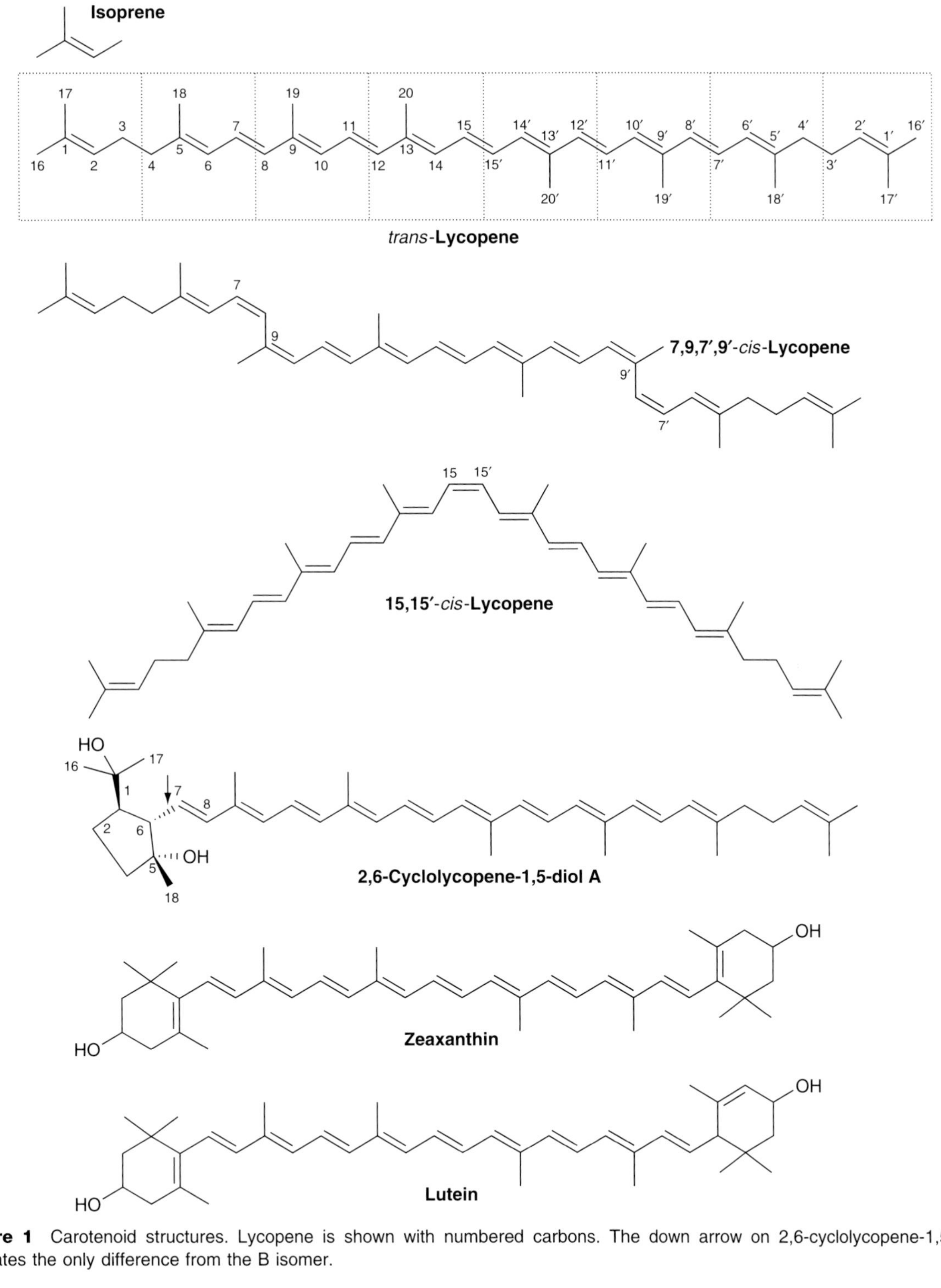

Figure 1 Carotenoid structures. Lycopene is shown with numbered carbons. The down arrow on 2,6-cyclolycopene-1,5-diol A indicates the only difference from the B isomer.

chromophore affects the amount of energy needed to excite the π-electrons. The longer the conjugated system, the easier it is to excite, so longer wavelengths of light can be absorbed. The result is that phytoene, having three conjugated double bonds is colorless, and phytofluene, having five, is colorless, but fluoresces green under UV light.

Zeta-carotene has seven, absorbs light at ~400 nm and appears yellow, while neurosporene has nine, absorbs light at ~451, and appears orange, and lycopene has eleven conjugated double bonds, absorbs at ~472, and appears red. The polyene chain also allows transfer of singlet or triplet energy.

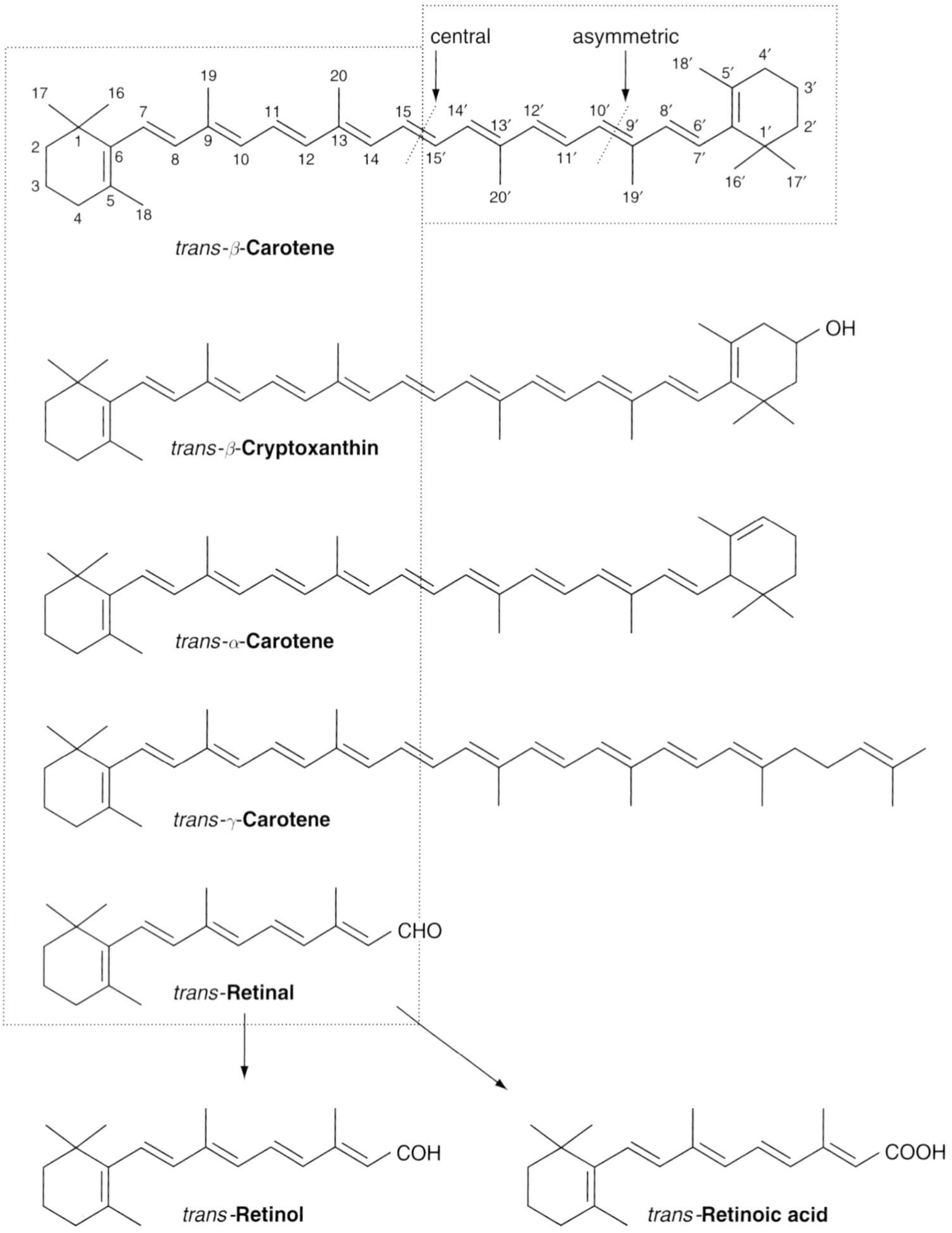

Figure 2 Provitamin A carotenoids. Dotted lines indicate the provitamin A moiety.

Reactions

Light and Chemical Energy

The basic energy-transfer reactions are assumed to be similar in plants and animals, even though environments differ. Excess light can cause excitation of porphyrin molecules (porphyrin triplets). These triplet-state porphyrin molecules can transfer their energy to oxygen-forming singlet oxygen, $^1O_2$. Singlet oxygen can damage DNA and cause lipid peroxidation, thereby killing the cell. Carotenoids, having nine or more conjugated double bonds, can prevent damage by singlet oxygen through: (1) transfer of

triplet energy from the excited porphyrin to the carotenoid, forming a carotenoid triplet, which would be too low in energy for further transfer and would simply dissipate as heat; or (2) singlet oxygen energy could transfer to the carotenoid, also forming a triplet carotenoid, dissipating heat, and returning to the ground state. This ability to quench sensitized triplets has been useful in treating protoporphyria (PP) and congenital erythropoietic porphyria (CEP) in humans. Porphyrias are disorders resulting from a defect in heme biosynthesis. Precursor porphyrins accumulate and can be sensitized to the singlet state and drop to the lower triplet state. The triplet state is longer-lived and thus more likely to react with other molecules such as oxygen to form singlet oxygen, which can cause cellular damage. Because β-carotene can transfer and dissipate either sensitized triplet or singlet oxygen energy it has been used to treat these disorders.

Light absorption and possibly scavenging of destructive oxygen species by the xanthophylls lutein and zeaxanthin are also important in the macula of the primate eye. Lutein and two isomers of zeaxanthin are selectively accumulated in the macula, creating a yellow area of the retina responsible for high visual acuity (smaller amounts are also found in the lens). Both carotenoids absorb light of about 450 nm 'blue light,' thus filtering light to the light receptors behind the carotenoid layer in the macula. Filtering blue light can reduce oxidative stress to retinal light receptors and chromatic aberration resulting from the refraction of blue light. A similar filter effect may occur in the lens, but the concentration of the xanthophylls is much lower, and further protection occurs with age when the lens yellows. Whether scavenging of destructive oxygen species by these carotenoids is useful here is unproven, but the retina is an area of higher blood flow and light exposure than other tissues.

Cleavage to Vitamin A

Provitamin A carotenoids are sources of vitamin A. Of the 50–60 carotenoids having provitamin A activity, β-carotene, β-cryptoxanthin, and α-carotene are the major sources of vitamin A nutrition in humans, β-carotene being the most important (**Figure 2**). Vitamin A (retinol) and its derivatives retinal and retinoic acid perform vital functions in the vertebrate body. Retinal (11-*cis* retinal) combined with opsin functions in the visual system in signal transduction of light reception. Retinol and retinoic acid function in reproduction (spermatogenesis), growth regulation (general development and limb morphogenesis), and cell differentiation. Provitamin A activity requires at least one unsubstituted β-ionone ring, the correct number and orientation of methyl groups along the polyene backbone, and the correct number of conjugated double bonds, preferably in the *trans*-isomer orientation. Two pathways for the formation of retinal from β-carotene have been proposed. First, central cleavage by which β-carotene 15,15'-mono- or dioxygenase catalyzes β-carotene cleavage to form two molecules of retinal, which can then be converted to retinol or retinoic acid (**Figure 2**). Some debate on the mechanism of the β-carotene central cleavage enzyme still exists, but evidence leans towards activity as a monooxygenase, not a dioxygenase. Alternatively, in

the eccentric cleavage pathway β-carotene can be cleaved at any of the double bonds along the polyene backbone (other than the 15-15'double bond). Products of these reactions (apocarotenals) are then further metabolized to retinoic acid and retinol. An asymmetric cleavage enzyme has recently been cloned that cleaves β-carotene at the 9'-10'-double bond to form β-ionone and β-apo-10'-carotenal. The discovery of this enzyme indicates at least some eccentric cleavage occurs in vertebrates. This eccentric cleavage process has been proposed to occur during more oxidative conditions, while central cleavage would predominate under normal physiological conditions. Central cleavage is considered to be the major pathway because of the scarcity of eccentric cleavage products detected *in vivo*.

Radical Reactions

Excess amounts of radicals, molecules having unpaired electrons, e.g., peroxyls (ROO·), can be created in tissues exogenously, e.g., by light exposure, or endogenously, e.g., by overexercising. Radicals react with lipids, proteins, and DNA causing damage, which possibly contributes to disease symptoms and aging. The special properties of the polyene chain make carotenoids susceptible to electrophilic attack, resulting in formation of resonance-stabilized radicals that are less reactive.

Three possible reactions can occur with carotenoids.

1. Adduct formation $(CAR + R^{\cdot} \rightarrow R\text{-}CAR^{\cdot})$; these products should be stable because of resonance in the polyene structure. If the radical were a lipid peroxyl, this reaction $(CAR + ROO^{\cdot} \rightarrow ROO\text{-}CAR^{\cdot})$ would prevent further propagation (chain-breaking).
2. Hydrogen atom abstraction $(CAR + R^{\cdot} \rightarrow CAR^{\cdot} + RH)$, where a hydrogen atom is taken from the carotenoid allylic to the polyene chain, leaving a resonance-stabilized carotenoid radical.
3. Electron transfer $(CAR + R^{\cdot} \rightarrow CAR^{\cdot +} + R^{-})$, which has been reported in plant and cyanobacterial photosystems using laser flash photolysis of Photosystem II.

In many cases, the products formed are colorless, thus revealing the bleaching effect of many oxidants on carotenoids. Further oxidation of the carotenoid or carotenoid radical can occur as in studies of soybean (*Glycine max*) and recombinant pea (*Pisum sativum*) lipoxygenase-mediated cooxidation of carotenoids and polyunsaturated fatty acids. Approximately 50 breakdown products of β-carotene were detected. This large number of products seems to indicate a random attack along the polyene chain of β-carotene by a linoleoylperoxyl radical. Studies using potassium permanganate, a metalloporphyrin (a P450 enzyme center mimic), and autooxidation have been performed with lycopene, resulting in formation of a number of apo-lycopenals and apo-lycopenones. However, only two metabolites of lycopene have been identified in human plasma, 2,6-cyclolycopene-1,5 diols A and B (**Figure 1**). Additionally, seven metabolites of the carotenoids lutein and zeaxanthin have been detected in human tissues.

Prooxidant Behavior

The ability to quench singlet oxygen, porphyrin triplet energies, and free radical reactions are examples of the antioxidant nature of carotenoids. An *in vitro* study showed that, at low partial pressures of oxygen (pO_2), β-carotene consumed peroxy radicals efficiently as in: $CAR + ROO^{\cdot} \rightarrow CAR^{\cdot+} + ROO^-$. At higher pO_2, however, β-carotene became a prooxidant through autooxidation. Recently, experiments in intact murine normal and tumor thymocytes showed that β-carotene lost its antioxidant potency at higher pO_2, and the effect was more pronounced in tumor cells. It is still unclear, however, whether some effects of carotenoid behavior at higher pO_2 are due to prooxidant activity or simply lack of antioxidant ability. Prooxidant effects of β-carotene have also been used to explain results from intervention trials of β-carotene supplementation in diets of smokers or individuals suffering from asbestosis where the incidence of carcinogenesis was higher in those individuals taking the β-carotene supplement. Generation of deleterious oxidation products from β-carotene reaction with reactive oxygen species in tobacco smoke or as a result of asbestosis has been proposed. Interference with retinoid signaling was also considered. However, whether those effects were due to prooxidant behavior or lack of antioxidant ability is still unclear.

Dietary Sources

Carotenoids cannot be synthesized by humans; therefore they must be obtained from dietary sources. These are primarily highly pigmented red, orange, and yellow fruits and vegetables. The carotenoid lycopene is red; however, not all red fruits and vegetables contain lycopene. For example, the red in strawberries, apples, and cherries is a result of their anthocyanin content; whereas, tomatoes, watermelon, and pink grapefruit derive their red color from lycopene. The carotenoids β-carotene, β-cryptoxanthin, lutein, zeaxanthin, and violaxanthin are yellow to orange, and phytoene and phytofluene are colorless. Green, leafy vegetables

also contain carotenoids, whose colors are masked by the green color of chlorophyll. **Table 1** lists carotenoids found in fruits and vegetables. Smaller amounts are also available from animal sources

Table 1 Carotenoid content (μg per g fresh weight) of fresh fruit and vegetables

Carotenoid	Concentration (μg per g fresh weight)	Source
Lycopene	380–3054	Gac (*Momordica cochinchinensis*, Spreng) aril
	179–483	Autumn olive (*Elaeagnus umbellate*)
	27–200	Tomato
	23–72	Watermelon
	53	Guava
	19–40	Papaya
	8–33	Grapefruit, pink
β-Carotene	101–770	Gac aril
	49–257	Carrot, orange
	16–216	Cantaloupe
	15–92	Kale
	0.5–92	Sweet potato
	47–89	Spinach
	46	Turnip greens
	26–64	Apricot
	22–58	Gac mesocarp
	3–70	Tomato
	42	Squash, butternut
	40	Swiss chard
	14–34	Mango
	33	Collards
	4–10	Grapefruit, pink
	0.51–1.2*	Orange (*blood)
Lutein	64–150	Kale
	6–129	Mango
	108	Parsley
	39–95	Spinach
	33–51	Collards
	15–28	Broccoli
	27	Chinese cabbage
	26	Watercress
	25	Pepper, orange
	24	Squash, butternut
	1–7	Tomato
Zeaxanthin	16–85	Pepper, orange
	43	Gou Qi Zi (*Lycium barabarum*)
	9	Gac aril
	22	Pepper, red
	7	Watercress
	1–5	Spinach
	5	Parsley
	5	Japanese persimmon
	1–3	Kale
	3	Squash, butternut
	0.4	Broccoli
	0.03–0.5	Tomato

Continued

Table 1 Continued

Carotenoid	Concentration (µg per g fresh weight)	Source
Lutein + zeaxanthin	71–3956	Kale
	119	Spinach
	84	Turnip greens
	26	Lettuce
	24	Broccoli
	21	Squash, zucchini
	16	Brussel sprouts
	8	Japanese persimmon
	7	Watercress
	6	Beans, green snap
	5	Tangerine
β-Cryptoxanthin	22	Pepper, sweet red
	14	Japanese persimmon
	11	Starfruit
	0.7–9	Pepper, chili
	2–8	Pepper, orange
	0.5–5	Tangerine
	4	Cilantro
	1.4	Papaya
	1	Watermelon
α-Carotene	20–206	Carrot
	8	Squash, butternut
	2	Collards
	1	Tomato
	0.7–0.9	Beans, green snap
	0.5	Swiss chard

such as ocean fish and dairy products. The pink color of salmon, for example, is derived from the xanthophylls, astaxanthin and canthaxanthin, which they obtain from eating small crustaceans and krill. Lutein imparts its yellow-orange color to eggs, and milk, butter, and cheese contain retinols and β-carotene. Carotenoids, such as lutein from marigolds and bixin (red color) from annatto, are also used widely as colorants in processed foods to make them more attractive.

Concentrations of carotenoids in fruit and vegetable sources vary, resulting from differences in conditions under which they are grown (temperature, amount of sunlight, degrees of stress from extremes in climate such as drought, heat, and cold), genotype, and maturity or ripeness. The carotenoid content in animal sources depends upon amounts contained in animal feeds and seasons of the year, which affect the availability of carotenoid-containing plants eaten by grazing animals.

Human diets and tissues contain six carotenoids in significant amounts (listed in **Table 1**). Lycopene is typically the carotenoid consumed in greatest amounts in Western diets. Per capita intakes in Europe and North America average from 1.6 to more

than 18 mg lycopene per day. More than 85% of the lycopene in North American diets comes from tomato products, which also contain significant amounts of other carotenoids (α- and β-carotene and lutein/zeaxanthin), as well as vitamins C, A, and E, and potassium and folic acid. (Flavonoids are also found in tomato skin; thus, cherry tomatoes contain higher concentrations.) In the US, the annual per capita consumption of tomatoes by 1999 averaged about 17.6 pounds of fresh and 72.8 pounds of processed tomatoes.

Effects of Storage and Processing

Carotenoids are susceptible to oxidative degradation and isomerization resulting from storage and processing conditions. These reactions result in both loss of color and biological activity and formation of often unpleasant volatile compounds. Degradation occurs upon exposure to oxygen and is accelerated by the presence of substances such as metals, enzymes, unsaturated lipids, and prooxidants; exposure to light; and conditions that destroy cell wall and ultrastructural integrity. Heating can promote isomerization of the naturally occurring all-*trans* to various *cis* isomers. This process then affects bioavailability of the carotenoid. Processing also affects bioavailability by macerating tissues, destroying or weakening cell ultrastructure, denaturing or weakening complexes with proteins, and cleaving ester linkages, thereby releasing carotenoids from the food matrix.

Processed foods are frequently fortified with carotenoids to increase nutritive value and/or enhance attractiveness. For example, annatto, an extract from the seeds of the *Bixa orella* tree, containing the carotenoids bixin and norbixin, is added to butter, margarine, and processed cheese to give a yellow-orange color to these products. Tomato oleoresin is added to processed tomato products, increasing lycopene content while enhancing their attractive red color.

Physiology

Digestion

Numerous factors affect the intestinal absorption of carotenoids. Digestion of food in the stomach increases accessibility of carotenoids for absorption by maceration in HCl and digestive enzymes. The acidic environment of the stomach helps to disrupt cell walls and other cellular ultrastructure of raw fruits and vegetables and causes further breakdown of cooked foods to release carotenoids from food matrices in which they are contained or bound.

Carotenoids in green leafy vegetables are found in chloroplasts; those in fruit are located in chromoplasts. Absorption studies comparing plasma levels of β-carotene and retinol after consuming fruit vs. green leafy vegetables showed that β-carotene is more efficiently absorbed from fruit, indicating that chloroplasts (or the bonds linking chloroplast proteins and carotenoids) are more resistant to disruption in the digestive tract than chromoplasts. Thus, the location of a carotenoid in the cell affects its accessibility.

Carotenoid isomerization can occur in the acidic gastric milieu. Lycopene present in fruits and vegetables occurs almost exclusively as the all-*trans* isomer, but is converted to *cis* isomers, which seem to be more bioavailable. Plasma and tissue profiles show that *cis* isomers make up more than 50% of the total lycopene present. On the other hand, studies show that no *trans/cis* isomerization of β-carotene occurs in the stomach. In fact, evidence has been found for transfer of a significant portion of both β- and α-carotene to the fat phase of the meal in the stomach, which would increase bioavailability of these carotenoids for absorption. No studies are available relating isomerization to bioavailability of other carotenoids.

Absorption and Transport

Because carotenoids are hydrophobic molecules, they are associated with lipophilic sites in cells, such as bilayer membranes. Polar substituents such as hydroxyl groups decrease their hydrophobicity and their orientation with respect to membranes. Lycopene and β-carotene are aligned parallel to membrane surfaces to maintain a hydrophobic environment, whereas the more polar xanthophylls lutein and zeaxanthin become oriented perpendicular to membrane surfaces to keep their hydroxyl groups in a more hydrophilic environment. These differences can affect the physical nature of a membrane as well as its function. Carotenoids can form complexes with proteins, which would aid them in moving through an aqueous environment. They can also interact with hydrophobic regions of lipoproteins. Carotenoproteins have been found mainly in plants and invertebrates, but intracellular β-carotene-binding proteins have been found in bovine liver and intestine and in livers of the rat and ferret. In addition, a xanthophyll-binding protein has been found in human retina and macula. Carotenoids are also present in nature as crystalline aggregates (lycopene in chromoplasts) or as fine dispersions in aqueous media (β-carotene in oranges).

In the intestinal lumen (**Figure 3**) where carotenoids are released from the food matrix, cleavage of carotenoproteins and fatty acid esters by carboxylic ester hydrolase, which is secreted by the pancreas, can occur. Carotenoids are then solubilized into lipid micelles. These hydrophobic compounds are thus more efficiently absorbed when accompanied by at least a small amount of fat. The amount of fat for optimal carotenoid absorption seems to differ among carotenoids. For example, lutein esters require more fat for optimal absorption than β-carotene. These differences have not been quantified for each carotenoid. In addition, the presence of a nonabsorbable, fat-soluble component was shown to decrease carotenoid absorption. Sucrose polyester, a nonabsorbable fat replacer decreased carotenoid

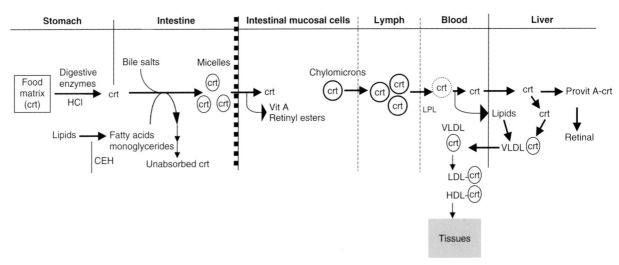

Figure 3 Factors affecting digestion, absorption, metabolism, and transport of carotenoids. crt, carotenoids; CEH, carboxylic ester hydrolase, secreted by the pancreas; LPL, lipoprotein lipase; VLDL, very low-density lipoprotein; LDL, low-density lipoprotein; HDL, high-density lipoprotein.

levels in plasma after ingestion by 20–120%. The extent of this inhibition depends upon the amount of nonabsorbable compound ingested, as well as the particular carotenoid under consideration. The mechanism for this inhibition is apparently similar to the action of fiber, i.e., sequestration. The type of fat that is ingested along with carotenoids will also affect carotenoid absorption. As macerated food passes into the intestinal lumen, carotenoids freed from the food matrix then become incorporated into micelles, consisting of free fatty acids, monoglycerides, phospholipids, and bile acids. Many other factors can affect intestinal absorption such as micelle size, phospholipid composition, solubilization of carotenoids into mixed micelles, and concentration of available bile salts, among others.

The presence of other carotenoids can affect the absorption of carotenoids into intestinal mucosal cells, since carotenoids can compete for absorption or facilitate the absorption of another. Data on carotenoid interactions are not clear. Human studies show that β-carotene decreases lutein absorption, while lutein has either no effect or a lowering effect on β-carotene absorption. Although not confirmed in humans, the inhibitory effect of lutein on β-carotene absorption might be partly attributed to the inhibition of the β-carotene cleavage enzyme by lutein shown in rats. Beta-carotene also seemed to lower absorption of canthaxanthin, whereas canthaxanthin did not inhibit β-carotene absorption. Studies showed that β-carotene increased lycopene absorption, although lycopene had no effect on β-carotene. Alpha-carotene and cryptoxanthin show high serum responses to dietary intake compared to lutein. In addition, cis isomers of lycopene seem to be more bioavailable than the all-trans, and selective intestinal absorption of all-trans β-carotene occurs, as well as conversion of the 9-cis isomer to all-trans β-carotene. It is clear, then, that selective absorption of carotenoids takes place into the intestinal mucosal cell.

Another complicating factor in the intestinal mucosal cell is the partial conversion of provitamin A carotenoids (β- and α-carotenes and cryptoxanthin) to vitamin A (primarily to retinyl esters). Therefore, in absorption studies these metabolic reactions must be accounted for in measuring intestinal transport. Nonprovitamin A carotenoids such as lycopene, lutein, and zeaxanthin are incorporated intact, although some cleavage can occur. Earlier studies on rats indicated that lycopene and β-carotene are absorbed by passive diffusion. However, recent evidence from the kinetics of β-carotene transport through Caco-2 cell monolayers indicates the involvement of a specific epithelial transporter that facilitates absorption.

In the intestinal mucosa, both carotenoids and retinyl esters are incorporated into chylomicrons and secreted into the lymph for transport to blood. In blood, lipoprotein lipase rapidly degrades the chylomicrons, and the liver sequesters the resulting carotenoid-containing fragments. The liver then secretes carotenoids back into the bloodstream in association with hepatic very low-density lipoproteins (VLDL). Most carotenoids in fasting plasma are carried by low-density lipoproteins (LDL) and high-density lipoproteins (HDL). Seventy-five per cent of the hydrocarbon carotenoids, e.g., lycopene and β-carotene, are associated with LDL, the rest is associated with HDL and, in smaller amounts, with VLDL. More polar carotenoids such as lutein and zeaxanthin are found equally distributed between HDL and LDL. After ingestion, carotenoids first appear in the bloodstream in chylomicrons, resulting from excretion from intestinal mucosal cells (4–8 h). HDL carotenoid levels peak in the circulation between 16 and 28 h; LDL carotenoid levels peak between 24 and 48 h. The bloodstream then transports carotenoids to different tissues (e.g., liver, prostate gland, fat, ocular macula) where they are sequestered by various mechanisms.

Distribution and Impact on Health

In general, carotenoid concentrations in serum reflect concentrations contained in the food that is ingested. Carotenoids have been found in various human organs and tissues. These include human liver, lung, breast, cervix, skin, and adipose and ocular tissues. The major storage organs are adipose tissue (probably because of its volume) and the liver. Tissues containing large amounts of LDL receptors seem to accumulate high levels of carotenoids, probably as a result of nonspecific uptake by lipoprotein carriers. Preferential uptake, however, is indicated in some cases. For example, unusually high concentrations of phytoene in the lung, ζ-carotene and phytofluene in breast tissue, lycopene in the prostate and colon, lycopene, β-carotene, and phytofluene in cervical tissue, and lutein and zeaxanthin in ocular tissues have been found.

The epidemiological findings that the ingestion of tomato and tomato products is strongly correlated with a reduced risk of several types of cancer, particularly prostate cancer, has stimulated a great deal of research on the protective effects of lycopene. Lycopene is the most efficient biological antioxidant. Hence, it has been assumed that it is this antioxidant activity that is responsible for the protection against prostate cancer. However, a recent study in which carcinogenesis was induced in rats using

N-methyl-N-nitrosourea showed that a diet containing whole tomato powder inhibited development of prostate cancer, but the same diet to which pure synthetic lycopene was added instead did not. These results indicate that lycopene alone was ineffective in reducing the incidence of prostate cancer. Therefore, either some other element in the tomato powder was the effective agent or the effect was obtained by lycopene working in concert with other tomato constituents. Obviously, more studies are required to determine which elements contained in tomato are responsible for the protective effect.

The finding that lutein and zeaxanthin are accumulated in the macula lutea of the eye has led to the hope that dietary supplementation might reduce the risk of age-related macular degeneration (AMD), which affects the central portion of the retina and is the most common cause of irreversible blindness in the Western world. Some studies have indicated benefits of diets supplemented with lutein and zeaxanthin from spinach in preventing AMD; others found no significant correlation between plasma levels of these carotenoids and reduced risk of AMD. Lutein, zeaxanthin, and a zeaxanthin stereoisomer 3R, 3′S(=meso)-zeaxanthin form the yellow pigment of the macula lutea. 3R, 3′S(=meso)-zeaxanthin is not found in either food or plasma in significant amounts. Also notable is that, in most food consumed in large quantities, the concentration of lutein is much greater than that of zeaxanthin (e.g., see **Table 1**, spinach, kale, broccoli, tomato). The yellow pigment of the macula is located in the center of the macula, covering the central fovea and overlapping the avascular zone. This location would allow the pigment to shield the photoreceptors from blue light. An environmental factor that seems to play a role in the development of age-related macular degeneration is ocular exposure to sunlight, in particular a history of exposure to blue light in the preceding 20 years. Light has been shown to induce oxidative damage in the presence of photosensitizers. Macular carotenoids are distributed in a pattern that is particularly advantageous. The two stereoisomers of zeaxanthin are concentrated in the central area and lutein in higher concentrations in the more peripheral regions. The lutein: zeaxanthin ratio in the center of the macula is about 0.8, in the peripheral regions about 2.4, but in plasma between 4 and 7. Therefore, the macula is able to concentrate lutein and zeaxanthin, change concentration ratios that are normally found in plasma, and invert the ratio to achieve higher zeaxanthin concentrations in the center of the macula lutea. The exact mechanism for this accumulation is not known; however, a specific membrane-associated, xanthophyll-binding protein was recently isolated from the human retina.

Carotenoids are believed to play a significant role in protecting skin from oxidative damage. *In vivo* measurements in humans of lycopene, β-, ζ-, γ-, and α-carotenes, lutein and zeaxanthin, phytoene, and phytofluene have shown that carotenoid concentrations are correlated with the presence or absence of skin cancer and precancerous lesions. Carotenoids are also believed to protect against several other types of cancer, cardiovascular diseases, and cataract formation and aid in immune function and gap-junction communication between cells, which is believed to be a protective mechanism related to their cancer-preventative activities.

Conclusions

Numerous studies indicate that carotenoids and their metabolites play a role in combating degradative reactions that are harmful to human health. Most of these functions seem to be related to their antioxidant nature and ability to dissipate energy from light and free radical-generating reactions. Obviously much research is still required to shed light onto mechanisms involved in these protective functions. Other fascinating roles in nature are also being discovered, for example, the signaling of apparent good health and consequently good potential parenting in birds by the red coloration of beaks, which seems to serve as an attractant to prospective mates.

See also: **Cancer**: Epidemiology and Associations Between Diet and Cancer. **Carotenoids**: Epidemiology of Health Effects. **Vitamin A**: Biochemistry and Physiological Role.

Further Reading

Borel P (2003) Factors affecting intestinal absorption of highly lipophilic food microconstituents (fat-soluble vitamins, carotenoids and phytosterols). *Clinical Chemistry and Laboratory Medicine* 41: 979–994.

Britton G (1995) Structure and properties of carotenoids in relation to function. *FASEB Journal* 9: 1551–1558.

Britton G, Liaaen-Jensen S, and Pfander H (eds.) (1995) *Carotenoids: Isolation and Analysis* vol. 1A and *Spectroscopy*, vol. 1B Basel, Boston, Berlin: Birkhåuser Verlag.

During A and Harrison EH (2004) Intestinal absorption and metabolism of carotenoids: insights from cell culture. *Archives of Biochemistry and Biophysics* 430: 77–78.

Frank HA, Young AJ, Britton G, and Cogdell RJ (1999) *The Photochemistry of Carotenoids*, (*Advances in Photosynthesis*, vol. 8). Dordrecht: Kluwer Academic Publishers.

Holden JM, Eldridge AL, Beecher GR, Buzzard IM, Bhagwat S, Davis CS, Douglass LW, Gebhardt S, Haytowitz D, and Schakel S (1999) Carotenoid content of U.S. foods: An update of the database. *Journal of Food Composition and Analysis* 12: 169–196.

Isler O (1971) *Carotenoids*. Basel: Birkhäuser-Verlag.

Khachik F, Carvalho L, Bernstein PS, Muir GJ, Zhao D-Y, and Katz NB (2002) Chemistry, distribution, and metabolism of tomato carotenoids and their impact on human health. *Experimental Biology and Medicine* 227: 845–851.

Krinsky NI, Mayne ST, and Sies H (eds.) (2004) *Carotenoids in Health and Disease* (Oxidative Stress and Disease Series vol. 15). New York: Marcel Dekker.

Rodriguez-Amaya B (1999) In *A Guide to Carotenoid Analysis in Foods*. Washington, DC: ILSI Press.

Schalch W (2001) Possible contribution of lutein and zeaxanthin, carotenoids of the macula lutea, to reducing the risk for age-related macular degeneration: a review. *HKJ Ophthalmology* 4: 31–42.

Yeum K-J and Russell RM (2002) Carotenoid bioavailability and bioconversion. *Annual Review of Nutrition* 22: 483–504.

Epidemiology of Health Effects

S A Tanumihardjo and Z Yang, University of Wisconsin-Madison, Madison, WI, USA

© 2005 Elsevier Ltd. All rights reserved.

Introduction

The colors of many fruits and vegetables are due to a class of compounds known as carotenoids. Over 600 carotenoids have been identified in nature. Humans are unique in that they can assimilate carotenoids from the foods that they eat whereas many other animals do not. Thus, carotenoids are an important class of phytochemicals. Phytochemicals are compounds derived from plants that may or may not have nutritional value. While many carotenoids circulate in humans, the most commonly studied ones are β-carotene, α-carotene, β-cryptoxanthin, lycopene, lutein, and zeaxanthin (**Figure 1**). The nutritional significance of carotenoids is that some are used by the body to make vitamin A. Indeed, approximately 50 carotenoids can be converted by the body into vitamin A and are known as provitamin A carotenoids. The three most abundant provitamin A carotenoids in foods are β-carotene, α-carotene, and β-cryptoxanthin. Provitamin A carotenoids, especially β-carotene, provide less than one-half of the vitamin A supply in North America but provide more than one-half in Africa and Asia.

Dietary recommendations for the intake of specific carotenoids have not been established due to lack of an adequate evidence base. To date, carotenoids are not considered essential nutrients. Dietary recommendations for vitamin A exist: 900 retinol activity equivalents (RAE) for men and 700 RAE for women. An RAE is equivalent to 1 μg of retinol. The recommendations for infants and children are less and range from 300 to 600 RAE depending on age. Consumers need to eat sufficient amounts of carotenoid-rich fruits and vegetables to meet their daily vitamin A requirement, and to achieve optimal dietary carotenoid intake to lower the risk of certain chronic diseases. In 2001, the Institute of Medicine revised the amount of carotenoids needed to provide vitamin A from foods as being approximately 12 μg of β-carotene or 24 μg of other provitamin A carotenoids to yield 1 RAE. Currently, high-dose pharmacological supplementation with carotenoids is not advised. Despite this, a tolerable upper intake level, the maximum daily amount of a nutrient that appears to be safe, has not been established for any individual carotenoid; however, supplemental β-carotene at 20 mg day^{-1} or more is contraindicated for use in current heavy smokers by the European Commission.

Because many factors affect the assimilation of carotenoids from foods (**Figure 2**), conversion factors need to be considered. This is especially important when most sources of vitamin A are from provitamin A carotenoids in the population. Bioavailability of preformed vitamin A, i.e., retinol and retinyl esters, is not a major concern because 80–95% of them are absorbed. However, foods that are high in preformed retinol (liver, eggs, and fortified milk) are not necessarily consumed by everybody. When discussing carotenoids from food, four terms need to be defined (see **Table 1**):

- bioaccessibility refers to how much carotenoid can be extracted from the food and is available for absorption;
- bioavailability is how much carotenoid is absorbed from the food and is available for physiological function;
- bioconversion relates to the provitamin A carotenoids and is defined as the amount of retinol that is formed from absorbed provitamin A carotenoids; and
- bioefficacy encompasses all of the biological processing of provitamin A carotenoids and is the amount of retinol formed from the amount of carotenoid contained in the food.

The study of carotenoid bioefficacy from foods is important in international health as the most frequently consumed sources of vitamin A are fruit and vegetables. A 100% bioefficacy means that 1 μmol of dietary β-carotene provides 2 μmol of retinol in the body; however, 100% bioefficacy does not actually occur in the process of digestion and carotenoid uptake by the body.

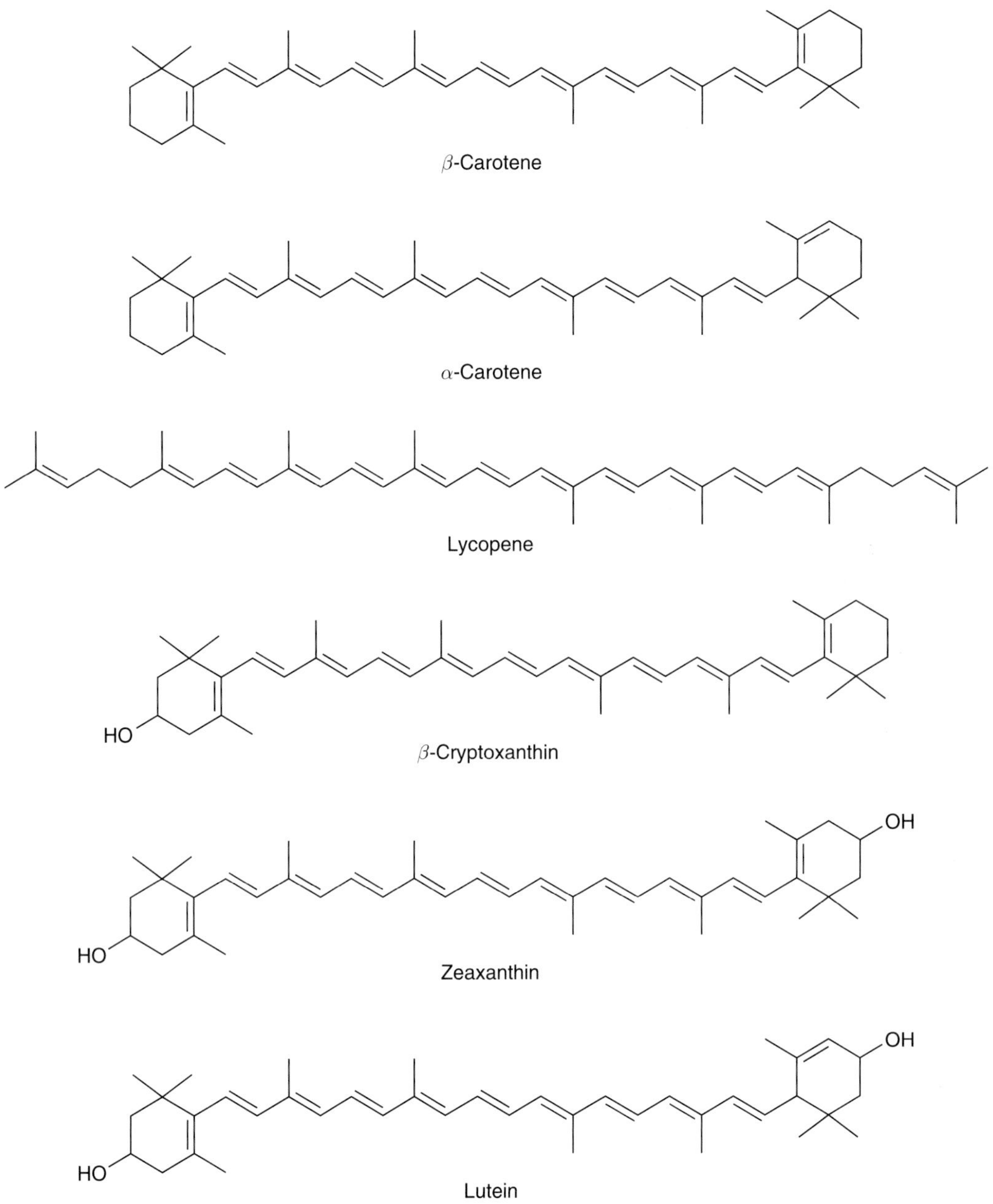

Figure 1 The structures of the most common carotenoids found in the human body. Three of them, β-carotene, α-carotene and β-cryptoxanthin, can be used by the body to make vitamin A. All carotenoids are antioxidants found in fruits and vegetables.

Once in the body, carotenoids can act as potent antioxidants, which are substances that neutralize free radicals formed from the natural metabolic processes of cells. Free radicals damage tissues and cells through oxidative processes. While free radical formation is a natural process in the body, environmental factors such as smoking and pollution can increase free radical load and thus disease risk. Carotenoids may counter these influences by functioning as an antioxidant and quenching oxygen-containing free radicals. In high- and low-density lipoproteins and cell membranes, carotenoids may

also regenerate the antioxidant form of vitamin E as well as protect vitamin E from oxidation.

At the whole-body level, some population studies have indicated that certain carotenoids from either dietary intake or blood concentration data are associated with better immune response, lower rates of age-related macular degeneration (AMD) and cataract, as well as lower risk for certain cancers and cardiovascular disease. β-Carotene may increase immunological functions by enhancing lymphocyte proliferation independent of its provitamin A functions. The associations between specific carotenoids

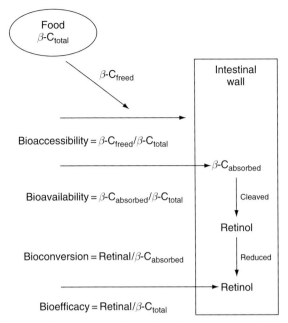

Figure 2 A schematic outlining the path of β-carotene (β-C) as it moves out from the food into the intestinal wall. The definition of terms associated with understanding β-carotene release, absorption, and conversion to retinol are illustrated: bioaccessibility, bioavailability, bioconversion, and bioefficacy. (Reproduced with permission from Tanumihardjo SA (2002) Factors influencing the conversion of carotenoids to retinol: Bioavailability to bioconversion to bioefficacy. *International Journal of Vitamin and Nutrition Research* **72**: 40–45.)

Table 1 Terms that are associated with the β-carotene vitamin A value of foods and subsequent utilization as retinol

Term	Definition	100%
Bioaccessibility	$\dfrac{\beta\text{-Carotene freed}}{\beta\text{-Carotene in food}}$	$\dfrac{1\ \mu\text{mol freed}}{1\ \mu\text{mol in food}}$
Bioavailability	$\dfrac{\beta\text{-Carotene absorbed}}{\beta\text{-Carotene in food}}$	$\dfrac{1\ \mu\text{mol absorbed}}{1\ \mu\text{mol in food}}$
Bioconversion	$\dfrac{\text{Retinol formed}}{\beta\text{-Carotene absorbed}}$	$\dfrac{2\ \mu\text{mol formed}}{1\ \mu\text{mol absorbed}}$
Bioefficacy	$\dfrac{\text{Retinol formed}}{\beta\text{-Carotene in food}}$	$\dfrac{2\ \mu\text{mol formed}}{1\ \mu\text{mol in food}}$

and decreased risk of various diseases are summarized in **Table 2**.

Blood levels of specific carotenoids are often used as biomarkers of fruit and vegetable intake to strengthen or replace dietary intake data. A wide variation in analytical methods exists and standardization between laboratories does not routinely occur. Nonetheless, higher blood concentrations have been favorably correlated with certain disease states. For example, vitamin A and carotenoid concentrations in serum were measured in middle-aged women who later developed breast cancer. Median concentrations of β-carotene, lycopene, lutein, and total carotenoids were significantly lower in women with breast cancer compared with case-control women who had not developed breast cancer. In contrast, vitamin A concentrations were either not different or showed a mixed response between cohorts, suggesting that carotenoids may be protective against breast cancer. Furthermore, the Nurses' Health Study, which included a cohort of over 83 000 women, also showed a significant inverse association between dietary β-carotene intake and breast cancer risk. This was especially strong for premenopausal women with a family history of breast cancer or high alcohol consumption. However, other prospective studies have had mixed results.

Hydrocarbon Carotenoid: β-Carotene

β-Carotene is one of the most widely studied carotenoids – for both its vitamin A activity and its abundance in fruits and vegetables. Epidemiological studies have often pointed to an abundance of carotenoids in the diet being protective against many diseases. Diets rich in fruits and vegetables are recommended to reduce the risk of cardiovascular disease and some forms of cancer. However, when β-carotene is removed from the plant matrix and administered as a supplement, these benefits sometimes disappear. For example, because lung cancer is

Table 2 A summary of epidemiologic and/or clinical studies where carotenoids and a significant association to a specific disease risk has been shown in at least one study[a]

Carotenoid	Cardiovascular disease	Cataract	Macular degeneration	Lung cancer	Prostate cancer
β-Carotene	Yes	–	–	Yes[b]	–
α-Carotene	Yes	–	–	Yes	–
β-Cryptoxanthin	–	–	–	Yes	–
Lycopene	Yes	–	–	Yes	Yes
Lutein/zeaxanthin	Yes	Yes	Yes	Yes	–

[a]For a more complete discussion of the association of specific carotenoids to disease please refer to: Krinsky NI, Mayne SI, and Sies H, (eds.) (2004) *Carotenoids in Health and Disease.* New York: Marcel Dekker.
[b]The opposite finding has been observed in clinical trials.

the leading cause of cancer death in many developed countries, the β-Carotene and Retinol Efficacy Trial (CARET) in the 1990s set out to test whether β-carotene conferred protection against cancer. CARET was based on a number of observational studies that showed high levels of β-carotene from food sources were protective against lung cancer. However, the CARET trial was halted for showing an increased risk for lung cancer in the treatment group over the control. Subsequent studies in ferrets showed that the amounts of β-carotene commonly consumed from fruit and vegetables were protective against lung damage but higher amounts, equivalent to those in CARET, increased the formation of abnormal tissue in the lung.

A similar outcome was observed among smokers in the α-Tocopherol β-Carotene (ATBC) Study Group. Although evidence clearly exists showing an association between β-carotene and enhanced lung function, as in the CARET study, the ATBC trial also found an increase in lung cancer rates among smokers. It is plausible that the lung cancer had already been initiated in the smokers and supplementation with β-carotene could not prevent the development of cancer. The ATBC study also showed an increased incidence of angina pectoris, a mild warning sign of heart disease characterized by chest pain, among heavy smokers. This may have been due to low blood levels of vitamin C in the study group leading to the inability of the individuals to quench β-carotene radicals, but this relationship requires more research.

In both the CARET and ATBC intervention trials, much higher doses of β-carotene were used than could be obtained from the diet, and the blood levels attained were two to six times higher than the 95th percentile level of β-carotene in a survey of a representative sample of the US population. Thus, it remains unclear whether β-carotene is a procarcinogen or an anticarcinogen. The associations for lower disease risk observed in epidemiologic studies may reflect other protective dietary agents or an interaction between dietary components. Furthermore, people with higher intake of fruits and vegetables may have healthier lifestyles that contribute to their lower risk of chronic diseases. The higher disease risk observed in the clinical trials may be correlated with the use of high doses of β-carotene where the mechanisms have not yet been identified, the limited duration of treatment, and/or the timing of the interventions was too late for cancers that were already present due to a history of heavy smoking. More research on β-carotene's biological actions is needed to explore the mechanisms involved. Current consensus is that the beneficial effects of β-carotene are associated with dietary consumption, whereas the harmful effects in some subpopulations are with pharmacological supplements.

Another explanation for a lack of a beneficial outcome with β-carotene supplementation may be that not all people respond to the same degree to β-carotene treatment, some being low- or nonresponders. Some researchers believe that individuals who do not respond to β-carotene supplementation may be better at converting it to vitamin A. Blood response to β-carotene supplementation is also inversely related to body mass index (BMI), which may be due to increased sequestration of lipophilic β-carotene by the larger amount of fat stores present in people with larger BMI. This theory may not hold true as individuals with larger BMIs do not necessarily have a high body fat percentage, but rather increased lean muscle mass.

Excellent food sources of β-carotene include carrots, winter squash, red-orange sweet potato, and various types of dark green leafy vegetables. No deficiency or toxicity has been observed from dietary β-carotene intake, although very rarely high intakes can be associated with yellow pigmentation of the skin as carotenoids are stored in adipose tissue. Supplements containing β-carotene are common. In the Women's Health Initiative, the largest observational/intervention study in postmenopausal women to date, approximately 50% reported using a supplement containing β-carotene. This trial included both a clinical trial and observational study involving more than 160 000 women. The Physicians' Health Study II also included β-carotene as one of its interventions to determine the balance of risks and benefits of this carotenoid with cancer, cardiovascular disease, and eye disease.

Hydrocarbon Carotenoid: α-Carotene

α-Carotene, another carotenoid frequently present in food, also has provitamin A activity. Based on its structure, it is only converted to one molecule of biologically active retinol after central cleavage. Like other carotenoids, it has antioxidant and possibly anticarcinogenic properties, and may enhance immune function as well. Some, but not all, epidemiological studies observed that higher α-carotene intake was associated with lower risk of cardiovascular disease and cancer, whereas others did not. Clinical trials to test α-carotene influences in humans have not been conducted to date. This is probably because α-carotene is usually associated with ample amounts of β-carotene when found in fruits and vegetables and singling out α-carotene is difficult.

α-Carotene's concentration is especially high in orange carrots. Low or high dietary intake of α-carotene alone has not been associated with any specific disease outcome or health condition.

Xanthophyll: β-Cryptoxanthin

β-Cryptoxanthin is one of the lesser known carotenoids that also has provitamin A activity and appears to have a protective health role. Several epidemiological studies suggest that dietary β-cryptoxanthin is associated with lower rates of lung cancer and improved lung function in humans. A large prospective study on dietary intake and cancer, which included an interview on dietary habits and life style, identified β-cryptoxanthin as protective against lung cancer after correcting for smoking. However, the beneficial effects for β-cryptoxanthin suggested by these results could be merely an indicator for other antioxidants and/or a measure of a healthy life style that are more common in people with high dietary intakes of β-cryptoxanthin. In tissue culture, β-cryptoxanthin has a direct stimulatory effect on bone formation and an inhibitory effect on bone resorption. Studies of these beneficial effects in humans have not been conducted.

No deficiency or toxicity has been observed from dietary β-cryptoxanthin intake. The best food sources for β-cryptoxanthin are oranges, papaya, peaches, and tangerines. Tropical fruit intake is directly proportional to β-cryptoxanthin blood concentrations.

Hydrocarbon Carotenoid: Lycopene

Lycopene, while having no provitamin A activity, is a potent antioxidant with twice the activity of β-carotene for quenching singlet oxygen and 10 times the antioxidant activity of α-tocopherol in some model systems. The antioxidant potential of food chemicals varies widely according to location in the body and the presence of other body chemicals. The primary sources of dietary lycopene are tomatoes and tomato products. Epidemiological evidence shows an inverse association between lycopene consumption and the incidence and development of certain cancers. This association is especially strong for prostate cancer, which is the most common cancer among men in Western countries and the second leading cause of cancer death in American men. Prostate cancer rates in Asian countries are much lower, but appear to be increasing rapidly. Lycopene is localized in prostate tissue. The current consensus is that a high consumption of tomatoes or high circulating concentrations of lycopene are associated with a 30–40% risk reduction for prostate cancer, especially the most aggressive forms. Recent studies in rats show that tomato products are more protective against prostate cancer than isolated lycopene.

Epidemiologic studies have also observed lower rates of bladder, cervical, and breast cancers as well as cancers of the gastrointestinal tract among people with high intake of lycopene. The discovery of significant concentrations of lycopene in specific tissues in the body, i.e., plasma, testes, adrenal glands, liver and kidney, suggests that lycopene may play a role in these tissues.

While the body of evidence seems strong, several studies have found either no or weak associations between lycopene consumption and disease. Some of this may be explained by the fact that blood lycopene concentrations were much lower in these studies than in those that showed a beneficial effect. Thus, future dietary based studies need to include blood sampling to further define the range of blood concentrations of lycopene in the population, ideally with method standardization so that studies can be directly compared. The prostate cancer association is usually stronger for cooked tomato products rather than raw tomatoes or total lycopene intake. This too supports the idea that it is the whole food, with a broad array of nutrients and nonnutritive bioactive components, that is important for overall health rather than isolated compounds. It is possible that the beneficial effects of tomatoes are increased by preparing a concentrated product that enhances the nutrient bioavailability, as processed and cooked tomatoes are more closely associated to decreased risk of disease than either raw tomatoes or tomato juice.

Because lycopene is a potent antioxidant, it may be protective against heart disease by slowing down the oxidation of polyunsaturated fats in the low-density lipoprotein particles in the blood. Epidemiological and clinical studies show that higher blood lycopene concentrations are associated with lower risk and incidence of cardiovascular disease. Higher fat stores of lycopene have also been associated with lower risk of myocardial infarction. The most profound protective effect is in nonsmokers. The evidence for protective cardiovascular effects is compelling, as studies have shown a 20–60% improvement in cardiovascular parameters with higher blood concentrations of lycopene. Furthermore, higher intake of fruits and vegetables is associated with better lung function. In particular, high tomato intake is associated with higher timed expiratory volume.

The major food source of lycopene globally is tomatoes and tomato products. In the US, more than 80% of dietary lycopene comes from tomatoes.

Other sources include watermelon, pink grapefruit, and red carrots.

Xanthophylls: Lutein and Zeaxanthin

The structural isomers lutein and zeaxanthin are non-provitamin A carotenoids that are also measurable in human blood and tissues. Lutein and zeaxanthin have been identified as the xanthophylls that constitute the macular pigment of the human retina. The relative concentration of lutein to zeaxanthin in the macula is distinctive. Zeaxanthin is more centralized and lutein predominates towards the outer area of the macula. A putative xanthophyll-binding protein has also been described, which may explain the high variability among people to accumulate these carotenoids into eye tissues. Increased lutein intake from both food sources and supplements is positively correlated with increased macular pigment density, which is theorized to lower risk for macular degeneration. AMD is the leading cause of irreversible blindness in the elderly in developed countries. AMD adversely affects the central field of vision and the ability to see fine detail. Some, but not all, population studies suggest lower rates of AMD among people with higher levels of lutein and zeaxanthin in the diet or blood. Possible mechanisms of action for these carotenoids include antioxidant protection of the retinal tissue and the macular pigment filtering of damaging blue light.

Free radical damage is also linked to the development of cataracts. Cataracts remain the leading cause of visual disability in the US and about one-half of the 30–50 million cases of blindness throughout the world. Although cataracts are treatable, blindness occurs because individuals have either chosen not to correct the disease or do not have access to the appropriate medical treatment. Several epidemiological studies have shown inverse associations between the risk of cataracts and carotenoid intake. However, these studies also present inconsistencies with regard to the different carotenoids and their association with cataract risk. Lutein and zeaxanthin are found in the lens and are thought to protect cells in the eye against oxidative damage, and consequently prevent formation of cataracts. However, to date, there is no evidence that any carotenoid supplement can protect against cataract development. Eating plenty of fruits and vegetables, good sources of many antioxidants including carotenoids, is a preventative measure for many diseases.

Because lutein and zeaxanthin may be involved in disease prevention, much needs to be learned regarding human consumption of these carotenoids. One complicating factor that requires better understanding is the bioavailability of lutein from food sources and supplements. The food matrix is an important factor influencing lutein bioavailability and the amount and type of food processing generally influences the bioavailability of all carotenoids. For example, the processing of spinach does not affect bioavailability of lutein, but it does enhance that of β-carotene. Such studies have been conducted with lutein supplements and/or foods containing lutein fed to human subjects. In humans, lutein from vegetables seems to be more bioavailable than β-carotene; however, this may be partially explained by bioconversion of β-carotene to vitamin A. Competition between carotenoids, such as lutein and β-carotene, for incorporation into chylomicra has been noted in humans consuming vegetables and supplements. The amount of fat consumed with the lutein source also affects bioavailability, as higher fat increases the bioavailability of lipid-soluble carotenoids. Decreased plasma lutein concentrations are noted when alcohol is consumed, but the mechanism is poorly defined.

Lutein may also protect against some forms of cancer and enhance immune function. Lutein may work in concert with other carotenoids such as β-carotene to lower cancer risk due to their antimutagenic and antitumor properties. Because of these potential health benefits, lutein supplements are sold commercially and incorporated into some multivitamins. However, the amount provided in multivitamins (about 10–20% of the level in an average diet) is likely to be too low for a biological influence. Levels of lutein available as a single supplement vary widely and neither benefit nor safety of lutein supplements has been adequately studied. Major dietary sources of both lutein and zeaxanthin in the diet include corn, green leafy vegetables, and eggs. Lutein tends to be the predominant isomer in foods. Lutein supplements are often derived from marigold flowers.

Summary

Most of the epidemiological evidence points to carotenoids being a very important class of phytochemicals. While some of the effects may be attributable to a diet high in fruits and vegetables, and an overall healthy lifestyle, the presence of specific carotenoids localized in different areas of the human body lend evidence to their overall importance in the human diet. As methods are developed to assess carotenoid levels noninvasively in humans, large-scale studies that determine carotenoid levels in blood, skin, and the eye may lead to a better understanding of their importance in human health and disease prevention. Additional epidemiologic studies to further strengthen the associations that have been observed in populations are needed.

It must be kept in mind that study design and statistical analyses vary across published work and no one study can give conclusive evidence. An integrated multidisciplinary approach to study the functions and actions of carotenoids in the body is necessary to understand fully the role of carotenoids in health and disease prevention. This includes comparisons of carotenoids in whole fruits and vegetables and their effect on human health and well being. High fruit and vegetable intake is associated with a decreased risk of cancer, cardiovascular disease, diabetes, AMD, and osteoporosis. Removing any one class of phytochemicals from the intricate matrix of the whole plant may not give the same beneficial outcome in terms of human health. Considering that the average intake of fruits and vegetables is still less than that recommended by health professionals, programs that promote the consumption of more fruit and vegetables may be more effective at preventing disease in the long-term than using individual pharmacological carotenoid supplements.

A question that remains is whether or not carotenoids can be considered nutrients. A variety of phytochemicals contained in fruits and vegetables including carotenoids are assumed to be needed for optimal health and reduction of chronic disease risk, but have not been classified as nutrients. Indeed, in 2000, the Institute of Medicine was unable to recommend a daily reference intake for any carotenoid. Several factors have been defined that categorize substances as nutrients: substances that must be obtained from the diet because the body cannot synthesize the active form, and are used in the body for growth, maintenance, and tissue repair. In addition, to being classified as a nutrient, further studies must be done to determine the essentiality of the substance and its specific function in the body. Other criteria for defining a nutrient include concentration in specific tissues, consumption, and/or supplementation resulting in tissue concentration increases and improved tissue function. Lastly, a daily established dosage needs to be defined and a biomarker identified to assess status.

A large body of observational studies suggests that high blood concentrations of carotenoids obtained from food are associated with chronic disease risk reduction. However, there is little other evidence of their specific role in the body. Lutein and zeaxanthin are the only carotenoids found in a specific tissue (the macular region of the retina) that seem to have a specific function. Providing lutein in the diet increases macular pigment in humans. Animal studies show that a diet low in lutein can deplete macular pigment, but the influence on the health of the eye is not yet well understood. To further our understanding, large randomized prospective intervention trials need to be conducted to explore the essentiality of lutein supplementation for reducing ocular disease risk in humans. Thus, to date, no one specific carotenoid has been classified as an essential nutrient.

See also: **Antioxidants**: Diet and Antioxidant Defense; Observational Studies; Intervention Studies. **Bioavailability**. **Cancer**: Epidemiology and Associations Between Diet and Cancer; Epidemiology of Lung Cancer; Effects on Nutritional Status. **Carotenoids**: Chemistry, Sources and Physiology. **Coronary Heart Disease**: Prevention. **Fruits and Vegetables**. **Lycopenes and Related Compounds**. **Older People**: Nutrition-Related Problems. **Phytochemicals**: Epidemiological Factors. **Supplementation**: Dietary Supplements.

Further Reading

Alves-Rodrigues A and Shao A (2004) The science behind lutein. *Toxicology Letters* **150**: 57–83.
Christen WG, Gaziano JM, and Hennekens CH (2000) Design of Physicians' Health Study II – a randomized trial of beta-carotene, vitamins E and C, and multivitamins, in prevention of cancer, cardiovascular disease, and eye disease, and review of results of completed trials. *Annals of Epidemiology* **10**: 125–134.
Giovannucci E (2002) A review of epidemiologic studies of tomatoes, lycopene, and prostate cancer. *Experimental Biology of Medicine* **227**: 852–859.
Hwang ES and Bowen PE (2002) Can the consumption of tomatoes or lycopene reduce cancer risk? *Integrative Cancer Therapies* **1**: 121–132.
Institute of Medicine, Food and Nutrition Board (2000) *Dietary Reference Intakes for Vitamin C, Vitamin E, Selenium, and Carotenoids*. Washington, DC: National Academy Press.
Johnson EJ (2002) The role of carotenoids in human health. *Nutrition in Clinical Care* **5**: 56–65.
Krinsky NI, Landrum JT, and Bone RA (2003) Biologic mechanisms of the protective role of lutein and zeaxanthin in the eye. *Annual Review of Nutrition* **23**: 171–201.
Krinsky NI, Mayne SI, and Sies H (eds.) (2004) *Carotenoids in Health and Disease*. New York: Marcel Dekker.
Mares-Perlman JA, Millen AE, Ficek TL, and Hankinson SE (2002) The body of evidence to support a protective role for lutein and zeaxanthin in delaying chronic disease. *Journal of Nutrition* **132**: 518S–524S.
Rapola JM, Virtamo J, Haukka JK et al. (1996) Effect of vitamin E and beta-carotene on the incidence of angina pectoris. A randomized, double-blind, controlled trial. *Journal of the American Medical Association* **275**: 693–698.
Tanumihardjo SA (2002) Factors influencing the conversion of carotenoids to retinol: Bioavailability to bioconversion to bioefficacy. *International Journal of Vitamin and Nutrition Research* **72**: 40–45.
The Alpha-Tocopherol Beta Carotene Cancer Prevention Study Group (1994) The effect of vitamin E and beta carotene on the incidence of lung cancer and other cancers in male smokers. *New England Journal of Medicine* **330**: 1029–1035.

CEREAL GRAINS

R W Welch, University of Ulster, Coleraine, UK

© 2005 Elsevier Ltd. All rights reserved.

Introduction

Cereal grains are dietary staples that provide a very substantial proportion of the dietary energy, protein, and micronutrients for much of the world's population. The major cereal crops are rice, maize (corn), wheat, barley, sorghum, millets, oats, and rye. Worldwide, these cereals are subjected to a very diverse range of traditional and technologically advanced processes before consumption. Thus, cereal-based foods vary enormously in their structural, storage, and sensory characteristics. Cereal-based foodstuffs also vary in nutritional value owing to inherent differences in nutrient content and to changes as a result of processing, which may be beneficial or detrimental. Cereals are also the raw materials for the production of alcoholic beverages and food ingredients including starches, syrups, and protein and fiber isolates. Furthermore, very substantial quantities of cereal enter the food chain as livestock feed.

Types of Cereal and Their Role in the Diet

Cereal grains are the seeds of cultivated annual species of the grass family (Gramineae). Cultivated cereal species have evolved with humankind and include a range of types differing widely in their environmental adaptation and their utility for food or other uses. Some cereals are adapted to tropical or subtropical regions, others are adapted to temperate climates, while some can withstand sub-zero temperatures. The type of cereal grown is largely determined by climatic and edaphic factors, although economic and cultural factors are also important. Total world cereal production is about 2 billion tonnes (**Table 1**). The major cereals produced are rice, maize (corn), wheat, barley, sorghum, millets, oats, and rye. Some of these are single species; others include a number of species with different agronomic and utilization characteristics. Each species comprises a range of cultivars (varieties or genotypes), which also differ in characteristics. Minor cereals include triticale (*Triticosecale*; a wheat–rye hybrid), buckwheat (*Fagopyrum esculentum*), and quinoa (*Chenopodium quinoa*). Buckwheat and quinoa are not Gramineae and are thus pseudocereals. All cereals are used for human nutrition. However, the forms in which they are consumed and their dietary significances vary substantially across cereal types and regions.

Grain Characteristics

The harvested grain of some cereals (wheat, maize, rye, sorghum, and some millets) comprises, botanically, a caryopsis. In other cereals (barley, oats, rice, and some millets) the harvested grain generally includes a hull (or husk) that encloses the caryopsis. The hull is tough and very high in fiber. It is unsuitable for human nutrition and is removed in primary

Table 1 World production of cereals 2000; figures are in thousands of tonnes

	Total	Rice[a]	Maize	Wheat	Barley	Sorghum	Millets	Oats	Rye	Other[b]
World	2 063 578	602 610	591 988	585 297	134 421	56 044	27 636	26 394	19 642	19 546
Asia (excluding China and the Russian Federation)	592 016	359 375	42 707	154 299	15 021	8 538	10 999	516	389	172
North and Central America	427 528	10 917	279 404	90 780	20 826	18 265	166	6 063	473	634
China	407 328	189 814	106 180	99 636	3 346	2 608	2 126	650	650	2 318
Europe (excluding the Russian Federation)	320 442	2 567	61 782	149 039	70 383	685	439	10 677	12 544	12 326
Africa	112 149	17 649	44 409	14 328	2 081	18 630	12 679	194	30	2 149
South America	104 275	20 583	55 407	20 199	1 543	5 083	48	1 128	135	149
Russian Federation	64 342	586	1 500	34 500	14 100	116	1 122	6 000	5 400	1 018
Oceania	35 498	1 119	599	22 516	7 121	2 119	57	1 166	21	780

[a]Paddy (rough) rice.
[b]Includes other cereals, pseudocereals, mixed grains, and their products not accounted for elsewhere.
Source: Food and Agriculture Organisation, FAOSTAT data at http://faostat.fao.org/accessed May 2003.

processing. The caryopsis is the edible part of the cereal grain. Cereal caryopses all have the same basic structure. The major part is the endosperm (63–91% of the total). The endosperm is high in starch and contains nutritionally significant amounts of protein. Enclosing the endosperm are cell layers, amounting to 5–20% of the caryopsis, which form the bran that is often separated from the endosperm during milling processes. The embryo, which is found at one end of the caryopsis, accounts for 2.5–12% of its weight. The embryo is the major component of the germ fraction, which is separated in some milling processes.

At harvest, cereal grains have a low moisture content (12–16%), and they are hard and inedible without processing. Some grain types may be subjected to simple milling procedures and made into palatable unleavened products; others are subjected to more complex milling procedures and further processed into leavened, extruded, or fermented products using technologically advanced processes.

Food use of cereals is shown in **Table 2**. From this it can be seen that rice and wheat are the major world food cereals, and maize is important in some regions. However, the data in **Table 2** represent food use of the crops. Since varying proportions of these crops will be lost in milling, the actual consumption levels may be substantially less.

Rice

World rice production exceeds 600 million tonnes annually (**Table 1**), and over 85% of the crop is used for human nutrition. Rice is a dietary staple for over half the world's population, and over 90% of the crop is produced and consumed in Asia and China. The per capita supply of paddy rice exceeds $600\,g\,day^{-1}$ in six countries (Myanmar, $847\,g\,day^{-1}$;

Laos, $707\,g\,day^{-1}$; Viet Nam $686\,g\,day^{-1}$; Cambodia, $668\,g\,day^{-1}$; Bangladesh, $643\,g\,day^{-1}$; and Indonesia, $611\,g\,day^{-1}$), and exceeds $400\,g\,day^{-1}$ in Thailand ($448\,g\,day^{-1}$), Guinea-Bissau ($422\,g\,day^{-1}$), the Philippines ($418\,g\,day^{-1}$), Côte d'Ivoire ($412\,g\,day^{-1}$), Nepal ($409\,g\,day^{-1}$), and Madagascar ($402\,g\,day^{-1}$). Rice makes a modest contribution to the diets in most industrialized countries, except Japan where rice is the major dietary cereal with a per capita supply of $244\,g\,day^{-1}$. Rice (*Oryza sativa*) can be grown in a wide range of environments, under water or on dry land. The subspecies *indica* is grown in the tropics, and the subspecies *japonica* is grown mainly in warm temperate regions. Harvested rice, known as paddy (or rough) rice, has a hull. Removal of the hull yields brown rice, which can be rendered edible by prolonged boiling. However, the type of rice preferred in most regions is white polished rice, in which the outer bran layers are removed by milling. The yield of edible milled rice from paddy rice is about 66%. Types of rice vary in grain morphology and in cooking characteristics. When boiled, short-grain *indica* types generally become soft and sticky and aggregate, whereas long-grain *japonica* types remain relatively firm and separated. A small proportion of rice is processed to flour. However, the absence of gluten precludes its general use in leavened products.

Maize

World production of maize (corn; *Zea mays*) is nearly 600 million tonnes annually (**Table 1**). About 20% is used directly for human food, and about 10% is used in industrial processing to yield oil and other products including starch, syrups, flour, and grits for food and other uses. Maize is grown in tropical and warm temperate regions.

Table 2   Food use of cereals, 2000; figures are per capita supply in grams per day

	Total	Rice[a]	Maize	Wheat	Barley	Sorghum	Millets	Oats	Rye	Other[b]
World	503	236	51	187	3.0	10.8	9.8	1.3	2.9	2.2
Asia (excluding China and the Russian Federation)	584	350	35	181	2.1	6.4	8.3	0.2	0.4	1.3
North and Central America	364	46	111	197	1.1	3.1	0.0	2.9	0.5	3.0
China	622	366	44	203	1.2	2.5	2.5	0.4	0.5	2.1
Europe(excluding the Russian Federation)	365	19	19	294	4.3	0.0	1.7	4.3	21.7	1.1
Africa	421	78	115	125	8.3	51.2	35.9	0.4	0.1	7.3
South America	347	128	60	150	1.3	0.0	0.0	5.9	0.1	1.0
Russian Federation	415	20	1	355	2.5	0.0	6.5	3.3	25.5	0.3
Oceania	251	65	9	168	0.2	1.5	0.0	3.3	1.0	2.5

[a]Paddy (rough) rice.
[b]Includes other cereals, pseudocereals, mixed grains, and their products not accounted for elsewhere.
Source: Food and Agriculture Organisation, FAOSTAT data at http://faostat.fao.org/accessed May 2003.

Maize is a dietary staple in parts of Africa. Food use is highest in Lesotho (427 g day^{-1} per person) and is 300–400 g day^{-1} per person in other southern and eastern African countries (Malawi, Zambia, Zimbabwe, and South Africa) and in Mexico, where it has a pre-Colombian tradition. Food use is 200–300 g day^{-1} per person in Moldova, Bosnia and Herzegovina, Guatemala, Kenya, El Salvador, and Honduras and 100–200 g day^{-1} per person in Benin, Bolivia, Botswana, Burkina Faso, Cameroon, Columbia, Egypt, Ethiopia, Georgia, Ghana, North Korea, Mozambique, Nepal, Nicaragua, Paraguay, Romania, Swaziland, Tanzania, Togo, and Venezuela. A harvested grain of maize is a caryopsis. There is a wide range of types varying in grain size, color, and endosperm characteristics. These include white, yellow, and red types and types with endosperms ranging from soft and floury to hard and flinty textures. Sweetcorn is generally regarded as a vegetable; it is harvested before the grain is mature and has a high water content (70–90%).

Wheat

World wheat production is nearly 600 million tonnes annually (**Table 1**). Worldwide, over 70% of the wheat supply is used for food, and it is the major dietary cereal in all regions except Asia and China (**Table 2**). Consumption levels are highest in western Asia (Turkmenistan, Kyrgyzstan, Azerbaijan, and Turkey) and North Africa (Algeria and Tunisia), where supplies for food use exceed 500 g day^{-1} per person. Although other species are grown in some regions, the major species are common or bread wheat (*Triticum aestivum*) and durum wheat (*Triticum durum*). Of these two species, common wheat accounts for about 95% of total production. Common wheat can be grown across widely diverse geographical regions including subtropical, warm temperate, and cool temperate climates, where it can withstand frosts. There is an extensive range of genotypes, varying in agronomic adaptability and grain quality. Quality is usually assessed in terms of suitability for milling and baking. The whole grain comprises about 82% endosperm and 18% bran. The aim of milling white flour is to separate the starchy endosperm from the darker coarser bran. Wheat bran is used as a fiber source in some foodstuffs including ready-to-eat cereals. The yield of white flour will depend on milling efficiency, but extraction rates of 75–81% are usually achieved. Wheat grains are classified as hard or soft and as strong or weak. The terms hard and soft indicate milling quality; hard wheats have superior milling characteristics. The terms strong and weak refer to bread-baking quality. Strong flours yield bread with a large loaf volume and good crumb structure. The quantity and quality of the viscoelastic gluten proteins are important for bread quality. Weak flours produce poor bread products but can be blended with strong flours in bread making or used to make other products. Durum wheat is hard and vitreous. It is used almost exclusively for the production of pasta in Europe, the Americas, and elsewhere, but in the Middle East and North Africa 85% of durum wheat is used to produce breads, couscous, and other non-pasta products.

Barley

World barley production is over 130 million tonnes annually (**Table 1**). Barley (*Hordeum vulgare*) is grown mainly in temperate regions and can withstand sub-zero temperatures. About 17% of the total crop is used industrially, primarily to produce malt, which is used mainly in brewing and distilling. Only about 5% of the total is used for food. The highest food usage is in Morocco (104 g day^{-1} per person), followed by the Baltic States (Estonia, Latvia, and Lithuania) and Moldova, where food usage is 86, 57, 55, and 55 g day^{-1} per person, respectively. Most barley grain has a fibrous hull that adheres closely to the caryopsis. However, naked or hull-less types are grown in some regions. Barley is processed for human use by removing the hull and polishing to yield pearl barley, which is used in soups and other foods. Pearl barley is also ground to a coarse meal and cooked as a gruel or ground to barley flour for making flat breads. Barley flours and brans, for ingredient use, are produced from pearl or hull-less barley.

Sorghum

World production of sorghum (*Sorghum bicolor*) is 56 million tonnes per year (**Table 1**), and about 40% of this is used for food. Sorghum is grown in semi-arid zones and is especially important in tropical and sub-tropical regions. Food use of sorghum is highest in Africa. The food supply in grams per head per day in the major consuming countries is: Sudan, 248 g day^{-1}; Burkino Faso, 192 g day^{-1}; Nigeria, 143 g day^{-1}; Chad, 142 g day^{-1}; Eritrea, 124 g day^{-1}, and Mali, 124 g day^{-1}. Food use is between 60 g day^{-1} and 75 g day^{-1} per person in a further six African countries (Botswana, Cameroon, Ethiopia, Mauritania, Niger, and Togo). Both sorghum and millets are generally milled by traditional methods to yield grits and flours, which are used to make a variety of traditional foodstuffs including porridges, steamed products, breads, and pancake products.

Millets

Annual production of millets is over 27 million tonnes. About 77% of production is used for food, and millets are very important food crops in semi-arid regions of Africa. There are at least nine species of millet. In production terms, the most important is pearl or bulrush millet (*Pennisetum glaucum*) (about 53% of the total). Foxtail millet (*Setaria italica*), proso millet (*Panicum miliaceum*), and finger millet (*Eleusine coracana*) contribute about 17%, 14%, and 12%, respectively, to world production. Other species, which include Japanese or barnyard millet (*Echinochloa crus-galli*), kodo millet (*Paspalum scrobiculatum*), teff (*Eragrostis tef*), fonio (*Digitaria exilis* and *D. iburua*), and little millet (*Panicum sumatrense*), contribute the remaining 4% of production. Pearl millet is a dietary staple in Niger, where the supply for food use is 426 g day^{-1} per person, providing over 70% of the total dietary cereal. High consumption levels are found in other African countries (Burkina Faso, Mali, Gambia, Namibia, Nigeria, Senegal, and Chad), where the supply for food use ranges from 100 g day^{-1} to 200 g day^{-1} per person.

Oats

World oat production is about 26 million tonnes annually (**Table 1**). Oats (*Avena sativa*) require a temperate climate and thrive in cool wet conditions but are less cold tolerant than rye, wheat, or barley. Approximately 11% of world production is used for food. Formerly a dietary staple in Northern and Western Europe, oats now contribute modestly to diets worldwide (**Table 2**). Dietary intakes are highest in Belarus, Estonia, and Finland, where supplies for food use are 24, 20, and 18 g day^{-1} per person, respectively. However, these data are for oat grain,

which includes 18–36% of fibrous inedible hull, which is removed in the first stages of milling to yield caryopses (groats). Naked or hull-less types also exist. Groats are further processed by cutting, rolling, or grinding to yield a range of oatmeal, oat-flake, and oat-flour products. These are wholemeal products with a composition similar to the groats. Oat bran, which is less structurally distinct than wheat bran, is made by sieving coarse-milled groats. Oat-mill products can be used for traditional porridge and oatcakes, as an ingredient in baby foods, and in breakfast cereals. Oats cannot be used to make good quality bread, but oat flour can be incorporated at 20–30% in wheat breads.

Rye

Rye (*Secale cereale*) is grown in temperate regions and is the most cold-tolerant of the cereals. World rye production is about 20 million tonnes annually (**Table 1**). About 33% of rye production is used for food and about 15% for industrial use, including whisky production. Food intakes are highest in Eastern and Central Europe, the Baltic states, and Scandinavia. Per capita supplies for food use in these countries are: Belarus, 110 g day^{-1}; Poland, 108 g day^{-1}; Austria, 39 g day^{-1}; Ukraine, 36 g day^{-1}; Slovakia, 31 g day^{-1}; Lithuania, 57 g day^{-1}; Estonia, 54 g day^{-1}; Finland, 46 g day^{-1}; Denmark, 36 g day^{-1}, and Sweden, 35 g day^{-1}. Harvested rye is a caryopsis, and it is milled to extractions ranging from 65% to wholemeal (100%). Rye flour is used to make crispbreads and yeast-leavened breads, where it is often mixed with wheat flour.

Energy, Macronutrient, and Fiber Content

Tables 3–6 show the water, energy, macronutrient, and fiber contents of cereals and cereal products. The macronutrients (carbohydrate, protein, and fat) and dietary fiber comprise the bulk of the dry

Table 3 Water, energy, macronutrient, and fiber contents of rice and maize (corn) products; representative values per 100 g

	Brown rice, uncooked	White rice, uncooked	Brown rice, boiled	White rice, boiled	White rice, flour	Maize meal	Cornflour	Cornflakes[a]
Water (g)	13.9	11.7	56.0	69.9	11.9	12.2	12.5	3.0
Energy (kJ)	1518	1536	599	522	1531	1517	1508	1515
Energy (kcal)	357	361	141	123	366	357	354	355
Carbohydrate (g)	81.3	86.8	32.1	29.6	80.1	77.2	92.0	84.9
Protein (g)	6.7	6.5	2.6	2.2	6.0	9.4	0.6	7.9
Fat (g)	2.8	1.0	1.1	0.3	1.4	3.3	0.7	0.6
Dietary fiber (g)	1.9	0.5	0.8	0.2	2.4	2.2	0.1	0.9

[a]Ready-to-eat cereal.

Table 4 Water, energy, macronutrient, and fiber contents of wheat products; representative values per 100 g

	Wholemeal flour	White bread-making flour	Bran	White bread	Wholemeal bread	Uncooked pasta[a]	Boiled pasta[a]
Water (g)	14.0	14.0	8.3	37.3	38.3	9.7	75.9
Energy (kJ)	1320	1452	872	1002	915	1473	411
Energy (kcal)	310	341	206	236	215	346	97
Carbohydrate (g)	63.9	75.3	26.8	49.3	41.6	74.9	20.9
Protein (g)	12.7	11.5	14.1	8.4	9.2	12.0	3.2
Fat (g)	2.2	1.4	5.5	1.9	2.5	1.9	0.6
Dietary fiber (g)	9.0	3.1	36.4	1.5	5.8	3.0	1.0

[a]Mean of lasagne, macaroni, and white spaghetti.

Table 5 Water, energy, macronutrient, and fiber contents of barley, oat, and rye products; representative values per 100 g

	Pearl barley, uncooked	Pearl barley, boiled	Oatmeal	Oatmeal porridge[a]	Oat bran	Wholemeal rye flour	Rye crispbread	Rye bread
Water (g)	10.6	69.6	8.5	87.4	9.5	15.0	6.4	37.4
Energy (kJ)	1535	510	1644	210	1478	1268	1367	937
Energy (kcal)	360	120	388	50	349	298	321	220
Carbohydrate (g)	83.6	27.6	69.4	9.0	53.5	65.9	70.6	45.8
Protein (g)	7.9	2.7	11.8	1.5	19.8	8.2	9.4	8.3
Fat (g)	1.7	0.6	9.0	1.1	7.7	2.0	2.1	1.7
Dietary fiber (g)	5.9	2.0	7.0	0.8	15.1	11.7	11.7	4.4

[a]Made with water and salt.

Table 6 Water, energy, macronutrient, and fiber contents of sorghum and millets; representative values per 100 g

		Millets					
	Sorghum	Pearl	Foxtail	Proso	Finger	Japanese	Fonio
Water (g)	12.0	11.0	11.3	13.5	11.7	11.1	10.0
Energy (kJ)	1422	1468	1364	1491	1377	1382	1541
Energy (kcal)	335	346	321	351	323	326	363
Carbohydrate (g)	69.9	68.1	67.8	70.7	76.0	65.4	75.8
Protein (g)	10.7	11.8	9.9	11.6	6.4	10.4	8.5
Fat (g)	3.3	4.8	3.0	4.4	1.4	4.3	3.5
Dietary fiber (g)	7.5	6.9	n/a	n/a	n/a	n/a	8.5

n/a, no data available.

matter of cereals. Carbohydrates are the major constituent, and there is a nutritionally significant amount of protein. Cereals can also be an important source of dietary fiber. However, most cereals are low in fat.

Dietary Energy

Dietary energy values are inversely related to water contents and also depend on the relative amounts of the macronutrients (digestible carbohydrate, protein, and fat). Fat has over twice the energy per gram of carbohydrate or protein, and thus differences in dietary energy are largely determined by variations in the levels of fat, water, and indigestible components (principally fiber). Energy values are higher when fat is higher and lower when water or fiber contents are higher (**Tables 3–6**). Higher fiber contents are found in whole-grain and bran-rich products, while water and fat contents may be changed during processing.

Carbohydrates

Digestible carbohydrate, in the form of starch, is the major dry-matter component of all cereals (**Tables 3–6**). Sugars, which usually account for much less than 1% of cereal grain, may be added in processing; cornflakes, for example, have about 7% sugars. Cornflour is a milling product with a very high starch content (**Table 3**). Most cereal starches are 20–30% amylose, the rest being amylopectin. However, there are types of rice, maize, and barley with up to 80% amylose or with up to 100% amylopectin (waxy types). In some cereal products a small proportion of the starch (up to 3%) exists as resistant starch, which resists enzymatic digestion. Digestible starch yields glucose. However, the rate of digestion and absorption is influenced by the degree of processing among other factors. Thus, there can be substantial variations in the post-prandial blood glucose responses following ingestion of equivalent digestible-carbohydrate loads from different cereal products.

Protein

Protein is the major nitrogen-containing component of cereal grains, and most protein data are based on nitrogen determination, followed by multiplication by a nitrogen-to-protein conversion factor. The general factor is 6.25, but factors vary from 5.7 to 6.31 for cereal products. Representative values for protein content (**Tables 3–6**) show that levels are lowest in rice, barley, and finger millet and highest in wheat, oats, pearl millet, and proso millet. However, the protein content of cereals can vary substantially, and greater than 2-fold ranges in protein content are found in crops of the same species. This variation is due partly to genetic differences, but agronomic factors are of greater importance. This variation is of little significance when crops are handled in bulk, as in modern milling and processing, but it may be important in less-developed regions. Although not usually considered a good protein source, many cereals provide an adequate amount, relative to energy, for adults. However, protein quality must also be considered, since cereal-based diets tend to be deficient in one or more essential amino-acids (see below).

Protein quality Cereal protein consists predominantly of endosperm storage proteins, which are low in dietary essential (indispensable) amino-acids. These amino-acids are required in differing amounts, and thus quality can be considered only in relation to requirements. Furthermore, requirements can differ. The most notable differences are related to age: the young have higher requirements for both protein and essential amino-acids than do adults. The first limiting essential amino-acid in cereals is generally lysine. However, there are variations between cereals. In oats, rice, and finger millet the deficiency in lysine may be only

Table 7 Amino-acid composition of rice, maize, wheat, barley, oats, and rye; representative values in grams per 100 g protein

Amino-acid	Rice	Maize	Wheat	Barley	Oats	Rye
Essential						
Histidine	2.4	2.6	2.3	2.1	2.1	2.2
Isoleucine	3.8	3.6	3.5	3.5	3.8	3.5
Leucine	8.2	11.1	6.7	6.7	7.2	6.2
Lysine	3.7	2.3	2.7	2.6	3.7	3.4
Methionine	2.1	1.6	1.2	1.6	1.8	1.4
Cysteine	1.6	2.0	2.5	2.2	2.7	1.9
Phenylalanine	4.8	4.4	4.6	5.1	5.0	4.5
Tyrosine	4.0	3.5	1.7	3.0	3.4	1.9
Threonine	3.4	3.3	2.8	3.4	3.4	3.4
Tryptophan	1.3	0.7	1.5	1.6	1.3	1.1
Valine	5.8	4.0	4.3	5.0	5.1	4.8
Non-essential						
Alanine	5.8	8.2	3.5	4.2	4.5	4.3
Arginine	7.5	4.4	4.3	4.8	6.2	4.6
Aspartic acid	9.6	7.2	4.9	5.6	7.7	7.2
Glutamic acid	19.2	18.6	32.1	23.5	21.0	24.2
Glycine	4.3	3.9	4.0	3.8	4.6	4.3
Proline	4.6	8.8	10.7	10.9	5.1	9.4
Serine	4.6	4.6	4.5	4.0	4.6	3.8

marginal, while in sorghum, maize, and other millets it is more pronounced (**Tables 7** and **8**). Tryptophan is also limiting in maize and some millets, while threonine and methionine may also be limiting in some cereals. Protein quality must be considered in relation to total protein content. Furthermore, as protein content is increased, for example by the use of nitrogenous fertilizer, the relative amounts of the essential amino-acids tend to decline as percentages of the protein. High-lysine types of maize, barley, and sorghum have been identified. However, their lower grain yield precludes their wide use.

Fat

Cereals are generally very low in fat, most containing only 2–4% (**Tables 3–6**). However, some types of maize and oats have more than 10% fat. The distribution of fat within the grain is variable. In oats the fat is distributed throughout the endosperm; in maize it is concentrated in the germ, from which it can be extracted after separation, while rice bran contains 15–20% oil depending on production conditions. Fat is often added in processing, for example in baked products.

Fatty acid composition Cereal fat is liquid at room temperature; it is high in unsaturates and is more correctly described as oil. The major fatty acids in cereal oils are oleic acid (monounsaturated), linoleic acid (polyunsaturated), and palmitic acid

Table 8 Amino-acid composition of sorghum and millets; representative values in grams per 100 g protein

Amino-acid	Sorghum	Millets					
		Pearl	Foxtail	Proso	Finger	Japanese	Fonio
Essential							
Histidine	2.2	2.2	2.3	2.2	2.6	1.9	2.2
Isoleucine	4.1	4.4	5.0	4.5	5.1	4.5	4.1
Leucine	14.6	12.2	13.3	12.9	13.5	11.5	10.8
Lysine	2.2	3.3	2.1	2.2	3.7	1.7	2.2
Methionine	1.4	2.2	2.6	2.0	2.6	1.8	4.3
Cysteine	1.7	1.5	1.4	1.7	1.6	1.5	2.5
Phenylalanine	5.0	5.2	5.3	5.2	6.2	5.9	5.9
Tyrosine	3.2	3.2	2.7	3.9	3.6	2.7	3.7
Threonine	3.3	3.9	3.9	3.4	5.1	2.7	3.7
Tryptophan	1.1	1.6	1.5	0.9	1.3	1.0	1.6
Valine	5.4	5.7	5.2	5.1	7.9	6.1	5.5
Non-essential							
Alanine	9.1	8.5	8.9	9.3	8.0	9.2	9.4
Arginine	4.3	4.8	6.1	4.4	5.2	3.2	3.6
Aspartic acid	6.4	8.7	6.9	5.5	7.9	6.3	9.0
Glutamic acid	22.6	21.2	18.8	20.5	27.1	20.7	22.3
Glycine	3.2	3.6	2.9	2.2	4.8	2.7	3.0
Proline	7.6	7.2	10.6	7.2	6.7	10.3	7.2
Serine	4.2	4.9	5.8	6.3	6.9	5.8	5.4

(saturated), and representative values for the fatty-acid compositions of cereals are given in **Table 9**. Stearic and linolenic acids are present in small but significant amounts, and a range of other fatty acids are present in trace amounts.

Dietary Fiber

Although it is not a nutrient, dietary fiber is being increasingly recognized as important in the prevention or alleviation of disease. Fiber can also yield some dietary energy from short-chain fatty acids produced by fermentation in the large intestine. Fiber is concentrated in the outer bran layers of cereals, and thus levels are higher in bran and whole-grain products than in refined milling products (**Tables 3–5**). Dietary fiber includes cellulose and other insoluble and soluble non-starch polysaccharides. Resistant starch, lignin, and other minor components are included in some definitions. A significant amount of soluble fiber (3–5%) occurs as β-glucan gum in oats and barley. A minimum of 5.5% β-glucan is found in oat bran. This gum is the major factor responsible for the reductions in serum cholesterol that result from diets high in these cereals. Wheat bran, which improves gut function, is high in total fiber (40%) but contains only 3–4% soluble fiber.

Table 9 Fatty-acid composition of cereals; representative values in grams per 100 g total fatty acids (total includes 2–3% of trace fatty acids)

	Palmitic acid (16:0)	Stearic acid (18:0)	Oleic acid (18:1)	Linoleic acid (18:2)	Linolenic acid (18:3)
Rice	22	2	34	38	2
Maize	12	2	32	50	2
Wheat	18	2	18	56	3
Barley	22	1	13	56	5
Sorghum	13	2	34	46	2
Pearl millet	20	4	26	44	3
Foxtail millet	10	3	17	64	3
Proso millet	9	2	21	64	2
Finger millet	24	2	46	24	1
Kodo millet	18	2	36	40	2
Oats	19	2	36	38	2
Rye	15	1	17	58	7

Micronutrient Content

Micronutrients comprise the inorganic mineral elements and the vitamins. Ash (inorganic mineral matter) comprises 1–3% of grain dry matter. Major mineral elements (potassium, sodium, calcium, phosphorus, and magnesium) and minor or trace elements (iron, zinc, copper, manganese, etc.) are found in all cereals. However, there are significant variations due to processing and other factors (**Tables 10–13**). There can also be substantial variations in the levels of trace minerals between crops due primarily to differences in their availability from the soil.

All cereals provide vitamin E (tocopherols and tocotrienols; tocols), thiamin, riboflavin, niacin, vitamin B$_6$, pantothenate, folate, and biotin (**Tables 10–13**). Vitamin A (retinol) is not found in cereals. However, carotenes and cryptoxanthins, which yield retinol and thus have provitamin A activity, are found in maize, pearl millet, and sorghum. Levels of provitamin A are variable, with the highest amounts in yellow endosperm types and negligible amounts in white endosperm types. Typical values for retinol equivalents in maize, pearl millet, and sorghum are 44, 42, and 8 µg 100 g^{-1}, respectively. Brown rice contains a trace amount (0–11 µg 100 g^{-1}, and most of this is lost on milling. Vitamin A deficiency can be a major problem in areas where rice is a dietary staple. In an effort to combat this, rice has recently been genetically modified to produce so called 'golden rice' with provitamin A levels of about 160 µg 100 g^{-1}. Vitamins B$_{12}$, C, and D are not found in unfortified cereals.

Effects of Processing

Vitamin and mineral contents may be profoundly influenced by processing. Vitamins and minerals are found at the highest concentrations in the outer bran layers. Comparison of the various whole-grain and milled products in **Tables 10–12** shows that bran is richer in vitamins and minerals, while flour and meal fractions are depleted. Sodium may be substantially increased by the addition of salt (**Tables 10–12**), leavening agents, or other additives. Other minerals and vitamins are often added as fortification to replace, standardize, or augment the levels naturally present. Although white bread made from fortified flour has a lower mineral and vitamin content than wholemeal bread (**Table 11**), wholemeal bread contains higher levels of phytic acid, which will influence availability (see below). Cornflour contains low levels of minerals and only traces of vitamins. Cornflakes are fortified with a number of minerals and vitamins, including vitamins B$_{12}$ and D (**Table 10**). The fortification of breads and other cereal foodstuffs with folic acid has recently become increasingly common.

Table 10 Mineral and vitamin contents of rice and maize (corn) products; representative values per 100 g fresh weight (water contents as per **Table 3**)

	Brown rice, uncooked	White rice, uncooked	Brown rice, boiled[a]	White rice, boiled[a]	White rice, flour	Maize meal	Cornflakes[b]
Sodium (mg)	3	6	1	2	5	40	1110
Potassium (mg)	250	110	99	38	76	350	100
Calcium (mg)	10	4	4	1	10	20	15
Magnesium (mg)	110	13	43	4	35	140	14
Phosphorus (mg)	310	100	120	34	98	290	38
Iron (mg)	1.4	0.5	0.5	0.2	0.4	3	6.7
Zinc (mg)	1.8	1.3	0.7	0.5	0.8	2	0.3
Copper (mg)	0.85	0.18	0.33	0.06	0.13	0.40	0.03
Manganese (mg)	2.30	0.87	0.90	0.30	1.20	0.60	0.08
Vitamin E (mg)	0.80	0.10	0.30	0.02	0.13	0.50	0.40
Thiamin (mg)	0.59	0.08	0.14	0.01	0.14	0.40	1.00
Riboflavin (mg)	0.07	0.02	0.02	0.01	0.02	0.11	1.50
Niacin (mg)	5.3	1.5	1.3	0.3	2.6	2.2	16.0
Vitamin B$_6$ (mg)	0.70	0.30	0.30	0.10	0.44	0.53	1.80
Pantothenate (mg)	1.2	0.6	0.4	0.2	0.8	0.6	0.3
Folate (µg)	40	20	10	3	4	40	250
Biotin (µg)	7	3	2	1	n/a	10	2

[a]Unsalted water.
[b]Ready-to-eat cereal, fortified.
n/a, no data available.

Table 11 Mineral and vitamin content of wheat products; representative values per 100 g fresh weight (water contents as per **Table 4**)

	Wholemeal flour[a]	White flour[a]	Bran	White bread[b]	Wholemeal bread[a]	Uncooked pasta[c]	Boiled pasta[c,d]
Sodium (mg)	3	3	28	520	550	8	1
Potassium (mg)	340	130	1160	110	230	237	24
Calcium (mg)	38	15	110	110	54	24	6
Magnesium (mg)	120	31	520	24	76	52	14
Phosphorus (mg)	320	120	1200	91	200	190	45
Iron (mg)	3.9	1.5	12.9	1.6	2.7	1.8	0.5
Zinc (mg)	2.9	0.9	16.2	0.6	1.8	1.5	0.5
Copper (mg)	0.45	0.18	1.34	0.20	0.26	0.30	0.09
Manganese (mg)	3.14	0.68	9.00	0.45	1.90	0.87	0.25
Vitamin E (mg)	1.40	0.30	2.60	trace	0.20	trace	trace
Thiamin (mg)	0.50	0.10	0.90	0.21	0.34	0.30	0.03
Riboflavin (mg)	0.09	0.03	0.36	0.06	0.09	0.05	0.01
Niacin (mg)	5.7	0.7	29.6	1.7	4.1	2.8	0.5
Vitamin B$_6$ (mg)	0.50	0.15	1.38	0.07	0.12	0.13	0.01
Pantothenate (mg)	0.8	0.3	2.4	0.3	0.6	0.3	trace
Folate (μg)	57	22	260	30	40	30	4
Biotin (μg)	7	1	45	1	6	1	trace

[a]Unfortified.
[b]Made from UK fortified white flour containing 140 mg calcium, 2.1 mg iron, 0.32 mg thiamin, 2.0 mg niacin per 100 g.
[c]Means of lasagne, macaroni, and white spaghetti.
[d]Unsalted water.

Availability

The presence of micronutrients does not ensure availability for metabolic processes. Mineral availability is reduced by the presence of phytic acid and phytates. Phytic acid (myoinositol 1,2,3,4,5,6-hexakis dihydrogen phosphate) accounts for a substantial proportion (usually over 50%) of the total phosphorus in cereals, and this phosphorus is not fully available for digestion and absorption. Phytic acid accounts for about 1% of whole-grain cereals. However, phytic

Table 12 Mineral and vitamin contents of barley, oat and rye products; representative values per 100 g fresh weight (water contents as per **Table 5**)

	Pearl barley, uncooked	Pearl barley, boiled[a]	Oatmeal	Oatmeal, porridge[b]	Oat bran	Wholemeal rye flour	Rye crispbread	Rye bread
Sodium (mg)	3	1	21	560	4	1	220	580
Potassium (mg)	270	92	360	46	586	410	500	190
Calcium (mg)	20	7	54	7	79	32	45	80
Magnesium (mg)	65	22	110	18	241	92	100	48
Phosphorus (mg)	210	71	380	47	723	360	310	160
Iron (mg)	3.0	1.0	4.0	0.5	6.1	2.7	3.5	2.5
Zinc (mg)	2.1	0.7	3.3	0.4	4.2	3.0	3.0	1.3
Copper (mg)	0.40	0.14	0.36	0.03	0.31	0.42	0.38	0.18
Manganese (mg)	1.30	0.44	3.80	0.46	5.80	0.68	3.50	1.00
Vitamin E (mg)	0.40	0.10	1.60	0.21	3.30	1.60	0.50	1.20
Thiamin (mg)	0.12	0.02	0.70	0.06	1.10	0.40	0.28	0.29
Riboflavin (mg)	0.05	0.01	0.10	0.01	0.18	0.22	0.14	0.05
Niacin (mg)	2.5	0.5	0.9	0.1	0.9	1.0	1.1	2.3
Vitamin B$_6$ (mg)	0.22	0.04	0.23	0.01	0.15	0.35	0.29	0.09
Pantothenate (mg)	0.5	0.1	1.1	0.1	1.0	1.0	1.1	0.5
Folate (μg)	20	3	60	4	37	78	35	24
Biotin (μg)	n/a	trace	21	2	38	6	7	n/a

[a]Unsalted water.
[b]Made with water and salt.
n/a, no data available.

Table 13 Mineral and vitamin contents of sorghum and millets; representative values per 100 g fresh weight (water contents as per Table 6)

	Sorghum	Millets					
		Pearl	Foxtail	Proso	Finger	Japanese	Fonio
Sodium (mg)	20.5	7.4	6.8	9.4	15.9	n/a	15.0
Potassium (mg)	285	432	243	215	367	n/a	160
Calcium (mg)	28	39	22	14	321	32	30
Magnesium (mg)	156	125	116	104	129	n/a	40
Phosphorus (mg)	291	335	268	220	251	330	175
Iron (mg)	5.1	8.4	5.3	4.7	4.6	4.3	6.0
Zinc (mg)	2.2	3.2	1.9	1.6	1.3	n/a	3.0
Copper (mg)	0.98	0.50	0.71	1.15	0.53	n/a	1.6
Manganese (mg)	1.84	1.45	1.87	1.64	1.19	n/a	3.0
Vitamin E (mg)	1.13	1.69	2.75	1.94	n/a	n/a	n/a
Thiamin (mg)	0.35	0.34	0.51	0.39	0.35	0.33	0.47
Riboflavin (mg)	0.15	0.17	0.10	0.19	0.10	0.10	0.10
Niacin (mg)	3.8	2.0	3.1	1.3	4.0	n/a	1.9
Vitamin B_6 (mg)	0.50	n/a	n/a	n/a	n/a	n/a	n/a
Pantothenate (mg)	1.2	1.1	0.7	1.0	n/a	n/a	n/a
Folate (μg)	19	63	18	n/a	n/a	n/a	n/a
Biotin (μg)	42	n/a	n/a	n/a	n/a	n/a	n/a

n/a, no data available.

acid is concentrated in the bran and germ fractions. Wheat bran and germ contain 3–4% phytic acid, while white endosperm flour contains 0.1–0.2%. Phytic acid reacts with calcium, magnesium, iron, zinc, and copper to form phytates, a process that renders these minerals unavailable for absorption.

Vitamin B_6 and niacin in cereals are also of limited availability. The niacin deficiency disease pellagra may develop where maize grits are the dietary staple. However, niacin, which is present in a bound form, is made available by alkali treatment in traditional maize tortilla production. Niacin can also be synthesized in the body from tryptophan; 60 mg of tryptophan yields 1 mg of niacin.

Dietary Contribution

Data on the relative amounts of minerals and vitamins present in cereals are useful for comparative purposes. However, data on availability and requirements are needed to give a fuller evaluation. Relative to energy content, whole-grain cereals have the potential to contribute significantly to intakes of potassium, magnesium, phosphorus, iron, copper, zinc, vitamin E, thiamin, riboflavin, niacin, vitamin B_6, and folic acid. Significant dietary selenium may also be provided, although levels depend on its availability in the soil.

Non-Nutrients of Potential Benefit

In addition to dietary fiber, cereals contain a number of other non-nutrient components, present in minor amounts, that have the potential to exert beneficial physiological effects. Some of these phytochemicals, which include phytic acid, sterols, phenolics, and flavonoids, have been shown to have *in vitro* antioxidant and oestrogen-like activities. Fiber and phytochemicals are found at their highest levels in bran and unrefined grain. Thus, these components may play an important role in the protective effects against heart disease and certain cancers that are conferred by diets rich in whole grains.

Potential Adverse Effects

Cereals do not have any intrinsic non-specific toxins. However, acrylamide, a carcinogen and potential neurotoxin, has recently been found at levels up to 120 μg $100\,g^{-1}$ in baked and fried foods, including breads and processed cereals. Research is ongoing, but the early indications are that acrylamide from these sources is unlikely to increase cancer risk. Detrimental effects may be caused by antinutrients in cereals and, in susceptible individuals, by adverse immune responses (celiac disease, food allergies). Cereals may also be a source of toxins of fungal origin (mycotoxins) or of toxic environmental, agricultural, or industrial contaminants.

Antinutrients

Phytic acid and phytates are antinutrients that are found in all cereals. They reduce mineral availability (see above). Tannins are polyphenolic compounds that are found in most cereals. Tannins can bind to protein, reducing its digestibility. Tannins can also inhibit the activity of digestive enzymes. In addition, cereals contain specific protease inhibitors, but the levels are low in comparison with those found in some seed legumes. The tannins and protease inhibitors are unlikely to have any significant adverse effects in human nutrition. However, pearl millet contains phenolic flavonoids, which have been implicated in the onset of goitre, a symptom of iodine deficiency.

Adverse Immune Responses

Many natural products, including cereals and other common foodstuffs, induce allergic responses in susceptible individuals. In such cases, after appropriate diagnosis, the individual should avoid the foodstuff responsible. Celiac disease (gluten enteropathy) is a condition characterized by a severe adverse immunological gastrointestinal reaction to gliadin, which is a component of gluten, the viscoelastic protein found in wheat and other cereals. Celiac disease is prevalent in all regions where wheat is commonly consumed, and its incidence may reach 0.5% of the population. Celiac patients must exclude gluten from their diets. Thus, products containing wheat, rye, barley, and triticale are not permitted. Although oats were originally proscribed, it is now becoming increasingly clear that they are safe for celiac patients.

Mycotoxins

Mycotoxins are produced by fungi, which may infect growing crops and stored grain. Ergot (*Claviceps purpurea*) infects rye and other temperate cereals and produces alkaloid toxins. If ingested in sufficient amounts, these alkaloids induce mental derangement, gangrene, and other symptoms. Aflatoxin, a toxin and potent carcinogen, is produced by the fungus *Aspergillus flavus*, which may occur in maize crops and stored grain. Other fungal toxins include ochratoxin, produced by *Penicillium* species, and trichothecenes, produced by *Fusarium* species. Mycotoxins are less of a problem in cereals than in seed legumes and nuts. Mycotoxin levels can be controlled by correct agronomy and storage, and crops are monitored to ensure that safe levels are not exceeded.

Contaminants

Cereals have the potential to be contaminated with toxic environmental, agricultural, or industrial chemicals in the field and during storage and processing.

However, the use of these chemicals is strictly controlled, and incidents of hazardous contamination are rare.

See also: **Bioavailability**. **Cancer**: Epidemiology and Associations Between Diet and Cancer. **Celiac Disease**. **Coronary Heart Disease**: Prevention. **Dietary Fiber**: Physiological Effects and Effects on Absorption. **Folic Acid**. **Food Fortification**: Developed Countries; Developing Countries. **Food Intolerance**. **Food Safety**: Other Contaminants. **Legumes**. **Niacin**. **Nuts and Seeds**. **Pellagra**. **Phytochemicals**: Classification and Occurrence. **Protein**: Deficiency. **Vitamin A**: Biochemistry and Physiological Role. **Whole Grains**.

Further Reading

Anderson JW (2002) Whole-grains intake and risk for coronary heart disease. In: Marquart L, Slavin JL, and Fulcher RG (eds.) *Whole Grain Foods in Health and Disease*, pp. 187–200. St Paul: American Association of Cereal Chemists.

Betschart AA (1988) Nutritional quality of wheat and wheat foods. In: Pomeranz Y (ed.) *Wheat: Chemistry and Technology*, 3rd edn, vol. II, pp. 91–130. St Paul: American Association of Cereal Chemists.

Bhatty RS (1993) Nonmalting uses of barley. In: MacGregor AW and Bhatty RS (eds.) *Barley: Chemistry and Technology*, pp. 355–417. St Paul: American Association of Cereal Chemists.

Dendy DAV (2001) Sorghum and millets. In: Dendy DAV and Dobraszczyk BJ (eds.) *Cereals and Cereal Products: Chemistry and Technology*, pp. 341–366. Gaithersburg: Aspen Publishers Inc.

Haq N and Ogbe FD (1995) Fonio (*Digitaria exilis* and *D. iburua*). In: Williams JT (ed.) *Cereals and Pseudocereals*, pp. 225–245. London: Chapman & Hall.

Juliano BO (1985) Production and utilization of rice. In: Juliano BO (ed.) *Rice: Chemistry and Technology*, 2nd edn, pp. 1–16. St Paul: American Association of Cereal Chemists.

Juliano BO and Bechtel DB (1985) The rice grain and its gross composition. In: Juliano BO (ed.) *Rice: Chemistry and Technology*, 2nd edn, pp. 17–57. St Paul: American Association of Cereal Chemists.

Klopfenstein CF and Hoseney RC (1995) Nutritional properties of sorghum and the millets. In: Dendy DAV (ed.) *Sorghum and Millets: Chemistry and Technology*, pp. 125–168. St Paul: American Association of Cereal Chemists.

Lorenz KJ (1991) Rye. In: Lorenz KJ and Kulp K (eds.) *Handbook of Cereal Science and Technology*, pp. 331–371. New York: Marcel Dekker.

McIntosh GH and Jacobs DR (2002) Cereal-grain foods, fibers and cancer prevention. In: Marquart L, Slavin JL, and Fulcher RG (eds.) *Whole Grain Foods in Health and Disease*, pp. 201–232. St Paul: American Association of Cereal Chemists.

Obilana AB and Manyasa E (2002) Millets. In: Belton PS and Taylor JRN (eds.) *Pseudocereals and Less Common Cereals*, pp. 177–217. Berlin: Springer Verlag.

Pomeranz Y (1988) Chemical composition of kernel structures. In: Pomeranz Y (ed.) *Wheat: Chemistry and Technology*,

3rd edn, vol. I, pp. 97–158. St Paul: American Association of Cereal Chemists.

Poutanen K, Liukkonen K, and Adlercreutz H (2002) Whole grains, phytoestrogens, and health. In: Marquart L, Slavin JL, and Fulcher RG (eds.) *Whole Grain Foods in Health and Disease*, pp. 259–268. St Paul: American Association of Cereal Chemists.

Rooney LW and Serna-Saldivar SO (1987) Food uses of whole corn and dry-milled fractions. In: Watson SA and Ramstad PE (eds.) *Corn: Chemistry and Technology*, pp. 399–429. St Paul: American Association of Cereal Chemists.

Serna-Saldivar S and Rooney LW (1995) Structure and chemistry of sorghum and millets. In: Dendy DAV (ed.) *Sorghum and Millets: Chemistry and Technology*, pp. 69–124. St Paul: American Association of Cereal Chemists.

Shewry PR and Bechtel DB (2001) Morphology and Chemistry of the Rye Grain. In: Bushuk W (ed.) *Rye: Production, Chemistry and Technology*, pp. 69–127. St Paul: American Association of Cereal Chemists.

Taylor JRN and Belton PS (2002) Sorghum. In: Belton PS and Taylor JRN (eds.) *Pseudocereals and Less Common Cereals*, pp. 25–91. Berlin: Springer Verlag.

Watson SA (1987) Structure and composition. In: Watson SA and Ramstad PE (eds.) *Corn: Chemistry and Technology*, pp. 53–82. St Paul: American Association of Cereal Chemists.

Welch RW (1995) Oats in Human Nutrition and Health. In: Welch RW (ed.) *The Oat Crop – Production and Utilization*, pp. 433–479. London: Chapman & Hall.

Welch RW (1995) The Chemical Composition of Oats. In: Welch RW (ed.) *The Oat Crop – Production and Utilization*, pp. 279–320. London: Chapman & Hall.

Cheese *see* **Dairy Products**

CHILDREN

Contents
Nutritional Requirements
Nutritional Problems

Nutritional Requirements

M Lawson, Institute of Child Health, London, UK

© 2005 Elsevier Ltd. All rights reserved.

Nutrition is particularly important in childhood because nutrients are required not only for general health and maintenance of body composition but also for linear growth, neurological development, body maturation, and as a basis for long-term health. There is considerable evidence of an association between early nutrition and later risk of diseases such as cardiovascular disease, obesity, and type 2 diabetes.

Two major factors affect nutrient requirements during infancy, childhood, and adolescence: body size and growth velocity. Growth velocity varies according to age, and age is used as a general proxy for weight velocity. Nutritional requirements for children should therefore be expressed in terms of units of body weight for each age throughout childhood. Nutrient requirements per unit of body weight are highest at birth and reduce as growth velocity decreases.

The pattern of nutrient requirement changes and is not constant per unit of body weight as body composition changes throughout the growing period from birth until the end of puberty. This is illustrated in **Figure 1**, which shows the changes in energy and protein requirements per kilogram body weight between birth and 15 years. Nutrient requirements are therefore both quantitatively and qualitatively different from those of adults.

For infants, breast milk is used as a model for assessing nutrient requirements. However, although breast milk is the 'gold standard' on which infant formulas are based, the physiological actions of nutrients and other components of breast milk and

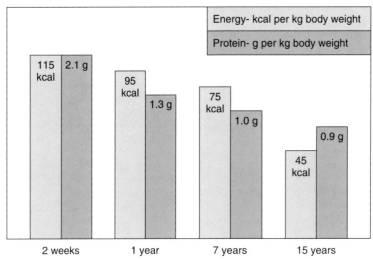

Figure 1 Changes in protein and energy requirements during infancy and childhood.

bioavailability of nutrients are quite different between breast milk and infant formula. In addition, breast milk composition changes during the duration of a feed and it is difficult to estimate the usual volumes of breast milk consumed. Dietary reference values are therefore only applicable to artificially fed infants: An adequate quantity of breast milk is assumed to meet all nutrient requirements for the majority of infants up until the age of approximately 6 months.

Estimates of physiological requirements are used to make dietary recommendations, which depend on the usual diet of the country or area. Again, estimates cannot be 'scaled down' versions of adult requirements because bioavailability of many nutrients varies with age, physiological state, and nutritional status. For example, iron absorption is poor during the first 6 months of life, increases during later infancy, and is greatest during adolescence.

Requirements for children are estimated from a limited number of direct studies of body composition and body content of children at different ages. Most of these were carried out on children living in unfavorable environments and very little data exist on normally nourished children, particularly those aged between 1 and 5 years. Recommendations are often extrapolated from adult studies. For most nutrients, energy and protein requirements are not known with any great precision and are expressed as units per day.

Discrepancies between recommendations published by different countries or authorities are due to a number of factors: Different assumptions are made about weight at a particular age, growth velocity, and age of onset of puberty, and different age groupings are used by different authorities. Some countries give recommendations for each year of life, whereas others aggregate several years together, giving an overestimation for the youngest ages and underestimation for older children in each age band. Some countries separate recommendations for males and females as early as the second year; others separate them at a later age or only during adolescence. **Table 1** illustrates the framework on which different recommendations and reference values are based. Diets of varying composition will affect bioavailability and, as a consequence, recommendations for dietary intake. Therefore, it is difficult to compare recommendations from different authorities and very large discrepancies exist in recommendations for some nutrients.

Energy

Most energy recommendations for infants and children are based on the 1985 FAO/WHO/UNU report and are shown in **Tables 2** and **3**. The FAO/WHO data have been reviewed recently and it is likely that a number of revisions to the 1985 document are required in light of additional information and the development of new assessment techniques such as doubly labeled water. Energy requirements expressed in terms of body weight are highest during the first few months of life, decrease fairly sharply after the age of 1 year, and then show a gradual decline until the onset of puberty, when they increase. This mirrors the growth velocity seen at different ages.

Table 1 Terminology for nutritional recommendations

Authority	Mean − 2SD	Mean	Mean + 2SD	Less evidence-based data	Upper limit of intake
United Kingdom	Lower Reference Nutrient Intake (LNRI)	Estimated Average Requirement (EAR)	Reference Nutrient Intake (RNI)	Estimated Safe + Adequate Dietary Intake (ESADI)	
European Union	Lowest Threshold of Intake (LTI)	Average Requirement (AR)	Population Reference Intake (PRI)	Acceptable Ranges	
USA/ Canada	—	Estimated Average Requirement (EAR)	Recommended Dietary Allowance (RDA)	Adequate Intake (AI)	Tolerable Upper Intake Level (TUL)
FAO/WHO	—	Estimated Average Requirement (EAR)	Recommended Dietary Intake (RDI)	—	Upper Tolerable Nutrient Intake (TUL)

The review suggests that the 1985 recommendations for dietary energy are too high for children younger than 5 years and possibly those younger than 7 years of age, whereas recommendations for adolescent boys and pubertal girls appear to be set too low, particularly in developing countries. The 1985 recommendations increased reported energy intakes by a factor of 5% to accommodate a 'desirable' level of physical activity. This may not be realistic in the increasingly sedentary environment seen in industrialized countries, and it has been suggested that recommendations for energy intake should be accompanied by recommendations for activity levels.

The proportion of dietary energy that is required to sustain normal growth varies according to the growth velocity at that particular age. **Figure 2** shows the percentage of the energy requirement that is needed for maintenance and growth at different ages. When estimating the likely energy requirement for a child who is unusually inactive (e.g., children with mobility difficulties), the estimate, based on the Estimated Average Requirement for age, should be reduced by the percentage of dietary energy normally required for activity (e.g., 29% at age 4 or 5 years). There is evidence that formula-fed

Table 2 Recommended energy intakes for infants (kJ/kg body weight/day)

Age (months)	UK EAR	Europe AR	USA EAR	FAO/WHO EAR
0–3	480	465	450	480
4–6	420	440	450	420
7–9	400	410	410	400
10–12	400	405	410	400

Table 3 Recommended energy intakes for Children (MJ/day)

Age (years)	Sex	UK EAR	Europe AR	USA EAR	FAO/ WHO EAR
2	M	4.9	5.0	5.4	5.9
	F	4.9	4.8	5.4	5.5
3	M	6.2	6.0	5.4	6.5
	F	5.7	5.6	5.4	6.0
4	M	6.7	6.6	7.5	7.1
	F	6.1	6.2	7.5	6.4
5	M	7.2	7.1	7.5	7.6
	F	6.5	6.8	7.5	6.8
6	M	7.6	7.7	7.5	7.9
	F	6.8	7.1	7.5	7.1
7	M	7.9	81	8.4	8.3
	F	7.0	7.3	8.2	7.4
8	M	8.2	8.3	8.4	8.7
	F	7.3	7.4	8.2	7.6
9	M	8.5	8.6	8.4	9.0
	F	7.5	7.4	8.2	0.79
10	M	8.2	8.7	8.4	10.5
	F	7.3	7.6	8.2	9.6
11	M	9.3	9.2	10.5	10.9
	F	7.7	8.0	9.0	9.8
12	M	9.3	9.8	10.5	11.3
	F	7.7	8.3	9.0	10.0
13	M	9.3	10.6	10.5	11.7
	F	7.7	9.0	9.0	10.2
14	M	9.3	10.9	10.5	12.1
	F	7.7	8.7	9.0	10.4
15	M	11.5	11.4	12.5	12.5
	F	8.8	8.9	9.2	10.5
16	M	11.5	11.9	12.5	12.8
	F	8.8	9.0	9.2	10.1
17	M	11.5	12.0	12.5	13.0
	F	8.8	9.0	9.2	9.8
18	M	11.5	11.9–12.5[a]	12.5	13.0
	F	8.8	8.3–10.6[a]	9.2	9.8

[a]Depends on physical activity level.
F, female; M, male.

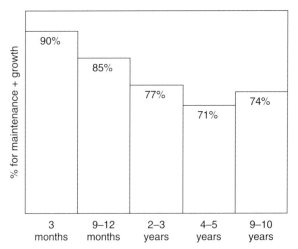

Figure 2 Energy required for maintenance and growth as percentage of total energy expenditure.

infants require a slightly increased energy intake to achieve the same growth velocity as breast-fed infants; children suffering from malnutrition have also been reported as having an increased energy expenditure and therefore may have a higher energy requirement than normal for their age.

Protein

Most recommendations for the protein intake of children are based on the 1985 FAO/WHO report, although much of the data were collected from studies on formula-fed infants. Because of differences in growth rates, efficiency of protein utilization, and the amino acid pattern of breast and cow's milk, these recommendations are likely to be an overestimation of true requirements. More recent data compiled on breast-fed infants give lower estimates of requirements. The Dewey estimates of minimum and

safe protein intakes plus recommendations from other authorities are shown in **Tables 4** and **5**. The minimum and safe intakes refer to a diet based on high biological value proteins such as breast milk or eggs. Adjustments need to be made for infants receiving an alternative source of protein (e.g., soya or a protein hydrolysate) and for older children consuming a mixed diet.

Protein requirements are highest during the first month of life and decrease thereafter. The proportion of protein intake that is required for growth decreases from 64% of requirement during the first month of life to 35% at age 3–6 months, 16% at age 1–2 years, and 11% at age 2–5 years.

Essential amino acid requirements are dependent on the growth rate of the infant and the rate of protein deposition, which changes throughout infancy. Some nonessential amino acids, including creatine, taurine, glycine, cysteine histidine, and arginine, cannot be synthesized in adequate quantities to meet the demands of the very rapid protein deposition that occurs during the first month of life, and these are considered to be semiessential during early infancy. It is likely that part of the nonprotein nitrogen portion of breast milk, such as choline, carnitine, and nucleotides, is used in metabolism and for amino acid synthesis and may also be conditionally essential.

Some countries express protein as a percentage of the estimated energy requirements, with a range of 8–15% energy from protein (i.e., 2–3.75 g protein per 100 total kilocalories). The protein: energy ratio is approximately 7.5% in human milk and 8–8.5% in infant formulas. These ratios are adequate for a normal rate of growth, although it may be argued that the more rapid growth rate seen in young formula-fed infants indicates that the ratio has been set too high in infant formulas.

Table 4 Recommended protein intakes for infants (g/kg body weight/day)

Age (months)	UK RNI	Europe PRI	USA Recommended Dietary Allowance	FAO/WHO[a]	
				Minimum requirements[b]	Safe minimum intake[c]
0–1	2.11		2.16	1.99	2.69
1–2	2.11		2.16	1.54	2.04
2–3	2.11		2.16	1.19	1.53
3–4	1.65		2.16	1.06	1.37
4–5	1.65	1.81	2.16	0.98	1.25
5–6	1.65	1.81	2.16	0.92	1.19
7–9	1.55	1.64	1.55	0.85	1.09
10–12	1.54	1.50	1.55	0.78	1.02

[a]From Dewy et al. (1996).
[b]Statistically will only meet requirements of 50% of the population.
[c]Should meet the requirements of 97.5% of the population.

Table 5 Recommendations for protein intake for children

Age (years)	Sex	UK RNI (g/day)	Europe PRI (g/day)	USA RDA (g/day)	WHO[a] Minimum requirements (g/kg/day)[b]	Safe minimum intake (g/kg/day)[c]
2	M + F	14.5	15.5	16.0	0.74	0.92
3	M + F	14.5	17.0	16.0	0.72	0.90
4	M + F	19.7	18.5	24	0.71	0.88
5	M + F	19.7	20.0	24	0.69	0.86
6	M + F	19.7	22.0	24	0.69	0.86
7	M + F	28.3	24.5	28	0.69	0.86
8	M + F	28.3	27.5	28	0.69	0.86
9	M + F	28.3	29.5	28	0.69	0.86
10	M	28.3	32.5	28	0.69	0.86
	F	28.3	34.0	28	0.69	0.86
11	M	42.1	36.0	45	0.69	0.88
	F	41.2	37.0	46	0.69	0.86
12	M	42.1	41.0	45	0.71	0.88
	F	41.2	41.5	46	0.69	0.86
13	M	42.1	45.5	45	0.71	0.88
	F	41.2	45.0	46	0.69	0.86
14	M	42.1	51.0	45	0.69	0.86
	F	41.2	45.5	46	0.68	0.84
15	M	55.2	53.5	59	0.69	0.86
	F	45.4	45.5	44	0.66	0.82
16	M	55.2	46.5	59	0.68	0.84
	F	45.4	45.0	44	0.66	0.81
17	M	55.2	55.5	59	0.67	0.83
	F	45.4	43.5	44	0.63	0.78
18	M	55.2	56.0	59	0.65	0.81
	F	45.4	47.0	44	0.63	0.78

[a]From Dewey et al. (1996).
[b]Statistically will only meet the requirements of 50% of the population.
[c]Should meet the requirements of 97.5% of the population.
F, female; M, male.

An increase in the protein:energy ratio is necessary for infants and children who are wasted or stunted and who need to grow at an increased velocity in order to catch up. Malnutrition during the first year of life, whether a result of a poor environment or because of conditions such as malabsorption or cystic fibrosis, is more serious than wasting and stunting later in childhood. Although the potential for catch-up growth remains until the end of puberty, deficits during early life can lead to permanent impairment of cognitive function. Estimates of requirements for malnourished infants and children should be based on the height age (i.e., the age at which the child's measured height falls on the 50th centile) because estimations based on normal requirements for chronological age are likely to be difficult to achieve and may lead to obesity. The increase in protein requirement for catch-up growth is proportionally greater than the increase in energy requirement and is dependent on age and growth velocity. For example, a child aged 1 year who is growing at twice the normal rate has a 5% increase in energy requirements and a 32% increase in protein requirements. When designing regimens for infants and children who need to catch up, a protein:energy ratio of at least 10% and possibly up to 15% is necessary. Ratios less than this will result in changes in body composition, with greater amounts of fat and water and lower amounts of lean tissue being deposited.

Water

The water content of the body is highest at birth (70%) and declines gradually to the adult value of 60% of body composition. The proportion of the fluid requirement that is needed for growth is small—approximately 5% soon after birth, decreasing to 1% at age 1 year. Fluid intake in infants is particularly important: They are unable to signify thirst, renal function is immature during the first few months of life, resulting in high obligatory losses of water, and extrarenal losses are high due to the high surface area of infants and young children. Physiological requirements for water are quite variable, are likely to be higher than adult requirements, and depend on climate, physical activity, and habitual diet.

Water is rarely on the list of nutrients for which dietary recommendations exist, and only one authority (Austria/Germany/Switzerland) recommends intakes that are based on energy intake and urine osmolality. Where recommendations do exist, they are usually approximately 1 ml water per kilocalorie of energy intake and are the same for both children and adults.

Fat, Carbohydrate, Fiber, and Recommendations for Healthy Eating

The transition from the high-fat, milk-based diet of the young infant to the generally accepted adult recommendations for healthy eating should be gradual, beginning from the onset of weaning. There is little consensus as to when qualitative adult intakes should be achieved, although dietary modification is not recommended by any authority for children younger than the age of 2 years and most agree that an adult-type diet is appropriate from the age of 5 years. Some authorities recommend a gradual change between the ages of 3 and 5 years, whereas others suggest that for most children a low-fat, cereal/vegetable predominant diet is suitable from age 2 years. If changes toward 'healthy eating' are made at too young an age, there is a danger that an inadequate energy and nutrient intake will result because infants and young children find it difficult to consume adequate quantities of such a bulky diet.

Fat

Fat contributes more than 50% of the energy intake in infants and is necessary to deliver the infant's high energy requirement in a small volume. Fat continues to be important during the first and second years of life because of the relatively high energy requirements per unit of weight. The United Kingdom, United States/Canada, and FAO/WHO do not recommend a specific fat:energy ratio for young children; some countries allow for higher fat intakes in young children, whereas other European countries suggest 25–30% energy from fat from the age of 2 years. Guidance on the intakes of fatty acids varies considerably throughout the world, and there are considerable differences in the way that recommendations are expressed where they do exist. Saturated fatty acids, where recommendations exist, are usually limited to a maximum of 10% total energy intake. For polyunsaturated fatty acids, recommendations for children are similar to those for adults

(5–10% of energy intake), except for infants, for whom a higher percentage is often deemed desirable, similar to quantities in breast milk. Many countries do not make a recommendation for omega-3 and omega-6 fatty acids. Where recommendations exist, they are usually the same as for adults: 2–4% and 0.5% of total energy intake for omega-6 and omega-3, respectively. Some authorities recommend a ratio of <5:1 omega-6:omega-3 for adult intakes, but it is unclear whether this recommendation is appropriate for children.

Carbohydrate

Few countries set reference values for carbohydrates for children. Young infants, particularly those born preterm, have a limited capacity for glucose synthesis and require approximately 40% of their energy from simple sugars in order to maintain adequate blood glucose levels. Breast milk and infant formulas normally contain approximately 7 g carbohydrate per 100 ml. For older children there is no reason to believe that requirements for carbohydrates are different from those for adults. Where recommendations for total carbohydrates and for simple or nonmilk extrinsic sugars are set, they are usually the same as those for adults.

Fiber

A lack of agreement on the definition of fiber and differences in analytical techniques make it difficult to compare recommendations from different sources, and there appears to be a 10-fold variation in recommendations worldwide. Some authorities (United Kingdom, European Union (EU), and FAO/WHO) set no reference values for children. Estimations of desirable fiber intakes are based on adult data corrected for body weight and energy requirement. A popular concept (which is not evidence-based) is the 'age + 5' concept. This recommendation states that children older than the age of 2 years consume an amount of fiber equivalent to their age in years plus 5 g daily. Thus, fiber recommendations increase by 1 g per year until adult values are reached at age 15–18 years. Infants consume a very low-fiber diet, although oligosaccharides in breast milk are thought to have fiber-like properties. fiber should be introduced gradually into the weaning diet from age 6 months, but the use of large quantities of whole grain cereals and pulses or nuts is not recommended in infancy because they are likely to affect the bioavailability of micronutrients and result in a bulky low-energy diet.

Mineral Elements

Requirements for mineral elements should be expressed per unit of body weight since excess minerals are excreted by the kidney. In addition, requirements are directly proportional to growth rates: Sodium and potassium increments reflect the amount of water retained during cellular growth; calcium, phosphorus, and magnesium requirements are in proportion to bone growth and maturation. However, few countries express recommendations in terms of body weight, reflecting the lack of direct data for infants and children.

Sodium and Potassium

Recommendations for sodium and potassium intakes are given in **Table 6**. Young infants are less efficient at excreting sodium than older children, and hypernatremic dehydration can occur in infants being fed a high-sodium milk (such as unmodified cow's milk) if they have any extrarenal water losses such as diarrhea. Many countries do not give recommendations for sodium or potassium. Recommendations that do exist are often based on usual sodium intakes, which in Western countries are far in excess of requirement. Because of the relationship between hypertension and sodium intake in populations, most Western countries recognize that a decrease in sodium and a concurrent increase in potassium intake are desirable. In the United Kingdom, in 2003 the Scientific Advisory Committee on Nutrition set target recommendations for salt intake in children. Infants younger than the age of

1 year should take 17 mmol or less per day; for ages 1–3, 4–6, 7–10, and 11–14 years, the targets are 34, 51, 85, and 102 mmol per day, respectively. The target recommendations are higher than the UK Reference Nutrient Intake but below estimated intakes of infants and children in the United Kingdom and below the upper limit of the EU acceptable range.

Calcium, Phosphorus, and Magnesium

Recommendations for calcium, phosphorus, and magnesium intakes are given in **Table 7**. A low calcium intake is rarely a cause of rickets, although calcium deficiency has been reported in children who have no milk or dairy products in their diet. An adequate calcium intake in childhood is particularly important in order to maximize bone density. There is some controversy over the optimum calcium intake during childhood in order to achieve maximum bone density, with US and FAO/WHO

Table 6 Recommendations for sodium and potassium intake, infants and children (mmol/day)

Nutrient	Age	UK LNRI	EU acceptable range	USA minimum requirement
Sodium	0–6 months	6	—	—
	6–12 months	9	—	—
	1–3 years	9	—	13
	4–6 years	12	25–152	13
	7–10 years	15	25–152	17.5
	11–14 years	20	25–152	22
	15–18 years	25	25–152	22
		RNI	EU PRI	USA RDA
Potassium	0–3 months	20	—	12.8
	4–6 months	22	—	18
	7–12 months	08	20	26
	1–3 years	20	20	36
	4–6 years	28	28	36
	7–10 years	50	41	41
	11–14 years	80	51	51
	15–18 years	90	51	51

Table 7 Recommendations for minerals for infants and children (mg/day)

Nutrient	Age	UK RNI	Europe PRI	USA RDA	FAO/ WHO RDI
Calcium	0–6 months	525	—	440	500
	6–12 months	525	400	600	600
	1–3 years	350	400	500	500
	4–6 years	450	450	800	600
	7–10 years	550	550	800	700
	11–14 years				
	M	1000	1000	1300	1300
	F	800	800	1300	1300
	15–18 years				
	M	1000	1000	1300	1300
	F	800	800	1300	1300
Phosphorus	0–6 months	400	—	300	—
	6–12 months	400	300	500	—
	1–3 years	270	300	460	—
	4–6 years	350	350	500	—
	7–8 years	200	450	500	—
	9–10 years	450	450	1250	—
	11–18 years				
	M	775	775	1250	—
	F	625	625	1250	—
Magnesium	0–6 months	60		40	
	6–12 months	80		60	
	1–3 years	85	85	80	60
	4–6 years	120	120	130	76
	7–8 years	200	200	130	100
	9–10 years	200	200	240	100
	11–14 years				
	M	280	280	240	230
	F	280	280	240	220
	15–18 years				
	M	300	300	410	230
	F	300	300	350	220

F, female; M, male.

recommendations set higher than EU and UK ones. Most countries differentiate between boys and girls at adolescence to account for greater bone mass in males.

Recommendations for phosphorus intakes show a similar variation. Estimates of requirements assume that there is an optimum ratio of calcium:phosphorus in the diet, so phosphorus recommendations are based on those for calcium. The optimum molar calcium:phosphorus ratio during childhood is assumed to be 1:1. The recommended ratio in infant formulas ranges from 1.3:1 to 2.1:1; the ratio in human milk is approximately 2.3:1.

There are limited data on magnesium requirements during infancy and childhood, and this is reflected in the variation of recommendations worldwide. Magnesium deficiency is rarely reported in healthy children and recommendations are largely based on normal intakes.

Trace Elements

Recommendations for trace element intakes in infancy and childhood are shown in **Tables 8** and **9**. In general, there are few data on trace element requirements in young children, although some studies have been carried out in infants. In the manufacture of breast milk substitutes, quantities available in breast milk are considered to be adequate, although the bioavailability of trace elements added to cow's milk-based formula has not been fully elucidated. Preterm infants are born with low stores of trace elements. They require supplements of iron until age 1 year. Deficiencies of selenium and copper have also been described in preterm and low-birthweight infants. Several authorities do not set dietary recommendations for molybdenum, manganese, and chromium, although all are essential for growth development and health. Recommendations for selenium have been set by the United Kingdom, EU, United States, and WHO. Where data for infants exist, recommendations for children are set between those for infants and those for adults. No reference values have been set for fluorine by any authority, although the effect of fluorine on the inhibition and reversal of caries progression is well accepted and is particularly important during tooth eruption and growth during infancy and childhood.

Iron

Recommendations for iron intake in infancy and childhood are shown in **Table 8**. Term infants are born with sufficient stores of iron to last until they have approximately doubled their birth weight.

Table 8 Recommendations for iron intake in infants and children (μmol/day)

Age	Sex	UK RNI	EU PRI	USA RDA	FAO/ WHO RNI
0–3 months	M + F	30	—	105	—
4–6 months	M + F	80	—	105	150
7–12 months	M + F	140	105	180	150
1–2 years	M + F	120	70	130	90
2 years	M	120	70	120	70
	F	120	70	128	70
3 years	M	120	70	135	70
	F	120	70	130	70
4 years	M	110	70	140	75
	F	110	70	145	75
5 years	M	110	70	145	75
	F	110	70	150	75
6 years	M	110	70	170	75
	F	110	70	160	75
7 years	M	160	107	185	105
	F	160	107	180	105
8 years	M	160	107	200	105
	F	160	107	190	105
9–10 years	M + F	160	107	140	105
11–14 years	M	200	180	140	270
	F	260	320–390	140	285
15–18 years	M	200	230	195	225
	F	260	320–390	270	370

F, female; M, male.

There is controversy over whether healthy infants have a requirement for dietary iron until the age of 4–6 months. Although most infant formulas are fortified with iron, there are some unfortified ones reflecting the uncertainty over requirements in very young infants. After the age of 4–6 months or when birth weight has doubled, iron requirements are very high. Levels of iron in breast milk are low, although bioavailability is high. Nevertheless, infants exclusively breast-fed after the age of 6 months have lower iron stores than those who receive a fortified formula or iron-containing complementary foods. Cow's milk is low in iron and the iron is poorly absorbed. Infants fed on cow's milk as a main drink younger than the age of 1 year or who consume large quantities of cow's milk after the age of 1 year are at risk of developing iron deficiency. Iron is required in early life not only for adequate growth but also because it is important in brain growth, and iron deficiency during infancy may lead to irreversible changes in mental and motor development. It is estimated that 43% of infants and children worldwide suffer from iron deficiency in infancy and childhood, most commonly between the ages of 6 and 24 months. The problem is worse in developing countries: The prevalence in Western industrialized countries is

Table 9 Recommendations for trace minerals

Nutrient	Age	UK RNI	Europe PRI	USA RDA	FAO/WHO RDI
Zinc (mg/day)	0–6 months	4.0	—	5.0	3.1–5.3[a]
	6–12 months	4.0	4.0	5.0	5.6
	1–3 years	5.0	4.0	3.0	5.5
	4–6 years	6.5	6.0	5.0	6.5
	7–10 years	7.0	7.0	5.0–8.0	7.5
	11–14 years				
	M	9.0	9.0	8.0	12.1
	F	9.0	9.0	8.0	10.3
	15–18 years				
	M	9.5	9.0	11.0	13.1
	F	7.0	7.0	9.0	10.2
Copper (mg/day)	0–6 months	0.2–0.3	—	0.4–0.6[b]	0.33–0.62
	6–12 months	0.3	0.3	0.6–1.0	0.6
	1–3 years	0.4	0.4	1.0–1.5	0.56
	4–6 years	0.6	0.6	1.0–2.0	0.57
	7–10 years	0.7	0.7	1.0–2.0	0.75
	11–14 years				
	M	0.8	0.8	1.5–2.5	1.0
	F	0.8	0.8	1.5–2.5	1.0
	15–18 years				
	M	1.0	1.0	1.5–3.0	1.33
	F	1.0	1.0	1.5–3.0	1.15
Selenium (μg/day)	0–6 months	10–13	—	10	6–9
	6–12 months	10	8	15	12
	1–3 years	15	10	20	20
	4–6 years	20	15	20	24
	7–10 years	30	25	30	25
	11–14 years				
	M	45	35	40	36
	F	45	35	45	30
	15–18 years				
	M	70	45	50	40
	F	60	45	50	30
Iodine (μg/day)	0–6 months	56–60	—	40	50
	6–12 months	60	50	50	50
	1–3 years	70	70	70	90
	4–6 years	100	90	90	90
	7–10 years	110	100	120	120
	11–14 years				
	M	130	120	150	150
	F	130	120	150	150
	15–18 years				
	M	140	130	150	150
	F	140	130	150	150

[a]Assuming diets of moderate bioavailability.
[b]USA Adequate Intake (not RDA).
F, female; M, male.

approximately 10% in children younger than the age of 2 years. Immigrant groups to Western countries, particularly those of Asian origin, have a higher prevalence rate than Caucasian children. This may in part be accounted for by differences in sources of dietary iron. Absorption varies according to the composition of the diet. Recommendations from FAO/WHO take this into consideration and give reference values for four absorption levels: 5, 10, 12, and 15%, with a 3-fold difference in recommendations between the lowest and highest level. Throughout the world, there is considerable variation in iron intake recommendations, part of which is due to differences in dietary composition. Most countries include two reference intakes for adolescent girls, depending on whether or not they have reached menarche.

Zinc

Breast milk provides adequate zinc for term infants until birth weight has approximately doubled. Requirements for zinc are particularly high in infancy because of the demands of growth, and zinc-containing complementary foods or a fortified infant formula is needed to meet requirements after the age of approximately 6 months. Zinc deficiency in childhood is common in developing countries, leading to slow weight gain in infancy and impaired linear growth in children. In unfavorable environments, zinc supplementation of infants and young children is associated with improvements in growth and a reduction of up to 25% in the incidence of diarrhea and 40% reduction in the incidence of pneumonia. Recommendations for zinc intakes vary considerably throughout the world. Zinc absorption is dependent on the composition of the diet and, as with iron, FAO/WHO reference intakes give three values for each age group for low, medium, and high bioavailability.

Copper

Although levels of copper in breast milk appear to be low, it is readily absorbed. Breast-fed term infants obtain adequate copper to meet requirements from stores in the liver and from breast milk until they have approximately doubled their birth weight. Unmodified cow's milk is particularly low in copper and does not meet the requirements for infants if used as a main drink under the age of 1 year; modified infant formulas are fortified with copper. Deficiency has been reported in infants and young children who consume a diet containing large quantities of cow's milk and few complementary foods. Most recommendations for copper intake in children have been extrapolated from infant and adult data and recommendations vary considerably worldwide.

Iodine

Adequate thyroid function is essential for optimal growth and development, and hypothyroidism due to iodine deficiency is seen in many developing countries and some areas of Eastern Europe. The breast milk of mothers who are iodine deficient does not provide an adequate intake for infants, and WHO has described childhood iodine deficiency as the most common cause of preventable brain damage in the world. Infants and children consuming vegetarian and vegan diets have a lower intake than children who consume dairy products. There is little recent data on iodine requirements in infants and children, and most data are extrapolated from adult requirements. Recommendations worldwide for desirable iodine intakes are similar with little variation.

Water-Soluble Vitamins

Recommendations for dietary intakes of water-soluble vitamins are shown in **Table 10**. Recommendations vary throughout the world. There are few direct data on infants and children and most recommendations are extrapolated from adult data. Recommendations for children for thiamine and for some other B vitamins are set relative to energy intakes; vitamin B_6 recommendations are expressed in terms of protein intake and are the same as for adults. The ratio of vitamins to macronutrients is set lower for infants younger than the age of 1 year, reflecting the relative quantities in breast milk. However, there are very few data on the bioavailability and efficiency of utilization of these nutrients in fortified infant formula and in complementary foods. Few countries set recommendations for biotin and pantothenic acid. Recommendations for some other B vitamins are expressed as safe intakes because there is insufficient data on which to base estimates of requirements or recommendations.

Deficiencies of water-soluble vitamins are rare in European and other Westernized countries. Infants are born with small stores of folate and can quickly become depleted if breast milk levels are low. A deficiency of folic acid is the most common cause of megaloblastic anemia in childhood. Infants of vegan mothers also have small stores of vitamin B_{12} and breast milk levels are likely to be low. Children consuming a macrobiotic or strict vegan diet are at risk of not meeting requirements for vitamin B_{12} unless they receive a supplement or a fortified infant soya formula.

Vitamin C is particularly important in childhood not only because of its functions as a vitamin but also because it improves the absorption of non-heme iron. Failure to consume foods rich in vitamin C at the same time as vegetable sources of iron plays a part in the etiology of iron deficiency in childhood. Levels of vitamin C in cow's milk are low and infantile scurvy has been reported in infants receiving unmodified cow's milk as a main drink. Infant formulas are fortified with vitamin C. Estimates of requirements are generally extrapolated from adult data. Intakes of vitamin C that were low (but that met current recommendations) have been associated with increased prevalence of asthma in childhood.

Table 10 Recommendations for water-soluble vitamins

Nutrient	Age	UK RNI	Europe PRI	USA RDA	FAO/WHO RDI
Thiamine (mg/day)	0–6 months	0.2	—	0.3	0.3
	6–12 months	0.3	0.3	0.4	0.3
	1–3 years	0.5	0.5	0.7	0.5
	4–6 years	0.7	0.7	0.9	0.6
	7–10 years	0.7	0.8	1.0	0.9
	11–14 years				
	M	0.9	1.0	1.3	1.2
	F	0.7	0.9	1.2	1.1
	15–18 years				
	M	1.1	1.1	1.1	1.2
	F	0.8	0.9	1.0	1.1
Riboflavin (mg/day)	0–6 months	0.4	—	0.4	0.5
	6–12 months	0.4	0.4	0.5	0.5
	1–3 years	0.6	0.8	0.5	0.5
	4–6 years	0.8	1.0	0.6	0.6
	7–10 years	1.0	1.2	0.6–0.9	0.9
	11–14 years				
	M	1.2	1.4	0.9	1.3
	F	1.1	1.2	0.9	1.0
	15–18 years				
	M	1.3	1.6	1.3	1.3
	F	1.1	1.3	1.0	1.0
Niacin (NE/day)[a]	0–6 months	3	—	5	5.4
	6–12 months	4–5	5	6	5.4
	1–3 years	8	9	6	6
	4–6 years	11	11	8	8
	7–10 years	12	13	8–12	12
	11–14 years				
	M	15	15	12	16
	F	12	14	12	16
	15–18 years				
	M	18	18	16	16
	F	14	14	14	16
Vitamin B_6 (mg/day)	0–6 months	0.2	—	0.3	0.3
	6–12 months	0.3–0.4	0.4	0.6	0.6
	1–3 years	0.7	0.7	0.5	0.5
	4–6 years	0.9	0.9	0.6	0.6
	7–10 years	1.0	1.1	0.6–1.0	1.0
	11–14 years				
	M	1.2	1.3	1.0	1.3
	F	1.2	1.1	1.0	1.2
	15–18 years				
	M	1.5	1.5	1.3	1.3
	F	1.5	1.1	1.2	1.2
Vitamin B_{12} (μg/day)	0–6 months	0.3	—	0.3	0.3
	6–12 months	0.4	0.5	0.5	0.5
	1–3 years	0.5	0.7	0.9	009
	4–6 years	0.8	0.9	1.2	1.2
	7–10 years	1.0	1.0	1.2–1.8	1.8–2.4
	11–14 years				
	M	1.2	1.3	1.8	2.4
	F	1.2	1.2	1.8	2.4
	15–18 years				
	M	1.5	1.4	2.4	2.4
	F	1.5	1.4	2.4	2.4
Folate (μg/day)	0–6 months	50	50	50	50
	6–12 months	50	50	50	50
	1–3 years	70	100	150	100
	4–6 years	100	130	200	130
	7–10 years	150	150	200–300	150

Continued

Table 10 Continued

Nutrient	Age	UK RNI	Europe PRI	USA RDA	FAO/WHO RDI
	11–14 years				
	M	200	180	300	180
	F	200	180	300	180
	15–18 years				
	M	200	200	400	200
	F	200	200	400	200
Vitamin C (mg/day)	0–6 months	25	—	20	20
	6–12 months	25	20	20	20
	1–3 years	30	25	15	30
	4–6 years	30	25	25	30
	7–10 years	30	30	25–45	35
	11–14 years				
	M	35	35	45	40
	F	35	35	45	40
	15–18 years				
	M	40	45	75	40
	F	40	40	65	40

[a]NE, nicotinic acid equivalent: 1 mg = 60 mg tryptophan.
F, female; M, male.

Fat-Soluble Vitamins

Recommendations for fat-soluble vitamins are shown in **Table 11**. There are few direct data on requirements for infants and children, and many of the recommendations are derived from adult data.

Vitamin A

Breast milk content of vitamin A is dependent on the mother's status, and term infants who are breast fed by a well-nourished mother will meet their requirements until approximately 6 months of age. The United Kingdom recommends a supplement of vitamin A for breast-fed infants between the ages of 6 months and 5 years because it is difficult to obtain adequate quantities from weaning foods. Clinical vitamin A deficiency is a major cause of childhood blindness in developing countries but is rarely seen in Western countries. There is growing evidence that mild or subclinical vitamin A deficiency is associated with increased susceptibility to infection.

Vitamin D

Vitamin D requirements in adults and older children are met by the exposure of the skin to sunlight, but infants and young children and those who may not receive adequate exposure have a dietary requirement for vitamin D. Breast milk content depends on maternal status, but breast milk and body stores should provide sufficient vitamin D to meet requirements until the age of 6 months. After this age, several countries recommend a supplement for breast-fed infants. Formula milks are fortified with

vitamin D. Deficiency of vitamin D in childhood causes rickets. In Western countries dark-skinned immigrant groups, particularly preschool children and adolescent Asian groups, are especially at risk of low levels of vitamin D because they require more sunlight exposure to synthesise adequate amounts of vitamin D compared to fairer skinned groups. The use of sun-block creams for children in Western countries reduces skin synthesis of vitamin D and may contribute to low levels. Recommendations for dietary intakes of children vary throughout the world. Some authorities make a recommendation but indicate that it may only apply to those without access to sunlight. Others make no general recommendations for children older than the age of 2 years except for those at risk of low skin synthesis.

Vitamin E

Vitamin E is particularly important for preterm infants because placental transfer is low and stores at birth are poor. Preterm infants are subjected to high levels of oxidative stress, and deficiency of vitamin E is associated with hemolytic anemia and bronchopulmonary dysplasia. Recommendations for vitamin E intakes are often expressed in relation to dietary polyunsaturated fatty acid intake. Recommendations for dietary intakes for infants and children are fairly consistent throughout the world.

Vitamin K

There are few recommendations for vitamin K since the major source of the vitamin is gastrointestinal

Table 11 Recommendations for fat-soluble vitamins

Nutrient	Age	UK RNI	Europe PRI	USA RDA	FAO/WHO RDI
Vitamin A (μg retinol equivalent/day)	0–6 months		—	350	350
	6–12 months		—	350	350
	1–3 years		400	300	400
	4–6 years		400	400	450
	7–10 years		500	400–600	500
	11–14 years				
	M		600	600	600
	F		600	600	600
	15–18 years				
	M		700	900	600
	F		600	700	600
Vitamin D (μg/day)	0–6 months		10–25	5[a]	5
	6–12 months		10	5	5
	1–3 years		10	5	5
	4–6 years		0–10	5	5
	7–10 years		1–10	5	5
	11–14 years				
	M		0–15	5	5
	F		0–15	5	5
	15–18 years				
	M		0–15	5	5
	F		0–15	5	5
Vitamin E (mg/day)	0–6 months	0.4 PUFA[c]	0.4 PUFA	6	—
	6–12 months	0.4 PUFA	0.4 PUFA	6	
	1–3 years	—	0.4 PUFA	6	—
	4–6 years	—	—	7	—
	7–10 years	—	—	7–11	—
	11–14 years				—
	M	>4	>4	11	
	F	>3	>3	11	
	15–18 years				—
	M	>4	>4	15	
	F	>3	>3	15	

[a]USA Adequate Intake (not RDA).
[b]FAO/WHO Recommended Safe Intake.
[c]UK Safe Intake.
F, female; M, male.

bacteria. Infants are born with a limited ability to synthesize vitamin K from this source, and hemorrhagic disease of the newborn, due to vitamin K deficiency, has a prevalence of 1 in 200–400 live births in Western countries. A single intravenous or intramuscular injection of vitamin K or an oral dose is usually offered to all neonates in many countries.

See also: **Amino Acids**: Chemistry and Classification. **Breast Feeding**. **Calcium**. **Carbohydrates**: Requirements and Dietary Importance. **Children**: Nutritional Problems. **Copper**. **Dietary Fiber**: Physiological Effects and Effects on Absorption. **Infants**: Nutritional Requirements. **Iodine**: Physiology, Dietary Sources and Requirements. **Iron**. **Magnesium**. **Phosphorus**. **Potassium**. **Protein**: Requirements and Role in Diet. **Sodium**: Physiology. **United Nations Children's Fund**. **Vitamin A**: Biochemistry and Physiological Role; Deficiency and Interventions.

Vitamin B₆. **Vitamin D**: Rickets and Osteomalacia. **Vitamin E**: Metabolism and Requirements; Physiology and Health Effects. **Vitamin K**.

Further Reading

Aggett P, Bresson J, Haschke F et al. (1997) Recommended Dietary Allowances (RDAs), Recommended Dietary Intakes (RDIs), Recommended Nutrient Intakes (NRIs) and Population Reference Intakes (PRIs) are not "recommended intakes." Journal of Pediatric Gastroenterology and Nutrition 25: 236–241.

Butte NF (1996) Energy requirements of infants. European Journal of Clinical Nutrition 50(supplement 1): S24–S36.

Department of Health (1991) Report on Health and Social Subjects, No. 41. Dietary Reference Values for Food Energy and Nutrients for the United Kingdom. London: HMSO.

Dewey KG, Beaton G, Fjeld C et al. (1996) Protein requirements of infants and children. European Journal of Clinical Nutrition 50(supplement 1): S119–S150.

FAO/WHO/UNI Expert Consultation (1985) *Energy and Protein Requirements*, Technical Report Series 724. Geneva: WHO.

Jackson AA (1990) Protein requirements for catch-up growth. *Proceedings of the Nutrition Society* 49: 507–516.

Torun B, Davies PS, and Livingstone MB (1996) Energy requirements for 1–18 year olds. *European Journal of Clinical Nutrition* 50(supplement 1): S37–S81.

Nutritional Problems

E M E Poskitt, London School of Hygiene and Tropical Medicine, London, UK

© 2005 Elsevier Ltd. All rights reserved.

Introduction

Good nutrition is needed for normal growth and development. However, it is not only provision of food that is necessary for energy and nutrients to be consumed, absorbed, and utilized optimally by the body: physical and mental health, emotion, and the overall environment in which children are fed affect what is eaten and how food is utilized. As a result complex interactions involving 'nature' and 'nurture' influence nutrition in children who are essentially healthy and those who are ill.

'Child' and 'children' are not specific terms, as the age at which individuals are defined as adults rather than children varies with the circumstances. Children under 1 year of age, or infants, are considered separately in this encyclopedia, as is nutrition in adolescents. In the following discussion, the term 'children' refers to individuals between infancy and the onset of puberty, i.e., roughly between 1 and 10 years of age.

Feeding Young Children

Nutritional needs for growth are unique to infants, children, and adolescents. Growth rates fall rapidly in early life. By 1 year of age, energy needs for growth have fallen to <3% of total energy requirements but relatively high proportions of protein and micronutrients per unit of energy are still required for growth. These needs must be reflected in the quantity and quality of foods offered to young children.

High nutrient and energy needs per kilogram body weight make it difficult for young children to consume sufficient food with only two meals a day. Frequent feeding, perhaps three significant meals and two to three snacks interposed between these meals, should overcome the problems posed by the large volumes of food per kilogram body weight needed daily. As children grow, mature, and their growth rates slow, the volumes of food needed decline. Growing independence and, with this, the ability to obtain and consume frequent snacks increase with age. By the end of their first year children are consuming foods similar to the rest of the family. The consistency of their food will still be different since their inexperience of chewing and biting off appropriately sized pieces of food means that most food requires chopping or mashing lightly.

Table 1 lists some feeding skills that develop after infancy. Young children need encouragement to practice the skills that enable them to progress from breast- and bottle-feeding to soft malleable foods in early weaning and to foods that require chewing by 9 months to 1 year. After 1 year they should be taking fluids (other than breast milk) predominantly from cups rather than bottles. Continuing to offer drinks from feeding bottles after 12 months can discourage children from accepting foods that need to be chewed. Persistent bottle-feeders may have excessively high fluid intakes because these provide their main nutrition. If the fluid is milk or infant formula, obesity may result. If fruit juices or carbonated drinks are fed, fluids may

Table 1 Developmental skills associated with feeding acquired after first year of life

Age	Relevant skills
12–15 months	Sits well and can move around in chair when feeding
	Keen to feed self
	Tries to feed with spoon but cannot manage rotation of wrist so food falls off spoon before reaching mouth
	Finger feeds well with thumb-first finger apposition
	Interested in emptying cups and throwing food and food containers from chair
	Will search for them after throwing
18 months	Manages to feed with rotation of wrist so food reaches mouth
	Hand preference beginning to show
	Drinks well without spilling
	Hands cup back to adult
21 months	Will ask for drink or food
	Follows family eating habits
2½ years	Very self willed and determined
	May be stubborn and rebellious
	Active – may not stay sitting throughout meal
3 years	Feeds with spoon and fork – rather messily
	Will carry utensils and can help lay table
5 years	Feeds with spoon and fork neatly
	Has clear and persistent likes and dislikes for foods
	Understands consequences of choice
	Greatly influenced by peer group preferences for foods

substitute for other more energy-dense foods. Failure to thrive may then result.

Everyday Feeding problems

Young children are usually determined to show their independence. This can be frustrating for carers. The children want to do things for themselves yet do not have the skills to succeed. Approaches such as letting young children attempt spoon-feeding whilst their carers feed them unobtrusively from other spoons are 'feeding skills' parents and carers develop. Young children are also easily distracted. It is wise to feed them away from active television sets and brothers and sisters at play if the family is not eating together. At family meals young children are likely to be slow eaters. They may eat in 'fits and starts' and continue to eat even when food has gone cold and is no longer palatable to adult tastes. Removing food as soon as a young child stops eating may be inappropriate since stopping eating is sometimes a temporary respite and not a sign that the child has had 'enough.' After a pause, eating may continue. Telling children to 'eat up,' nagging them to 'hurry up', or trying to force them to eat are not helpful and can lead to mealtime defiance, frantic carers, and impaired nutrition. Most parents become skilled at anticipating and forestalling mealtime problems in diverse ways.

If children refuse food at mealtimes or show no intention of finishing their meals, they probably do not need the food. This is particularly likely if they have recently had a snack. Small children are readily sated by amounts of food that seem very small to adults. Snacks should be timed closer to previous meals than to following meals – perhaps 2 h before the next meal. Children who eat poorly at one meal often eat much better at the next meal because by then they are hungry. Offering biscuits or confectionery in exchange for an unfinished meal ('because they have not had enough') is neither helpful nor usually necessary. Children learn very quickly that if they do not eat meals they may get foods that are, to them, more enjoyable. Mealtime organization begins to collapse. However, very young children have slight risk of hypoglycemia if they go for prolonged periods without food so it is advisable to feed them before bed if they have exhibited persistent food refusal earlier in the day.

The appetites of young children are very variable. Low intakes on one day are usually compensated by excellent intakes on other days. Carers should adopt organized, but relaxed, approaches to meals and eating. Mealtimes should be enjoyable occasions for positive parent–child interaction, not the battles that sometimes develop from parents' understandable anxieties because their children 'don't eat.'

Nutrient needs that are easily met in healthy children may be more difficult to achieve if children are offered, or accept, only a limited variety of foods or have poor appetites because of illness. Vegetarian diets for young children can provide adequate nutrition but some nutritional knowledge is advisable for those managing children on such diets. Plant proteins do not individually contain all the amino acids so mixing of protein sources is important for the provision of the amino acids needed for optimal nutrition and growth. Provided breast-feeding continues, or children take significant amounts of other milk or formula (cows' milk-based or soy-based infant formulas or, after 1 year, neat cows' milk), amino acid requirements can be met from milk or formula and little other protein is needed from plant or animal sources.

WHO recommends that breast-feeding continues as part of a mixed diet into the second year of life. Milk in some form is recommended for young children. It provides a ready source of calcium throughout childhood. Before 1 year of age, European Union (EU) recommendations are for infant formula rather than neat cows' milk. After the first year of life whole cows' milk is appropriate. In the UK National Diet and Nutrition Survey 1992/3, 83% of children aged $1\frac{1}{2}$–$4\frac{1}{2}$ years were taking some whole cows' milk and for 68% of children this was as a drink. Twenty-six per cent of food energy, on average, came from milk and milk products whereas in the $3\frac{1}{2}$–$4\frac{1}{2}$ years age group this figure was only 16%. In a similar study by Gregory and Lowe, 7–10-year-old children were still consuming, on average, close to 1 l of whole milk a week providing around 12% of total daily energy. Fat-reduced milks should only be used as drinks in children under 5 years if the rest of the diet is varied and 'balanced' with other sources of fat-soluble micronutrients, in which case semi-skimmed milk may be used as a drink from the age of 2 years onwards.

Nutrient Interactions

Nutrient–nutrient interaction in the process of digestion and absorption is more important for child than adult nutrition. The requirements for micronutrients are high in childhood because of the need to form new tissues in growth. However, phytates from cereal and vegetable foods bind minerals, particularly calcium, vitamin D and iron, in the bowel and reduce absorption. Asian children in northern latitudes on high-phytate traditional diets are at risk of developing vitamin D deficiency rickets. This is partly due to poor absorption of both calcium and vitamin D because they are bound with phytates in the small intestine and absorption is reduced. Inadequate synthesis of vitamin D from precursors in the skin because of low sunlight exposure will exacerbate poor vitamin D nutrition and further impair calcium absorption. Thus, whilst nonstarch polysaccharides (NSP) from unrefined cereals, whole fruits, and vegetables should be an increasing proportion of the diets of children as they grow, NSP intakes should only be gradually increased to perhaps $15\,g\,day^{-1}$ by 10 years of age.

Nutrient–nutrient interactions are not necessarily disadvantageous. Vitamin C, through its reducing power, maintains iron in the ferrous state in the gastrointestinal tract and thus facilitates absorption of this important micronutrient. Vitamin C also facilitates absorption of a number of other micronutrients. Each meal should contain a good source of vitamin C to optimize utilization of other micronutrients.

Assessment of Nutrition in Children: Anthropometry

After the first year of life, children usually follow very predictable gains in weight and height over time. Growth as gain in weight and height remains, with activity, the aspect of energy consumption that the body can reduce if energy intakes are inadequate for all needs. The wide range of normal weights for age in a population means that a single weight in an individual child is not a good indicator of over or under nutrition. Nevertheless, weight change over time is the most widely used parameter for judging nutritional status. Failure to gain weight at the expected rate is often the first evidence of declining nutritional status. Where inadequate nutrition is prolonged, linear growth faltering also occurs. Growth curves showing weights and heights plotted against age with trajectories for mean and standard deviation or centile distributions of a population are the basis of growth assessment in childhood. In infancy, crossing the centiles upwards or downwards is quite common as infants express their genetic potential for growth in a postnatal environment of different constraints from those *in utero*. In adolescence, growth may diverge from population patterns because of the timing of the pubertal growth spurt in relation to the reference population. Between these two periods of apparent growth instability, the majority of children follow very stable growth trajectories in relation to population distribution for age. This is particularly so for height. The obesogenic environment enveloping so many children in westernized societies today may be causing children's weights to move up across the centiles much more frequently than in the past.

Failure to Thrive

Failure to thrive is failure to gain in height and weight at the expected rate, the expected rate usually being that indicated by charts for height and weight related to age and sex in reference populations. Since it is often easier to measure weight than height in small children and since weight can be lost as well as not gained, whereas height gain can only be absent or slowed, assessment of failure to thrive is frequently made on weight progress alone. Although a child may be low weight for height and age, this does not necessarily imply failure to thrive since some 'normal' children are always small, perhaps because of genetic endowment. They grow with normal velocity but at the lower extreme of normal population distribution. Thus, following weight gain over time is essential for diagnosis of failure to thrive (**Figure 1**).

Failure to thrive can result from a wide range of underlying medical problems as outlined in **Table 2**.

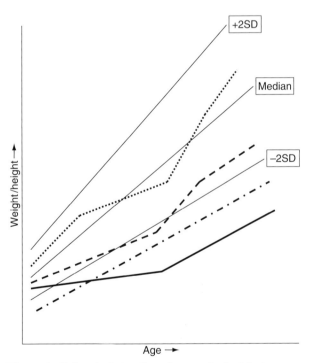

Figure 1 Failure to thrive: figurative growth chart for increase in either weight or height of four children with abnormal growth showing normal population growth as median and ± standard deviations (SD). ··············, failure to thrive in above average child with growth falling below the median and then showing complete catch up growth; — — — — —, failure to thrive in a child growing below the median with failure to thrive, falling below −2SD and then showing complete catch up; ——————, child with failure to thrive and failure to complete catch up so growth continues at about average rate but child remains below previous SD position; — · — · — ·, child gaining throughout at normal velocity but starting below −2SD and remaining below −2SD in size, i.e., 'small normal'.

Table 2 Some causes of failure to thrive according to pathophysiology

Basic cause of FTT	Clinical situation	Medical condition
Too little energy taken in	Inadequate food energy offered	Poverty; ignorance of child's needs; lack of understanding of progression of weaning process
	Significant feeding difficulties	Neurological and other conditions affecting motor coordination of chewing and swallowing, especially hypertonic cerebral palsy
	Energy density of food inappropriately low	Strict vegetarian diet; excessive and inappropriate parental concern to feed 'healthy diet'
	Poor appetite	Anorexia due to infection or other illness
	Vomiting	Esophageal reflux, infection, metabolic disturbance
Too much energy lost from the body	Energy lost as sugar in urine	Diabetes mellitus
	Protein lost as protein in urine	Nephrotic syndrome
	Protein lost through skin	Burns
		Severe eczema
Failure to absorb	Malnutrition syndromes	Gluten-sensitive enteropathy/celiac syndrome
		Cystic fibrosis
		Protein-losing enteropathy
		Lactose intolerance
Failure to utilize	Chronic illness	Chronic infection
		Urinary tract infection
		Other hidden infections
		Cyanotic congenital heart disease
		Inborn errors of metabolism
		Severe mental retardation
		Deficiency of other essential nutrients
Increased requirements	Elevated BMR	Thyrotoxicosis
		Congenital heart disease with left to right shunts and high output state
	Increased growth rates	Catch up growth following period of failure to thrive
	Increased activity as increased respiratory rate	Cystic fibrosis
		Congenital heart disease
	Increased activity	Uncontrolled hyperactive behavior

BMR, basal metabolic rate.

Some children have no recognizable pathological abnormalities and yet they fail to thrive. In some children inappropriate management of the feeding problems described earlier underlies poor growth. Others may be underfed because of poverty, ignorance, or incompetence amongst carers. Some parents, anxious to forestall obesity or cancer and cardiovascular conditions in later life, feed diets that are too restricted in nutrient quantity or variety for normal growth, or which follow rigidly the dietary recommendations intended for adults. In the so-called muesli belt syndrome, skimmed milk, wholemeal cereals, and low-sugar low-fat foods dominate.

Psychosocial Deprivation

Some children fail to thrive despite apparently adequate intakes and no evidence of underlying illness. Some are subject to physical and/or emotional abuse and have psychosocial deprivation (PSD), 'non-organic failure to thrive,' or 'emotional deprivation syndrome.' If children are not stimulated by face to face contact and communication with parents and carers, if they are verbally and/or physically abused, or if they are neglected and ignored, the silent response may be growth failure. Affected children may show other signs of emotional distress. They are withdrawn, developmentally delayed, rarely smile, and avoid eye to eye contact. Sometimes they seek attention through destructive, aggressive, and disturbing behavior or steal food, raid dustbins for food, or eat the leftovers on their schoolmates' plates, and yet show no weight gain.

The process inhibiting normal growth in PSD is likely to be multifactorial and to vary with individual circumstances. In some cases, affected children have not received sufficient food for normal growth. In other cases, food may have been offered but misery and fear prevented the children eating it thus subjecting them to further ridicule or punishment because of unfinished meals. Some children, who appear to have been given adequate food and yet fail to grow, may have elevated metabolic rates and increased energy needs secondary to anxiety and stress. A few studies suggest the growth problem in PSD can be linked to neuroendocrine abnormalities secondary to stress. Levels of growth hormone and adrenocorticotrophic hormone have been low in some children studied in their adverse environments. Changes to loving, caring, and stimulating environments result in rapid resolution of the endocrine abnormalities.

The treatment of nonorganic failure to thrive is to change the caring environment either by support and help for affected families or, in difficult cases, removal of affected children from their homes on a temporary or permanent basis. Proof of the diagnosis comes with rapid onset of vigorous catch up growth and positive changes in behavior following improvement in the home environment without other specific treatment.

Toddler Diarrhea

One troublesome diet-related problem occurring in preschool children is 'toddler diarrhea.' Young children are susceptible to gastrointestinal infections because of immature, inexperienced immune systems and poor hygiene from their habit of 'mouthing' almost everything they handle. Children are also prone to develop loose stools in response to minor nongastrointestinal infections. However, some children suffer frequent episodes of loose watery stools with or without increased stool frequency and without evidence of infection. These episodes of diarrhea may last weeks or months. Since it may be difficult to distinguish this diarrhea from other significant gastrointestinal pathology, affected children may be subjected to a lot of unrewarding clinical investigation.

Children with toddler diarrhea usually grow normally, unlike most children with significant gastrointestinal pathology. Typically, they are untroubled by their diarrhea although their parents are understandably very concerned – parents have to cope with loose stools in incontinent children! Investigation of toddler diarrhea should include stool microscopy and stool culture to look for evidence of infection and fat maldigestion. Results are usually normal although parents frequently state that the children's stools contain 'undigested food.' On questioning, 'undigested food' means tomato skins, bean husks, and other substances always present in stools but not obvious in formed stools. The fluid stools make these normal food residues more noticeable than usual.

The balance of macronutrients in affected children's diets may be at least partly responsible for toddler diarrhea. Young children who drink a lot of sugared fluids can have loose stools due to sugars reaching the large bowel and causing osmotic diarrhea particularly when fructose corn starch is used since the fructose is poorly absorbed without associated glucose. Sorbitol, sometimes used as a artificial sweetener, is also unabsorbed and can cause loose stools. In the 1992 National Diet and Nutrition Survey children aged $1\frac{1}{2}$–$4\frac{1}{2}$ years drank on average 1.5 l of sugar-containing drinks and 1 l of 'diet' drinks per week. Some drank much more. On average, 6% of food energy came from soft drinks in children $1\frac{1}{2}$–$4\frac{1}{2}$ years old. High intakes of food-derived refined carbohydrates add to osmotic diarrhea. Sugar, preserves, confectionery, and sweetened drinks contribute around 20% of the total energy intake of 4–10-year-olds in the UK.

Diets high in refined carbohydrates are commonly low in nonstarch polysaccharides (NSP) and in the proportion of energy derived from fat. Reducing the intake of refined sugars and carbohydrates, increasing the fat content of the diet to 30–35% total energy, and increasing the intake of unrefined carbohydrates and NSP usually result in less fluid stools. The improved continence that comes with age also helps resolution of toddler diarrhea. Most affected children are free of major symptoms by school age. Some retain tendencies to loose stools in response to infection and stress throughout life.

Anemia

Anemia is common in young children. It has many causes but nutritional deficiencies, i.e., inadequate nutrient intakes and anemia secondary to disease processes, explain much childhood anemia. Acceptable hemoglobin levels in children are lower on average than in adults. The World Health Organization (WHO) accepted lower limit of normal hemoglobin is $110\,\mathrm{g\,l^{-1}}$ for children 1–6 years old and $120\,\mathrm{g\,l^{-1}}$ for those over 6 years. Infants are born with relatively high hemoglobin levels which, whilst appropriate for the low oxygen tensions of intrauterine life, are unnecessary for postnatal life. The bone marrow therefore becomes quiescent and hemoglobin levels fall. Although erythropoeisis increases again after about 2 months of postnatal life, hemoglobin levels remain lower than in adults for most of childhood perhaps partly because erythropoeisis cannot keep up with the rapid expansion of the blood compartment as body size increases.

Nutritional anemia is most commonly due to iron deficiency. **Table 3** outlines some causes of iron deficiency. Iron absorption from foods other than breast milk is never very efficient although deficiency increases the proportion of iron absorbed from the

Table 3 Some causes of iron deficiency in children

Categorization of problem	Causative condition
Too little iron ingested	Diet poor in meats, dark green leaves, iron-fortified cereals
	Anorexia and low iron intakes
Too much iron lost from body	Hemorrhage from any cause if severe or chronic
	Insidious intestinal blood loss, e.g., cows' milk protein intolerance
	Crohn's disease
Failure to absorb	Vegetarian diets where no heme iron in diet
	Low fruit and vegetable intake so ferric iron not reduced in stomach by dietary vitamin C
	Lack of gastric acid: achlorhydria
	Pyrexia reducing absorption
	Malabsorption involving jejunum and upper ileum, e.g., celiac syndrome
Failure to utilize	Deficiency of other essential nutrients for formation of hemoglobin, e.g., vitamin A, riboflavin
	Chronic inflammatory conditions
Increased requirements	After blood loss
	In rapid catch up growth

jejunum. Absorption of iron in heme from meat is more efficient than as inorganic ferrous or ferric iron. Thus, vegetarian diets present increased risk of iron deficiency. However, most diets, even in affluent westernized countries, are marginal in the amount of iron in relation to population needs. All children are at risk of developing iron deficiency with minor disturbances in dietary quality, iron absorption and metabolism, or with blood loss. Iron absorption takes place in the jejunum and upper ileum so conditions such as gluten-sensitive enteropathy (celiac syndrome), where the brunt of intestinal damage is in the jejunum and upper ileum, may present as severe iron deficiency. Reduced iron absorption during pyrexial illness contributes to iron deficiency in children who suffer frequent infections.

Anemia is not easy to recognize clinically since pallor is a very nonspecific sign. Koilonychia (spoon-shaped nails) although fairly specific is not obvious in the small finger nails of children. Iron deficiency affects mentality and behavior making children irritable, uncooperative and anorexic, or tired and apathetic. Severe iron deficiency is associated with pica or desire for abnormal foods particularly those with metallic earthy tastes such as clay and coal.

Hypochromic, microcytic anemia is the end point of iron deficiency when stores have been exhausted, tissue iron levels are falling, and there is insufficient iron to meet the needs of red cell production. If severe, iron deficiency anemia (IDA) causes breathlessness, tiredness, poor appetite, and failure to thrive. Anemia develops slowly so there is physiological adaptation to the developing anemia and hemoglobin levels may be very low ($<40\,\mathrm{g\,l^{-1}}$) before symptoms are noticed. Oral iron therapy allows gradual return to normal physiology and is safer than blood transfusion even when hemoglobin levels are very low.

Worldwide, iron deficiency is possibly the commonest nutritional deficiency. Studies show that IDA is associated with poor outcomes in growth and intellectual capacity. The evidence that impaired growth and intellectual development can also result from iron deficiency without anemia is less definite and remains an area of research.

Circulating iron-binding factors such as transferrin are reduced in children with protein energy malnutrition. Normally, iron circulating in plasma and tissues is bound to proteins such as transferrin. When these proteins are reduced in quantity, iron in the tissues may be inadequately 'bound.' Unbound tissue iron encourages free radical damage in tissues and cells, counteracting immunological resistance and facilitating overwhelming infection. Iron supplements should not be given to malnourished children until they are showing signs of recovery by which time they will need the iron for catch up growth.

Zinc Deficiency

Zinc deficiency is associated with impaired growth and maturation. Zinc deficiency is common in those with frequent diarrhea since zinc concentrations in gastrointestinal secretions are high. Nevertheless, there is little consistent population evidence that children who show recurrent acute diarrhea or who have prevalent growth faltering are improved by zinc supplementation. Supplementation of children with diarrhea in zinc-deficient environments may reduce the duration of diarrhea and thus the risk of persistent diarrhea, but does not reduce the risk of children developing diarrhea.

The original reports of zinc deficiency referred to short boys in the Middle East who had delayed puberty that responded to zinc supplementation with maturation and growth acceleration. However, few studies provide good evidence that zinc has a significant effect on maturation in the vast majority of children with pubertal delay. Clinical signs of zinc deficiency are unusual apart from the nonspecific signs of poor growth. In children fed artificial diets deficient in zinc or in those with acrodermatitis enteropathica (congenital lack of zinc-binding intestinal ligand), zinc deficiency results in severe diarrhea, peeling eczematous skin, and death from overwhelming infection and/or malnutrition without supplementary zinc. Breast milk contains a zinc-binding ligand that facilitates the absorption of zinc, so clinical evidence of acrodermatitis enteropathica does not appear until breast-feeding ceases.

Calcium and Vitamin D

These micronutrients are discussed elsewhere (see 00033 and 00051). Childhood is an important time for deposition of bone mineral and the development of peak bone mass (PBM). Seventy-five per cent of bone mineral is deposited in childhood. Low PBM in late adolescence is a significant precursor of later osteoporosis. Much of the population variation in PBM is genetically determined, but low calcium and vitamin D together with a relatively sedentary lifestyle seem factors likely to contribute to low PBM and risks of osteoporosis later in life. Data from The Gambia show that in preadolescent children adequate calcium deposition takes place despite very low intakes of calcium. In some studies where milk-derived calcium phosphate was fed to children there was accelerated growth and maturation in the supplemented children. The Gambian studies showed no change in growth in the supplemented children although there was increased bone mineralization.

Vigorous calcium deposition in children in the tropics and subtropics despite very low calcium intakes may relate to higher circulating 25 hydroxy vitamin D derived from the action of sunlight on 7-dehydrocholesterol in the skin and to high levels of physical activity amongst these children. Deposition of calcium in bone is significantly affected by the weight-bearing activity of the individual. Where children are less active and vitamin D levels lower, dietary calcium intakes may have a greater determining effect on bone mineralization. In northerly temperate climates, such as the UK, children's diets should provide a good source of calcium and there should be reasonable exposure to summer sunshine (a slightly controversial area in view of current concerns about increased skin cancer risk from UVL). An active lifestyle is also important for optimal bone mineralization and high PBM, particularly in those where there is reason to suspect genetic predisposition to low PBM.

Other Micronutrients

Table 4 and **Table 5** outline some of the micronutrient deficiency problems that can arise in childhood. Most of these conditions are rare in their overt form in westernized countries because of the variety of children's diets. There remain questions as to whether levels of micronutrient nutrition that do not lead to clinical deficiency syndromes may nevertheless have effects on immunity, growth, and development in children. This seems possible for iron deficiency and psychoneurological functioning and is proven for folic acid and embryological development. For other micronutrients the evidence is less strong. Similarly, there is currently no good evidence that raising children's micronutrient intakes above recommended levels incurs any particular benefit to health or intellectual development.

Allergy

Food allergy is discussed elsewhere (see 00122 and 00123). It is a frequent diagnosis in childhood. Diarrhea, rashes, and wheezing are common symptoms caused by infection probably more commonly than by food allergy. Parental desire to explain a child's frequent illness may lead to food being wrongly blamed for recurrent symptoms. Vague associations between food and the development of symptoms can result in many foods being unnecessarily excluded and children reduced to diets of very limited variety. For example, whilst 14% of children may be described as allergic to some food, as few as 5% may have had this diagnosis confirmed by their medical practitioners.

Much publicity has surrounded the idea that 'fast foods' and carbonated drinks influence behavior. Even so, there is very little hard scientific evidence to support the widely held view that food additives are harmful to children's behavior. A few studies have shown a minority of children where food does seem to be directly associated with behavioral change, particularly when tartrazine is considered. However, the organization and discipline necessary to eliminate certain foods from young children's diets may be as influential in improving behavior as removal of a food from the diet. The area remains a confused one but there seems little justification for the use of most food colorants, texturizers, and even preservatives, irrespective of their effects on behavior.

Promoting Good Nutrition for Children

Good nutrition is only one aspect of the positive life style that promotes sustainable physical, mental, and social well-being. But the diets and life styles learnt in childhood are likely to influence adult life and

Table 4 Vitamin deficiency problems that may occur in childhood

Vitamin	Condition	Features
Vitamin A – retinol, carotene	Xerophthalmia	Minor: night blindness
		Major: total destruction of eye and blindness
		Nutritional stunting
		Increased infection; severe infection
Vitamin B_1 – thiamine	Beriberi	Mental changes: apathy, irritability, depression
		Cardiac failure
		Peripheral neuritis
Vitamin B_2 – riboflavin	Anemia	Hypochromic, microcytic anemia
		Dry skin; seborrhoeic dermatitis in skinfolds; angular stomatitis; raw red tongue
Vitamin B_3 – niacin	Pellagra	Cracked, dry, peeling, or blistering light-sensitive dermatitis
		Apathy, depression, confusion
		Diarrhea
Vitamin B_6 – pyridoxine	Convulsions	Unusual except in inborn errors of metabolism involving pyridoxine
		Peripheral neuritis
		Convulsions
		Anemia
Vitamin B_{12} – cyanocobalamin	Pernicious megaloblastic anemia	Megaloblastic macrocytic anemia
	Subacute combined degeneration of the spinal cord	Anesthesia and loss of position sense and motor weakness in limbs
		Encephalopathy
Folic acid	Anemia	Megaloblastic anemia
	Growth faltering	Folic acid deficiency may develop whenever there is rapid growth. It may also cause impaired catch up growth or growth faltering
Vitamin C – ascorbic acid	Scurvy	Bleeding, bruising with painful bleeding subperiosteally
		Anemia
		Osteoporosis
Vitamin D – calciferol	Rickets	Painful deformity of weight-bearing bones with bowed legs; swollen ends to shafts of long bones and ribs giving Harrison's sulcus at attachment of diaphragm to lower ribs and 'rickety rosary' effect; bossed skull
		Poor growth and increased infection
		Rarely, hypocalcemic tetany
Vitamin E – tocopherol	Hemolytic anemia	Unusual except in fat malabsorption conditions such as cystic fibrosis and abetalipoproteinemia
	Neurological degeneration	Loss of sensation and motor power in limbs similar to that with vitamin B_{12} deficiency

Table 5 Mineral deficiencies that can occur in childhood

Mineral	Condition	Features
Iron	Anemia	Hypochromic, microcytic anemia
	Impaired growth	Role of iron, as separate from anemia, in relation to poor growth not clear.
	Impaired cognition	Likewise role of iron independent of anemia in impaired cognition not clear
Iodine	Cretinism	Severity of iodine deficiency and age at which it occurs affect the damage caused
	Stunting	The younger the child the more likely there is permanent neurological damage
	Goiter	Goiter common when growth rapid in early life and at adolescence
Zinc	Loss of taste	Anorexia
	Growth impairment	Zinc deficiency is associated with growth faltering and delayed maturation
	Gastrointestinal effects	Acute diarrhea may be more likely to persist when there is zinc deficiency
Selenium	Keshan disease	Cardiomyopathy which may be precipitated by associated deficiency of vitamin E or perhaps by Coxsackie virus infection
	Kachin-Beck syndrome	Osteoarthritis affecting particularly lower limbs
Copper	Anemia	Microcytic hypochromic anemia
	Poor bone mineralization	Osteoporosis
Calcium	Rickets-like syndrome	Very low calcium diets can be associated with rickets-like condition but more usual for associated vitamin D deficiency as well
Magnesium	Often silent deficiency	Deficiency is very unusual except in severe malnutrition when it is universal
		Occasionally magnesium deficient convulsions

Table 6 Principles of good nutrition in childhood

Policy	Practice
Feed children appropriate to their developmental skills	Progress diet from soft mushy weaning diet to increasingly lumpy and then chewable foods Encourage biting and chewing Encourage new foods, textures, and tastes
Encourage recognition of satiety and hunger	Organize regular meals and snacks Eat as a family where possible Eat away from activities such as watching television Avoid snacking whilst occupied with television or computer or other absorbing activity
Encourage varied nutrient intake	Home prepared foods when possible so nutrient content is recognized Vary diet and recognize that children may not accept new foods on first tasting If possible use other members of the family to show how specific foods are enjoyable
Achieve nutrient needs by varied diet	Plan for an energy-dense staple, protein source, micronutrient source at each meal Aim for about 500 ml of milk or formula daily to provide a good calcium source Provide a source of vitamin C at each meal Aim towards five small portions of fruit and vegetable/day and gradually increase portion sizes (e.g., from few segments of an orange work up to a whole orange as the child's appetite grows)
Aim for diet that will protect as far as possible against chronic noncommunicable diseases as adult	Work towards recommendations for a healthy adult diet as child matures but avoid high fiber, low-fat diets in early childhood
Maintain active life style	Encourage activity both outside and inside the home Encourage children to take part in household chores Encourage children to take an interest in and understand food preparation and food choice

should optimize opportunities for health and social well being throughout life.

It is unlikely that the Western world, with its working mothers and busy parents, can return to a society where all meals are consumed as families. Eating and socializing over meals are nevertheless important for child development since they may encourage children to recognize satiety during the time spent eating. Further, the communication and stimulation that should take place during family meals develops children's social skills. Even when family meals are not practical, eating should be organized, and to some extent formalized, preferably away from distractions such as television, which may detract from awareness of the quantity of food consumed. Snacking should be at specific times rather than an activity that happens because food is available or because there is nothing else to do. **Table 6** outlines some of the principles to be followed when trying to develop good eating and nutritional habits in childhood.

A healthy diet needs to be accompanied by plenty of exercise, out of doors whenever possible. Young children are naturally extremely active and should be encouraged to explore and develop their physical skills under supervision. Sedentary interests, particularly watching television, should occupy only a very small portion of the day although as children grow older, homework, which is usually fairly sedentary, inevitably occupies part of the after school hours. At home children can be kept active helping around the

house, playing games, and pursuing varied hobbies. Overcoming sedentariness may involve parents as well as children, but that should be good for parents' health also.

Eating and drinking opportunities at school can run counter to the good nutritional practices parents may be pursuing. For example, in schools, water dispensers could replace those selling carbonated drinks although drinks sales are often significant sources of revenue for schools. Many countries now have guidelines, such as making fruit available at lunch, for healthy eating programs in schools. Nevertheless, diet is only one, admittedly important, area for action when developing life styles that should sustain normal nutrition throughout the life cycle.

Conclusion

The common nutritional problems in children on varied Western diets are mostly fairly minor feeding-related difficulties in the very young, failure to thrive, or the concerning modern problem of obesity (see 00210). However, childhood nutrition can influence health in later life. Good nutritional practice should be a continuum running from infancy through to old age. Childhood is an important stage in setting such practice.

See also: **Anemia**: Iron-Deficiency Anemia. **Behavior**. **Calcium**. **Children**: Nutritional Requirements. **Dietary Fiber**: Role in Nutritional Management of Disease.

Food Allergies: Etiology; Diagnosis and Management.
Growth and Development, Physiological Aspects.
Iron. Malnutrition: Secondary, Diagnosis and
Management. **Obesity**: Childhood Obesity. **Vegetarian
Diets. Vitamin D**: Rickets and Osteomalacia.
Zinc: Physiology.

Further Reading

Anon (1997) Guidelines for school health programs to promote lifelong healthy eating. *Journal of School Health* **67**: 9–26.

Black RE and Sazawal S (2001) Zinc and childhood infectious disease morbidity and mortality. *British Journal of Nutrition* **85** (supplement) 2: S125–S129.

Dibba B, Prentice A, Ceesay M *et al.* (2000) Effect of calcium supplementation on bone mineral accretion in Gambian children accustomed to a low calcium diet. *American Journal of Clinical Nutrition* **71**: 544–549.

Gregory JR, Collins DL, Davies PSW, Hughes JM, and Clarke PC (1995) *National Diet and Nutrition Survey: Children Aged 1½–4½*, pp. 27–48. London: HMSO.

Gregory J and Lowe S (2000) *National Diet and Nutrition Survey: Young People Aged 4 to 18 Years, Volume 1: Report of the Diet and Nutrition Survey*, pp. 45–105. London: HMSO.

Prasad AS, Miale A, Farid Z, Schulert A, and Sandstead HH (1963) Zinc metabolism in patients with iron deficiency anaemia, hypogonadism and dwarfism. *Journal of Laboratory and Clinical Medicine* **61**: 537–549.

Rayner PH and Rudd BT (1973) Emotional deprivation in three siblings associated with functional pituitary growth hormone deficiency. *Australian Paediatric Journal* **9**: 79–84.

Rowe KS and Rowe KJ (1994) Synthetic food coloring and behavior: a dose response effect in a double blind, placebo controlled, repeated measure study. *Journal of Pediatrics* **125**: 691–698.

WHO (1972) *Nutritional Anemia*. WHO Technical Report Series Number 3. Geneva: WHO.

Cholecalciferol *see* **Vitamin D**: Physiology, Dietary Sources and Requirements; Rickets and Osteomalacia

---

CHOLESTEROL

Contents
Sources, Absorption, Function and Metabolism
Factors Determining Blood Levels

Sources, Absorption, Function and Metabolism

D J McNamara, Egg Nutrition Center, Washington, DC, USA

© 2005 Elsevier Ltd. All rights reserved.

The intestinal absorption of cholesterol, its transport through the vascular system, its utilization for synthesis of steroids and bile acids, and its fecal excretion represent a complex interplay between two metabolic processes: the absorption of exogenous dietary cholesterol and endogenous cholesterol synthesis by body tissues. From the initial mixing of dietary and biliary cholesterol in the small intestine to the excretion of fecal neutral and acid steroids, there are two sources of cholesterol, which combine to determine the overall dynamics of whole-body cholesterol metabolism and the ability of the metabolic regulatory processes to maintain tissue cholesterol homeostasis as well as a steady-state plasma cholesterol level. It is the balance between dietary cholesterol intake and absorption, endogenous cholesterol synthesis, and fecal steroid excretion that determine overall cholesterol homeostasis in the body (**Table 1**).

Absorption, Transport, and Storage

Cholesterol Absorption

Cholesterol in the intestinal lumen typically consists of one-third dietary cholesterol and two-thirds biliary cholesterol. The average daily diet contains 300–500 mg of cholesterol obtained from animal

Table 1 Average cholesterol metabolism values for a 70-kg adult

Cholesterol pools and flux	Mass
Cholesterol pool (70-kg adult)	160 g
Plasma cholesterol pool	8 g
Dietary cholesterol intake	300 mg/day
Absorption (average 60%)	180 mg/day
Synthesis (12 mg/kg/day)	840 mg/day
Total cholesterol input	1020 mg/day
Bile acid synthesis (= fecal excretion)	250 mg/day
Neutral steroid excretion	770 mg/day

products. The bile provides an additional 800–1200 mg of cholesterol throughout each day as gallbladder contractions provide a flow of bile acids, cholesterol, and phospholipids to facilitate lipid digestion and absorption. Dietary cholesterol is a mixture of free and esterified cholesterol, whereas biliary cholesterol is nonesterified and is introduced into the small intestine as a cholesterol–bile salt–phospholipid water-soluble complex. The only other source of intraluminal cholesterol is mucosal cell cholesterol, derived from either sloughed mucosal cells or cholesterol secreted by the mucosal cells into the intestinal lumen. Measurements of exogenous and endogenous cholesterol absorption in humans indicate that there is probably very little direct secretion of newly synthesized cholesterol from mucosal cells into the intraluminal contents.

Cholesterol absorption occurs primarily in the duodenum and proximal jejunum of the small intestine and is dependent on the presence of bile salts. In the absence of bile secretion, or in the presence of bile acid-binding resins, there is virtually no intestinal absorption of cholesterol. On average, humans absorb 50–60% of the intestinal contents of cholesterol, but there is a large interindividual variance in absorption, with values ranging from as low as 20% to as high as 80%. Intestinal transit time is related to cholesterol absorption, with slower transit times resulting in higher fractional absorption rates. Dietary factors that affect the relative percent absorption of cholesterol include the total mass of dietary cholesterol, the concentration of plant sterols in the diet, and the type and amount of dietary fiber. Studies suggest that the ratio of polyunsaturated to saturated fat (P:S) in the diet has little effect on cholesterol absorption rates in humans, nor does the amount of dietary fat.

Two interesting, and as yet undefined, aspects of cholesterol absorption are that it decreases as the mass of cholesterol increases above an intake of 1500 mg per day, and that the fractional absorption below this level is relatively constant for an individual. For example, at a daily cholesterol intake of 800 mg a subject may absorb 60% or 480 mg per day, whereas at a daily intake of 400 mg the absorption remains at 60%, equaling 240 mg per day absorbed. The quandary is that if the system can accommodate absorption of 480 mg at the high cholesterol intake, then why is the amount absorbed 240 mg at the low intake? Clearly, the upper value of cholesterol absorption is achievable, yet at the lower intake level the absorption rate stays at a fixed fractional value. The mechanisms controlling this aspect of cholesterol absorption have not been defined.

Experimental evidence indicates that biliary cholesterol and dietary cholesterol are absorbed equally; however, the pattern of exogenous and endogenous cholesterol absorption differs along the length of the intestinal lumen. Dietary cholesterol enters the small intestine solubilized in the oil phase of the stomach digest, whereas the binary cholesterol enters in the micelle phase of the bile. This differential distribution results in a greater absorption of biliary cholesterol in the upper portion of the small intestine, with dietary cholesterol absorption increasing as the oil phase of the intestinal contents are hydrolyzed. As the oil phase is reduced, dietary cholesterol moves from the oil phase to the aqueous micelle phase and becomes available for absorption. In the case of cholesteryl esters in the diet, it is necessary that the esters are hydrolyzed by pancreatic cholesterol esterase (CEase) before the cholesterol is available for absorption. Pancreatic CEase requires the presence of bile salts for activity and may play a key role in the actual absorption process.

The process, and selectivity, of sterol absorption involves a complex interplay of regulated transporters, transporting sterols into and out of the enterocyte, and the assembly and secretion of chylomicrons into the lymph. The enterocyte takes up both cholesterol and phytosterols from the intestinal lumen by what appears to be a common sterol transporter or permease in the brush border membrane. Preliminary studies suggest that the Neiman–Pick C1 like 1 (NPC1L1) protein is involved in this process. Once the sterols enter the enterocyte, the ATP binding cassette (ABC) hemitransporters ABCG5 and ABCG8 function in the apical excretion of sterols back into the intestinal lumen. The selectivity of this process accounts for the higher absorption rates of cholesterol (50–60%) compared to the phytosterols, which are very poorly absorbed. Loss of ABCG5/G8 function results in excessive absorption of both cholesterol and phytosterols. Studies in mice have shown that ABCG5/G8 are expressed primarily in the liver and intestine, are coordinately upregulated at the transcriptional level by dietary cholesterol intake, and require the liver X receptor-α (LXR-α), a nuclear receptor that regulates the expression of a number of key genes involved in lipid metabolism.

Evidence is accumulating that the fractional cholesterol absorption rates are regulated by one or more genetic determinants. The apolipoprotein (apo) E phenotype has a significant effect on fractional cholesterol absorption and appears to play a major role in determining the plasma lipoprotein response to changes in dietary cholesterol intake. Men with the *apoE4* allele have a high cholesterol absorption rate, whereas those with the *apoE2* allele have a low cholesterol absorption efficiency. The absorption values for the more common *apoE3/3* fall between the *apoE2* and *apoE4* patterns. Polymorphisms of the apolipoprotein A-IV and of the low-density lipoprotein (LDL) receptor gene have also been related to differences in fractional cholesterol absorption. These genetic variants affecting cholesterol absorption no doubt play a significant role in determining an individual's fractional absorption of cholesterol as well as accounting for much of the heterogeneity of plasma lipid responses to changes in dietary cholesterol intakes.

Exogenous Cholesterol Transport

Cholesterol is absorbed in the unesterified state, whereas the cholesterol secreted into the lymph is 70–80% esterified. This esterification process generates a concentration gradient of free cholesterol within the mucosal cell that may facilitate absorption rates. Cholesterol is esterified in intestinal mucosal cells by acyl-coenzyme A:cholesterol acyltransferase-2 to form cholesteryl esters, which are secreted from the basolateral surface of the enterocyte as part of the chylomicrons. At this stage, it is assumed that cholesterol molecules from exogenous and endogenous sources are indistinguishable and have similar effects on endogenous cholesterol and lipoprotein metabolism. Chylomicrons are large particles (>70 nm in diameter) composed mainly of triacylglycerols (95% by weight) and contain 3–7% cholesterol by weight, with the esterified cholesterol localized in the hydrophobic core and the free cholesterol primarily in the hydrophilic outer layer. The data indicate that the amount of dietary cholesterol consumed has little effect on the cholesterol content of chylomicrons. The chylomicrons are released from the intestinal cells, enter the lymphatic system, and are transported via the lymphatics (thoracic duct) to the bloodstream. Since chylomicrons are too large to pass through the capillaries, this is the only mechanism by which they can enter the bloodstream.

In the plasma compartment, the chylomicrons pick up a number of apolipoproteins, which are required for intravascular metabolism of the particles. The initial metabolism of chylomicrons involves hydrolysis of the associated triacylglycerols by endothelial cell lipoprotein lipase (LPL) located in adipose, muscle, and heart tissues, which results in production of chylomicron remnants. The chylomicron remnants, depleted of triacylglycerol and enriched with cholesteryl ester, are taken up by the liver via the LDL receptor-related protein (LRP). The ligand for hepatic uptake of the chylomicron remnant appears from various transgenic mouse studies to be the apo-E moiety of the particle. The clearance of chylomicrons from the bloodstream is rapid, with particles having a half-life of less than 1 h. The liver cannot take up native chylomicrons but rather takes up the chylomicron remnant, which has lost approximately 90% of its triacylglycerol content and become relatively enriched in free and esterified cholesterol through the actions of the plasma cholesteryl ester transfer protein (CETP), which transfers cholesteryl ester from high-density lipoprotein (HDL) to the apo-B-containing lipoproteins.

The chylomicron remnants taken up by the liver are subjected to lysosomal hydrolysis, resulting in the release of the absorbed dietary and biliary cholesterol into the hepatocyte as free cholesterol. The influx of cholesterol contained in the chylomicron remnant has the ability to affect a number of regulatory sites of hepatic cholesterol metabolism that function to maintain cholesterol homeostasis in the liver. The liver has four primary fates for the newly delivered cholesterol: catabolism to bile acids, secretion as biliary cholesterol, storage in lipid droplets as cholesteryl ester, or incorporation into very low-density lipoprotein (VLDL) for secretion from the liver.

Tissue Uptake and Storage

The body pool of cholesterol is approximately 145 g, with one-third of this mass localized in the central nervous system. The remainder of the metabolically active cholesterol pool exists in the plasma compartment (7.5–9 g) and as constituents of body tissues. In humans, tissue cholesterol levels are relatively low, averaging 2 or 3 mg/g wet weight. Little information exists regarding changes in hepatic and extrahepatic tissue cholesterol concentrations with changes in dietary cholesterol intake. Animal studies, which are usually carried out using very high levels of dietary cholesterol, have shown that hepatic cholesterol can increase from 2-fold up to 10-fold, depending on the species and other dietary constituents, when dietary cholesterol is increased.

Biosynthesis

Tissue Cholesterol Synthesis

Cholesterol biosynthesis occurs in every nucleated cell in the body. Although it is often thought that the majority of cholesterol synthesis occurs in the liver, studies have shown that the bulk tissues of the body account for the overwhelming majority of endogenous cholesterol production. Hepatic cholesterol synthesis in humans is thought to contribute 10–20% of the total daily synthesis rate. Since the majority of cholesterol synthesis in the body occurs in extrahepatic tissues, and since the only quantitatively significant site for excretion and catabolism of cholesterol is the liver, approximately 600–800 mg of cholesterol each day must be transported from peripheral tissues through the plasma compartment to the liver to account for daily cholesterol catabolism and binary secretion. Approximately 9 mg cholesterol per kilogram body weight is synthesized by peripheral tissues every day and must be moved to the liver for catabolism via a process termed 'reverse cholesterol transport' (RCT).

RCT describes the metabolism, and important antiatherogenic function, of the HDL-mediated efflux of cholesterol from nonhepatic cells and its subsequent delivery to the liver and steroidogenic organs for use in the synthesis of lipoproteins, bile acids, vitamin D, and steroid hormones. A cellular ABC transporter (ABCA1) mediates the first step of RCT involving the transfer of cellular cholesterol and phospholipids to lipid-poor apolipoproteins. Lecithin:cholesterol acyltransferase-mediated esterification of cholesterol generates spherical particles that continue to expand with ongoing cholesterol esterification and phospholipid transfer protein-mediated particle fusion and surface remnant transfer. Larger HDL_2 particles are converted into smaller HDL_3 particles when CETP facilitates the transfer of cholesteryl esters from HDL onto apoB-containing lipoproteins. The scavenger receptor B1 (SR-B1) promotes selective uptake of cholesteryl esters into liver and steroidogenic organs, whereas hepatic lipase- and LPL mediate hydrolysis of phospholipids and triglycerides. SR-B1 mediates the selective uptake of cholesteryl esters from HDL and also LDL into hepatocytes and steroid hormone-producing cells without internalizing HDL proteins, which can recycle through the RCT sequence moving cholesterol from peripheral tissues to the liver.

Regulation of Synthesis

The rate-limiting enzyme in cholesterol biosynthesis is 3-hydroxy-3-methylglutaryl coenzyme A (HMG-CoA) reductase, a microsomal enzyme that converts HMG-CoA to mevalonic acid in the polyisoprenoid synthetic pathway. Peripheral tissue cholesterol synthesis is much less responsive to regulatory factors compared to the liver, which is controlled by a variety of dietary, hormonal, and physiological variables. Studies indicate that endogenous cholesterol synthesis is significantly increased in obesity and in patients with the metabolic syndrome. Obesity, insulin resistance, and diabetes have pronounced effects on both cholesterol absorption and synthesis. Findings in type 1 diabetes appear to be related to low expression of ABCG5/G8 genes, resulting in high absorption and low synthesis of cholesterol. Cholesterol absorption efficiency is lower and cholesterol synthesis is higher in obese subjects with type 2 diabetes compared to obese subjects without diabetes, suggesting that diabetes modulates cholesterol metabolism to a greater extent than obesity alone. Similarly, low cholesterol absorption and high synthesis appear to be part of the insulin resistance (metabolic) syndrome.

Research shows that in most individuals, dietary cholesterol alters endogenous cholesterol synthesis and that this feedback regulation can effectively compensate for increased cholesterol input from dietary sources. The precision of these regulatory responses depends on a number of genetic factors, and data suggest that multiple genetic loci are involved. For example, family studies have shown that in siblings of low cholesterol absorption families, cholesterol absorption percentages are significantly lower and cholesterol and bile acid synthesis, cholesterol turnover, and fecal steroids are significantly higher than in siblings of high absorption families.

Metabolism and Excretion

The body's metabolic processes cannot break the sterol rings of cholesterol and therefore must either catabolize cholesterol to other products, which can be excreted in the urine or feces, or directly excrete cholesterol in the bile, with a fraction of the biliary cholesterol lost daily as fecal neutral sterols. In humans, the major route of excretion is as biliary cholesterol (two-thirds of the total lost each day), with catabolism to bile acids and bile acid excretion being the second most important route, accounting for approximately one-third of the daily turnover.

For all practical purposes, the body must excrete daily an amount of neutral and acidic sterols equivalent to the combined inputs of total dietary and newly synthesized cholesterol. Given an average fecal excretion of 1020 mg per day with 250 mg as acidic sterols, it can be calculated that the 770 mg per day excreted as neutral steroids comes from unabsorbed biliary

(650 mg) and unabsorbed dietary (120 mg) cholesterol (Table 1) It is easy to see that even small changes in the daily balance between a cholesterol input and output value of 1020 mg per day could, over years, result in significant tissue cholesterol accumulation.

Bile Acid Synthesis

The results from numerous sterol balance studies carried out in subjects fed diets low or high in cholesterol indicate that in humans, dietary cholesterol has little effect on fecal bile acid excretion rates. This finding is in striking contrast to results from studies of some rodent models that show that intake of pharmacological doses of dietary cholesterol can result in severalfold increases in bile acid synthesis and excretion. In contrast, some rodent species and nonhuman primates have little, if any, increase in bile acid excretion with increased intakes of cholesterol. Although there have been a few reports of enhanced bile acid excretion on a high-cholesterol diet in some patients, this does not appear to be a major regulatory response in humans.

Biliary Cholesterol Secretion

The majority of cholesterol entering the intestinal tract is biliary cholesterol. Biliary cholesterol secretion averages 1000 mg per day as part of the bile system and enters as free cholesterol already solubilized with bile acids and phospholipids. Both cholesterol absorption by enterocyte and biliary cholesterol secretion by hepatic cells are regulated by expression of the half-transporters ABCG5 and ABCG8. Studies in animals have shown that treatment with a LXR agonist decreases cholesterol absorption, increases biliary cholesterol secretion, and increases fecal neutral sterol excretion. Studies in transgenic mouse models demonstrate that increased expression of ABCG5 and ABCG8 increases biliary neutral sterol secretion and reduces intestinal cholesterol absorption, leading to increased neutral sterol excretion and cholesterol synthesis.

Fecal Excretion

The only route of significant cholesterol excretion is through fecal excretion of neutral sterols. The combination of unabsorbed biliary and dietary cholesterol accounts for the total neutral sterol output and under most conditions is 750–850 mg per day. Dietary patterns or drugs that interfere with intestinal cholesterol absorption result in increased fecal neutral steroid excretion. In the colon, intestinal bacteria are able to metabolize cholesterol to a variety of neutral steroids as well as to nonsteroid end products. Some studies have suggested that the intestinal metabolism of cholesterol by bacteria, which can be altered by diet and drugs, can influence endogenous cholesterol metabolism as well as plasma cholesterol levels. What these relationships may be and the mechanisms involved have not been defined.

Metabolic Function

Steroid Hormones

Daily production of steroid hormones is quantitatively a very small fraction of the daily turnover of dietary and newly synthesized cholesterol in the body. For men, the average daily excretion of steroid hormones is approximately 50 mg per day, whereas for women the value can be substantially higher depending on the menstrual phase.

Bile Acid Synthesis

The enterohepatic circulation of bile acids is essential for fat and cholesterol digestion and absorption. Each day, the bile acid pool (approximately 3–5 g) cycles through the intestine 6–10 times. The absorption of bile acids by the ileum is very effective and 98 or 99% of bile acids secreted in the bile are returned to the liver via the portal vein. The small amount of bile acids lost each day as fecal acidic steroids are replaced through the conversion of hepatic cholesterol to the primary bile acids, cholic acid and chenodeoxycholic acid. This catabolism of cholesterol can be as little as 250 mg per day up to 500 mg per day depending on the diet. The bile acids represent the only major catabolic product of cholesterol metabolism and in humans account for approximately 25–30% of the daily loss of cholesterol from the body.

Very Low-Density Lipoprotein Synthesis

The endogenous pathway for cholesterol transport focuses on the liver with the synthesis and secretion of VLDL particles. Cholesterol in these triacylglycerol-rich particles comes from multiple sources: endogenous synthesis, diet, and plasma lipoproteins. Catabolism of VLDL by LPL leads to formation of intermediate-density lipoproteins (IDLs), which can either be taken up by the liver or undergo further metabolism to form LDL. Low-density lipoproteins contain apo-B_{100} and account for 60–80% of the plasma cholesterol in most individuals. During lipolysis of VLDL triacylglycerol, the lipoproteins containing apo-B become enriched with cholesteryl ester through the plasma CETP-catalyzed net transfer of cholesteryl ester from HDL. This process, called reverse cholesterol transport, moves cholesterol from extrahepatic tissues to HDL to VLDL–IDL–LDL and eventual uptake by the liver.

Approximately 70% of the LDL degraded each day is degraded by the hepatic LDL receptor pathway.

Dietary Cholesterol and Plasma Cholesterol

The effect of dietary cholesterol on plasma cholesterol levels has been an area of considerable debate. In 1972, the American Heart Association recommended that dietary cholesterol intake should average less than 300 mg per day as part of a 'heart-healthy,' plasma cholesterol-lowering diet. Since that initial recommendation, a number of other public health dietary recommendations in the United States have endorsed the 300 mg daily limit. Interestingly, few dietary recommendations from other countries contain a dietary cholesterol limitation. The evidence for a relationship between dietary cholesterol and plasma cholesterol indicates that the effect is relatively small, and that on average a change of 100 mg per day in dietary cholesterol intake results in a $0.057 \, \text{mmol} \, l^{-1}$ ($2.2 \, \text{mg} \, dl^{-1}$) change in plasma cholesterol concentrations. Studies have also shown that the majority of individuals are resistant to the plasma cholesterol-raising effects of dietary cholesterol 'nonresponders' and have less than the predicted response. In contrast, a segment of the population (estimated to be between 15 and 25%) is sensitive to dietary cholesterol 'responders' and exhibits a greater than expected plasma cholesterol response to a change in dietary cholesterol intake. To date, there are no defined physiological or clinical characteristics to differentiate responders from nonresponders, but studies suggest that the apoE phenotype plays a role, as does the clinical condition of combined hyperlipidemia. Data also suggest that sensitivity to dietary cholesterol is associated with sensitivity to dietary fat, and that overall adiposity may also play a role. Although on a population basis the plasma cholesterol response to dietary cholesterol is relatively small, and in most epidemiological analyses not related to hypercholesterolemia, some individuals are sensitive to dietary cholesterol changes and, if hypercholesterolemic, would experience plasma cholesterol reduction with dietary cholesterol restrictions. For the majority, however, dietary cholesterol restrictions have little effect on plasma cholesterol levels.

Dietary Sources

Dietary Cholesterol Intake Patterns

Dietary cholesterol intakes in the United States have been declining, from an average of 500 mg per day in men and 320 mg per day in women in 1972 to levels in 1990 of 360 mg per day in men and 240 mg per day in women. This decline is due in part to dietary recommendations to the US public to reduce total and saturated fat intake and to reduce dietary cholesterol daily intake to less than 300 mg and in part from the increased availability of products with reduced fat and cholesterol content. Major efforts in the early 1970s by public health agencies and advertising emphasized reducing dietary cholesterol as a means to lower plasma cholesterol levels, leading to a high degree of consumer concern regarding cholesterol-containing foods and demand for low-cholesterol products. Today, practically all foods sold in the United States are labeled for their cholesterol content and their percentage contribution to the daily value of 300 mg for cholesterol.

Major Dietary Sources

The major sources of cholesterol in the diet are eggs, meat, and dairy products. A large egg contains approximately 215 mg of cholesterol and contributes approximately 30–35% of the total dietary cholesterol intake in the United States. Meat, poultry, and fish contribute 45–50%, dairy products 12–15%, and fats and oils 4–6%. In the United States, the range of dietary cholesterol intake is 300–400 mg per day for men and 200–250 mg per day for women; thus, for much of the population the national goal of a dietary cholesterol intake of less than 300 mg per day has been met.

See also: **Coronary Heart Disease**: Hemostatic Factors; Lipid Theory; Prevention. **Fats and Oils**. **Fatty Acids**: Metabolism. **Hyperlipidemia**: Overview; Nutritional Management. **Lipids**: Chemistry and Classification; Composition and Role of Phospholipids.

Further Reading

Dietschy JM, Turley SD, and Spady DK (1993) Role of liver in the maintenance of cholesterol and low density lipoprotein homeostasis in different animal species, including humans. *Journal of Lipid Research* **34**: 1637–1659.

Gylling H and Miettinen TA (2002) Inheritance of cholesterol metabolism of probands with high or low cholesterol absorption. *Journal of Lipid Research* **43**: 1472–1476.

McNamara DJ (1987) Effects of fat-modified diets on cholesterol and lipoprotein metabolism. *Annual Review of Nutrition* **7**: 273–290.

McNamara DJ (1990) Relationship between blood and dietary cholesterol. *Advances in Meat Research* **6**: 63–87.

McNamara DJ (2000) Dietary cholesterol and atherosclerosis. *Biochimica et Biophysica Acta* **1529**: 310–320.

Millatt LJ, Bocher V, Fruchart JC, and Staels B (2003) Liver X receptors and the control of cholesterol homeostasis: Potential therapeutic targets for the treatment of atherosclerosis. *Biochimica et Biophysica Acta* **1631**: 107–118.

Oram JF (2003) HDL apolipoproteins and ABCA1—Partners in the removal of excess cellular cholesterol. *Arteriosclerosis Thrombosis and Vascular Biology* **23**: 720–727.

Ordovas JM and Tai ES (2002) The babel of the ABCs: Novel transporters involved in the regulation of sterol absorption and excretion. *Nutrition Reviews* **60**: 30–33.

Sehayek E (2003) Genetic regulation of cholesterol absorption and plasma plant sterol levels: Commonalities and differences. *Journal of Lipid Research* **44**: 2030–2038.

Thompson GR, Naumova RP, and Watts GF (1996) Role of cholesterol in regulation of apolipoprotein B secretion by the liver. *Journal of Lipid Research* **37**: 439–447.

Wilson MD and Rudel LL (1994) Review of cholesterol absorption with emphasis on dietary and biliary cholesterol. *Journal of Lipid Research* **35**: 943–955.

Yu LQ, Li-Hawkins J, Hammer RE *et al.* (2002) Overexpression of ABCG5 and ABCG8 promotes biliary cholesterol secretion and reduces fractional absorption of dietary cholesterol. *Journal of Clinical Investigation* **110**: 671–680.

Factors Determining Blood Levels

S M Grundy, University of Texas Southwestern Medical Center, Dallas, TX, USA

© 1999 Elsevier Ltd. All rights reserved.

This article is reproduced from the previous edition, pp. 376–382, © 1999, Elsevier Ltd.

Introduction

A high blood (serum) cholesterol level is a major risk factor for atherosclerotic coronary heart disease (CHD). Consequently, there has been much interest in the causes of elevated serum cholesterol concentrations. Although the serum cholesterol can be measured as a single entity, in fact cholesterol is carried in the bloodstream by several independent entities called lipoproteins. Each lipoprotein has its own characteristics, and the concentrations of each are affected by different factors. Several of these factors are related to diet, i.e., dietary cholesterol, certain fatty acids, and energy imbalance resulting in obesity. Other factors also modify lipoprotein metabolism, including advancing age, the postmenopausal state in women, and genetics. Consideration of each of the factors regulating serum cholesterol concentrations first requires a description of the different lipoprotein species.

Serum Lipoproteins

Lipoproteins are macromolecular complexes that consist of discrete particles and are composed of both lipids and proteins. The lipids include cholesterol, phospholipids, and triacylglycerols (TAG). A portion of serum cholesterol is esterified with a fatty acid; the remainder is unesterified. The protein components go by the name of apolipoproteins. The major forms of apolipoproteins and their functions

Table 1 Apolipoproteins of serum lipoproteins

Apolipoprotein	Function
A-I	Major apolipoprotein of HDL
	Activator of LCAT
A-I	Structural apolipoprotein of HDL (other functions unknown)
A-IV	Apolipoprotein of chylomicrons (other functions unknown)
B-48	Chylomicron assembly and secretion
B-100	VLDL assembly and secretion
	Ligand for LDL receptor unknown
C-I	Unknown
C-II	Activator of LPL
C-III	Inhibitor of LPL
E	Apolipoprotein of remnant lipoproteins
	Ligand for LDL receptor
	Promotes hepatic uptake of remnants

Abbreviations: HDL, high-density lipoproteins; LDL, low-density lipoproteins; VLDL, very low-density lipoproteins; LCAT, lecithin cholesterol acyl transferase; LPL, lipoprotein lipase.

are listed in **Table 1**. Four categories of lipoproteins that carry cholesterol in the serum are chylomicrons, very low-density lipoproteins (VLDL), low-density lipoproteins (LDL), and high-density lipoproteins (HDL). The characteristics and metabolism of each lipoprotein will be reviewed briefly.

Chylomicrons

Dietary cholesterol enters the intestine together with fat, which is predominantly TAG. The latter undergoes hydrolysis by pancreatic lipase and releases fatty acids and monoacylglycerols. In the intestine, these mix with bile acids, phospholipids, and cholesterol from the bile. The mixture of hydrolyzed lipids associates with phospholipids and bile acids to form mixed micelles. Fatty acids, monoacylglycerols, and cholesterol are taken up by the intestinal mucosa. In the mucosal cells, the fatty acids and monoacylglycerols are recombined by enzymatic action to form TAG, which are incorporated with the cholesterol into lipoprotein particles called chylomicrons. Most of the cholesterol in chylomicrons is esterified with a fatty acid. The major apolipoprotein of chylomicrons is apo B-48; other apolipoproteins – apo Cs, apo Es and apo As – attach to the surface coat of chylomicrons and aid in metabolic processing. In the mucosal cells, microsomal lipid transfer protein (MTP) facilitates the transfer of TAG and cholesterol ester into chylomicron particles. The presence of MTP is required for the secretion of chylomicrons from mucosal cells.

Chylomicrons are secreted by intestinal mucosal cells into the lymphatic system; from here they pass through the thoracic duct into the systemic circulation. When chylomicrons enter the peripheral circulation they come into contact with an enzyme, lipoprotein lipase (LPL), which is located on the endothelial surface of capillaries. LPL is activated by apo C-II on chylomicrons; this process is modulated by apo C-III, an inhibitor of LPL activity. Nonetheless most chylomicron TAG is hydrolyzed by LPL; a residual lipoprotein particle, named chylomicron remnant, is released into the circulation and is rapidly removed by the liver. Hepatic uptake of chylomicron remnants is believed to be mediated by binding of remnants with a glycoprotein on the surface of liver cells. Almost all newly absorbed cholesterol thus enters the liver in association with chylomicron remnants.

Very Low-Density Lipoproteins

The liver also secretes a TAG-rich lipoprotein called VLDL. Fatty acids used in synthesis of TAG in the liver are normally derived from circulating nonesterified fatty acids (NEFA); even so, the liver has the capacity to synthesize fatty acids when the diet contains mainly carbohydrate. MTP inserts TAG into newly forming VLDL particles. The surface coat of VLDL contains unesterified cholesterol, phospholipids, and apolipoproteins. The major apolipoprotein of VLDL is apo B-100. Other apolipoproteins, notably apo Cs and apo Es, also are present. As VLDL circulate they acquire cholesterol esters from HDL. Circulating VLDL particles lose TAG through interaction with LPL in the peripheral circulation; in this process, VLDL are transformed into VLDL remnants. The latter can have two fates: hepatic uptake or conversion to LDL. Hepatic uptake of VLDL remnants may occur via two mechanisms: interaction with glycoproteins or interaction with LDL receptors. Both glycoproteins and LDL receptors are located on the surface of liver cells.

Low-Density Lipoproteins

Conversion of VLDL remnants to LDL appears to be largely the result of hydrolysis of remaining TAG by hepatic triacylglycerol lipase (HTGL). Normally about two-thirds of cholesterol is carried by LDL, most of this LDL cholesterol existing in the form of esters. The only apolipoprotein in LDL is apo B-100. LDL is removed from the circulation largely by hepatic LDL receptors. The level of expression of LDL receptors is a major determinant of serum LDL cholesterol concentrations. The synthesis of LDL receptors is regulated in large part by the liver's content of cholesterol. An increase in hepatic cholesterol content suppresses LDL receptor synthesis and raises serum LDL cholesterol; conversely, a decrease in hepatic cholesterol stimulates receptor

synthesis and lowers serum LDL cholesterol. The mechanism whereby hepatic cholesterol controls LDL receptor synthesis is through a regulatory protein called sterol regulatory element-binding protein (SREBP). When hepatic cholesterol content falls, SREBP is activated and stimulates the synthesis of LDL receptors.

The regulatory form of cholesterol in the liver cell is unesterified cholesterol, not cholesterol ester. The hepatic content of unesterified cholesterol depends on several factors including the amounts of cholesterol derived from chylomicrons and other lipoproteins, hepatic synthesis of cholesterol, secretion of cholesterol into bile, conversion of cholesterol into bile acids, esterification of cholesterol, and secretion of cholesterol into serum with VLDL. Factors that influence each of these processes can alter serum LDL cholesterol concentrations by modifying the hepatic content of unesterified cholesterol and thereby expression of LDL receptors.

High-Density Lipoproteins

HDL consist of a series of lipoprotein particles of relatively high density, all of which contain apo A-I. A proportion of HDL particles also contain apo A-II. Some HDL species (HDL$_3$) are denser than others (HDL$_2$). HDL particles are composed largely of by-products of catabolism of TAG-rich lipoproteins. The surface coats of HDL particles contain phospholipids and unesterified cholesterol, apo A-I with or without apo A-II, and other apolipoproteins (apo Cs and apo Es). Their particle cores consist largely of cholesterol esters, although small amounts of TAG are also present. The cholesterol esters of HDL are formed by esterification with a fatty acid through the action of an enzyme, lecithin cholesterol acyl transferase (LCAT); the substrates for this reaction derive either from unesterified cholesterol released during lipolysis of TAG-rich lipoproteins or from the surface of peripheral cells. After esterification of cholesterol, the cholesterol esters of HDL are transferred back to TAG-rich lipoproteins and eventually are removed by the liver through direct uptake of remnant lipoproteins or LDL. Whether whole HDL particles can be directly removed from the circulation is uncertain. Some investigators believe that the HDL components are dismantled and removed piecemeal.

Dietary Regulation of Serum Lipoproteins

A large body of research has shown that diet has a major impact on the concentrations and composition of serum lipoproteins, and hence on serum cholesterol concentrations. Three major factors affect cholesterol and lipoprotein concentrations: (1) dietary cholesterol, (2) the macronutrient composition of the diet, particularly dietary fatty acids, and (3) energy balance, as reflected by body weight. The influence of each of these factors can be considered.

Dietary Cholesterol

All dietary cholesterol is derived from animal products. The major sources of cholesterol in the diet are egg yolks, products containing milk fat, animal fats, and animal meats. Many studies have shown that high intakes of cholesterol will increase the serum cholesterol concentration. Most of this increase occurs in the LDL cholesterol fraction. When cholesterol is ingested, it is incorporated into chylomicrons and makes its way to the liver with chylomicron remnants. There it raises hepatic cholesterol content and suppresses LDL receptor expression. The result is a rise in serum LDL cholesterol concentrations. Excess cholesterol entering the liver is removed from the liver either by direct secretion into bile or by conversion into bile acids; also, dietary cholesterol suppresses hepatic cholesterol synthesis. There is considerable variability in each of these steps in hepatic cholesterol metabolism; for this reason the quantitative effects of dietary cholesterol on serum LDL cholesterol levels vary from one person to another. For every 200 mg of cholesterol per day in the diet, serum LDL cholesterol is increased on average by about $6 \, \text{mg} \, \text{dl}^{-1}$ ($0.155 \, \text{mmol} \, \text{l}^{-1}$).

Macronutrient Composition of the Diet

Dietary fat and fatty acids Most of the fat in the diet consists of TAG that are composed of three fatty-acid molecules bonded to glycerol. The contribution of TAG to total energy intake varies among individuals and populations, ranging from 15% to 40% of total nutrient energy. The fatty acids of TAGs are of several types: saturated, *cis*-monounsaturated, *trans*-monounsaturated, and polyunsaturated fatty acids. All fatty acids affect lipoprotein levels in one way or another. **Table 2** lists the major fatty acids of the diet and denotes their effects on serum lipoproteins. Also shown are the effects of carbohydrates, which also influence serum lipoprotein metabolism. It should be noted that all lipoprotein responses are compared with and related to those of *cis*-monounsaturated fatty acids, which are widely accepted to be neutral, or baseline.

Saturated fatty acids The saturated fatty acids are derived from both animal fats and plant oils. Rich sources of dietary saturated fatty acids include butter fat, meat fat, and tropical oils (palm oil, coconut oil, and palm kernel oil). Saturated fatty acids are straight-chain organic acids with an even number of carbon atoms (**Table 2**). All saturated fatty acids that have from eight to 16 carbon atoms raise the serum LDL cholesterol concentration when they are consumed in the diet. In the USA and much of Europe, saturated fatty acids make up 12–15% of total nutrient energy intake.

Table 2 Macronutrient effects on serum lipoprotein cholesterol

Nutrient	Symbol[a]	VLDL cholesterol[a]	LDL cholesterol	HDL cholesterol
Fatty acids				
Saturated				
Palmitic	$C_{16:0}$	$-$[b]	$\uparrow\uparrow$	$-$
Myristic	$C_{14:0}$	$-$	$\uparrow\uparrow\uparrow$	$\downarrow$
Lauric	$C_{12:0}$	$-$	$\uparrow$	$-$
Caproic	$C_{10:0}$	$-$	$\uparrow$	$-$
Caprilic	$C_{8:0}$	$-$	$\uparrow$	$-$
Stearic	$C_{18:0}$	$-$	$-$	or $\downarrow$
trans-Monounsaturated	*trans* $C_{18:1 \, n-9}$	$-$	$\uparrow$ or $\uparrow\uparrow$	$\downarrow$
cis-Monounsaturated	*cis* $C_{18:1 \, n-9}$	$-$	$-$	$-$
Polyunsaturated				
n-6[d]	$C_{18:2 \, n-6}$	$-$ or $\downarrow$	$-$ or $\downarrow$	$-$ or $\downarrow$
n-3[d]	DHA, EPA[e]	$\downarrow\downarrow\downarrow$	$-$ or $\downarrow$	$-$
Carbohydrate		$\uparrow\uparrow\uparrow$	$-$	$\downarrow\downarrow$

[a]First number denotes number of carbon atoms; second number denotes number of double bonds.
[b]The dash ($-$) indicates that there is no change in level compared with that produced by *cis*-monosaturated fatty acids (oleic acid) ($C_{18:1 \, n-9}$). All the lipoprotein responses to oleic acid are considered 'neutral', i.e., no effect.
[c]The letter 'n' and number indicates at which carbon atom, numbered from the terminal methyl group, the first double bond appears. Abbreviations: VLDL, very low-density lipoproteins; LDL, low-density lipoproteins; HDL, high-density lipoproteins; DHA, docosahexanoic acid ($C_{22:6 \, n-3}$); EPA, eicosapentanoic acid ($C_{20:5 \, n-3}$).

The mechanisms whereby saturated fatty acids raise LDL cholesterol levels are not known, although available data suggest that they suppress the expression of LDL receptors. The predominant saturated fatty acid in most diets is palmitic acid ($C_{16:0}$); it is cholesterol-raising when compared with *cis*-monounsaturated fatty acids, specifically oleic acid ($C_{18:cis1\ n-9}$), which is considered to be 'neutral' with respect to serum cholesterol concentrations. In other words, oleic acid is considered by most investigators to have no effect on serum cholesterol or lipoproteins. Another saturated fatty acid, myristic acid ($C_{14:0}$), apparently raises LDL cholesterol concentrations somewhat more than does palmitic acid, whereas other saturates – lauric ($C_{12:0}$), caproic ($C_{10:0}$), and caprylic ($C_{8:0}$) acids – have a somewhat lesser cholesterol-raising effect. On average, for every 1% of total energy consumed as cholesterol-raising saturated fatty acids, compared with oleic acid, the serum LDL cholesterol level is raised about $2\,\mathrm{mg\,dl}^{-1}$ ($0.025\,\mathrm{mmol\,l}^{-1}$).

One saturated fatty acid, stearic acid ($C_{18:0}$), does not raise serum LDL cholesterol concentrations. The main sources of this fatty acid are beef tallow and cocoa butter. The reason for its failure to raise LDL cholesterol concentrations is uncertain, but may be the result of its rapid conversion into oleic acid in the body.

***Trans*-monounsaturated fatty acids** These fatty acids are produced by hydrogenation of vegetable oils. Intakes of *trans*-monounsaturates vary from one country to another depending on consumption of hydrogenated oils. In many countries they contribute between 2% and 4% of total nutrient energy intake. A series of *trans* acids are produced by hydrogenation: most are monounsaturated. For many years, it was accepted that *trans*-monounsaturated fatty acids were neutral with respect to LDL cholesterol concentrations. However, recent studies have shown that they raise LDL cholesterol concentrations to a level similar to that of palmitic acid when substituted for dietary oleic acid. In addition, they cause a small reduction in serum HDL cholesterol concentrations. Thus, *trans*-monounsaturates must be placed in the category of cholesterol-raising fatty acids.

***Cis*-monounsaturated fatty acids** The major fatty acid in this category is oleic acid ($C_{18:cis1\ n-9}$). It is found in both animal and vegetable fats, and typically is the major fatty acid in diet. Intakes commonly vary between 10% and 20% of total energy. Oleic acid intake is particularly high in the Mediterranean region where large amounts of olive oil are consumed. Other sources rich in oleic acid are rapeseed oil (canola oil) and high-oleic forms of safflower and sunflower oils. Peanuts and pecans also are high in oleic acid. Animal fats likewise contain a relatively high percentage of oleic acid among all their fatty acids; even so, these fats also tend to be rich in saturated fatty acids. When high-carbohydrate diets are consumed, the human body can synthesize fatty acids; among these, oleic acid is the predominant fatty acid produced.

As indicated before, oleic acid generally is considered to be the 'baseline' fatty acid with respect to serum lipoproteins levels, i.e., it does not raise (or lower) LDL cholesterol or VLDL cholesterol concentrations, nor does it lower (or raise) HDL cholesterol concentrations. It is against this 'neutral' fatty acid that responses of other fatty acids are defined (**Table 2**). For example, when oleic acid is substituted for cholesterol-raising fatty acids, the serum LDL cholesterol concentration will fall. Nonetheless, oleic acid is not designated a cholesterol-lowering fatty acid, but instead, this response defines the cholesterol-raising potential of saturated fatty acids.

Polyunsaturated fatty acids There are two categories of polyunsaturated fatty acids: n-6 and n-3. The major n-6 fatty acid is linoleic acid ($C_{18:2,n-6}$). It is the predominant fatty acid in many vegetable oils, e.g., corn oil, soya bean oil, and high linoleic forms of safflower and sunflower seed oils. Intakes of linoleic acid typically vary from 4% to 10% of nutrient energy, depending on how much vegetable oil is consumed in the diet. The n-3 fatty acids include linolenic acid ($C_{18:3,n-3}$), docosahexanoic acid (DHA) ($C_{22:6,n-3}$), and eicosapentanoic acid (EPA) ($C_{20:5,n-3}$). Linolenic acid is high in linseed oil and present in smaller amounts in other vegetable oils. DHA and EPA are enriched in fish oils.

For many years, linoleic acid was thought to be a unique LDL cholesterol-lowering fatty acid. Recent investigations suggest that earlier findings overestimated the LDL-lowering potential of linoleic acid. Even though substitution of linoleic acid for oleic acid in the diet may reduce LDL cholesterol levels in some people, a difference in response is not consistent. Only when intakes of linoleic acid become quite high do any differences become apparent. At high intakes, however, linoleic acid also lowers serum HDL cholesterol concentrations. Moreover, compared with oleic acid, it may reduce VLDL cholesterol levels in some people. Earlier enthusiasm for high intakes of linoleic acid to reduce LDL cholesterol levels has been dampened for several reasons: for example, its LDL-lowering ability does not offset potential disadvantages of HDL lowering, and other concerns include possible untoward side effects such as promoting oxidation of LDL and suppressing cellular immunity to cancer.

The n-3 fatty acids in fish oils (DHA and EPA) have a powerful action to reduce serum VLDL levels. This action apparently results from suppression of the secretion of VLDL by the liver. The precise mechanism for this action is not known. However, these fatty acids do not reduce LDL cholesterol concentrations relative to oleic acid. They have been used for treatment of some patients with elevated VLDL concentrations, although drug treatment generally is employed when it is necessary to lower serum VLDL levels.

Carbohydrate   When carbohydrates are substituted for oleic acid in the diet, serum LDL cholesterol levels remain unchanged. However, VLDL cholesterol concentrations usually rise and HDL cholesterol concentrations fall on high-carbohydrate diets. Thus, a lack of difference in total serum cholesterol concentrations during the exchange of carbohydrate and oleic acid is misleading. The two categories of nutrients have different actions on lipoprotein metabolism. The differences in response to dietary carbohydrate and oleic acid provide a good example of how measurements of serum total cholesterol fail to reveal all of the changes that are occurring in the lipoprotein fractions.

Energy Balance

Obesity   When energy intake exceeds energy expenditure, the balance of energy is stored in adipose tissue in the form of TAG. When the TAG content of adipose tissue becomes excessive (body mass index 30 or above), a state of obesity is said to exist. In some obese persons, excessive accumulations of TAG occur in other tissues than adipose tissue. Two such tissues are skeletal muscle and liver. High contents of TAG in muscle and liver arise primarily because of continuous leakage of excessive quantities of NEFA from adipose tissue. In the presence of desirable body weight, normal insulin levels are sufficient to suppress hydrolysis of TAG in adipose tissue, and NEFA release is low. On the other hand, in obese persons NEFA release is excessive, and skeletal muscle and liver are flooded with high serum NEFA concentrations. The result is engorgement of these organs with TAG. When skeletal muscle is overloaded with TAG, insulin-mediated glucose uptake is impaired. This condition is called insulin resistance. When liver is packed with TAG, hepatic metabolism is altered and insulin action on the liver is deranged. As a result,

there is an overproduction of VLDL; this leads to high VLDL cholesterol concentrations and, because LDL is a product of VLDL, to higher LDL cholesterol levels. In addition, obesity is accompanied by a reduction in HDL cholesterol concentrations. Thus obesity is responsible for multiple alterations in lipoprotein metabolism; it has significant effects on three major lipoprotein species – VLDL, LDL, and HDL. These changes appear to be the result of a combination of excessive hepatic TAG as a substrate for VLDL formation and failure of insulin to exert its usual action to curtail VLDL secretion.

Exercise   Many of the adverse metabolic effects of obesity are reversed by exercise. Increased energy expenditure through regular and sustained exercise helps to prevent accumulation of excessive quantities of TAG in adipose tissue. In addition, increased muscle metabolism produced by exercise burns off NEFA and prevents TAG accumulation in the liver. Hence, increased and sustained energy expenditure favourably modifies the lipoproteins, particularly by lowering VLDL cholesterol concentrations and raising serum HDL cholesterol. Effects of exercise on LDL cholesterol concentrations are more modest, but in some people exercise produces a reduction.

Other Factors Affecting Serum Lipoproteins

Advancing Age

Between the ages of 20 and 50 years, there is a gradual rise in serum cholesterol concentrations. In the USA, for example, the serum cholesterol increases on average about $50 \, \text{mg} \, \text{dl}^{-1}$ ($1.295 \, \text{mmol} \, \text{l}^{-1}$). This change may be related in part to increasing obesity, according to the mechanisms described above. However, even in people who do not gain weight with advancing age, serum cholesterol concentrations usually rise to some extent. Available evidence indicates that this rise results from a decrease in expression of LDL receptors. The reasons for a decline in receptor synthesis with aging are not known, but may reflect 'metabolic' aging. However, in men, after age 50 years, there is little further rise in serum cholesterol. This observation suggests that the impact of weight gain, which occurs mostly between the ages of 20 and 50 years, may be greater than generally recognized.

Postmenopausal State in Women

In women, there is a further rise in serum cholesterol concentrations after age 50 years. This rise is believed to be due largely to loss of oestrogens after the menopause. Oestrogens are known to stimulate the synthesis of LDL receptors, and, consequently, receptor expression declines after the menopause. This increment in cholesterol levels can be largely reversed by oestrogen replacement therapy.

Genetics

Family studies and research in twins indicate that about 50% of the variation of serum cholesterol concentrations in the general population can be explained by genetic polymorphisms. Presumably this variation is related to factors that regulate lipoprotein concentrations. In some cases, specific genetic defects are severe, resulting in marked changes in lipoprotein concentrations. When this occurs, the affected individual is said to have a monogenic disorder. In other cases, multiple genetic modifications are present that combine to alter lipoprotein concentrations. When a few modifications are present, the condition is called oligogenic, but when many modifications combine to change lipoprotein concentrations, the condition is named polygenic. Several monogenic disorders have been identified; a few oligogenic conditions have been described, but there are very few instances in which complex polygenic traits have been unravelled. A question of great interest is whether nutritional and genetic factors ever interact synergistically to alter lipoprotein concentrations. Undoubtedly, dietary factors and genetic changes can be additive in their effects on serum lipoproteins, but synergistic interaction has been difficult to prove. In what follows, consideration will be given to the impact of modification of some of the key gene products regulating lipoprotein metabolism.

LDL receptors The most severe elevations in LDL cholesterol levels occur in patients who have mutations in the gene encoding for LDL receptors. About one in 500 people are heterozygous for these mutations. Their condition is called heterozygous familial hypercholesterolemia. LDL cholesterol concentrations are essentially twice the normal level in this condition. Very rarely patients are homozygous for mutation in the LDL receptor gene and thus have homozygous familial hypercholesterolemia. Their LDL cholesterol levels are approximately four times normal. Individuals with this condition develop severe premature atherosclerosis.

Many other people appear to have a reduction in LDL receptor expression on a genetic basis, but they do not have as severe elevations of serum LDL cholesterol as patients with familial hypercholesterolemia. Presumably, these people have genetic modifications in factors that regulate transcription of the LDL receptor gene. Although such genetic modifications may be relatively common, they are poorly defined. Again, an important but unanswered question is whether some people are genetically susceptible to the cholesterol-raising effects of dietary cholesterol and saturated fatty acids. If so, they may possess modifications in the genetic control of LDL receptor expression.

Apolipoprotein B-100 structure About one in 500 people also have a mutation in the primary structure of apo B that interferes with its binding to LDL receptors. This mutation gives rise to the disorder called familial defective apolipoprotein B-100. The consequence is an elevation of LDL cholesterol concentrations, and the clinical pattern resembles that of familial hypercholesterolemia.

Apolipoprotein B synthesis Rare patients have mutations in the gene encoding for apo B that impair the synthesis of this apolipoprotein. Such patients usually have very low LDL cholesterol concentrations. These individuals are said to have familial hypobetalipoproteinemia. In other rare cases, the intracellular TAG transport protein called MCT is genetically absent; when this occurs, no lipoprotein particles containing apo B can be formed. LDL cholesterol is absent from serum, and the disorder is called familial abetalipoproteinemia.

Some researchers speculate that serum elevations in VLDL cholesterol and LDL cholesterol can result from excessive synthesis and/or secretion of apo B-containing lipoproteins by the liver. When this occurs on a genetic basis, the disorder is designated familial combined hyperlipidemia. However, a monogenic basis of this clinical phenotype has not yet been identified. Therefore, most investigators have concluded that familial combined hyperlipidemia probably represents an oligogenic or polygenic disorder. In this disorder, lipoprotein elevations appear to be worsened by nutritional factors – particularly by obesity.

Apolipoprotein E This apolipoprotein is present on TAG-rich lipoproteins and it facilitates removal of remnant lipoproteins by LDL receptors in the liver. When apo E is affected by mutation, this enabling action is curtailed and hepatic uptake of remnant lipoproteins is impaired. The result is an accumulation of chylomicron remnants and VLDL remnants in the circulation. The accumulation is accentuated by the coexistence of other disorders of metabolism of TAG-rich lipoproteins. When remnant accumulation occurs on a genetic basis, the disorder is called familial dysbetalipoproteinemia.

Apolipoprotein C There are two forms of apo C – apo C-II and apo C-III. Apo C-II is required for activation of LPL; when it is genetically absent, affected patients develop severe elevations of TAG-rich lipoproteins. Apo C-III inhibits the activity of LPL. In certain metabolic disorders, notably insulin resistance, synthesis of apo C-III is increased; an elevated apo C-III can lead to impaired function of LPL and increases in serum concentrations of TAG-rich lipoproteins.

Apolipoprotein A-I This is the major apolipoprotein of HDL. Rare patients have mutations in apo A-I that result in very low concentrations of HDL cholesterol. However, most people in whom HDL cholesterol concentrations are moderately reduced show increased catabolism of apo A-I. The mechanism for this change has not been fully determined, but one important cause may be an overexpression of HTGL.

Lipoprotein lipase This enzyme is required for lipolysis of TAG in TAG-rich lipoproteins. Rare patients are homozygous for mutations in LPL that impair its function. In such patients, serum concentrations of chylomicrons are markedly increased. The accumulation of chylomicrons in serum is greatly accentuated by the presence of fat in the diet. Only by severe dietary fat restriction is it possible to prevent severe TAG elevations in serum.

Genetic regulation of HDL cholesterol Family and twin studies reveal that about 50% of the variation in serum HDL cholesterol levels in the general population is explained by genetic factors. However, the regulation of HDL cholesterol concentrations is complex, and HDL cholesterol levels are determined by many factors, e.g., serum TAG concentrations, activity of HTGL, production rates of apo A-I, and activities of cholesterol ester transfer protein and LCAT. Genetic factors undoubtedly affect each of these regulating factors.

See also: **Eggs**. **Exercise**: Beneficial Effects; Diet and Exercise. **Fatty Acids**: Metabolism; Monounsaturated; Omega-3 Polyunsaturated; Omega-6 Polyunsaturated; Saturated; *Trans* Fatty Acids. **Lipoproteins**.

Meat, Poultry and Meat Products. **Obesity**: Definition, Etiology and Assessment.

Further Reading

Bonanome A and Grundy SM (1988) Effect of dietary stearic acid on plasma cholesterol and lipoprotein levels. *New England Journal of Medicine* **318**: 1244–1248.

Cater NB, Heller HJ, and Denke MA (1997) Comparison of the effects of medium-chain triacylglycerols, palm oil, and high oleic sunflower oil on plasma acylglycerol fatty acids and lipid and lipoprotein concentrations in humans. *American Journal of Clinical Nutrition* **65**: 41–45.

Connor WE (1988) Effects of omega-3 fatty acids in hypertriglyceridemic states. *Seminars in Thrombosis and Hemostasis* **14**: 271–284.

Denke MA, Sempos CT, and Grundy SM (1993) Excess body weight: an underrecognized contributor to high blood cholesterol levels in white American men. *Archives of Internal Medicine* **153**: 1093–1103.

Dietschy JM, Turley SD, and Spady DK (1993) Role of liver in the maintenance of cholesterol and low density lipoprotein homeostasis in different animal species, including humans. *Journal of Lipid Research* **34**: 1637–1659.

Ericsson S, Eriksson M, Vitols S *et al.* (1991) Influence of age on the metabolism of plasma low density lipoproteins in healthy males. *Journal of Clinical Investigation* **87**: 591–596.

Expert Panel on Detection, Evaluation, and Treatment of High Blood Cholesterol in Adults (S M Grundy, chairman) (1994) National Cholesterol Education Program: Second Report of the Expert Panel on Detection, Evaluation, and Treatment of High Blood Cholesterol (Adult Treatment Panel II). *Circulation* **89**: 1329–1445.

Grundy SM (1986) Comparison of monounsaturated fatty acids and carbohydrates for lowering plasma cholesterol. *New England Journal of Medicine* **314**: 745–748.

Grundy SM (1991) Multifactorial etiology of hypercholesterolemia: implications for prevention of coronary heart disease. *Arteriosclerosis and Thrombosis* **11**: 1619–1635.

Grundy SM and Denke MA (1990) Dietary influences on serum lipids and lipoproteins. *Journal of Lipid Research* **31**: 1149–1172.

Hegsted DM, McGandy RB, Myers ML, and Stare FJ (1965) Quantitative effects of dietary fat on serum cholesterol in man. *American Journal of Clinical Nutrition* **17**: 281–295.

Innerarity TL, Mahley RW, Weisgraber KH *et al.* (1990) Familial defective apolipo-protein B-100: a mutation of apolipoprotein B that causes hypercholesterolemia. *Journal of Lipid Research* **31**: 1337–1349.

Keys A, Anderson JT, and Grande F (1965) Serum cholesterol response to changes in the diet. IV. Particular saturated fatty acids in the diet. *Metabolism* **14**: 776–787.

Mattson FH and Grundy SM (1985) Comparison of effects of dietary saturated, monounsaturated, and polyunsaturated fatty acids on plasma lipids and lipoproteins in man. *Journal of Lipid Research* **26**: 194–202.

Mensink RP and Katan MB (1990) Effect of dietary *trans* fatty acids on high-density and low-density lipoprotein cholesterol levels in healthy subjects. *New England Journal of Medicine* **323**: 439–445.

CHOLINE AND PHOSPHATIDYLCHOLINE

X Zhu and S H Zeisel, University of North Carolina at Chapel Hill, Chapel Hill, NC, USA

© 2005 Elsevier Ltd. All rights reserved.

Introduction

Choline, an essential nutrient for humans, is consumed in many foods. It is part of several major phospholipids (including phosphatidylcholine – also called lecithin) that are critical for normal membrane structure and function. Also, as the major precursor of betaine it is used by the kidney to maintain water balance and by the liver as a source of methyl groups for the removal of homocysteine in methionine formation. Finally, choline is used to produce the important neurotransmitter acetylcholine (catalyzed by choline acetyltransferase in cholinergic neurons and in such non-nervous tissues as the placenta). Each of these functions for choline is absolutely vital for the maintenance of normal function.

Although there is significant capacity for biosynthesis of the choline moiety in the liver, choline deficiency can occur in humans. Male adults deprived of dietary choline become depleted of choline in their tissues and develop liver and muscle damage. Premenopausal women may not be sensitive to dietary choline deficiency (unpublished data). No experiments have been conducted to determine if this occurs in similarly deprived pregnant women, infants, and children.

Endogenous Formation of Choline Moiety as Phosphatidylcholine

Unless eaten in the diet, choline can only be formed during phosphatidylcholine biosynthesis through the methylation of phosphatidylethanolamine by phosphatidylethanolamine *N*-methyltransferase (PEMT) using *S*-adenosylmethionine as the methyl donor. This enzyme is most active in the liver but has been identified in many other tissues including brain and mammary gland. At least two isoforms of PEMT exist: PEMT1, localized to the endoplasmic reticulum and generating the majority of PEMT activity, and PEMT2, which resides on mitochondria-associated membranes. Both enzymes are encoded by the same gene but differ either because of post-translational modification or alternative splicing. This gene is very polymorphic and functional

SNPs (single nucleotide polymorphisms) in humans may exist and, if so, would influence dietary requirements for choline. In mice in which this gene is knocked out, the dietary requirement for choline is increased and they get fatty liver when eating a normal choline diet. Estrogen induces greater activity of PEMT perhaps explaining why premenopausal women require less choline in their diets. In addition to formation of choline, this enzyme has an essential role in lipoprotein secretion from the liver.

Choline, Homocysteine, and Folate are Interrelated Nutrients

Choline, methionine, methyltetrahydrofolate (methyl-THF), and vitamins B_6 and B_{12} are closely interconnected at the transmethylation metabolic pathways that form methionine from homocysteine. Perturbing the metabolism of one of these pathways results in compensatory changes in the others. For example, as noted above, choline can be synthesized *de novo* using methyl groups derived from methionine (via *S*-adenosylmethionine). Methionine can be formed from homocysteine using methyl groups from methyl-THF, or using methyl groups from betaine that are derived from choline. Similarly, methyl-THF can be formed from one-carbon units derived from serine or from the methyl groups of choline via dimethylglycine. When animals and humans are deprived of choline, they use more methyl-THF to remethylate homocysteine in the liver and increase dietary folate requirements. Conversely, when they are deprived of folate, they use more methyl groups from choline, increasing the dietary requirement for choline. There is a common polymorphism in the gene for methyltetrahydrofolate reductase that increases dietary requirement for folic acid; 15–30% of humans have this mutation. In mice in which this gene is knocked out, the dietary requirement for choline is increased and they get fatty liver when eating a normal choline diet.

Choline in Foods

Choline, choline esters, and betaine can be found in significant amounts in many foods consumed by humans (see **Figure 1** and **Figure 2**); some of the choline and betaine is added during processing (especially in the preparation of infant formula).

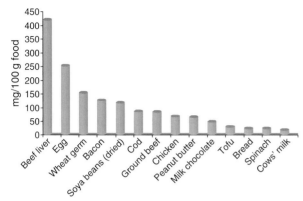

Figure 1 Total choline content of some common foods. Foods, which had been prepared as normally eaten, were analyzed for choline, phosphocholine, glycerophosphocholine, phosphatidyl-choline, and sphingomyelin content using an HPLC mass spectrometric method. (Modified from Zeisel SH, Mar M-H, Howe JC, and Holden JM (2003) Concentrations of choline-containing compounds and betaine in common foods. *Journal of Nutrition* 133: 1302–1307.)

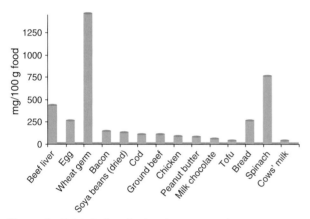

Figure 2 Total choline plus betaine content of some common foods. For methyl donation choline must be converted to betaine, thus the methyl donor capacity is best expressed as total choline and betaine content, assayed as in **Figure 1**. Several vegetable and grain products contain significant amounts of betaine (Modified from Zeisel SH, Mar M-H, Howe JC, and Holden JM (2003) Concentrations of choline-containing compounds and betaine in common foods. *Journal of Nutrition* 133: 1302–1307.)

Though the different esters of choline have different bioavailability, it is likely that choline in all forms is fungible; therefore, total choline content is probably the best indicator of food choline content. Betaine should also be considered, as it spares the use of choline for methyl donation.

A number of epidemiologic studies have examined the relationship between dietary folic acid and cancer or heart disease. It may be helpful to also consider choline intake as a confounding factor because folate and choline methyl donation can be interchangeable.

Dietary Recommendations

The Institute of Medicine, USA National Academy of Sciences, recommended an adequate intake (I) of 550 mg/70 kg body weight for choline in the diet. This amount may be influenced by gender, and it may be influenced by pregnancy, lactation, and stage of development (**Table 1**).

Amino acid-glucose solutions used in total parenteral nutrition of humans lack choline. The lipid emulsions that deliver extra calories and essential fatty acids during parenteral nutrition contain choline in the form of lecithin (20% emulsion contains 13.2 mmol l^{-1}). Humans treated with parenteral nutrition require 1–1.7 mmol of choline-containing phospholipid per day during the first week of parenteral nutrition therapy to maintain plasma choline levels.

Human milk, which contains approximately 200 mg l^{-1} choline and choline esters, is an especially good source of choline. An infant consuming 500 ml breast milk in a day ingests 50 mg choline. Human milk is not a static food; its choline composition changes over time postnatally. The choline composition of infant formulas can differ greatly from that present in human milk. It is essential that variations in the bioavailability and utilization of choline, phosphocholine, glycerophosphocholine, and lecithin in milk be considered when milk substitutes are developed.

Functional Effects of Varying Choline in the Diet

Fatty Liver

The triacylglycerol (TG) produced by the liver is mainly delivered to other tissues as very low-density

Table 1 Recommended adequate intakes (AI) for choline

Population	Age	AI (mg day^{-1})
Infants	0–6 months	125
	6–12 months	150
Children	1 through 3 years	200
	4 through 8 years	250
	9 through 13 years	375
Males	14 through 18 years	550
	19 years and older	550
Females	14 through 18 years	400
	19 years and older	425
Pregnancy	All ages	450
Lactation	All ages	550

From Institute of Medicine, National Academy of Sciences USA (1998) Dietary reference intakes for folate, thiamin, riboflavin, niacin, vitamin B$_{12}$, panthothenic acid, biotin, and choline, vol. 1. Washington DC: National Academy Press.

lipoprotein (VLDL) of which lecithin is a required component. In choline deficiency, the diminished ability of liver cells to synthesize new lecithin molecules results in the intracellular accumulation of TG. Treating malnourished patients with high-calorie total parenteral nutrition (TPN) solutions that contain little or no choline will deplete choline stores and cause fatty liver and hepatic dysfunction that can be reversed by treatment with phosphatidylcholine.

Liver Cell Death

When deprived of dietary choline, healthy male subjects have diminished plasma concentrations of choline and phosphatidylcholine, and they develop liver cell death (elevated plasma alanine aminotransferase). In similarly deprived animal models, the liver cell death is caused by apoptosis, a regulated form of cell suicide. In an ongoing study of choline deficiency in humans, muscle cell death (elevated plasma creatine phosphokinase, MM form) has also been noted.

Liver Cancer

Dietary deficiency of choline in rodents causes development of hepatocarcinomas in the absence of any known carcinogen. Choline is the only single nutrient for which this is true. It is interesting that choline-deficient rats not only have a higher incidence of spontaneous hepatocarcinoma but also are markedly sensitized to the effects of administered carcinogens. Several mechanisms are suggested for the cancer-promoting effect of a choline-devoid diet. A progressive increase in cell proliferation that is related to regeneration after parenchymal cell death occurs in the choline-deficient liver. Cell proliferation and its associated increased rate of DNA synthesis could be the cause of the heightened sensitivity to chemical carcinogens. Methylation of DNA is essential to the regulation of expression of genetic information, and the undermethylation of DNA observed during choline deficiency (despite adequate dietary methionine) may be responsible for carcinogenesis. Choline-deficient rats experience increased lipid peroxidation in the liver. Lipid peroxides in the nucleus are a possible source of free radicals that could modify DNA and cause carcinogenesis. Choline deficiency activates protein kinase C signaling, usually involved in growth factor signaling in hepatocytes. Finally, a defect in cell suicide (apoptosis) mechanisms may contribute to the carcinogenesis of choline deficiency.

Kidney Function

Renal function is compromised by choline deficiency, which leads to abnormal concentrating ability, free-water reabsorption, sodium excretion, glomerular filtration rate, renal plasma flow, and gross renal hemorrhage. The deterioration in renal function may be related to changes in acetylcholine release by nerves that regulate blood flow to the kidney. Additionally, the renal glomerulus uses the choline-metabolite betaine as an osmolyte to assist cells in maintaining their volume in the presence of concentrated salts in urine.

Brain Development

During the fetal and neonatal period, the availability of choline to tissues fluctuates because of the varied dietary intake of choline among neonates and the slower oxidation of choline during the first weeks of life. However, ensured availability of this amine appears to be vital to infants because organ growth, which is extremely rapid in the neonate, requires large amounts of choline for membrane biosynthesis. Choline is also particularly important during the neonatal period because it appears to change brain function. There are two sensitive periods in rat brain development during which treatment with choline produces long-lasting enhancement of spatial memory that is lifelong and has been detected in elderly rats. The first occurs during embryonic days 12–17 and the second, during postnatal days 16–30. Choline supplementation during these critical periods elicits a major improvement in memory performance at all stages of training on a 12-arm radial maze.

The choline-induced spatial memory facilitation correlates with altered distribution and morphology of neurons involved in memory storage within the brain, with biochemical changes in the adult hippocampus and with electrophysiological changes in the adult hippocampus. It also correlates with changes in proliferation, apoptosis, and migration of neuronal precursor cells in the hippocampus during fetal brain development. When pregnant rats were treated with varying levels of dietary choline between day 12 and 18 of gestation, it was found that choline deficiency significantly decreased the rate of mitosis in the neuroepithelium of fetal brain adjacent to the hippocampus. An increased number of apoptotic cells were found in the region of the dentate gyrus of choline-deficient hippocampus compared to controls. Modulation of dietary choline availability changed the distribution and migration of precursor cells produced on embryonic day 16 in the fimbria, primordial dentate gyrus, and Ammon's horn of the fetal hippocampus. Choline deficiency also decreased the migration of newly proliferating cells from the neuroepithelium into the lateral septum, thus indicating that the sensitivity of fetal brain to choline availability is not restricted to the hippocampus. The expression of TOAD-64 protein, an early neuronal differentiation marker, increased in the hippocampus of choline-deficient day E18 fetal brains compared to controls. These findings show that dietary choline availability during pregnancy alters the timing of mitosis, apoptosis, migration, and the early commitment to neuronal differentiation by progenitor cells in fetal brain hippocampus and septum, two regions known to be associated with learning and memory.

A disruption in choline uptake and metabolism during neurulation produces neural tube defects in mouse embryos grown *in vitro*. Exposing early somite staged mouse embryos *in vitro* with an inhibitor of choline uptake and metabolism, 2-dimethylaminoethanol (DMAE) causes craniofacial hypoplasia and open neural tube defects in the forebrain, midbrain, and hindbrain regions. Embryos exposed to an inhibitor of phosphatidylcholine synthesis, 1-O-octadecyl-2-O-methyl-rac-glycero-3-phosphocholine (ET-18-OCH$_3$) exhibit similar defects or expansion of the brain vesicles and a distended neural tube at the posterior neuropore as well as increased areas of cell death. Thus, choline like folic acid is important during neural tube closure.

Are these findings in rats likely to apply to humans? We do not know. Human and rat brains mature at different rates; rat brain is comparatively more mature at birth than is the human brain, but in humans synaptogenesis may continue for months after birth. Are we varying the availability of choline when we substitute infant formulas for human milk? Does choline intake in infancy contribute to variations in memory observed between humans? These are good questions that warrant additional research.

Brain Function in Adults

It is unlikely that choline acetyltransferase in brain is saturated with either of its substrates, so that choline (and possibly acetyl-CoA) availability determines the rate of acetylcholine synthesis. Under conditions of rapid neuronal firing acetylcholine release by brain neurons can be directly altered by dietary intake of choline. Based on this observation, choline has been used as a possible memory-improvement drug. In some patients with Alzheimer's disease, choline or phosphatidylcholine has beneficial effects, but this effect is variable. Both verbal and visual memory may be impaired in other patients who require long-term intravenous feeding and this may be improved with choline supplementation.

Measurement of Choline and Choline Esters

Radioisotopic, high-pressure liquid chromatography, and gas chromatography/isotope dilution mass spectrometry (GC/IDMS) methods are available for measurement of choline. However, these existing methods are cumbersome and time consuming, and none measures all of the compounds of choline derivatives. Recently, a new method has been established for quantifying choline, betaine, acetylcholine, glycerophosphocholine, cytidine diphosphocholine, phosphocholine, phosphatidylcholine, and sphingomyelin in liver, plasma, various foods, and brain using liquid chromatography/electrospray ionization-isotope dilution mass spectrometry (LC/ESI-IDMS).

Acknowledgments

Supported by the National Institutes of Health (DK55865, AG09525, DK56350).

See also: **Brain and Nervous System. Cancer:** Epidemiology and Associations Between Diet and Cancer. **Folic Acid. Homocysteine. Liver Disorders. Vitamin B$_6$.**

Further Reading

Albright CD, Tsai AY, Friedrich CB, Mar MH, and Zeisel SH (1999) Choline availability alters embryonic development of the hippocampus and septum in the rat. *Brain Research. Developmental Brain Research* 113: 13–20.

Buchman AL, Dubin M, Jenden D, Moukarzel A, Roch MH, Rice K, Gornbein J, Ament ME, and Eckhert CD (1992) Lecithin increases plasma free choline and decreases hepatic steatosis in long-term total parenteral nutrition patients. *Gastroenterology* 102: 1363–1370.

da Costa KA, Badea M, Fischer LM, and Zeisel SH (2004) Elevated serum creatine phosphokinase in choline-deficient humans: mechanistic studies in C2C12 mouse myoblasts. *Am J Clin Nutr* 80: 163–70.

Institute of Medicine, National Academy of Sciences USA (1998) *Dietary Reference Intakes for Folate, Thiamin, Riboflavin, Niacin, Vitamin B12, Panthothenic Acid, Biotin, and Choline,* vol. 1. Washington DC: National Academy Press.

Koc H, Mar MH, Ranasinghe A, Swenberg JA, and Zeisel SH (2002) Quantitation of choline and its metabolites in tissues and foods by liquid chromatography/electrospray ionization-isotope dilution mass spectrometry. *Analytical Chemistry* **74**: 4734–4740.

Meck WH and Williams CL (1997) Simultaneous temporal processing is sensitive to prenatal choline availability in mature and aged rats. *Neuroreport* **8**: 3045–3051.

Montoya DA, White AM, Williams CL, Blusztajn JK, Meck WH, and Swartzwelder HS (2000) Prenatal choline exposure alters hippocampal responsiveness to cholinergic stimulation in adulthood. *Brain Research. Developmental Brain Research* **123**: 25–32.

Niculescu MD and Zeisel SH (2002) Diet, methyl donors and DNA methylation: interactions between dietary folate, methionine and choline. *Journal of Nutrition* **132**: 2333S–2335S.

Zeisel SH and Blusztajn JK (1994) Choline and human nutrition. *Annual Review of Nutrition* **14**: 269–296.

Zeisel SH, daCosta K-A, Franklin PD, Alexander EA, Lamont JT, Sheard NF, and Beiser A (1991) Choline, an essential nutrient for humans. *FASEB Journal* **5**: 2093–2098.

Zeisel SH, Mar M-H, Howe JC, and Holden JM (2003) Concentrations of choline-containing compounds and betaine in common foods. *Journal of Nutrition* **133**: 1302–1307.

CHROMIUM

R A Anderson, US Department of Agriculture, Beltsville, MD, USA

© 2005 Elsevier Ltd. All rights reserved.

Chromium (Cr) in the trivalent form is an essential nutrient that functions primarily in sugar and fat metabolism. Dietary intake of Cr by humans and farm animals is often suboptimal. Insufficient dietary intake of Cr is associated with increased risk factors associated with type 2 diabetes mellitus (DM) and cardiovascular diseases. Chromium functions in glucose and insulin metabolism primarily via its role in the improvement of insulin activity. Improved insulin function is also associated with an improved lipid profile. People with type 2 diabetes have a more than twofold increased incidence of cardiovascular diseases compared to control subjects.

Chromium in foods and dietary supplements is trivalent, whereas Cr often found in paints, welding fumes, and other industrial settings is hexavalent and is severalfold more toxic than the trivalent nutritional Cr. Trivalent Cr is one of the safest nutrient supplements based on the ratio of the amount that is needed relative to the amount that can be consumed over a lifetime with no adverse effects. An expert panel of the US Food and Nutrition Board was unable to set an upper level of safe intake since none of the levels of intake tested showed any signs of toxicity. Toxicity is also alleviated by the low level of absorption, usually less than 2%.

Essentiality and Metabolic Functions of Chromium

The essentiality of trivalent Cr in human nutrition was documented in 1977 when diabetic signs and symptoms of a patient on total parenteral nutrition (TPN) were reversed by supplemental Cr. Diabetic symptoms, including elevated blood glucose, weight loss, impaired nerve conduction, brain disorders, and abnormal respiratory quotient, that were refractory to exogenous insulin were reversed following increased intake of the essential nutrient Cr. Upon daily addition of supplemental Cr to the patient's TPN solution for 2 weeks, diabetic symptoms were alleviated and exogenous insulin requirement declined from 45 units per day to zero. These findings have been repeated and documented in the scientific literature on several occasions.

Signs and symptoms of Cr deficiency listed in **Table 1** are not limited to subjects on TPN. Improvements in glucose and/or lipid concentrations have been reported in children with protein calorie malnutrition; the elderly; people with type 1 and type 2 DM, hypoglycemia, and marginally impaired glucose tolerance; and numerous animal species.

The hallmark sign of marginal Cr deficiency is impaired glucose tolerance. The effects of Cr on people with high, low, and normal glucose tolerance as well as diabetes are illustrated in **Figure 1**. Chromium leads to a decrease in blood glucose in people with elevated blood sugar and an increase in those with low blood sugar due to its role in normalizing insulin. In the presence of Cr in a physiologically active form, insulin is more efficient and much lower levels of insulin are required. During periods of elevated blood glucose, more efficient insulin leads to a decrease in blood glucose. In people with low blood sugar, reactive hypoglycemia, more efficient insulin leads to a rapid rise in response to a glucose challenge and a more rapid return to baseline values. This leads to less of a decline in

Table 1 Signs and symptoms of Cr deficiency

Function	Animals
Impaired glucose tolerance	Human, rat, mouse, squirrel monkey, guinea pig, cattle
Elevated circulating insulin	Human, rat, pig, cattle
Glycosuria	Human, rat
Fasting hyperglycemia	Human, rat, mouse
Impaired growth	Human, rat, mouse, turkey
Hypoglycemia	Human
Elevated serum cholesterol and triglycerides	Human, rat, mouse, cattle, pig
Increased incidence of aortic plaques	Rabbit, rat, mouse
Increased aortic intimal plaque area	Rabbit
Nerve disorders	Human
Brain disorders	Human
Corneal lesions	Rat, squirrel monkey
Ocular eye pressure	Human
Decreased fertility and sperm count	Rat
Decreased longevity	Rat, mouse
Decreased insulin binding	Human
Decreased insulin receptor number	Human
Decreased lean body mass	Human, pig, rat
Elevated percent body fat	Human, pig
Impaired humoral immune response	Cattle
Increased morbidity	Cattle
Gestational diabetes	Human
Steroid-induced diabetes	Human
Atypical depression	Human

Adapted from Anderson RA (1998) Chromium, glucose intolerance and diabetes. *Journal of the American College of Nutrition* **17**: 548–555.

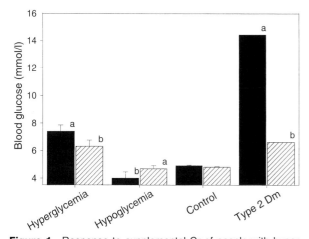

Figure 1 Response to supplemental Cr of people with hyperglycemia, hypoglycemia, optimal glycemia (control), and type 2 diabetes mellitus (DM). The minimal amount of Cr usually showing beneficial effects in people with high or low blood sugar is 200 μg per day. People with diabetes require 400–600 μg per day or more. Bars with different superscripts denote differences at $p < 0.05$.

hypoglycemic glucose values. Supplemental Cr also leads to increased insulin binding and increased insulin receptor number, and evidence suggests that Cr may be involved in the phosphorylation–dephosphorylation of the insulin receptor proteins. Chromium activates insulin receptor kinase, the enzyme that phosphorylates the insulin receptor, leading to activation of insulin function, and it appears to inhibit the phosphatase enzyme that deactivates insulin function.

Recent advances in Cr nutrition research include the demonstration of an inverse relationship between toenail Cr and cardiovascular disease (CVD) in studies from the United States and Europe, supporting studies indicating that people with CVD tend to have lower levels of serum and tissue Cr and also substantiating the beneficial effects of supplemental Cr on blood cholesterol, triglycerides, and high-density lipoprotein cholesterol. Supplemental Cr as chromium picolinate (the most common form of supplemental Cr) was shown to be effective in the treatment of depression. Preliminary studies suggest that the effects of Cr are greater than those of any drugs used in the treatment of atypical depression. Supplemental Cr is also free of side effects associated with drugs, which are often quite serious in the treatment of depression. Studies also show that Cr is beneficial in the reversal of polycystic ovarian syndrome, gestational diabetes, and steroid-induced associated with administration of steroids such as prednisone given as antiinflammatory agents in the treatment of arthritis, asthma, allergies, and related diseases.

Response to Cr is due to not only the Cr status of the subjects but also the forms and amount of Cr consumed. Subjects with diabetes or glucose intolerance who consume 200 μg daily of supplemental Cr or less often do not respond to supplemental Cr, but they may respond to 400–600 μg daily or more. A dose response to Cr for subjects with type 2 DM is shown in **Figure 2**. Subjects had been diagnosed with diabetes for approximately 5 years and had taken no Cr supplements. There was a progressive decline in the hemoglobin A1c after 2 and 4 months of consuming 200 or 1000 μg daily of Cr as Cr picolinate, respectively. There were also dose-dependent improvements in glucose, insulin, and cholesterol. These results were confirmed in a separate double-blind, placebo-controlled study.

The responses to Cr are difficult to predict and the phenotypic characteristics of the individual may be important. Phenotype is also important in insulin signaling and may explain, in part, the wide range

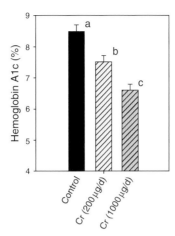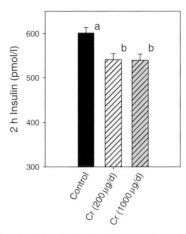

Figure 2 Chromium effects on hemoglobin A1C and 2-h insulin. The study involved chromium supplementation (200 or 1000 μg/day) for 4 months in 180 people with type 2 diabetes mellitus. Bars with different superscripts denote differences at $p < 0.05$. (Adapted from Anderson RA, Cheng N, Bryden NA et al. (1997) Elevated intakes of supplemental chromium improve glucose and insulin variables in individuals with type 2 diabetes. *Diabetes* **46**: 1786–1791.)

of individual responses to Cr supplementation. Data demonstrate that Cr has beneficial effects in insulin-resistant obese but not lean JCR:LA corpulent rats, which are used as a model for insulin resistance. Although Cr had no effect on the weight of lean and obese rats, obese rats consuming supplemental Cr displayed lower insulin, improved glucose control, and increased phosphoinositol-3-kinase activity. This work documents a specific effect of Cr in a key control site in the insulin signaling pathway, which is the system responsible for the overall control of sugar, fat, and energy metabolism.

Chromium and Stress

Stresses that have been shown to alter Cr metabolism in humans are glucose loading, high simple sugar diets, lactation, infection, acute exercise, chronic exercise, and physical trauma. Urinary losses can be used as a measure of the response to stress since once Cr is mobilized in response to stress it is not reabsorbed by the kidney but is lost in the urine. The degree of stress as measured by the stress hormone, cortisol, is correlated with the amount of Cr lost in the urine.

The administration of glucocorticoids also leads to increased urinary Cr losses as well as insulin resistance. These steroids are often employed as antiinflammatory agents in the treatment of common chronic diseases, such as asthma, allergies, and arthritis, and they are also administered following organ transplantation, but a side effect of glucocorticoid administration is steroid-induced diabetes.

The mechanisms responsible for steroid-induced diabetes are unknown, but decreased insulin sensitivity is an overlying cause. Impaired Cr metabolism also appears to be a related cause since supplementation of 50 people who had uncontrolled steroid-induced diabetes with Cr for 10 days resulted in the reversal of the steroid-induced diabetes in 47 of these patients, with no adverse side effects, and a decrease of at least 50% of the medication needed prior to the supplementation of Cr.

Dietary Intake and Requirements of Chromium

A panel on micronutrients convened by the Institute of Medicine defined an adequate intake for Cr of 25 μg for women and 35 μg for men 19–50 years old and 20 μg for women and 30 μg for men older than age 50 years. Adequate intake is "the recommended average daily intake based on observed or experimentally determined approximations or estimates of nutrient intake by a group (or groups) of apparently healthy people that are assumed to be adequate—used when an RDA cannot be determined." The adequate intake for Cr is nearly identical to the average Cr intake but much lower than earlier committee recommendations.

It is unclear why the adequate intake for Cr should be lower for people older than 50 years when the primary function of Cr is to combat problems associated with insulin and glucose metabolism, which tend to increase with age. Indices of Cr status, such as the Cr content of hair, sweat, and urine, were shown to decrease with age in a study of more than 40 000 people. The recommended intakes in France are higher and more in line with studies demonstrating that a large segment of the population may not be consuming adequate Cr. The French Conseil National d'Etudes et de Recherche sur la nutrition et l'Alimentation has proposed daily intakes of 55 μg for adult French women 19–65 years old and 60 μg/day for those older than 65 years and 65 and 70 μg, respectively, for men. Since Cr losses are increased by high intake of simple sugars such as glucose, sucrose, and fructose, modern diets high in these sugars appear to be increasing the requirements for Cr.

More than 34 studies have reported beneficial effects of supplemental Cr for people with blood glucose values ranging from hypoglycemia to diabetes when consuming diets of average Cr content. In a controlled diet study, consumption of diets in the lowest quartile of normal Cr intakes, but near the new adequate intakes, led to detrimental effects on glucose and insulin in subjects with marginally impaired glucose tolerance (90-minute glucose between 5.6 and 11.1 mmol/l or 100–200 mg/dl) following an oral glucose load of 1 g/kg body weight. The average person older than 25 years of age has blood glucose in this range. Consumption of these same diets by people with good glucose tolerance (90-minute glucose less than 5.6 mmol/l) did not lead to changes in glucose and insulin variables. This is consistent with previous studies demonstrating that the requirement for Cr is related to the degree of glucose intolerance and demonstrates that an intake of 20 μg Cr per day is not adequate for people with decreased insulin sensitivity, such as those with marginally impaired glucose tolerance, and certainly not for those with impaired glucose tolerance or diabetes.

Absorption, Transport, Storage, and Excretion

Absorbed Cr is excreted primarily in the urine, and only small amounts of Cr are lost in the hair, perspiration, and bile. Therefore, urinary Cr excretion can be used as an accurate estimation of absorbed Cr. At normal dietary Cr intakes (10–40 μg per day), Cr absorption is inversely related to dietary intake. Chromium absorption is approximately 0.5% at a daily intake of 40 μg and increases to 2% when intake decreases to 10 μg. Therefore, the amount of absorbed Cr over this range is approximately 0.2 μg and is reflected in the urinary Cr losses of approximately 0.2 μg/day. This inverse relationship of Cr

intake and absorption appears to be a basal control mechanism to maintain a minimal level of absorbed Cr. Intakes higher than 40 μg result in corresponding increases in total Cr absorbed. There is no direct evidence that Cr absorption involves active transport.

Chromium absorption in young and old normal subjects is similar, but people with type 1 DM absorb two- to fourfold more Cr than other groups tested. People with diabetes appear to have an impaired ability to convert inorganic Cr to a useable form. Diabetic mice also lose the ability to convert Cr to a useable form. People with diabetes require additional Cr and the body responds with increased absorption, but the absorbed Cr cannot be utilized effectively and is excreted in the urine. Chromium content in tissues of people with diabetes is also lower.

Chromium absorption and incorporation into tissues are also dependent on the form of Cr ingested. An accurate estimation of Cr absorption and utilization in animal studies can be achieved by measuring Cr incorporation into tissues. The tissue with the greatest Cr concentration is the kidney, followed by the spleen, liver, lungs, heart, and skeletal muscle.

Tissue Cr is an accurate method to assess Cr absorption and utilization and is also a measure of Cr storage. The kidney, which is one of the primary sites of tissue Cr storage, is also one of the best sources of insulin potentiating forms of Cr. Chromium is transported to the tissues primarily bound to transferrin, the same protein that transports iron. There are two metal binding sites on transferrin—one primarily for iron and a second involved in Cr transport. During conditions of high iron excess or iron overload, such as in iron storage diseases (hemosiderosis and hemochromatosis), all the metal transport sites on transferrin are occupied by iron. This may explain the high incidence of diabetes in hemochromatosis patients that may be due in part to Cr deficiency.

Dietary Sources

Dietary Cr content of foods varies widely, and there are no comprehensive databases to calculate dietary Cr intake. Chromium content of foods is often erroneously high due to Cr contamination during collection and analyses. For example, stainless-steel blender blades are often used in the homogenization of foods, but stainless steel is approximately 18% Cr. In the presence of acidic foods, more Cr may leach from the blender blades than is present originally in the foods.

Table 2 Daily intakes of chromium from various food groups

Food group	Average daily intake (μg/day)	Comment
Cereal products	3.7	55% from wheat
Meat	5.2	55% from pork; 25% from beef
Fish and seafoods	0.6	
Fruits, vegetables, nuts, and mushrooms	6.8	70% from fruits and berries
Dairy products, eggs, and margarine	6.2	85% from milk
Beverages, confectionaries, sugar, and condiments	6.6	45% from beer, wine, and soft drinks
Total	29.1	

From Anderson RA (1988) Chromium In: Smith K (ed.) *Trace Minerals in Foods*, pp. 231–247. New York: Marcel Dekker.

Chromium is present in several food groups but at low levels. The distribution is similar among fruits, vegetables, dairy products, beverages, and meats, with lesser amounts from cereal products and small amounts from fish and seafood (**Table 2**). Chromium content of foods is a combination of the endogenous Cr present in the foods and the Cr introduced during the various stages of growing and processing. For example, fruit juices are often high in Cr since Cr may leach from containers during processing and storage under acidic conditions.

Safety of Chromium

Trivalent Cr, the form of Cr found in foods and nutrient supplements, is one of the least toxic nutrients. The reference dose established by an expert panel of the US Environmental Protection Agency (EPA) is 350 times the upper limit of the estimated safe and adequate daily dietary intake. The newer adequate intakes are lower and would have a safety ratio of approximately 2000. The reference dose is defined as "an estimate (with uncertainty spanning perhaps an order of magnitude) of a daily exposure to the human population, including sensitive subgroups, that is likely to be without an appreciable risk of deleterious effects over a lifetime." This conservative estimate of safe intake has a much larger safety factor for trivalent Cr than almost any other nutrient. The ratio of the EPA reference dose to the requirements is approximately two to five for other trace elements, such as zinc and manganese, and five to seven for selenium. Chromium in the form of both Cr chloride and Cr picolinate fed to rats at

several thousand times the current adequate intake (based on body weight) resulted in no detectable signs of toxicity.

Conclusion

Dietary intake of Cr may be suboptimal for most humans and farm animals. Increased intake of trivalent Cr often leads to improved glucose and lipid metabolism. The physiological role of Cr appears to be primarily through the improved function of insulin. Increased intake of Cr leads to increased insulin binding, increased insulin receptor number, and increased phosphorylation of the insulin receptor proteins, leading to increased insulin sensitivity and function and lower glucose and lipids. Chromium is a nutrient and not a therapeutic agent, and only subjects whose impaired glucose and insulin function is related to suboptimal intake of Cr will benefit from additional Cr. Although a significant number of subjects often respond to supplemental Cr, there are also a significant number of subjects who do not respond to improved Cr nutrition. This is likely due to the amount and form of Cr consumed and glucose tolerance and Cr status of the subjects. No negative effects of supplemental Cr have been reported in any of the Cr supplementation studies involving daily Cr intakes of up to 1000 μg per day.

See also: **Diabetes Mellitus**: Etiology and Epidemiology; Classification and Chemical Pathology; Dietary Management. **Glucose**: Chemistry and Dietary Sources. **Lipoproteins**.

Further Reading

Althuis MD, Jordan NE, Ludington EA, and Wittes JT (2002) Glucose and insulin responses to dietary chromium supplements: A meta-analysis. *American Journal of Clinical Nutrition* 76: 148–155.

Anderson RA (1994) Stress effects on chromium nutrition of humans and farm animals. In: Lyons TP and Jacques KA (eds.) *Proceedings of Alltech's Tenth Symposium on Biotechnology in the Feed Industry*, pp. 267–274. Nottingham, UK: University Press.

Anderson RA (1998a) Chromium, glucose intolerance and diabetes. *Journal of the American College of Nutrition* 17: 548–555.

Anderson RA (1998b) Effects of chromium on body composition and weight loss. *Nutrition Review* 56: 266–270.

Anderson RA (2000) Chromium in the prevention and control of diabetes. *Diabetes and Metabolism* 26: 22–27.

Anderson RA (2003) Chromium and insulin resistance. *Nutrition Research Review* 16: 267–275.

Anderson RA, Cheng N, Bryden NA et al. (1997) Elevated intakes of supplemental chromium improve glucose and insulin variables in individuals with type 2 diabetes. *Diabetes* 46: 1786–1791.

Anonymous (2001) *Dietary Reference Intakes for Vitamin A, Vitamin K, Arsenic, Boron, Chromium, Copper, Iodine, Iron,*

Manganese, Molybdenum, Nickel, Silicon, Vanadium and Zinc, pp. 197–223. Washington, DC: National Academy Press.

Cefalu WT, Wang ZQ, Zhang XH, Baldor LC, and Russell JC (2002) Oral chromium picolinate improves carbohydrate and lipid metabolism and enhances skeletal muscle Glut-4 translocation in obese, hyperinsulinemic (JCR-LA corpulent) rats. Journal of Nutrition 132: 1107–1114.

Gunton JE, Hams G, Hitchman R, and McElduff A (2001) Serum chromium does not predict glucose tolerance in late pregnancy. American Journal of Clinical Nutrition 73: 99–104.

Heimbach JT and Anderson RA (2005) Chromium: Recent studies regarding nutritional roles and safety. Nutrition Today.

Morris BW (1999) Chromium action and glucose homeostasis. Journal of Trace Element in Experimental Medicine 12: 61–70.

Ravina A, Slezak L, Mirsky N, and Anderson RA (1999) Control of steroid-induced diabetes with supplemental chromium. Journal of Trace Elements in Experimental Medicine 12: 375–378.

Vincent JB (2000) The biochemistry of chromium. Journal of Nutrition 130: 715–718.

COBALAMINS

R Green, University of California, Davis, CA, USA

© 2005 Elsevier Ltd. All rights reserved.

Introduction

The cobalamins are a group of closely related and interconvertible compounds with a complex structure that are collectively known by the common name of vitamin B_{12}. Recommended biochemical nomenclature restricts the term 'vitamin B_{12}' for the particular form of cobalamin known as cyanocobalamin. All cobalamins belong to the broader family of corrinoids, which share the characteristic of consisting of a planar four-member pyrrole ring (corrin ring) containing a central cobalt atom. Cobalamins are distinguished from other corrinoids by possessing both alpha (lower) and beta (upper) axial ligands that are attached to the central cobalt atom (**Figure 1**). The lower ligand consists of a base (5,6-dimethylbenzimidazole) attached to a sugar (ribose), which in turn is attached to a phosphate and an amino-propyl group that ultimately is tethered back to the corrin ring. In the naturally occurring cobalamins the upper ligand is variably a cyano-, hydroxo-, aquo-, methyl-, or adenosyl- group, giving rise to the correspondingly named chemical forms of the vitamin. Of these, methylcobalamin and deoxyadenosylcobalamin are the forms that function as coenzymes for metabolic reactions. These are sensitive to destruction by light. Cyanocobalamin is a stable form and is therefore used in therapeutic preparations. Hydroxo- or

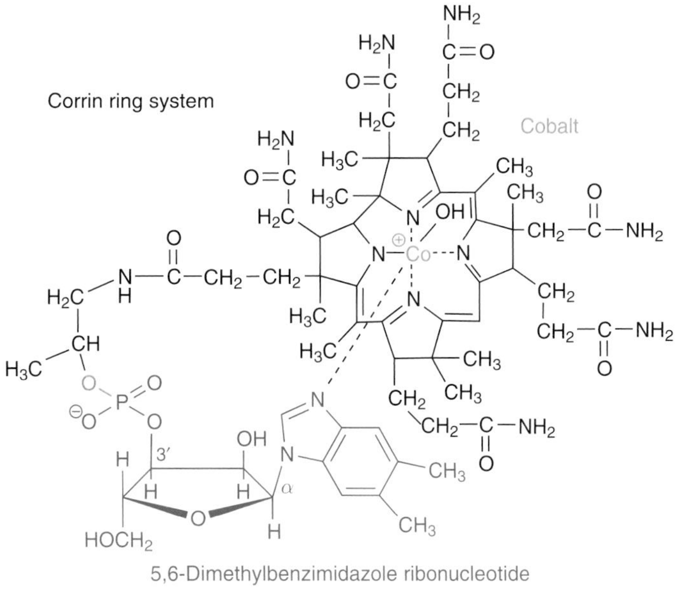

Figure 1 Chemical structure of cobalamin (vitamin B_{12}).

aquocobalamin are intermediates formed during the synthesis of the coenzyme forms. Other forms including sulfito-, nitrite-, and glutathionyl- derivatives of cobalamin have also been described but their role in metabolism is not known.

Biochemistry and Metabolic Functions

Only two reactions in humans and other animals are known to require cobalamin (**Figure 2**). One is isomerization of methylmalonyl coenzyme A (CoA), which requires deoxyadenosylcobalamin, is catalyzed by the enzyme methylmalonyl CoA mutase, and is

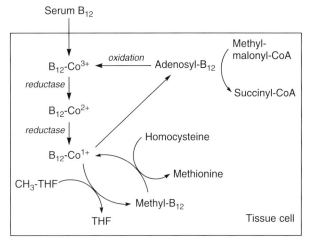

Figure 2 Reactions in humans and other animals known to require cobalamin.

mitochondrial. The other reaction is the transmethylation of homocysteine by 5-methyl-tetrahydrofolate to methionine, catalyzed by the enzyme methionine synthase (N^5-methyltetrahydrofolate:homocysteine methyltransferase) which requires methylcobalamin as coenzyme and is located in the cytosol. It is through their essential roles in this important metabolic reaction that cobalamin and folate interact and are linked with respect to their importance in nutrition. In addition, there are major similarities in the effects of their deficiencies in humans. These will be discussed below. Considering this 'metabolic crossroad' for the two vitamins, it may be pointed out that without adequate supplies of both nutrients, the synthesis of methionine and its derivative S-adenosylmethionine (SAM) is disrupted, with consequent profound effects on normal cellular function. Methionine is a key and essential amino acid and normal supply depends critically on recycling through the remethylation pathway (**Figure 3**). Moreover, SAM is the universal methyl donor, essential for over 100 transmethylation reactions involving amino acid, nucleotide, neurotransmitter, and phospholipid metabolism as well as detoxification reactions.

Apart from methionine the other product of the methionine synthase reaction, which is almost completely irreversible, is tetrahydrofolate (THF); this constitutes the first step by which folate enters bone marrow and other cells from plasma, for its conversion into the various intracellular forms of reduced folate containing a series of one-carbon substituents (see 00119 and **Figure 3**). The active forms of these

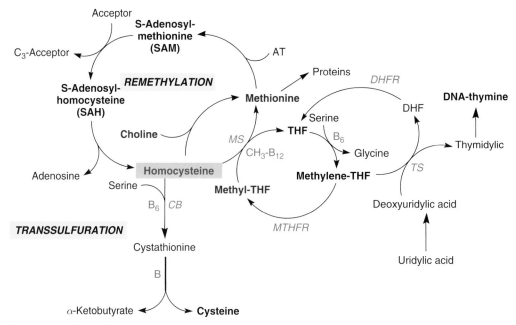

Figure 3 The remethylation pathway.

folate congeners are all polyglutamated by an enzyme, folate polyglutamate synthetase, that cannot use methyl-THF as substrate. Tetrahydrofolate is the obligate substrate for polyglutamate addition. Consequently, when the methionine synthase reaction is blocked as a result of cobalamin deficiency, there is 'THF starvation.' Methyl-THF accumulates in the plasma, while intracellular folate concentrations fall due to failure of formation of the critical intracellular folate polyglutamates because of 'methyl-folate trapping.' This theory explains the abnormalities of folate metabolism that occur in cobalamin deficiency (high concentrations of serum folate, low red cell folate) and also why the anemia that occurs in cobalamin deficiency will temporarily or partially respond to folic acid in large doses. The explanation of why the serum cobalamin falls in folate deficiency may also be related to impairment of the methionine synthase reaction resulting in reduced formation of methylcobalamin, the predominant circulating form of cobalamin in plasma.

Physiology

The recommended daily allowance (RDA) for cobalamin in adults proposed by the Food and Nutrition Board of the National Academy of Sciences/National Research Council in 1997 is 2.4 μg. Cobalamins do not occur in plants but are synthesized by certain bacteria, fungi, and algae, which constitute the ultimate source of all cobalamin found in nature. Cobalamins enter the food chain through herbivorous animals that harbor cobalamin-producing microorganisms in their upper gastrointestinal tract (e.g., the 'first stomach' of ruminants). Consumption of the meat or products of these animals supplies cobalamin in the diet for other animals. Dietary sources of cobalamin in humans are restricted to meat, poultry, fish, shellfish, eggs, and dairy products. Cobalamin is resistant to destruction by cooking, unlike the heat labile folates. On account of the exceedingly small daily requirement for cobalamin, in the order of 2 to 3 μg, and the relatively large body store of the vitamin (3000–5000 μg in developed countries) complete absence of intake or absorption of cobalamin is preceded by a long lag of up to 3–5 years before depletion of body cobalamin stores reaches a critical point that results in the manifestations of cobalamin deficiency. This is not the case in developing countries where the onset of depletion may be much more rapid because of initially lower stores. Still, complete lack of dietary intake of cobalamin is somewhat rare and occurs only in strict vegans who shun all animal foods, including dairy products and eggs.

Cobalamin absorption is a complex mechanism that consists of several steps and involves several protein chaperones and receptors, defects of which can result in reduced or absent uptake of dietary cobalamin. The related and continuous processes of ingestion, digestion, and absorption of cobalamin comprising the assimilation of the vitamin are arbitrarily divided into six steps. During the first step of mastication and swallowing of food, dietary cobalamin becomes mixed with a binding protein derived from saliva belonging to the family of cobalamin-binding proteins known as haptocorrins. Cobalamin in foods is generally complexed to proteins that must first be digested to release the bioavailable vitamin. In the second step release of cobalamin takes place largely in the stomach, under the influence of gastric hydrochloric acid and proteolytic digestion by pepsin. It is during this process and in the acid environment of the stomach that salivary haptocorrin preferentially binds and protects food cobalamin. Another specific cobalamin-binding protein, known as intrinsic factor, is secreted by the parietal cells of the stomach, but is unable to bind the cobalamin still tightly complexed to haptocorrin. During the third step, which occurs in the duodenum, cobalamin is released from its complex with haptocorrin through the combined effects of pancreatic bicarbonate, which neutralizes the gastric acid, and the proteolytic action of the enzymes trypsin and chymotrypsin that digest haptocorrin and thus enable the binding of the free cobalamin by gastric intrinsic factor. In the fourth step, the intrinsic factor–cobalamin complex, having traversed the full length of the small intestine, arrives at the luminal surface of the terminal ileum. There, it comes in contact with specialized receptors. In the presence of calcium, the complex attaches to the receptor consisting of two distinct proteins, cubulin and a recently identified protein known as amnionless that is necessary to complete the assimilation process. Both proteins are essential for the internalization of the intrinsic factor–vitamin B_{12} complex through a process known as receptor-mediated endocytosis. Through this process, cobalamin together with intrinsic factor and escorted by the receptor are taken into lysosomes where the intrinsic factor–cobalamin complex is released and intrinsic factor is degraded through the action of acid hydrolysis of peptidases. The final fifth step is poorly understood but involves first the release from lysosomes and then the metabolism of cobalamin to its methyl and deoxyadenosyl derivatives. It is primarily in the form of methylcobalamin that the vitamin finally enters the plasma. The assimilation of food vitamin

B_{12} is a lengthy process, as evidenced by the 6–8 h taken for orally administered cobalamin to first appear in the plasma and several additional hours for the process to be completed.

When cobalamin enters the plasma, it is bound to the cobalamin-binding protein transcobalamin (previously known as transcobalamin II to distinguish it from transcobalamins I and III, which, together with the salivary cobalamin-binding protein and other binders present in secretions are now referred to collectively as the haptocorrins). The properties of transcobalamin and the haptocorrins are summarized in **Table 1**. The fraction of cobalamin bound to transcobalamin accounts for only 20–30% of the total plasma cobalamin. The major residual fraction of the plasma cobalamin is attached to haptocorrins. The function of haptocorrins is not known, but rapidly proliferating cells including bone marrow precursors can obtain cobalamin only from transcobalamin. Consequently, the critical fraction of the serum cobalamin is the transcobalamin-bound portion, known as holo-transcobalamin. Conditions that alter the amount or distribution of cobalamin on these binding proteins can critically affect its delivery and transport. Therefore, conditions that lead to an increase in haptocorrins, such as chronic granulocytic leukemia (haptocorrins are produced in granulocytes), can give rise to an apparently normal serum cobalamin level even in patients who have pernicious anemia or some other cause of cobalamin deficiency. Conversely, a decrease in holo-transcobalamin can result in cobalamin deficiency even if the serum cobalamin level is apparently normal. This occurs in infants and children affected by congenital transcobalamin deficiency, which is associated with severe megaloblastic anemia. Levels of transcobalamin, which is produced mainly in endothelial cells, may be affected by a number of factors. Lowering of holo-transcobalamin can result in tissue cobalamin deficiency with a normal serum cobalamin level. Although holo-transcobalamin has been measured, and appears to correlate well with serum metabolite levels and other parameters of cobalamin deficiency, routine assays sufficiently sensitive to measure the small fraction of cobalamin that occurs as holo-transcobalamin have only recently become available.

Causes and Effects of Cobalamin Deficiency and Mechanisms

There are a number of causes of cobalamin deficiency that range in severity and frequency of occurrence. These are summarized in **Table 2**. In general, causes of cobalamin deficiency can be divided into those caused by absent or markedly reduced dietary intake and chemical inactivation (both rare) and those caused by malabsorption, either gastric or ileal. The most frequent cause of clinically important cobalamin deficiency is malabsorption of the vitamin and, in particular, pernicious anemia, caused by an autoimmune

Table 1 Properties of human plasma cobalamin binding proteins

	Haptocorrins (transcobalamin I + III)	Transcobalamin II
Source	Granulocytes	Endothelial cells
Transport functions	Storage, excretion of vitamin B_{12} analogs, antimicrobial	Cellular vitamin B_{12} uptake
Binding specificity	Low specificity, binds vitamin B_{12} analogs	Binds vitamin B_{12} with higher specificity
Membrane receptors	Nonspecific asialoglycoprotein receptors on hepatocytes	Specific receptors on most cells
Saturation	High (mainly 'holo')	Low (mainly 'apo')
Fraction of total vitamin B_{12}	80–90%	10–30%
Plasma clearance	Slow ($t_{1/2} \approx 10$ days)	Rapid ($t_{1/2} \approx 6$ min)
Molecular weight (Daltons)	60 000	38 000–45 000

Table 2 Causes of cobalamin deficiency

1. Dietary
   Veganism
2. Gastric
   - Atrophic gastritis and food cobalamin malabsorption
   - Autoimmune gastritis/gastric atrophy (classical pernicious anemia)
   - Extensive gastric disease or resection
3. Ileal
   - Extensive ileal disease (Crohn's, inflammatory bowel disease, tuberculous enteritis) or resection for these diseases
   - Luminal disturbances (chronic pancreatic disease, gastrinoma) and parasites (giardiasis, bacterial overgrowth, fish tapeworm)
4. Chemical/drug
   - Nitrous oxide
   - PAS, oral antidiabetic agents, colchicine
5. Congenital/inherited
   - Intrinsic factor deficiency/defect ('juvenile' pernicious anemia)
   - Intrinsic factor receptor deficiency/defect (Immerslund-Grasbeck syndrome)
   - Transcobalamin II deficiency
   - Cobalamin mutants (C-G)

destruction of the gastric mucosa with consequent failure of intrinsic factor production. Another more common cause of malabsorption of cobalamin is so-called food cobalamin malabsorption, caused by atrophy of the stomach lining that often occurs with increasing age. The mechanism of malabsorption in this condition is caused by a failure of complete food digestion and hence release of cobalamin for binding to intrinsic factor rather than a failure of intrinsic factor production itself. Food cobalamin malabsorption *per se* does not appear to result in clinically important cobalamin deficiency but may set the stage for greater susceptibility to the onset of deficiency when other conditions completely abrogate cobalamin absorption.

In all situations resulting from impairment of cobalamin absorption, the time to onset of deficiency depends on several factors, including the size of the body store, the extent of impairment of absorption (partial or complete), and, in diseases like pernicious anemia and others affecting all of the intestine, the rate of progression of the disease. In general, however, cobalamin deficiency resulting from malabsorption develops sooner (2–5 years) than is the case in the dietary deficiency encountered among vegans (10–20 years). This difference may be explained by the existence of a considerable enterohepatic recirculation of cobalalmin. Biliary cobalamin is efficiently reabsorbed in vegans compared with patients who have pernicious anemia or other forms of malabsorption.

Deficiency of cobalamin, when severe, affects all rapidly growing (DNA synthesizing) tissues, particularly in the bone marrow, with resulting production of larger abnormal cells with nuclei that bear evidence of impaired maturation. These marrow precursor cells then give rise to reduced numbers of blood cell progeny that are, in turn, abnormally large and show the stigmata of disrupted development. Resulting macrocytic anemia together with neutrophil leucocytes that have, on average, more nuclear lobes than normal (hypersegmented neutrophil leucocytes) are the usual telltale signs of megaloblastic anemia seen in cobalamin, as well as folate, deficiency. After the marrow, the next most affected tissues are the epithelial cell surfaces of the mouth, stomach, and the small intestine. Affected cells are also large, with increased numbers of multinucleated and dying cells. The gonads are also affected and infertility is common in patients with deficiency. Cobalamin deficiency may also be associated with skin hyperpigmentation and has been described in association with reduced bone-derived alkaline phosphatase and osteocalcin in the plasma.

Cobalamin deficiency may also cause nervous system complications including bilateral peripheral neuropathy or degeneration (demyelination) of the posterior and pyramidal tracts of the spinal cord, and, less frequently, atrophy of the optic nerve or cerebral symptoms. Cobalamin-deficient patients typically display sensory disturbances or paraesthesiae, muscle weakness, difficulty in walking, and sometimes dementia, psychotic disturbances, or visual impairment. Long-term nutritional cobalamin deficiency in infancy leads to poor brain development and impaired intellectual development. The effects of cobalamin deficiency on the blood and on the nervous system may occur separately or in combination and their severity is often inversely rather than directly correlated. The biochemical basis for cobalamin neuropathy, however, remains obscure. Its occurrence in the absence of methylmalonic aciduria in transcobalamin II deficiency, and in monkeys given the anesthetic agent nitrous oxide, suggests that the neuropathy is related to a defect in homocysteine–methionine conversion. Accumulation of S-adenosylhomocysteine in the brain resulting in inhibition of transmethylation reactions has been suggested.

Psychiatric disturbance is common in cobalamin deficiencies. Like the neuropathy, this has been attributed to a failure of the synthesis of SAM, due to reduced conversion of homocysteine to methionine. SAM is needed in the methylation of biogenic amines (e.g., dopamine), as well as of proteins, phospholipids, and neurotransmitters in the brain. A reduced ratio of SAM to S-adenosyl-homocysteine is postulated to result in reduced methylation. In cobalamin deficiency there is an intriguing inverse correlation between the degree of anemia, on the one hand, and the severity of the myeloneuropathy, on the other hand.

Diagnosis of Cobalamin Deficiency

Cobalamin deficiency is suspected in individuals who display the typical manifestations of deficiency of the vitamin as described in the section above on the effects of deficiency. In addition to the symptoms that may be experienced by individuals that are related to anemia (easy fatigue, shortness of breath, palpitations) and neuropathy (sensory and motor disturbances and memory loss) there are features that may be detected by a physician, including skin pallor (from anemia), abnormalities in neurological examination (sensory loss, abnormal balance and reflexes, mental changes), and epithelial changes (skin pigmentation, smooth tongue). On the basis of any combination of such changes, cobalamin deficiency may be suspected but confirmation is necessary using laboratory tests because other conditions may give rise to effects that closely resemble cobalamin deficiency. This need to confim suspected cobalamin deficiency applies also in individuals who have abnormalities in their blood count results with anemia and macrocytosis (larger than normal red blood cells).

The standard screening test for cobalamin deficiency consists of direct measurement of circulating levels of cobalamin. Serum levels less than $150 \, \text{pmol} \, l^{-1}$ are considered deficient and $150–250 \, \text{pmol} \, l^{-1}$ are considered borderline. Serum or plasma cobalamin concentration can be measured in several ways and this has evolved from early microbial growth assays through competitive binding assays that were first radioisotopic and are now enzyme-linked or based on chemiluminescence detection. The sensitivity and specificity of these assays is imperfect, such that measurement of serum cobalamin levels does not always detect the presence of deficiency, nor does the finding of a low serum cobalamin always connote true deficiency. There are several reasons for this including the distribution of cobalamin between the binding proteins in circulation (**Table 1**), imperfections in the assays for its measurement, and various poorly understood factors relating to exchange of cobalamin between cellular and circulatory compartments. Regarding the distribution of cobalamin between plasma-binding proteins, since transcobalamin is responsible for cobalamin delivery to cells, the fraction of the total cobalamin that is associated with transcobalamin (holoTC), even though small in comparison with the haptocorrin-associated fraction, is more likely to be indicative of cobalamin status than is the total serum cobalamin. Some studies bear this out, although technical difficulties with measuring holoTC levels have only recently been overcome.

The other approach to identification of cobalamin deficiency is indirect, based on the detection of raised levels of compounds in the blood or urine that require adequate tissue levels of cobalamin for their metabolic disposal. The compounds most commonly measured for identification of possible cobalamin deficiency are methylmalonic acid and homocysteine. These are the substrates in two cobalamin-dependent reactions shown in **Figure 2**. Since the identification of these metabolic roles for cobalamin, it has been apparent that deficiency of cobalamin or disturbances in its metabolism would result in accumulation of these substances and a variety of assays for these metabolites is now available. Of the two compounds, elevation of the levels of methylamalonic acid is the more specific for identification of cobalamin deficiency; however, renal insufficiency can cause raised levels of methylmalonate in the blood. In addition to cobalamin deficiency, several other conditions also can cause raised homocysteine levels in the blood, including deficiencies of folate and of vitamin B_6, lack of thyroid hormone, and renal insufficiency (see 00151).

Table 3 shows the idealized usefulness of the various tests commonly available for detection of cobalamin deficiency.

Inborn Errors of Cobalamin Metabolism

There are several known but rare inherited molecular defects resulting in absence or structural defects in proteins required for normal absorption, transport. or metabolism of cobalamin. These include the intestinal binding proteins gastric intrinsic factor and its ileal receptor complex cubulin and amnionless, the plasma binders transcobalamin and haptocorrin, the enzymes that are required for conversion of cobalamin to its coenzymatically active methyl and deoxyadenosyl forms, and enzyme complexes involved in the catalysis of the two cobalamin-dependent reactions responsible for conversion of homocysteine to methionine and methylmalonate to succinate, respectively. Individuals who inherit a defective gene from each parent for any one of these proteins that are critical for cobalamin metabolism suffer from varying degrees of impairment of normal cobalamin-related status (see **Table 4**), closely mimicking the various

Table 3 Laboratory identification of cobalamin deficiency

Test	Finding	Major limitations
Serum/plasma cobalamin concentration	Low ($<150 \, \text{pmol} \, l^{-1}$)	Normal levels in some deficient subjects; slight to moderately low levels may not connote deficiency
Serum/plasma holotranscobalamin (holo TC II)	Low ($<35 \, \text{pmol} \, l^{-1}$)	Test not yet widely available; insufficient validation of usefulness
Serum/plasma or urine methylmalonic acid	Raised ($>350 \, \text{nmol} \, l^{-1}$)	Levels raised in renal insufficiency
Plasma homocysteine	Raised ($>12 \, \mu\text{mol} \, l^{-1}$)	Levels raised in folate and in vitamin B_6 deficiencies, renal insufficiency, hypothyroidism

Table 4 Inherited disorders affecting cobalamin metabolism and their effects

Cobalamin protein	Effects of deletion or mutation
Intrinsic factor	Cobalamin malabsorption (juvenile pernicious anemia)
Cubulin/amnionless complex	Cobalamin malabsorption (Immerslund-Grasbeck syndrome)
Transcobalamin	Severe cobalamin deficiency
Haptocorrin	No apparent abnormality
Cobalamin reducing and activating enzymes (mut$^+$ and mut$^-$, cobalamin mutants C-G)	Varying degrees of disruption in one or both cobalamin-dependent pathways

manifestations of cobalamin deficiency described above. These disorders usually become manifest at an early age.

See also: **Amino Acids**: Chemistry and Classification; Metabolism; Specific Functions. **Anemia**: Iron-Deficiency Anemia; Megaloblastic Anemia. **Folic Acid**. **Homocysteine**. **Inborn Errors of Metabolism**: Classification and Biochemical Aspects.

Further Reading

Carmel R (2000) Current concepts in cobalamin deficiency. *Annual Review of Medicine* 51: 357–375.
Carmel R, Green R, Rosenblatt DS, and Watkins D (2003) Update on cobalamin, folate, and homocysteine. *Hematology (American Society of Hematology Education Program)*: 62–81.
Green R and Kinsella LJ (1995) Current concepts in the diagnosis of cobalamin deficiency. *Neurology* 45: 1435–1440.
Stabler SP and Allen RH (2004) Vitamin B12 deficiency as a worldwide problem. *Annual Review of Nutrition* 24: 299–326.
Stover PJ (2004) Physiology of folate and vitamin B12 in health and disease. *Nutrition Reviews* 62: S3–12.

CELIAC DISEASE

V Nehra, E Marietta and J Murray, The Mayo Clinic College of Medicine, Rochester, MN, USA

© 2005 Elsevier Ltd. All rights reserved.

Introduction

Celiac disease is the end result of a collision between the human immune system and the widespread cultivation of wheat, where the point of contact is the lining of the small intestine. This collision results in inflammatory and architectural changes of the absorptive mucosa in those susceptible to celiac disease. The inflammation leads to the destruction and eventual loss of the absorptive surface (villi), increased net secretion, and malabsorption, leading to a multitude of consequences. Celiac disease predominantly affects Caucasians, and it is relatively rare in peoples from sub-Saharan Africa and the Far East, which may be due to different genetic backgrounds and/or the absence of wheat from the diet. The disease occurs in people who carry the particular tissue types HLA-DQ2 or HLA-DQ8, which appear to play an essential role in the disease pathogenesis. The inflammation usually resolves completely with the exclusion of gluten from the diet, will recur if gluten is reintroduced, and, as such, is regarded as permanent. While once thought to be a rare disease, it is recognized as a common chronic disorder that affects as many as 1% of some Western populations. Indeed, in some populations, it is regarded as the most common genetic disease that affects the gastrointestinal tract. It is now frequently detected by the presence of circulating autoantibodies against tissue transglutaminase, which is released in the damaged intestine. The final diagnosis of celiac disease is defined by biopsy evidence of the characteristic inflammatory changes in the small intestine and ultimately a response to the gluten-free diet.

Pathogenesis

Established celiac disease is characterized by an inflammatory response in the proximal small intestine. This inflammation consists of increased numbers of lymphocytes, plasma cells, and macrophages in the lamina propria and increased lymphocytes in the surface layer of the epithelium, called intraepithelial lymphocytes. The surface enterocytes are shorter and wider than normal and have poorly ordered nuclei. The normally tall thin villi are shortened and flattened. The cryptal layer is increased in depth. These changes may be patchy and affect variable lengths of the proximal small intestine (**Figure 1**).

The lamina propria is packed with T cells, many of which are CD4+ cells that respond to gliadin molecules in a manner that is DQ2 or DQ8 restricted. These cells are thought to be crucial in

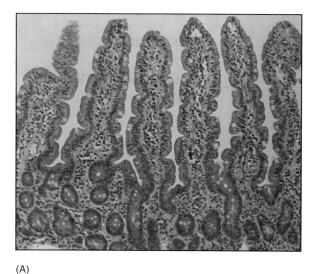
(A)

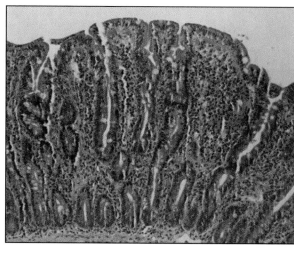
(B)

Figure 1 Inflammatory response in proximal small intestine. Proximal small intestinal tissue from a normal control (A) and from a celiac patient (B) was stained with hematoxylin and eosin. Shortened and flattened villi, shorter and wider enterocytes, increased numbers of intraepithelial lymphocytes, and a cryptal layer with increased depth are all present in (B) but not in (A).

the actual pathology of the lesion, and clones derived from such cells have been used to characterize the response to gliadin. Lymphocytes in the intraepithelial layer are also increased in number in untreated celiac disease, many of which bear the $\gamma\delta$ TCR. These cells slowly decrease when gluten is removed. An early event in the pathology is an increased expression of class II HLA molecules by enterocytes and antigen-presenting cells such as the macrophages within the lamina propria. These molecules are involved in the presentation of the exogenous and possibly the endogenous antigens that are released in the setting of inflammation.

In addition to the pathological changes in the small bowel mucosa, a potent humoral response occurs in untreated celiac disease. In the intestinal mucosa there are increased numbers of plasma cells secreting IgA, IgG, and IgM directed against gluten peptides and other plasma cells secreting antibodies directed against connective tissue autoantigens, particularly tissue transglutaminase. Those antibodies are found in the intestinal juice and the serum. The dynamics of the humoral response seems to parallel the dynamics of cellular injury, although antibodies may rise prior to mucosal relapse and disappear prior to healing.

There is also increased permeability of the small intestine to macromolecules. It is not clear if this increased permeability precedes the development of gliadin sensitivity. It may persist after healing of the microscopic lesions has occurred. Family members without the disease may have increased permeability. Recently, it has been suggested that gluten itself may rapidly cause an increase in paracellular permeability due to the uncoupling of intercellular tight junctions via the release of zonulin.

Adaptive Immune Response to Gluten

Celiac disease is characterized by an immune response to the storage proteins of wheat, rye, and barley, with wheat as the most immunogenic. Wheat gluten is composed of glutenin and gliadin, and evidence suggests that the gliadin fraction induces disease. Information gathered from T cell clones derived from chronic lesions of the small intestines of celiac patients with established disease demonstrate that gliadin peptides are presented by HLA class II molecules to CD4+ T cells. Several studies have suggested that unaltered native gliadin peptides were antigenic but lacked the negatively charged amino acids needed to bind to the recognition sites of the DQ2 or DQ8 molecules. It has since been recognized that the gliadin peptides are made more antigenic by tissue transglutaminase, and it is these altered (deamidated) peptides that either perpetuate or cause gluten sensitivity in celiac disease.

It is thought that tissue transglutaminase is released by fibroblasts in the setting of intestinal inflammation, since tissue transglutaminase is normally involved in cell to cell signaling and extracellular matrix formation. Released tissue transglutaminase would then bind to its preferred substrate, gliadin, and convert (deamidate) the specific glutamine residues in gliadin to glutamic acid, resulting in improved binding of gliadin peptides to specific pockets in the DQ molecule. Interestingly, this release of tissue transglutaminase into the inflamed celiac gut also results in a strong autoimmune response to tissue transglutaminase with high levels of circulating anti-tTG IgA present in untreated celiac patients. Thus, the main characteristics of celiac disease are the DQ2/DQ8 restricted responses to gliadin peptides, the strong intestinal T cell response to deamidated gliadin peptides, and the production of circulating autoantibodies against tissue transglutaminase. However, it has been observed that some native gliadin peptides can also induce strong T cell proliferation. The 11-mer native peptide of gliadin, amino acids 206–216, was observed to induce proliferation in DQ8 T cell lines, and when instilled into the jejunum of a patient with celiac disease, induced jejunal inflammation.

Observations in the DQ8 mouse support the notion that both native gliadin peptides and deamidated gliadin peptides can evoke T cell responses in a DQ restricted fashion. Also of interest is that T cell cultures derived from the biopsies of children, who presumably would have had a recent onset of disease, responded to native gluten peptides and a narrower range of gliadin peptides than those derived from adults. Thus, it is possible that naturally occurring (native) epitopes of gliadin may be involved in the initiation of gluten sensitivity, whereas the deamidation process is involved in the perpetuation and amplification of the process.

Innate Immune Response

Many of the studies on gut responses to gluten have been performed in the established chronic lesion. Little is known of innate responses that can elicit effects within minutes to hours of exposure to gluten. *In vitro* studies demonstrated an increase in the expression of HLA antigen on the cells in the surface layers of the intestinal mucosa occurring within 2–4 h after exposure to gluten. Gluten also causes the production of the proinflammatory cytokine IL-15 at the surface epithelium. IL-15 expressed by the surface enterocytes activates NK-like T cells to recognize gluten presented by MHC class 1a molecules in the context of the NKG-2D receptor. The NK-like T cell may be a key player in both the damage to the surface epithelium and be a proinflammatory influence on adaptive response that occurs in the underlying lamina propria. This induction of innate immune responses by gluten may have important consequences. Since the gluten peptides enter into the epithelial compartment and paracellular regions, the Peyer's patch pathway is not the exclusive route for the introduction of the gluten peptides to the immune system. As such, the bypass of the Peyer's patches may lead to a loss of tolerance

and even an induction of sensitization, resulting in an uncontrolled immune response in the intestinal mucosa. The stimulation of the surface layer not only explains the substantial changes that occur in the surface but may well condition the inflammatory response beneath. Thus, both arms of the immune system, the innate and the adaptive, play a role in the development of celiac disease, even though most attention has so far been focused on the adaptive arm.

Triggers for Loss of Tolerance

Celiac disease only develops in a minority of DQ2+ individuals. How the consumption of gluten generates an inflammatory state in these individuals can be theorized as follows. First, there may be a trigger of the innate immune response, such as a viral infection or physical injury (surgery) that initiates inflammation and later permeability. Enough triggers repeated over time will alter the immune milieu of the mucosal compartment and perturb gut homeostasis, potentially altering the levels of the regulatory cytokines IL-10 and TGF-β and increasing the levels of inflammatory cytokines like IFN-γ and ILNA.

Determining which factors lead to the loss of tolerance to gluten in DQ2+ individuals who later develop celiac disease will be crucial in understanding the pathogenesis of celiac disease. Possible factors that may lead to the loss of tolerance are recurring gastrointestinal infections, surgery, or pregnancy. The way in which children are first exposed to gluten may also affect whether tolerance to gluten or an inflammatory response develops. Quantity and timing of exposure to gluten during childhood may affect the development of tolerance to gluten. Interestingly, the aging process has also been implicated in the loss of tolerance to gluten. More recently, it has become apparent that most celiac patients initially present with disease as adults, possibly due to an increased propensity to autoimmunity associated with advanced age.

The mechanism of response to gluten in celiac disease is quite different from that of IgE-mediated food allergies. IFN-γ, a potent inflammatory cytokine, is characteristically produced in celiac disease as well as TNF-α. IL10 and TGF-β, which are both counterinflammatory regulatory cytokines for the intestine, are also expressed in celiac disease, although they are apparently inadequate to prevent the substantial inflammation that occurs.

Overall then, it is thought that environmental triggers, which may be nonspecific, the innate responses to gluten, and finally the adaptive responses to gluten combine to result in the enteropathy that characterizes celiac disease. This process

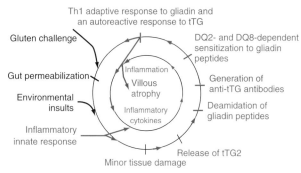

Figure 2 Maelstrom of celiac disease. An initial perturbation of the mucosal immune system would activate the innate immune response, increase epithelial permeability, and inflame the mucosal environment, resulting in overexpression of MHC class II molecules and the presentation of gliadin peptides to CD4+ T cells. tTG produced by fibroblasts in the damaged lining would deamidate gliadin peptides and amplify the CD4+ T cell response to gliadin. The released tTG would subsequently be targeted by the humoral immune response as an autoantigen, further advancing the mucosal immune system down a spiraling pathway towards self-destruction and villous atrophy.

can be best described as a 'maelstrom' of immune activity that leads to celiac disease if unchecked (**Figure 2**). Removal of gluten, the major instigator, will result in the reversal of this process and healing of the intestine. However, reintroduction of gluten will often result in a prompt recurrence of the disease, demonstrating that celiac disease is a permanent intolerance to gluten.

Epidemiology of Celiac Disease

Celiac disease is one of the most common, chronic genetic gastrointestinal conditions affecting just under 1% of Caucasian individuals. Whilst it was initially recognized in Northern Europeans, celiac disease will affect Caucasians wherever they live. It can affect people of mixed ethnic background. It is apparently rare in Southeast Asia and sub-Saharan Africa. While celiac disease was once considered primarily a childhood disease, in many geographic locations, celiac disease is more commonly diagnosed in adulthood. The median age in one study in the US was 50 years of age. Even in childhood, the age at diagnosis is now increased from early infancy to later in childhood or adolescence. The spectrum of disease has also changed with an increasing proportion of patients being diagnosed with mono-symptomatic or less severe celiac disease. Many of these patients would not have been diagnosed in the past, but their symptoms described as functional disorders. It is not uncommon to diagnose celiac disease in those of advanced age. Patients in their 80s may be diagnosed for the first

time with celiac disease, some of these having symptoms that persist for many years prior to diagnosis. The delay time to diagnosis may be anywhere between 8 and 11 years from the time of first clinical presentation to the actual diagnosis being made.

Diagnosed celiac disease appears to be more common in women than men. However, in those individuals who are identified by population-based screening, the prevalence of the disease appears to be equal between genders. The explanation for this is unclear, however, presentation of disease may be more common in women because of the nutritional challenges posed by pregnancy and menstruation, especially when producing iron deficiency anemia. The predisposition of women to autoimmune disease may also increase the likelihood of the occurrence of symptomatic celiac disease.

The sister condition of celiac disease is dermatitis herpetiformis, which is the skin manifestation of gluten-sensitive enteropathy. It is an extremely itchy immunobullous disease that affects the extensor surfaces of elbows, knees, buttocks, the hairline, and the torso and is much less common than celiac disease. Probably the ratio between the two in geographic areas where both have been estimated is approximately 10:1. However, in countries where there has traditionally been less celiac disease awareness, such as North America, the ratio may be closer to 3:1.

The incidence of celiac disease and the prevalence of celiac disease have been estimated in a number of geographic locations. These have shown incidence estimates of approximately between 1 and 9 cases per 100 000 person years and prevalence rates of anywhere from 1 in 2000 to 1 in 300. The latter high estimate is based on geographic locations where there have been active case findings such as Tampere in Finland. The lower rates are the prevalence based on clinically diagnosed cases. However, these measures may greatly underestimate the true prevalence of celiac disease in the community. Two specific lines of research would suggest this. One is a systematic follow-up of birth cohorts for the occurrence of celiac disease by using serologic screening. In one geographic location in Denver, Colorado, almost 1% of children became persistently seropositive for markers for celiac disease by 7 years of age. This cumulative prevalence is remarkably similar to population-based studies in both Europe and North America that suggest prevalence in an adult general population of approximately 1 in 133. The estimates of the prevalence of celiac disease in most Caucasian studies have been remarkably similar, varying from 1 in 300 to 1 in 87.

All the studies so far have been carried out in predominantly Caucasian populations. No studies have been carried out that have incorporated substantial numbers of African-Americans, nor have systematic studies been carried out in sub-Saharan Africa. Areas of North Africa are at least as commonly affected as Europe. Individuals from Southeast Asia very rarely develop celiac disease.

The major effect of these screening studies has been to illustrate the wide spectrum of disease that incorporates celiac disease. Many individuals are completely asymptomatic. Others may be severely ill, presenting at an early age. It is possible that some individuals who have developed celiac disease may have no symptoms whatsoever despite the presence of demonstrable serologic and histopathological changes of celiac disease.

Associated Disorders

Dermatitis herpetiformis This is characterized by an extremely pruritic papulovesicular eruption, which usually occurs symmetrically on the elbows, knees, buttocks, and back. About 80% of patients with dermatitis herpetiformis have small intestine histology indistinguishable from celiac sprue. The diagnosis is established by skin biopsy demonstrating granular IgA deposits in areas of normal appearing skin. A majority of patients with the skin lesion who undergo small bowel biopsy have intestinal mucosal changes of celiac disease. The skin lesions, as well as small bowel histology, improve on a gluten-free diet. Dapsone is an effective short-term treatment for dermatitis herpetiformis; however, it does not have any impact on management of small bowel enteropathy. Also, those with dermatitis herpetiformis who are not compliant with the gluten-free diet are at higher risk for malignancy, as are those with celiac disease.

Celiac disease has also been associated with other autoimmune as well as nonautoimmune disorders. It has been reported that the longer there is exposure to gluten in patients with celiac disease, the greater the occurrence of other autoimmune diseases. There is evidence for a strong association between type 1 diabetes and celiac disease. About 8% of patients with type 1 diabetes have the characteristic features of celiac sprue on small bowel biopsy. When the two diseases coexist, 90% have the diagnosis of diabetes before celiac disease. Among the symptoms that may be suggestive of coexisting celiac disease, in addition to those considered classical for celiac disease, are delayed puberty, hypertransaminasemia, anemia, iron deficiency, arthralgias, dental enamel defects, hypoglycemia, and unexplained reduction in insulin requirements. Treatment with a gluten-free diet may improve diabetic control and decrease the occurrence of hypoglycemia episodes.

There is also a strong association between selective IgA deficiency and celiac sprue. Studies including adults and children in Ireland and Italy reported the frequency of selective IgA deficiency in celiac sprue to be about 2%, and 5–11% of IgA-deficient individuals have celiac disease.

There is a strong association between Down's syndrome and celiac disease. Individuals with Down's syndrome and celiac disease more commonly have gastrointestinal manifestations such as intermittent diarrhea, failure to thrive, anemia, and low serum iron and calcium. The prevalence of celiac disease in patients with Down's syndrome varies between 5 and 12%. An increased prevalence of celiac sprue has also been reported in individuals with Turner's syndrome and Williams syndrome.

Clinical Presentation

Celiac disease may present in a wide variety of ways (**Table 1**). In children, the onset of celiac disease is classically described as occurring within the first to seventh year of life with the introduction of cereals to the diet. Symptoms may vary with the age of the child at onset of disease. Young children may develop chronic diarrhea, failure to thrive, muscle wasting, abdominal distension, vomiting, and abdominal pain. Older children may present with anemia, rickets, behavioral disturbances, or poor performance in school. In some children constipation, pseudo-obstruction, and intussusception may be seen. It has been estimated that 2–8% of children with unexplained short stature may have celiac disease. Dental enamel defects involving secondary dentition as well as

Table 1 Presentations of celiac disease

Gastrointestinal presentations
- Classic malabsorption syndrome – diarrhea, steatorrhea, weight loss, bloating, failure to thrive, multiple deficiencies
- Monosymptomatic – anemia, diarrhea, lactose intolerance, constipation
- Acute abdomen – abdominal pain, intussusception, vomiting, obstruction perforation, lymphoma

Nongastrointestinal presentations
- Neurological diseases – migraine, ataxia, peripheral neuropathy, dementia, depression, epilepsy
- Autoimmune diseases – dermatitis herpetiformis, pulmonary hemosiderosis
- Diseases associated with nutritional deficiencies – bruising, epistaxis, chronic fatigue, infertility, bone disease, short stature

neurological syndrome and epilepsy with intracranial calcification have also been reported in children with celiac disease.

In adults, celiac disease may be overt in presentation with classic gastrointestinal symptoms of diarrhea, weight loss, and abdominal pain. The presence of diarrhea and/or steatorrhea, which occurs in about 50% of patients, indicates severe disease and malabsorption. Often celiac disease is diagnosed in adults with nongastrointestinal symptoms including iron deficiency anemia, abnormal liver tests, osteopenic bone disease, neurological symptoms, or menstrual abnormalities. Anemia is common in both children and adults with celiac disease and may be secondary to iron deficiency, folate deficiency, or a combination of the two. Iron deficiency is frequently associated with celiac disease. Six to ten per cent of patients with unexplained iron deficiency anemia when evaluated by upper endoscopy with small bowel biopsy were diagnosed with celiac sprue in the absence of any other features suggestive of the disease.

Unexplained elevated serum transaminases (ALT, AST) should also raise the suspicion of undiagnosed celiac disease. Up to 9% of adults with unexplained elevated serum transaminases have been diagnosed with celiac disease based on serological testing or small bowel biopsy. Liver biopsies in these individuals may show reactive hepatitis. In this setting, adherence to a gluten-free diet results in improvement or normalization of the liver enzyme levels. The prevalence of celiac sprue is higher in adults with autoimmune liver disease than in the general population. Volta *et al.* demonstrated a 4% prevalence of celiac sprue in 181 patients with autoimmune hepatitis. Similarly, a high prevalence of celiac disease has been reported in other autoimmune liver disorders such as primary biliary cirrhosis, autoimmune cholangitis, and primary sclerosing cholangitis.

Patients with untreated celiac disease are at increased risk for the development of osteoporosis and low bone mineral density. Celiac disease can result in malabsorption of calcium and vitamin D. Malabsorption of calcium results from impaired transport by the diseased small bowel as well as precipitation of the ingested calcium with unabsorbed intraluminal fats to form insoluble soaps that are then excreted in the stool. Untreated, patients with celiac disease have been observed to have increased bone turnover and elevated levels of 1,25 dihydroxycholecalciferol because of secondary hyperparathyroidism that helps maintain a positive calcium balance. This results in diminished bone densities associated with increased risk of fractures in patients with classical celiac disease. Untreated patients with celiac sprue are at risk for developing low bone mineral density and osteoporosis reported that 34% of their study population with celiac disease had fractures in the peripheral skeleton. For those with classical celiac symptoms, the odds ratio for fracture was 5.2 compared to those without celiac disease. Although the reduced bone mineral density improves on a gluten-free diet, adults with celiac sprue may be at increased risk for the development of peripheral bone fractures, although this is not universally agreed.

Infertility and recurrent spontaneous abortions have been reported in women with celiac disease. Male infertility has also been observed in patients with untreated celiac disease. Restoration of fertility both in males and females has been observed following treatment with a strict gluten-free diet and may be unexpected in some couples who have been unable to become pregnant before this time.

Patients with celiac disease may in addition present with neurological symptoms such as ataxia, muscle weakness, paresthesias, weight sensory loss, epilepsy, and bilateral parieto-occipital calcification. Symptoms of depression, epilepsy, and migraine have been reported in 30% of patients with celiac disease.

Diagnosis

Small bowel biopsy remains the gold standard for diagnosis of celiac disease. Over the past decade the diagnostic criteria for celiac sprue have changed. Based on the 1990 revised criteria of the European Society of Paediatric Gastroenterology and Nutrition, the diagnosis of celiac sprue can be made with a diagnostic small bowel biopsy in a patient with highly suggestive clinical symptoms, followed by an objective clinical response to a gluten-free diet. Endoscopic biopsies from the distal duodenum are preferable because the presence of Brunner glands in the duodenal bulb and proximal second portion of the duodenum may affect histologic interpretation. The original criteria requiring a series of three biopsies, i.e., first to confirm the diagnosis, second for demonstration of response to a gluten-free diet and the third for deterioration after gluten challenge, are only required in those few patients in which there is still some diagnostic uncertainty.

Endoscopic features observed in patients with celiac disease include scalloped or fissured folds, absence of folds when the duodenum is inflated, and visible submucosal blood vessels; however, these findings are unreliable in diagnosing celiac disease as only roughly half of the patients will have the findings detected endoscopically. Other causes of atrophy are indistinguishable from celiac disease.

Characteristic histologic changes described are partial or total villous atrophy, elongation of crypts, a decreased villous:crypt ratio, and increased intraepithelial lymphocytes (>30 per 100 enterocytes). Marsh and colleagues proposed a classification for the spectrum of histologic changes ranging from type 0 or preinfiltrative/normal, type1 or infiltrative lesion (increased intraepithelial lymphocytes), type 2 or hyperplastic lesion (presence of crypt hyperplasia), type 3 or destructive lesion (variable degree of villous atrophy), and type 4 or the hypoplastic lesion (total villous atrophy with crypt hypoplasia).

The role of radiological studies in the initial diagnosis of celiac sprue is limited. The findings of flocculation and segmentation of barium representing excessive fluid secretion in the lumen of the small intestine, thickened mucosal folds, and dilation of the small intestine are nonspecific and insensitive for celiac disease. Reversal of the fold patterns between the jejunum and ileum may also be seen. Computerized tomography techniques may be useful in diagnosing the complications of celiac sprue such as development of lymphoma, malignancy, hyposplenism, or cavitating mesenteric lymphadenopathy. CT enterography techniques are currently under investigation and may become an accepted diagnostic test in the future.

Serological Screening Tests

Serological tests are helpful in detecting celiac disease in individuals with nongastrointestinal symptoms, and high-risk groups who may or may not have signs of disease. The clinicians often use the serological results to triage those who need small bowel biopsy. The high-risk groups include first-degree relatives of confirmed cases of celiac disease, those with type 1 diabetes mellitus, Down's syndrome, Turner's syndrome and unexplained dental enamel deficits, and children with unexplained short stature. Serological tests are also used to monitor progress after diagnosis as well as in prevalence studies in unselected populations. The serological tests utilized in current clinical practice include the endomysial antibody, tissue transglutaminase antibody, and the anti-gliadin antibodies (IgA and IgG).

An enzyme-linked immunosorbent assay (ELISA) for both the IgA and IgG subclass of antibodies to gliadin has been used for the diagnosis of celiac disease. Their role in diagnosis is limited because of moderate sensitivity and specificity. The antigliadin antibodies are found in intestinal secretions as well as in serum of patients with untreated celiac disease. However, these antibodies are also found in a variety of autoimmune disorders including rheumatoid arthritis, Sjögren's syndrome, sarcoidosis, inflammatory bowel disease, and cows' milk protein intolerance. IgA antigliadin antibodies have sensitivity of 75–90% and specificity of 82–95%. The IgG antigliadin antibodies range in sensitivity from 69% to 85% and have specificity of 73–90%; they are useful in the diagnosis of celiac patients with IgA deficiency. Other than this use gliadin antibodies have fallen from favor as a screening test for celiac disease (National Institute of Health consensus panel).

The IgA antiendomysial antibody (EMA) assay is directed against the connective tissue protein found in the collagenous matrix of human and monkey tissue. This antibody is found in association with celiac sprue. The test is based on immunofluorescence techniques using monkey esophagus or human umbilical cord as a substrate. Although quite sensitive (85–98%) and specific (97–100%), the test has several limitations including false-negative results in 23% of patients with celiac disease who have selective IgA deficiency. Other factors that have an impact on the sensitivity and specificity of this test include laboratory variations and disease severity. In a study of 101 patients with untreated celiac disease the sensitivity of the endomysial antibody in those with total villous atrophy was excellent (100%), but decreased remarkably (31%) in patients with partial villous atrophy. The endomysial antibody performed by the indirect immuno-flourescent assay (IFA) technique is technically challenging and is being replaced by the tissue transglutaminase antibody test.

Tissue transglutaminase (tTG) is a cytosolic protein released by damaged epithelial cells. This is the autoantigen recognized by the endomysial antibody indirect immunofluorescence assay in patients with celiac disease. The advantages of this test are that it is performed using ELISA techniques, which makes it easier to perform, is widely available, and less costly. It eliminates the use of monkey esophagus as well as the subjective interpretation of immunofluorescence analysis of the endomysial antibody test. Though the tTG test is comparable to EMA in sensitivity, there is loss of specificity in patients with autoimmune disorders, hence it is important to confirm the diagnosis with small intestine biopsy.

In some patients biopsies are taken during an endoscopy that has been performed for another reason. In these patients serological tests can be useful to help confirm the diagnosis if there is some uncertainty with an equivocal biopsy, while negative serology in this circumstance may indicate another cause. Celiac disease may occur in the absence of antibodies however.

Treatment

Once the presumptive diagnosis of celiac disease is made then treatment may be commenced. It is important that the patient does not start to restrict their diet until each of the steps including the biopsy have been completed. Once confirmed, the responsibility for directing the management of the patient lies with the physician.

The treatment starts with an explanation of the condition and its cause. It is important that the patient understands that this is a chronic inflammatory condition of the gut and not a simple food allergy, that it is permanent eventhough the intestine will heal, and that the central and indeed only treatment at present is a gluten-free diet for life. The clinician should expect shock and even a fully expressed grief reaction on the part of the patient. Disbelief that something as basic to the Western diet as wheat is responsible is common. Some patients are overwhelmed both by the realization of having a chronic illness and others by relief that an explanation for their suffering has been found. The tone that the physician sets is crucial to the patient's success. A positive and upbeat though serious demeanor on the part of the doctor is appropriate, as most patients will do very well so long as they stick to the diet. Probably the most important thing that the doctor can do beyond diagnosis is to refer the patient for professional dietary advice that is up to date on how to achieve a gluten-free life style.

Patients should be encouraged to join both local and national support groups as an essential adjunct to management. The feeling of isolation so common in newly diagnosed patients in the past can be quickly dispelled by participation in an active support group.

It is important to identify and to correct deficiencies with nutritional supplementation. Deficiencies of the fat-soluble vitamins (D, E, A, and K), iron, folate, B_{12}, and even zinc or selenium are common. Baseline bone mineral density should be measured, as osteoporosis and osteomalacia are common.

Occasionally, intensive nutritional support and fluid replacement may be needed in very ill patients. Coexisting malignancy/autoimmune disease should be considered especially in elderly or ill patients.

Follow-up of patients to ensure response to gluten-free diet and compliance is crucial to ensure long-term compliance as well as detecting potential complications of the disease. Screening of at-risk family members should be considered.

The Gluten-Free Diet

The term 'gluten' as it is used in the context of celiac disease refers to the storage proteins of wheat (gliadins and glutenin) and of barley (prolamines), and rye (hordeins), and oats (avedins). Gluten is defined in the setting of celiac disease as any protein-containing derivative of the offending grains or their derivatives. Grains that should be avoided are as follows:

1. wheat;
2. barley;
3. rye;
4. spelt;
5. kamut; and
6. triticale.

To achieve healing and maintain health, a well-balanced, interesting dietary life style that avoids gluten should be adopted. However, it is not enough to simply avoid gluten; patients need to be enabled to explore dietary alternatives and strategies that minimize impact on their life style.

The role of oat toxicity in celiac disease is still controversial. Several recent, well-constructed studies have demonstrated no ill effects when a moderate amount of oat products have been included in the diet of either newly diagnosed or already treated celiac patients. These recent studies have clearly demonstrated that oats are nontoxic for most patients with celiac disease, however, the concern is that contamination of oat products by gluten is taking place during the growing, milling, or processing of oat products. When completely gluten-free oats become available then it will probably be safe to recommend them to most celiac patients. A small number of patients may still react to oats, some markedly so. Where a patient intends to include oats in their diet they need to have a careful and informed medical follow-up.

While foods such as bread, cookies, biscuits, and pasta are obvious sources of gluten, many other seemingly 'safe' foods contain hidden gluten. It is important to enquire if a food has any ingredients that are in any way derived from, or processed with, wheat, barley, or rye. This part of the diet is not self evident, and the patient needs both expert counseling from a dietitian as well as being versed with and up to date on the gluten-free diet with ongoing support from a local or national support group. Nonfood items, such as medications and communion wafers, may also be unappreciated sources of gluten, as are fat substitutes and food contaminants. Ingredients that should be viewed with suspicion include:

1. malt or malt flavoring;
2. hydrolyzed vegetable protein (HVP);
3. modified food starch (and starch in foreign foods);
4. natural flavorings;
5. vegetable gum; and
6. fat substitutes.

It is important that the most up to date instruction manuals are used. Older manuals may contain out of date or even misleading information.

Some ostensibly gluten-free foods may become contaminated with gluten during processing, packaging, transport, handling in the store, or even preparation in the patient's own kitchen.

Home testing kits for gluten are now available but generally are not helpful or practical for most patients. Large listings of the commercially available processed foods that are gluten free are available but must be updated at least yearly and must be tailored to geographic location. Patients should not rely on the self test of reaction to gluten as a means of detecting gluten in foods as symptoms may be delayed.

Bone Metabolism

Osteomalacia is a well-recognized, although uncommon, complication of celiac disease, with bone pain and pseudofractures as features. It is associated with elevated alkaline phosphotase and often normal levels of calcium and phosphate. It usually responds well to a gluten-free diet and calcium and vitamin D supplementation.

Osteoporosis, which is common in adults with celiac disease, affects both men and women, and the exact mechanisms are not clear. The prevalence of osteoporosis is even higher in refractory sprue compared to gluten-free-diet-responsive patients. Diagnosis depends on bone mineral density testing with a T-score less than 2.5 SD below mean peak value in young adults. The primary treatment for the osteoporosis in a celiac is the strict gluten-free diet with adequate calcium (1500 mg day^{-1} and vitamin D). Other measures directed at preserving or building bone density may be necessary if the boss mineral loss has been substantial or does not recover with a gluten-free diet.

Complications

Nonresponsive Celiac Disease

Whilst most patients with celiac disease respond appropriately to a gluten-free diet, usually with responses to symptoms occurring within days to weeks of institution of the diet, a small proportion of patients (approximately 5%) do not have the expected complete response to a gluten-free diet or they have a relapse of symptoms while apparently on a gluten-free diet. This scenario termed 'nonresponsive celiac disease' is multifactorial in nature.

The single most common cause of continued or relapsing symptoms in patients with celiac disease is that of inadvertent gluten ingestion. There are many ways in which gluten can get into the diet, and in one series the most common source was commercial cereal in which minor ingredients were derived from the offending grains. However, other sources such as communion wafers and environmental contamination with flour, particularly of baked goods, are also possible.

In patients whose serologic tests have returned to normal and where a careful dietary review, including a detailed food record, does not reveal any potential source of gluten contamination, the occurrence of a second associated disease or a complication of celiac disease must be considered. A common associated disorder would be microscopic colitis, either lymphocytic or collagenous. Typically, these patients will have watery diarrhea whereas symptoms related to malabsorption such as weight loss, bloating, and steatorrhea will have resolved. The patient will continue to have watery diarrhea or may, indeed, develop watery diarrhea while on a gluten-free diet. The taking of biopsies from the colon can readily identify this condition. Whilst in some patients adhering to a strict gluten-free diet may improve the colitis, in many circumstances, it does not or it has not sufficed. The use of empiric therapy such as Pepto-Bismol®, loperamide, or, in some circumstances, delayed release budesonide may be valuable. Another cause of continued diarrhea is disaccharidase deficiency such as lactose intolerance. In most patients with celiac disease, the lactose intolerance that occurs is secondary to the injury and resolves its treatment. In a few unfortunate patients there may be a genetic predisposition to lactose intolerance. Avoidance of lactose or the use of lactase enzyme supplementation may suffice for correction of symptoms. In patients who have continued steatorrhea but in whom small bowel biopsies are found to have become normal, pancreatic exocrine insufficiency or bacterial overgrowth syndrome might be considered.

Where the small intestine has failed to recover histologically, particularly in patients who have continued symptoms and signs of malabsorption, the diagnosis of refractory sprue is made. This condition is often associated with severe illness, significant bone disease, and hypoalbuminemia. These patients are particularly prone to ulceration in the proximal small intestine, so-called ulcerative jejunitis. Some have clonal expansion of T cells within their intestine. These patients are probably entering a pre-lymphoma state and the mortality in these circumstances is high with a relatively poor response to immunosuppression; many will progress to lymphoma within 5 years. Other patients appear to have refractory sprue but without clonality, and they tend to respond much better to immunosuppression. This probably represents a now self-perpetuating autoimmune process within the intestine. The rare case of collagenous sprue, which has features similar to celiac disease but is characterized by a thick layer of collagen in the intestine subepithelial layer in the colon, typically responds poorly to all therapies and often require long-term nutritional support.

The approach to diagnosing and treating nonresponsive celiac disease is outlined in **Figure 3**.

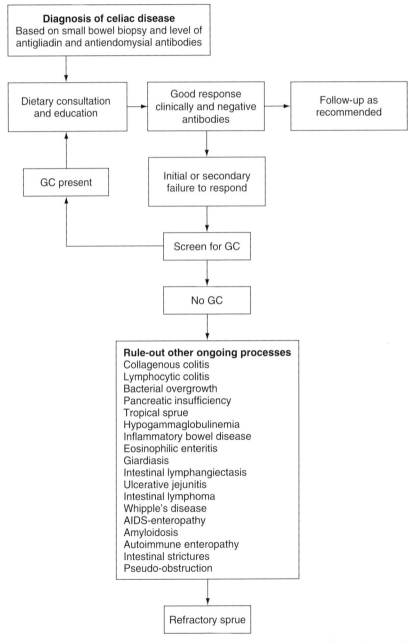

Figure 3 Flow chart for diagnosing and treating celiac patients. The proper procedure for diagnosing a patient who potentially has celiac disease, education and treatment of that patient, followed by the steps that need to be taken in the event that the patient is not responsive to a gluten-free diet are illustrated in a flow chart. GC, gluten challenge.

Malignant Complications of Celiac Disease

The complications of celiac disease can be divided into malignant and nonmalignant complications. In addition, the malignant complications of celiac disease are most commonly that of non-Hodgkin's lymphoma of a T cell variety. This particular tumor occurs in patients who have not been compliant with the diet or within 3 years of diagnosis. The risk of lymphoma or other malignancies appears to drop once a gluten-free diet has been instituted. While the relative risk of malignancy in celiac disease is greatly increased for specific diseases, the actual absolute risk is relatively small. The presentation of lymphomas in the small intestine can be acute with a surgical emergency such as obstruction, perforation, and bleeding, or gradual with insidious return or progress of severe malabsorptive symptoms, often associated with hypoalbuminemia and severe weight loss and malnutrition. The treatment for lymphoma is often unsuccessful. Those patients presenting acutely and managed surgically appear to do better than those who have a slow insidious onset. Occasional cases of response to stem cell transplantation have been reported.

The second most common malignancy occurring in celiac disease is that of adenocarcinoma of the small intestine. This adenocarcinoma seems to occur in the setting of the chronic inflammation of celiac disease. It is associated with defects and mismatch repair and whilst this is an unusual tumor, the survival with aggressive surgical therapy may be better than that for small bowel adenocarcinomas that occur sporadically. Usually, these patients present with iron deficiency anemia, gastrointestinal bleeding, obstruction, or pain. Other malignancies such as esophageal cancer or melanoma are increased in frequency in celiac disease, though again the absolute risk is low. Some recent evidence suggests that risk of breast cancer may be reduced in patients with celiac disease, though this is yet to be confirmed.

Nonmalignant Complications of Celiac Disease

Nonmalignant complications of celiac disease include ulcers and structuring within the intestine that occasionally may present with small bowel obstruction and/or bleeding, and recurrent acute pancreatitis as the result of inflammation, probably of the sphincter of Oddi. Nongastrointestinal complications are usually the consequence of malnutrition or specific deficiencies. However, others such as neurological problems including ataxia, peripheral neuropathy, or dementia are of uncertain mechanism and perhaps autoimmune in nature. Other consequences of celiac disease have been discussed in the section on atypical or nongastrointestinal presentations (**Table 1**). Many, but not all, of these nonmalignant complications of celiac disease will respond to a gluten-free diet.

See also: **Cereal Grains**. **Cytokines**. **Handicap**: Down's Syndrome. **Osteoporosis**. **Vitamin D**: Rickets and Osteomalacia.

Further Reading

Abdo A, Meddings J, and Swain M (2004) Liver abnormalities in celiac disease. *Clinical Gastroenterology and Hepatology* **2**: 107–112.

Abdulkarim AS, Burgart LJ, See J, and Murray JA (2002) Etiology of nonresponsive celiac disease: results of a systematic approach. *American Journal of Gastroenterology* **97**: 2016–2021.

Ackerman Z, Eliakim R, Stalnikowicz R, and Rachmilewitz D (1996) Role of small bowel biopsy in the endoscopic evaluation of adults with iron deficiency anemia. *American Journal of Gastroenterology* **91**: 2099–2102.

Farrell RJ and Kelly CP (2002) Celiac sprue. *New England Journal of Medicine* **346**: 180–188.

Farrell RJ and Kelly CP (2001) Diagnosis of celiac sprue. *American Journal of Gastroenterology* **96**: 3237–3246.

Holmes GK (2002) Screening for coeliac disease in type 1 diabetes. *Archives of Disease in Childhood* **87**: 495–498.

Marsh MN (1992) Gluten, major histocompatibility complex, and the small intestine. A molecular and immunobiologic approach to the spectrum of gluten sensitivity ('celiac sprue'). *Gastroenterology* **102**: 330–354.

Murray JA, Watson T, Clearman B, and Mitros F (2004) Effect of a gluten-free diet on gastrointestinal symptoms in celiac disease. *American Journal of Clinical Nutrition* **79**: 669–673.

Pengiran-Tengah DS, Wills AJ, and Holmes GK (2002) Neurological complications of coeliac disease. *Postgraduate Medical Journal* **78**: 393–398.

Schuppan D (2000) Current concepts of celiac disease pathogenesis. *Gastroenterology* **119**: 234–242.

Sollid LM (2000) Molecular basis of celiac disease. *Annual Review of Immunology* **18**: 53–81.

Sulkanen S, Halttunen T, Laurila K et al. (1998) Tissue transglutaminase autoantibody enzyme-linked immunosorbent assay in detecting celiac disease. *Gastroenterology* **115**: 1322–1328.

Anonymous (1990) Working Group of European Society of Paediatric Gastroenterology and Nutrition: Revised criteria for diagnosis of coeliac disease. *Archives of Disease in Childhood* **65**: 909–911.

COFACTORS

Contents

Inorganic

E D Harris, Texas A&M University, College Station, TX, USA

© 2005 Elsevier Ltd. All rights reserved.

Introduction

In the next article, a cofactor is defined as any non-enzyme component that promotes the catalytic prowess of an enzyme. The definition emphasizes function rather than structure. Since nearly a third of all enzymes require metal ions for catalytic function, it is apparent that inorganic components make up a substantial number of cofactors. Most of the trace metals have a common denominator in their intimate involvement with enzymes. Many are active site components that bind substrates, accept electrons, stabilize tertiary and quaternary structures, or even regulate the pace of metabolic pathways. In this article, the individual metal ion cofactors are discussed.

History

The nutritional history of the mineral elements, unlike the vitamins, had little early focus on humans. Rather, it was domestic livestock eating forage from mineral-poor soils that exhibited deficiency symptoms (thought at first to be due to toxicity). Typical signs were the crimping of wool in sheep, aortic rupture in pigs and cattle, and loss of myelin in brains of newborn lambs. Symptoms were lessened sharply by supplementing the feed with salts of metal ions such as $CuSO_4$, $Fe(NH_4)_2(SO_4)_2$, and $ZnCl_2$. Reversing symptoms and reestablishing optimal growth to livestock provided the first evidence for essential metals. In time, biochemical studies led to the isolation of enzymes that required metal ions for function, and soon after that specific enzymes could be linked to the deficiency symptoms. Metal ion interactions were viewed as detrimental as well as valuable to the system. An early study by Hart *et al.* showed that copper potentiated the effects of iron in alleviating an anemia condition in laboratory rats fed milk-based diets. That observation was repeated in chicks and pigs and soon attracted the attention of clinicians who adopted a similar bimetal protocol in the treatment of anemic humans. Coupled with the advent of semipurified diets in that same era, the science of nutrition stood on the threshold of major discoveries as to the roles of the essential mineral elements.

General Properties

Mineral cofactors comprise a large group of inorganic substances the bulk of which are the metal ions. The domain of metal ions include macro metals, such as Na^+, K^+, Ca^{2+} and Mg^{2+}, trace metal ions, including Fe^{2+}, Zn^{2+}, Cu^{2+} and Mn^{2+}, and metalloids, such as Se, Si and B (**Table 1**). In seeking a reason for their necessity, one must realize that metal ions are suited to the task of executing dangerous chemical reactions on enzyme surfaces, reactions that would otherwise harm the more sensitive organic side chains of amino acids in an enzyme. For example, redox metals such as iron, manganese, and copper can accept electrons into their structure, hold them temporarily, and then donate them to oxygen, forming water as a way to dispose of the electrons safely. In essence, one should consider a metal cofactor as extending the

Table 1 Inorganic cofactors

Metal	Common biological form or valence
Iron	Fe^{2+}, Fe^{3+}
Zinc	Zn^{2+}
Copper	Cu^+, Cu^{2+}
Manganese	Mn^{2+}, Mn^{4+}
Cobalt	Co^+, Co^{2+}, Co^{3+}
Vanadium	VO^{2+}
Molybdenum	MoO_2^{2+}, MoO_4^{2-}
Nickel	Ni^{2+}
Selenium	Selenocysteine, selenomethionine
Silicon	$Si(OH)_4$, SiO_2
Potassium	K^+
Sodium	Na^+
Calcium	Ca^{2+}
Magnesium	Mg^{2+}
Boron	$B(OH)_3$

repertoire of catalytic functions available to and performed by enzymes.

Metal-Activated Enzymes versus Metalloenzymes

Enzymes that depend on metal ions as cofactors fall into two categories: metal-activated enzymes and metalloenzymes. As the name implies, metal-activated enzymes are prompted to greater catalytic activity by the presence of a mono- or divalent metal ion exterior to the protein (in the assay medium). The metal may activate the substrate (e.g., Mg^{2+} with ATP), engage the enzyme directly, or enter into equilibrium with the enzyme exploiting its ionic charge to render a more favorable substrate binding or catalytic environment. Therefore, metal-activated enzymes require the metal to be present in excess, perhaps 2–10 times more than the enzyme concentration. Because the metal cannot be bound in a more permanent way, metal-activated enzymes typically lose activity during purification. An example is pyruvate kinase, which has a specific requirement for K^+ and is inactivated by dialysis (diffusion through a semiporous membrane). Other examples of metal-activated enzymes are shown in **Table 2**.

Metalloenzymes, in contrast, have a metal cofactor bound firmly to a specific region on the protein surface. Some may even require more than one metal ion and in rare instances could be two different metals as, for example, in Cu_2,Zn_2 superoxide dismutase. With few exceptions, trace metals fit into the picture as cofactors for metalloenzymes. Fe, Zn, Cu, and Mn, referred to as first transition series metals, are the most common. Their counterparts,

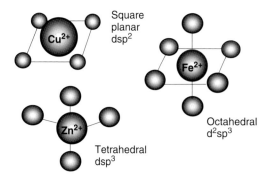

Figure 1   Some common geometries of metal complexes.

Mg, K, Ca, and Na, are not considered 'trace' and only in rare instances are these so-called macroelements strongly bound to the surface of enzymes. Tight binding precludes loss of the metal ion by dialysis or loss to weakly dissociating agents. Metalloenzymes, however, can lose their metal cofactor and hence be rendered inactive when treated with metal chelators that have a stronger binding affinity than the enzyme and out compete the enzyme protein for the metal ion. As prosthetic groups, metals in metalloenzymes have a stoichiometric relationship (metal ion–enzyme protein ratio) represented by a whole integer. Metalloenzymes seldom are primed to greater activity by adding its conjugate metal ion to the enzyme. Spatial geometry is also a concern. Metals in the first transition series metals (Mn, Fe, Co, Ni, Cu, Zn) must adhere to strict geometric configurations around the metal-binding site. Examples of the more common geometrical arrangements are shown in **Figure 1**. For metals in the first transition series one takes note of the $3d$ and $4s$ orbitals in assigning valence states and likely geometric shapes. Apart from those with Zn, enzymes with first transition series metals tend to be highly colorful; for example, the beautiful red color of hemoglobin (iron) or the blue color of ceruloplasmin (whose name means heavenly blue) associated with copper. **Table 3** gives some examples of metalloenzymes and the specific metal each requires.

Individual Metal Cofactors

Iron

Most iron enzymes engage iron either as heme or as a special arrangement of iron with sulfur groups referred to as iron-sulfur centers (Fe_nS_n). Iron in heme bears a striking resemblance to the magnesium ion in chlorophyll (**Figure 2**). Heme, which is basically a porphyrin ring system with iron positioned in the center, is the most common form of iron in

Table 2   Metal-activated enzymes and metalloenzymes

Metal or metal cofactor	Enzyme	Function
Metal-activated enzymes		
K^+	Pyruvate kinase	Synthesize pyruvate
Mg^{2+}	Hexokinase	Phosphorylate glucose
	DNase	Cleave DNA
	RNase	Cleave RNA
	ATPase	Cleave ATP
Metalloenzymes		
Cu^{2+}, Zn^{2+}	Superoxide dismutase	Destroy superoxide anion
Fe	Catalase	Destroy H_2O_2
Zn	Alcohol dehydrogenase	Metabolize alcohol
	DNA polymerase	Synthesize DNA
Mn	Pyruvate carboxylase	Synthesize oxaloacetate
	Arginase	Synthesize urea
Ca	Alpha amylase	Cleave glycogen, starch

Table 3 Important iron enzymes

Enzyme	Source	Function	Form of iron
Cytochrome c oxidase	Mitochondria	Electron transport	Heme
Aconitase	Mitochondria	Krebs cycle	Fe_4S_4
Succinate dehydrogenase	Mitochondria	Krebs cycle	Fe_4S_4
Catalase	Peroxisomes	H_2O_2 destruction	Heme
Peroxidase	Peroxisomes	Peroxide destruction	Heme
Prolyl hydroxylase	Cytosol	Collagen synthesis	Fe^{2+}
Ribonucleotide reductase	Cytosol	DNA synthesis	Fe-O-Fe
Cytochrome P450	Microsomes	Sterol synthesis	Heme

biological proteins. In cytochrome *c*, a common heme protein in the mitochondria, the axial ligands to the iron are occupied by histidine and methionine from the protein. Heme enzymes include calalase and peroxidase. As components of iron-sulfur centers, iron enters into multiple cluster arrangements with cysteine residues on enzymes that offer a more direct contact with the protein. These centers differ in their complexity from the simple 2Fe-2S to the more elaborate 4Fe-4S (**Figure 3**). Iron in these centers binds substrates as well as transfer electrons and takes part in reactions involving dehydrations and rearrangements. Enzymes with iron-sulfur centers include xanthine oxidase, succinate dehydrogenase, aconitase, and nitrogenase. A third class, represented by ribonucleotide reductase, has a FeO_2 cluster with a dioxygen as a peroxide anion O_2^{2-} straddled between two iron centers (**Figure 4**). This arrangement allows the enzyme to remove a hydrogen atom

from a very stable C—H bond. No metal can replace iron in these complexes. Enzymes with a heme group generally are reddish-brown in color (depending on the oxidation state of the iron). The color led to early interest in these proteins and was the motivating factor behind naming heme proteins in the mitochondria 'cytochromes.' Although only a relatively few soluble enzymes have iron as a cofactor, iron is especially prominent in membrane-bound proteins that comprise electron transport pathways. Examples of the latter include the cytochromes in the mitochondria, endoplasmic reticulum, and photosystem I, II in chloroplasts. Perhaps the most unusual iron protein is ferritin, a huge multisubunit iron storage protein that has the capacity to bind more than 2500 iron atoms in its structure.

Reactivity The redox property of iron carries over to much of its chemistry as a cofactor. Iron is nearly always involved with the transfer of electrons and many times donates the electrons to a molecule of oxygen. Two important properties that fit that role are: (1) an iron atom that can readily undergo reversible valence changes from Fe^{2+} to Fe^{3+}, which allows facile exchange of electrons; and (2) the ferrous-ferric ion pair has a relatively low electrochemical potential (-0.1 V), which allows iron to be on the high (reducing) end of an electron transport chain. In cytochrome P450 a single oxygen atom is transferred to the substrate after O_2 binds to Fe(II). In the mechanism the Fe(II)–O_2 complex is converted into FeO, which features an Fe(V) species that attacks the substrate and incorporates the single oxygen atom into its structure. Although higher valence states such as Fe(IV) and Fe(VI) are formed by removing additional 3*d* electrons, only rarely are these higher valences of iron seen in biological

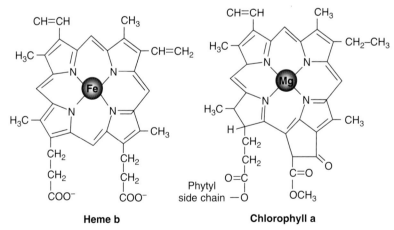

Figure 2 Heme iron in hemoglobin. Heme is a porphyrin ring with iron in the center. Four heme b groups are present in hemoglobin, the iron protein in erythrocytes. A similar structural arrangement is seen with magnesium in chlorophyll a from plants.

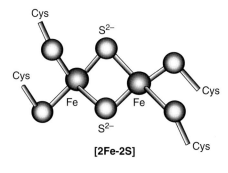

[2Fe-2S]

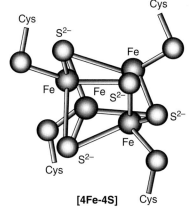

[4Fe-4S]

Figure 3 Iron-sulfur clusters. Both the Fe_2S_2 and Fe_4S_4 clusters are bound to the protein via cysteine residues. The iron in these complexes either engages a substrate or holds and passes electrons.

systems. As noted above, catalase and peroxidase, two heme enzymes, use iron to engage dangerous oxidants. Both enzymes are located in the cytosol and in peroxisomes where harmful oxidation reactions occur during the course of normal metabolic events. Perhaps the most familiar iron-containing

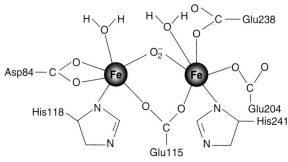

Figure 4 Fe-O-Fe center in ribonucleotide reductase. The two iron atoms are in close juxtaposition to bind dioxygen as the peroxide-anion O_2^{2-}. Side chains of aspartic and glutamic acid residues as well as two histidine residues assist in linking the center to the protein. The center assists in the formation of a free radical that forms on a neighboring tyrosine residue. (After Fraústo da Silva JJR and Williams RJP (1991) *The Biological Chemistry of the Elements. The Inorganic Chemistry of Life.* Oxford: Oxford University Press.)

enzyme is cytochrome *c* oxidase, the terminal electron acceptor in the mitochondrial electron transport chain and the enzyme capable of splitting a molecule of oxygen to form water.

$$4 \text{ cytochrome } c \text{ (Fe}^{2+}) + O_2 + 4H^+$$
$$\rightarrow 4 \text{ cytochrome c (Fe}^{3+}) + 2H_2O$$

Zinc

Zinc is perhaps the most ubiquitous and versatile of all metal cofactors. More than 300 enzymes have a zinc cofactor. **Table 4** lists some of the important zinc enzymes. Zinc-binding proteins that engage DNA, the so-called zinc finger proteins, attest to the versatility of zinc in biological systems. Approximately 3% of the genome of mammals codes for zinc finger protein. As a cofactor, zinc can perform both structural and catalytic functions. In carbonic anhydrase, for example, zinc enters into a coordinate bond with the CO_2 substrate (**Figure 5**). In carboxypeptidase, zinc takes an active part in the cleavage of the peptide bond (**Figure 6**). Multisubunit enzymes such as aspartate transcarbamylase use zinc to coordinate the positions of the catalytic and regulatory subunits, a structural role. Cu_2,Zn_2 superoxide dismutase requires zinc to position the copper atom in the channel accessed by the substrate $HO_2^{\cdot}$, another structural role. In zinc finger proteins, Zn^{2+} contributes to the stability of the loop structure that contacts the major and minor grooves of DNA. These examples illustrate why zinc is an important companion to enzymes and proteins.

Reactivity Zinc is considered a bland metal because it behaves as a divalent cation with no special geometric preference. It is perhaps this blandness that allows zinc to adapt to so many different enzyme environments. Zinc exists in one

Table 4 Important zinc enzymes

Enzyme	Source	Function	Zn/ protein
Alcohol dehydrogenase	Liver	Alcohol metabolism	4
Alkaline phosphatase	Placenta	Unknown	4
Carbonic anhydrase	Erythrocyte	CO_2 hydration	1
Carboxypeptidase	Pancreas	Protein catabolism	1
Glutamate dehydrogenase	Liver	Glutamate synthesis	2–6
Leucine aminopeptidase	Intestine	Peptide catabolism	4–6

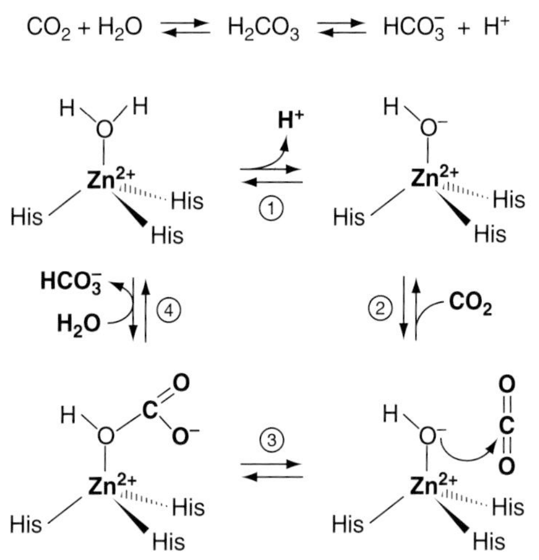

$$CO_2 + H_2O \rightleftharpoons H_2CO_3 \rightleftharpoons HCO_3^- + H^+$$

Figure 5 Zinc in carbonic anhydrase. Zinc in the enzyme 'activates' a water molecule (1) creating a better nucleophile to attack the CO_2 (2). Once formed (3) the hydrated CO_2 as HCO_3^- is displaced from the enzyme via a second water molecule (4) regenerating the active enzyme.

valence state, Zn^{2+}, and hence has no redox properties. The Zn^{2+} ion is configured as a $3d^{10}$, which denotes a filled $3d$ orbital. For that reason, zinc complexes lack color and zinc itself behaves mostly as a cation. Zn^{2+} is a good electron acceptor (Lewis acid) that can enter into a coordinate bonding arrangement that polarizes groups to which it binds. This property allows zinc to increase the susceptibility of a chemical bond to attack. For example, Zn^{2+} polarizes water:

$$Zn^{2+} + H_2O \rightleftharpoons Zn^{2+}(OH^-) + H^+$$

This makes the water behave more like a hydroxide ion and be more effective in attacking the CO_2 to form HCO_3^- in the reaction catalyzed by carbonic anhydrase. Another example is the use of zinc to polarize the ester or amide bonds thus promoting nucleophilic attack of water on the bond as in reactions catalyzed by carboxypeptidase and aminopeptidase.

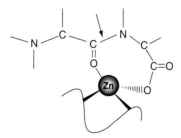

Figure 6 Zinc in carboxypeptidase. In carboxypeptidase, the zinc atom forms a binary complex with groups on the C-terminal end of the protein. Arrow shows bond that will be cleaved with water. Only the C-terminus residue is released from the protein.

Copper

Copper, like iron, is a redox metal. Like iron, copper exists in multiple valence states; Cu^+ and Cu^{2+}(cuprous and cupric) are the most common. Copper enzymes, while not nearly as numerous as zinc, fill important biological functions, mostly within the cytosol. Many fit the category of oxidoreductases, or more specifically 'oxidases,' meaning they catalyze reactions in which electrons from the substrate are transferred to O_2. Copper enzymes can be simple or complex, depending on the number of Cu atoms in the enzyme. Simple enzymes generally contain one Cu per subunit. The more complex enzymes include the multicopper oxidases, which may have as few as four, e.g., laccase, or as many as eight copper atoms per enzyme, e.g., dopamine-β-monooxygenase. Copper in these enzymes exists in three different chemical environments referred to as type 1, type2, and type 3 copper sites. Ceruloplasmin, for example, contains 6–7 Cu atoms in three distinct sites. The type 1 copper site gives a blue color to ceruloplasmin and other blue copper proteins. The copper-binding sites in a multicopper oxidase form a triad consisting of one type two and two type 3 coppers arranged as an isosceles triangle. Oxygen binds to the two type 3 coppers at the base of the triangle. Examples of copper enzymes include cytochrome c oxidase, lysyl oxidase, and ascorbate oxidase (**Table 5**).

Reactivity Because it is prone to accept electrons, copper is a powerful oxidant in biological systems. The copper sites in ceruloplasmin have the capacity to oxidize Fe^{2+} to Fe^{3+}, which prepares ferric ions to bind to transferrin and deliver iron to the organs and tissues. This reaction links iron with copper metabolism and could explain how an absence of copper in the diet impairs the transport of iron and causes anemia in humans. In Cu_2, Zn_2 superoxide dismutase, the Cu^{2+} at the active site removes the single nonbonding electron from one superoxide anion (O_2^-) and transfers it to another:

$$O_2^- + O_2^- + 2H^+ \rightarrow H_2O_2 + O_2$$

Seldom is copper destined to perform only a structural role and many enzymes that possess copper as a cofactor use the metal at the active site. More recent studies have linked copper ions with the formation of blood vessels or angiogenesis. One of the more exciting discoveries yet to be fully understood is that depriving an animal or human of copper delays or even inhibits the growth of cancerous tumors. From a nutritional perspective, this could

Table 5 Important copper enzymes

Enzyme	Source	Function	Cu/protein
Ascorbate oxidase	Squash	Ascorbate catabolism	8
Ceruloplasmin	Plasma	Iron oxidation	6–7
Cytochrome c oxidase	Mitochondria	Electron transport	2
Dopamine-β-monooxygenase	Adrenal	Noradrenaline synthesis	8
Lysyl oxidase	Aorta	Collagen, elastin synthesis	1
Superoxide dismutase	Erythrocyte	Superoxide radical destruction	2

mean that copper is essential for the development of the microvascular system.

Manganese

Whereas zinc may be the most common transition metal in enzymes, manganese is perhaps the least common. Part of the reason is that complexes of manganese with proteins tend to be weakly stable and dissociate readily. Notable manganese metalloenzymes include pyruvate carboxylase and manganese superoxide dismutase in the mitochondria and arginase in the urea cycle. Manganese can also function as a metal-activating cofactor for many enzymes that require magnesium.

Reactivity Although manganese is not considered a redox metal based on reactivity, it nonetheless can exist in six oxidation states (Mn^{2+} to Mn^{7+}), three of which (Mn^{5+} to Mn^{7+}) are not seen in biological systems. The most common form of manganese is Mn^{2+}. The highest number of multiple valences of manganese occurs in the water splitting enzyme that is found in chloroplasts of plants as part of photosystem II.

Cobalt

The role of cobalt as a cofactor is limited to its presence in vitamin B_{12}. Cobalt can exist in three valence states, Co^{+}, Co^{2+}, and Co^{3+} with Co^{2+} being the most common in 5' deoxyadenosylcobalamin, the familiar form of vitamin B_{12} coenzyme. Cobalt is bound by a planar ring system analogous to heme but with very special features (see 00059). Cobalt and nickel are ions that may have figured more prominently in primitive systems when the atmosphere contained H_2 and CH_4 as common environmental gases. The argument has been made that as biological systems gradually adapted to O_2 the necessity for these two metals became less.

Reactivity Cobalt in the structure of vitamin B_{12} resembles iron in heme by being bound in a square planar arrangement to a ring (corrin). Unlike heme, however, cobalt has two axial ligands that are free from the protein, which allows nonprotein groups to

access the central metal from above and below the plane. In the octahedral complex, one axial position (the fifth coordinate) is normally occupied by a benzimidazole and the other by a methyl group (as in methyl cobalamin). The arrangement is unique and allows cobalt to form carbon–metal bonds with the potential for two different reactivities. The methyl group, for example, may be removed as a carbonium ion retaining both electrons on the cobalt, which then reverts to a less stable Co(I). This is typical of the reaction in which vitamin B_{12} acts as a methyl donor. In positional rearrangements, cobalt retains only one electron and forms a stable Co(II) or d^7 ion with the release of a free radical. Free radicals are highly reactive and overcome energy barriers that would stymie other reactants. Thus, cobalt's chemical properties transfer groups as carbonium ions or highly reactive carbon-centered radicals. Both products are possible and hence explains the necessity for cobalt as a cofactor for a reaction that proceeds via a free radical mechanism. An example of the latter is the intramolecular rearrangement of methylmalonyl-CoA to succinyl-CoA as catalyzed by methylmalonyl-CoA mutase.

Vanadium

Although a defined biochemical function for vanadium in higher animals and humans is yet to be described, recent reports of vanadium in bacteria and algae have provided clues as to the functional necessity of this metal in enzyme catalysis. About 10 years ago, vanadium was found to be essential for the activity of bromoperoxidase, an enzyme found in brown and red algae. Shortly thereafter, a vanadium-dependent iodoperoxidase was characterized. Vanadium was also found in high concentrations in mushrooms and was shown to accumulate in large quantities in ascidians, specifically the blood cells (vanocytes) of these organisms. Speculation as to the function of vanadium in microorganisms ranges from antimicrobial action to electron transfer and the trapping of oxygen. In higher animals, however, vanadium has been shown to have insulin-mimetic properties and to stimulate cell proliferation and differentiation. It is also believed to regulate phosphorylation and dephosphorylation reactions through control of ATPases, phosphatases, and adenylcyclase, which have widespread effects on cell functions. These are the most plausible theories to date. However, it should be emphasized that vanadium has not been shown to be a specific activator (or inhibitor) of any enzyme in humans.

Reactivity Vanadium is like molybdenum (see below) in being able to form both oxyanions and oxycations, VO_4^{2-} (MoO_4^{2-}), VO_2^+ (MoO^{2+}, MoO_2^+, and MoO_2^{2+}), as well as sulfur centers, e.g., VS_4^{3-} (MoS_4^{2-}). Vanadate differs from molybdate in being a rather strong oxidizing agent ($E \sim +0.5$ V at pH 7), which may relate to its electron transfer function in lower life forms but has questionable significance in humans.

Calcium

Calcium is a cofactor for a limited number of important enzymes apart from the more familiar actin–myosin complex in muscle; alpha amylase and thermolysin are two of the most familiar. As a free ion or working through calmodulin, calcium is better understood as an activator of enzymes in hormone-dependent cell signaling pathways. Enzymes that have been referred to as Ca-ATPases and H^+/Ca-ATPases should not be mistaken for calcium-dependent enzymes. This is a misnomer in that the Ca^{2+} is the object of the enzyme's action rather than the cofactor for activity. The ATPases comprise a large group of membrane-bound enzymes that either pump Ca^{2+} from the cytosol into the endoplasmic reticulum or expel calcium from the cell through membrane channels.

Reactivity As a group IIa metal, calcium is limited to a 2+ valence state and serves primarily as a divalent cation in its interactions with enzymes. The role of Ca^{2+} is limited mainly to structure stability.

Molybdenum

Molybdenum is widely distributed in plants and animals. The metal exists in three valence states: Mo^{4+}, Mo^{5+}, and Mo^{6+}. A limited number of redox reactions exploit the multivalence states. Molybdenum-dependent enzymes are found in pathways that metabolize purines, pyrimidines, pterins, aldehydes, and sulfites. A cofactor structure for molybdenum has been proposed (**Figure 7**) and is referred to as molybdopterrin. Enzymes that use the cofactor include xanthine oxidase, sulfite oxidase,

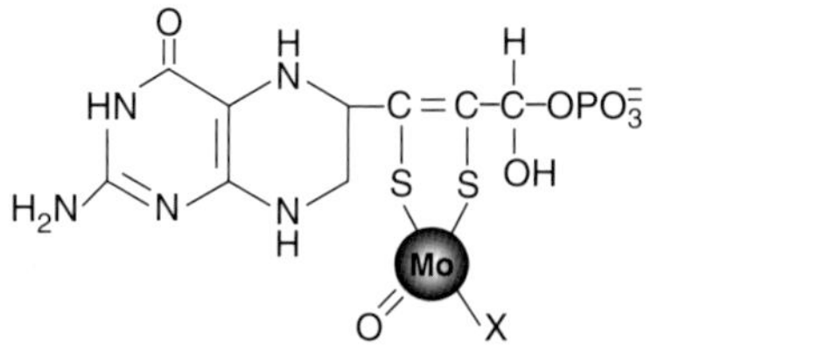

Figure 7 Proposed structure for the molybdenum cofactor in nitrogenase. This center consists of a special pterin cofactor, a relative of tetrahydrofolate. The molybdenum engages two sulfur atoms as a dithiolate complex.

and aldehyde oxidase. In microorganisms, molybdenum is a key metal for the fixation of nitrogen. Xanthine oxidase is the enzyme with importance relevance to a mammalian system.

Reactivity A major nutritional concern of molybdenum is its ability to antagonize copper. Indiscriminant spraying of soils with molybdenum has been shown to affect the growth and productivity of ruminants. The effect relates to the formation of thiomolybdates in the rumen. The thiomolybdates interact and bind copper preventing its absorption from the rumen. Thiomolybdates have a very high affinity for copper almost to the exclusion of other metal ions. Lately, thiomolybdates have been used to control copper toxicity in Wilson's disease, a genetic disease of copper poisoning in humans.

Nickel

As a cofactor, nickel occurs infrequently. About the only known occurrence of nickel is in microbial and plant enzymes such as urease from jack bean, soy bean, rice, and tomatoes. There are roughly two gram-atoms of nickel per mole of the 96 000 Da subunits of the enzyme. Other metalloenzymes containing nickel include Factor F430 found in the membrane of methanogenic bacteria, carbon monoxide dehydrogenase, and hydrogenases I and II. Nickel has drawn the attention of nutritionists because of the observation that nickel concentrations in the serum of women rise sharply immediately after parturition.

Reactivity Some consider nickel the 'metal that was.' As biosystems evolved and moved from an atmosphere of no oxygen to one rich in oxygen, where methane and H_2 have tended to be minimized as energy substrates, metals that formed a major cofactor in the anaerobic environment and were used by the more primitive organisms such as archaebacteria have been replaced in favor of a metal or cofactor more suitable to the present day environment. Thus, nickel, like cobalt, may have had its greatest era in enzymes that catabolized CH_4 or H_2.

Other

The sodium ion is generally not considered a specific cofactor because one has yet to demonstrate an enzyme whose catalysis depends strictly on sodium ions. Sodium-activated enzymes often respond to surrogate metal cofactors such as Li^+ or even divalent cations. The magnesium ion is required by a large number of enzymes referred to as kinases, enzymes that transfer the terminal phosphate group of ATP to a substrate. Kinase enzymes figure prominently in many biochemical pathways such as glycolysis (hexokinase, fructose-6-phosphate kinase, pyruvate kinase), hormone responses mediated by cyclic AMP, cell signaling, and regulation of cell division. The potassium ion is a specific cofactor for pyruvate kinase in the glycolysis pathway. Both potassium and magnesium form no permanent bonds with their respective enzymes and hence act more in the capacity of activators.

Although chromium, tin, arsenic and strontium have been postulated by some investigators to be essential for optimal growth and health of organisms, as well as having a positive influence on biological systems, cofactor functions for their ions have not been assigned because specific enzymes that may require them for activity have not been found.

Nonmetal Mineral Cofactors

Selenium

Selenium belongs to the category of redox nonmetals. Selenium is included in the same class as sulfur (sometimes referred to as metalloids), which implies that selenium should be able to substitute for sulfur in biological complexes. As a congener of sulfur, selenium becomes part of a protein's structure as selenocysteine and selenomethionine, not as a selenium atom ligated directly to the protein as a prosthetic group. The former are the active cofactors in selenium enzymes.

Reactivity Although a selenium ion is clearly capable of redox reactions, there is still little information available as to how selenium functions as a cofactor. Enzymes such as glutathione peroxidase are soluble enzymes that transfer electrons to and from substrates. Replacing the selenium with sulfur in the enzyme negates the activity. With only a few selenoenzymes available, there is little information as to the precise catalytic role of selenium.

Glutathione peroxidase in the reduced (resting) form is believed to contain an ionized selenol that can react with either organic peroxides or H_2O_2 according to the reaction (a) below:

$$\text{(a) Enz-Se}^- + \text{ROOH} \rightarrow \text{Enz-SeOH} + \text{ROH}$$

$$\text{(b) Enz-Se}^- + \text{RI}_4 \rightarrow \text{Enz-SeI} + \text{RI}_3$$

A selenol enzyme is also believed to be an intermediate in the reaction (b) catalyzed by $5'$ deiodinase, the enzyme that catalyzes the removal of iodine from thyroid hormone. The enzyme–selenenic acid complex (Enz-SeOH) is regenerated by reduced glutathione (GSH), which forms a mixed selenide sulfide intermediate (Enz-Se-S-G). This intermediate then reacts with a second GSH to restore Enz-Se$^-$ and releases oxidized glutathione (GSSG) as a product. Regeneration of the Enz-SeI of $5'$ deiodinase also requires a reducing agent whose identity is still uncertain although dithiothreitol can perform the reduction *in vitro*.

Silicon

There is still some question as to whether silicon is a cofactor. It is included here because of the importance of silicon in a number of biochemical reactions leading to the synthesis of glycoproteins and polysaccharides in the extracellular matrix of connective tissue ground substance. Silicon as $Si(OH)_4$ is very abundant in soils and minerals and is as common in human tissues as magnesium. In plants, especially grasses, silicon is a major component of a mineral skeleton and has a metabolic turnover nearly on a par with carbon. In humans, the highest concentrations of silicon occur in connective tissues such as aorta, trachea, tendon, bone, and skin. Lesser amounts are found in liver, heart, and muscle. The epidermis and hair are significantly high in silicon.

Reactivity Silicon, as silicic acid, has been shown to be required for maximal activity of prolyl hydroxylase, the enzyme that converts proline residues to hydroxyproline in collagen. High levels (0.2–2.0 mM) are needed to stimulate the enzyme, which catalyzes a rate-determining factor in collagen biosynthesis.

Boron

Manipulating the boron content of a diet leads to a wide number of metabolic responses, which is testament to the potential importance of boron in human nutrition. Early studies reported increased levels of steroid hormones, testosterone, and estradiol in animals supplemented with boron. Further studies suggest that boron has a regulatory role in the metabolism of other minerals such as calcium and may affect bone metabolism. In a comparative way the role of boron is well established in vascular plants, diatoms, and marine algal flagellates. Zebra fish deprived of boron tend to suffer developmental defects. These data have prompted investigations into the biological functions of boron in higher vertebrates. To date, however, few studies have supported boron's essential role in vertebrates. In a comparison to Zebra fish, pregnant rats fed one-fiftieth the level of boron as control rats exhibited no impairment in fetal growth or development. Fewer two-cell embryos from the deficient rats, however, reached the blastocyst stage when cultured *in vitro*, suggesting boron deprivation did have an impact at a very early stage of development. Perhaps the strongest hold-up to accepting boron as essential is the failure to define and link a specific organoboron compound with a physiological function. A report of boron associated with a naturally occurring antibiotic is an exception. The data, however, tend to support the notion that boron complexes with biological components are too unstable to be isolated and studied. This clearly has put a damper on the forward thrust of establishing boron's precise metabolic function.

Conclusions

The mineral cofactors described above may be thought of as representing a special subset of the biominerals. Rather than contributing to skeletal mass and fluid homeostasis, however, mineral cofactors are subtler and are devoted specifically to enzymes. The words 'mineral' and 'cofactor' combine to designate an inorganic component required by an enzyme in order to achieve optimum catalytic efficiency. In seeking a reason for mineral confactors, one must consider that to meet its functional obligations, an enzyme faces many challenges. The protein surface can easily be modified chemically through interaction with substrates and the enzyme protein can readily lose its biological form through denaturation. Electrons and groups that are transferred to and from substrates have the potential to permanently modify the enzyme. This happens frequently and instead of undergoing repair, old enzymes are replaced by new ones. The mineral cofactors fit into the daily wear and tear by making the enzyme better able to stand up to the harsh environment of their existence. They also have been shown to be effective binders of substrate and to interact with oxidants and reductants in a facile manner. Some

trace metals such as zinc can accept electron pairs in forming a covalent attachment that polarizes and facilitates rupture of the chemical bonds in the substrate. Other metals such as copper and iron can accept electrons from the substrate and pass them to oxygen. Catalysis and structure stability are the two primary functions of metals in enzymes. Many organic factors serve as electron-capturing and group-transferring agents (see 00059). This suggests that metalloenzymes may back up enzymes with organic cofactors. This view is rather narrow and oversimplified since there are many enzyme-catalyzed reactions where only a metal will suffice, such as in the metalloenzymes that catalyze the destruction of oxygen radicals. In biology seldom does one factor become indispensable. What nutritionists refer to as essential metals are on the same level as vitamins in that they are needed in very small quantities to maintain the status quo in a system and, like vitamins, are available strictly through the diet. Therefore, one must conclude that essential minerals and vitamins have common ground in the enzymes, which they literally permit to function.

See also: **Calcium. Cofactors:** Organic. **Copper. Iron. Magnesium. Manganese. Potassium. Selenium. Zinc:** Physiology.

Further Reading

Berthon G (1995) *Handbook of Metal Ligand Interactions in Biological Fluids. Bioinorganic Medicine*, vols I and II. New York: Marcel Dekker.

Eichhorn GL (1973) *Inorganic Biochemistry*, vols 1 and 2. Amsterdam: Elsevier Scientific Publishing.

Fraústo da Silva JJR and Williams RJP (1991) *The Biological Chemistry of the Elements. The Inorganic Chemistry of Life.* Oxford: Oxford University Press.

Harris ED (2003) Basic and clinical aspects of copper. *Critical Reviews of Clinical and Laboratory Sciences* 40: 547–586.

King TE, Mason HS, and Morrison M (1988) *Oxidases and Related Redox Systems: Progress in Clinical and Biological Research*, vol. 274. New York: Alan R. Liss.

Lanoue L, Taubeneck MW, Muniz J, Hanna LA, Strong PL, Murray FJ, Nielsen FH, Hunt CD, and Keen CL (1998) Assessing the effects of low boron diets on embryonic and fetal development in rodents using *in vitro* and *in vivo* model systems. *Biological Trace Element Research* 66: 271–298.

Mertz W (1987) *Trace Elements in Human and Animal Nutrition*, 5th edn, vols I and II, New York: Academic Press.

Prasad AS (1993) *Essential and Toxic Trace Elements in Human Health and Disease: An Update.* New York: Wiley-Liss.

Stadtman TC (1996) Selenocyteine. *Annual Reviews of Biochemistry* 65: 83–100.

Stryer L (1995) *Biochemistry*, 4th edn. New York: WH Freeman & Co.

Organic

E D Harris, Texas A&M University, College Station, TX, USA

© 2005 Elsevier Ltd. All rights reserved.

Introduction

Cofactors are important accessories to biochemical processes. Generally present as small organic compounds or metal ions, cofactors empower enzymes to functional at maximal catalytic effectiveness or endurance. A related term, coenzymes, relates to a subgroup of cofactors whose structure in part is derived from water-soluble B vitamins. Historically, cofactors were often inadvertently removed during purification and had to be added back to restore enzyme activity. Today, we regard a cofactor as an obligatory component of the catalytic mechanism. Compounds meeting the criteria are either: (1) small organic molecules that bind directly to the enzyme surface forming an active site for the substrate to bind or interact, or assist in these events indirectly, or (2) inorganic ions that bind to specific groups on an enzyme surface and aid in substrate binding, catalysis, stabilizing the transition state, or contributing to the overall stability of the enzyme's structure. Practically speaking, any substance in an assay medium that promotes the catalytic activity or stability of an enzyme is a candidate for its cofactor.

As will be illustrated in this and was in the last article, cofactors are indispensable adducts of the catalytic machinery of the body and have provided nutritionists with the strongest insights into the essential role of vitamins and trace elements. It is still fashionable to consider coenzymes as vitamin derivatives that bind loosely to enzymes or serve as transient active sites. Cofactors and coenzymes are terms that are used interchangeably. It is important to note, however, that the prefix 'holo' is used to refer to an enzyme and its coenzyme together as a catalytic unit and 'apo' when the coenzyme is missing. Apoenzymes are functionless and are of no benefit to the organism.

History

Early studies of vitamins found that many, especially the water-soluble B vitamins, formed the nucleus of compounds that partook in enzyme catalysis. The discovery established a bridge between nutrition and the fledgling science of biochemistry. Indeed, many early biochemical investigations were devoted to learning the biological functions of essential nutrients, which included the vitamins. A general principle that emerged at the time was that a vitamin had to be changed to another compound in order to be metabolically functional. With the diet as the only source, it was possible to learn the specific effects of individual vitamins by omission studies. With deeper insights into biological processes, it was soon realized that canceling an enzyme in a critical biochemical pathway was behind many of the vitamin deficiency diseases such as beriberi, pellagra, and pernicious anemia. This put dramatic new emphasis on enzyme functions and the search for enzymes that depended on vitamins for function.

Cofactors in Biochemical Pathways

Table 1 lists vitamins and nonvitamins that are known to give rise to many of the organic cofactors in humans. **Figure 1** provides a glimpse into their importance by showing the location of organic cofactors in the biochemical pathway for oxidizing glucose and other biocompounds to CO_2 and H_2O. That overall reaction for glucose is:

$$C_6H_{12}O_6(glucose) + 6O_2 \rightarrow 6CO_2 + 6H_2O$$

One sees that at least seven distinct B vitamin-derived coenzymes are needed to complete the transition. Nicotine adenine dinucleotide (NAD^+), derived from niacin, is required for the oxidation of glucose to pyruvate and thiamine pyrophosphate (TPP) derived from the vitamin thiamine (sometimes written as thiamin), flavin adenine dinucleotide (FAD) from riboflavin, panthothenic acid from pantothene, and lipoic acid all take part in the oxidation of pyruvate to acetyl-coenzyme A in the middle stage. In addition, flavinmononucleotide (FMN) also from riboflavin and coenzyme Q from ubiquinone take part in completing the oxidation to CO_2 and H_2O in the oxidative-phosphorylation pathway in the mitochondria. All told, some 20 organic cofactors engage enzymes in the various biochemical pathways of humans. Below is a brief description of each coenzyme/cofactor. **Table 2** summarizes the list of key enzymes known to be associated with each coenzyme.

Specific Vitamins as Cofactors

Thiamine (Vitamin B₁)

Best known as the anti-beriberi factor and called at first simply vitamin B by McCollum, thiamine was shown to be involved in the decarboxylation of pyruvate to acetaldehyde in alcohol fermentation and was named 'cocarboxylase' in 1932.

Table 1 Vitamins and nonvitamin cofactors[a]

Name of vitamin[a]	Related coenzymes	Biochemical function
Thiamine, thiamin B_1	Thiamine-pyrophosphate	Carbonyl group transfer
Riboflavin B_2	FMN, FAD	Redox reactions
Niacin (nicotinamide) B_3	NAD, NADP	Redox reactions
Pantothenic acid B_5	Coenzyme A	Acyl group transfer
Pyridoxine B_6	Pyridoxal 5′ phosphate	Amine group transfer
Folic acid (folacin) B_9	Tetrahydrofolates	One-carbon transfer
Cobalamin B_{12}	5′ Deoxyadenosyl cobalamin	Methylation, rearrangement reactions
L-Ascorbic acid C	Dihydroascorbate	Collagen, adrenaline synthesis
Calciferol D	None	Calcium absorption
Tocophoral E	None	Antioxidant
Biotin H	Biocytin	CO_2 fixation
Phylloquinone K	None	Prothrombin synthesis
Bioflavonoids P	None	Antioxidant
Nonvitamin cofactors		
p-Aminobenzoate	Tetrahydrofolate	One-carbon transfer
α-Lipoic acid	None	Acetyl group transfer
Betaine	None	Methylating agent
Coenzyme Q	Ubiquinone	Electron transfer
PQQ	None	Oxidation reactions
Topaquinone	None	Oxidation reactions
Carnitine	None	Fatty acid transfer
Inositol	None	Membrane lipids
S-adenosyl methionine	None	Methylation reactions
Glutathione	None	Group transfer, anitoxidant
3′ Phosphoadenosine-5′ phosphosulfate	None	Sulfate esterification

[a]Although codified in vitamin literature at one time, B_4, B_{10}, and B_{11} have since been abandoned.

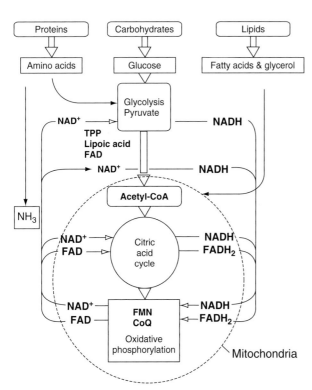

Figure 1 Occurrence of organic cofactors in energy metabolism. Only a few key intermediates in the pathway are shown. Dotted circle shows reactions taking place in the mitochondria. Note how coenzymes NAD^+ and FAD cycle between oxidized and reduced forms.

Confirmation of its structure as TPP came 5 years later. Its name is meant to signify a vitamin containing sulfur (*thios* in Greek).

Reactions

1. Pyruvate dehydrogenase complex in mitochondria.
2. α-Ketoglutarate dehydrogenase complex in mitochondria.
3. Branch chain dehydrogenase.
4. Transketolase reactions in pentose pathway and in reductive pentose pathway of photosynthesis.

Reactivity The structure of thiamine has two rings bridged by a methylene group as seen in **Figure 2A**. The coenzyme (TPP) arises via an ATP-dependent pyrophosphorylation of the primary alcohol group (**Figure 2B**). What may be called the active site of the coenzyme is the carbon in position 2 (C-2) of the smaller five-member thiazolium ring (arrow). A favorable positioning of C-2 between atoms of nitrogen and sulfur causes C-2 hydrogen to exchange protons with water, indicating C-2 can ionize to a carbanion. As a carbanion, C-2 is able to engage positive centers such as carbonyl carbons of α-keto acids and keto sugars. In the reaction with pyruvate, α-ketoglutarate, or branch-chain α-keto acids from valine, leucine, or isoleucine, a carboxyl group is

Table 2 Sample of enzymes associated with each of the coenzymes derived from vitamins

Coenzyme	Enzyme
1. Thiamine-pyrophosphate	Pyruvate dehydrogenase complex
	α-Ketoglutarate dehydrogenase complex
	Transketolase
	Branch chain dehydrogenase
2. NAD$^+$, NADH	Glyceraldehyde-3-PO$_4$ dehydrogenase
	Pyruvate dehydrogenase complex
	Alcohol dehydrogenase
	Lactate dehydrogenase
3. NADP$^+$, NADPH	Glucose-6-PO$_4$ dehydrogenase
	Glutamate dehydrogenase
	β-Ketoacyl-ACP synthase
4. FAD, FADH$_2$	Glucose-6-PO$_4$ dehydrogenase
	Succinate dehydrogenase
	Fatty acyl-CoA dehydrogenase
5. Pyridoxal-5$'$ phosphate	Aminotransferases
	Glycogen phosphorylase
6. Tetrahydrofolate	Glycine synthase
	Homocysteine methyltransferase
7. Biocytin	Pyruvate carboxylase
	Acetyl-CoA carboxylase
	Propionyl-CoA carboxylase
8. Coenzyme A (pantothenic acid)	Pyruvate dehydrogenase complex
	Acetyl-CoA carboxylase
	Citrate synthase
9. Cobalamin	Homocysteine methyltransferase
	Methylmalonyl-CoA mutase
10. L-Ascorbate	Prolyl and lysyl hydroxylase
	Dopamine-β-monooxygenase

expelled as CO_2 and the electrons remain with the 'active aldehyde' on the C-2 position. Attack on a keto sugar cleaves the first two carbons as a unit, which then attaches to C-2 as an 'active glycoaldehyde' adduct. Yeast disengage active aldehyde as acetaldehyde later to be reduced to ethanol by alcohol dehydrogenase. Bacteria convert 'active aldehyde' to acetyl-phosphate. In the mitochondria of higher organisms, however, active aldehyde is oxidized by an FAD-containing enzyme (part of the pyruvate dehydrogenase complex) and transferred to lipoic acid (see **Figure 10**), which transfers the highly energetic acetyl group to the thiol group of coenzyme A. As a coenzyme for transketolases in the pentose pathway, TPP takes part in the formation of ribose-5-phosphate, glyceraldehyde-3-phosphate, and erythrose-4-phosphate from sedohepulose-7-phosphate, xyulose-5-phosphate, and fructose-6-phosphate, respectively. Each sugar phosphate donates an 'active glycoaldehyde' to an aldose acceptor.

TPP is also the coenzyme for branch chain dehydrogenase, the enzyme that catalyzes the oxidative decarboxylation of α-keto acids derived from leucine, isoleucine, and valine, three essential amino acids. The reaction follows a scheme similar to pyuvate oxidation, only this time the carbon skeleton of the amino acid condenses with coenzyme A (CoA).

Riboflavin (Vitamin B$_2$)

The first hint that McCollum's vitamin B was in reality a multifactor complex came when yeast void of antineuritis activity still retained growth-stimulating activity. Originally called vitamin G, riboflavin was renamed vitamin B$_2$ when it was recognized to be part of the yeast B complex. The name riboflavin followed the discovery in 1935 of its association with green fluorescent pigment of whey. Today, we regard riboflavin and niacin as the two principal vitamins that give rise to coenzymes that function with enzymes known as oxidoreductases. Both coenzymes transport electrons to and from substrates and in so doing form oxidized or reduced products. The two are referred to as 'redox' (an abbreviation for oxidation-reduction) coenzymes for that reason. Riboflavin was identified as the biochemical compound that gave the color to Warburg's 'yellow enzyme,' glucose-6-phosphate dehydrogenase (G6PDH). G6PDH was observed to catalyze the transfer of electrons from nicotinamide adenine dinucleotide phosphate (NADPH) to methylene blue, a redox sensitive dye that lost color upon reduction, suggesting that riboflavin probably mediated the electron exchange. G6PDH is a key entrance point for glucose into the pentose pathway and a major contributor of NADPH for the biosynthesis of fatty acids and other fats. The reaction is:

$$\text{Glucose-6-phosphate} + 2\text{NADP}^+ + \text{H}_2\text{O}$$
$$\rightarrow \text{ribose-5-phosphate} + \text{CO}_2 + 2\text{NADPH} + 2\text{H}^+$$

Riboflavin (**Figure 2C**) is associated with two coenzymes, FMN and FAD. FMN is formed by phosphorylating the primary alcohol on the sugar moiety of riboflavin, an ATP-dependent reaction. FAD results from a further condensation of FMN with the 5$'$ AMP moiety of ATP (**Figure 2D**). What may be considered the active site is the isoalloxazine ring, which can exist in both oxidized and reduced states depending on whether electron pairs are absent or present, respectively. Enzymes that contain FAD or FMN are referred to as flavoproteins. FMN is limited to the membrane proteins of the mitochondria electron transport system whereas FAD is found in both membrane-bound and soluble

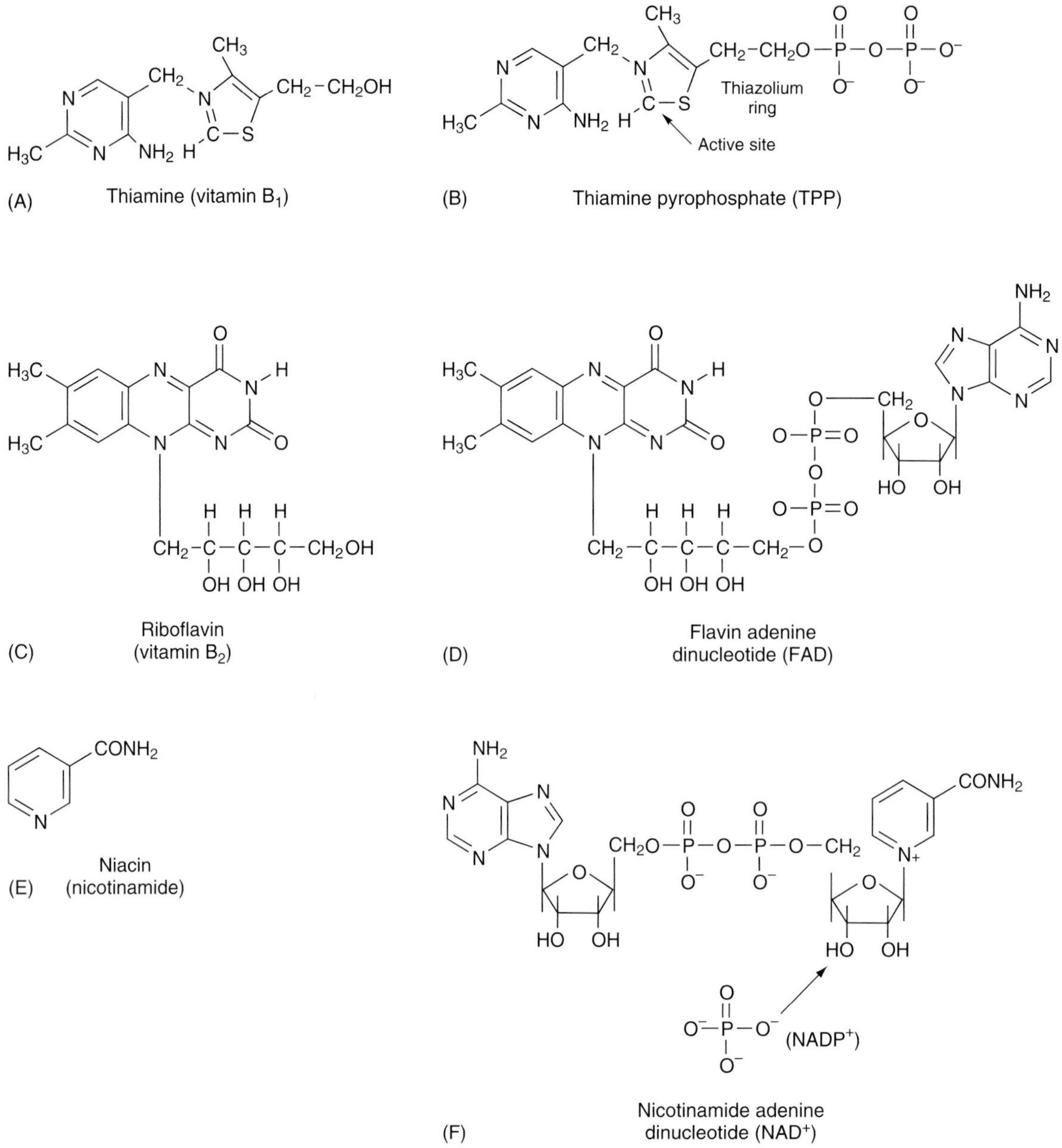

Figure 2 Structural relationship of vitamin-coenzyme for (A) thiamine (B_1), (C) riboflavin (B_2), and (E) niacin. In the left column is the structure of the vitamin, in the right column the coenzyme derived from the vitamin. Note the pyrophosphate group in the coenzyme derived from thiamine (B) and the prevalence of phosphate and adenyl groups in the coenzymes derived from riboflavin (D) and niacin (F), showing the necessity for ATP in their synthesis.

enzymes. The flavin cofactor is bound covalently to the structure preventing disengagement during purification procedures.

Reactions Flavin enzymes are designed to remove (and add) electrons to and from substrates. In general, flavin coenzymes are stronger oxidizing agents than the pyrimidine coenzymes (NAD^+, $NADP^+$) and tend to participate in more complex reactions. Also, flavin coenzymes can accept single electrons from a donor, forming a semiquinone and allowing

flavoproteins to take part in reactions that form free radicals. Having a single electron also allows favins to bind molecular oxygen as a hydroperoxyl complex.

Niacin (Nicotinic acid, Nicotinamide)

Niacin presents an unusual twist in that its parent compound, nicotinic acid, had been known for about 70 years (ca. 1867) before its activity as a vitamin first become known (ca. 1937). If thiamine (vitamin B_1) is the anti-beriberi factor, niacin (vitamin B_3) is the anti-pellagra factor. Pellagra is a disease characterized by a rash or dermatitis on areas of the skin exposed to sunlight as well as swelling in the legs from the knee on down and a painful flush and rash. Niacin (also called nicotinic acid or nicotinamide), its amide derivative (**Figure 2E**), is the active component of the second major redox coenzyme nicotinamide adenine dinucleotide and its phosphate (NAD^+ and $NADP^+$, respectively; **Figure 2F**). As with FMN and FAD, NAD^+ and $NADP^+$ arise by phosphorylation and condensation of the basic vitamin structure with ATP. NAD^+ differs from $NADP^+$ by having a phosphate group on the 3' position of the pentose nearest to the adenine (**Figure 2F**). NAD^+ and NADH were discovered in dialyzable extracts of yeast, meaning these coenzymes readily disengaged from the enzyme that bound them. The ability to come on and come off an enzyme is fundamental to the electron delivery scheme shown in **Figure 1**.

Reactivity With few exceptions, the redox-related reactions of NAD^+ and $NADP^+$ are with dehydrogenase enzymes, i.e., enzymes that catalyze the removal and addition of electrons (as hydride ions) to substrates. A typical reaction in which NAD^+ is the oxidizing agent is the conversion of L-lactic acid to pyruvate:

$$\text{L-Lactate} + NAD^+ \rightleftarrows \text{pyruvate} + NADH + H^+$$

Therefore, the coenzyme is a major participant in energy-yielding catabolic reactions. $NADP^+$ performs less of a catabolic role, but its reduced form, NADPH, is a major reductant in anabolic reactions, especially the biosynthesis of fatty acids and other lipids.

The active site of both NAD^+ and $NADP^+$ is the nicotinamide ring. The oxidized form of nicotinamide has a quaternary nitrogen (four attaching bonds) that is written as a positive charge (**Figure 2F**). The oxidized ring accepts two electrons and one proton from a substrate (literally a hydride

ion, H^-) reducing the ring and abolishing the positive charge on the nitrogen:

$$NAD^+ + 2e^- + 2H^+ \rightarrow NADH + H^+$$
$$NADP^+ + 2e^- + 2H^+ \rightarrow NADPH + H^+$$

More than 200 enzymes are known to catalyze reactions in which NAD^+ or $NADP^+$ accepts a hydride ion from a substrate. Moreover, there is a strong stereospecificity to this reaction. Addition of an H^- to the ring can either be in front (A-type) or in back (B-type), depending on the enzyme. Reducing the ring weakens it bonding to the enzyme and causes the NADH (NADPH) to dissociate and engage other cell components for the purpose of transferring the electrons.

NAD^+ is also a source of 5' adenosine monophosphate (5' AMP) in a limited series of activation or inhibition reactions. The transferred 5' AMP becomes a leaving group for subsequent bond formation. In DNA ligase in bacteria, for example, the 5' AMP is transferred to a lysine on the enzyme to form an unusual phosphoamide adduct that subsequently is transferred to one of the DNA strands. Attack by the 3' hydroxyl group on the adjacent DNA strand releases the 5' AMP concomitant with forming a phosphodiester bond and sealing the two DNA strands together. A related reaction, referred to as an ADP-ribosylation results in the nicotinamide group being split from the NAD^+ and the ribose moiety forming a covalent glycosylamine bond with a protein. ADP-ribosylation of sensitive proteins is one of the deadlier effects of bacteria toxins such as cholera toxin, diphtheria toxin, or pertussis toxin.

Pyridoxine (Vitamin B₆)

Vitamin B_6 was discovered in the 1930s and named pyridoxine because of its structural resemblance to pyridine (**Figure 3**). Pyridoxine's principal involvement is with a family of enzymes known collectively as amino transferases. These enzymes exchange amine groups from amino acids to α-keto acids. Familiar names include serum glutamate-oxalate transaminase (SGOT). The coenzyme, pyridoxal-5'

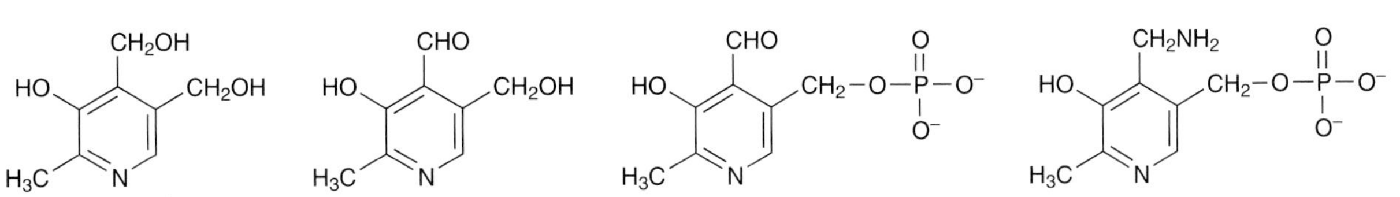

Figure 3 Pyridoxine (vitamin B_6) and its coenzymes. The coenzyme form is capable of receiving (pyridoxal) and donating (pyridoxamine) NH_3 groups.

phosphate (PLP), is the predominant form and is synthesized in a two-step reaction involving the oxidation of the hydroxymethyl group in the para position on the pyridine ring to an aldehyde, and the phosphorylation of the hydroxymethyl group on the 5 position. PLP is also a coenzyme for glycogen phosphorylase and ornithine decarboxylase. With tetrahydrofolate (see below), PLP takes part in serine to glycine interconversion. On the enzyme surface, the reactive species is not an aldehyde, but rather an aldamine formed by a Schiff base bond between the aldehyde and an ε-amino group of lysine in the active site.

Reactivity The reactivity of PLP is due to a number of features. First, the carbonyl (aldehyde) on the ring is positioned to engage the amino groups from amino acids and tether the amino acid to the enzyme. Through a series of electron rearrangements promoted by the PLP, the nitrogen on the amino acid substrate is disengaged and the carbon skeleton (an α-keto acid) is set free retaining the amine group on the coenzyme (pyridoxamine-5' phosphate). The enzyme then binds a second α-keto acid and transfers the amino group generating a new amino acid and restoring the carbonyl function on the PLP. Other changes can also occur to a tethered structure. An electron rearrangement can result in the loss of a carboxyl group (as CO_2) or a molecule of H_2O. Thus, PLP enzymes also take part in decarboxylation and dehydration reactions. In the glycogen phosphorylase reaction, the phosphate group of the coenzyme acts as a general catalyst, promoting the attack of phosphate on the glycosidic bond of glycogen.

Folic Acid

Folic acid was first recognized as the yeast or liver factor that could cure a severe megoblastic anemia in chicks, monkeys, and humans. Later proof that the active substance was a growth factor for certain bacteria such as *Lactobacillus casei* and *Streptococcus faecalis* provided a rapid bioassay for isolating, identifying, and eventually synthesizing the vitamin and its coenzymes. The name folic acid was given in 1941 in recognition of its abundance in leafy green vegetables or 'foliage' and its structure was confirmed as monopterylglutamic acid in 1946. Today, we recognize folic acid as one of our most complex vitamin coenzymes because of its presence in many biochemical forms. Despite such enormous complexity, however, the biochemical role of folic acid narrows down to a specific set of synthetic reactions whose common denominator is one-carbon units.

The structure of folic acid (*N*-pteroyl-L-glutamic acid) can be pictured as a composite of three covalently linked molecules: a methylated pteridine ring attached to *p*-aminobenzoic acid (PABA), which in turn is linked via the carboxyl group to the α nitrogen of glutamic acid (**Figure 4A**). The coenzyme form is tetrahydrofolate (FH_4) formed in mammals by adding four electrons and four hydrogens to the pteridine ring (**Figure 4B**). The reduction is catalyzed by dihydrofolate reductase with NAPDH as the electron donor. The addition of one or more glutamic acid residues completes the structure. In the reductive step, a new asymmetric center is generated at C-6 and appears to be critical to the biological role since only one stereoisomer of this center

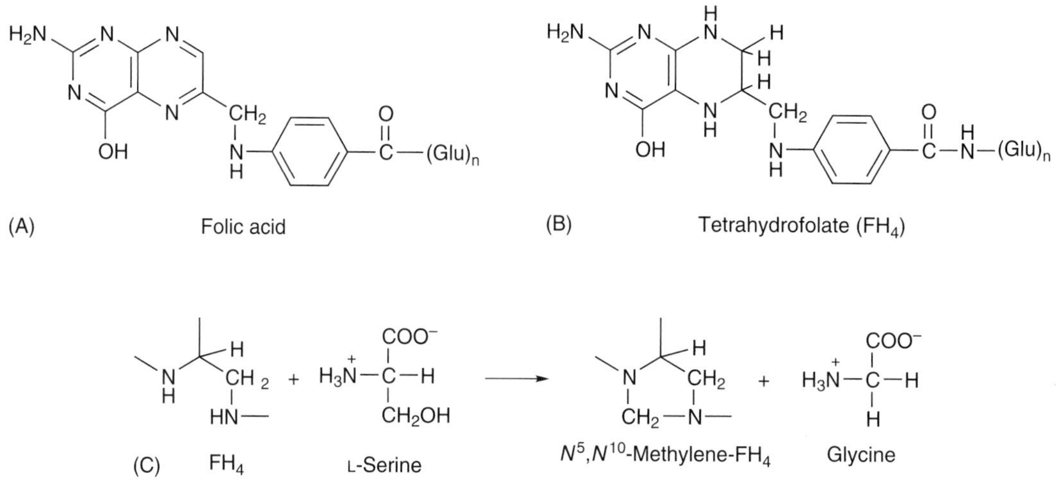

Figure 4 Folic acid (A) and its coenzyme form. Activation requires folic acid to be converted into its tetrahydrofolate derivative (B). (C) Specific function of one of the tetrahydrofolate derivatives, N^5,N^{10}-methylene-FH_4, in the synthesis of glycine from serine. Serine is thus able to donate a carbon to the coenzyme for a subsequent one-carbon transfer reaction.

is active. FH_4 may have up to seven glutamic acid residues and exist in many different chemical forms, most of which are interconvertible.

The basic reactions take part at the N^5 and N^{10} positions on the molecule, which serve as attachment points for one-carbon units in transit (**Figure 4C**). N^{10}-formyl- and N^5,N^{10}-methenyl-FH_4 are two synthetic forms that are biologically active. Complexes of N^5-formyl-FH_4 (folinic acid) transfer formyl groups to specific substrates. Active folic acid derivatives have carbon in the oxidation state of formate as well as formaldehyde (methylene) and a methyl derivative, N^5-methyl-FH_4, is known to take part in the enzymatic conversion of homocysteine to methionine. These observations reveal that the family of folic acid coenzymes is quite complex but all seem to involve the attachment of a single carbon atom to the substrate.

Reactivity Enzymes that require folic acid participate in what is referred to as 'one-carbon metabolism.' This takes the form of group transfers involving methyl groups, formyl groups, formimino groups, and methylene groups. Folic acid does not take part in acetylations or carboxylations. A typical reaction in higher vertebrates is the synthesis of glycine by the enzyme glycine synthase:

$$CO_2 + NH_4^+ + NADH + H^+ + N^5,$$

$$N^{10}\text{-methenyl-}FH_4 \rightarrow glycine + NAD^+ + FH_4$$

In perhaps its only major requirement as a methyl group donor, N^5-methyl-FH_4 is needed by the enzyme homocysteine methyltransferase to synthesize (regenerate) methionine from homocysteine. This reaction also uses a methylated derivative of vitamin B_{12} (see below) to mediate the group transfer. Another important reaction is the interconversion of serine and glycine. As shown in **Figure 4C**, the reaction requires the N^5,N^{10}-methylene-FH_4 derivative. Today, the list of folate-catalyzed reactions is quite large and includes one-carbon units in

the synthesis of a purine ring of nucleic acids, methylation of DNA and RNA, thymidine biosynthesis, choline and *S*-adenosylmethionine biosynthesis, and histidine and tyrosine catabolism.

Biotin

Early interest in biotin involved the so-called egg white injury factor. When it was confirmed that egg white injury was caused by a deficiency and not a toxicity, pursuit of the missing substance led eventually to the discovery of biotin. Research on the vitamin brought a new concept to nutrition, that of the 'antivitamin' or substances capable of negating the action of vitamins before their use as cofactors. In the case of biotin, the 'antivitamin' turned out to be the protein avidin, which bound biotin tenaciously and limited its intestinal absorption.

Reactivity Biotin can be thought of as another one-carbon cofactor, but for biotin this is CO_2. Thus, biotin-requiring enzymes catalyze carboxylation, decarboxylation, or transcarboxylation reactions. The active form of biotin is 'biocytin' (ε-N-biotinyl L-lysine), which is formed by the covalent attachment of the biotin side chain to the ε-amino group of a lysine residue on the apoenzyme as catalyzed by a specific synthetase (**Figure 5B**). The condensation requires ATP and proceeds via a biotinyl-AMP intermediate with the apoenzyme catalyzing formation of the amide bond. The resulting unique structure combines the aliphatic chains or biotin and lysine permitting the ring structure of biotin to extend about 14 Å from the enzyme's surface (**Figure 5B**).

The active site on the biotinyl group is one of the N in the 5-member ring (**Figure 5C**). An N-carboxyl derivative serves as a donor of CO_2 to an appropriate substrate acceptor. The reaction occurs in two steps and requires an ATP-dependent formation of a carboxy biotinyl enzyme. If the enzyme is a carboxylase, there are two main substrate types: (1) acyl-CoA derivatives, which include acetyl-CoA,

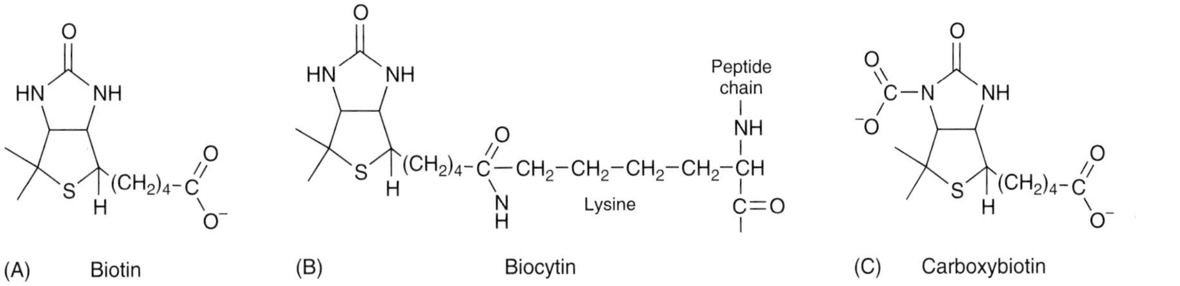

Figure 5 Biotin and its coenzyme. (A) Biotin as a vitamin, (B) biotin attached to the ε-amino group of lysine to form the coenzyme biocytin, and (C) the carboxy derivative of biotin prepared to donate CO_2 to a substrate.

propionyl CoA; and (2) simple α-keto acids such as pyruvate. Each substrate must contain a carbonyl group adjacent to or conjugated with the carbon receiving the carboxyl group from carboxy biocytin. Perhaps the most familiar biotin carboxylase enzymes in mammalian systems are acetyl-CoA carboxylase in fatty acid biosynthesis, propionyl CoA carboxylase in odd-chain fatty acid catabolism, pyruvate carboxylase in gluconeogenesis, and β-methylcrotonyl CoA carboxylase in leucine catabolism.

Pantothenic Acid

Pantothenic acid was named by Roger Williams who recognized its ubiquitous (greek, *pantothene*, from all quarters) occurrence in tissues of all organisms and all food sources. There are two twists to the story of its discovery. First is that the coenzyme form, CoA, was discovered long before the vitamin and, second that investigations of the substructure of CoA led to an understanding of how the coenzyme was synthesized. CoA was known to be a dialyzable cofactor essential for the acetylation of sulfonilamide and choline. Indeed, the 'A' designation in CoA recognized the importance of the acetylation reactions. The first clue to the vitamin's structure came when digests of CoA with intestinal phosphatase and liver extracts were found to contain β-alanine and pantothenic acid as hydrolysis products. Treating CoA with a specific 3' nucleotidase inactivated the coenzyme and a specific pyrophosphatase cleaved the coenzyme to a panthothene-containing product that could be restored to CoA by adenylation with ATP. These studies showed that pantothenic acid was an essential component of CoA and had been locked into the structure of a rather complex coenzyme (**Figure 6**).

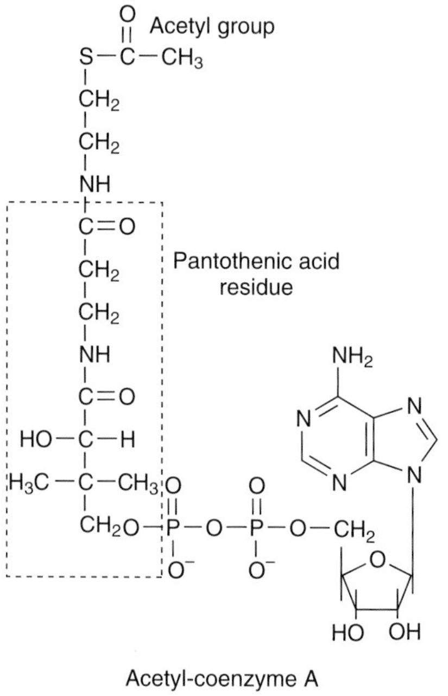

Reactivity As a major component of CoA and its derivatives, pantothenic acid is involved in acetylation reactions, which include the synthesis of acetoacetyl-CoA, a precursor of cholesterol, and the biosynthesis of citrate from acetate. CoA can engage in acyl thiotransfer reactions such as accepting the acetyl groups from lipoic acid and forming acetyl-CoA as well as fatty acyl CoAs. Pantothene is also found as a prosthetic group (4'-pantothene) attached to a serine residue of acyl carrier protein (ACP), which plays a prominent role in the biosynthesis of fatty acids.

Cobalamin (Vitamin B$_{12}$)

Few vitamins have been more challenging to structure–function studies than vitamin B$_{12}$. Among its many unique features, B$_{12}$ is the only vitamin-

Figure 6 Pantothenic acid in the structure of coenzyme A.

coenzyme known to have a transition metal ion (cobalt) coordinated to its structure. The metal allows some usual chemistry (see 00058). The vitamin is present in a variety of foods but is almost totally lacking in plants. Although the vitamin can be synthesized *de novo* by intestinal flora, the absorption site anatomically is prior to the synthesis site in the gut, which means little benefit is derived from endogenous synthesis. Isolating the active form of the vitamin meant developing an *in vitro* assay for 'pernicious anemia,' one of the deficiency symptoms. In 1950, Shive introduced an assay in which homocysteine was converted to methionine in a B$_{12}$-dependent reaction. A second assay showed that the derivative 5-deoxyadenosyl cobalamin was essential for the interconversion of L-glutamate and β-methyl aspartate. The latter discovery led to the isolation of 5' adenosylcobalamine, the principal active form of the vitamin.

Reactivity The core of the vitamin consists of a corrin ring with a central cobalt atom. Corrin contains four pyrrole rings linked together, which vaguely resembles structurally the porphyin ring in heme (**Figure 7**). An inactive form of the vitamin contains a displaceable CN group bound to the cobalt; hence the early name cyanocobalamin for one of its more familiar forms (**Figure 7**). The cobalt atom in the ring can have a +1, +2, or +3 oxidation state. The fifth valence (below the ring plane) has a dimethylbenzimidazole attached to the cobalt and the six can be either a methyl group, an –OH

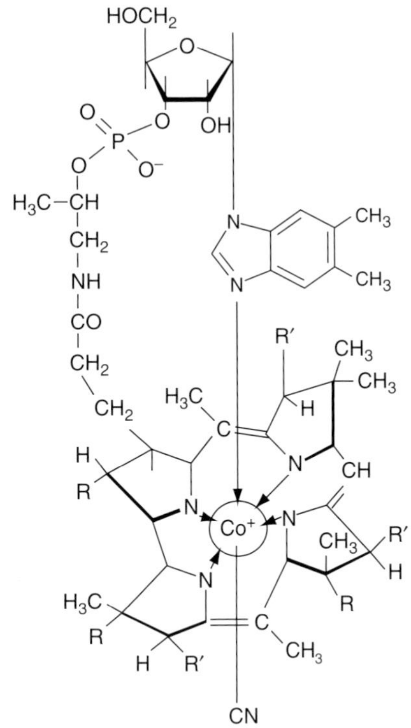

Figure 7 Cyanocobalamin, one of the forms of vitamin B12. Shown are the corrin ring and the attachment of the dimethylbenzimidazole to the cobalt above the ring. The cyano group is shown attached to the cobalt below the plane of the ring.

group, or a 5′ deoxyadenosyl group depending on the reaction or enzyme. As noted, 5′ deoxyadenosylcobalamin is the most common form of the coenzyme. The 5′ deoxyadenosylcobalamine arises by an attack on the 5′ carbon of ATP by Co^+, which displaces the triphosphate group of ATP, a rare action in biochemistry. Known enzymes that require B12 fit one of two functional categories: those that transfer methyl groups from the coenzyme to the substrate, and those that take part in positional rearrangements of neighboring groups on the substrate, or group transfer reactions.

As noted above, methylation reactions in mammalian systems that involve B12 are limited to the transfer of a methyl group to homocysteine to form methionine. Recall, N^5-methyl-THF is the methyl group donor in the reaction and B12 mediates the transfer. Restoring the methyl group on methionine primes the system to further methylation since methionine itself, acting through its active form, S-adenosylmethionine (see below), is a primary donor of methyl groups to other substrates.

Of late, there has been considerable interest in vitamin B12 reactions that have free radicals as intermediates. This may be one of the principal advantages of the coenzyme, i.e., the ability to form and retain a stable free radical in its structure. The stability of the free radical is due to the unusual chemistry of the cobalt ion.

Ascorbic Acid

The vitamin (L-ascorbic acid) linked with scurvy is known to be a cofactor for two enzymes that take part in the biosynthesis of collagen, the major connective tissue protein; the formation of hydroxyproline and hydroxylysine residues as catalyzed by prolyl hydroxylase and lysyl hydroxylase enzymes, respectively (**Figure 8**). Collagen is an essential component of the extracellular matrix. As a cofactor for dopamine-β-monooxygenase, L-ascorbic acid is also required for the synthesis of adrenaline (epinephrine) and noradrenaline (epinephrine) in the adrenal medulla. Another important noncofactor role of L-ascorbate is as an antioxidant in cells and blood.

Vitamin K

The antihemorrhagic role of vitamin K had been established long before it was realized that the vitamin with no structural modification was essential for the biosynthesis of functional prothrombin. The two forms of the vitamin, phylloquinoine (vitamin K_1) and menadione (vitamin K_2), differ only in the structure of their side chains (**Figure 9**).

Reactivity Vitamin K takes part in an extensive series of carboxylation reactions involving all the glutamic acid residues in the first half of prothrombin, a blood-clotting factor. The carboxyglutamic acid residues or 'gla' that occupy this region of the prothrombin molecule are able to bind the calcium ions needed to catalyze formation of thrombin. Carboxylation is dependent on oxygen and uses the hydroquinone form of the vitamin as the driving force. Warfarin, a clotting inhibitor, interferes with the carboxylation reaction, which explains the basic mechanism of this inhibitor. A synthetic substrate, Pro-Leu-Glu-Glu-Val, has been found to substitute for prothrombin in the reaction, opening the way to learning the finer details of the reaction mechanism and the specific role of vitamin K.

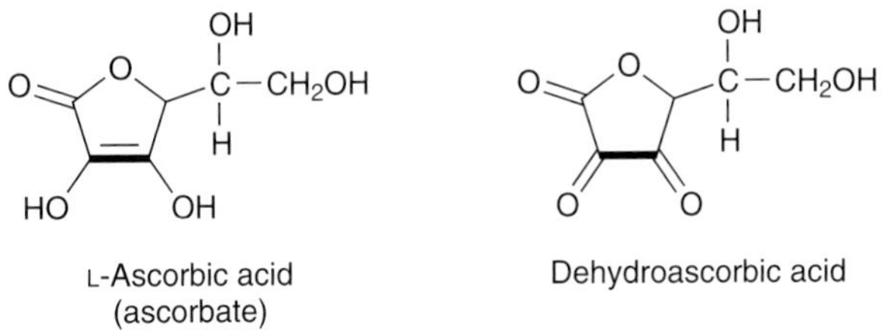

Figure 8 Vitamin C in its reduced (dihydro) and oxidized (dehydro) forms.

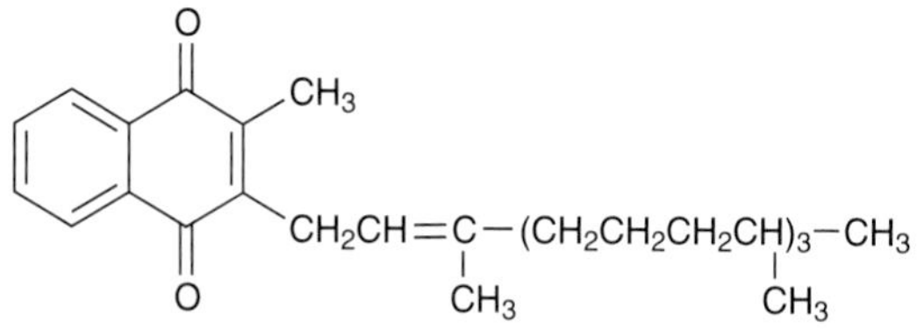

Figure 9 Phylloquinone, one of the active forms of vitamin K (Vitamin K$_1$).

Nonvitamin Cofactors

In addition to the above vitamin-coenzymes, there is a list of cofactors that do not fit the general category of vitamin-derived cofactors. Nonetheless, these organic cofactors are essential components of the catalytic mechanisms of important enzymes or membrane-bound enzyme systems.

Lipoic Acid

Lipoic acid's role as a growth factor for microorganisms and as a cofactor for biochemical reactions in all organisms is well established. The cofactor was discovered originally in the conversion of pyruvate to acetate and as a factor essential for the oxidation of pyruvate. Lipoic acid is known to occur in α-keto acid dehydrogenases from a variety of organisms. It is normally bound to the ε-amino group of a lysine residue (analogous to biotin) allowing the cofactor to extend out and away from the enzyme surface as a 'swinging arm.'

Reactivity The reactions taking place in the pyruvate dehydrogenase complex best reveal the cofactor function of lipoic acid. As a cofactor, lipoic acid (6,8 dithiooctanoic acid) exists in both an oxidized (disulfide) and reduced form (**Figure 10**). The disulfide form oxidizes active acetaldehye bound to TPP simultaneously with the transfer of the acetate product to one of the -SH groups of the now reduced lipoic acid. As a thioester, the acetate group is subsequently transferred to coenzyme A forming acetyl-CoA and regenerating a free -SH group on lipoic acid. The reduced lipoic acid, which still contains the electrons, is then oxidized by a flavoprotein (FAD) restoring the disulfide group of lipoic acid for another round of catalysis. Eventually, FADH$_2$ passes the electrons to NAD$^+$,

which links to the electron transport chain of the mitochondria. Lipoic acid is thus an oxidizing agent and a carrier of acetate in the reaction. One can picture the long arm of the cofactor swinging between sites on the subunits of the pyruvate dehydrogenase complex in order to perform the multiple reactions in synchrony with the catalytic events taking place.

Carnitine

Carnitine is readily synthesized from lysine. As a cofactor, carnitine takes part in the membrane-bound enzyme system that transports fatty acids into the mitochondria for energy oxidation. Two enzymes, carnitine acyl transferase I and carnitine acyl transferase II, comprise a cycle that delivers the fatty acid as an acyl carnitine derivative to the interior of the mitochondria and returns the carnitine to the cytosolic side for further transport (**Figure 11**). The structure of carnitine with its hydroxyl group on C-3 is ideally suited for forming an acyl bound with a fatty acid.

Coenzyme Q (Ubiquinone)

First detected in lipid extracts of mitochondria and identified as a quinone, coenzyme Q (CoQ) was so named to signify its cofactor role in oxidation reactions. A second group of investigators discovered a cofactor that had ubiquitous occurrence in oxidative processes, which they named ubiquinone. In time, CoQ and ubiquinone were found to be the same compound. Early studies on the electron transport chain of mitochondria showed at least three complexes required CoQ and recognized its essential role in the electron transfer process overall. CoQ can be synthesized in man from tyrosine in a rather complex synthesis.

Reactivity CoQ and its reduced form CoQH$_2$ are designed to handle electron pairs in transit in oxidation-reduction reactions. A third form, semiquinone (CoQH·), exists as a stable radical and is capable of a one-electron transfer (**Figure 12**). Because of its ability to deal with electrons on a single or paired base, CoQ takes part in electron transport chains where one- and two-electron transfers are essential. Its lipid nature allows the cofactor to bind firmly to

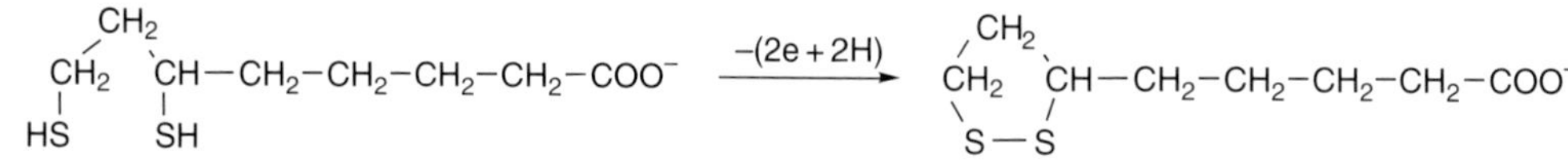

Figure 10 Lipoic acid in its reduced (sulfhydryl) and oxidized (disulfide) forms. The carboxyl group on the end is attached to a lysine group on the enzyme thus forming a swinging arm that is designed to transverse remote donor-acceptor sites across the surface of the enzyme.

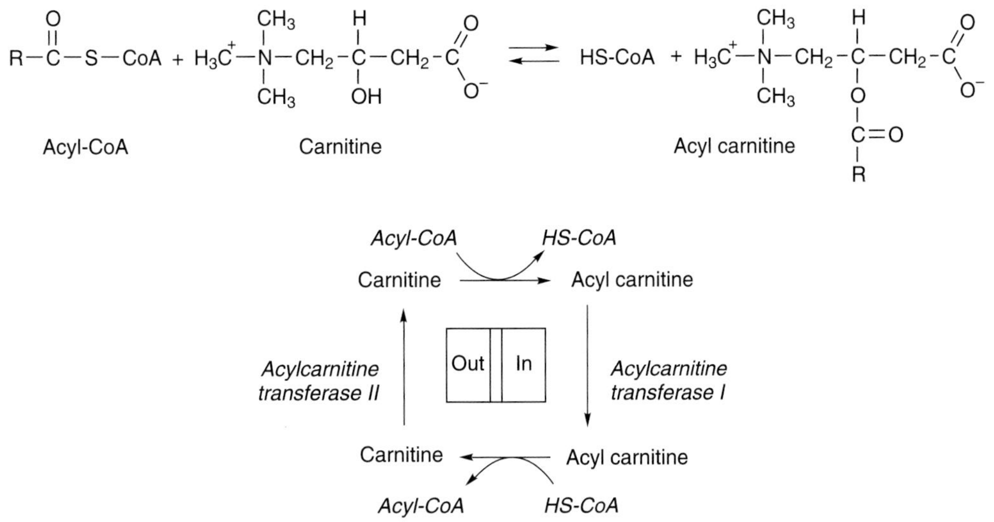

Figure 11 Carnitine-dependent transfer of fatty acyl groups. Two juxtaposed membrane transferase enzymes, acylcarnitine transferase I,II, are designed to transport a fatty acyl carnitine complex into the mitochondria and return the carnitine for additional reactions. Note that the acyl group is transferred to the carnitine from CoA and returned to CoA inside the mitochondria.

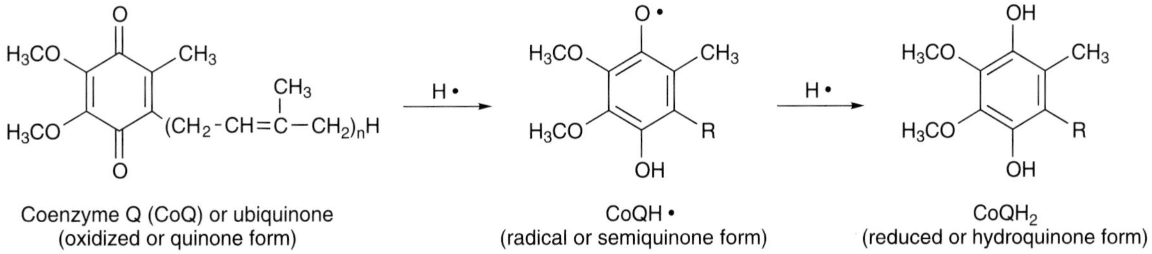

Coenzyme Q (CoQ) or ubiquinone
(oxidized or quinone form)

CoQH •
(radical or semiquinone form)

CoQH$_2$
(reduced or hydroquinone form)

Figure 12 Coenzyme Q (ubiquinone) as an electron carrier. The coenzyme is a mobile electron carrier that moves between protein complexes in the mitochondria membrane. Shown are single (semiquinone) and dual (hydroquinone) forms that permit one- and two-electron transport, respectively.

the mitochondria inner membrane. Besides being a prominent carrier of electrons in the electron transport chain of mitochondria, CoQ is known to be a source and mediator of protons that are pumped across the inner mitochondria membrane to form the high-energy proton gradient associated with oxidative phosphorylation.

Pyrroloquinoline Quinone (PQQ) and 6-Hydroxydopa (topa) Quinone

A cofactor known to be present in methylogenic bacteria and other microorganisms, PQQ was considered at first to be a cofactor for mammalian copper amine oxidases and other copper enzymes. Its essential nature led some workers to consider PQQ an undiscovered vitamin. This, however, turned out not to be the case and PQQ as a cofactor has now been relegated to the world of microorganisms.

What at first was thought to be PQQ in copper oxidases turned out to be a cofactor with quinone

properties that was derived by modifying a tyrosine residue in the enzyme (Figure 13). The synthesis of 6-hydroxy (topa) quinone, a derivative of tyrosine, requires copper in an apparently autocatalytic reaction. Though rare and limited, this most unusual biochemical reaction opens a new chapter on cofactors by showing that some enzymes have a limited but specific capacity

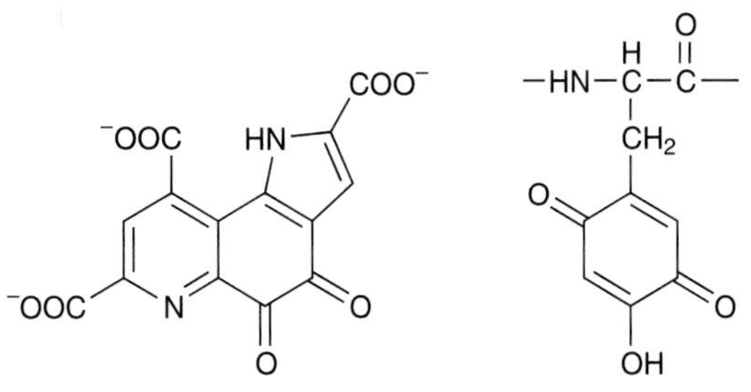

PQQ

6-Hydroxydopa (topa) quinone

Figure 13 Comparison of structures of pyrroloquinoline quinone (PQQ) with topa quinone. Cofactor on the right has been identified in mammalian systems.

to synthesize cofactors on their surface through modification of existing amino acid side chains.

Other

There are a number of natural organic compounds that do not quite fit the description of cofactors, yet have been identified as being involved with stabilizing enzymes or taking part in a select series of reactions. We include them here with the caveat that some may behave more as substrates than cofactors.

Glutathione

Glutathione is a naturally occurring tripeptide that is known to exist in millimolar quantities in cells. The reduced form (GSH) has exposed -SH groups associated with an internal cysteine residue that has been shown to figure prominently in the stability of enzymes that have -SH groups at the active site. Glutathione partakes in many biological reactions such as amino acid transport, heavy metal transport, and antioxidant activity. Its cofactor role, however, should not be overlooked since GSH has been shown to activate many enzymes or retain their catalytic effectiveness during assays. One suspects, with justification, that this could be one of the functions of GSH *in vivo*.

Betaine

Betaine *(N,N,N-trimethylglycine)* arises from choline by an oxidation reaction. The structure is a trimethyl derivative of glycine. Betaine occurs in very small quantities in cells and has been shown to be a methyl donor for a limited number of reactions, notably synthesis of methionine from homocysteine.

S-Adenosylmethionine

To consider *S*-adenosylmethionine (SAM, also known as adomet) a cofactor is to recognize its role in a multitude of reactions that transfer methyl groups to substrates. Thus, SAM is involved in an extensive series of methylation reactions that surpass methylations of either N^5-methyl-FH$_4$ or methyl cobalamin combined. The methyl group transferred is the terminal carbon of methionine. To activate the methyl group, methionine reacts with ATP, adding an adenosyl group to the sulfur atom and causing a high-energy methyl-donating species to form (**Figure 14**). Although SAM is perhaps more of a substrate than a cofactor, its inclusion here is to denote the importance of methionine and its reactive

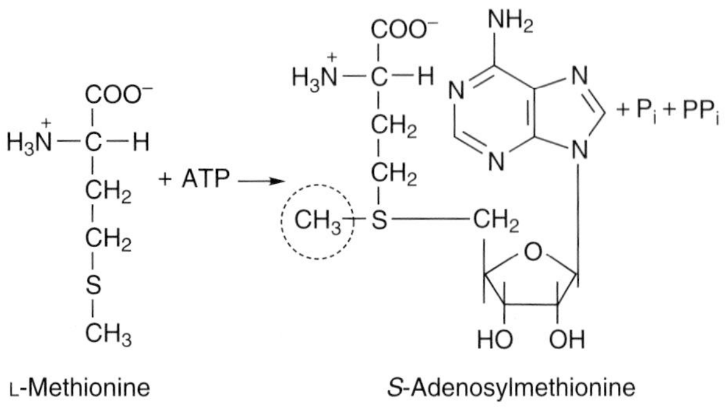

Figure 14 Synthesis of *S*-adenosylmethionine from methionine. Note the favorable positioning of the methyl group of methionine (dotted circle) as a result of the condensation with ATP.

form, SAM, in a series of extremely important biosynthetic reactions.

3′ Phosphoadenosine-5′ Phosphosulfate (PAPS)

PAPS is a cofactor for sulfation reactions, a process confined largely to plants and bacteria, but an important metabolic reaction in humans. PAPS serves as an active agent for sulfate esterification, as in the synthesis of sulfated polysaccharides such as chondroitin sulfate, keratin sulfate, and heparin.

Conclusions

Of the 20 or so organic cofactors that have been discovered over the years, the structures of more than half are derived from the nucleus of vitamins, primarily the water-soluble B vitamins. As companions to enzymes, organic cofactors relate to all forms of life. While we may think of vitamins as being needed by only higher organisms, many organic factors were designed to serve exclusively with enzymes and imperfections in enzyme systems that gave vitamins an essential character were revealed in bacteria and yeast systems long before they became known in humans. The carryover between cofactor-dependent reactions in microorganisms and humans has been remarkable, an illustration of the structure-function principle of biochemistry. Still, we must not overlook the fact that the study of cofactors has brought a sharper focus to the role of dietary components in human health and nutrition. Whereas mutated bacteria may fail to grow for want of a vitamin synthesized *de novo*, a susceptible human will develop a deficiency symptom. Both need the vitamin factor in a failing enzyme system in order for that system to perform at a healthy capacity. Nutritionists are challenged to learn the function of all cofactors because that information provides fundamental insights into a chemical blueprint that applies to a wide spectrum of different organisms at the molecular level.

See also: **Anemia**: Megaloblastic Anemia. **Ascorbic Acid**: Physiology, Dietary Sources and Requirements; Deficiency States. **Biotin. Cobalamins. Cofactors**: Inorganic. **Folic Acid. Niacin. Pantothenic Acid. Riboflavin. Thiamin**: Physiology; Beriberi. **Vitamin A**: Deficiency and Interventions. **Vitamin B₆. Vitamin D**: Rickets and Osteomalacia. **Vitamin K**.

Further Reading

Brown DE, McGuir MA, Dooley DM, Jane SM, Mu D, and Klinman JP (1991) The organic functional group in copper-containing amine oxidases. Resonance Raman spectra are consistent with the presence of TOPA quinone (6-hydroxy quinone) in the active site. *Journal of Biological Chemistry* 266: 4049–4051.

Carpenter KJ (2003) A short history of nutritional science: Part 3 (1912–1944). *Journal of Nutrition* 133: 3023–3032.

Freedland RA and Briggs S (1977) *A Biochemical Approach to Nutrition.* London: Chapman and Hall.

Harris ED (1992) The pyrroloquinoline quinone (PQQ) coenzyme: a case of mistaken identity. *Nutrition Reviews* 50: 263–267.

Jukes TH (1977) Adventures with vitamins. In: Klemm WR (ed.) *Discovery Processes in Modern Biology,* pp. 152–170. New York, NY: Krieger.

Kutsky JK (1973) *Handbook of Vitamins & Hormones.* London: Van Nostrand Reinhold.

Marks J (1975) *A Guide to the Vitamins. Their Role in Health and Disease.* Baltimore: University Park Press.

Mathews CK and van Holde KE (1990) *Biochemistry.* Redwood City, CA: Benjamin Cummings.

Shive W and Lansford EM Jr. (1980) Roles of vitamins as coenzymes. In: Alfin-Slater RB and Kritchevsky D (eds.) *Human Nutrition. A Comprehensive Treatise: Nutrition and the Adult, Micronutrients,* vol. 3B, ch. 1, pp. 1–71. New York: Plenum Press.

Coffee *see* **Caffeine**

COLON

Contents
Structure and Function
Disorders
Nutritional Management of Disorders

Structure and Function

A Maqbool, The Children's Hospital of Philadelphia, Philadelphia, PA, USA

© 2005 Elsevier Ltd. All rights reserved.

The colon is a dynamic organ involved in the absorption of salts, fluids, and nutrients, and it has a primary role in defecatory function. Additionally, the colon is an immunologically active tubular cavity playing an important part in host immune responses and defense from pathogens.

Gross Morphology

The colon is a continuous structure originating at the ileocecal valve and extending to the anus. The cecum is the first part of the colon, which lies in a posterior position at the right iliac fossa and has an ovoid-like shape. This cavity is more generous in proportion than other compartments of the colon. The appendix (a blind-ending out pouching) originates in the cecum and its opening is usually visible during colonoscopy.

The ascending colon runs cephalad and anteriorly from the cecum to just inferior to the liver, to the hepatic flexure, emerging into the peritoneum. The transverse colon continues from the hepatic flexure to the splenic flexure, from which it travels distally and once again posteriorly to the sigmoid colon, an S-shaped, tortuous, narrow peritoneal structure. At the peritoneal reflection, the rectum arises and, closely following the sacral curve, leads to the anal canal. The rectum is a vault-like structure that can distend in order to accommodate fecal load. The anal canal bears two sphincters, an internal and an external anal sphincter. The internal sphincter is composed of inner circular smooth muscle fibers and a distal external fiber on the other side of a muscular pelvic diaphragm. The fibers of the external sphincter are intertwined with those of the levator ani, tethered anteriorly and posteriorly to the perineal body and the coccyx, respectively.

With respect to colonic mobility within the abdominal, peritoneal, and pelvic cavities, the cecum and flexures are less mobile, with the sigmoid colon being the most mobile. The transverse colon supports the greater omentum and has a variable degree of mobility.

Cross-sectionally, the colon has an external longitudinal muscle and an inner layer of circular musculature, the former of which has coalescence of fibers forming band-like structures known as taeniaecoli. These taeniae are particular to the large intestine, are located at one-third of the circumference from each other, and run continuously from one end of the colon to the other. Haustra are hemilunar-like outpouchings present between taeniae. The more proximal rectal taenial fibers surround the rectum; the inner fibers form the internal anal sphincter. The external fibers are intertwined with those of the levator ani and sandwiched between fibers running anterior to posterior from the peroneal body to the coccyx, forming the external sphincter.

Vasculature

The ascending colon and portions of the transverse colon are perfused by branches of the superior mesenteric artery, with the remainder of the colon receiving arterial blood from tributaries of the inferior mesenteric artery. Distal iliac arterial branches perfuse the anal canal. Venous drainage is achieved via the superior and inferior mesenteric veins laying in close proximity to their arterial counterparts and subsequently dumping into the portal vein.

Additional gross morphologic structures include lymphatic vessels, in close approximation to the vasculature, leading to lymph nodes in the celiac, superior, and inferior preaortic regions. Perianal drainage is via the inguinal lymph nodes.

Innervation

Parasympathetic innervation to the proximal colon is provided via the vagus nerve; the distal colon and rectum are innervated via pelvic parasympathetic fibers. The sympathetic nervous system innervates the proximal colon via lower thoracic fibers and the distal colon and rectum via lumbar fibers. Prevertebral sympathetic vertebrae receive fibers from neurons projecting out of the gut.

Histology

Cross-sectionally, the intestinal wall is divided into four layers, with the serosa, a monolayer of mesothelial cells comprising the outermost layer, followed by the muscularis externa. These muscle layers comprise an external longitudinal layer and an internal circular layer. Sandwiched between these two layers lies Auerbach's (myenteric) plexus. The submucosa is the next more medial layer. A rich admixture of cells, including structural elements such as fibroblasts and dense connective tissue, immunologically important cells (plasma cells, lymphocytes, macrophages, eosinophils, and mast cells), and vascular tissue and innervation to Meissner's plexus (ganglion cells) and lymphatics comprise this layer. The muscularis mucosa, a thin sheet of smooth muscle, separates the deeper submucosa from the mucosa. The lamina propria runs interior to this layer, is composed of connective tissue, and is lined by the luminal epithelium (**Figure 1A**).

The intestinal epithelium is a tight monolayer of cells that function to absorb nutrients, electrolytes, and liquids as well as to secrete mucous and fluids. The epithelial surface is punctuated by numerous tightly packed crypts, which contain epithelial precursor cells, enterendocrine cells, other undifferentiated cells, and Paneth cells. Goblet cells, which secrete mucin, are also located in the crypt (**Figures 1B** and **1C, Table 1**). As undifferentiated and precursor cells mature, they migrate superiorly to the surface to the monolayer of absorptive cells present in crypts. The average life span of a colonocyte is 3–6 days.

The absorptive colonocyte develops short microvilli while in the colonic crypt, which elongate during its migration to the surface. The hydrophobic lipid bilayer of the colonocyte epithelium prevents passive transport of charged particles. The epithelial membrane contains specific protein transporters, carrier proteins, and channels allowing electrolyte transport. The electrochemical gradient formed by active transport facilitates passive flow across cell membranes.

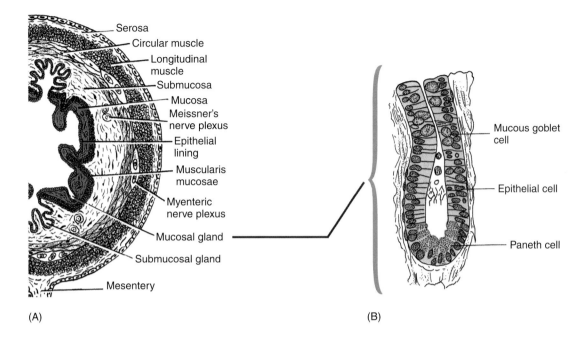

(A)   (B)

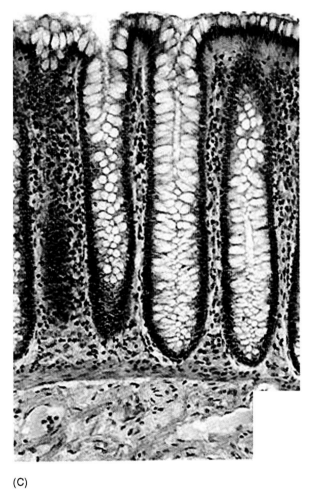

(C)

Figure 1   (A) Cross section of the gut and (B) a colonic crypt. (Reproduced with permission from Guyton (1991) *Guyton's Textbook of Medical Physiology*, 8th edn. Philadelphia: WB Saunders.) (C) Histology H&E stain of a colonic crypt, with prominence of mucin-containing goblet cells. (Reproduced with permission from Burkett HG, Young B, and Heath JW (1993) *Wheater's Functional Histology*, 3rd edn. London: Churchill Livingstone.)

Table 1 Colonic cell types

Cell type	Location	Function(s)
Stem cells	Crypt (base) Nonmigratory until differentiated	Pluripotent
Undifferentiated crypt cell	Crypt	Secrete water and chloride into intestinal lumen
Paneth cells	Crypt base Nonmigratory Basophilic cytoplasm Proximal one-third of colon only	Growth factor secretion, digestive enzyme synthesis Antimicrobial peptide synthesis and release
Goblet cells	Colonic crypt Most common cell type in the colon	Mucin release
Enteroendocrine cells	Mostly in small intestine Basolateral membrane	Receptor-mediated epithelial cell function modulators
Enterocytes	Predominantly small intestinal; present in the colon	Digestive enzyme synthesis (small intestine) Ion transporters and channels involved in fluid and electrolyte transport
M cells	Small and large intestines Overlying lymphoid follicles	Bind, process, and present antigens to components of the mucosal lymphoid immune system
Intraepithelial lymphocytes	Small and large intestines Basolateral membranes	Memory T cells Mucosal immune defense

Electrolyte Transport: Ion Channels

Fluids and electrolytes are absorbed via either the transcellular or the paracellular pathway. Active and passive transport systems exist via both of these pathways.

There is a clear polarity to the distribution of protein transporters, channels, and pumps distinguishing the apical from the basolateral membrane. Active transport utilizes a transcellular, energy-driven protein pump or channel to facilitate passage of an electrolyte from an area of low concentration to one of high concentration (electrochemical gradient). A prime example of this is the NA-K ATPase pump, the principal pump present along the basolateral membrane. The net effect of the three Na ions expelled for every two K ions accepted into the cell is a lowered intracellular Na content and resultant net negative charge. The negative charge formed by this active transport creates an electrochemical gradient facilitative to the passive flow for other ions across the cell membrane—a process known as secondary active transport (**Figure 2**).

Ion transporters may be subclassified into symporters, in which ions move in the same direction, or antiporters, in which ions move in opposite directions across the cell membrane (**Figure 3**). Cotransport of ions occurs with other molecules, such as Na and glucose. The intracellular concentration of glucose is regulated both by uptake at the apical surface and by exit through the basolateral membrane, allowing for conditions favorable to uptake from the lumen. The Na-glucose transporter system allows for therapeutic interventions, such as the use of oral rehydration solution in cases of severe diarrhea related to cholera or other processes. Similar cotransporters are linked to the transport of bile salts and amino acids (**Table 2**).

Whereas sodium is the primary cation involved in ion transport, short-chain fatty acids constitute the primary anion in the colon and the primary metabolic fuel for colonocytes. Their transport is postulated to be linked to Na-H transporters and pH, specific bicarbonate-linked transporters, and the concentration gradient across cell membranes. Chloride transport occurs via both active and passive processes, and it is the major intestinal anion involved in intestinal secretion of fluids.

Colonic smooth channels also possess ion channels and are involved in active and secondary ion

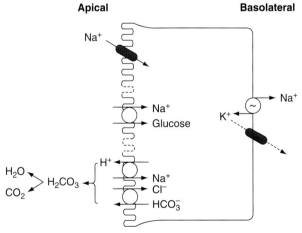

Figure 2 Electrolyte transport at the colonocyte level. (From Despopoulos A and Silbernagl S, *Color Atlas of Physiology*. New York: Thieme; 2000. Reprinted with permission.)

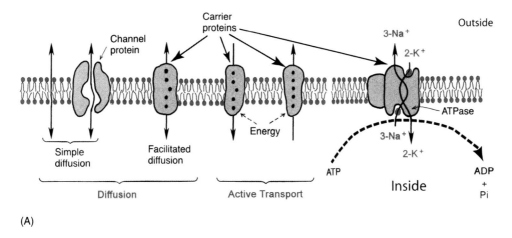

(A)

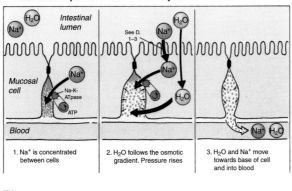

(B)

Figure 3 Electrolyte transport across the cell membrane and the different types of tranporters. (Reproduced with permission from Guyton (1991) *Guyton's Textbook of Medical Physiology*, 8th edn. Philadelphia: WB Saunders.)

transport processes involving calcium. The electrochemical gradient formed by the activity of these ion channels facilitates the function of smooth muscle action potential generation upon depolarization. With the generation of smooth muscle action potentials attaining threshold voltage, contractility of the smooth muscle is possible. The efflux of calcium into these active transport channels activates the process of contraction. Interaction with the enteric nervous system stimulates the release of calcium ions in intracellular stores. The function of ion channels can be modified by calcium channel-blocking drugs. This contractile activity, when it occurs in a coordinated fashion and is modulated by neurotransmission, effects peristalsis and colonic motility.

Fluid Transport

There is heterogeneity to the mucosal epithelium in several aspects dependent on the location in the alimentary canal. The type, variety, and number of ion transporters, channels, and carrier proteins vary from region to region (e.g., from jejunum to colon). Additionally, the nature of interepithelial cell junctions varies from the proximal to distal intestinal tract, influencing the 'leakiness' of the respective regions. Finally, a clear gradient in cell composition and function between colonic crypt cells and those on the surface exists. Physiologic heterogeneity follows the aforementioned patterns, defining tissue function in these respective areas. For example, the colonic crypts serve more of a secretory function, whereas the villus structures seen most notably in the jejunum exhibit greater absorptive function. This heterogeneity is key in understanding changes in intraluminal osmolality and fluid shifts that occur in the intestine.

Approximately 98% (9 l per day) of the daily fluid load handled by the intestine is reabsorbed. Of this, the jejunum absorbs 85%, and the colon absorbs approximately 13% (1.5 l).

Passive reabsorption of water occurs in the intestines, regulated primarily by electrolyte transport (i.e., following an osmotic gradient). Na-driven or -related transport mechanisms are the primary driving force

Table 2   Electrolyte transport

Ion	Transporter	Location	Type	Function(s)
Na	Na-K-ATPase	Basolateral membrane	Active; antiport	Principal ion involved in water absorption
	Na-H exchangers	Apical and basolateral membrane	Secondary; antiport	
Na and Cl	NaCl	Apical	Antiport; passive; electrochemically neutral	
Cl	Protein channel	Apical	Diffusion; passive (secretion) and some active transport proteins at the apical surface (absorption and secretion), including CFTR	Principal ion involved in water secretion
				Basal rate of secretion influenced by several mediators (endocrine, paracrine, neural, luminal, etc.)
Cl	Protein channel			
K	Protein channel		Antiport; active transport (basolateral membrane)	
			Active secretion at the apical membrane; linked to Cl transport function	
			Absorptive active apical K-ATPase pumps in distal colon	
HCO$_3$		Apical and basolateral channels	Alkaline phosphatase linked	
			Passive transport mechanisms	
			Na-HCO$_3$ cotransporter postulated	
			CFTR-synchronized apical channel and Cl-HCO$_3$ exchanger postulated	
Short-chain fatty acids	Apical		Postulated link to NA-H ion transport	Principal anion of the colon

allowing water absorption. This osmotic gradient facilitates water absorption via both transcellular and paracellular pathways.

Transcellular water transport mechanisms such as aquaporins, or water channels, have been described. The paracellular pathway of water transport has been studied extensively, a process often described as 'solvent drag' (**Figure 4A**).

The leakiness of paracellular pathways, which varies by location in the lower alimentary tract (more prominent in the jejunum, with subsequent decrease distally), and the magnitude of the osmotic gradient (also affected by dietary Na content) are important factors affecting solvent drag. The nature of the intercellular junctions in a particular region of the colon determines the permeability or leakiness of that particular epithelial area. Several intercellular structures have been described, including the zona accludens (tight junction), desmosomes (connections between cells), and the zona adherens, which functions in cell adhesion and contributes to maintaining cellular polarity across the membrane. Zona occuldens are more apical in location and form junctional complexes between cells. It has been postulated that these junctional complexes may be more dynamic

than previously believed, responding to signaling mechanisms and subject to regulation, thereby influencing their function and resultant permeability characteristics (**Figure 4B**).

The Enteric Nervous System and Gastrointestinal Motility

The enteric nervous system (ENS) operates both in conjunction with and independent of the peripheral nervous system. As discussed previously, nerve plexi exist within the bowel wall, with Auerbach's plexus sandwiched between longitudinal and circular muscle layers, and Meissner's plexus located more medially in the submucosa. The ENS is the largest component of the autonomic nervous system, based on nerve cell number.

Interstitial cells of Cajal, a cell type unique to the alimentary tract, are present medial to the inner smooth muscle layer. These specialized cells interact with myenteric neurons and are thought to exhibit independent electrical activity, generating and transmitting slow waves to smooth muscle, functioning as pacemakers for colonic motility. The ENS

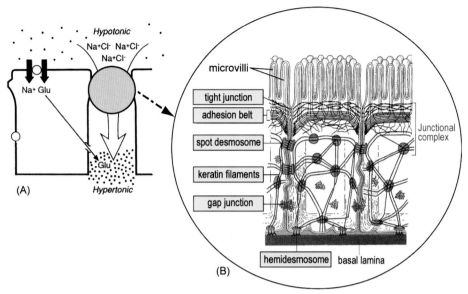

Figure 4 (A) Fluid transport across the cell membrane. (Reproduced with permission from Shils ME, Olson JA, Shike M, and Ross AC (1999) *Modern Nutrition in Health and Disease*, 9th edn. Baltimore: Lippincott Williams & Wilkins.) (B) Intercellular junctions. (Reproduced with permission from Alberts B, Bray D, Lewis J, Raff M, Roberts K, and Watson JD (1989) *Molecular Biology of the Cell*, 2nd edn. Garland Publishing, NY.

functions independent of the central nervous system, with reflex activity in response to luminal stimuli, including muscle contraction and coordination (i.e., motility, blood flow, and glandular secretion). Modulation of the ENS is via the sympathetic and parasympathetic nervous system.

Colonic Motility

The colon functions to delay passage of luminal contents to allow for water absorption and for mixing of luminal contents with the mucosa, to store fecal matter prior to defecation, and, at the time of defecation, to propel contents forward.

The frequency and duration of propagative, high-pressure waves in the colon in part are determined by pressure exerted by intraluminal contents (mechanical) and the degree of stretch stimulation, the (chemical) composition of the contents, and other stimuli interacting with the colon.

The gastrocolic reflex, an anterograde postperistaltic process, occurs following a meal, originating proximally and propagating anterograde. Both the caloric content and the fat composition of the meal influence colonic peristalsis. Gastric distention by food contents, water, or gas also has a stimulatory effect. Gastrointestinal hormones secreted in response to a meal, such as cholecystokinin, are thought to mediate peristaltic responses to a (fatty) meal. Irritant laxatives also stimulate peristalsis, even when administered rectally. Opiates are

known to inhibit the ENS and, as a consequence, retard peristalsis. Colonic motility diminishes significantly during sleep, resuming upon awakening.

Motor activity varies by colonic region; in degree, frequency, amplitude, and velocity; in being propagative versus nonpropagative (the latter is more common in the distal colon); in relative distance of propagation; and in direction of propagation (anterograde versus retrograde, the latter most commonly seen in the proximal colon). Approximately one-third of these colonic peristaltic waves are propulsive, and those associated with propulsion of stool tend to be slower but greater in amplitude.

Defecation involves the integration of peristaltic activity in the majority of colonic regions, not exclusively to that solely in the anorectal region. In the predefecatory phase, approximately 1 h prior to actual defecation, the majority of the colon exhibits an increase in propulsive peristaltic waves, first in the proximal colon and then advancing distally.

The sensation of defecatory urge is not evident until approximately 15 minutes prior to defecation. At that time, there is a marked increase in propagative peristaltic activity, originating more distally in the colon. Each of these late propagative waves successively originates proximate to the preceding one with greater amplitude and presents over a greater distance of colonic length.

Stool contact with the receptors in the upper anal canal can effect relaxation of the inner anal sphincter. In addition, stretch receptor stimulation of the

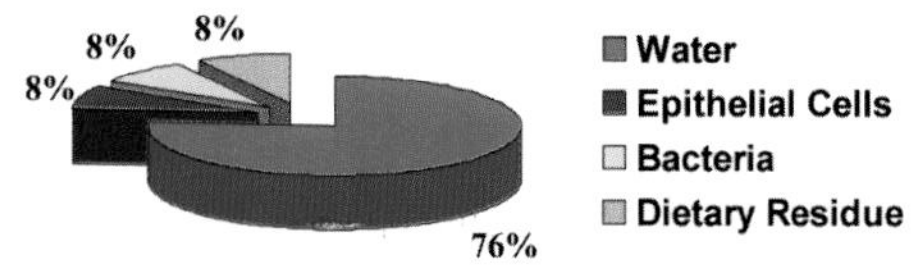

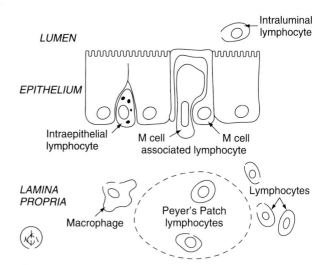

Figure 5 Composition of feces (60–80 g/day).

rectal vault walls results in the urge to defecate. Failure of relaxation of the external anal sphincter (which is under voluntary control) results in retrograde passage of stool into the rectum, with subsequent diminishing of more proximal peristaltic propagative waves, thereby maintaining continence when immediate defecation is not desirable or convenient.

Evacuation of the rectum and defecation require correcting the angle of the anal canal in the anterior–posterior plane, which is accomplished by assuming a squatting position. Contraction of the abdominal musculature and of the diaphragm, with a relaxed pelvic floor, facilitates defecation, even in the absence of colonic peristalsis.

Stool size and consistency vary based on diet, water intake, and transit time, as well as bacterial content (a major component of stool). Higher water content tends to result in larger, softer stools. The more fusiform-shaped the stool is, the less likely that its passage is associated with straining. The transit time through the colon is inversely related to the stool's water content and, hence, its consistency (**Figure 5**).

Colonic Immune Function and Colonic Bacterial Flora

The immune system of the gastrointestinal tract defends against infection (bacterial, viral, and parasitic) and luminal antigens ingested/formed by bacteria. Nonspecific and specific mechanisms exist.

The mucin secreted by colonic goblet cells serves a barrier function for the mucosal surface. Mucosal integrity is an important barrier to luminal pathogens. Interepithelial cell junctions function both to control permeability as pertains to fluid and electrolyte absorption and to prevent pathogen access beyond this layer.

The enteric immune system is vast and complex; it interacts with the rest of the immune system as well as with luminal contents. Gut-associated lymphoid tissue consists of both discretely organized tissue, such as Peyer's patches (lymphoid follicles with proliferative potential in response to antigen presentation) containing M cells, and the more diffuse lymphocytes and macrophages distributed among the submucosa, mucosa, and lamina propria (**Figure 6**). M cells function in antigen sampling of

Figure 6 Mucosal immunology. (Reproduced with permission from Shils ME, Olson JA, Shike M, and Ross AC (1999) Modern Nutrition in Health and Disease, 9th edn. Baltimore: Lippincott Williams & Wilkins.)

intraluminal contents by binding antigens, endocytosis, antigen processing, and subsequent interaction with lymphocytes and macrophages within Peyer's patches, eliciting host responses. The lymphocyte complement of Peyer's patches originate in either the bone marrow or the thymus, enter the systemic circulation to migrate to Peyer's patches, interact, return to the intestinal mucosa or, via mesenteric lymph nodes, re-enter the systemic circulation to other organs.

The gastrointestinal tract houses up to 80% of the body's immunoglobulin-producing cells. Intraepithelial T lymphocytes, plasma cells, macrophages, dendritic cells, eosinophils, and mast cells also function in a specialized manner (**Figure 7**).

Secretory IgA is an important host immune defense mechanism. Unlike the monomeric, systemic form of IgA, intestinal secretory IgA is polymeric (specifically, dimeric) in nature. This dimeric immunoglobulin is secreted by B lymphocytes situated in the lamina propria, and it contains a unique 'J' chain instrumental in polymer formation. This IgA binds to the Ig receptor of the epithelial cell on the basolateral membrane and, following endocytosis and transport across the cell, is secreted from the apical side.

Secretory IgA binds to intraluminal antigens, including dietary ones, and functions in preventing their absorption. Additionally, secretory IgA has the ability to bind to microorganisms, thus preventing adherence, colonization, and invasion. Secretory IgA is secreted in breast milk, and in breast-fed neonates and infants it confers a degree of passive immunity to infection by limiting luminal contents from interacting with, or directly binding to or invading, the mucosa.

Interaction of intraluminal bacteria with the immune system may affect intestinal permeability, and it may modulate the intestinal immune system. Certain bacterial species are believed to interact with other enteric flora as well as with the host immune system to effect a healthier gastrointestinal tract and enhance nutrient digestion. Organisms studied include Lactobacillus, *Vibrio* species, and sacromyces. These findings, among others beneficial to the host, have prompted investigation into oral supplementation of single and multiple species of these probiotics for prevention and treatment of antibiotic-associated diarrhea, bacterial overgrowth in short bowel syndrome, and as an adjuvant therapy for inflammatory bowel disease, as well as for the treatment and prevention of recurrent clostridium difficile colitis.

Regulation of the quantity of bacteria, in addition to the specific profile of bacterial species present, is dependent on a host of factors, including gastric acid output, gastrointestinal motility, luminal contents, and the milieu created therein. Additionally, the intraluminal environmental milieu is affected by the specific properties of different species of bacteria and their interactions with other luminal species and with the host.

The colon accommodates the largest number of enteric flora, on the order of 10^{10}–10^{12}—more than 100 000 flora and more than 100-fold greater diversity of species than in any other location in the alimentary canal. Efflux of bacteria into the ileum is hindered by the ileocecal valve, which functions to restrict several of these bacterial species to the large intestine. The majority of these colonic bacteria are anaerobic in nature (**Table 3**).

Table 3 Colonic enteric flora

Bacterial genus	Prevalence (%)	Total count (CFU/g or ml)
Anaerobes		10^9–10^{12}
Bacteroides	100	
Porphyromonas	100	
Bifidobacterium	30–70	
Lactobacillus	20–60	
Clostridium	25–35	
Peptostreptococcus	—	
Peptococcus	—	
Methanogens	—	
Facultative aerobes		10^2–10^9
Enterococcus	100	
Escherichia coli	100	
Staphylococcus	30–50	
Other Enterobacteriaceae	40–80	

Table 4 Examples of biochemical reactions by intestinal flora

Reaction type	Reaction	Example substrate
Hydrolysis	Amides	Methotrexate
	Glucuronides	Estradiol-3-glucuronide
Dehydroxylation	Decarboxylation	Amino acids
	Deamination	Amino acids
	Dehydrogenase	Bile acids, cholesterol
Reduction	Double bonds	Unsaturated fatty acids
	Acetylation	Histamine

From Klein S, Cohn SM and Alpers DH (1999) The alimentary tract in nutrition. In: *Modern Nutrition in Health & Disease*, 9th edn, pp. 605–631. Baltimore: Williams & Wilkins.

The enteric flora plays several important roles. It interacts with the enteric immune system, effecting cellular immune activity; it is associated with the size and number of Peyer's patches present, influencing intestinal motility; and it has nutritively important functions, including bile salt deconjugation (facilitating enterohepatic circulation of bile salts), bilirubin metabolism (deconjugation and urobilin formation, allowing excretion), mucin degradation, and lipid metabolism (generation of short-chain fatty acids). Androgens and estrogens are hydrolyzed, facilitating resorption and conservation of these sterols, whereas cholesterol is processed into coprostanol, a nonabsorbed sterol. Ammoniagenesis via protein and urea degradation may play a role in hepatic encephalopathy (**Table 4**).

Consumption of lipids, carbohydrates, and protein also occurs by colonic bacteria, in addition to that of vitamins (vitamin B_{12} and folic acid are consumed; vitamin K and biotin are produced by these bacteria).

Dietary Fiber and the Colon

Nondigestible carbohydrates, traditionally defined as deriving from plant sources (but recently encompassing some non-plant-derived polysaccharides), that escape digestion and reach the colon nearly 100% intact compromise dietary fiber.

The metabolic fate of this fiber is influenced primarily by the colonic bacterial complement, which, depending on its structure, may render it susceptible to fermentation (such as pectin and oat bran). Common by-products of colonic fermentation include carbon dioxide, methane (in addition to other gases), oligofructases (among the classes of compounds of oligosaccharides termed prebiotics because of their nutritive support for the sustainment of certain colonic bacteria thought to be beneficial to human health—the so-called probiotics), and short-chain fatty acids.

The common short-chain fatty acids produced by fermentation include acetate, butyrate, and proprionate. The pattern of short-chain fatty acid production is dependent on several dynamic factors, including the type of fiber or oligosaccharide present in the diet, the transit time and exposure to bacteria, and the bacteria flora to which the substrate is being exposed. Short-chain fatty acids influence colonic physiology by stimulating colonic blood flow as well as fluid and electrolyte uptake. Butyrate in particular is thought to be preferred fuel for the colonocyte. This short-chain fatty acid is thought to have a role in maintaining the normal phenotype in these cells (i.e., in decreasing the risk of dyplasia by promoting differentiation and apoptosis of these cells). Because there is a lack of agreement on the *in vivo* and *in vitro* effects of the latter chemopreventive role of butyrate, it is commonly referred to the 'butyrate paradox.' Comparisons between these two models may have to do with the assumptions made with respect to environment and conditions. These include duration and patterns of exposure of the colonic to butyrate, interactions with other dietary components (such as the omega-3 dietary fats), and the confounding effect of dietary fiber that is resistant to digestion as well as to fermentation by the colon.

Nondigestible dietary fiber is also thought to play an important role in chemoprevention by diluting toxins, carcinogens, and tumor promoters; by decreasing transit time, thereby decreasing colonic mucosal exposure; and by promoting their expulsion in the fecal stream.

Dietary fiber resistant to colonic degradation may also play a role in maintaining and promoting stool bulk and in the regulation of intraluminal pressure/colonic wall resistance, disordered colonic motility, or both. These consequences of lack of dietary fiber have been linked to constipation as well as to the development of diverticulosis. Epidemiologically, the observed pattern of diverticulosis is striking: A dichotomy between the industrialized world and developing countries is clearly noted, and it is believed to be very closely linked to dietary fiber content. The nutrition transition and changes in lifestyle may impact dietary fiber intake and, as a consequence, may eventually be reflected by changing patterns of incidence and prevalence of processes linked to low dietary fiber intake, as mentioned previously.

See also: **Colon**: Disorders; Nutritional Management of Disorders. **Diarrheal Diseases**. **Dietary Fiber**: Physiological Effects and Effects on Absorption; Potential Role in Etiology of Disease; Role in Nutritional Management of Disease. **Electrolytes**: Water–Electrolyte Balance. **Fatty Acids**: Metabolism. **Microbiota of the Intestine**: Prebiotics; Probiotics. **Potassium**. **Small Intestine**: Structure and Function. **Sodium**: Physiology.

Further Reading

Feldman (2002) *Sleisenger & Fordtran's Gastrointestinal & Liver Disease*, 7th edn. Philadelphia: WB Saunders.

Food and Nutrition Board (2001) *Dietary Reference Intakes: Proposed Definition of Dietary Fiber*, A report of the Panel on the Definition of Dietary Fiber and the Standing Committee on the Scientific Evaluation of Dietary Reference Intakes. Institute of Medicine. Washington DC: National Academy Press.

Klein S, Cohn SM, and Alpers DH (1999) The alimentary tract in nutrition. In: *Modern Nutrition in Health & Disease*, 9th edn, pp. 605–631. Baltimore, MD: Williams & Wilkins.

Netter FH (1999) *Netter's Interactive Atlas of Human Anatomy*, version 2.0 East Hanover, NJ: Novartis Pharmaceuticals Medical Education Division.

Walker WA, Durie PR, Hamilton JR, Walker Smith JA, and Watkins JB (eds.) (2000) *Pediatric Gastrointestinal Disease: Pathology, Diagnosis, Management*, 3rd edn. Hamilton, Ontario, Canada: BC Decker.

Willie R and Hyams J (1999) *Pediatric Gastrointestinal Disease*, 2nd edn. Philadelphia: WB Saunders.

Disorders

A Maqbool, The Children's Hospital of Philadelphia, Philadelphia, PA, USA

© 2005 Elsevier Ltd. All rights reserved.

Diarrhea

Diarrhea is defined as a decrease in stool consistency and/or an increase in stool frequency and volume. It results from a complex interplay between colonic epithelial cell function, luminal factors, intestinal motility, and other factors.

Stool consistency and volume are determined partly by dietary factors (e.g., fiber intake) and fluid and electrolyte transport. Electrolyte transport mechanisms and diffusion processes in the small intestine render the fluid milieu isotonic. Active (primary and secondary) electrolyte transport mechanisms create an electrochemical gradient by which means cotransport of additional electrolytes can occur. Sodium is the major cation involved in the process of fluid absorption. Chloride constitutes the major anion that plays a significant role in fluid transport, and its active export into the intestinal lumen is an important mechanism of intestinal fluid secretion. Potassium and bicarbonate also play a role in intestinal absorption and secretion mechanisms. Water transport is facilitated by this osmotic gradient. It is then absorbed by processes of transcellular passage facilitated by aquaporins as well as by solvent drag via paracellular pathway; paracellular permeability is regulated by junctional complexes. Glucose transport is linked to sodium transport, as is the case for certain amino acids. Electrolyte transporter function can be influenced by glucocorticoids and mineralocorticoids.

Intestinal motility also influences stool volume and consistency. The enteric nervous system, with some modulation by the autonomic nervous system, is the primary regulator of gastrointestinal motility. Neuropeptides, gastrointestinal hormones, and luminal stimuli, such as dietary factors and interactions with bacteria, influence colonic motility.

Mechanisms of diarrhea can also be viewed from the perspective of absorptive capacity of the small intestine and colon. Of the 8–10 l of fluid processed by the small and large intestines daily (composed of intake as well as gastrointestinal secretions), the smaller intestine absorbs 80–90% of the net load. The normal adult colon absorbs approximately 1 l of fluid per day but has a capacity to absorb 3 or 4 l per day; diarrhea results when this threshold is exceeded.

From a pathophysiological perspective, four mechanisms of diarrhea are traditionally described: osmotic, secretory, motility, and inflammatory. A degree of overlap occurs between these different types of diarrhea.

Osmotic diarrhea occurs when the failure to absorb a solute (usually a carbohydrate) in the proximal small intestine occurs, thus rendering the fluid hypertonic rather than isotonic, as would regularly occur. Whereas electrolytes may be reabsorbed, the carbohydrate is not; rather, a portion of it is metabolized by enteric flora to short-chain fatty acids, carbon dioxide, hydrogen, and methane. With sodium and other electrolytes absorbed readily by the colon, and resultant low-sodium concentration in the lumen, compounded by the presence of nonabsorbed carbohydrate, the high osmotic gradient draws fluid into the lumen and results in diarrhea. This type of diarrhea is characterized by a significant osmotic gap that can be calculated; an additional clinically significant feature of this type of diarrhea is that it diminishes upon cessation of enteral intake. Malabsorbed carbohydrate and its metabolites effect a lowering of the pH of the stool as well. Lactose deficiency is a good example of osmotic diarrhea in both children and adults. Ingestion

of nonabsorbable sugars, such as sorbitol, can also lead to osmotic diarrhea. In children, excess intake of fruit beverages or of carbohydrates when recovering from a bout of acute gastroenteritis can occur, which resolves upon cessation of consumption of the carbohydrate.

Secretory diarrhea occurs when the net secretion of fluids and electrolytes from the colon exceeds their absorption. This type of diarrhea exists independent of eating and is not influenced by fasting or bowel rest. The prototypical example of pure secretory diarrhea (i.e., in the absence of inflammation or blood present in the stool) is of congenital chloride transport defects and of gastrointestinal hormonal disorders, such as in Zollinger–Ellison syndrome and disorders of vasoactive intestinal peptide or in other neuroendocrine tumors (**Figure 1**).

Cholera occurs when the toxin interacts with the colonocyte stimulating chloride, potassium, and bicarbonate secretion via toxin A stimulation of cyclic adenosine monophopshate; some degree of inflammation may accompany this. Oral rehydration solution, which contributes fluid, sodium, and glucose, relies on cellular mechanisms to effect rehydration and is the mainstay of therapy.

Motility disorders influence intestinal function as pertains to absorption; whereas decreased transit enhances absorption of nutrients, significant decreases in motility can result in stasis. Deconjugation of bile acids by enteric flora can result in malabsorption and inflammation. Increases in motility can occur in the clinical picture of an inflamed colon, such as can occur in infants and adults. Acute hormonal influences are more common in the adult population, such as those seen with thyrotoxicosis

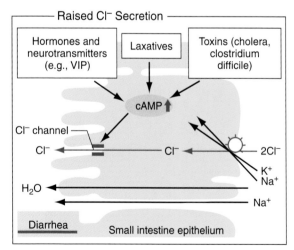

Figure 1 Chloride mechanisms of secretory diarrhea. (Reproduced with permission from Silbernagl S and Lang F (2000) p. 151 *Color Atlas of Pathophysiology*, p. 333. New York: Thieme.)

and carcinoid syndrome. Pharmacological agents or substance abuse can also influence motility.

Inflammatory diarrhea results in secretion of mucus, typically with the presence of blood in the lumen, which is also a cathartic agent. The integrity of the epithelial barrier is often compromised, with resultant exudation of water and proteins. Bacterial invasion of the mucosa may occur and is one example of inflammatory diarrhea. Additional disorders that may cause inflammatory diarrhea include allergic colitis and inflammatory bowel disease (IBD).

Lastly, diarrhea can be categorized clinically into acute and chronic forms, with the latter being defined as persistence of symptoms for more than 3 weeks. Each type of diarrhea can be further clinically divided based on age with respect to likelihood of cause.

Constipation

Constipation is defined as the infrequent, painful passage of large, hard stools; the frequency of defecation may be variable. Breast-fed infants may stool more than five times per day or as little as once every 3 days. Children age 2 years average two stools per day. Adults stool between three times a day and three times per week on average. The colon functions to store stool as well as to absorb fluids.

Eating triggers the gastrocolic reflex, mediated by the enteric nervous system and gastrointestinal hormones to stimulate propogative peristalsis. Stool traverses the colon and accumulates, filling the rectum. The stretch upon the rectal walls stimulates reflexive relaxation of the internal anal sphincter, which is sensed by the individual. If defecation is desired, relaxation of the external anal sphincter and correction of the angle of the rectum with respect to the anus (achieved by relaxation of the puborectalis muscle, the Valsalva maneuver, and proper posturing) allow for passage of stool. Abnormalities in sensation, conditions in which paradoxical contraction of the puborectalis muscle occurs instead of relaxation (anismus), pelvic floor muscle dyssenergia, and congenital absence of innervation of the rectal vault (Hirschprung's disease) also result in constipation. Anatomical structural defects, such as an anteriorly displaced anus, or an imperforate anus present as constipation in childhood.

Stool frequency and consistency are influenced by dietary factors. Fats decrease intestinal motility and facilitate greater absorption of nutrients. Dietary fiber acts as a stool bulking agent and is a major determinant of stool weight, size, and transit time; larger, fiber-laden stools are defecated more frequently than smaller ones. Additional factors, including physical activity level, stress, and functional changes in the environment, can influence stooling frequency. Medical conditions, such as spinal cord injuries, abdominal surgery, and hypothyroidism, as well as the use of pharmacological agents such as opioid derivatives, can decrease colonic motility and result in constipation. Transit time for stool through the colon varies greatly by age, with 8 or 9 h being the average for infants and 1.5 to 2 days for adults.

Encopresis is chronic fecal incontinence with frequent fecal soiling seen in children with otherwise normal colonic anatomy and physiology, usually triggered by a social stressor as opposed to an event such as painful passage of a large stool. The passage of this large, painful stool may result in rectal tearing, and, as a consequence, behaviors regarding defecation and its avoidance may occur, leading to stool withholding. The rectal vault is capable of accommodating stool, and, with time, the stretch receptors will diminish nerve stimulation. The stool present undergoes desiccation as more stool is propagated to the rectum, distending the rectal vault further. Liquid stool may pass the perimeter of stool and continue caudally, resulting in anal leakage. Rectal vault distension may reach a threshold at which defecatory urge may be diminished or lost.

Diagnosis of constipation and encopresis is based on a thorough history and physical examination, with additional laboratory and radiological testing as indicated. Correction of the underlying condition, and correction of dietary composition, and pharmacological therapy usually improve constipation; an initial disimpaction and colonic clean-out may also be warranted. For encopresis, additional behavioral therapy is often required. Conditions such as anismus may require additional modalities, such as anorectal manometry to diagnose and biofeedback training to aid in correcting.

Inflammatory Disorders of the Colon

Infections and Enteric Parasites

For viral and bacterial agents to cause inflammatory disease involving the gastrointestinal tract, nonspecific host defense factors of gastric acidity, gastrointestinal motility, enteric flora, barrier functions of mucus secretion and mucosal integrity (in some cases), and specific enteric mucosal immunity and systemic immune mechanisms have to be overcome.

These infections can results in vomiting, diarrhea, and abdominal pain, in addition to systemic effects such as fever. Clinical symptoms vary according to pathogen.

Bacterial virulence is facilitated by enterotoxin secretion (which may be site specific in it action, secreted prior to introduction or while within in the lumen), adherence and invasion of the mucosa, and cytotoxin production, which function to disrupt mucosal and cellular function.

Bacteria can be classified based on their pathological mechanism (Table 1) as well as by their site of activity and the nature of clinical signs and symptoms manifest. Signs and symptoms vary significantly by pathogen and age at presentation, with some forms presenting as crampy abdominal pain with watery diarrhea of relatively short duration, bloody diarrhea, systemic signs and symptoms of inflammation with frank sepsis, and shock. Common bacterial, viral, and parasitic infections involving the colon are outlined in Tables 2 and 3.

Polyps

Intestinal polyps are intraluminal protuberant tumors characterized by their gross morphological appearance, location(s), number, size, and presence (pedunculated) or absence (sessile) of a stalk. Additional salient features include specific histological features used to discriminate between types and to aid in predicting malignant potential. Extraintestinal manifestations are also associated with specific polyposis syndromes.

Age of occurrence is important with respect to clinical significance and malignant potential. Family history of polyps or polyposis syndromes can also be predictive of disease evolution and aid in screening and surveillance of family members.

In children, juvenile polyps account for approximately 90% of colonic polyps. They can be classified as hamartomatous or inflammatory and are also commonly referred to as retention polyps. Grossly, they are large (up to 3 cm), mostly pedunculated, erythematous, and friable. Fluid-filled cysts on the surface can be appreciated endoscopically; microscopically, this corresponds to dilated, mucous-laden cystic glands and some inflammatory cells (Figure 2).

This type of polyp is not in itself neoplastic; however, focal areas of adenomatous and epithelial changes indicate a risk of carcinoma. The presence of these findings in an index case also confers increased risk of carcinoma in first-degree relatives. The age of the subject, family history and inheritance patterns, number and location of polyps, and histology guide the frequency of surveillance colonoscopy. Symptoms of rectal bleeding usually bring these children to the attention of a physician. Polyps can cause clinically significant, but often painless, bleeding so as to cause anemia, and they can be linked to abdominal pain, rectal prolapse, or lead points associated with intussusceptions.

Syndromes associated with juvenile polyps are summarized in Table 4. Other intestinal polyposis syndromes are outlined in Table 5.

Adenomas are composed by immature cells, with the growth rate exceeding regenerative/replacement needs of the colonic crypt. Three features of these polyps aid in detecting malignant potential. Regarding size, adenomatous polyps less than 1 cm have a 2% incidence of being malignant; larger ones have a risk more than 2.5 times that of colorectal carcinoma for the general population. Regarding histology, the degree of cellular atypia defines the degree of irregularity; this can vary from region to region even within a single polyp. Villous structures are associated with the highest risk group, followed by tubulovillous types (Figure 3), with simple tubular types conferring the lowest risk of dysplasia. Smaller polyps tend to display a tubular nature.

Adenomatous polyps are much more common in adults than in children and bear significant malignant potential. They are usually inherited in an autosomally dominant manner. When they occur in children, it is usually in the context of familial adenomatous polyposis–neoplastic polyps that appear gradually, rarely in the first decade of life. Adenomatous polyps may be singular and isolated, multiple, limited to the colon or spread throughout the gastrointestinal tract, or occur in a syndromic manner. Gardner's syndrome, Turcot's syndrome, and Cronkhite–Canada syndrome are all adenomatous in nature.

Lymphoid hyperplasia may be mistaken for polyps and consists of sessile projections. Histologically,

Table 1 Bacterial pathogens grouped by pathogenic mechanism

Adherent	Invasive	Toxigenic	Cytotoxic
Enteropathogenic *Escherichia coli*	Shigella	Shigella	Shigella
Enterohemorrhagic *E. coli*	Salmonella	Enterotoxigenic *E. coli*	Enteropathogenic *E. coli*
Enteroaggregative *E. coli*	*Yersinia enterocolitica*	*Yersinia enterocolitica*	Enterohemorrhagic *E. coli*
Diffuse-adherent *E. coli*	*Campylobacter jejuni*	Aeromonas	*Clostridium difficile*
	Vibrio parahemolyticus	*Vibrio cholerae*	

Table 2 Bacterial enteric infections

Name	Epidemiology and pathogenesis	Clinical features	Diagnosis and treatment

Shigella
  S. dysentriae
  S. sonnei
  S. flexneri
  S. boydii
	Acute infection
	Highly contagious; low infective
	  dose (10–100 organisms)
		Bacterial dysentery
		  Crampy abdominal pain
		    and watery stools
		  Progressive to bloody,
		    mucoid, pus-laden stools
		  Tenesmus
		  Fever
		  Meningismus
		  Febrile seizures in
		    younger patients
		  Hemolytic uremic
		    syndrome (HUS) possible
			Diagnosis
			  Crypt abscesses
			  Lymphatic hypertrophy
			  Necrosis
			  Elevated WBC count
			  Stool culture
			Treatment
			  Fluid and electrolyte
			    replacement
			  Hand washing to prevent
			    transmission
			  Limited role of antibiotics

Salmonella
  S. typhi
  S. paratyphi
  S. enteritidis
	Infective load: 10^3–10^5 organisms
	Reservoirs: poultry and eggs,
	  lizards, amphibians
	Raw/undercooked foods
	Mucosal invasion (jejunum
	  and colon
	Inflammatory response with
	  active secretion
		Five clinical syndromes
		  Acute gastroenteritis
		    (12- to 72-h incubation)
		  Focal, nonintestinal
		    infection
		  Bacteremia
		  Asymptomatic carrier state
		  Enteric fever
		Abdominal cramping, nausea
		Vomiting
		Bloody, mucoid stools
		Rose spots on the trunk
		Leucopenia
		Prolonged excretion possible,
		  variable by age
		Carrier state not uncommon
			Diagnosis
			  Stool culture
			Treatment
			  Supportive
			  Very limited role for
			    antibiotics

Campylobacter	Transmission by contaminated
	  foods (poultry, eggs, milk;
	  water; domestic animals)
	Initial site(s): jejunum colon
		Incubation period of
		  2–11 days
		Fever prodrome
		Severe diarrhea
		Tenesmus
		Abdominal pain
			Diagnosis
			  Incubation for culture
			Treatment
			  Supportive
			  Role for antibiotics for limiting
			    excretion period and
			    duration of illness

Clostridium
  C. difficile
	Enteric flora
	Toxin A (enterotoxin: alters
	  permeability; inflammation
	  mediator)
	Toxin B (cytotoxin)
	Pseudomembranes
		Antibiotic-associated diarrhea
		May be restricted to the right
		  colon
			Diagnosis
			  Stool C. difficile toxins
			    A and B
			  ELISA
			Endoscopy and histology
			  Pseudomembranes (mucin,
			    fibrin, polymorphonuclear
			    lymphocytes, necrotic
			    debris)
			  Erythema
			  Edema
			  Friability
			  Apthous ulcers
			Treatment
			  Supportive therapy
			  Cessation of offending
			    antibiotic
			  Metronidazole as first-line agent
			  Vancomycin secondary agent
			  Probiotics useful in relapse
			    prevention

Yersinia
  Y. enterolytica
	Transmission
	  Contaminated pork,
	  Enterotoxin elaboration
			Diagnosis
			  Cultures not very accurate

Continued

Table 2 Continued

Name	Epidemiology and pathogenesis	Clinical features	Diagnosis and treatment

			Endoscopy
			  Mucosal ulcerations,
			    friability throughout
			    colon, and terminal ileum
			    possible
			Histology
			  Lamina propria infiltration
			    of inflammatory cells
			  Ulcerative and necrotic
			    areas
			  Dilated crypts
			Treatment
			  Antibiotics

Aeromonas
  A. hydrophila
	Water contaminants	Three syndromes
		  Mild watery diarrhea
		  Bloody diarrhea
		  Persistent diarrhea
			Diagnosis
			  Stool culture
			Treatment
			  Antibiotics

Escherichia coli			

Enteropathogenic
    E. coli (EPEC)
	Localized adherence to
	  enterocytes
	Signal transduction
	Intimate adherence and
	  effacement
		Diarrhea
		Vomiting
		Malaise
		Fever
		Mucoid, nonbloody stools
		Two-week duration
			Diagnosis
			  Presence of adherent
			    organisms on small
			    intestinal/rectal biopsy
			Treatment
			  Antibiotics

Enterotoxigenic E. coli
    (ETEC)
	Enterotoxin elaboration
	  Heat labile (LT) toxin
	  Heat stable (ST) toxin
	  Fimbriae-based attachment
	  Stimulate adenylate cyclase
	  (LT) and guanylate cyclase
	  (ST) to secrete fluid
		Nausea
		Abdominal pain
		Watery diarrhea
		Traveler's diarrhea
			Diagnosis
			  Bioassays
			  Immunoassays
			  Gene probes for ST or LT
			Treatment
			  Supportive
			  Antibiotics decrease duration
			    of excretion; not
			    recommended for children

Enteroinvasive E. coli
    (EIEC)
	Colonize colon
	Invade tissue
	Replicate within cells
	Secretory enterotoxins
		Shigella-like
		  Watery diarrhea
		  Then, bloody mucoid,
		    pus-laden diarrhea
		  Tenesmus and fever
		    possible
			Diagnosis
			  Bioassays
			  Serotyping
			  ELISA
			Treatment
			  Supportive
			  Limited antibiotic role

Enterohemorrhagic
    E. coli (EHEC)
	Part of normal enteric flora in
	  healthy animals
	Cytotoxin similar to Shiga toxin
	Adherence
	O157:H7 prototypical
	Transmission
	  Contaminated, undercooked
	    meat
	  Unpasteurized apple cider
	  Children and the elderly more
	    prone to HUS
		Hemorrhagic colitis
		  Crampy abdominal pain
		  Watery diarrhea
		    progressing to bloody
		    stools
		  Absence of fever
		  HUS
			Diagnosis
			  Serotyping
			  Serum antibody tests
			  Cytotoxin bioassays
			  DNA hybridization
			  PCR-based tests
			  ELISA
			Treatment
			  No effective therapy
			  Supportive care
			  Dehydration correction
			  Management of electrolyte
			    abnormalities
			  Blood transfusions as
			    necessary

Enteroaggregative
    E. coli (EAEC)
	Localized adherence likely
	  (HEp-2 or HeLa cells)
	Enterotoxin
	Increased intestinal mucus
	  secretion
		Diarrhea
		  Watery
		  Mucoid
		  Persistent
			Diagnosis
			  DNA probes

Diffuse adherent E. coli
    (DAEC)
	Diffuse adherence likely (HEp-2
	  or HeLa cells)
		Diarrhea	Diagnosis
			  DNA probes

Table 3 Additional colonic pathogens

Name	Pathogenesis	Clinical symptoms	Diagnosis and treatment
Amoeba *Entamoeba histolytica*	Travel to endemic areas a risk factor Large intestinal commensal organism Transmission Person-to-person contact Contaminated food/water (cysts) Cysts transform into trophozoytes at the terminal ileum Invade mucosa and submucosa	Acute onset Fulminant colitis Bloody, mucoid diarrhea Abdominal distention Abdominal pain Perforation possible Hepatic abscesses possible	Diagnosis Histopathology: Hyperemia and edema Acute inflammation Microulceration Flask ulcer formation (Fresh) stool examination for cysts or trophozoites Treatment Iodoquinol Metronidazole
Helminths *Trichuris trichura* (whipworm)	Primarily colonic	Heavy infestations associated with (bloody) diarrhea Rectal prolapse	Diagnosis Stool assays Treatment Thiabendazole Mebendazole
Schistosomiasis *S. mansoni*	Snail as pathogen Contaminates fresh water	Dysenteric-like illness Bloody diarrhea Perianal fistulas	Diagnosis Endoscopic Focal and diffuse fibrosis Intraluminal Granulamatous masses (bilharziomas) Stool exam for viable eggs Treatment Praziquantal

hyperplastic lymphoid follicles are present; it is not uncommon for ulcerations to overlie these areas.

Inflammatory polyps (also referred to as pseudopolyps) can be seen during the recovery phase from inflammation or in inflammatory diseases, and they are often seen in the context of IBD. They can be

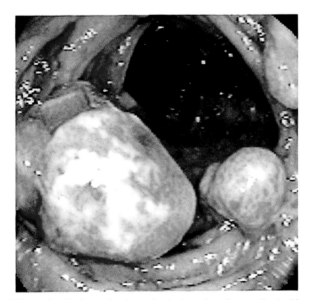

Figure 2 Endoscopic view of colonic polyps in a patient with juvenile polyposis col. (Reproduced with permission from Kleinman RE, Gilger MA, Braverman RM, Finegold MS, Hawkins EP, and Klish WJ (eds.) (1998) *Atlas of Pediatric Gastrointestinal Disease*. Hamilton Ontario: Decker.)

associated with phases of regeneration and are pleimorphic in nature.

Inflammatory Bowel Disease

The term inflammatory bowel disease encompasses ulcerative colitis and Crohn's disease. Indeterminate colitis is a diagnosis attributed to a condition in which clear distinction cannot be made between the two aforementioned forms of IBD, as opposed to a heterogeneous group of diseases that present over a wide clinical and histological spectrum.

Epidemiology

IBD presents in a bimodal manner as pertains to age, first in late adolescence or early adulthood and a smaller peak in the fifth decade of life. The sexes are equally affected by ulcerative colitis; in adults, the incidence of Crohn's disease is 20–30% higher in women.

In terms of trends in disease over time, the incidence of ulcerative colitis remained stable during the second half of the twentieth century; Crohn's disease has demonstrated a marked increase across all age groups since 1950. Although IBD can affect all races, Caucasians are affected significantly more than Africans or people of African origin.

Table 4 Hamartomatous intestinal polyps

Syndrome	Location of polyps	Pathology	Extraintestinal abnormalities	Cancer risk
Juvenile polyposis	Colon; some small intestinal	Up to 3 cm Mucus retention and inflammatory cells in the lamina propria cysts Mostly pedunculated		Colonic; low risk
Peutz–Jeghers	Mostly small intestinal; some gastric and colonic	1–3 cm Either sessile or pedunculated Glandular epithelium and smooth muscle branching	Macular pigmentation on hands, lips, and mouth	Up to 18 times versus the general population; lower than other polyposis syndromes
Cowden's syndrome	Colon and stomach	Multiple polyps Hamartomatous	Lipomas Papillomas Orocutaneous hamartomas	Fibrocystic or fibroademomatous, ductal breast cancer Nodular thyroid hyperplasia or follicular adenoma

Table 5 Polyposis syndromes

Type/syndrome	Location(s)	Histology	Clinical features	Cancer risk
Familial polyposis coli	Colonic; fundic gland hyperplasia (stomach)	Thousands of adenomas Elevated ornithine decarboxylase levels APC gene	Apparent after puberty Diarrhea most common symptom Abdominal pain Hypertrophic retinal lesions	Thyroid cancer Pancreatic cancer Risk of colon cancer 100% by 55 years of age
Gardner's syndrome	Colon, stomach, duodenum, small intestine	2–5 mm Sessile mostly Adenomas in the antrum and periampular regions More than 1000 over time	Triad of: Polyps Osteomas Soft tissue tumors Also dental abnormalities	Duodenal tumors at highest risk Associated risk of Pancreatic carcinoma Ampullary cancer Hepatoblastoma
Turcot's syndrome	Colonic	Adenomatous polyps	Presents in adolescents with cancer; family history Autosomal recessive	Associated neural tumors Medulloblastmas Gliomas
Cronkhite–Canada syndrome	Throughout gastrointestinal tract	Adenomatous lesions within adenomatous polyps	Alopecia Nail dystrophy Brown macular skin lesions Edema related to protein-losing enteropathy	5% of cases evolve into gastrointestinal carcinomas
Inflammatory polyposis	Colonic; pseudopolyps	Pleiomorphic Regenerative tissue	Systemic signs and symptoms of inflammation	Colonic; risk of cancer from inflammatory bowel disease (Crohn's disease and ulcerative colitis)

Ashkenazi Jews have a markedly increased risk of IBD compared to other Jewish groups. The incidence in the Ashkenazi Jewish population roughly parallels that of the respective geographical community in which they reside, albeit at a level that can be three or four times that of the general population, suggesting a genetic predisposition. The majority of individuals affected by these disorders reside in North America and northern Europe. The remainder of Europe, Latin America, and Australia have lower incidence rates, and rare cases occur in Africa and Asia.

Etiology

The exact etiology of IBD is unclear and an area of active research. A multifactorial interaction between genetic predisposition, environmental stimuli, endogenous triggers, immunological dysregulation, and modifying factors is postulated.

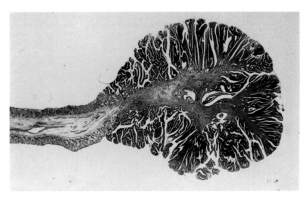

Figure 3 Polyp histology: tubullovillous adenoma. (Reproduced with permission from Wheater PR, Burkitt HG, Stevens A, and Lowe JS (1991) *Basic Histopathology*, 2nd edn. Churchill Livingston, UK.)

Genetics

A positive family history confers significant risk (10–20%) of disease occurrence of either disease type in a first-degree relative. The roles of race and ethnicity were discussed previously, with northern European and North American populations, particularly the Ashkenazi Jewish population globally, having the highest risk of disease.

A high rate of concordance among Swedish monozygotic twins versus dizygotic twins has been reported for Crohn's disease (44 vs 3.8%). In the same study, the incidence rate observed in monozygotic twins for ulcerative colitis was 6.3%. These data, although supportive of a genetic role, show less than 100% penetrence, suggesting that although genetics are more important in Crohn's disease than in ulcerative colitis, environmental influences play a significant role. Simple Mendelian models of inheritance are inadequate to address the complex inheritance patterns of IBD. Candidate gene studies have suggested modest HLA associations that differ in different populations. Systemic genome searches performed on families with several members with IBD have employed linkage analyses. Evidence that the *NOD-2* gene on chromosome 16 is involved in Crohn's disease has led to it being labeled the *IBD1* gene locus. This gene is involved with the encoding of a protein associated with monocytic nuclear factor-κB; this protein and pathway are involved in the interaction of monocytes with bacterial peptidoglycans. Note that only approximately 30% of individuals with Crohn's disease are positive for this particular gene mutation.

Environmental Influences

Because of the rapid increase in Crohn's disease during the past 50 years, increasing trends in immigrant populations, as well as incomplete genotype–phenotype associations, attention has focused on environmental factors. In particular, the search to identify an antigenic trigger for the enteric immune system has been pursued by several investigators. Postulated microbial intraluminal triggers include mycobacterium and viruses. Dietary antigens or toxins have not been identified; Westernized diet has been explored and remains an active area of research. Exposures early in the life cycle (birth environment) and nutritive factors (breast vs formula feeing; the former confers protective effects) have also been considered. Additional modulating factors include smoking and the use of oral contraceptives.

Pathogenesis

The interactions between the enteric immune system and the intestinal lumen are dynamic; some degree of inflammation in response is always present in the normal mucosal lamina propria of the colon and small intestine, which handle a very large antigenic load daily. An intact mucosal barrier, in addition to normally functioning immunoregulatory mechanisms, prevents this interaction from progressing to the level at which tissue injury occurs.

Current chronic, inflammatory relapsing disease processes may represent an inappropriate persistent immune response to a luminal antigen/stimulus versus an appropriate immune response to a persistent, abnormal stimulus or perhaps a prolonged immune response to a ubiquitous stimulus.

Enteric flora may play a role in this process, although no evidence strongly indicates a single pathogen. Defective mucosal barrier function and increased intestinal permeability may also be involved, with the latter being documented in patients with IBD and in up to 10% of nonaffected first-degree relatives.

The immune response is primarily T cell mediated and of a Th-1 nature—interleukin-12, interferon-gamma, and tumor necrosis factor-alpha (TNF-α). White blood cells respond to these inflammatory mediators and proliferate the immune response. These recruited cells synthesize agents such as arachidonic acid metabolites, platelet activating factor, proteases, and free radicals such as reactive oxygen species—all of which cause direct injury to cells and the mucosa.

Pathology

Pathology differs between these two disorders in terms of anatomical distribution and tissue involvement. Ulcerative colitis is limited to the colon and rectum, usually beginning distally in the rectum and extending to varying lengths proximally in a continuous manner (**Figure 4**). Usually, a clear distinction

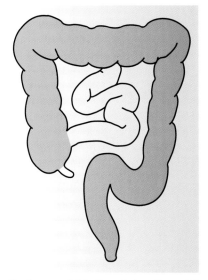

Figure 4 Continuous distribution of ulcerative colitis.

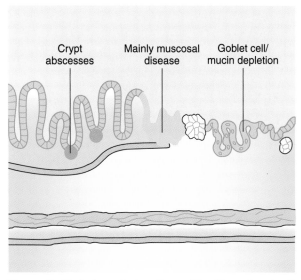

Figure 5 Illustration of ulcerative colitis. (Reproduced with permission from Kelly DA and Booth IW (1996) *Pediatric Gastroenterology & Hepatology*. London: Mosby–Wolfe.)

can be made where disease ends and normal mucosa can be appreciated grossly or endoscopically. The gross appearance of the mucosa is dependent on the severity of the disease process. Mild disease presents with a diffuse erythema and loss of the characteristic appearance of the vasculature. Numerous small, superficial ulcerations, exudates, and bleeding are seen in moderate disease; larger, deeper ulcerations, increased exudates, and the development of pseudopolyps are seen in severe disease, with loss of normal gross architectural landmarks such as the folds. Microscopically, ulcerative colitis is limited to the mucosa; with more severe disease, deeper layers may show a degree of involvement, with inflammatory cell infiltrates, shortening, branching, and decreases in the number of crypts as well as crypt abscesses (**Figure 5**).

Crohn's disease may involve any part of the alimentary tract from the mouth to the anus, and it frequently does so in a discontinuous manner, leaving 'skip areas'—regions that are grossly and histologically normal; in the colon, this lends a cobblestone appearance. Macroscopically, wall thickening is evident in longstanding disease. By definition, this disease is a transmural process (**Figure 6**). With chronic disease, fibrostenosis occurs, narrowing the intestinal lumen. Stricturizing disease may follow fibrosis of superficial and deeper layers of the intestinal wall, evident on radiographic studies (**Figure 7**).

The mesentery may also demonstrate inflammation, with resutant adhesion and fixation of the colon. Adjacent loops of bowel may become matted

together. As luminal diameter narrows, intraluminal pressure may increase; in the case of nonabating inflammation, this transmural process may lead to fistula formation. Enteroenteric fistulas are limited to the bowel; enterovaginal, enterovesicular, and enterocutaneous fistulization may occur. Inflammatory intraabdominal masses called phlegmons may also form by this fistulization process.

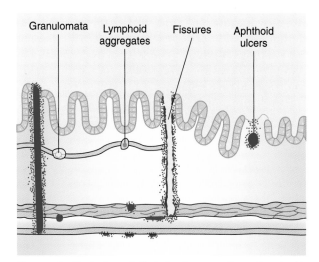

Figure 6 Illustration of Crohn's disease. (Reproduced with permission From Kelly DA and Booth IW (1996) *Pediatric Gastroenterology & Hepatology*. London: Mosby–Wolfe.)

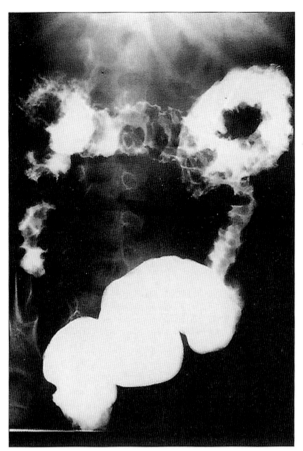

Figure 7 Barium enema in a patient with colonic Crohn's disease. Note the bowel wall ulcerations, structuring, and asymmetric bowel wall edema. (Reproduced with permission from Kelly DA and Booth IW (1996) *Pediatric Gastroenterology & Hepatology*. London: Mosby–Wolfe.)

thus indicating that examination of the entire alimentary canal and surveillance biopsies are required prior to arriving at a diagnosis.

IBD and the Terminal Ileum

The terminal ileum is one of the most commonly involved sites in the intestine in Crohn's disease, often originating at the lymphoid follicle; strictures may form. A phenomenon of ileal involvement has been postulated in cases of apparent ulcerative colitis that involve the ileum, in which cecal inflammation is postulated to 'backwash' into the ileum; this finding being consistent with ulcerative colitis is controversial.

Extraintestinal manifestations are common in both Crohn's disease and ulcerative colitis, including ophthalmologic manifestations (uveitis), joint involvement (arthralgias and arthritis of the large joints), and manifestations of the skin, hepatobiliary system, pancreas, renal system, and vascular system. Anemia and weight loss are common at the time of presentation. Growth and pubertal delay are very common at the time of presentation in children; short stature occurs in up to 50% of children. Some of these findings relate to the inflammatory process; others are linked to malnutrition associated with IBD. Perianal disease with fistulization and/or skin tags is perhaps the most common extraintestinal abnormality associated with Crohn's disease.

Nutritional Consequences of IBD

Malnutrition includes weight loss acutely, partly attributable to anorexia associated with inflammation and partly to the disease process (i.e., inadequate intake as well as excessive (malabsorptive) losses). These deficiencies can evolve from frank losses as well as be malabsorptive in nature. An example delineating all of these mechanisms is anemia, which can result from frank blood loss from associated gastrointestinal bleeding, anemia of chronic disease mediated by the inflammatory mediators, anorexia with decreased dietary iron intake, and, as in the case of duodenal and jejunal disease activity (as can occur in Crohn's disease), anorexia with decreased absorption.

Intestinal disease can result in both decreased nutrient absorption and disruption of the mucosal barrier, resulting in exudation of proteins, a process known as protein-losing enteropathy (PLE). The latter can result in hypoalbuminemia; third spacing of fluids as a result of decreased intravascular oncotic pressure can occur. Increased energy expenditure as

The endoscopic appearance of Crohn's disease varies by location and time relative to disease evolution. Intestinal Crohn's disease may initially present with apthous ulceration overlying Peyer's patches in the colon. Ulcerations eventually grow, with frankly friable, exudative lesions.

Histological findings of affected areas include intense inflammatory cell infiltrates extending into the crypts, with shortening and forking of these structures, and associated abscesses. The inflammation is transmural; fibrosis and histiocyte proliferation are also seen. Noncaseating granulomatous submucosal and mucosal lesions, which are a hallmark of this disease, are not found in a majority of biopsy specimens. Granulomas can also be seen in intestinal infections, such as in intestinal tuberculosis and sacoidosis. Even macroscopically appearing normal tissue may yield histological findings of inflammation compatible with Crohn's disease, a consequence of inflammation is noted, particularly in the febrile state or with sepsis. Inflammation and discomfort also contribute to decreased enteral intake—factors contributory to a catabolic state.

In addition to iron, other mineral and trace element deficiencies are noted in IBD. Iron deficiency was discussed previously. Zinc is closely associated with gut mucosa and is susceptible to deficiency; low albumin levels resulting from PLE and increased intestinal epithelial cell turnover probably represent a significant source of zinc depletion. Vitamin B_{12} and folic acid deficiency has also been documented among the water-soluble vitamins, particularly when the terminal ileal disease is noted. Vitamin D deficiency is the most common among the fat-soluble vitamins.

Treatment of IBD

Several antiinflammatory treatment modalities have been employed in the treatment of IBD. Their use is dictated by disease type, location, extent, and severity. Steroids provide the cornerstone of initial therapy for acute inflammation. Five aminosalicylate derivatives, antimetabolites such as azothioprine and 6-mercaptopurine methotrexate, and newer biological agents including anti-TNF-α are currently employed.

Nutritional therapies including semielemental enteral feedings or parenteral therapy have a role in the management of IBD. Although enteral therapy is not considered a first-line therapy for ulcerative colitis in the United States, its use as such is popular in Europe and Canada and allows for steroid sparing/ avoidance. The time to onset of remission using enteral therapy in Crohn's disease is much less with steroids than with enteral therapy, however, with the former occurring typically within 2 weeks and the latter taking usually 6–8 weeks to achieve similar clinical remission. Smaller studies have been conducted employing low-fat diets and less processed sugar foods. The latter has shown promise in studies of Crohn's disease, thought to be secondary to the immunomodulatory effects of these fatty acids. Another approach under investigation is enteral therapy containing TGF-β, which is thought to modulate the enteric immune response. Also under investigation are dietary fiber, short-chain fatty acids, and influencing the colonic flora with the use of prebiotics and probiotics.

Surgical treatment is indicated in ulcerative colitis when acute, fulminant disease does not respond to medical therapy or when persistent chronic disease is refractory to medical (steroid) therapy and the diagnosis has been confirmed (i.e., Crohn's disease has been ruled out). Colectomy is curative in this instance.

Crohn's disease is more complex, and surgical intervention, limited to involved segments only, is not curative. Failure of medical therapy to reduce inflammation, critical stenosis of the involved segments with fibrosis leading to obstruction, perforation, fistulization, and/or abscess formation not amenable to medical therapy, and frank gastrointestinal hemorrhage are indications for surgical intervention. Reactivation of disease can occur postoperatively at the site of anastomoses or elsewhere.

The natural history of IBD is such that long-standing disease increases the risk of colonic dysplasia, particularly in the case of ulcerative colitis, even though it is a curative intervention, making colectomy more attractive in the older patient. Ileoanal continuity can be achieved by means of surgical anastomoses. Pouchitis secondary to bacterial overgrowth, smoldering pockets of disease activity that may not have been resected or become evident after resection, and loss of continence are common complications of these procedures.

See also: **Colon**: Structure and Function; Nutritional Management of Disorders. **Diarrheal Diseases**. **Dietary Fiber**: Physiological Effects and Effects on Absorption; Potential Role in Etiology of Disease; Role in Nutritional Management of Disease. **Small Intestine**: Structure and Function; Disorders.

Further Reading

Balfour R (2002) Mucosal immunology & mechanisms of gastrointestinal inflammation. In: Feldman M, Friedman LS, and Sleisenger MH (eds.) *Sleisenger & Fordtran's Gastrointestinal and Liver Disease: Pathophysiology, Diagnosis Management*, 7th edn, pp. 21–54. Philadelphia: WB Saunders.

Bayless TM and Hanauer S (eds.) (2001) *Advanced Therapy of Inflammatory Bowel Disease*. Hamilton, Ontario, Canada: BC Decker.

Griffiths AM and Bueller HB (2000) Inflammatory bowel disease. In: Waker WA, Durie P, Hamilton R, Watkins J, and Walker-Smith J (eds.) *Pediatric Gastroenterology: Pathophysiology, Diagnosis, Management*, 3rd edn, pp. 28–38. Hamilton, Ontario, Canada: BC Decker.

Guandalini S (2000) Acute diarrhea. In: Waker WA, Durie P, Hamilton R, Watkins J, and Walker-Smith J (eds.) *Pediatric Gastroenterology: Pathophysiology, Diagnosis, Management*, 3rd edn. Hamilton, Ontario, Canada: BC Decker.

Homer DH and Gorbach SL (2002) Infectious diarrhea and bacterial food poisoning. In: Feldman M, Friedman LS, and Sleisenger MH (eds.) *Sleisenger & Fordtran's Gastrointestinal and Liver Disease: Pathophysiology, Diagnosis Management*, 7th edn, pp. 1864–1932. Philadelphia: Saunders.

Pickering LK and Cleary TG (1998) Approach to patients with gastrointestinal tract infections and food poisoning. In: Feigin RD and Cherry JD (eds.) *Textbook of Pediatric Infectious Diseases*, 4th edn, pp. 567–600. Philadelphia: WB Saunders.

Shashidhar S and Mobassaleh M (1998) Bacterial infections. In: Altshuler S and Liacouras C (eds.) *Clinical Pediatric Gastroenterology*, pp. 131–142. Philadelphia: Churchill Livingstone.

Steffen R and Loering-Burke V (1999) Constipation and encopresis. In: Willie R and Hyams J (eds.) *Pediatric Gastroenterology*, 2nd edn, pp. 43–50. Philadelphia: WB Saunders.

Yamada F, Alpers DH, Laine L, Owyang C, and Powell DW (eds.) (1999) *Textbook of Gastroenterology*, 3rd edn. Philadelphia: Lippincott, Williams & Wilkins.

Nutritional Management of Disorders

D M Klurfeld, US Department of Agriculture, Beltville, MD, USA

© 2005 Elsevier Ltd. All rights reserved.

The primary functions of the colon are to absorb water and to form and store feces for excretion. The length of the large intestine in an adult is approximately 1.5 m; several divisions and landmarks of the colon are shown in **Figure 1**. Disturbances in colonic function are symptoms of diseases or disorders, including constipation, diarrhea, diverticular disease, irritable bowel syndrome, and inflammatory bowel diseases; due to surgical treatment of inflammatory bowel diseases, stomas are often created. Symptoms of these conditions range from mild discomfort to life-threatening emergencies, although most are chronic and can benefit from nutritional

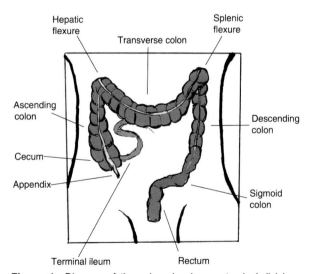

Figure 1 Diagram of the colon showing anatomical divisions and landmarks. Intestinal chyme enters via the ileum, ferments in the proximal ascending portion of the colon, and becomes feces, which is stored in the transverse and distal descending portions for elimination.

management. Although pharmacological therapy in some of these conditions may often be indicated, nutritional management is recognized as the first choice and is particularly effective in preventing and treating some of these disorders. As in many issues related to nutrition, there is a tremendous amount of misinformation believed by many. For example, there is no basis for the claims that meat remains undigested in the colon for years or that colonic cleansing with enemas or herbal preparations is of any value.

Constipation

Constipation can be defined as the slow movement of feces through the large intestine that results in the passage of dry, hard stool. Another acceptable definition is the infrequent passage of small, dry, hard feces accompanied by discomfort or pain. Many individuals self-diagnose the condition based on perceived deviations from 'normal' bowel habits; this often leads to unnecessary use of chemical laxatives that can irritate the colon and eventually lead to dependence on such preparations for evacuation. Normal bowel habits are generally deemed as at least three stools per week to no more than three per day. Constipation is often accompanied by symptoms of distension and flatulence. Diverticular disease is characterized by thinning and outpouching of the colonic wall. The diverticula are generally asymptomatic but can become infected with the potential for rupture. The major complications of this condition are bleeding and bacterial infection; the latter may result in abscess formation or perforation of an existing diverticulum with subsequent peritonitis. Although past practices were to prescribe low-residue diets to rest the bowel, it is now known that high-fiber diets are effective in the treatment and prevention of diverticular disease as well as for reducing the complication rate.

In the early 1970s, it was proposed that reduced fiber consumption in Western countries resulted in an incidence of diverticular disease that approximated 50% beyond the age of 70 years, whereas this condition was almost nonexistent in sub-Saharan Africa. Since that time, there have been contradictory studies on this point, and it seems that dietary fiber may not be the only factor that influences the development of diverticular disease. However, several explanations for some of the contrary findings in this area are evident. First, many factors in the diet are correlated; that is, a diet low in fiber tends to be high in meat and fat. Second, the measurement of dietary fiber in many studies has not included total dietary fiber, thereby suffering from measurement bias. Third, not all sources of dietary fiber have a therapeutic effect and the benefit varies according to the specific type of food or fiber supplement along with the amount of water available.

Despite past controversy, it now seems clear that diets high in dietary fiber will prevent the development of diverticular disease, can be used successfully for symptomatic treatment, and reduce the risk of infection of the diverticula. It must be understood that once formed, diverticula do not spontaneously resolve, and surgery is the only means of removing them. Recommended dietary modifications are increases in water and dietary fiber, particularly wheat bran or psyllium. Although fruits and vegetables also contribute to the prevention or reduction of symptoms, there is controversy about including those that have seeds. Seeds often pass through the gastrointestinal tract undigested; these have been found in infected diverticula, and it was assumed that they were the nidus for infection. Therefore, many practitioners have prohibited patients from consuming foods with small seeds, such as raspberries, cranberries, and blueberries, or larger seeds, such as tomatoes, peppers, and cucumbers. In addition, seeds added to foods, such as caraway, sesame, and poppy, have been proscribed. Some do not prohibit consumption of these seed-containing foods but there is little evidence to demonstrate the safety of abandoning this advice.

Diarrhea

Diarrhea is generally defined as loose, watery stools occurring more than three times a day and is a symptom of an underlying condition. It is estimated that the average adult has four episodes of diarrhea each year. Most events are self-limited and resolve within 24–48 h; it is presumed that the majority of these are viral in etiology and numerous agents have been implicated. Bacterial causes include *Campylobacter*, *Escherichia coli*, and, less commonly, *Salmonella* or *Shigella*. The latter organism is prevalent in tropical areas of the world and one species of *Shigella* is responsible for dysentery, which is characterized by profuse, watery diarrhea particularly in children and the elderly. Parasitic infections with *Giardia lamblia*, *Entamoeba histolytica*, or *Cryptosporidium* are often linked to chronic diarrhea. Alterations of normal colonic flora secondary to antibiotic therapy may result in diarrhea; the best studied organisms that overgrow the normal bacteria are *Clostridium* species. Noninfectious causes of diarrhea may be lactose intolerance, excess consumption of

sugar alcohols, irritable bowel syndrome, inflammatory bowel disease, or celiac disease.

Clearly, the underlying cause of chronic diarrhea needs to be established and proper therapy instituted. Although most episodes of diarrhea will resolve spontaneously without specific therapy, nutritional management of diarrhea is primarily concerned with replacement of lost fluid. Copious or chronic diarrhea increases the need for electrolytes. Any episode of diarrhea in young children or the elderly may require electrolytes in addition to fluid replacement; this is easily obtained from oral rehydration therapy solutions made for this purpose if diarrhea is severe or protracted. Such solutions contain starch, proteins, and electrolytes and have been shown to reduce stool volume significantly. In less severe cases, maintenance of, or return to, the usual diet after 24 h is recommended. Four foods traditionally recommended for children—bananas, rice, applesauce, and toast—and referred to as the BRAT diet were thought useful because they do not irritate the colon since they are low in fiber and residue. However, this diet is no longer recommended by some pediatrics organizations because it is low in energy density, protein, and fat. During bouts of diarrhea, it is generally recommended that individuals avoid spicy foods, fatty foods, high-sugar foods, or high-fiber foods. Milk is sometimes proscribed, but evidence suggests that 80% of children with diarrhea can tolerate full-strength milk so most do not need to avoid this food, which provides more energy and protein than alternative fluid sources. Clear broth or soup is often recommended. Although clear fruit juices or soft drinks are sometimes recommended, these should be not be used or they should be diluted to avoid an osmotic effect of the sugars drawing more fluid into the intestine. There is considerable controversy regarding the consumption of specific foods during or just after a bout of diarrhea. Some studies justify use of complex carbohydrates (rice, wheat, potatoes, bread, and cereals), lean meats, yogurt, fruits, and vegetables because they are well tolerated even during active diarrhea. Many health professionals recommend a more limited diet of toast, rice, bananas, cooked carrots, and skinless chicken until symptoms abate. The choice of specific foods will depend on the tolerance of an individual, keeping in mind the fluid and energy needs of that person. Research suggests that repopulating the colonic bacteria through consumption of yogurt may provide more healthful organisms (Lactobacilli, Bifidobacteria, and *Streptococcus thermophilus*) and a quicker return of the total flora to normalcy, particularly in antibiotic-induced diarrhea.

Irritable Bowel Syndrome

Irritable bowel syndrome (IBS) is also called spastic colon or mucus colitis, and it is one of the most common causes for referral to gastroenterologists. Symptoms include abdominal pain, bloating, constipation and/or diarrhea, heartburn, belching, and mucus in the stool. IBS is diagnosed by eliminating other diagnoses or organic causes and, therefore, treatment is aimed at alleviating symptoms. Women are affected twice as frequently as men, and it is estimated that as much as 8% of the US population is afflicted with this condition. Although stress and other psychological factors seem to play a significant role in IBS, a number of dietary interventions have been suggested. Although dietary fiber has been advocated for alleviation of the symptoms of IBS, it is clear that some patients will benefit but others will get worse, so individual trial and error may be the logical therapeutic plan. Patients with abdominal distension or excessive flatulence should reduce consumption of gas-provoking foods, such as beans, lentils, cabbage, broccoli, onions, garlic, raw fruits and juices, bananas, and nuts. Caffeinated, alcoholic, and carbonated beverages cause exacerbations in some patients. In addition, high-fat foods, such as deep-fried foods, processed meats, gravies, and chocolate, as well very spicy or pickled foods, may increase symptoms of IBS. Since many IBS patients are also lactose intolerant, reduction of milk products is often recommended empirically but should probably be done based on a patient's response to these food products. Sweeteners such as sorbitol and fructose are often associated with increased diarrhea, so products containing these should be tested for effects on symptoms. In patients with constipation, the addition of fiber to the diet along with increased fluid intake will help to alleviate this symptom. The most commonly recommended types of fiber are wheat bran and psyllium. In patients with diarrhea, some have benefited from the addition of wheat bran, pectin, or kaolin to the diet, but other patients seem to do better with a low-fiber diet. Individualized trials of dietary intervention seem to be indicated for IBS. In addition to nutritional therapy, drug treatment to reduce intestinal transit and emotional or psychological support are major parts of therapy for IBS. Aerobic exercise, consumption of smaller, more frequent meals, relaxation techniques, cessation of cigarette smoking, and a variety of other environmental changes have been tried with varying degrees of efficacy.

Inflammatory Bowel Diseases

Inflammatory bowel disease (IBD) refers to a group of conditions in which inflammation involves portions of the small or large intestines. The ileum and colon are most commonly affected. The types of IBD are Crohn's disease and ulcerative colitis (UC). Although the two conditions have many common features, they can be distinguished based on clinical, x-ray, and pathological findings. Symptoms include chronic abdominal pain, cramps, rectal bleeding, or bloody stools; diarrhea and rectal bleeding are more common in UC. The diagnosis is usually made in adults younger than age 30 years and there is a preponderance of cases among whites, especially Jews. There is familial clustering of these conditions, indicating that genetic predisposition is important; approximately 20% of patients have a close relative with the same diagnosis. The onset of either disease can be acute or insidious, and the course is protracted. Both are characterized by exacerbations and remissions, sometimes of long duration. The international epidemiology of Crohn's disease suggests that it is uncommon in developing countries and has become more common in Western countries, where fiber intakes are lower and consumption of refined carbohydrates is high, but there is no direct evidence that diet plays a role in its etiology. Much research has focused on the etiology, but no clear-cut factors have been identified. Infectious and immunological mechanisms have been most thoroughly investigated with no conclusive evidence. Cigarette smoking has been strongly linked to Crohn's disease but not to UC.

As a result of chronic abdominal pain and diarrhea, many patients lose large amounts of weight. Since oral intake is often limited, there are frequently protein and multiple micronutrient deficits. It is important to replenish these nutrients, but often the early nutritional intervention for IBD relies on bowel rest. Total parenteral nutrition (TPN) accomplishes this best, but enteral liquid formulae can be used in some cases. In fact, TPN often results in short-term remission of symptoms in Crohn's disease. Unfortunately, long-term remissions are not maintained in most patients by this intervention.

Crohn's disease may involve any portion of the gastrointestinal tract but is most commonly found in the terminal ileum, often with extension to the proximal colon. In the majority of patients, multiple areas of the intestine are involved, usually separated by areas of normal intestine. The inflammatory changes are nonspecific but tend to be granulomatous and involve all layers of the intestinal wall. Because inflammation involves the entire thickness of the intestinal wall, there is a high propensity for development of fistulae into adjacent structures that are often infected by the bacteria from the colon. Bowel obstruction from strictures or adhesions tends to occur more frequently in Crohn's disease than in UC.

Ulcerative colitis often begins in the distal colon or rectum and progresses to involve most or all of the colon. Approximately one-fourth of cases have involvement of the terminal ileum, usually in continuity with the colonic manifestations. Ulcerative colitis involves primarily the mucosal layer. The chronic inflammation often leads to shortening and narrowing of the muscle layer in which the colon has been likened to resembling a garden hose. The ulcers tend to undermine portions of the mucosa and this frequently gives rise to pseudopolyps. The incidence of colon cancer is greatly increased in patients with chronic UC; tumors are often multiple and tend to have a poorer prognosis than in sporadic colon cancer. Thus, prophylactic subtotal colectomy is required in approximately 30% of patients who have persistent signs of colonic dysplasia. One of the surgical developments in the therapy of UC is the production of an ileoanal reservoir or 'J pouch,' which becomes a functional rectum, allowing a patient to defecate through the rectum rather than via a colostomy. Some patients with this type of surgery continue to have many bowel movements per day, so limitation of dietary fiber or fruits and vegetables is often required; gas-inducing foods should be avoided. A complication of this surgery is infection of the reservoir or pouchitis. Although no foods or food groups have been identified as contributing to this condition, it is recommended that patients pay attention to foods that may be associated with episodes of pouchitis.

In acute phases of IBD, bland low-residue or elemental diets are recommended; sometimes, total bowel rest is required and TPN is prescribed. Malabsorption of many nutrients has been documented in patients with IBD; the estimation of macronutrient needs is not difficult, but the determination of vitamin and mineral losses is problematic. In UC, elimination of milk products is often advised to reduce the amount of fermentable carbohydrate (lactose) entering the colon, which contributes to bloating, cramps, and diarrhea. In Crohn's disease, intestinal strictures are often found; these are contraindications to high-fiber diets because of the possibility of intestinal obstruction, which is a fairly common complication of the condition. The current consensus is to use low-fiber, low-milk, low-fat diets in patients with IBD; however, controlled studies have found little significant benefit of dietary intervention. This is because some dietary components are beneficial in certain patients but have no,

or detrimental, effects in others. It is important for the patient to receive nutritional counseling to avoid deficiencies of calories and most nutrients. However, there is little specific nutritional therapy available for these conditions. Some patients find that spicy foods or alcoholic beverages exacerbate symptoms; in others, wheat bran or raw fruits have the same effect. The only hard and fast rule is to avoid foods that provoke symptoms while maintaining as nutritious and balanced a diet as possible.

Research studies in which UC patients were treated with short-chain fatty acid (SCFA) enemas generally showed considerable improvement in symptoms. Because dietary fiber is fermented to SCFA, this suggests that high-fiber diets may be beneficial. If this turns out to be the case, it is likely that specific types of dietary fiber will be recommended to achieve defined concentrations of one or more of the SCFAs.

Surgery and drug treatments are the mainstays of therapy, but there is no cure. In fact, surgical removal of an affected portion of the intestine must be weighed quite seriously because the disease may recur in previously normal tissue. Immunosuppressive medications are the standard therapy for these conditions. Because fish oils, rich in n-3 fatty acids, have immunosuppressive properties, these products have been studied and found to have benefit in treating Crohn's disease that is approximately equal in effectiveness to immunosuppressive drugs, but side effects of indigestion and bad breath were major limiting factors in acceptance of the fish oil. The best study done in this area was conducted in Italy, and it is unknown if the fat types and amounts in the Italian diet play some interacting role with the fish oil treatment. In addition, because Crohn's disease is heterogeneous, it is not clear if all patients will benefit from this treatment.

Sublingual vitamin B_{12} has been recommended by some for patients with Crohn's disease because absorption of this vitamin occurs in the ileum, which is the segment of gut frequently affected. However, the absence of the specific transport system for absorption of the vitamin and intrinsic factor, produced in the stomach, call into question the benefit of the route of administration. The efficacy of sublingual vitamin B_{12} is primarily a result of swallowing the vitamin, with subsequent intestinal absorption. Patients should have regular blood counts and intramuscular injection of vitamin B_{12} may be necessary if macrocytic anemia develops.

One of the complications in patients with Crohn's disease who have had ileal resections is increased formation of calcium oxalate kidney stones. This is due to enhanced absorption of oxalate. Since limiting dietary sources of oxalate is considered too restrictive, calcium supplementation and increased fluid intake are recommended. The calcium will decrease oxalate absorption if taken with meals, and the increased fluids will dilute the urine. Since ascorbic acid increases urinary oxalate, supplements and dietary sources rich in vitamin C should be used judiciously, if at all.

Stomas

Although the creation of a surgical stoma is associated with some dietary restrictions, many patients find that there are fewer prohibited foods following the creation of the stoma than prior to surgical resection. Jejunostomies are usually indicated for treatment of Crohn's disease. Ileostomies are created when the colon is removed typically due to a disorder such as ulcerative colitis or bypassed due to trauma (usually short term and reversible). Continent ileostomies are made by creating an internal reservoir that is drained by the patient several times a day via a tube inserted through the stoma; this avoids the necessity of wearing an external appliance. Colostomies are made by attaching a portion of the colon to the abdominal wall, often as a treatment for cancer, IBD, or trauma. The site of the colostomy often determines the nutritional modifications a patient requires; a stoma in the proximal colon (**Figure 1**) produces more liquid feces, whereas one placed distally results in more solid fecal material. Intestinal excreta are collected into a plastic bag attached to a device around the stoma. Postsurgical diets reflect a transition from clear liquids through low-fiber diets to a relatively unrestricted diet. A number of concerns regarding patients with stomas are reflected in nutritional management.

One of the more important complications of bowel resection and stoma placement is the development of short bowel syndrome. Patients with this condition have reduced absorption of most nutrients, which is accompanied by diarrhea. The degree of symptoms depends on the portion and length of intestine resected. Postsurgical nutritional management usually consists of TPN to reduce an osmotic effect of food in the remaining gut. There is concern about long-term bowel rest inducing intestinal atrophy and allowing bacterial translocation; this is based almost exclusively on studies in animals but there are few data from humans. Formula diets given enterally are indicated if the length of the remaining small bowel is insufficient for adequate digestion and absorption of a normal diet. Combinations of enteral, parenteral, and normal feeding

may be required. Specific advice depends on the length of remaining intestine and which portions were resected.

Since one of the primary physiological functions of the colon is reabsorption of water and electrolytes, surgical removal of this organ can result in excessive losses. Many patients voluntarily restrict their fluid intake in the mistaken belief that this will reduce effluent volume; however, excess water intake is eliminated primarily via the kidneys. In addition, the typical patient will need to be reminded to consume adequate sodium and potassium. When stomal losses exceed oral intake, parenteral fluids and minerals are required. Absorption of most trace elements and vitamins can also be reduced and, when needed, these are also supplied parenterally. A number of foods have been found to influence the amount of effluent. Those that increase volume are beans, cabbage, broccoli, spinach, raw fruits and juices, many spicy foods, red wine, and beer. Foods that are associated with decreased effluent volume include rice, bananas, applesauce, cooked milk, and peanut butter. Limited research indicates that pectin supplements can control excessive ileal effluent. Often, there are differences in the way individuals react to specific foods or combinations of them, so a food diary is highly recommended to relate changes in effluent to diet.

Because the diameter of a surgical stoma can be less than that of the intestine, certain foods can cause problems if chewed insufficiently. Therefore, chewing food thoroughly is an important part of the nutritional advice for a patient with a stoma. Some high-fiber foods are also relatively undigested and may need to be reduced or eliminated to control fecal volume and viscosity. These include corn, popcorn, nuts, coconut, celery, and raw fruits, particularly the skins and seeds.

Foods that are associated with gas production should be avoided if the patient is concerned with odor or flatulence from the stoma, which are common problems with this type of surgery. Such foods include the cabbage family, onions, beans, nuts, peppers, chocolate, carbonated beverages, eggs, and alcoholic beverages. Habits that encourage swallowing of air should also be minimized, such as gum chewing or drinking through a straw.

Weight control is important for patients with stomas to avoid some of the complications involving the skin surrounding the stoma. There is also a tendency for patients to gain weight once their primary gastrointestinal disease is treated successfully. There are a number of support groups for patients that provide nutrition advice, but it is important to distinguish between claims based on hype and soundly conducted studies. Nutritionists with proper academic credentials are generally the best source of accurate information.

See also: **Colon**: Structure and Function; Disorders. **Diarrheal Diseases. Nutritional Support**: Adults, Enteral; Adults, Parenteral; Infants and Children, Parenteral.

Further Reading

Beers MH and Berkow R (eds.) (1999) *The Merck Manual of Diagnosis and Therapy*, 17th edn. Whitehouse Station, NJ: Merck.

Coulston AM, Rock CL, and Monsen ER (eds.) (2001) *Nutrition in the Prevention and Treatment of Disease*. San Diego: Academic Press.

Haubrich WS, Shaffner F, and Berk JE (1995) *Bockus Gastroenterology*, 5th edn. Philadelphia: WB Saunders.

Kinney JM, Jeejeebhoy KN, Hill GL *et al.* (eds.) (1988) *Nutrition and Metabolism in Patient Care*. Philadelphia: WB Saunders.

Lewis JD and Fisher RL (1994) Nutrition support in inflammatory bowel disease. *Medical Clinics of North America* **78**: 1443–1456.

Nightingale JM (1995) The short-bowel syndrome. *European Journal of Gastroenterology and Hepatology* 7: 514–520.

Ozick LA, Salazar CO, and Donelson SS (1994) Pathogenesis, diagnosis, and treatment of diverticular disease of the colon. *Gastroenterologist* **2**: 299–310.

Sax WC and Souba WW (1993) Enteral and parenteral feedings. Guidelines and recommendations. *Medical Clinics of North America* **77**: 863–880.

Shils ME, Olson JA, Shike M *et al.* (eds.) (1999) *Modern Nutrition in Health and Disease*, 9th edn. Baltimore: Williams & Wilkins.

Spíller GA (ed.) (1993) *CRC Handbook of Dietary Fiber in Human Nutrition*, 2nd edn. Boca Raton, FL: CRC Press.

Zeman FJ and Ney DM (1996) *Applications in Medical Nutrition Therapy*, 2nd edn. Englewood Cliffs, NJ: Prentice Hall.

COMPLEMENTARY FEEDING

K G Dewey, University of California—Davis, Davis, CA, USA

© 2005 Elsevier Ltd. All rights reserved.

Introduction

Complementary feeding has been defined as

> ...the process starting when breast milk alone is no longer sufficient to meet the nutritional requirements of infants, and therefore other foods and liquids are needed, along with breast milk.
>
> (PAHO/WHO, 2003, p. 8)

In the past, such foods were often called 'weaning foods.' However, the term 'complementary foods' is preferred because weaning implies the cessation of breastfeeding, whereas the goal is that such foods should complement breast milk, not replace it. Breast milk alone is generally sufficient to meet the nutrient needs of infants during the first 6 months of life, but after that time infants need additional sources of nutrients. The World Health Organization (WHO) recommends exclusive breastfeeding for 6 months and continued breastfeeding thereafter (along with the provision of safe and appropriate complementary foods) until 2 years of age or beyond. Therefore, the period of complementary feeding usually refers to the age range of 6–24 months. This is a critical time because it is the peak age for growth faltering, deficiencies of certain micronutrients, and common childhood illnesses such as diarrhea.

In 1998, WHO and UNICEF jointly published a document entitled *Complementary Feeding of Young Children in Developing Countries: A Review of Current Scientific Knowledge*, which provided background information to assist in the development of scientifically based feeding recommendations and intervention programs. In 2003, an update to that document was published (see Further Reading), and a separate document entitled *Guiding Principles for Complementary Feeding of the Breastfed Child* was published by the Pan American Health Organization and WHO (see **Table 1**). This chapter will summarize the information presented in these three documents.

Age of Introduction of Complementary Foods

In 2001, the WHO Expert Consultation on the Optimal Duration of Exclusive Breastfeeding reviewed the evidence regarding the age of introduction of complementary foods and concluded that exclusive breastfeeding for 6 months is beneficial for both the infant and the mother. Risks arising from the early introduction of complementary foods include reduced breast-milk intake and a higher incidence of infant gastrointestinal infections. On a population basis, there is no adverse effect on infant growth of waiting to

Table 1 Guiding principles for complementary feeding of the breastfed child

1. *Duration of exclusive breastfeeding and age of introduction of complementary foods*
   Practice exclusive breastfeeding from birth to 6 months of age, and introduce complementary foods at 6 months of age (180 days) while continuing to breastfeed.
2. *Maintenance of breastfeeding*
   Continue frequent on-demand breastfeeding until 2 years of age or beyond.
3. *Responsive feeding*
   Practice responsive feeding, applying the principles of psychosocial care. Specifically: (a) feed infants directly and assist older children when they feed themselves, being sensitive to their hunger and satiety cues; (b) feed slowly and patiently, and encourage children to eat, but do not force them; (c) if children refuse many foods, experiment with different food combinations, tastes, textures, and methods of encouragement; (d) minimize distractions during meals if the child loses interest easily; (e) remember that feeding times are periods of learning and love – talk to children during feeding, with eye-to-eye contact.
4. *Safe preparation and storage of complementary foods*
   Practice good hygiene and proper food handling by (a) washing caregivers' and children's hands before food preparation and eating, (b) storing foods safely and serving foods immediately after preparation, (c) using clean utensils to prepare and serve food, (d) using clean cups and bowls when feeding children, and (e) avoiding the use of feeding bottles, which are difficult to keep clean.
5. *Amount of complementary food needed*
   Start at 6 months of age with small amounts of food and increase the quantity as the child gets older, while maintaining frequent breastfeeding. The energy needs from complementary foods for infants with 'average' breast-milk intake in developing countries are approximately 200 kcal day^{-1} at 6–8 months of age, 300 kcal day^{-1} at 9–11 months of age, and 550 kcal day^{-1} at 12–23 months of age. In industrialized countries these estimates differ somewhat (130, 310, and 580 kcal day^{-1} at 6–8, 9–11, and 12–23 months, respectively) because of differences in average breast-milk intake.
6. *Food consistency*
   Gradually increase food consistency and variety as the infant gets older, adapting to the infant's requirements and abilities. Infants can eat puréed, mashed, and semi-solid foods from the age of 6 months. By 8 months most infants can also eat 'finger foods' (snacks that can be eaten by children alone). By 12 months, most children can eat the types of foods consumed by the rest of the family (keeping in mind the need for nutrient-dense foods, as explained in #8 below). Avoid foods that may cause choking (i.e., items that have a shape and/or consistency that may cause them to become lodged in the trachea, such as nuts, grapes, and raw carrots).
7. *Meal frequency and energy density*
   Increase the number of times that the child is fed complementary foods as he/she gets older. The appropriate number of feedings depends on the energy density of the local foods and the usual amounts consumed at each feeding. For the average healthy breastfed infant, meals of complementary foods should be provided two or three times per day at 6–8 months of age and three or four times per day at 9–11 and 12–24 months of age. Additional nutritious snacks (such as a piece of fruit or bread or chapatti with nut paste) may be offered once or twice per day, as desired. Snacks are defined as foods eaten between meals – usually self-fed, convenient, and easy to prepare. If energy density or amount of food per meal is low, or the child is no longer breastfed, more frequent meals may be required.
8. *Nutrient content of complementary foods*
   Feed a variety of foods to ensure that nutrient needs are met. Meat, poultry, fish, or eggs should be eaten daily, or as often as possible. Vegetarian diets cannot meet nutrient needs at this age unless nutrient supplements or fortified products are used (see #9 below). Fruits and vegetables rich in vitamin A should be eaten daily. Provide diets with adequate fat content. Avoid giving drinks with low nutrient value, such as tea, coffee, and sugary drinks such as soda. Limit the amount of juice offered to avoid displacing more nutrient-rich foods.
9. *Use of vitamin–mineral supplements or fortified products for infant and mother*
   Use fortified complementary foods or vitamin–mineral supplements for the infant, as needed. In some populations, breastfeeding mothers may also need vitamin–mineral supplements or fortified products, both for their own health and to ensure normal concentrations of certain nutrients (particularly vitamins) in their breast milk. (Such products may also be beneficial for pre-pregnant and pregnant women.)
10. *Feeding during and after illness*
    Increase fluid intake during illness, including more frequent breastfeeding, and encourage the child to eat soft, varied, appetizing, favorite foods. After illness, give food more often than usual and encourage the child to eat more.

Reproduced from Pan American Health Organization/World Health Organization (2003) *Guiding Principles for Complementary Feeding of the Breastfed Child.* Washington, DC: Pan American Health Organization.

introduce complementary foods until 6 months, and the risk of micronutrient deficiencies is very low among full-term infants of normal birth weight whose mothers are well-nourished. Although iron deficiency may occur prior to the age of 6 months in infants whose iron reserves at birth are low (e.g., low-birth-weight infants and those whose mothers were iron deficient during pregnancy), the recommended approach is to provide medicinal iron drops from 2–3 months of age to such infants, rather than introducing complementary foods. Zinc status may also be marginal in low-birth-weight infants, and deficiency can be prevented by using zinc supplements. When the mother's diet is poor, the concentrations of certain vitamins (e.g., vitamin A and many of the B vitamins) and trace elements (e.g., iodine and selenium) in breast milk may be lower than desirable. In such situations, improving the mother's diet or giving her micronutrient supplements are the preferred approaches, rather than providing complementary foods to the infant before the age of 6 months.

At 6 months of age, infants are developmentally ready to consume complementary foods and can benefit from the additional nutrients that they provide. Continued breastfeeding is recommended because breast milk remains an important source of energy, fat, protein, and several micronutrients. In addition, continued frequent breastfeeding beyond 6 months protects child health by reducing the risk of diarrhea and other infections in disadvantaged populations and by delaying maternal fertility (thereby increasing the interval before the next pregnancy among women who do not use other forms of contraception).

Nutrient Needs from Complementary Foods

The amounts of nutrients provided by breast milk can be estimated by multiplying average breast-milk intake by the concentration of each nutrient in human milk. By subtracting these values from the total recommended nutrient intakes (RNIs) one can derive estimates of the amounts of nutrients needed from complementary foods after 6 months of age. Using this approach, **Table 2** lists these estimates for three age ranges: 6–8 months, 9–11 months, and 12–23 months. In this table, the RNIs for energy and protein are taken from the update report on complementary feeding published in 2003, and the RNIs for micronutrients are taken from the most recent FAO/WHO estimates or the US dietary reference intakes. The estimated amount of each nutrient provided by breast milk is based on the average milk intake during each of the age intervals, calculated separately for infants in developing countries and in industrialized countries, using data from the studies compiled in the 1998 WHO/UNICEF document. Because of differences between developing and industrialized countries in average milk intake and in the assumed breast-milk concentration of vitamin A, the estimated amount of each nutrient provided by breast milk may vary. Within each column of **Table 2**, the first value listed refers to developing countries, and the second value refers to industrialized countries.

The first row of **Table 2** shows the total energy requirements and the estimated amounts of energy obtained from breast milk and required from complementary foods at each age. In developing countries, the average expected energy intake from complementary foods is approximately 200 kcal (837 kJ) at 6–8 months, 300 kcal (1256 kJ) at 9–11 months, and

550 kcal (2302 kJ) at 12–23 months. These values represent 33%, 45%, and 61% of total energy needs, respectively. In industrialized countries, the corresponding values are approximately 130 kcal (544 kJ) at 6–8 months, 310 kcal (1298 kJ) at 9–11 months, and 580 kcal (2428 kJ) at 12–23 months (21%, 45%, and 65% of total energy needs, respectively). Of course, these values will differ if the child is consuming more or less breast milk than the average.

The second row of **Table 2** shows the same estimates for protein. Assuming average breast-milk intake, the amount of protein needed from complementary foods increases from about $2 \, g \, day^{-1}$ at 6–8 months to 5–$6 \, g \, day^{-1}$ at 12–23 months, with the percentage from complementary foods increasing from 21% to about 50%. The remaining rows show the estimates for the key vitamins and minerals. For vitamin B_{12} and selenium, the amounts needed from complementary foods prior to 12 months are zero because human milk contains generous amounts of these nutrients if the mother is adequately nourished. For the other micronutrients, the percentage of the RNI needed from complementary foods varies widely. At 6–8 months, for example, complementary foods need to provide less than 30% of the RNI for vitamin A, folate, vitamin C, copper, and iodine but more than 70% of the RNI for niacin, vitamin B_6, vitamin D, iron, and zinc. The values for the amount of niacin needed from complementary foods are high in all age intervals (75–88% of the RNI), but, because niacin needs can also be met by the contribution of tryptophan in the diet, niacin is not likely to be a limiting nutrient among infants who receive adequate protein. Similarly, the percentage of vitamin D needed from other sources is very high (more than 92%) because there is relatively little vitamin D in human milk; however, it should be noted that adequate exposure to sunlight can meet the child's needs for vitamin D even if complementary foods are not rich in this nutrient.

Complementary foods need to provide relatively large amounts (at least 80% of the RNI in all age intervals) of iron, zinc, and vitamin B_6. Because the amount of iron in human milk is very low (even though what is present is well absorbed), it is likely to be one of the first limiting nutrients in the diets of infants who rely predominantly on breast milk.

Fat is not listed in **Table 2** because there is uncertainty about the optimal intake of fat during the first 2 years of life. Dietary lipids are important not only as a source of essential fatty acids but also because they influence dietary energy density and sensory qualities. Breast milk is generally rich in fat (approximately 30–50% of energy) relative to most complementary foods, so as breast-milk intake

Table 2 Recommended nutrient intakes, average amount provided by breast milk, and amount needed from complementary foods at 6–8 months, 9–11 months, and 12–23 months

	6–8 months				9–11 months				12–23 months			
	RNI[a]	Amount from breast milk[b]	Amount needed from CF[c]	% from CF[c]	RNI[a]	Amount from breast milk[b]	Amount needed from CF[c]	% from CF[c]	RNI[a]	Amount from breast milk[b]	Amount needed from CF[c]	% from CF[c]
Energy (kcal d⁻¹)	615	413;486	202;129	33;21	686	379;375	307;311	45	894	346;313	548;581	61;65
Protein (g d⁻¹)	9.1	7.2	1.9	21	9.6	6.5;5.6	3.1;4.0	32;42	10.9	5.8;4.7	5.1;6.2	47;57
Vitamin A (µg RE d⁻¹)	400	337;461	63;0	16;0	400	308;354	92;46	23;12	400	275;300	125;100	31;25
Folate (µg d⁻¹)	80	58	22	28	80	52;45	28;35	35;44	160	47;38	113;122	71;76
Niacin (mg d⁻¹)	4	1	3.0	75	4	0.9;0.8	3.1;3.2	78;80	6	0.8;0.7	5.2;5.3	87;88
Riboflavin (mg d⁻¹)	0.40	0.24	0.16	40	0.40	0.22;0.19	0.18;0.21	45;53	0.50	0.19;0.16	0.31;0.34	62;68
Thiamin (mg d⁻¹)	0.30	0.14	0.16	53	0.30	0.12	0.18	60	0.50	0.11	0.39	78
Vitamin B₆ (mg d⁻¹)	0.30	0.06	0.24	80	0.30	0.06	0.24	80	0.50	0.05	0.45	90
Vitamin B₁₂ (µg d⁻¹)	0.50	0.66	0	0	0.50	0.60;0.51	0	0	0.90	0.53;0.47	0.37;0.43	41;48
Vitamin C (mg d⁻¹)	30	28	2	7	30	25;21	5;9	17;30	30	22;18	8;12	27;40
Vitamin D (µg d⁻¹)	5	0.4	4.6	92	5	0.3	4.7	94	5	0.3;0.2	4.7;4.8	94;96
Calcium (mg d⁻¹)	270	191	79	29	270	172;148	172;148	36;45	500	154;125	346;375	69;75
Copper (mg d⁻¹)	0.20	0.17	0.03	15	0.20	0.14	0.06	30	0.30	0.14;0.11	0.16;0.19	53;63
Iodine (µg d⁻¹)	90	75	15	17	90	68;58	22;32	24;36	90	60;49	30;41	33;46
Iron[d] (mg d⁻¹)	9.3	0.2	9.1	98	9.3	0.2	9.1	98	5.8	0.2;0.1	5.6;5.7	97;98
Magnesium (mg d⁻¹)	54	24	30	56	54	22;19	32	59	60	19;16	41;44	68;73
Phosphorus (mg d⁻¹)	275	95	180	65	275	86;74	189;201	69;73	460	77;63	383;397	83;86
Selenium (µg d⁻¹)	10	14	0	0	10	12	0	0	17	11	6	35
Zinc (mg d⁻¹)	3	0.6	2.4	80	3	0.5;0.4	2.5;2.6	83;87	3	0.4;0.3	2.6;2.7	87;90

[a]Recommended nutrient intakes, from FAO/WHO (2002) except for energy and protein (from Dewey and Brown, 2003) and calcium, copper, phosphorus, and zinc (from the US-Canada Dietary Reference Intakes).

[b]Based on average milk volumes of 674, 616, and 549 ml d⁻¹ in developing countries and 688, 529, and 448 ml d⁻¹ in industrialized countries for 6–8, 9–11, and 12–23 months, respectively (WHO 1998) and milk nutrient concentrations from the Institute of Medicine (IOM 1991, *Nutrition During Lactation*, Washington, DC: National Academy Press), except for vitamin A in milk of women from developing countries (WHO 1998) and zinc (Krebs NF *et al. Am J Clin Nutr* 1995; **61**: 1030–1036). For each nutrient, the first value refers to developing countries and the second value (after the semicolon) refers to industrialized countries, whenever there is a difference between the two.

[c]CF, complementary foods. For each nutrient, the first value refers to developing countries and the second value (after the semi-colon) refers to industrialized countries, whenever there is a difference between the two.

[d]Assuming medium bioavailability of iron.

declines with age, total fat intake is also likely to decline. If one assumes that the percentage of energy from fat in the total diet should be at least 30% and that the concentration of fat in breast milk averages $38 \, \mathrm{g \, l^{-1}}$, the amount of fat needed from complementary foods (assuming average breast-milk intake) is zero at 6–8 months, approximately $3 \, \mathrm{g \, d^{-1}}$ at 9–11 months, and 9–$13 \, \mathrm{g \, d^{-1}}$ at 12–23 months, or 0%, 5–8%, and 15–20% of the energy from complementary foods, respectively. As infants decrease their intake of breast milk they also need other good sources of essential fatty acids, such as fish, egg, liver, nut pastes, and most vegetable oils.

Meal Frequency, Energy Density, and Consistency of Complementary Foods

The frequency with which complementary foods need to be fed (i.e., the number of meals per day) depends on the total amount of food required and the amount of food that a child can consume at a single meal (gastric capacity). The total amount of food required is a function of the amount of energy needed from complementary foods (which varies with age and breast-milk intake) and the energy density of the foods (i.e., $\mathrm{kcal \, g^{-1}}$). The functional gastric capacity of infants and young children is assumed to be $30 \, \mathrm{g \, kg^{-1}}$ reference body weight. Thus, for a given age interval and level of breast-milk intake, calculating the recommended number of meals requires information about the energy density of the foods. To cover the needs of nearly all children, these calculations use as a starting point the average total energy requirement plus two standard deviations (25%). For children with average breast-milk intake who consume complementary foods with an energy density of at least $0.8 \, \mathrm{kcal \, g^{-1}}$, the number of meals required is two at 6–8 months and three thereafter. Children who consume less breast milk or who consume complementary foods with a lower energy density would need a greater number of meals. These calculations assume that children are fed to their gastric capacity at each meal, which may not be the case. For this reason, the guidelines recommend that additional nutritious snacks be offered once or twice per day, as desired (see guiding principle 7, **Table 1**).

A meal frequency greater than necessary may lead to excessive displacement of breast milk and may also require more time and effort by caregivers. Thus, it is useful to adapt meal-frequency guidelines to the characteristics of the target population.

The consistency of complementary foods needs to be appropriate for the child's stage of neuromuscular development. Semi-solid or puréed foods are needed at first because young infants do not have the ability to chew and swallow food of thick or solid consistency. By the age of 8 months most infants can also eat 'finger foods,' and by 12 months they can generally consume 'family foods' of a solid consistency. Thus, there should be a gradual change in the consistency of foods offered between 6 and 12 months, to match the infant's developmental progression (see guiding principle 6, **Table 1**).

Meeting Nutrient Needs During the Period of Complementary Feeding

As described above and shown in **Table 2**, breastfed infants need considerable amounts of certain nutrients from complementary foods after 6 months of age. It is a challenge to meet nutrient needs at this age because the amount of food consumed is relatively small, yet nutrient requirements during infancy (per unit of body weight) are very high because of the rapid rate of growth. Thus, nutrient-dense complementary foods are needed. The desired nutrient density (e.g., the amount of nutrient per 100 kcal of food) can be calculated by dividing the amount of each nutrient needed from complementary foods by the amount of energy expected to come from complementary foods (as shown in **Table 2**). When the desired nutrient densities are compared with the actual nutrient densities of the typical complementary foods consumed in various populations, protein density is generally seen to be adequate but several micronutrients are 'problem nutrients.' In most developing countries, iron, zinc, and vitamin B_6 are problem nutrients, and even in industrialized countries these nutrients may be limiting. Intake of iron is likely to be marginal in all populations unless iron-fortified products or substantial amounts of meat are consumed. Riboflavin, niacin, thiamin, folate, calcium, vitamin A, and vitamin C may also be problem nutrients, depending on the local mix of complementary foods. At present there is insufficient information to determine the extent to which some of the other micronutrients, such as vitamin E, iodine, and selenium, may be problem nutrients. Guiding principles 8 and 9 (**Table 1**) provide general recommendations to help ensure that the nutrient density of complementary foods will be adequate. It is difficult to develop more specific dietary 'prescriptions' to be used globally because of the great variability across populations in the types of complementary foods available. However, it is clear that predominantly vegetarian diets cannot meet the nutrient needs of breastfed infants unless nutrient supplements or fortified products are used. Part of the reason for this is that plant-based diets are often high in phytate, which greatly reduces the bioavailability of iron and zinc. Therefore, it is recommended that meat, fish, poultry, or egg be offered daily, if possible. Iron-fortified infant cereals are a good source of iron, but meats can also provide adequate iron if consumed in large enough quantities, and they have the added advantage of being rich in zinc. When the amount of animal-source food available locally is limited, the amounts of iron and zinc absorbed from the diet can be enhanced by, first, reducing the phytate concentrations of the staple complementary food through germination, fermentation, and/or soaking, second, reducing the intake of polyphenols (e.g., from coffee and tea), which are known to inhibit iron absorption, and, third, increasing the intake of enhancers of iron and zinc absorption, such as vitamin C (for iron) and other organic acids (for iron and zinc). Adequate calcium can be obtained from cheese, yoghurt, and other dairy products, but feeding fresh unheated cow's milk is not recommended before 12 months because it is associated with fecal blood loss and lower iron status. Some vegetables can also provide modest amounts of calcium, but the bioavailability of calcium from foods with high amounts of oxalate (such as spinach) is very low. Fruits and vegetables rich in vitamin A are recommended daily because of the importance of preventing vitamin A deficiency, which has been linked with excess child mortality and other adverse outcomes. The bioavailability of pro-vitamin A carotenoids can be enhanced by finely chopping or puréeing the food and serving it with a source of fat to facilitate absorption. Beverages with low nutrient density (e.g., sugary drinks) should be avoided and the amount of juice should be limited because such beverages can displace more nutrient-dense foods and potentially contribute to child obesity.

In most populations, designing a diet that satisfies the requirements for all the 'problem nutrients' without the use of fortified foods is difficult, because, even when animal-source foods are available, infants typically eat very small quantities. One option that is currently being investigated is the addition of micronutrients, in the form of 'sprinkles' or fat-based products, to home-prepared foods.

Preparation and Feeding of Complementary Foods

Complementary feeding involves not only what to feed but also how to feed infants and young children. The first issue is the safe preparation and storage of complementary foods (see guiding principle 4, **Table 1**). Attention to hygienic practices during food preparation and feeding is essential for preventing gastrointestinal illness. In developing countries, the age range of 6–24 months is when diarrhoea is most prevalent, largely because of microbial contamination of complementary foods. Feeding bottles can be a major source of contamination because they are difficult to keep clean, and thus in resource-poor populations it is recommended that they be avoided. The other recommendations in guiding principle 4 stress the importance of washing hands and feeding utensils carefully, serving food immediately, and storing leftovers safely.

The second issue involves the interaction between caregiver and infant during feeding (see guiding principle 3, **Table 1**). Appropriate feeding behavior is termed responsive feeding and is more sensitive to the child's hunger and satiety cues than either a laissez-faire style of feeding (the caregiver rarely encourages the child to eat) or, at the opposite extreme, a controlling style of feeding (the caregiver determines when and how much the child will eat, even to the point of force feeding). Responsive feeding also involves feeding slowly and patiently, minimizing distractions during meals, and positive interactions with the child while feeding. Although there is little evidence to date regarding the impact of promoting responsive feeding, it is hypothesized that it will enhance dietary intake, child growth, and possibly behavioral development.

The third issue regarding behavioral aspects of complementary feeding involves feeding during and after illness (see guiding principle 10, **Table 1**). The need for fluids is often greater during illness, and for this reason it is recommended that breastfeeding frequency be increased and other fluids be offered as needed. During illness, children prefer breast milk over other foods, so frequent breastfeeding is critical for maintaining nutrient intake. Although appetite may be reduced, continued consumption of complementary foods is recommended to enhance recovery. After illness, the child needs more food than usual to make up for nutrient losses during illness and to allow for catch-up growth.

See also: **Breast Feeding**. **Calcium**. **Diarrheal Diseases**. **Fatty Acids**: Metabolism; Monounsaturated; Omega-3 Polyunsaturated; Omega-6 Polyunsaturated; Saturated; *Trans* Fatty Acids. **Fertility**. **Fish**. **Hunger**. **Infants**: Nutritional Requirements; Feeding Problems. **Iron**. **Obesity**: Prevention. **Protein**: Requirements and Role in Diet. **United Nations Children's Fund**. **Vitamin D**: Rickets and Osteomalacia. **World Health Organization**. **Zinc**: Physiology.

Further Reading

Caulfield LE, Huffman SL, and Piwoz EG (1999) Interventions to improve intake of complementary foods by infants 6 to 12 months of age in developing countries: impact on growth and on the prevalence of malnutrition and potential contribution to child survival. *Food and Nutrition Bulletin* 20: 183–200.

Dewey KG (2001) Nutrition, growth and complementary feeding of the breastfed infant. *Pediatric Clinics of North America* 48: 87–104.

Dewey KG (2002) Success of intervention programs to promote complementary feeding. In: Black R and Michaelsen KF (eds.) *Public Health Issues in Infant and Child Nutrition*, pp. 199–212. Nestle Nutrition Workshop Series, Pediatric Program, vol. 48, Nestec Ltd. Philadelphia: Vevey/Lippincott Williams & Wilkins.

Dewey KG and Brown KH (2003) Update on technical issues concerning complementary feeding of young children in developing countries and implications for intervention programs. *Food and Nutrition Bulletin* 24: 5–28.

FAO/WHO Joint Expert Consultation (2002) *Vitamin and Mineral Requirements in Human Nutrition*. Geneva: World Health Organization.

Gibson RS, Ferguson EL, and Lehrfeld J (1998) Complementary foods for infant feeding in developing countries: their nutrient adequacy and improvement. *European Journal of Clinical Nutrition* 52: 764–770.

Lutter CL and Dewey KG (2003) Proposed nutrient composition for fortified complementary foods. *Journal of Nutrition* 133: 3011S–3020S.

Pan American Health Organization/World Health Organization (2003) *Guiding Principles for Complementary Feeding of the Breastfed Child*. Washington, DC: Pan American Health Organization.

World Health Organization (2001) *The Optimal Duration of Exclusive Breastfeeding: A Systematic Review*. WHO/NHD/01.08; WHO/FCH/CAH/01.23. Geneva: World Health Organization.

World Health Organization/London School of Hygiene and Tropical Medicine (2000) *Complementary Feeding: Family Foods for Breastfed Children*. WHO/NHD/00.1; WHO/FCH/CAH/00.6. Geneva: World Health Organization.

World Health Organization/UNICEF (1998) *Complementary Feeding of Young Children in Developing Countries: A Review of Current Scientific Knowledge*. WHO/NUT/98.1. Geneva: World Health Organization.

COPPER

X Xu, S Pin, J Shedlock and Z L Harris, Johns Hopkins Hospital and School of Medicine, Baltimore, MD, USA

© 2005 Elsevier Ltd. All rights reserved.

Introduction

Transition metals occupy a special niche in aerobic physiology: as facile electron donors and acceptors, they are essential participants in oxidation/reduction reactions throughout the cell. These unique properties of transition metals are largely dependent on the electronic configuration of the electrons in the outer shell and in the penultimate outer shell. These metals can exist in different oxidation states, which is critical for their usefulness as catalysts. However, it is during these same committed reactions essential for aerobic metabolism that toxic reactive oxygen species can be generated. As such the transition metals are chaperoned as they traffic through the body and are regulated tightly. Subtle disruptions of metal homeostasis culminate in disease and death. Iron, copper, and zinc are the most abundant and well-studied transition metals. Copper is the oldest metal in use: copper artifacts dating back to 8700BC have been found. The physiology, requirements, and dietary sources of copper are described here with an emphasis on the role of copper in human health and disease.

Copper, as a trace metal, can be found in all living cells in either the oxidized Cu(II) or reduced Cu(I) state. Copper is an essential cofactor for many enzymes critical for cellular oxidation. These include: cytochrome *c*-oxidase, which is essential for mitochondrial respiration as the terminal enzyme in the electron transport chain; superoxide dismutase, a potent antioxidant defense mechanism; tyrosinase, which is critical for melanin production; dopamine B-hydroxylase, a prerequisite for catecholamine production; lysyl oxidase, which is responsible for collagen and elastin cross-linking; ceruloplasmin, a ferroxidase/metallo-oxidase; hephaestin, a ferroxidase/metallo-oxidase; and peptidylglycine α-amidating monooxygenase, a peptide processor (**Table 1**). Mice that lack the copper transport protein Ctr1 are embryonic lethal, which confirms the importance of copper in enzyme function and normal cellular homeostasis.

Copper Homeostasis

Dietary intake of copper is approximately $5\,\text{mg day}^{-1}$ with an equivalent amount being excreted by bile in stool. Approximately $2\,\text{mg day}^{-1}$ are directly absorbed across the gastrointestinal tract daily and incorporated into blood, serum, liver,

Table 1 Mammalian copper enzymes

Enzyme	Function
Cytochrome *c*-oxidase	Mitochondrial respiration
cu,zn-Superoxide dismutase	Antioxidant defense
Tyrosinase	Melanin production
Dopamine B-hydroxylase	Catecholamine production
Lysyl oxidase	Collagen and elastin cross-linking
Ceruloplasmin	Ferroxidase/metallo-oxidase
Hephaestin	Ferroxidase/metallo-oxidase
PAM	Peptide processing

Table 2 Copper content of various foods

Food	Copper concentration (μg wet wt)	Size of typical serving (g)	Copper/ serving (mg g^{-1})
Fish	0.61	120	0.070
Turkey	0.71	120	0.090
Chicken	0.34	120	0.040
Hamburger	0.95	120	0.110
Roast beef	0.82	120	0.100
Steak	1.2	120	0.140
Sheep liver	157.05	120	18.850
Pork liver	141.14	120	16.940
Egg	0.8	40	0.030
Single sliced cheese	0.43	120	0.050
Whole wheat	1.07	30	0.030
Scallops	6.08	120	0.030
Clams	7.39	120	0.730
Crab	1.75	120	0.890
Shrimp	1.75	120	0.210
Oysters	2.89	120	0.350
Smoked oysters	15	120	1.800
Mussels	4.75	120	0.570
Lobster	36.6	120	4.390
Candy bar	1.18	15	0.020
Milk	0.33	120	0.040
Peas	2.38	120	0.290
Soy beans	109	120	0.130
Applesauce (can)	0.2	120	0.020
Avocado	1.68	120	0.200
Raisins	1.68	30	0.050
Peanut butter	8.53	30	0.260

brain, muscle, and kidney. An equal amount is excreted and maintains the sensitive copper balance (**Figure 1**). The main sources of copper are seeds, grains, nuts, beans, shellfish, and liver (**Table 2**). Drinking water no longer contributes significantly. When copper pipes were commonly used for plumbing, copper toxicity was a more recognized phenomenon.

It is difficult to define specific dietary copper requirements because of the lack of suitable indices to assess copper status. As such, knowledge of factors affecting the bioavailability of dietary copper is limited. Ceruloplasmin contains 95% of the copper found in serum and is frequently used as a marker of copper status. However, ceruloplasmin levels vary with pregnancy and inflammation and ceruloplasmin mRNA is regulated by estrogen, infection, and hypoxia among other factors. Currently, investigators are searching for genetic biomarkers in intestinal, liver, and lymphocyte cells that respond to copper levels and may serve as better markers of copper status. Whole-body

copper metabolism is difficult to study in human subjects. However, isotopic tracers and kinetic modeling have added a dimension to what can be learned in humans by direct measurement. These studies suggest that the efficiency of copper absorption varies greatly, depending on dietary intake. Mechanisms regulating total body copper seem to be strong, given the relatively small and constant body pool, but they are not yet well understood. Changes in efficiency of absorption help to regulate the amount of copper retained by the body. In addition, endogenous excretion of copper into the gastrointestinal tract depends heavily on the amount of copper absorbed. When dietary copper is high and an excess is absorbed, endogenous excretion increases, protecting against toxic accumulation of copper in the body. When intake is low, little endogenous copper is excreted, protecting against copper depletion. Regulation is not sufficient with very low amounts of dietary copper ($0.38\,\text{mg day}^{-1}$) and appears to be delayed when copper intake is high.

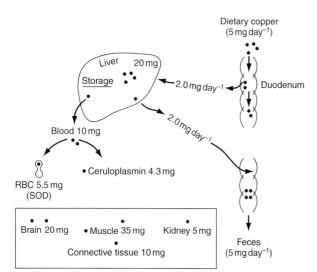

Figure 1 Mammalian copper metabolism: daily copper cycle including oral absorption, tissue distribution, and excretion. Values are for adult men (mg day^{-1}). An equal amount of copper is absorbed and excreted to maintain copper balance.

Recommended Intakes

The Tolerable Upper Intake Limit (UL) for adults is 10 mg daily, based on degree of liver damage associated with intake. UL for children vary with age: 1–3 years/1 mg daily, 4–8 years/3 mg daily, 9–13 years/ 5 mg daily, 14–18 years/8 mg daily (irrespective of pregnancy or lactation status). UL for children under the age of 1 year are not possible to establish. There are no official recommended daily allowances (RDAs) for copper in children. The RDA for adult males and females is a daily intake of 0.9 mg. Measurements of the dietary requirements for copper in adult men have shown the requirement to range from about 1.0 to 1.6 mg daily. A review of nutrient intakes in the US from 1909 to 1994 confirms that intake varied between 1.5 mg day^{-1} (1965) to 2.1 mg day^{-1} (1909). These trends reflect a diet higher in copper-rich potatoes and grain predominating in 1909 versus a decline in potato popularity in 1965. Daily intake recommendations for children vary with age (see **Table 3**). Persons who consume diets high in zinc and low in protein are at risk of copper deficiency. High intakes of dietary fiber apparently increase the dietary requirement for copper. Diets in Western countries provide copper below or in the low range of the estimated safe and adequate daily dietary intake. Copper deficiency is usually a consequence of low copper stores at birth, inadequate dietary copper intake, poor absorption, elevated requirements induced by rapid growth, or increased copper losses.

Bioavailability

The issue of bioavailability from food sources and the interactions between food groups and copper availability remains a critical question. Lonnerdal *et al.* demonstrated that heat treatment of cows'

milk formula decreases the copper bioavailability. Transitional complexes form in the milk upon heating that have a similar configuration to copper and thereby directly inhibit copper absorption. High doses of zinc also reduce copper bioavailability, as does combined iron and zinc supplementation. The dilemma is how to prepare an infant formula containing adequate copper, iron, and zinc that will meet the RDA for copper. Other nutrients dramatically affect copper absorption from foods. Soy protein-based diets promote less copper retention in tissues than lactalbumin-based diets. However, it is unclear if this effect is solely due to the soy protein composition or to the higher zinc in these soy-based formulas. In animals, phytate causes a drop in serum copper but human stable isotope studies reveal no effect on copper absorption in adult men. Patients with low copper indices need to be evaluated for the copper content of their diets, other foods ingested at the same time, and other mineral supplements that may be given.

Absorption and Excretion

Dietary copper is absorbed across the small intestine. It diffuses through the mucous layer that covers the wall of the bowel via the divalent metal transporter DMT1. Copper is thus released into the serum and presumably is transported bound to either albumin or histidine to the multiple sites that require copper or to storage tissues. The liver is the primary storage organ for copper followed by muscle and bone. Not all of the copper ingested is absorbed and gastrointestinal cells that hold on to the excess copper are 'sloughed' when the lining of the gut is turned over every 24–48 hs. Copper bound to albumin or histidine enters the hepatocyte via the high-affinity mammalian copper transporter, hCtr1. Initially identified in yeast by functional complementation studies, this protein has subsequently been cloned in mice and humans. Human Ctr1 has a high homology to the yeast proteins Ctr1 and Ctr3 involved in high-affinity copper uptake. The N-terminus of the protein is rich in histidine and methionine residues, which presumably bind the copper and move it into the cell. Characterization of hCtr1 confirms its localization on the plasma membrane consistent with its role as a copper transporter. *In vitro* work has also identified a vesicular perinuclear distribution for hCtr1 that is copper concentration dependent. Redistribution of the hCtr1 suggests that under different copper states, copper moves through the membrane transporter and into a vesicular compartment for further 'assignment' within the cell.

Table 3 Recommended dietary allowances for copper (mg day^{-1})

Age	RDA (daily)
Infants	
<6 months	0.2 (30 mcg/kg)
6–12 months	0.2–0.3 (24 mcg/kg)
Children	
1–3 years	0.34
4–8 years	0.44
9–13 years	0.7
14–18 years	0.89
Adult	
19+ years	0.9
Pregnant women	1
Nursing women	1.3

hCtr2, a low-affinity copper uptake transporter, has also been identified. This low-affinity copper transporter is unable to complement the respiratory defect seen in yeast strains lacking copper transport capabilities. Once inside the cell, copper has one of four fates: (1) bind to and be stored within a glutathione/metallothionein pool; (2) bind to CCS, the copper chaperone for Cu, Zn - SOD; (3) bind to cox 17 for delivery to mitochondrial cytochrome *c*-oxidase; or (4) bind to HAH1 (human Atox1 homolog) for subsequent copper delivery to either the Wilson disease P-type ATPase or the Menkes' P-type ATPase. Copper from HAH1 is incorporated into ceruloplasmin, the most abundant serum cuproprotein, within the trans golgi network (TGN). How the protein unfolds within the TGN to accept copper and how the copper is incorporated into ceruloplasmin is still under study. Ceruloplasmin is then secreted into the serum, and any excess copper not incorporated into ceruloplasmin is recycled in vesicles containing either the Wilson disease P-type ATPase or Menkes' P-type ATPase, and excreted into bile or stored in the liver. Recent characterization of a new protein, Murr1, suggests that this protein regulates copper excretion into bile such that mutations in the Murr1 gene are associated with normal copper uptake but severe defects in exporting copper from hepatocytes.

Approximately 15% of the total copper absorbed is actually transported to tissues while the remaining 85% is excreted. Of that copper pool, 98% is excreted in bile with the remaining 2% eliminated in the urine. The liver is the predominant organ responsible for regulating copper homeostasis at the level of excretion. Whereas copper import is highly conserved between yeast and humans, copper export in vertebrates involves a complex vesicular system that culminates in a lysosomal excretion pathway 'dumping' copper into the bile for elimination. At steady state, the amount of copper excreted into the biliary system is directly proportional to the hepatic copper load. In response to an increasing copper concentration within the hepatocyte, biliary copper excretion increases. There is no enterohepatic recirculation of copper and once the unabsorbable copper complex is in bile it is excreted in stool. Localization studies reveal redistribution of the ATP7b from the TGN to a vesicular compartment that migrates out to the biliary epithelium in response to increasing copper concentrations. Alternatively, under conditions of copper deficiency, the ATP7b remains tightly incorporated with the TGN for maximal copper incorporation into ceruloplasmin.

The highly homologous Wilson disease P-type ATPase (ATP7b) and the Menkes's P-type ATPase (ATP7a) differ only in their tissue expression and both function to move copper from one intracellular compartment to another. The ATP7a is predominantly located in the placenta, blood–brain barrier, and gastrointestinal tract and hence any mutation in the Menkes's P-type ATPase results in a copper deficiency in the fetus, brain, and tissues. In contrast, the Wilson's disease P-type ATPase is expressed in the liver and mutations in this culminate in profound copper overload of the liver because of the inability to shuttle copper into the trans golgi network for incorporation into ceruloplasmin. The excess copper is stored in the liver and eventually leaks out in the serum where it is deposited within sensitive tissues: the eye and brain. The psychiatric illnesses ascribed to Wilson's disease are a result of hepatocyte-derived copper 'leaking' out of the liver and accumulating within the basal ganglia. Similarly, Kayser-Fleischer rings arise from copper deposition in the cornea. The toxic copper in the liver eventually results in cirrhosis and hepatic fibrosis as a result of oxyradical damage. Menkes's syndrome has an incidence of 1:300 000 while Wilson's disease has an incidence of 1:30 000. Expression of these diseases may differ considerably among affected family members.

The recognition of a novel disorder of iron metabolism associated with mutations in the copper-containing protein ceruloplasmin revealed an essential role for ceruloplasmin as a ferroxidase and regulator of iron homeostasis. Patients and mice lacking the serum protein ceruloplasmin have normal copper kinetics: normal absorption, distribution, and copper-dependent activity. These data suggest that although under experimental conditions ceruloplasmin may donate copper, ceruloplasmin is not a copper transport protein. The six atoms of copper are incorporated into three type 1 coppers, one type 2 copper, and a type 3 copper. The type 1 coppers provide the electron shuttle necessary for the concomitant reduction of oxygen to water that occurs within the trinuclear copper cluster comprised of the type 2 and type 3 copper. This reaction is coupled with the oxidation of a variety of substrates: amines, peroxidases, iron, NO, and possibly copper. The recent observation that Fet3, the yeast ceruloplasmin homolog, also has critical cuprous oxidase activity in addition to ferroxidase activity has prompted renaming some of the multicopper oxidases (ceruloplasmin, Fet3, hephaestin) as 'metallo-oxidases' rather than ferroxidases.

Copper Deficiency

Reports of human copper deficiency are limited and suggest that severe nutrient deficiency coupled with malabsorption is required for this disease state to occur. Infants fed an exclusive cows' milk diet are at risk for copper deficiency. Cows' milk not only has substantially less copper than human milk but the bioavailability is also reduced. High oral intake of iron or zinc decrease copper absorption and may predispose an individual to copper deficiency. Other infants at risk include those with: (1) prematurity secondary to a lack of hepatic copper stores; (2) prolonged diarrhea; and (3) intestinal malabsorption syndromes. Even the premature liver is capable of impressive copper storage. By 26 weeks' gestational age the liver already has 3 mg of copper stored. By 40 weeks' gestational age, the hepatic liver has 10–12 mg copper stored with the majority being deposited in the third trimester. Iron and zinc have been shown to interfere with copper absorption and further complicate the picture of copper deficiency. The most frequent clinical manifestations of copper deficiency are anemia refractory to iron treatment, neutropenia, and bone demineralization presenting as fractures.

The anemia is characterized as hypochromic and normocytic with a reduced reticulocyte count, hypoferremia, and thrombocytopenia. Bone marrow aspirate reveals megaloblastic changes and vacuolization of both erythroid and myeloid progenitor lineages. It is believed that a profound copper deficiency results in a multicopper oxidase deficient state and as such bone marrow demands are unmet by the lack of ferroxidase activity. Bone abnormalities are common and manifest as osteoporosis, fractures, and epiphyseal separation. Other manifestations of copper deficiency include hypopigmentation, hypotonia, growth arrest, abnormal cholesterol and glucose metabolism, and increased rate of infections.

Multiple factors associated with copper deficiency are responsible for the increased rate of infection seen. Most copper-deficient patients are malnourished and suffer from impaired weight gain. The immune system requires copper to perform several functions. Recent research showed that interleukin 2 is reduced in copper deficiency and is probably the mechanism by which T-cell proliferation is reduced. These results were extended to show that even in marginal deficiency, when common indexes of copper are not affected by the diet, the proliferative response and interleukin concentrations are reduced. The number of neutrophils in human peripheral blood is reduced in cases of severe copper deficiency. Not only are they reduced in number, but their ability to generate superoxide anion and kill ingested microorganisms is also reduced in both overt and marginal copper deficiency. This mechanism is not yet understood.

Copper Excess

Excess copper is the result of either excessive copper absorption or ineffective copper excretion. The most common diseases associated with copper excess are: (1) Wilson's disease, a genetic disease resulting in mutations in the Wilson's disease P-type ATPase and excessive hepatocyte copper accumulation; (2) renal disease, in patients on hemodialysis due to kidney failure when dialysate solutions become contaminated with excess copper; and (3) biliary obstruction. Excessive use of copper supplements may also contribute to copper toxicity and is clinically manifested by severe anemia, nausea and vomiting, abdominal pain, and diarrhea. Copper toxicosis can rapidly progress to coma and death if not recognized. Current management of most diseases associated with copper toxicity includes a low-copper diet, a high-zinc diet (competitively interferes with copper absorption), and use of copper chelators such as penicillamine and trientine. Affected individuals should have their tap water analyzed for copper content and drink demineralized water if their water contains more than 100 µg/liter. Given that the liver is the most significant copper storage organ, any activity that can affect hepatic cellular metabolism needs to be monitored. Hence, alcohol consumption is strongly discouraged.

There are reports of chronic copper exposure resulting in toxic accumulation. Fortunately, these events appear to be geographically restricted. Indian childhood cirrhosis (ICC), also known as Indian infantile cirrhosis or idiopathic copper toxicosis, has been associated with increased copper intake from contaminated pots used to heat up infant milk. The milk is stored and warmed in brass (a copper alloy) or copper containers. It is interesting to note that the increased copper absorption alone is not critical for disease formation but rather this occurs in infants that already have prenatal liver copper stores in excess of adult values. How the neonatal liver is able to compartmentalize this toxic metal so effectively is unknown. Perhaps in ICC, this delicate balance is disrupted. Tyrolean liver disease, occurring in the Austrian Tyrol, despite having a Mendelian pattern of inheritance suggestive of an autosomal recessive trait, appears related to use of copper cooking utensils. However, recent reports describe how a persistent percentage of the German population remains susceptible to copper toxicosis despite adjustments in cooking utensils. Perhaps a genetic susceptibility exists in this population that has yet to be determined.

Conclusion

Adult copper homeostasis rests on the foundation of an adequate copper balance in early life. Copper deficiency, either due to inadequate intake or abnormal absorption, may result. While the clinical stigmata of severe copper deficiency are easy to identify, the subtle changes in neurobehavioral development associated with mild copper deficiency are unknown. Given the high copper concentration in the brain, one could postulate that critical copper deficiency during development could lead to significant central nervous system deficits. Recent evidence suggesting that copper metabolism may be involved as an epigenetic factor in the development of Alzheimer's disease (AD) highlights the importance of balance. In this scenario, elevated central nervous system copper, as seen in AD, may initiate increased oxyradical formation and hasten damage. In fact, some are advocating that serum copper might be a good biomarker for AD. Copper is an essential trace metal critical for normal development. The goal of future studies will be to develop sensitive biomarkers for copper status. Only with these tools can we adequately assess copper status and treat copper-deficient and copper excess states appropriately.

See also: **Bioavailability**. **Zinc**: Physiology.

Further Reading

Araya M, Koletzko B, and Uauy R (2003) Copper deficiency and excess in infancy: developing a research agenda. *Journal of Pediatric Gastroenterology and Nutrition* 37: 422–429.

Bush AI and Strozyk D (2004) Serum copper: A biomarker for Alzheimer disease. *Archives of Neurology* 61: 631–632.

Gitlin JD (2003) Wilson disease. *Gastroenterology* 125: 1868–1877.

Klein CJ (2002) Nutrient requirements for preterm infant formulas. *Journal of Nutrition* 132: 1395S–1577S.

Lutter CK and Dewey KG (2003) Proposed nutrient composition for fortified complimentary foods. *Journal of Nutrition* 133: 3011S–3020S.

Prohaska JR and Gybina AA (2004) Intracellular copper transport in mammals. *Journal of Nutrition* 134: 1003–1006.

Rees EM and Thiele DJ (2004) From aging to virulence: forging connections through the study of copper homeostasis in eukaryotic microorganisms. *Current Opinion in Microbiology* 7: 175–184.

Schulpis KH, Karakonstantakis T, Gavrili S *et al.* (2004) Maternal-neonatal serum selenium and copper levels in Greeks and Albanians. *European Journal of Clinical Nutrition* 1: 1–5.

Shim H and Harris ZL (2003) Genetic defects in copper metabolism. *Journal of Nutrition* 133: 1527S–1531S.

Tapiero H, Townsend DM, and Tew KD (2003) Trace elements in human physiology. Copper. *Biomedicine & Pharmacotherapy* 57: 386–398.

Uauy R, Olivares M, and Gonzalez M (1998) Essentiality of copper in humans. *American Journal of Clinical Nutrition* 67(S): 952S–959S.

Wijmenga C and Klomp LWJ (2004) Molecular regulation of copper excretion in the liver. *Proceedings of the Nutrition Society* 63: 31–39.

CORONARY HEART DISEASE

Contents
Hemostatic Factors
Lipid Theory
Prevention

Hemostatic Factors

W Gilmore, University of Ulster, Coleraine, UK

© 2005 Elsevier Ltd. All rights reserved.

Introduction

The two major processes that contribute to the pathogenesis of coronary heart disease (CHD) and stroke are atherosclerosis and thrombosis. These, in turn, involve inflammation and hemostasis; two pathways that are linked both at the molecular and cellular levels. In addition to stimulating the inflammatory response, the proinflammatory cytokines, chiefly interleukin-1beta (IL-1β) and tumor necrosis factor alpha (TNFα), may promote the initiation of hemostasis by upregulating tissue factor (TF) on endothelial cells and the blood monocytes. The explosion of interest in the role of cholesterol in vascular diseases in the latter half of the twentieth century led to a decrease in interest in the role of hemostatic factors in this group of diseases. However, the efficacy of thrombolytic drugs in the treatment of acute myocardial infarction together with the demonstration that clots were involved in sudden ischemic death renewed interest in the role of the blood clotting pathways in these disorders. Hemostasis is part of the body's normal defense system and response to injury. The advancement, by Russell Ross, of the response to injury hypothesis of vascular disease has directed attention towards hemostasis again. Hemostasis involves the interaction between cells of the immune system, blood platelets, smooth muscle cells, endothelial cells, and the blood clotting proteins. The blood clot is eventually broken down by the fibrinolytic mechanism and the normal tissue repair processes promote wound healing. A balance between the processes of hemostasis and fibrinolysis has always been thought necessary to prevent blood loss, on the one hand, and thrombosis, on the other. Many of the components of the hemostatic mechanism have been identified as risk factors for vascular disease and these include: increased plasma levels of the blood clotting proteins fibrinogen and factor VII, increased platelet aggregation, and elevated plasma levels of the inhibitor of plasmin activation, plasminogen activator inhibitor-1 (PAI-1).

Nutrition plays a central role in the activity of the blood coagulation factors with the requirement of vitamin K in the posttranslational carboxylation of glutamic acid residues on key blood clotting proteins and some of their physiological inhibitors. In addition to this involvement of vitamin K in the biosynthesis of biologically active blood clotting proteins other nutrients may modify components of the blood coagulation pathway. However, results from many intervention studies still often yield conflicting results. This article will concentrate on a description of hemostasis, as we currently understand it, rather than an exhaustive account of the studies on dietary factors and hemostasis. This may enable the reader to discern the most appropriate aspects of hemostasis for study by nutrition scientists.

Hemostasis

Platelets

When trauma occurs platelets can form a small primary hemostatic plug that is sufficient to stop bleeding from a small nick in the skin. Platelets are very easily activated and, therefore, difficult to study. They are formed from megakaryocytes in the bone marrow and, to a lesser extent, in the peripheral blood and lungs. Platelets are small ($0.2-3.5\,\mu m$ in diameter) buds off these large megakaryocytes. They have a volume of about $10\,fl$ and number $100-400 \times 10^9\,l^{-1}$ in peripheral blood. When viewed under light microscopy, they have little structure; however, electron microscopy reveals abundant subcellular organelles. Platelets contain large quantities of lipids; their plasma membrane is highly involuted and their cytoplasm contains numerous membrane-bound granules. These granules are of two types: electron-dense granules that contain, *inter alia*, ADP, Ca^{2+} and serotonin, and the so-called specific alpha-granules that contain some blood coagulation proteins and growth factors such as platelet-derived growth factor (PDGF) and transforming growth factor-beta (TGF-β), which promote wound healing.

When activated, platelets express the adhesion molecule P-selectin (CD62P), which, in unactivated platelets, is present in the alpha-granules. Activated platelets stick to damaged endothelium, a process known as platelet adhesion, and then stick to each other, a process known as platelet aggregation. Adhesion molecules form important molecular components of this process. Platelet aggregation can be measured in the laboratory by simple photometric techniques. This *in vitro* aggregation is stimulated by adrenaline, collagen, ADP, and the toxic antibiotic risocetin and has been widely applied in studies of the effect of nutrients on platelet function. However, adhesion and aggregation may only be minor biological functions of platelets. The main function of these tiny fragments seems to be in their ability to release a vast array of biologically active substances. In particular, they release phospholipid from their membranes to participate in the coagulation cascade. Platelets release serotonin, a powerful vasoconstrictant. They also release PDGF and TGF-β both of which are growth factors intimately involved in wound healing and tissue regeneration. Low platelet numbers will lead to an increased bleeding tendency and, interestingly, to a decrease in the integrity of the blood vessel walls. Therefore, platelets have two main functions in the body: they participate in hemostasis, and are responsible for the repair and maintenance of the blood vessel walls.

The products of cyclooxygenases play a crucial role in the action of blood platelets. The substrates of these enzymes are the n-6 and n-3 long-chain polyunsaturated fatty acids. Platelets cannot synthesize these from the short-chain precursors and so must rely on direct incorporation of the long-chain polyunsaturated fatty acids into their cellular membranes. In platelets, cyclooxygenases and other enzymes convert arachidonic acid (C20:4n-6) to thromboxane A_2, which potentiates platelet aggregation, whereas the less potent thromboxane A_3 is generated when eicosapentaenoic acid (C20:5n-3) is the substrate. The endothelial cells constitutively synthesize the arachidonic acid (C20:4n-6)-derived eicosinoid, prostaglandin I$_2$ (PGI$_2$) which is antiaggregatory in its action and thus the normal endothelium provides a surface that prevents blood clotting.

The Coagulation Cascade

Blood coagulation factors are proteins, most of which were discovered when a genetically inherited bleeding disorder was discovered in patients. A newly discovered coagulation factor was often named after the patient in whom it was first recognized, but nowadays the Roman numerals I through to XIII are designated and accepted names of these proteins. A suffix, 'a' indicates an activated coagulation factor. The components of the blood coagulation pathways are mostly serine proteases that sequentially activate each other in turn, giving rise to a fibrin clot. Some, however, act as cofactors in some of the reactions, e.g., factors Va and VIIIa. There are two different mechanisms whereby blood clotting may be initiated (**Figure 1**). The principal mechanism, known as the tissue factor (TF) pathway or the extrinsic coagulation cascade, involves the expression of TF (thromboplastin or factor III) on the cells of the intima of the damaged blood vessel. TF is only expressed on the cells that are not in contact with the peripheral blood. The exposure of blood to TF, in turn, leads to the sequential activation of the blood clotting factors, and the generation of the fibrin clot. The only cells in day-to-day contact with blood that can be stimulated to

produce TF are endothelial cells and monocytes when the proinflammatory cytokines and bacterial endotoxins stimulate these cells to express this cell membrane-bound protein. The presence of a NFκB binding site in the promoter region of the tissue factor gene on chromosome 1 further indicates involvement of hemostasis in inflammatory processes.

TF is an integral membrane protein of 263 amino acids and molecular weight 47 000. It has been assigned CD142 by the VIth International Workshop and Conference on Human Leukocyte Differentiation Antigens held in Kobe, Japan, in 1996. The ligand for this cell surface protein is factor VII or factor VIIa. There are relatively small amounts of factor VIIa constantly present in normal blood. However, only when factor VIIa binds to TF does it become significantly potent as an activator of blood coagulation. A TF:Ca^{2+}:factor VIIa complex is formed and this activates both factor X to factor Xa and factor IX to factor IXa, which forms a complex with factor VIIa, Ca^{2+}, and platelet phospholipids to activate further molecules of factor X. The activated factor X forms a factor Xa:Ca^{2+}:factor Va complex, which converts prothrombin to thrombin. Thrombin acts on fibrinogen molecules to convert them to fibrin monomers. These monomers form an instantaneous clot by associating via noncovalent bonds. The clot is then stabilized in a reaction catalyzed by factor XIIIa by crosslinking the fibrin molecule by covalent bonds between glutamic acid and lysine residues of adjacent fibrin monomers. Thrombin plays a central role in hemostasis in that it not only converts fibrinogen to fibrin but also activates other key players in the pathways; in particular, factor VII, factor XI, and the copper-dependent factors V and VIII. The major physiological activator of factor VII remains unidentified but, in addition to thrombin; factor Xa, factor XIa, and factor XIIa are capable of converting factor VII to factor VIIa.

TF is inhibited by a specific inhibitor of the TF:Ca^{2+}:factor VIIa complex (**Figure 3**). This inhibitor, designated tissue factor pathway inhibitor (TFPI), is a 276 amino acid polypeptide that has three Kunitz-like regions. Therefore, this belongs to the Kunitz-type protease inhibitors whilst most other inhibitors of blood coagulation are serpins. In peripheral blood this inhibitor is associated with the lipid fractions and is, like tissue factor, synthesized by activated endothelial cells and monocytes. The TFPI remains inactive until sufficient amounts of activated factor X (i.e., factor Xa) can bind. The TFPI:factor Xa complex then inactivates the TF:Ca^{2+}:factor VIIa complex.

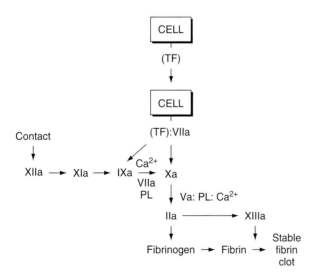

Figure 1 The tissue factor pathway and contact activation pathways of blood coagulation. PL, platelet phospholipids; TF, tissue factor.

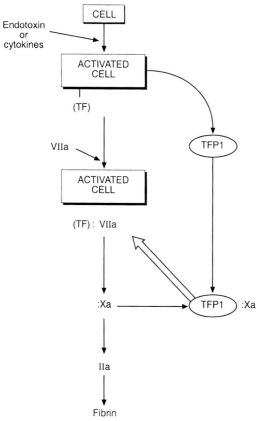

Figure 2 The action of tissue factor pathway inhibitor (TFPI). TF, tissue factor.

In the second mechanism of initiation, the contact activation pathway (**Figure 1** and **Figure 2**), blood coagulation may be triggered by activation upon contact with collagen and other highly charged surfaces, including glass or plastic test tubes. Contact with collagen leads to activation of factor XII and, in turn, factor XIIa activates factor XI. Factor XIa activates factor IX, which together with Ca^{2+}, platelet phospholipid, and factor VIIIa activates factor X to factor Xa. The contact activation pathway merges with the tissue factor pathway

at this point and, as before, the factor Xa, together with Ca^{2+}, platelet phospholipid, and factor Va activates prothrombin to thrombin, which converts fibrinogen to fibrin. The existence of this second pathway means that fibrin production remains switched on as long as the blood remains in contact with external surfaces despite the fact that the tissue factor pathway may, at this point, be closed down by the action of TFPI and factor Xa. The formation of factor XIIa has important consequences for other processes involved in the response of the body to injury. For example; high-molecular-weight kininogen and prekallikrein are activated to the kinins and to kallikrein, mediators of inflammation that can activate the contact pathway (**Figure 3**). In addition, fibrinolysis and the complement pathway are both activated by factor XIIa. It is probable that the physiological role of factor XIIa is to act as a mediator in many of the processes involved in the defense of the body during trauma and its role in the activation of blood coagulation may be of minor importance.

The coagulation process is inhibited by nonspecific mechanisms such as blood flow and by the presence in plasma of general serine protease inhibitors such as alpha2-macroglobulin. In addition, unique molecular systems will specifically inhibit blood coagulation and one of these involves heparin, a sulfated glycosaminoglycan. Heparin combines with antithrombin III in a one to one molar ratio and the resultant complex inhibits factor Xa and thrombin. Another specific control mechanism involves the vitamin K-dependent proteins, protein S and protein C, which combine with each other in molar ratios to form a complex with cellular membranes that inhibits the activity of factors Va and VIIIa. The complex also inhibits the action of PAI-1 thereby promoting fibrinolysis. Interestingly, a normal factor V molecule is essential for the inhibitory properties of this complex since mutation of factor V will cause a malfunction of the complex and result in a tendency to form clots (thrombophilia). This is the basis of the action of factor V Leiden, a mutant of factor V that causes familial thrombophilia.

Fibrinolysis, Fibrinogen, and the Acute Phase Response

The breakdown of the fibrin clot is initiated by activators of plasminogen, mainly tissue plasminogen activator (tPA) (**Figure 4**). This protein is produced by endothelial cells and activates plasminogen by converting it to plasmin. The plasmin then acts on fibrin to form the fibrin split

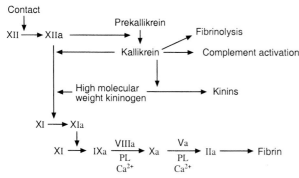

Figure 3 Contact activation pathway. PL, platelet phospholipids.

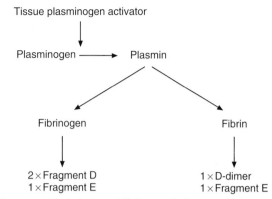

Figure 4   Fibrinolysis and fibrinogenolysis.

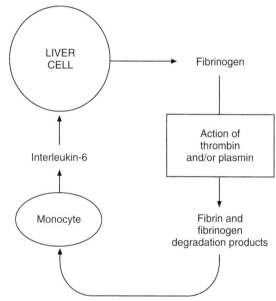

Figure 5   The role of interleukin-6 in fibrinogen synthesis.

products, a D-dimer and a fragment E from each fibrin monomer, and on fibrinogen to form the fibrinogen degradation products, two molecules of fragment D and one of fragment E. These breakdown products act as inhibitors of thrombin. They also stimulate the release of interleukin-6 (IL-6) from blood monocytes; the IL-6 then acts on the liver parenchymal cell to stimulate the synthesis of fibrinogen. The presence of this regulatory loop demonstrates the direct link between a proinflammatory cytokine, interleukin-6, and the production of a protein (fibrinogen) of the so-called acute phase response (**Figure 5**). Fibrinolysis is inhibited by PAI-1 and alpha2-antiplasmin.

Thrombosis

Thrombosis is a major cause of mortality and morbidity in Western societies. Deep venous thrombosis, myocardial infarction, pulmonary embolism, and acute thromboembolic stroke are, probably, all consequences of inappropriate blood coagulation or fibrinolysis. Fibrin formation is instantaneous and therefore clots can quickly occlude an artery and thereby precipitate an acute cardiac or cerebral event. This usually, but not exclusively, occurs in atherosclerotic blood vessels where plaques may rupture and cause thrombus formation.

The expression of tissue factor on cells and their subsequent exposure to blood is probably the major initiator of thrombus formation *in vivo*. It has been demonstrated that the blood monocytes from unstable angina and myocardial infarction patients express increased amounts of tissue factor when compared to healthy controls. Furthermore, it has been shown that monocytes from atherosclerotic plaques from unstable angina patients express increased amounts of tissue factor when compared to controls, thereby further implicating plaque rupture in the pathology of heart disease.

Hemostatic Factors and Risk of Coronary Heart Disease

Elevated plasma coagulation factor levels are risk factors for coronary heart disease. Fibrinogen synthesis in the liver is stimulated by the proinflammatory cytokine interleukin-6 and, therefore, elevated levels are found during the acute phase response. It has been argued that it may be difficult to assign elevated plasma fibrinogen as a definitive risk factor since the pathology of CHD involves inflammation and the acute phase response, which will lead to increased fibrinogen anyway. The same argument has been used in the case of elevated white cell counts, which is also a risk factor for coronary events. However, it has been demonstrated that if fibrinogen and/or white blood cell count remain high after a vascular event then there is greater risk of subsequent events. Therefore, increased plasma fibrinogen and elevated white cell count are now considered a major risk factor for CHD.

Further studies have indicated that other blood clotting factors may act as risk factors for CHD. For example, a prospective study, The Northwick Park Heart Study, identified factor VII as a risk factor for CHD and showed that plasma levels of factor VII were predictive of CHD in a dose-dependent manner. Another study has shown that factor VIII may be a risk factor for cardio-vascular disease. Increased levels of PAI-1 and decreased plasma levels of plasminogen activators have also been identified as risk factors for coronary heart disease.

Dietary Effects on Hemostatic Function

Dietary vitamin K profoundly affects the activity of the blood clotting factors II, VII, IX, and X and the inhibitory molecules, protein C and protein S. These proteins are synthesized in the liver and contain a region or module of the protein that contains modified glutamic acid residues (gamma carboxy glutamic acid) (Gla). Gla formation requires vitamin K and so a deficiency state will cause abnormal bleeding. A dietary deficiency of vitamin K is rare and nearly always occurs in the neonate leading to hemorrhagic disease of the newborn. However, the oral anticoagulant drugs based on warfarin are vitamin K analogs and thus prevent the synthesis of a biologically active coagulation protein.

Fibrinogen levels are elevated in obese individuals although many studies have failed to demonstrate any relationship between plasma fibrinogen levels and dietary fat. Active men have lower fibrinogen levels and a number of studies have demonstrated an inverse relationship between alcohol consumption and plasma fibrinogen. A high-fiber diet was also shown to correlate negatively with plasma fibrinogen. A few studies on the effects of antioxidant vitamins show that they may lower fibrinogen. For example, the Swedish MONItoring CArdiovascular disease (MONICA) study found that high levels of plasma retinol were associated with lower fibrinogen levels. However, plasma tPA levels were also lowered indicating that the fibrinolytic pathway was compromised in these subjects. Fish oil was shown to lower fibrinogen levels when the oil contained vitamin E.

Dietary fat profoundly affects the activity of factor VII. A high fat intake is associated with increased amounts of factor VIIa. Indeed, the post-prandial levels of this active blood coagulation factor have been shown to be elevated after a high-fat meal. If exposed to tissue factor, these increased levels of factor VIIa would have major consequences for thrombogenesis. Platelet aggregation is often

affected by diet and fish oils can reduce platelet aggregation.

The influence of diet on the components of the coagulation pathway is well recognized by the requirement of vitamin K. However, the role that diet plays in modulating the levels of coagulation factors that are, or may be, risk factors for coronary heart disease is unclear and the results are often conflicting. For example, in intervention studies examining the effects of fish oils on monocyte TF production, one study reported a decrease in expression whilst other studies showed no effect. The study where the positive effects were reported was carried out in Italy and it has been suggested that the Mediterranean diet of the Italians was a contributory factor in these findings. Obviously, more work is required to establish the effects of fish oils on TF expression.

Hemostasis is an exciting and important area of medicine and our knowledge of the molecular and cellular interactions that bring about clot formation is now at an advanced stage. Many of the studies on diet and hemostasis may have used inappropriate laboratory techniques. For example, blood platelets are easily activated making aggregation data difficult to interpret. The advent of automated coagulometers means that the clotting factors may be easily measured. There are commercially available immunoassays for many of the components of hemostasis described in this article. Using flow cytometry, TF can be measured on monocytes and P-selectin may be detected on activated platelets. Since thrombosis is a major cause of acute coronary events the rewards of studies on diet and hemostasis may be great.

See also: **Cholesterol**: Sources, Absorption, Function and Metabolism; Factors Determining Blood Levels. **Coronary Heart Disease**: Lipid Theory; Prevention. **Vitamin K**.

Further Reading

Hutton RA, Laffan MA, and Tuddenham EGD (1999) Normal haemostasis. In: Hoffbrand AV, Lewis SM, and Tuddenham EGD (eds.) *Postgraduate Haematology*, pp. 550–580. Oxford: Butterworth Heinemann.

Laffin MA and Manning RA (2001) Investigation of haemostasis. In: Lewis SM, Bain BJ, and Bates I (eds.) *Practical Haematology*, pp. 339–413. London: Churchill Livingstone.

Ross R (1993) The pathogenesis of atherosclerosis: a perspective for the 1990's. *Nature* **362**: 801–809.

Lipid Theory

D Kritchevsky, Wistar Institute, Philadelphia, PA, USA

© 2005 Elsevier Ltd. All rights reserved.

Introduction

Arteriosclerosis is a group of conditions characterized by thickening and stiffening of the arterial wall. Atherosclerosis is characterized by the formation of atheromas (lipid-laden plaques) in medium to large arteries. These are associated with calcifications of the arterial wall along with other changes. Eventually, the arterial lumen is reduced and the restricted blood flow due to these changes leads to clinical symptoms. Over the years there have been varying theories about the development of arterial lesions and these theories become more complex as our biochemical and molecular biological skills and knowledge increase.

Arterial fatty streaks are ubiquitous in humans and appear early in life. The fatty streak is comprised of lipid-rich macrophages and smooth muscle cells. Macrophages that accumulate lipid and are transformed into foam cells may be involved in the transformation of the fatty streak to an atherosclerotic lesion. In susceptible persons the fatty streaks may progress to fibrous plaques. Fibrous plaques, at their core, consist of a mixture of cholesterol-rich smooth muscle and foam cells. This core may contain cellular debris, cholesteryl esters, cholesterol crystals, and calcium. The fibrous cap consists of smooth muscle and foam cells, collagen, and lipid. The final stage in this process is the complicated plaque, which can obstruct the arterial lumen. Rupture of the cap may lead to clot formation and occlusion of the artery.

There are several theories of atherogenesis and these may eventually be shown to be interactive. The lipid hypothesis suggests that persistent hyperlipidemia leads to cholesterol accumulation in the arterial endothelium. Hypercholesterolemia may activate protein growth factors, which stimulate smooth muscle cell proliferation.

The lipid infiltration hypothesis proposes that elevated LDL levels increase LDL infiltration which, in turn, increases uptake of epithelial cells, smooth muscle cells, and macrophages. This cascade leads to cholesterol accumulation and, eventually, atheroma formation. The endothelial injury may arise from the action of oxidized lipid.

The endothelial injury hypothesis may help to explain the focal distribution of atheromas, which is not adequately accounted for by the lipid hypothesis. The endothelial injury hypothesis asserts that plaque formation begins when the endothelial cells that cover fatty streaks separate thus exposing the underlying lesion to the circulation. This may lead to smooth muscle proliferation, stimulated by circulating mitogens, or may cause platelet aggregation leading to mural thrombosis.

Another hypothesis relating to atherogenesis is the response-to-injury hypothesis. In this hypothesis the injury may be due to mechanical factors, chronic hypercholesterolemia, toxins, viruses, or immune reactions: these increase endothelial permeability, and lead to monocyte adherence to the epithelium or infiltration and platelet aggregation or adherence at the site of the injury. Injury releases growth factors that stimulate proliferation of fibrous elements in the intima. These growth factors may arise from the endothelial cell, monocyte, macrophages, platelet, smooth muscle cell, and T cell. They include epidermal growth factor, insulin-like growth factors, interleukins 1 and 2, platelet-derived growth factors, transforming growth factors α and β, and tumor necrosis factors α and β, among others. Monocytes and smooth muscle cells carry the 'scavenger' receptor, which binds oxidized but not native low-density lipoprotein (LDL) in a nonsaturable fashion. Uptake of oxidized LDL converts macrophages and smooth muscle cells into foam cells. Another theory of atherogenesis suggests that it begins as an immunological disease, which starts by an autoimmune reaction against the heat stress protein, hsp60. There have been suggestions that oxidized LDL may be an underlying cause of arterial injury.

The term 'atherosclerosis' is derived from the Greek words *athere*, meaning gruel, and *skleros*, meaning hardening. The term was coined by Marchand in 1904 to describe the ongoing process beginning with the early lipid deposits in the arteries to the eventual hardening. The World Health Organization (WHO) definition describes atherosclerosis as a 'variable combination of changes in the intima of the arteries involving focal accumulation of lipids and complex carbohydrates with blood and its constituents accompanied by fibrous tissue formation, calcification, and associated changes in the media' – a decidedly more complex concept than attributing it all to the dietary cholesterol.

Discussions of the etiology of heart disease always describe it as a life-style disease and list a number of risk factors, which include family history, hypercholesterolemia, hypertension, obesity, and cigarette smoking. Having listed these factors, discussion generally reverts to blood cholesterol and its control.

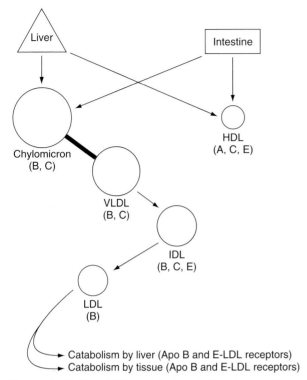

Figure 1 Outline of lipid metabolism. Letters in parentheses refer to apolipoproteins (apo). HDL, high-density lipoprotein; VLDL, very-low-density lipoprotein; IDL, intermediate-density lipoprotein; LDL, low-density lipoprotein.

The fasting blood plasma of a healthy individual is a clear, straw-colored liquid, which may contain 400–800 mg of lipids per 100 ml. This clear solution, which is high in lipids, is made possible by the water-soluble complex of lipids with protein, the lipoproteins. A generalized view of lipoprotein metabolism is provided in **Figure 1**. The existence of soluble lipid–protein complexes in serum was suggested about a century ago. Precipitation of a lipoprotein from horse serum was achieved in 1929 and classes of lipoproteins were adduced from studies using moving boundary electrophoresis. The critical experiments were carried out by Gofman and his group in the 1950s. They demonstrated that classes of lipoprotein complexes could be identified by their flotation characteristics in the analytical ultracentrifuge. These complexes were separable because they possessed different hydrated densities and they were defined initially by Svedberg units of flotation (S_f). The lipoproteins vary in chemical composition and although it is common to provide tables describing lipoprotein composition, the values are generally average values. This is so since the lipoproteins exist in a dynamic state exchanging their lipid components with those of tissues or other lipoproteins. Since identification is made according to a physical property, i.e., hydrated density, it is evident that different agglomerates of lipid and protein may have similar hydrated densities. In general, the lipoproteins are a series of macromolecules that, as they progress from low to high density, display decreasing triacylglycerol content and increasing cholesteryl ester, phospholipid, and protein.

Table 1 describes the major lipoproteins. Their chemical composition is described in **Table 2**.

As research continues and as analytical methodology becomes more precise we find a higher resolution of some lipoprotein classes and better definition of their roles. One example is lipoprotein (a) (lp(a)), first described in 1963. Lipoprotein (a) is an LDL whose normal apoprotein (apo B) is linked to an additional protein, apoprotein a, via a disulfide bridge. Lipoprotein (a) interferes with normal fibrinolysis leading to an increased prevalence of blood clots, and is thought to present an especially high risk for myocardial infarction. Characteristics and functions of lipoproteins are described in **Table 3**.

Molecular size influences the ease with which LDL particles can enter the arterial wall. Diabetic rabbits have greatly elevated plasma lipid levels but display surprisingly little atherosclerosis. The reason

Table 1 Major plasma lipoproteins

Lipoprotein class	Size (nm)	Mol. wt	Density (g ml^{-1})	Electrophoretic mobility	Origin	Major apoproteins
Chylomicron	100–400	10^6–10^7	<0.95	Origin	Intestine	A-I, B-48, C-II, C-III, E
VLDL	40–70	5×10^3	0.95–1.006	Prebeta	Liver	B-100, C-II, C-III, E
IDL	30–40	4.5×10^3	1.006–1.019	Between prebeta and beta	Catabolism of VLDL	B-100, C-II, C-III, E
LDL	22.5–27.5	2×10^3	1.019–1.063	Beta	Catabolism of VLDL and IDL	B-100
HDL	7.5–10	0.4×10^3	1.063–1.210	Alpha	Liver, intestine	A-I, A-II, C-II, C-III, E

VLDL, very-low-density lipoprotein; IDL, intermediate-density lipoprotein; LDL, low-density lipoprotein; HDL, high-density lipoprotein.

Table 2 Plasma lipoprotein composition

Lipoprotein	Composition (wt%)				
	FC	CE	TAG	PL	PROT
Chylomicron	1	3	90	4	2
VLDL	7	14	55	16	8
IDL	6	22	30	24	18
LDL	7	48	5	20	20
HDL	4	15	4	27	50

FC, free cholesterol; CE, cholesteryl ester; TAG, triacylglycerol; PL, phospholipid; PROT, protein; VLDL, very-low-density lipoprotein; IDL, intermediate-density lipoprotein; LDL, low-density lipoprotein; HDL, high-density lipoprotein.

for this apparent discrepancy is that the lipoproteins of diabetic rabbits are rather large in size and do not penetrate the artery. Since 1982 we have known of an array of LDL particles ranging from small and dense to large and comparatively light. An LDL pattern characterized by an excess of small, dense particles is associated with a threefold increased risk of myocardial infarction, independent of age, sex, or body weight. Commonly, LDL is known as the 'bad' cholesterol and high-density lipoprotein (HDL) as the 'good' cholesterol. These recent findings indicate the presence of 'good, bad' cholesterol and 'bad, good' cholesterol.

Among the apolipoproteins, polymorphism of apoprotein E apparently dictates a subject's chances for successful treatment of lipidemia. The apoE alleles are designated as E2, E3, and E4. The most common pattern (55%) is homozygosity for E3, which gives rise to the E3/E3 phenotype. The next most common phenotype is E3/E4 (26%). The least frequently observed phenotype is E2/E (1%), which is often associated with type III hyperlipoproteinemia. There is some evidence suggesting that subjects bearing the E4 allele have higher levels of LDL than those with the E3/E3 pattern; they may also be more prone to Alzheimer's disease. **Tables 4** and **5** list primary and secondary dyslipoproteinemias.

Cholesterol and Cholesterolemia

In 1913 Anitschkow showed that it was possible to establish atherosclerosis in rabbits by feeding cholesterol. Since then virtually all research on atherosclerosis has centered on cholesterol – circulating cholesterol and dietary cholesterol. The epidemiological data suggest a role for

Table 3 Characteristics and functions of major apolipoproteins

Apolipoprotein	Lipoprotein	(Approximate molecular weight (kD))	Source	(Average plasma) concentration (mg dL^{-1})	(Physiologic) function
A-1	HDL, chylomicrons	28	Liver, intestine	100–120	Structural apoprotein of HDL, cofactor for LCAT
A-II	HDL, chylomicrons	17	Intestine, liver	35–45	Structural apoprotein of HDL, cofactor for hepatic lipase
A-IV	HDL, chylomicrons	46	Liver, intestine	10–20	Unknown
Apo (a)	Lp(a)	600	Liver	1–10	Unknown
B-48	Chylomicrons	264	Intestine	Trace	Major structural apoprotein, secretion and clearance of chlylomicrons
B-100	VLDL, LDL	550	Liver	100–125	Ligand for LDL receptor, structural apoprotein of VLDL and LDL
C-I	Chylomicrons, VLDL, HDL	5.80	Liver	6–8	Cofactor for LCAT
C-II	Chylomicrons, VLDL, HDL	9.10	Liver	3–5	Cofactor for LCAT
C-III	Chylomicrons, VLDL, HDL	8.75	Liver	12–15	Inhibitor of LPL, involved in lipoprotein remnant uptake
E-2	Chylomicrons, VLDL, HDL	35	Liver, peripheral tissues	4–5	Ligand for cell receptor
E-3	Chylomicrons, VLDL, HDL	35	Liver, peripheral tissues	4–5	Ligand for cell receptor
E-4	Chylomicrons, VLDL, HDL	35	Liver, peripheral tissues	4–5	Ligand for cell receptor

HDL, LDL, VLDL, high-, low-, and very-low-density lipoprotein; LCAT, lecithin-cholesterol acyltransferase; LPL, lipoprotein lipase.

Table 4   The primary dyslipoproteinemias

Type	Changes in plasma		Apparent genetic disorder	Biochemical defect
	Lipids	Lipoproteins		
I	TAG ↑	CM ↑	Familial LPL deficiency	Loss of LPL activity
II-a	C ↑	LDL ↑	Familial hypercholesterolemia	Deficiency of LDL receptor and activity
II-b	C ↑, TAG ↑	LDL, VLDL ↑	Familial combined hyperlipidemia	Unknown
III	C ↑, TAG ↑	β-VLDL ↑	Familial type III hyperlipidemia	Defect in TAG-rich remnant clearance
IV	TAG ↑	VLDL ↑	Familial hypertriacylglycerolemia	VLDL synthesis ↑, catabolism ↓
V	TAG ↑, C ↑	VLDL ↑, CM ↑	Familial type V hyperlipoproteinemia	Lipolysis of TGA-rich LP ↓, Production of VLDL TAG ↑
Hyper Lp(a)	C ↑	Lp(a) ↑	Familial hyper apo(a) lipoproteinemia	Inhibits fibrinolysis
Hyperapobeta-lipoproteinemia	TAG ↑	VLDL, LDL ↑	Familial type V hyperlipoproteinemia	CETP deficiency
Familial hypobeta-lipoproteinemia	C ↓, TAG ↓	CM ↓, VLDL ↑, LDL ↓	?	Inability to synthesize apo B-48 and apo B-100
A-beta-lipoproteinemia	C ↓, TAG ↓	CM ↓, VLDL ↓, LDL ↓	?	Apo B-48 and apo B-100 not secreted into plasma
Hypo-alphalipoproteinemia	C ↓, TAG ↓	HDL ↓	?	LCAT deficiency
Tangier disease				Apo A-I ↓, apo C-III ↓
Fish eye disease				Abnormal apo A-I, and apo A-II metabolism

C, cholesterol; CM, chylomicrons; CETP, cholesteryl ester transfer protein; HDL, LDL, VLDL, high-, low-, and very-low-density lipoprotein; LCAT, lecithin-cholesterol acyltransferase; LPL, lipoprotein lipase; TAG, triacylglycerol.

dietary fat, and hypercholesterolemia has been established as a principal risk factor for atherosclerosis. The lipid hypothesis was developed from the data obtained in the Framingham study, which suggested a curvilinear relationship between risk of atherosclerosis and plasma or serum cholesterol levels. However, studies of actual cholesterol intake as it affects cholesterol levels have yielded equivocal results.

Several studies have shown that the addition of one or two eggs to their daily diet did not influence serum cholesterol levels of free-living subjects. Data

from the Framingham study show no correlation between cholesterol intake and cholesterol level. So we are left with the anomalous situation that blood cholesterol is an indicator of susceptibility to coronary disease but it is relatively unaffected by dietary cholesterol. It is of interest to point out that we are also seeing a correlation between low plasma or serum cholesterol levels and noncoronary death.

The type of fat in the diet has a strong influence on serum or plasma cholesterol levels. Rabbits fed saturated fat develop more severe atherosclerosis

Table 5   Secondary dyslipoproteinemias

Type	Associated disease	Lipoproteins elevated	Apparent underlying defect
I	Lupus erythematosis	Chylomicrons	Circulating LPL inhibitor
II	Nephrotic syndrome, Cushing's syndrome	VLDL and LDL	Overproduction of VLDL particles, defective lipolysis of VLDL triglycerides
III	Hypothyroidism, dysglobulinemia	VLDL and LDL	Suppression of LDL receptor activity, overproduction of VLDL triglycerides
IV	Renal failure, diabetes mellitus, acute hepatitis	VLDL	Defective lipolysis of triglyceride-rich VLDL due to inhibition of LPL and HL
V	Noninsulin dependent diabetes	VLDL	Overproduction and defective lipolysis of VLDL triglycerides

HDL, LDL, VLDL, high-, low, and very-low-density lipoprotein; HL, hepatic lipase; LPL, lipoprotein lipase.

than do rabbits fed unsaturated fat. In 1965 the groups of Keys and Hegsted independently developed formulae for predicting changes in cholesterol levels based on changes in the diet. Their formulae were based upon changes in quantity of saturated and unsaturated fat and in dietary cholesterol, but the last value makes a very small contribution to the overall number. The Keys formula is:

$$\Delta C = 1.35(2\Delta S - \Delta P) + 1.5\Delta Z$$

where ΔC represents the change in cholesterol level, ΔS and ΔP represent changes in levels of saturated and unsaturated fat, and Z is the square root of dietary cholesterol in mg per 1000 kcal of diet. The Hegsted formula is:

$$\Delta C_P = 2.16\Delta S - 1.65\Delta P + 0.168\Delta C_D + 85$$

where ΔC_P is change in plasma cholesterol and ΔC_D is change in dietary cholesterol in mg per 1000 kcal.

Both studies found that changes in dietary stearic acid did not fit the formula. Since those formulae were introduced a number of newer formulae have appeared, which provide a coefficient for every individual fatty acid, but the original formulae are still used most frequently. Under metabolic ward conditions it has been shown that lauric ($C_{12:0}$), myristic ($C_{14:0}$), and palmitic ($C_{16:0}$) acids raise both LDL and HDL cholesterol levels, and that oleic ($C_{18:1}$) and linoleic ($C_{18:2}$) acids raise HDL and lower LDL levels slightly. Thus, the type of fat is the determining factor in considering dietary fat effects on serum cholesterol. Experiments in which subjects were fed low or high levels of cholesterol in diets containing high or low ratios of saturated to polyunsaturated fat have been reported. When the fat was homologous, changing from low to high dietary cholesterol raised serum cholesterol concentration by 2%. However, even under conditions in which low levels of cholesterol were fed, changing from saturated to unsaturated fat raised serum cholesterol levels by 10% or more.

In nature most, but not all, unsaturated fatty acids are in the *cis* configuration. The major source of fats containing *trans* unsaturated fatty acids (*trans* fats) in the diet of developed nations is hydrogenated fat, such as is present in commercial margarines and cooking fats. Interest in *trans* fat effects on atherosclerosis and cholesterolemia was first evinced in the 1960s. In general, *trans* fats behave like saturated fats and raise serum cholesterol levels, but have not been found to be more atherogenic than saturated fats in studies carried out in rabbits, monkeys, and swine. Studies have also shown that *trans* fat effects may be relatively small if the diet contains sufficient quantities of essential fatty acids.

Studies, clinical and epidemiological, on the influence of *trans* unsaturated fats on the risk of coronary heart disease have continued. The evidence is that *trans* fats may influence the chemical indicators of heart disease risk but final proof must rest on verification by clinical trial. The concerns relative to *trans* fat effects have led to recommendations that the levels of *trans* fats present in the diet be reduced as much as possible. The availability of *trans*-free margarines and other fats may render the entire argument obsolete.

Protein

The type of protein in the diet also influences cholesterolemia and atherosclerosis. In animal studies in which the sole source of protein is of animal or plant origin, the former is more cholesterolemic than atherogenic. However, a 1:1 mix of animal and plant protein provides the higher-grade protein of animal protein and the normocholesterolemic effects of plant protein. The results underline the need for a balanced diet.

Fiber

Dietary fiber may influence lipidemia and atherosclerosis. Substances designated as insoluble fibers (wheat bran, for instance) possess laxative properties but have little effect on serum lipid levels. Soluble fibers (gel-forming fibers such as pectin or guar gum) influence lipidemia and glycemia. Oat bran, which contains β-glucans, which are soluble fibers, will lower cholesterol levels despite its designation.

Variations in Cholesterol Levels

Ignoring the differences of technique involved in cholesterol measurement in the laboratory – variations that are amenable to resolution – there are physiological considerations that should be recognized. Age, gender, genetics, adiposity, and personality traits can affect cholesterol levels, as can diseases unrelated to coronary disease. Stress (job stress, deadlines, examinations) can lead to increased cholesterol levels.

A definite seasonal variation in cholesterol levels (usually higher in winter months) has been seen in a number of studies. Scientists from the National Institutes of Health in the US carried out one of

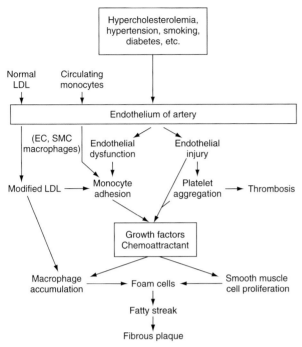

Figure 2 Factors involved in formation of the atherosclerotic plaque.

the finest studies in this area. They examined carefully the data from the 10 American Lipid Research Clinics. They observed that the etiology of their findings was unknown but they found the total and LDL cholesterol levels varied inversely with length of day. The level of HDL cholesterol varied much less, but its variation was correlated directly with ambient temperature. The foregoing does not reduce the importance of measuring cholesterol levels but makes it important to take into consideration the subjects' physical and mental state as well as time of year.

Figure 2 attempts to summarize the many factors now considered to play a role in the formation of the atherosclerotic plaque.

See also: **Cholesterol**: Sources, Absorption, Function and Metabolism; Factors Determining Blood Levels. **Coronary Heart Disease**: Hemostatic Factors; Prevention. **Diabetes Mellitus**: Etiology and Epidemiology. **Fats and Oils**. **Fatty Acids**: *Trans* Fatty Acids. **Hyperlipidemia**: Overview; Nutritional Management. **Lipids**: Chemistry and Classification. **Lipoproteins**.

Further Reading

Ginsburg HN (1998) Lipoprotein physiology. *Endocrinology Metabolism Clinics of North America* 27: 503–519.

Gold P, Grover S, and Roncari DAK (eds.) (1992) *Cholesterol and Coronary Heart Disease – The Great Debate*. Park Ridge, NJ: CRC Press.
Libby P (2002) Inflammation in atherosclerosis. *Nature* 420: 868–874.
Lusis AJ (2000) Atherosclerosis. *Nature* 407: 233–241.
McNamara (2000) Dietary cholesterol and atherosclerosis. *Biochimica Biophysica Acta* 1529: 310–320.
Nicolosi RJ, Kritchevsky D, and Wilson TA (1999) Pathobiology of hypercholesterolemia and atherosclerosis. In: Rippe JM (ed.) *Lifestyle Management and Prevention of Cardiovascular Disease*, pp. 25–39. London: Blackwell Science Press.
Ross R (1999) Atherosclerosis – an inflammatory disease. *New England Journal of Medicine* 340: 115–126.
Tabas T (2002) Cholesterol in health and disease. *Journal of Clinical Investigation* 110: 583–589.
Velican C and Velican D (1989) *Natural History of Coronary Atherosclerosis*. Boca Raton, FL: CRC Press.
White RA (1989) *Atherosclerosis and Arteriosclerosis*. Boca Raton, FL: CRC Press.

Prevention

K Srinath Reddy, All India Institute of Medical Sciences, New Delhi, India

© 2005 Elsevier Ltd. All rights reserved.

Introduction

Coronary heart disease (CHD) is the leading cause of death in the world. While it is well established as the foremost contributor to mortality in most developed countries, it is also a major and rapidly rising cause of death in many developing countries. Global health transitions, which have seen substantial changes in age-specific coronary mortality rates across the world, in the past half a century, have also been associated with changes in nutrition, which explain a large part of the rise or fall of CHD-related death rates.

Diet and nutrition have been extensively investigated as risk factors for CHD. Many dietary factors have been linked directly to an increased or decreased risk of CHD or to major established risk factors of CHD like high blood pressure, disordered blood fats (dyslipidemia), diabetes and metabolic syndrome, overweight and obesity, and also to emerging risk factors like inflammatory markers and homocysteine. Nutrition influences atherogenesis, thrombosis, and inflammation – all of which are interconnected pathways that lead to CHD.

Observational epidemiological studies and clinical trials have contributed to a wide body of knowledge of the role that some nutrients (like saturated and *trans* fats, salt, and refined carbohydrates) play in increasing the risk of CHD and of the protective effect of other nutrients (such as fruit and vegetables, polyunsaturated fats, nuts, and fish) against CHD. This knowledge has been successfully applied both in public health and in clinical practice to reduce the risk of CHD in populations as well as in individuals. The present state of that knowledge, as relevant to prevention of CHD, is summarized below.

Global Trends in CHD as a Reflection of Nutrition Transition

Coronary heart disease accounted for 7.2 million deaths in 2002, which forms a large fraction of not only the total number of deaths worldwide due to cardiovascular diseases (16.6 million) but also of the global total number of deaths from any cause (57 million). While age-specific coronary mortality rates have declined in the industrial countries over the past three decades, the absolute burdens of CHD continue to be high. CHD death rates are rising in the developing countries, where about half of these deaths occur below the age of 70 years. In Eastern and Central Europe CHD mortality rates rose sharply in the 1980s and 1990s and have only recently shown signs of stabilization, albeit at high levels.

These changes in CHD mortality rates have accompanied well-documented or clearly discernible shifts in the nutritional state of the populations. The decline of CHD mortality in Western and Northern Europe was linked to a reduction in the consumption of unhealthy fats (saturated fats and *trans* fats) and salt as well as an increased consumption of fruits and vegetables. This is best documented in The Netherlands and Finland. Similarly, the recent decline of CHD mortality in Poland was explained by the increase in fruit and vegetable consumption and growing substitution of vegetable fats for animal fats. Similar evidence of a favorable nutrition transition preceding the decline in CHD mortality rates is available from other developed countries like the US, Canada, Australia, and New Zealand.

The developing countries have, however, witnessed a recent transition in the opposite direction. China, for example, has experienced a large increase in fat consumption over the past two decades, accompanied by a progressive rise in the mean plasma cholesterol levels of the population as well as in the CHD mortality rates. Other developing countries are also increasingly adopting unhealthy dietary patterns that augment the risk of CHD.

Understanding the Links between Nutrition and CHD

The pathogenesis of CHD is mediated through the interconnected pathways of atherogenesis (fat deposition in the walls of the coronary arteries to form plaques), thrombosis (blood clotting over disrupted plaques) and inflammation (which initially damages the blood vessel walls and continues to destabilize the plaques). Nutrition has a major role in influencing each of these pathways and often provides the connecting link between them.

Major coronary risk factors include an abnormal blood lipid profile (especially plasma cholesterol and its subfractions), high blood pressure, and diabetes. Overweight and obesity (both the general and central patterns) are also associated with an increased risk of CHD. Nutrition has a powerful influence on all of these risk factors, with an unhealthy diet pattern tending to elevate them and a healthy diet pattern reducing the levels of risk. Diet becomes especially important in the context of the metabolic syndrome (a complex of central obesity, high blood pressure, dyslipidemia, and glucose intolerance), an entity which is being increasingly identified as a major risk factor for CHD. Nutrition is also linked to the propensity to develop cardiac arrhythmias, in the setting of CHD, and is an important predictor of sudden cardiac death. These links between dietary patterns and several specific nutrients not only manifest as fat deposition in the arteries, plaque growth, plaque instability, and thrombosis but are evident much earlier in the natural history of CHD, as endothelial dysfunction (inability of the arteries to dilate normally), elevated levels of inflammatory markers (such as C reactive protein), and increased intimal medial thickness of arterial walls. These precede and predict the clinical manifestation of CHD.

Nutrients and CHD

Dietary Fats: Cholesterol

The relationship between dietary fats and cardiovascular disease (CVD), especially CHD, has been extensively investigated, with strong and consistent associations emerging from a wide body of evidence accrued from animal experiments, as well as observational studies, clinical trials, and metabolic studies conducted in diverse human populations. This relationship was initially considered to be mediated mainly through the atherogenic effects of plasma lipids (total cholesterol, lipoprotein fractions, and triglycerides). The effects of dietary fats on thrombosis and endothelial function as well as the relationship of plasma and tissue lipids to the pathways of inflammation have been more recently understood. Similarly, the effects of dietary fats on blood pressure have also become more evident through observational and experimental research.

Cholesterol in the blood and tissues is derived from two sources: diet and endogenous synthesis. Dairy fat and meat are major dietary sources. Dietary cholesterol raises plasma cholesterol levels. Although both high-density lipoprotein (HDL) and low-density lipoprotein (LDL) fractions increase, the effect on the total/HDL ratio is still unfavorable, but small. The upper limit for dietary cholesterol intake has been prescribed, in most guidelines, to be $300 \, \text{mg day}^{-1}$. However, as endogenous synthesis is sufficient to meet the physiological needs, there is no requirement for dietary cholesterol and it is advisable to keep the intake as low as possible. If intake of dairy fat and meat are controlled, then there is no need for severe restriction of egg yolk intake, although some limitation remains prudent.

Saturated Fatty Acids (SFAs)

The relationship of dietary saturated fat to plasma cholesterol levels and to CHD was graphically demonstrated by the Seven Countries Study involving 16 cohorts, in which saturated fat intake explained up to 73% of the total variance in CHD across these cohorts. In the Nurses' Health Study, the effect of saturated fatty acids was much more modest, especially if saturates were replaced by carbohydrates. The most effective replacement for saturated fatty acids in terms of CHD prevention is by polyunsaturated fatty acids (PUFAs). This agrees with the outcome of large randomized clinical trials, in which replacement of saturated and *trans* fats by polyunsaturated vegetable oils effectively lowered CHD risk.

Trans-Fatty Acids (*t*-FAs)

t-FAs (*Trans*-Fatty Acids) are geometrical isomers of unsaturated fatty acids that assume a saturated fatty acid-like configuration. Partial hydrogenation, the process used to create *t*-FAs, also removes essential fatty acids such as LA (Linoleic Acid) and ALNA (Alpha Linolenic Acid). Metabolic studies have demonstrated that *t*-FAs render the plasma lipid profile even more atherogenic than SFAs, by not only elevating LDL cholesterol to similar levels but also decreasing HDL cholesterol. As a result, the ratio of LDL cholesterol to HDL cholesterol is significantly higher with a *t*-FA diet (2.58) than with a SFA diet (2.34) or an oleic acid diet (2.02). This

greatly enhances the risk of CHD. Evidence that intake of *t*-FAs increases the risk of CHD initially became available from large population-based cohort studies in the US and in an elderly Dutch population. Eliminating *t*-FAs from the diet would be an important public health strategy to prevent CHD. Since these are commercially introduced agents into the diet, policy measures related to the food industry practices would be required along with public education. *t*-FAs have been eliminated from retail fats and spreads in many parts of the world, but deep-fat fried fast foods and baked goods are a major and increasing source.

Monounsaturated Fatty Acids (MUFAs)

The only nutritionally important MUFA is oleic acid, which is abundant in olive and canola oils and also in nuts. The epidemiological evidence related to MUFAs and CHD is derived from studies on the Mediterranean diet (see below), as well as from the Nurses' Health Study and other similar studies in the US.

Polyunsaturated Fatty Acids (PUFAs)

PUFAs are categorized as *n*-6 PUFAs (mainly derived from linoleic acid) and *n*-3 PUFAs (mainly present in fatty fish and also derived from alpha-linoleic acid). Clinical trials, in which *n*-6 PUFAs (containing linoleic acid) were substituted for SFAs showed a greater impact on reduction of both plasma cholesterol and CHD risk, in contrast to trials where low-fat diets were employed.

Much of the epidemiological evidence related to *n*-3 PUFAs is derived from the study of fish consumption in populations or interventions involving fish diets in clinical trials. Fish oils were, however, used in a large clinical trial of 11 300 survivors of myocardial infarction. After 3.5 years of follow-up, the fish oil group ($1 \, \text{g day}^{-1}$) had a statistically significant 20% reduction in total mortality, 30% reduction in cardiovascular death, and 45% decrease in sudden death.

The Lyon Heart Study in France incorporated an *n*-3 fatty acid (alpha-linolenic acid) into a diet that was altered to develop a 'Mediterranean diet' intervention. In the experimental group, plasma ALNA and EPA (Eicosapentenoic Acid) increased significantly and the trial reported a 70% reduction in cardiovascular mortality at 5 years. Total and LDL cholesterol were identical in the experimental and control groups, suggesting that thrombotic and perhaps arrhythmic events may have been favorably influenced by *n*-3 PUFAs. Since the diet altered many other variables, such as fiber and antioxidants (by increasing fruit and vegetable consumption), direct attribution of benefits to *n*-3 PUFAs becomes difficult to establish.

The proportions of SFAs, MUFAs, and PUFAs as constituents of total fat intake and total energy consumption have engaged active attention, in view of the strong relationship of these fatty acids to the risk of CHD. The reduction of SFAs in the diet has been widely recommended, but its replacement has been an area of debate, as to whether the place of reduced SFAs should be taken by MUFAs, PUFAs, or carbohydrate. Both MUFAs and PUFAs improve the lipoprotein profile, although PUFAs are somewhat more effective. In view of this, several recent dietary recommendations suggested that SFAs should be kept below 10% of daily energy intake (preferably reduced to 7–8%), MUFAs should be increased to 13–15%, and PUFAs raised to 7–10% of daily energy, with the total fat contributing to less than 30% of all calories consumed. These may need to be adjusted for populations who consume less quantities of total fat, so as to ensure an adequate intake of MUFAs and PUFAs even under those circumstances. The emphasis is now shifting from the quantity of fat to the quality of fat, with growing evidence that even diets with 30–35% fat intake may be protective if the type of fats consumed are mostly from the MUFA and PUFA categories. Enhancing the nutritional quality of dietary fat consumption, to provide greater cardiovascular protection, may be attempted by decreasing the sources of saturated fats and eliminating *t*-FAs in the diet, increasing the consumption of foods containing unsaturated fatty acids (both MUFAs and PUFAs), and decreasing dietary cholesterol consumption.

Carbohydrates

Diets which are high in refined carbohydrates appear to reduce HDL cholesterol levels and increase the fraction of small dense LDL, both of which may impact adversely on vascular disease. This dyslipidemic pattern is consistent with the elevation of plasma triglycerides and is typical of the 'metabolic syndrome.' Carbohydrate diets with high glycemic index might adversely impact on glucose control, with associated changes in plasma lipids, and have been linked to an increased risk of CHD.

Fiber

Most soluble fibers reduce plasma total and LDL cholesterol concentrations, as reported by several trials. Fiber consumption strongly predicts insulin levels, weight gain, and cardiovascular risk factors like blood pressure, plasma triglycerides, LDL and HDL cholesterol, and fibrinogen. Several large cohort studies in the US, Finland, and Norway have reported that subjects consuming relatively large amounts of whole-grain cereals have significantly lower rates of CHD.

Antioxidants

Though several cohort studies showed significant reductions in the incidence of cardiac events in men and women taking high-dose vitamin E supplements, large clinical trials failed to demonstrate a cardioprotective effect of vitamin E supplements. Beta-carotene supplements also did not provide protection against CHD and, in some trials, appeared to increase the risk.

Folate

The relationship of folate to CVD has been mostly explored through its effect on homocysteine, which has been put forward as an independent risk factor for CHD. Reduced plasma folate has been strongly associated with elevated plasma homocysteine levels and folate supplementation has been demonstrated to decrease those levels. Data from the Nurses' Health Study in the US showed that folate and vitamin B_6, from diet and supplements, conferred protection against CHD (fatal and nonfatal events combined) and suggested a role for their increased intake as an intervention for primary prevention of CHD. Recommendations related to folate supplementation must, however, await the results of ongoing clinical trials. Dietary intake of folate through natural food sources may be encouraged in the meanwhile, especially in individuals at a high risk of arterial or venous thrombosis and elevated plasma homocysteine levels.

Flavonoids and Other Phytochemicals

Flavonoids are polyphenolic antioxidants, which occur in a variety of foods of vegetable origin, such as tea, onions, and apples. Data from several prospective studies indicate an inverse association of dietary flavonoids with CHD. The role of these and other phytochemicals (such as plant stanols and sterols) in relation to CHD needs to be elucidated further.

Sodium and Potassium

High blood pressure (HBP) is a major risk factor for CHD. The relative risk of CHD, for both systolic and diastolic blood pressures, operates in a continuum of increasing risk for rising pressure but the absolute risk of CHD is considerably modified by coexisting risk factors (such as blood lipids and diabetes), many of which are also influenced by diet. A cohort study in Finland observed a 51%

greater risk of CHD mortality with a 100 mmol increase in 24-h urinary sodium excretion. Several clinical trials have convincingly demonstrated the ability of reduced sodium diets to lower blood pressure. A meta-analysis of long-term trials suggests that reducing daily salt intake from $12\,g\,day^{-1}$ to $3\,g\,day^{-1}$ is likely to reduce CHD by 25% (and strokes by 33%). Even more modest reductions would have substantial benefits (10% lower CHD for a 3-g salt reduction). The benefits of dietary potassium in lowering blood pressure have been well demonstrated but specific effects on CHD risk have not been well studied. Keeping the dietary sodium:potassium ratio at a low level is essential to avoid hypertension.

Food Items

Fruits and Vegetables

A systematic review reported that nine of ten ecological studies, two of three case–control studies, and six of sixteen cohort studies found a significant protective association for CHD with consumption of fruits and vegetables or surrogate nutrients. In a 12-year follow-up of 15 220 male physicians in the US, men who consumed at least 2.5 servings of vegetables per day were observed to have a 33% lower risk for CHD, compared with men in the lowest category (<1 serving per day). A follow-up study of NHANES (National Health and Nutrition Examination Survey), a large national survey in the US, also reported a coronary protective effect of regular fruit and vegetable intake. Persons who consumed fruits and vegetables 3 or more times a day were at 24% lower risk than those who consumed less than one portion a day. A global study of risk factors of CHD in 52 countries (INTERHEART) also reported low consumption of fruit and vegetables to be a major risk factor, across all regions.

Fish

In the UK diet and reinfarction trial, 2-year mortality was reduced by 29% in survivors of a first myocardial infarction in those receiving advice to consume fatty fish at least twice a week. A meta-analysis of 13 large cohort studies suggests a protective effect of fish intake against CHD. Compared with those who never consumed fish or did so less than once a month, persons who ate fish had a lower risk of CHD (38% lower for 5 or more times a week, 23% lower for 2–4 times a week, 15% lower for once a week, and 11% lower for 1–3 times a month). Each $20\,g\,day^{-1}$ increase in fish consumption was related to a 7% lower risk of CHD.

Nuts

Several large epidemiological studies, the best known among them being the Adventist Health Study, demonstrated that frequent consumption of nuts was associated with decreased risk of CHD. The extent of risk reduction ranged from 18% to 57% for subjects who consumed nuts more than 5 times a week compared to those who never consumed nuts. An inverse dose–response relationship was demonstrated between the frequency of nut consumption and the risk of CHD, in men as well as in women. Most of these studies considered nuts as a group, combining many types of nuts (walnuts, almonds, pistachio, pecans, macadamia nuts, and legume peanuts).

Soy

Soy is rich in isoflavones, compounds that are structurally and functionally similar to estrogen. Several animal experiments suggest that intake of these isoflavones may provide protection against CHD, but human data on efficacy and safety are still awaited. Naturally occurring isoflavones, isolated with soy protein, reduced the plasma concentrations of total and LDL cholesterol without affecting the concentrations of triglycerides or HDL cholesterol in hypercholesterolemic individuals.

Dairy Products

Dairy consumption has been correlated positively, in ecological studies, with blood cholesterol as well as coronary mortality. Milk consumption correlated positively with coronary mortality rates in 43 countries and with myocardial infarction in 19 regions of Europe.

Alcohol

The relationship of alcohol to overall mortality and cardiovascular mortality has generally been J-shaped, when studied in Western populations in whom the rates of atherothrombotic vascular disorders are high. The protective effect of moderate ethanol consumption is primarily mediated through its effect on the risk of CHD, as supported by more than 60 prospective studies. A consistent coronary protective effect has been observed for consumption of 1–2 drinks per day of an alcohol-containing beverage but heavy drinkers have higher total mortality than moderate drinkers or abstainers, as do binge drinkers.

Composite Diets and CHD

The Mediterranean diet

The traditional Mediterranean diet has been described to have eight components:

1. high monounsaturated-to-saturated fat ratio;
2. moderate ethanol consumption;
3. high consumption of legumes;
4. high consumption of cereals (including bread);
5. high consumption of fruits;
6. high consumption of vegetables;
7. low consumption of meat and meat products; and
8. moderate consumption of milk and dairy products.

Most of these features are found in many diets in that region. The characteristic component is olive oil, and many equate a Mediterranean diet with consumption of olive oil.

A secondary prevention trial of dietary intervention in survivors of a first recent myocardial infarction (the Lyon Heart study), which aimed to study the cardioprotective effects of a 'Mediterranean type' of diet, actually left out its most characteristic component, olive oil. The main fat source was rapeseed oil. Vegetables and fruits were also increased in the diet. On a 4-year follow-up, the study reported a 72% reduction in cardiac death and nonfatal myocardial infarction. The risk of overall mortality was lowered by 56%. Large cohort studies in Greece and in several elderly European population groups have also recently reported a protective effect against CHD and better over all survival in persons consuming a Mediterranean type of diet. The protection was afforded by the composite diet rather than by any single component. Improvement in metabolic syndrome and reduction of inflammatory markers has also been observed with this diet, which may explain part of the protection against CHD.

DASH Diets

A composite diet, employed in the Dietary Approaches to Stop Hypertension (DASH) trials, has been found to be very effective in reducing blood pressure in persons with clinical hypertension as well as in people with blood pressure levels below that threshold. This diet combines fruits and vegetables with food products that are low in saturated fats. The blood pressure lowering effect is even greater when the DASH diet is modified to reduce the sodium content. Though the effects on CHD prevention have not been directly studied, the blood pressure and lipid-lowering effects of the low

salt-DASH diet are likely to have a substantial impact on CHD risk.

Vegetarian Diets

A reduced risk of CVD has been reported in populations of vegetarians living in affluent countries and in case–control comparisons in developing countries. Reduced consumption of animal fat and increased consumption of fruit, vegetables, nuts, and cereals may underlie such a protective effect. However, 'vegetarian diets' *per se* need not be healthful. If not well planned, they can contain a large amount of refined carbohydrates and t-FAs, while being deficient in the levels of vegetable and fruit consumption. The composition of the vegetarian diet should, therefore, be defined in terms of its cardioprotective constituents.

Prudent versus Western Patterns

In the Health professionals follow-up study in the US, a prudent diet pattern was characterized by higher intake of vegetables, fruits, legumes, whole grains, fish, and poultry, whereas the Western pattern was defined by higher intake of red meat, processed meat, refined grains, sweets and dessert, French fries, and high-fat dairy products. After adjustment for age and other coronary risk factors, relative risks, from the lowest to the highest quintiles of the prudent pattern score, were 1.0, 0.87, 0.79, 0.75, and 0.70, indicating a high level of protection. In contrast, the relative risks, across increasing quintiles of the western pattern, were 1.0, 1.21, 1.36, 1.40, and 1.64, indicating a mounting level of excess risk. These associations persisted in subgroup analyses according to cigarette smoking, body mass index, and parental history of myocardial infarction.

Japanese Diet

The traditional Japanese diet has attracted much attention because of the high life expectancy and low CHD mortality rates among the Japanese. This diet is low in fat and sugar and includes soy, seaweeds, raw fish, and a predominant use of rice. It has been high in salt, but salt consumption has recently been declining in response to Japanese Health Ministry guidelines.

Prevention Pathways

The powerful relationship of specific nutrients, food items and dietary patterns to CHD has been persuasively demonstrated by observational epidemiological studies (which indicate the potential for primary prevention in populations) and by clinical trials (which demonstrate the impact on secondary prevention in individuals).

Atherosclerotic vascular diseases (especially CHD) are multifactorial in origin. Each of the risk factors operates in a continuous manner, rather than across an arbitrary threshold. When multiple risk factors coexist, the overall risk becomes multiplicative. As a result of these two phenomena, the majority of CHD events occurring in any population arise from any individuals with modest elevations of multiple risk factors rather than from the few individuals with marked elevation of a single risk factor.

These phenomena have two major implications for CHD prevention. First, it must be recognized that a successful prevention strategy must combine population-wide interventions (through policy measures and public education) with individual risk reduction approaches (usually involving counseling and clinical interventions). Second, diet is a major pathway for CHD prevention, as it influences many of the risk factors for CHD, and can have a widespread impact on populations and substantially reduce the risk in high-risk individuals. Even small changes in blood pressure, blood lipids, body weight, central obesity, blood sugar, inflammatory markers, etc., can significantly alter the CHD rates, if the changes are widespread across the population. Modest population-wide dietary changes can accomplish this, as demonstrated in Finland and Poland. At the same time, diet remains a powerful intervention to substantially reduce the risk of a CHD-related event in individuals who are at high risk due to multiple risk factors, prior vascular disease, or diabetes.

A diet that is protective against CHD should integrate: plenty of fruits and vegetables (400–600 g day^{-1}); a moderate amount of fish (2–3 times a week); a small quantity of nuts; adequate amounts of PUFAs and MUFAs (together constituting about 75% of the daily fat intake); low levels of SFAs (less than 25% of the daily fat intake); limited salt intake (preferably less than 5 day^{-1}); and restricted use of sugar. Such diets should be culturally appropriate, economically affordable, and based on locally available foods.

National policies and international trade practices must be shaped to facilitate the wide availability and uptake of such diets. Nutrition counseling of individuals at high risk must also adopt these principles while customizing dietary advice to specific needs of the person. CHD is eminently preventable, as evident from research and demonstrated in practice across the world. Appropriate nutrition is a major pathway for CHD prevention and must be used more widely to make CHD prevention even more effective at the global level.

See also: **Alcohol**: Absorption, Metabolism and Physiological Effects; Disease Risk and Beneficial Effects; Effects of Consumption on Diet and Nutritional Status. **Antioxidants**: Diet and Antioxidant Defense; Observational Studies; Intervention Studies. **Cholesterol**: Sources, Absorption, Function and Metabolism; Factors Determining Blood Levels. **Coronary Heart Disease**: Hemostatic Factors; Lipid Theory. **Dietary Fiber**: Role in Nutritional Management of Disease. **Fatty Acids**: Monounsaturated; Omega-3 Polyunsaturated; Omega-6 Polyunsaturated; Saturated. **Fish**. **Folic Acid**. **Fruits and Vegetables**. **Nuts and Seeds**. **Potassium**. **Sodium**: Physiology; Salt Intake and Health. **Vegetarian Diets**.

Further Reading

Appel LJ, Moore TJ, Obarzanek E *et al.* (1997) A clinical trial of the effects of dietary patterns on blood pressure. DASH Collaborative Research Group. *New England Journal of Medicine* **336**: 1117–1124.

De Lorgeril M, Salen P, Martin JL *et al.* (1999) Mediterranean diet, traditional risk factors, and the rate of cardiovascular complications after myocardial infarction: final report of Lyon Diet Heart Study. *Circulation* **99**: 779–785.

He FJ and MacGregor GA (2003) How far should salt intake be reduced? *Hypertension* **42**: 1093–1099

He K, Song Y, Daviglus ML *et al.* (2004) Accumulated evidence on fish consumption and coronary heart disease mortality: a meta-analysis of cohort studies. *Circulation* **109**: 2705–2711.

INTERSALT Cooperative Research Group (1988) INTERSALT: an international study of electrolyte excretion and blood pressure. Results for 24 hr urinary sodium and potassium excretion. *British Medical Journal* **297**: 319–328.

Kris-Etherton P, Daniels SR, Eckel RH *et al.* (2001) Summary of the scientific conference on dietary fatty acids and cardiovascular health: conference summary from the nutrition committee of the American Heart Association. *Circulation* **103**: 1034–1039.

Ness AR and Powles JW (1997) Fruit and vegetables, and cardiovascular disease: a review. *International Journal of Epidemiology* **26**: 1–13.

Reddy KS and Katan MB (2004) Diet, nutrition and the prevention of hypertension and cardiovascular diseases. *Public Health and Nutrition* **7**: 167–186.

Sacks FM, Svetkey LP, Vollmer WM *et al.* (2001) Effects on blood pressure of reduced dietary sodium and the Dietary Approaches to Stop Hypertension (DASH) diet. DASH-Sodium Collaborative Research Group. *New England Journal of Medicine* **344**: 3–10.

Seely S (1981) Diet and coronary disease. A survey of mortality rates and food consumption statistics of 24 countries. *Medical Hypotheses* **7**: 907–918.

Trichopoulou A, Costacou T, Bamia C, and Trichopoulos D (2003) Adherence to a Mediterranean diet and survival in a Greek population. *New England Journal of Medicine* **348**: 2599–2608.

Verschuren WMM, Jacobs DR, Bloemberg BP *et al.* (1995) Serum total cholesterol and long-term coronary heart disease mortality in different cultures. Twenty-five year follow-up of the Seven Countries Study. *JAMA* **274**: 131–136.

World Health Organization (2003) Diet, nutrition and the prevention of chronic diseases. *Technical Report Series* **916**: 1–149.

World Health Organization (2002) *The World Health Report 2002. Reducing Risks, Promoting Healthy Life.* Geneva: WHO.

Yusuf S, Hawken S, Ounpuu S *et al.* (2004) INTERHEART study Investigators. Effect of potentially modifiable risk factors associated with myocardial infarction in 52 countries (the INTERHEART study): case-control study. *Lancet* **364**: 937–952.

CYSTIC FIBROSIS

J Dowsett and O Tully, St Vincent's University Hospital, Dublin, Ireland

© 2005 Elsevier Ltd. All rights reserved.

Definition and Etiology

Cystic fibrosis (CF) is a multisystem autosomal recessive disorder caused by the mutation of a single gene on the long arm of chromosome 7 that codes for the cystic fibrosis transmembrane regulator (CFTR). This protein regulates the passage of chloride through the membrane of secretory epithelia; the dysfunction of which results in an altered composition of epithelial secretions. Clinically, CF is characterized by chronic pulmonary infection with periods of acute exacerbation, pancreatic insufficiency and excessive losses of sweat electrolytes. The latter forms the basis for the diagnostic test. The mutated gene was identified in 1989 and since then over 800 CFTR mutations have been reported, the most common of these being △ F508.

Prevalence

Approximately 5% of the Caucasian North European and North American populations are carriers of the gene defect causing CF, leading to an approximate incidence of 1 in 2500 live births. This inheritance is illustrated in **Figure 1**. The incidence of CF in non-Caucasians is much lower and estimated to be around 1 in 100 000 in Oriental populations.

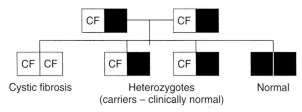

Figure 1 Mode of inheritance of CF: a Mendelian inherited recessive characteristic.

Prognosis

The median age of survival has dramatically risen from approximately 2 years in the 1940s to around 30 years in the 1990s. A current survival estimation following diagnosis is approximately 40 years. This improved prognosis can be attributed to a combination of factors including aggressive management of infections, effective antibiotics, improved nutritional management, modern physiotherapy techniques, and the centralization of treatment in specialist centers. The survival age for females with CF would appear to be less than that for males. This may be related to poorer nutritional status amongst female CF patients. Expert management started immediately after an early diagnosis of CF by neonatal screening results in an important beneficial effect on outcome and may be critical to the clinical course of the condition and long-term prognosis. Even though optimized nutrition, antibiotics, and chest physiotherapy remain the mainstay of CF management, new approaches to treatment are being developed that may add to the traditional medical therapy for CF. As prognosis and survival improves nutritional related issues become more prevalent including the effective management of pregnancy, diabetes, osteoporosis, and transplantation.

Clinical Features

The clinical features of CF are listed in **Table 1**.

Pathogenesis of Lung Disease

Pulmonary disease can be demonstrated within the first few months of life. Bacterial infection is characterized by high levels of neutrophils and mediators of infection in the form of interleukin 1, 8 and elastases. Mucous glands become dilated leading to obstruction, secondary infection, and progressive lung damage. Frequent periods of respiratory infection and exacerbation are common in CF with increased cough, increased sputum production, and shortness of breath. The immune response appears

Table 1 Clinical features of CF

Respiratory features of cystic fibrosis

Atelectasis	Incomplete expansion of a lung or part of a lung due to airlessness or collapse
Bronchiectasis	Chronic dilatation of the bronchi associated with coughing and expectoration of purulent mucus
Bronchitis	Inflammation of one or more bronchi
Pneumonia	Inflammation of the lungs with air spaces becoming filled with exudates
Pneumothorax	An accumulation of air in the pleural space

Gastrointestinal features of cystic fibrosis

Cholelithiasis	The presence or formation of gallstones
Cirrhosis	Liver disease characterized by loss of normal liver tissue and fibrosis
Distal intestinal obstruction syndrome	Blockage of the bowel with feces, mucus, and undigested food
Gastroparesis	Paralysis of the stomach or delayed gastric emptying
Malabsorption	Impaired intestinal absorption of nutrients
Maldigestion	Impaired intestinal digestion of nutrients
Meconium ileus	Blockage of the bowel with meconium
Osteoporosis/ Osteopenia	Reduction in bone mass
Pancreatic insufficiency	Reduction of enzyme production from the pancreas
Portal hypertension	High pressure in the portahepatic artery
Rectal prolapse	Protrusion of the rectal mucous membrane through the anus
Splenomegaly	Enlargement of the spleen

to be of great significance. Chronic inflammation has been cited as the cause of so much of the lung damage seen in CF. Steroidal anti-inflammatory drugs have been shown to be beneficial but have nutritional side effects such as hyperglycemia and osteoporosis. Nonsteroidal anti-inflammatory drugs such as ibuprofen have been used in some centers with positive results but their long-term effect on renal function is not yet known. The impact of malnutrition on lung disease and respiratory muscle function has been extensively studied in patients with CF. Malnutrition and deterioration of lung function are interdependent. Prevention of malnutrition from the time of diagnosis is associated with better lung function and improved survival.

Gastrointestinal Complications

Individuals with CF can develop a variety of gastrointestinal (GI) disorders related to the pathophysiological changes associated with CF. Pancreatic insufficiency, which is present in the majority of CF patients leads to many of the GI manifestations of CF including steatorrhea, abdominal pain, distal intestinal obstruction syndrome (DIOS), and rectal prolapse. Gastroesophageal reflux (GOR) occurs frequently in CF due to decreased lower esophageal sphincter pressure and is usually treated by proton pump inhibitors. In patients with advanced lung disease vomiting is common after strenuous bouts of coughing and this over time may lead to decline in nutritional status. Peptic ulcer disease, pancreatitis, and intussusception also occur to varying degrees in patients with CF. Crohn's disease and celiac disease occur more frequently in the CF population than in controls and gastrointestinal tumors, although rare, have an increased incidence in CF.

Meconium ileus is the presenting complaint in up to 15% of infants with CF. This is a condition in which the small intestine is blocked with tenacious meconium and surgical intervention is required to correct it. Excessive mucus in the small bowel of patients with CF can provide a physical barrier to the absorptive surface. Undigested or unabsorbed food in association with this mucus, and possibly a reduced gut motility, can lead to a partial or complete obstruction of the GI tract in older children and adults known as meconium ileus equivalent, or more accurately distal intestinal obstruction syndrome (DIOS). This is a condition specific to CF. The usual clinical presentation is one of abdominal pain, abdominal distension, and constipation. It can be precipitated by dehydration, change in eating habits, change in enzyme brand or dose, or immobility. DIOS is treated with a laxative regime and should have a diet and enzyme review.

CF-Related Diabetes Mellitus (CFRD)

Diabetes requiring insulin is the most common comorbidity in CF. The islets of Langerhan are the last cells to be damaged in the process of fibrosis of the pancreas. The incidence of diabetes in CF has been reported to be 8–15% but this may be underestimated due to lack of screening. It is estimated that 50% of patients over 30 years will have some degree of glucose intolerance. The primary cause of CFRD is insulin deficiency secondary to pancreatic fibrosis. Diagnostic criteria for CFRD are the same as for non-CF-related diabetes. Glucose metabolism is also affected by many factors including infection, malabsorption, abnormal intestinal transit time, and steroid use, all features of CF. While CFRD shares many of the characteristics of both type 1 and type 2 diabetes, it is itself a distinct clinical condition. Hyperglycemia may adversely influence weight and pulmonary function and as the age of survival increases may lead to the development of microvascular complications. Retrospective studies have shown in those presenting with overt diabetes mellitus, deterioration in weight and respiratory status for 2 years before diagnosis are reversed once insulin therapy is instituted. A program of multiple daily insulin injections and self-monitoring of blood glucose with the aim of normoglycemia is the preferred treatment with regular follow-up with the Endocrinology team. All patients with CF should be screened annually for CFRD using the oral glucose tolerance test. Minimal dietary restrictions are imposed on this group of patients in an attempt to maximize nutritional intake. See section on dietary management of CF.

Liver Disease

Another complication associated with increased longevity in CF is liver disease, which affects between 2 and 37% of adults with CF. The development of liver disease in CF has been attributed to the blockage of small bile ductules with thick secretions, and the subsequent development of progressive cholestasis, biliary fibrosis, and eventually biliary cirrhosis and portal hypertension. The persisting acidic conditions in the upper small bowel lead to bile salt precipitation and defective lipid emulsification. Unhydrolyzed fat and other products of maldigestion may interfere with bile acid reabsorption in the terminal ileum, thereby reducing the total bile salt pool. Fecal losses of primary and secondary bile acids leads to an imbalance of bile salts, which further increases the viscosity of the already tenacious bile. Treatment with ursodeoxycholic acid has led to an improvement in bile excretion and liver function tests. Complications of liver disease including ascites, gastro and esophageal varices may further exacerbate a patient's nutritional status. In a small number of patients liver failure may require liver transplantation. See section on dietary management of CF.

Nutritional Management

Aggressive nutritional management of patients with CF is key in their overall management. Nutritional management of CF involves maximizing dietary intake, minimizing malabsorption and maldigestion, monitoring vitamin intakes and serum levels, and adapting eating patterns in the event of diabetes, osteoporosis, DIOS, or liver disease. Nutritional support in the form of nocturnal gastrostomy feeding may be necessary if nutritional failure persists (BMI $< 18.5 \, \text{kg/m}^2$). It is well recognized that the malnutrition seen in CF is due to an energy imbalance caused by three main factors: decreased dietary intake, increased energy requirements, and increased energy losses. There appears to be a direct association between the degree of malnutrition and the severity of pulmonary disease, affecting overall prognosis. Many patients are capable of balancing these factors effectively and have a normal growth velocity and good nutritional status. However, as lung function deteriorates, energy requirement increases and appetite decreases leading to a loss of energy stores and lean tissue further contributing to progressive deterioration of lung function (see **Figure 2**).

Decreased Dietary Intake

People with CF are advised to consume a diet high in energy with no fat restriction. Prior to the development of enteric-coated enzymes in the mid 1980s, patients with CF were advised to follow a low-fat diet in an attempt to minimize fat malabsorption and steatorrhea. Unfortunately, older patients continue this practice as they have developed an aversion to fatty foods after many years of avoiding them. Decreased dietary intake secondary to anorexia is common in CF and can become more of a problem during recurrent chest infections. There have also been an increased number of reports of eating disorders and abnormal eating behavior in the CF population. In addition polypharmacy, repeated exacerbations of CF, organomegaly, gastrointestinal problems, food intolerance, and poor social circumstances can reduce oral intake.

Increased Energy Requirements

Energy requirements are increased during periods of infection by catabolism and fever and continue to increase with advanced pulmonary disease. It has been estimated that CF patients require 120–150% of the estimated average requirement for energy. As pulmonary function deteriorates, mobility also decreases and overall energy expenditure is reduced as a result. Owing to the heterogenicity of CF the energy requirements of individuals will vary and should be assessed on an individual basis. Energy losses through sputum may also be significant in a patient with a marginal energy intake. Salbutamol, often used as a bronchodilator in CF, can increase basal metabolic rate.

Increased Energy Losses

Pancreatic changes are caused by the obstruction of small ducts with thick secretions and cell debris.

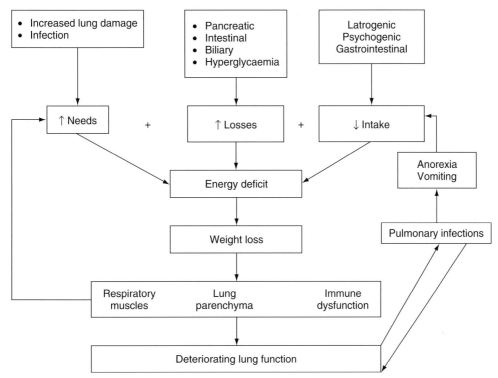

Figure 2 Interdependent factors that may give rise to progressive energy deficit as lung function deteriorates.

Functional tissue becomes replaced with fibrotic tissue leading to pancreatic exocrine insufficiency when more than 90% of the normal structure of the pancreas is lost. Pancreatic insufficiency is the most common gastrointestinal manifestation in CF, occurring in at least 95% of patients. The production of pancreatic secretions including enzymes and bicarbonate is reduced, necessitating pancreatic enzyme replacement therapy (PERT). PERT is supplied in the form of gelatin capsules containing microspheres, which are swallowed whole with food. The capsule dissolves within the stomach and releases the microspheres, which are protected from the gastric acid by an enteric coating. Enzymes should be taken immediately before or during a meal to maximize their efficacy. The microspheres mix with the stomach contents and pass through the pylorus into the duodenum where they become activated. Microspheres should be less than 1.5 mm in diameter to ensure they leave the stomach with food. Fibrosis of the pancreas tends to be a progressive process so increasing amounts of oral enzyme supplements are often required as patients get older. All people with CF have some level of pancreatic dysfunction but requirements of enzymes are variable and must be assessed individually. Clinically, the aim of PERT is to correct symptomatic steatorrhea, relieve any abdominal pain, reduce the mass and frequency of stool passed, and achieve weight gain within normal limits.

The enteric coating on enzyme supplements is designed to dissolve at a pH of 6, the optimal pH for pancreatic enzymatic action. Owing to the reduced production of bicarbonate and the resulting lower pH of the duodenum in patients with CF, the enteric coating of the enzyme may fail to dissolve so that the enzyme does not become activated at the absorptive surface of the small bowel. Increasing the duodenal pH by taking proton pump inhibitors may improve absorption. Changing the brand of enzyme may also improve absorption as dissolution characteristics of the enteric coating and proportions of enzymes contained within the microspheres vary. Patients should be dissuaded from chewing enzymes as this breaks the enteric coating and leads to deactivation in the acid medium of the stomach. Even with maximal PERT it has been estimated that between 10 and 20% of ingested fat will be malabsorbed. Colonic strictures known as fibrosing colonopathy (FC) in CF populations receiving high-potency enzymes with a more concentrated dose of lipase and protease per capsule have been reported The etiology of this FC remains unclear. Recently, it has been suggested that FC may be related to the presence of methacrylic acid copolymer (MAC) coating present in some preparations rather than actual enzyme strength. Some adult patients continue to take high-dose enzymes and are advised to do so within recommended levels. The working group on PERT use recommends that no more than 10 000 units of lipase per kilogram body weight be taken per day.

Dietary Management of CF

Patients with CF are encouraged to consume a diet providing 150% of the recommended intake for age and sex. However, this is only a guideline, since in practice the energy requirement for a patient with CF is that which maintains their ideal body weight when malabsorption has been controlled. Maximizing energy intake from everyday foods should be the initial step in the promotion of a high-energy diet. As fat is the most concentrated source of energy in the diet, liberal use of fat should be encouraged; this can best be achieved by recommending frequent consumption of high-fat meals and snacks including confectionery, desserts, and cakes. PERT should be dosed accordingly.

Dietary Supplements

The energy intake of many patients with CF is commonly suboptimal. Many patients find it difficult to eat sufficient food daily to attain or maintain their ideal body weight. During a respiratory exacerbation of CF, energy requirements are at a maximum, but appetite is often reduced. Dietary supplements in the form of sip feeds can be a useful adjunct to a high-energy diet. Care should be taken to ensure that supplements are used in addition to a diet and not as a substitute for normal foods.

Enteral Feeding

When diet and oral dietary supplements are undesirable or ineffective and nutritional failure persists, i.e., BMI <18.5 kg/m^2, enteral feeding should be considered. Research has demonstrated a sustained weight gain and a slowing decline in respiratory function associated with supplemental enteral feeding. Artificial nutritional support can be provided via nasogastric or gastrostomy tube depending on patient preference. Gastrostomy feeding is becoming more popular, whether passed endoscopically or under fluoroscopic guidance. The introduction of low-profile gastrostomy feeding tubes or 'button' tubes have made this method of nutritional support more acceptable of patients. The type of feed used and the PERT given with it, varies between centers. Feeds are usually administered overnight in an attempt to provide 30–50% of energy requirements and to allow for maximal oral intake during the day. Gastrostomy feeds can be used over longer periods during periods of acute pulmonary infection, loss of appetite, or in the severely malnourished patient. Patients with a previous poor intake should be monitored for refeeding syndrome.

Specific Dietary Considerations

There are some medical complications of CF that warrant particular nutritional attention.

Liver Disease

Patients with liver disease as a complication of their CF may have ascites, gastric, or esophageal varices, all of which may affect nutritional status and options for nutritional support. Dietary management of the patient with CF and liver disease centers on maximizing energy intake and is best achieved by encouraging small, frequent, energy-dense meals, snacks, and drinks. Suboptimal oral intake can arise in patients with hepatomegaly or splenomegaly, who often have a feeling of fullness after eating referred to as the 'small stomach syndrome.' The benefits of gastrostomy insertion should be carefully weighed in the patient with gastric varices or splenomegaly due to risk of bleeding. A moderate sodium restriction may alleviate ascites. If coagulation is impaired, supplementation with vitamin K may be indicated.

Treatment of liver disease in CF is with ursodeoxycholic acid, which has a positive effect on liver enzymes. Whether this improvement is associated with improvement in nutritional status is unknown.

Cystic Fibrosis-Related Diabetes (CFRD)

The dietary treatment of CF-related diabetes varies from standard diabetic dietary advice. The principle of the diet centers on maintaining caloric intake whilst ensuring glycemic control. The treatment of CFRD should enhance rather than impair a patient's nutritional status. This is done by encouraging a high-fat diet and confining the intake of refined carbohydrate to mealtimes. Insulin doses should be increased so as to maximize the flexibility of the diet, particularly in those patients who are already nutritionally compromised Patients taking oral nutritional supplements and/or overnight gastrostomy feeds need to have their insulin doses carefully monitored and adjusted accordingly.

Bone Disease in CF

Osteopenia and osteoporosis are now widely recognized in the CF population. There are a number of contributing factors to this early development of bone disease including steroid usage, malabsorption of calcium and, more importantly, vitamin D, poor nutritional status, decreased levels of physical activity, and a reduced peak bone mass in CF patients compared to healthy individuals. Assessment of bone health is by dual energy X-ray absorptiometry (DXA) scanning and there are a variety of treatment options available depending on the severity of disease ranging from dietary calcium and vitamin D supplementation to the use of bisphosphonate drugs, which aim to halt the progression of bone loss and promote bone formation.

Fertility Issues

As the number of people with CF of a reproductive age increases, so does the incidence of pregnancy in this group. Although almost all males with CF are infertile owing to the absence of the vas deferens, most females are fertile. Pregnancy in women with CF requires special nutritional attention with regular monitoring, particularly with respect to adequate weight gain, and vitamin and mineral status.

Body Composition Studies in CF

Studies of body composition in CF patients have shown deficits in total body mass, lean body mass, and body fat, which affect body density. As skinfold thickness percentiles are derived from body density, it has been suggested that the assessment of the body fat content of children with CF using, or derived from, body density such as skinfold thickness is invalid. Muscle function indices have been shown to respond to refeeding in malnourished patients with CF before body composition or biochemical indices of protein status improved, and so appear to be sensitive markers of nutritional status.

Assessment of Nutritional Status

Malnutrition in CF remains a major clinical problem. Growth and nutritional status should be monitored at each clinic visit to ensure early detection of any deterioration, and to prompt appropriate nutritional intervention. The many factors that complicate nutritional status in CF are shown in **Table 2**.

When weight falls to a BMI of less than $18.5 \, \text{kg/m}^2$ nocturnal enteral feeding should be considered. At diagnosis and when the patient shows clinical deterioration the following should be determined:

Table 2 Factors affecting nutritional status

- Variation in gene mutation
- Frequency of pulmonary exacerbations
- Gastroesophageal reflux
- Distal intestinal obstruction syndrome
- Pancreatitis
- Liver disease
- Diabetes mellitus
- Drug therapy
- Dietary dislikes and misconceptions
- Psychological problems/eating disorders
- Pregnancy
- Transplantation

electrolytes, serum albumin and other liver function tests, oral glucose tolerance test, full blood count, serum retinol, and alpha tocopherol. If there is any evidence of iron deficiency, iron status should be assessed. Other medical disorders should be considered in the evaluation of nutritional failure. These include diabetes mellitus, liver disease, Crohn's disease, celiac disease, chronic abdominal pain, DIOS, and esophagitis.

Vitamin Status in CF

At least 85% of CF patients have some level of pancreatic insufficiency leading to a degree of fat malabsorption. For this reason, unless supplemented, most patients are at risk of developing either clinical or subclinical deficiencies of the fat-soluble vitamins, vitamin A, D, E, and K. Those most at risk appear to be individuals with poorly controlled malabsorption, poor adherence to treatment, liver disease, bowel resection, or following a late diagnosis.

Vitamin A

Vitamin A should be supplemented at a dose of 4000–10 000 IU per day. However, low serum levels of retinol have been noted even at this dose. If retinol levels are persistently low despite adequate supplementation, an assessment of compliance, retinol-binding protein (RBP), and zinc levels should be checked. Special care should be given to vitamin A supplementation during pregnancy as high levels are reported to be teratogenic.

It is important to consider hepatotoxicity with large supplemental doses of vitamin A in a patient who may store vitamin A in the liver, yet shows low serum levels of retinol, and who may display ocular signs of deficiency. The free alcohol retinol is almost entirely attached to RBP, which is synthesized in the liver. Decreased levels of RBP, which may occur in up to 25% of patients with CF, may be due to an abnormality in its production by the liver, zinc deficiency, or protein energy malnutrition. Even with adequate vitamin supplementation and pancreatic enzyme replacement treatment, up to 20% of patients may have ocular signs of deficiency of retinol. Xerosis may improve by increasing the dose of vitamin A alone, or combined with zinc. It has been suggested that there may exist a specific defect in the handling of retinol in the GI tract of people with CF unrelated to the level of fat malabsorption. A correlation has been demonstrated between low levels of vitamin A and poor lung function.

Beta-Carotene

Beta-carotene is one of the carotinoids present in plasma and a precursor of vitamin A. It is effective as an antioxidant at lower oxygen saturation states than vitamin E. It has a biological role as a lipid-soluble chain-breaking antioxidant in biomembranes. Routine supplementation with beta-carotene could diminish lipid peroxidation and improve essential fatty acid status.

Vitamin D

Vitamin D deficiency may be caused by malabsorption, underexposure to sunlight or defects in metabolism due to liver disease. Even though skin exposure to sunlight is the major source of vitamin D, serum concentrations will vary between individuals depending on endogenous production in the skin. Rickets as a result of vitamin D deficiency is rare but has been described in CF. Osteopenia and retarded bone maturation have been reported in a number of CF patients, even with supplementation to recommended levels. Bone density has been shown to be significantly decreased in all sites compared with that of normal young adults. Other variables such as activity levels and nutritional status have not been adequately researched, although the incidence of osteoporosis was found to be higher in those patients with severe respiratory disease. To attain and maintain normal serum levels a daily dose of 400–2000 IU is generally required in adults.

Vitamin E

Cholestasis and a reduced enterohepatic circulation of bile acids contribute to the malabsorption of fat-soluble vitamins from the small intestine. Vitamin E is highly lipophilic and deficiency correlates with degree of fat malabsorption. Subclinical neuro-electrophysiological abnormalities are already present in about 40% of patients by 2 months of age. Neurological signs of vitamin E deficiency are responsive to supplementation if initiated early but are irreversible if treatment starts after the neurological lesions are present. As circulating alpha tocopherol is transported in the blood attached to lipid it is should be expressed as a ratio to total lipid to be correctly interpreted. Current recommendations are to monitor serum vitamin E levels annually and adjust supplementation accordingly. A daily dose of 400 IU per day should achieve normal serum levels in adults.

Vitamin K

A review of the literature provides conflicting opinions in the area of routine supplementation of vitamin K as the prevalence of vitamin K deficiency has not been established. Theoretically, the risk factors for patients developing vitamin K deficiency are pancreatic insufficiency, severe liver disease, extensive small bowel resection, and chronic broad-spectrum antibiotic use. Monitoring the coagulation system is advised, as vitamin K estimations are not generally routinely available. It seems prudent to prescribe vitamin K supplements to patients with the above risk factors. Vitamin K has recently been shown to play an important role in bone health. There are no specific guidelines on supplementation, but doses of 5–10 mg appear to be a prudent guide. Annual monitoring of fat-soluble vitamin levels should be carried out and doses of vitamins altered as appropriate.

Water-Soluble Vitamins

Supplementation with water-soluble vitamins is, in general, thought to be unnecessary in CF. In cases where dietary intake is poor or unbalanced, supplementation of vitamin C is advised. Supplementation with other water soluble vitamins is not routinely recommended.

Mineral Status in CF

Fat malabsorption can lead to the formation of insoluble fatty acid complexes with minerals in the gut, leading to a reduction in their absorption. CF may also be associated with intestinal mucosal defects, which may further retard the absorption of nutrients. Suboptimal levels of zinc, selenium, manganese, and iron have all been described in CF. Routine iron supplementation is not recommended as it has been suggested that *Pseudomonas aeruginosa* grows in tissues with a high concentration of iron. In addition, levels of iron may be suppressed as a normal body response in times of infection, and attempting to correct this is potentially harmful. Sodium and chloride do not need to be supplemented unless in very hot climates or during excessive exercise.

The Oxidant/Antioxidant Imbalance in CF

Patients with CF frequently exhibit increased oxygen free radical generation from activated neutrophils due to chronic lung inflammation. This, coupled with antioxidant deficiencies due to exocrine pancreatic insufficiency, results in an oxidant/antioxidant imbalance. Consequently, free radical attack on unsaturated fatty acids of lipid structures occurs leading to lipid peroxidation. An efficient antioxidant supply is suggested to control tissue damage by restoring the oxidant/antioxidant balance.

Conclusions

There is a complex relationship between physiological, environmental, and genetic variables leading to a great variability in energy requirements among individuals with CF. Despite advances in the treatment of CF the need for good nutritional strategies in CF will continue. Individually tailored nutritional advice for each patient with CF by a dietitian experienced in the area of CF is essential.

See also: **Diabetes Mellitus**: Etiology and Epidemiology; Classification and Chemical Pathology; Dietary Management. **Eating Disorders**: Anorexia Nervosa; Bulimia Nervosa. **Liver Disorders**. **Malnutrition**: Primary, Causes Epidemiology and Prevention; Secondary, Diagnosis and Management. **Nutritional**

Assessment: Anthropometry; Biochemical Indices; Clinical Examination. **Nutritional Support**: Adults, Enteral; Adults, Parenteral; Infants and Children, Parenteral. **Vitamin A**: Physiology; Biochemistry and Physiological Role; Deficiency and Interventions. **Vitamin D**: Physiology, Dietary Sources and Requirements; Rickets and Osteomalacia. **Vitamin K**.

Further Reading

Borowitz DS, Grand RJ, and Durie PR, and the Consensus Committee (1995) Use of pancreatic enzyme supplements for patients with cystic fibrosis in the context of fibrosing colonopathy. *Journal of Paediatrics* 127: 681–684.

Dodge JA (1992) Nutrition in cystic fibrosis: a historical overview. *Proceedings of the Nutrition Society* 51: 225–235.

McDonald A, Holden C, and Harris G (1991) Nutritional strategies in cystic fibrosis: current issues. *Journal of the Royal Society of Medicine* 84(supplement 18): 28–35.

Moran A, Hardin D, Rodman D, and Allen HF, and the consensus committee (1999) Diagnosis screening and management of cystic fibrosis related diabetes mellitus: A consensus conference report. *Diabetes Research and Clinical Practice* 45: 57–68.

Ramsey BW, Farrell PM, and Pencharz P, and the Consensus Committee (1992) Nutritional assessment and management in cystic fibrosis: a consensus report *American Journal of Clinical Nutrition* 55: 108–116

Rosenstein *et al.* (1998) The diagnosis of cystic fibrosis: A consensus statement. *Journal of Pediatrics* 132(4): 589–595.

Sinaasappel M, Stern M, Litttlewood J, Wolfe S, Steinkamp G, Harry, Heijerman HGM, Robberecht E, and Döring G (2002) Nutrition in patients with cystic fibrosis: a European Consensus. *Journal of Cystic Fibrosis* 1: 51–75.

Warner J (ed.) (1992) Cystic fibrosis. *British Medical Bulletin* 48(4): 717–978.

Zentler-Munro PI (1987) Cystic fibrosis: a gastroenterological cornucopia. *Gut* 28: 1531–1547.

CYTOKINES

R F Grimble, University of Southampton, Southampton, UK

© 2005 Elsevier Ltd. All rights reserved.

Chemistry and Classification

Cytokines comprise a wide range of proteins that are released mainly from cells of the immune system in response to invasion of animals by pathogens or severe injury. Cytokines induce a state of inflammation in the body and modulation in the activity of the immune system. Research shows that cytokine production is not restricted to cells in the immune system, but that fibroblasts, endothelial cells, adipocytes, and specialized tissues, such as the ovary, produce cytokines. Although largely influencing immune function, a number of cytokines act as growth factors and lead to the proliferation and differentiation of a wide range of cell populations in the body. Cytokines are proteins of low molecular weight. They act generally in an autocrine or paracrine fashion and are active in the subnanomolar range. Cytokines are subclassified as interleukins (ILs), tumor necrosis factors (TNFs), interferons, and colony-stimulating factors. Examples from the family of cytokines are detailed in **Table 1**. All influence cells of the immune system; however,

Table 1 Main properties of the pro-inflammatory cytokines

Cytokine	Mol. wt	Cell sources	Main cell targets	Main actions
Interleukin-1α Interleukin-1β	33 000 ⎱ 17 500 ⎰	Monocytes, macrophages, astrocytes, epithelial cells, endothelium, fibroblasts, dendritic cells	Thymocytes, neutrophils, T and B cells, skeletal muscle, hepatocytes	Immunoregulation, inflammation, fever, anorexia, acute-phase protein synthesis, muscle proteolysis, enhanced gluconeogenesis
Interleukin-6	20 000	Macrophages, T cells, fibroblasts, some B cells	T and B cells, thymocytes, hepatocytes	Acute-phase protein synthesis, immune cell differentiation
Tumor necrosis factor-α	50 000 (trimer)	Macrophages, lymphocytes	Fibroblasts, endothelium, skeletal muscle hepatocytes	As for IL-1

only three exert metabolic effects upon the host. These are denoted as pro-inflammatory cytokines IL-1, IL-6, and TNF-α. A summary of the cell sources, main cell targets, and actions of the proinflammatory cytokines is shown in **Table 1**.

Metabolism and Metabolic Functions

Widespread metabolic changes occur as a result of cytokine production (**Figure 1**). These responses are powerful, focused, and dangerous to both host and pathogens. A hostile environment for pathogens is created within the body by the release of oxidant molecules (superoxide, hydrogen peroxide, perchlorous acid, and nitric oxide) from phagocytes.

Nutrients are provided for the immune system as a result of wasting of peripheral tissues. Amino acids released as a consequence of increased proteolysis in muscle, skin, and bone provide substrate for the synthesis of cells in the system. Glutamine, released from muscle, and glucose, derived from increased hepatic gluconeogenesis of amino acids, are major sources of nutrition for the immune system. Likewise, increased lipolysis in adipose tissue provides fatty acids as metabolic fuel for the body. Zinc, an important cofactor in DNA synthesis, is released from peripheral tissues, incorporated into the zinc transporting protein metallothionein in liver and kidney, and subsequently utilised by the immune system. A loss of appetite often occurs. This may be purposeful in permitting a situation in which substrate is more closely tailored to the requirements of the immune system than would occur from the vagaries of habitual dietary intake. This concept, however, is a matter of debate. Nonetheless, it is important that the immune system receives a guaranteed source of nutrition immediately after the body is infected or damaged because bacterial cells

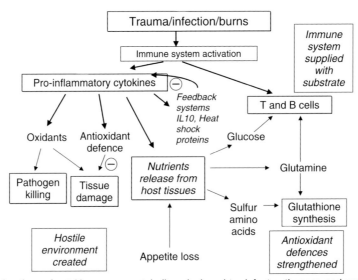

Figure 1 The coordinated actions of cytokines upon metabolism designed to defeat pathogens and protect the host. The resultant effects are shown in italics.

multiply at least 50 times more rapidly than T cells under favorable conditions. Under the actions of cytokines, the metabolic activity of the liver is greatly enhanced and modified. Large increases in the rates of gluconeogenesis, glycogen breakdown, and urea and fat synthesis occur. Blood glucose, urea, and triacylglycerol concentrations may rise. The increase in triacylglycerol levels may have functional importance due to the ability of these molecules to bind and neutralize endotoxin, thereby reducing the impact of this toxic bacterial product upon the host. Paradoxically, however, metabolism of xenobiotics is decreased due to a reduction in the activity of cytochrome P450. The profile of export proteins synthesized by the liver is changed, synthesis of albumin is reduced, and the synthesis of a group of proteins closely associated with inflammation (acute-phase proteins) is increased. Acute-phase proteins are multifunctional and include caeruloplasmin (an antioxidant and copper transport protein), C-reactive protein (to improve macrophage activity), fibrinogen (for blood clotting), complement proteins (for enhanced phagocytosis and pathogen destruction), and metallothionein (a zinc transport protein).

The antioxidant defences of the body are strengthened by increases in the activities of superoxide dismutase, catalase, glutathione peroxidase, and reductase and by increases in the hepatic synthesis of the reduced form of glutathione (GSH). The liver thus becomes the main focus for the synthesis of molecules for the nutrition, support, and direction of the immune system and for the protection of the body from the adverse effects of cytokine action. Indeed, when the ability of the liver of patients with sepsis (a severe clinical form of inflammation induced by infection) to extract amino acids from the circulation was assessed, it was found that the livers of patients who subsequently died had only half of that of livers of patients who survived.

A number of molecules synthesized in enhanced amounts when cytokines are produced are part of complex feedback systems that limit cytokine production and effects (**Figure 2**). These include GSH and some acute-phase proteins that suppress cytokine production and also cytokine receptor antagonist molecules for IL-1 and TNF. The first two types of molecule are derived from liver and the last two from lymphocytes and the cellular targets for TNF, respectively. Other molecules also moderate cytokine actions. Anti-inflammatory cytokines such as IL-10 and heat shock proteins exert an anti-inflammatory influence in the latter stages of the inflammatory response. This downregulation of inflammation, once the infectious agent has been defeated, is important for survival since the inflammatory process has a large capacity to deplete the body. The balance between the pro- and anti-inflammatory process is of key importance for survival since excessive production of IL-10 has been associated with increased mortality.

Role in Disease and Disease Processes

Despite the importance of cytokines in protecting the host from pathogens, the molecules may have damaging and even lethal effects on the host. Thus, the response of the host to a pathogen may play as significant a part in the demise of the host as the effects of the pathogen. Cytokines may also play a major role in tissue damage in chronic inflammatory disease, in which no infective agent is operating. Excessive or inappropriate cytokine production has been associated with increased morbidity and mortality in a wide range of diseases and conditions in which inflammation plays a role. These include

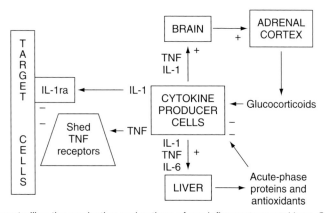

Figure 2 Innate systems for controlling the production and actions of pro-inflammatory cytokines. Stimulatory actions are indicated by plus signs and inhibitory actions by minus signs.

diseases where the immune system is clearly interacting with invading pathogens, such as malaria, meningitis, sepsis, and AIDS, and conditions such as asthma, inflammatory bowel disease, rheumatoid arthritis, and cancer, in which inflammatory disease develops without obvious involvement of pathogens. Furthermore, pro-inflammatory cytokines may be involved in the progression of disease processes such as plaque development in atherosclerosis and demylination in multiple sclerosis and Alzheimer's disease (**Figure 3**).

Damage may also be exerted on the host by release of free radicals and other oxidant molecules that are also released from phagocytic cells in response to the inflammatory stimulus and IL-1 and TNF. Furthermore, oxidant molecules upregulate production of IL-1, TNF, and IL-8 by activation of the transcription factor, nuclear factor-kappa B (NF-κB). The factor is normally held quiescent in the cytoplasm due to attachment of an inhibitory component (IκB) to it. In the presence of oxidants, IκB dissociates from NF-κB, migrates to the nucleus, and brings about the transcription of a large range of genes associated with the inflammatory process (**Figure 4**). Unfortunately, the human immunodeficiency virus (HIV) has an NF-κB response element on its genome. Thus, a by-product of the inflammatory response is increased replication of this virus and progression toward AIDS.

The fact that insulin resistance and disordering of lipid metabolism occur in obesity, diabetes mellitus, and during the inflammatory response has led to investigation of the possibility that obesity exerts an inflammatory influence on individuals. Large population studies show a strong association between indices of inflammation, abnormal lipid and carbohydrate metabolism, obesity, and atherosclerosis. This association is particularly strong in populations with a high incidence of obesity, diabetes, and cardiovascular disease (e.g., Pima Indians and Southeast Asians). TNF-α is produced not only by cells of the immune system but also by adipocytes and may provide the link between inflammation, insulin sensitivity, and the diseases associated therewith (**Figure 5**). TNF-α results in insulin insensitivity indirectly by stimulating stress hormone production and directly by down-regulating insulin receptor substrate-1 and by negative regulation of PPAR-γ, an important insulin-sensitising nuclear receptor. Adipose tissue produces both TNF-α and leptin. Production of the latter relates positively to adipose tissue mass and through its actions on immune function exerts a pro-inflammatory influence. It is unclear whether chronic inflammation is a trigger for chronic insulin insensitivity and conditions associated therewith or whether the reverse is the case. Evidence favours the former interpretation of the data.

Genetic factors play a role in the propensity of individuals to produce damaging or life-threatening amounts of cytokines during inflammation. Males and postmenopausal females possess a genetically determined propensity to produce high, medium, or low levels of cytokines in response to stimuli. Single base changes in the promoter regions of cytokine genes (single nucleotide polymorphisms (SNP)) result in these different levels of production. In the case of TNF-α, production of the cytokine is influenced by SNP in the TNF-α (*TNF2*) and TNF-β (*TNFB2*) genes. Individuals with the *TNF2* or *TNFB2* alleles produce higher amounts of TNF. In premenopausal women, the capacity to produce cytokines is influenced by the hormones of the oestrous cycle. Although the capacity for genetically determined levels of cytokines produces no apparent harm in healthy subjects, in disease, genetics has an impact on mortality. Studies in The Gambia showed that subjects who were homozygous for *TNF2* had a seven times higher rate of death or serious neural symptoms than subjects with one or no copies of the allele. Likewise, in patients with severe sepsis, possession of a *TNFB22* genotype resulted in 72% mortality in men compared with 42% mortality in men with a *TNFB11* genotype. Women were less severely affected by this genotypic influence. There is controversy about the reason for the retention of this lethal characteristic within the gene pool of the population. It is possible that in heterozygotes the presence of the genetic characteristic gives an immunological advantage. Homozygotes, who are less numerous than

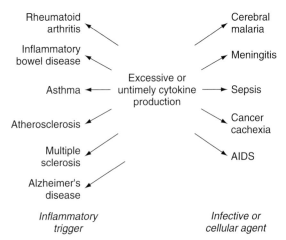

Figure 3 Diseases and conditions in which cytokines play a role.

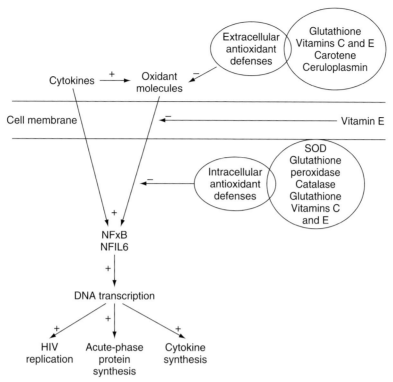

Figure 4 The interactions among oxidants, cytokines, and antioxidant defenses during inflammation. Minus signs indicate an inhibitory effect, and plus signs indicate a stimulatory effect. NF, nuclear factor; SOD, superoxide dismutase.

heterozygotes might pay the price for the advantageous retention of the genetic characteristic within the population. It is also interesting to note that in longevity studies a SNP that results in raised IL-10 production is more common in nonagenarians than in younger subjects, and conversely a SNP that results in raised production of IL-6 is rarer in the older than younger subjects. Thus, although it is an essential component of the ability of the body to combat pathogens, inflammation is inimical with longevity.

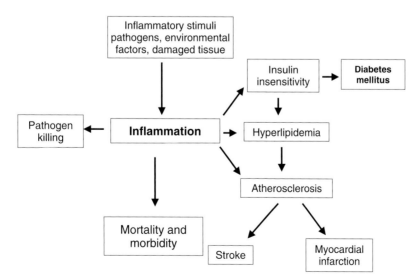

Figure 5 Linkage between inflammation as part of the defense against infection and as a factor in insulin insensitivity and disease processes.

Influence of Nutrients on Cytokine Biology

Proinflammatory cytokines exert widespread effects on metabolism, involving alterations in lipid, carbohydrate, and protein metabolism. In addition, there are substantial changes in micronutrient metabolism. A number of intracellular signaling pathways are activated by the actions of cytokines on target cells, including prostaglandins and leukotrienes, cyclic AMP, and protein kinase C. There are thus many levels at which nutrient intake can modify the intensity and characteristics of the response to inflammatory stimuli. The ability of nutrients to modify inflammation has been used in the treatment of diseases with an inflammatory basis. The interaction between nutritional status and inflammation is also important in public health because it determines the effects of infection on growth and well-being of populations with a poor nutrient intake.

The earliest indications that nutritional status could affect cytokine biology came from studies on malnourished hospital patients. White blood cells from patients had a reduced capacity to produce cytokines. The high mortality rates in these patients highlighted the importance of cytokines in the process of recovery from injury and infection. Protein supplements improved cytokine production and decreased the mortality rate. Since these observations were made, a large number of studies have been conducted in animals and human volunteers that show that fats, amino acids, and micronutrients change the ability of mammals to produce and respond to IL-1, IL-6, and TNF (**Figure 6**). Figure 6 indicates whether a change in the intake of a nutrient, or nutrient status, alters cytokine production or the response of target tissues to the actions of cytokines.

Influence of Fats on Cytokine Production and Effects

Dietary fats can be divided into four main types. Some are rich in n-6 polyunsaturated fatty acids (PUFAs); fats in this group include corn, sunflower, and safflower oils. Some are rich in n-3 PUFAs; these include fats from marine sources. Some are rich in monounsaturated fatty acids; these include olive oil and butter. Some fats are characterized by a high content of saturated fatty acids, usually accompanied by low concentrations of PUFAs; coconut oil, butter, suet, and lard are in this category.

The production and actions of pro-inflammatory cytokines are profoundly influenced by dietary fat intake. There are a number of levels at which fats may modify cytokine biology. Most relate to the ability of fats to change the fatty acid composition of membrane phospholipids. Subsequently, membrane fluidity may be changed, the types and amounts of prostaglandins and leukotrienes produced during inflammation may be altered, and the synthesis of a number of cellular mediators that arise from phospholipids (platelet activating factor, diacylglycerol, and ceramide) may also be changed. As a result of these changes, the binding of cytokines to target tissues and the intensity of the inflammatory response may be altered.

Phospholipids contain two fatty acid chains attached to the remainder of the molecule at positions designated sn1 and sn2. Normally, arachidonic acid (AA C20:4 n-60) is released from this position and provides the parent compound for prostaglandins and leukotrienes. However, the long-chain PUFA eicosapentaenoic acid (EPA C20:5 n-3) may compete with AA for insertion at sn2. Prostaglandins and leukotrienes with a much lower bioactivity may result. This biological effect may account in part for the anti-inflammatory effects of fish oil. Many animal studies indicate that fats rich in n-6 PUFAs exert a pro-inflammatory influence, whereas fats rich in monounsaturated fatty acids or n-3 PUFA have the opposite influence. In human studies, however, evidence for the influence of n-6 PUFA or monounsaturated fatty acids is not so clear-cut. It has been postulated that the major increase in inflammatory disease that has occurred in the past 40 years in industrialized countries is due to a major

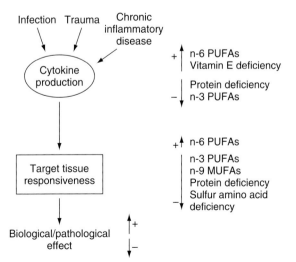

Figure 6 Summary of the effects of nutrients and nutritional conditions on cytokine biology. A stimulatory effect is indicated by a plus sign and an inhibitory influence by a minus sign.

increase in the intake of n-6 PUFAs during this time (from approximately 5 to 7% of dietary energy). It has also been postulated that the lower levels of inflammatory disease associated with the habitual consumption of a 'Mediterranean diet' are due in part to high intakes of monounsaturated fatty acids. The evidence for n-3 PUFAs producing an anti-inflammatory effect in humans is much stronger, however. Also, n-3 PUFAs have been shown to produce beneficial effects in inflammatory disease. In many double-blind, randomised controlled clinical trials, fish oil produced significant clinical benefit in patients with rheumatoid arthritis. A number of trials also report beneficial effects of fish oil in the treatment of Crohn's disease. The precise mechanisms for these effects is unclear. A number of studies have demonstrated the ability of fish oil to reduce pro-inflammatory cytokine production and to alter the production of eicosanoids. However, recent studies have indicated a genomic influence on the ability of fish oil to reduce TNF production, thus indicating that fish oil may not be universally effective as an anti-inflammatory agent. A fish oil and vitamin E intervention trial (GISSI) was carried out on 11,324 survivors of a myocardial infarct in Italy. Patients were given 1 g of n-3 PUFA and/or 300 mg vitamin E/d. In the GISSI trial, fish oil supplements were shown to reduce the chance of stroke or a second myocardial infarct by 15%. Because inflammation plays a role in atherosclerosis, it is interesting to note that a trial of fish oil in patients with severe atherosclerosis showed that a supplement of 6 g/day of fish oil for 7 weeks significantly reduced macrophage activity in plaques.

Modulation of Cytokine Biology by Amino Acid and Protein Intake

Substantial increases occur in protein synthesis as the result of infection. It has been estimated that approximately 45 g of protein is required to produce and maintain the increased quantities of white blood cells and acute phase proteins in an infected individual. This demand will have a considerable impact on the availability of amino acids for other processes in the body that involve protein synthesis. The inhibitory effect of infection on growth, pregnancy, and lactation is well recognized. Output of amino acids from skeletal muscle, skin, and bone provides substrate for the synthesis of cells and proteins associated with the response to infection and trauma, as indicated previously. However, the supply may not always match demand, as is evident from the decrease in plasma concentrations of a

number of amino acids. In particular, reductions occur in the concentrations of a metabolically related group of amino acids, including glycine, serine, and taurine. All three are metabolically related with the sulfur amino acids. Glycine and serine, together with the sulfur amino acids, are found in high concentrations in many compounds associated with the immune and inflammatory response, most notably comprising 66% of glutathione, 56% of metallothionein, and up to 25% of many acute-phase proteins. Experimental studies have shown that the production of cytokines, acute-phase proteins, and glutathione is influenced by the adequacy of both protein and sulfur amino acid intake. The partitioning of cysteine into glutathione and proteins in the liver may change if dietary sulfur amino acid intake becomes inadequate. This phenomenon is due to the biochemical properties of rate-limiting enzymes in both pathways. Whereas the K_m for γ-glutamyl cysteine synthetase (rate limiting for GSH synthesis) is 0.35 mM, that for amino acid activating enzymes (rate limiting for protein synthesis) is only 0.003 mM. This biochemical characteristic means that the GSH synthesis will fall below maximal rates at much higher intracellular cysteine concentrations than protein synthesis. Thus, at low sulfur amino acid intakes antioxidant defenses will become compromised. Low concentrations of GSH in tissues may have implications for the extent of inflammatory processes in the individual. In animal studies, decreased lung GSH concentrations are associated with the accumulation of inflammatory cells in tissues. In studies on HIV patients given N-acetyl cysteine, to improve GSH status, a decrease in plasma IL-6 concentrations has been noted indicating a reduction in inflammation. In view of the effects of NF-κB activation on HIV replication, it is interesting to note that the drug also brought about a reduction in HIV mRNA levels.

Modulation of Cytokine Biology by Micronutrients

Micronutrients play varied and complex roles in the response to infection and trauma. They are incorporated into substances that are synthesized in increased amounts during the response and into components of antioxidant defence, and they also modulate immune function. Trace elements are present in several acute-phase proteins and enzymes associated with antioxidant defense (**Figure 4**). These proteins include metallothionein (Zn), caeruloplasmin (Cu), superoxide dismutases (Mn, Cu, and Zn), and glutathione peroxidase (Se). Deficiencies in copper impair the ability of rats to increase superoxide dismutase and caeruloplasmin activities in response to inflammatory agents. Deficiencies in zinc impair the ability to increase metallothionein synthesis; furthermore, zinc deficiency has potent suppressive effects on lymphocyte proliferation. Iron status may influence inflammation and immune function in a number of ways. Normally, iron is tightly bound to transport proteins such as transferrin and ferritin. However, following tissue damage and infections such as malaria, which may destroy red blood cells, free iron may be released and exert a proinflammatory effect by catalyzing free radical production. The latter effect may activate NF-κB and upregulate cytokine production. Indeed, iron dextran infusion has been shown to exacerbate inflammatory symptoms in rheumatoid arthritis. Desferrioximine, an iron chelator, suppresses TNF and IL-1 production by rodent macrophages. Iron deficiency also decreases the ability of such cells to produce cytokines. Impairment of immunological defence is commonly found in iron-deficient animals and human populations. Defects occur in T cell proliferation and in the ability of macrophages to engulf and kill bacteria. The latter may relate to the role of iron as part of the NADPH oxidase complex that is responsible for the respiratory burst and generation of hydroxyl radicals that kill bacteria. Myeloperoxidase activity generates hypochlorous acid for bacterial killing, and myeloperoxidase is also a hemoprotein whose activity is decreased by iron deficiency.

Vitamins also exert a number of effects on cytokine biology. These effects may relate to the roles that some of these nutrients play as antioxidants and growth factors (**Figure 4**). Rats deficient in vitamin E exhibit an enhanced inflammatory response to endotoxin; addition of the vitamin to the diet will suppress this effect. In healthy subjects and smokers, a daily dose of 600 IU of vitamin E for 4 weeks reduces the ability of white blood cells to produce TNF and IL-1. Cigarette smoking enhances cytokine production and raises acute-phase protein concentrations. The extent of the elevation is inversely related to vitamin E. Strenuous exercise results in a small increase in plasma concentrations of IL-1 and IL-6; vitamin E supplementation will prevent this effect.

Vitamin A status also influences cytokine production, although the mechanism underlying the effect is unclear. Macrophages taken from Indian children who received a supplement of 100 000 IU of retinol produced seven times the quantity of IL-1 produced by cells of children who had not received supplementation. The effect may be more pharmacological than nutritional in nature. Mice given vitamin A at a dose that was 16 times their requirement had macrophages that produced twice as much IL-1 upon stimulation than cells from unsupplemented animals.

Hormone-like properties have been attributed to vitamin D in relation to its effects on calcium. It is apparent that endocrine effects of the vitamin extend to immune function. Macrophages treated with 1,25-dihydroxyvitamin D_3 produce increased amounts of TNF and were more effective at killing *Mycobacterium avium* than untreated cells.

Vitamin B_6 supplementation has been found to increase lymphocyte proliferation and production of IL-2 in elderly subjects. The effect of the vitamin on pro-inflammatory cytokine production is unknown. Little is known about the effects of other water-soluble vitamins on cytokine biology. Although no effects of vitamin C status on pro-inflammatory cytokine production have been reported, doses of the vitamin reduce the incidence of respiratory infections in long-distance marathon runners.

Conclusions

The objective of the response of the body to infection and trauma is to disadvantage and destroy invading organisms while simultaneously protecting healthy tissues from the damaging influence of compounds produced during the response. Cytokines play a central role in the protection of the animal from damage during the response. The close interrelationship between pro-inflammatory cytokines, oxidant molecules, and antioxidant defenses gives a biological advantage to the host (**Figure 7**).

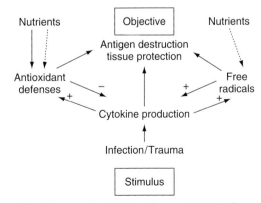

Figure 7 Influence of nutrients on the coordinated inflammatory events for destroying pathogens and protecting the host. Direct and indirect effects of nutrients are shown as solid and broken lines, respectively.

The essence of survival of an individual or species lies in the ability to prioritize physiological processes, particularly those processes that exert a large metabolic demand. Thus, at various times throughout the life cycle mammals will focus metabolic processes on achieving growth, the construction of placenta and fetus, the synthesis of milk components, or the repulsion of invasion by pathogens. For the infected individual, the marshalling of resources to combat the invading pathogen must assume a priority over all other physiological events. These other physiological processes can continue once the invasion has been repulsed and the damage done by the invader has been repaired.

The production of cytokines and other molecules associated with the inflammatory process carries risks of damage to the host as well as a survival advantage. The risk to the host is minimized by a sophisticated range of feedback control systems and synthesis of substances that protect the host. As discussed previously, nutrient intake modulates cytokine biology and the control and protective systems. A wide range of nutrients modulate cytokine biology at the level of production and sensitivity of target tissues (**Figure 6**). As a consequence of the modulation, the extent of depletion of nutrient stores and the risk of damage during the inflammatory response will be changed. The extent of tissue depletion and risk to the host will thus range from mild and transient in nature to severe, chronic, or lethal in effect.

See also: **Amino Acids**: Chemistry and Classification; Metabolism. **Diabetes Mellitus**: Classification and Chemical Pathology. **Fatty Acids**: Monounsaturated; Omega-3 Polyunsaturated; Omega-6 Polyunsaturated; Saturated. **Fish**. **Obesity**: Definition, Etiology and Assessment. **Vitamin A**: Biochemistry and Physiological Role. **Vitamin E**: Metabolism and Requirements. **Zinc**: Physiology.

Further Reading

Beutler B and Cerami A (1986) Tumor necrosis factor as two sides of the same biological coin. *Nature* **320**: 584–588.

Dinarello CA (1988) Biology of IL1. *FASEB Journal* **1**: 108–115.

Douglas RG and Shaw JHF (1989) Metabolic response to sepsis and trauma. *Bristish Journal of Trauma* **76**: 115–122.

GISSI-Prevenzione Investigators (1999) Dietary supplementation with n-3 polyunsaturated fatty acids and vitamin E after myocardial infarction: Results of the GISSI-Prevenzione trial. *Lancet* **354**: 447–455.

Grimble RF (1994) Nutritional antioxidants and the modulation of inflammation: The theory and the practice. *Critical Care Medicine* **2**: 175–185.

Grimble RF (1996) The interaction between nutrients, pro-inflammatory cytokines and inflammation. *Clinical Science* **91**: 121–130.

Grimble RF (2002) Inflammatory status and insulin resistance. *Current Opinion in Clinical Nutrition and Metabolic Care* **5**: 551–559.

Grimble RF (2003) Inflammatory response in the elderly. *Current Opinion in Clinical Nutrition and Metabolic Care* **6**: 21–29.

Grimble RF, Howell WM, O'Reilly G *et al.* (2002) The ability of fish oil to suppress tumor necrosis factor-alpha production by peripheral blood mononuclear cells in healthy men is associated with polymorphisms in genes which influence TNF-alpha production. *American Journal of Clinical Nutrition* **76**: 454–459.

Grunfeld C and Feingold KR (1992) Tumour necrosis factor, interleukin 1 and interferon induce changes in lipid metabolism as part of host defence. *Proceedings of the Society of Experimental Biology and Medicine* **200**: 214–227.

Heinrich PC, Castell JV, and Andus T (1990) Interleukin 6 and the acute phase response. *Biochemical Journal* **265**: 621–636.

Murray MJ and Murray AB (1980) Cachexia: A 'last ditch' mechanism of host defence. *Journal of the Royal College of Physicians (London)* **14**: 197–199.

Newsholme P and Newsholme EA (1989) Rates of utilisation of glucose, glutamine and oleate and end product production by mouse macrophages in culture. *Biochemical Journal* **261**: 211–218.

Paolini-Giacobino A, Grimble R, and Pichard C (2003) Genomic interactions with disease and nutrition. *Clinical Nutrition* **22**: 507–514.

Schreck R, Rieber P, and Baeurerle PA (1991) Reactive oxygen intermediates as apparently widely used messengers of NFκB transcription factor and HIV1. *EMBO Journal* **10**: 2247–2256.

Thies F, Garry JMC, Yaqoob P *et al.* (2003) Association of n-3 polyunsaturated fatty acids with stability of atherosclerotic plaques: A randomized trial. *Lancet* **361**: 477–485.

DAIRY PRODUCTS

J Buttriss, British Nutrition Foundation, London, UK

© 2005 Elsevier Ltd. All rights reserved.

Introduction

Dairy products are traditional dietary items in many parts of the world, in particular regions such as northern Europe where the cooler climate is especially suited to dairying. The history of milk as a food has been documented over the centuries and examples of early dairying are depicted in Egyptian friezes such as that from the sarcophagus of Queen Kawit from Der-al-Bahri, between Luxor and Karnak, dating back 4000 years. There is an even earlier Mesopotamian frieze from the temple of Ninkhasarg, near Ur, which is thought to be 1000 years older.

The popularity of milk as a staple food over the centuries must partly be due to its versatility. Early humans discovered that milk could be churned to make butter and fermented with bacterial cultures to produce cheese and yogurt, all of which were methods of preserving some or all of the nutrients in milk for consumption at a later date.

Variety

The range of dairy products on the market is immense. In most countries, a range of milks with differing fat contents is available. For example, in the UK consumers can choose between Channel Islands milk, with 4.9 g per 100 g fat, whole milk (3.9 g per 100 g), semiskimmed (1.6 g per 100 g fat), and skimmed milk, which has virtually no fat. Similarly, a wide range of cheeses exists with varying fat contents: at one end of the spectrum are soft fresh cheeses, made with skimmed milk, and at the other, hard cheeses such as Cheddar. Also available is cheese made with nonanimal rennet, suitable for vegetarians. In the UK alone, about two hundred different cheeses are produced, and cheese is particularly popular in countries such as France, where an even greater variety is available.

Fermented milk products such as yogurt, smetana, and kefir have always been popular in Middle Eastern countries, but their popularity, particularly that of yogurt, is increasing dramatically in Europe. Again, a wide range of yogurts exists, from very low-fat varieties to the creamier, whole milk or Greek-style product. Today, the range includes set yogurts, stirred yogurts, fruit yogurts, frozen yogurts, drinking yogurts, fromage frais, and the newer 'bio' yogurts with their milder flavor.

Traditional products such as cream and butter are still in demand, in spite of their high fat content, and are being joined by other 'luxury' products such as real dairy ice creams, fresh cream desserts, and luxury mousses. To meet the demand for a spread with a buttery flavor, products have been developed which incorporate butterfat for taste but often have a lower fat and energy content than butter.

A number of products also exist to which nutrients have been added, such as calcium-enriched milks and yogurts fortified with additional vitamins.

Nutrient Composition of Milk and its Products

Milk can be described as one of the most nutritionally complete foods. It provides a wide range of essential nutrients, in particular protein, and a range of vitamins and minerals (**Table 1**). It is, however, a poor source of iron and vitamin D, and contains no starch or dietary fiber. By volume, water is the major constituent of milk, comprising just over 87%. The remainder consists of milk fat and solids-not-fat (SNF)–principally comprising protein, lactose and minerals.

Protein

The principal proteins found in milk and its products are casein, lactalbumin, and lactoglobulin. Milk protein has a high biological value since it contains all of the eight essential amino acids, which cannot be synthesized in the body and so need to be provided by diet. In addition, milk can

Table 1 Nutrient composition per 100 g of pasteurized milk in the UK

	Whole milk	Skimmed milk	Semiskimmed milk	Channel Islands milk
Energy (kcal)	66	33	46	78
Energy (kJ)	275	140	195	327
Protein (g)	3.2	3.3	3.3	3.6
Carbohydrate (g)	4.6	4.8	4.8	4.6
Sugars (g)	4.6	4.8	4.8	4.6
Fat (g)	3.9	0.1	1.6	5.1
Saturates (g)	2.4	0.06	1.0	3.3
Monounsaturates (g)	1.1	Trace	0.5	1.3
Polyunsaturates (g)	0.1	Trace	Trace	0.1
Sodium (mg)	55	55	55	54
Dietary fiber (g)	Nil	Nil	Nil	Nil
Vitamin A (μg)	56	1	23	58
Thiamin (mg)	0.04	0.04	0.04	0.04
Riboflavin (mg)	0.17	0.18	0.18	0.19
Niacin (mg)	0.83	0.87	0.87	0.92
Vitamin B_6 (mg)	0.06	0.06	0.06	0.06
Folic acid (μg)	6	6	6	6
Vitamin B_{12} (μg)	0.4	0.4	0.4	0.4
Pantothenic acid (mg)	0.35	0.32	0.32	0.36
Biotin (μg)	1.9	2.0	2.0	1.9
Vitamin C (mg)	1	1	1	1
Vitamin D (μg)	0.03	Trace	0.01	0.03
Vitamin E (mg)	0.09	Trace	0.03	0.11
Calcium (mg)	115	120	118	130
Chloride (mg)	100	100	100	100
Copper (mg)	Trace	Trace	Trace	Trace
Iodine (μg)	15	(15)	(15)	N
Iron (mg)	0.05	0.05	0.05	0.05
Magnesium (mg)	11	12	11	12
Phosphorus (mg)	92	95	95	100
Potassium (mg)	140	150	150	140
Selenium (μg)	1	(1)	(1)	(1)
Zinc (mg)	0.4	0.4	0.4	0.4

N, no reliable information available; values in parentheses, estimated value.
Adapted from Holland *et al.* (1989) *Milk Products and Eggs*. Fourth supplement of *McCance and Widdowson's The Composition of Foods*, 4th edn. London: Royal Society of Chemistry/MAFF.

improve the overall protein quality of a meal when consumed with foods of lower protein quality such as cereals and pulses.

Carbohydrate

The carbohydrate in milk is in the form of lactose, a disaccharide comprising a molecule of glucose and a molecule of galactose. This sugar is found naturally only in milk and is much less sweet than sucrose (packet sugar).

In the small intestine, lactose is digested by the enzyme lactase to its two component monosaccharides, in readiness for absorption. This enzyme is present in babies, young children, and most European adults. However, in some adults enzymatic activity can decrease, making milk in quantity less well tolerated. Such individuals are described as being lactose intolerant. Most can tolerate small quantities of milk, and fermented milk products appear to be better

tolerated. Cheese is also usually well tolerated as it contains only trace amounts of lactose. In the UK, lactose intolerance is relatively rare in people of European descent but is more common in those of Asian, Far Eastern, and African descent, particularly first-generation members of these ethnic groups.

Fat

The fat in milk is in the form of minute droplets, which rise to the top when milk is left to stand. The principal component of milk fat is triacylglycerol, three fatty acids joined to a glycerol backbone. All triacylglycerols contain mixtures of three families of fatty acids: saturated, monounsaturated, and polyunsaturated. The contribution of these three types of fatty acid to milk fat in the UK is 61% saturated, 28% monounsaturated, and 3% polyunsaturated. The percentages do not add up to 100% because milk fat is not composed totally of fatty acids. When milk is skimmed, it is the amount rather than the type of fat that changes, and so the fatty acid profile remains the same. Milk fat contains small amounts of the two essential fatty acids, linoleic acid (1.4 g per 100 g fatty acids) and linolenic acid (1.5 g per 100 g fatty acids).

Vitamins

All of the known vitamins are to be found in whole milk (**Table 1**), although some are present in small quantities. Milk and milk products make a significant contribution to intakes of a number of these (**Table 2**). The fat-soluble vitamins – A, D, E and K – are removed with the fat when milk is skimmed. Consequently, they are present in only trace amounts in skimmed milk and in reduced amounts in semiskimmed milk. Whole milk is a good source of vitamin A, a pint (568 ml) providing 47% of the adult male and 55% of the adult female UK reference nutrient intake (RNI).

All of the three major types of cows' milk (whole, semiskimmed, and skimmed) are good sources of riboflavin (vitamin B_2) and vitamin B_{12}. Milk can also make an important contribution to intakes of thiamin (vitamin B_1), niacin, and ascorbic acid (vitamin C), particularly where the overall diet is poor.

Some vitamins are sensitive to heat and light. Over 90% of milk for liquid consumption is pasteurized, a mild heat treatment that causes little loss of vitamins other than vitamin C. In general vitamin losses are less than 10%. Milk that has undergone the ultra heat treatment (UHT) process keeps for longer, but the higher temperature used in the processing results in slightly greater losses (10–20%) of some vitamins, particularly vitamins B_6 and B_{12}, vitamin C, and folate. The sterilization process used for milk has a somewhat greater effect: about one-third of the thiamin and half the vitamin C, folate, and B_{12} are destroyed.

Some loss of vitamins is inevitable when milk is stored. The extent of these losses is dependent on the translucency and permeability to light of the container, and the length and conditions of exposure. Milk exposed to bright sunlight on the doorstep will readily lose its vitamin C. Loss of riboflavin is slower but after 4 h, half will be lost and only a third remains after 6 h. Therefore, measures should be taken to limit such exposure. There will also be gradual losses of some vitamins from UHT and sterilized milks, even under ideal storage conditions, because of reactions with small amounts of oxygen remaining in the pack or bottle. Boiling milk also reduces its vitamin content, ranging from a 5% reduction in vitamin B_{12} to a 50% reduction in vitamin C.

Table 2 Contribution of milk and milk products to daily nutrient intake from all food and drink in Great Britain

	Liquid milk		Cheese		All milk and milk products	
	Average amount provided	Percentage of total intake	Average amount provided	Percentage of total intake	Average amount provided	Percentage of total intake
Energy (kcal)	152	8.1	56	3.0	247	13.1
Protein (g)	9.3	14.8	3.5	5.6	14.1	22.4
Fat (g)	7.2	8.8	4.7	5.8	13.7	16.8
Saturates (g)	4.3	13.5	2.9	9.1	8.5	26.6
Monounsaturates (g)	2.1	7.0	1.3	4.3	3.9	13.0
Polyunsaturates (g)	0.2	1.4	0.2	1.4	0.5	3.6
Calcium (mg)	330	39.8	93	11.2	471	56.8
Iron (mg)	0.2	2.0	<0.1	0.4	0.3	3.0
Zinc (mg)	1.2	15.4	0.3	3.8	1.7	21.8
Magnesium (mg)	34	14.8	4.0	1.7	40.0	17.5
Potassium (g)	0.43	16.9	0.01	0.4	0.49	19.2
Thiamin (mg)	0.11	8.5	0.01	0.8	0.13	10.1
Riboflavin (mg)	0.5	31.1	0.04	3.9	0.63	39.1
Niacin (mg)	2.5	9.9	0.8	3.2	3.6	14.2
Vitamin B_6 (mg)	0.18	9.6	0.01	0.53	0.21	11.2
Vitamin B_{12} (μg)	1.1	22.9	0.2	4.2	1.4	29.2
Folate (μg)	16	6.6	5	2.1	25	10.4
Vitamin C (mg)	1.8	3.0	–	–	3.0	5.0
Vitamin A (μg)	96	9.3	50	4.8	174	16.9
Vitamin D (μg)	0.05	1.9	0.04	1.5	0.23	8.7

Adapted from Ministry of Agriculture, Fisheries and Food (1995) *National Food Survey 1994*. London: HMSO.

Minerals

Milk makes a contribution to human needs for virtually all the minerals and trace elements known to be essential for health. These are often present in a form that is well absorbed and utilized by the body (high bioavailability), e.g., calcium and zinc. For most people in the Western world, milk and milk products are a major source of calcium. Almost 60% of the calcium in the typical British diet is contributed by milk and milk products (**Table 2**). Milk alone contributes about 40% of the total. Although the contribution to zinc requirements made by milk is relatively low compared with meat (the major contributor), the zinc in milk is in a highly bioavailable form and there is evidence that the combination of milk (or meat) with vegetable foods, in which the zinc is less bioavailable, can enhance the bioavailability of zinc from the whole meal.

Cultural Significance of Milk and Milk Products

In countries where dairying has traditionally been a strong industry, milk and milk product consumption tends to be widespread and makes a significant contribution to nutrient needs. **Table 2** shows the contribution in Great Britain. The average daily intake of milk in the UK is a little under half a pint per person (271 ml). **Table 3** shows the contribution half a pint of whole milk makes to the nutrient and energy needs of a 4-year-old girl and a man. Skimmed or semi-skimmed milk would make smaller contributions to intakes of energy and fat-soluble vitamins.

In Scandinavian countries, where dairying is also traditional, liquid milk consumption is typically higher than in the UK. However, in warmer climates, in particular the Indian subcontinent, Africa and South America, climatic conditions lend themselves less readily to cows' needs, so that the development of dairying and, hence, milk-drinking habits has been far more patchy. Exceptions exist, such as the Masai in East Africa, whose culture is dominated by the cow. Similarly, in parts of India, cows have religious significance but have not, until recently, been intensively managed for their milk.

Being rich in calcium needed for skeletal development and maintenance, milk has traditionally been seen as an important food during childhood, pregnancy and lactation, when calcium requirements are particularly high. This view is still supported today. The Departments of Health in the UK advises milk (and water) to be the most suitable drinks for

Table 3 Contribution of 285 ml (half pint) of whole milk to nutrient needs

	Percentage of UK reference nutrient intake (RNIs)	
	Girls (4–6 years)	Adult men (19–50 years)
Energy[a]	12.5	7.6
Fat[a]	19.0	11.5
Saturates[a]	37.3	22.7
Monounsaturates[a]	14.3	8.6
Polyunsaturates[a]	2.7	1.7
Carbohydrate[a]	7.0	4.2
Protein	47.5	16.8
Nonstarch polysaccharide	–	–
Vitamin A	32.8	23.4
Thiamin	16.4	11.5
Riboflavin	62.5	38.5
Niacin	22.1	14.3
Vitamin B_6	19.4	12.5
Folic acid	17.5	8.8
Vitamin B_{12}	143.8	76.7
Vitamin C	10.0	7.5
Calcium	74.8	48.1
Sodium	23.9	10.4
Chloride	26.6	11.7
Copper	Trace	Trace
Iodine	44.0	31.4
Iron	2.4	1.7
Magnesium	26.7	10.7
Phosphorus	77.0	49.0
Potassium	37.3	16.4
Selenium	15.0	4.0
Zinc	17.7	12.1

[a]There is no RNI for these components of food. For energy, the estimated average requirement has been used in the calculation; for fat and carbohydrate, the desirable average intake has been used.

Figures for milk composition from Holland *et al.* (1989) *Milk Products and Eggs*. Fourth supplement of *McCance and Widdowson's The Composition of Foods*, 4th edn. London: Royal Society of Chemistry/MAFF. Figures for RNIs from Department of Health (1991) *Dietary Reference Values for Food Energy and Nutrients*. Report on Health and Social Subjects 41. London: HMSO.

children, both from a nutritional standpoint and in terms of dental health.

Availability of Subsidized and Free Milk in the UK

Under the school milk subsidy scheme, funded by the European Community (EC), primary school pupils are eligible to receive 250 ml of milk (whole or semiskimmed) each school day at a subsidized price. Until the spring of 1996, secondary school pupils were also eligible for this benefit and a subsidy was available for milk used in school catering (all age groups). Children under the age of 5 years, attending nursery schools or looked after by registered child minders, are eligible to a third of a pint of milk, free of charge, on each day they attend.

For families on income support, pregnant women, breast-feeding mothers, and children under the age of 5 years are entitled to a pint of milk a day, free of charge. For bottle-fed babies, tokens can be exchanged for infant formula. Others entitled to free milk (a third of a pint per school day) include children attending special schools.

Nutritional Significance of Milk and its Products in the Diets of Children

The benefits of milk fall into three main areas: general provision of a range of nutrients and energy; provision of calcium for bone health; and dental health benefits.

General Benefits

Dairy products such as yogurt, fromage frais, grated cheese, and small amounts of whole milk, e.g., in custard, can be given to babies as they begin to experience a wide range of foods (4–6 months onwards). As the child becomes established on 'solids,' quantities can be increased, e.g., cows' milk may be used to mix infants' cereals. However, cows' milk should not be introduced as a main drink until a child is 1 year old. This is because, unlike infant formulas, cows' milk is relatively low in iron and vitamin D, and there is growing concern about the iron status of older infants and preschool children.

Amounts consumed by babies may be small, but for preschool and school-age children, milk and products such as cheese and yogurt can make a significant contribution to nutrient needs (**Table 3**). In summary, as well as providing energy, milk is a good source of protein, calcium, zinc, and vitamins A (whole milk only), B_2 (riboflavin), and B_{12}. Milk also makes a valuable contribution to intakes of iodine, niacin (a B vitamin), and vitamin B_6.

Given its nutritional credentials, it is not surprising that milk has been made available free of charge or at a subsidized price to children (see above). A study in Scotland of children aged 7–8 years found generally adequate intakes of most vitamins and minerals, although intakes of sugar and fat were high compared with the adult guidelines (no specific guidelines exist for schoolchildren). However, they noted that the nutrient provision of the diet as a whole improved with the amount of milk consumed. There was no significant difference in the proportion of energy provided by fat when the high milk consumers (at least 3 L a week) were compared with the low milk consumers.

Calcium and Bone Health

There is abundant evidence that calcium plays a major role in the development and maintenance of skeletal strength. Achieving adequate intakes of calcium during growth is important to optimizes peak bone density in early adulthood, thus protecting against osteoporosis in later life.

Approximately 45% of the mineral in the adult skeleton is laid down during adolescence. By the age of about 17 years (earlier in girls), over 90% of the maximum amount of bone mineral (e.g., calcium) that will ever be present in the skeleton is already there. Calcium requirements are, therefore, particularly high during adolescence. Yet it is at this age that milk consumption often falls, frequently resulting in dramatic reductions in calcium intake. There is evidence from national UK surveys among schoolchildren and adults that 1 in 4 teenage girls and young women have wholly inadequate calcium intakes, i.e., below the lower reference nutrient intake (LRNI).

Dairy Products and Oral Health

Milk is kind to teeth and dental experts recommend that milk or water are the most suitable drinks for children. A recent national dental health survey in Britain among preschool children revealed that among those aged between $1\frac{1}{2}$ and $3\frac{1}{2}$ years, the main dietary measure differentiating children with and without dental decay was taking a drink containing non-milk sugars (e.g., fruit juice or squash) to bed, as opposed to not drinking in bed or having other kinds of drink (milk or water). A significantly higher proportion of children who consumed drinks containing non-milk sugars in bed had tooth decay (26%) than did children who drank water (11%) or milk (12%).

Cheese is also considered to be important. A number of studies have shown that chewing (not just swallowing) a small cube of cheese (5–10 g) can revert the reduction in pH in the mouth brought about by the acid produced during the fermentation of sugars by bacteria in the mouth. It is this production of acid that is associated with tooth decay. It is thought that this effect is achieved via cheese's ability to stimulate saliva flow. However, other mechanisms may also be important, including cheese's high concentration of calcium and other minerals needed by teeth, and the ability of the protein in cheese (and milk) to buffer acid.

Nutritional Significance of Milk and its Products for Adults

During pregnancy, especially the final months, requirements for a number of nutrients increase. Although the mother's efficiency at absorbing nutrients rises to help meet this need, dietary supply remains important. Milk is seen to have a major part to play here, given the broad range of nutrients it contains (see **Table 1**).

The needs for some nutrients, for example calcium, rise dramatically after the baby is born in women who choose to breast-feed. Dietary requirements for calcium almost double and consumption of several servings of dairy products daily is one of the few ways of easily achieving such intakes (in the UK the RNI is 1200 mg day^{-1}). Breast-feeding teenagers need even more calcium, as their own skeleton is still developing as well as that of the baby.

Milk and milk products remain a nutritional safeguard for other adults, especially those who choose to restrict their choice of foods because they are slimming or following a vegetarian diet. For elderly people, whose overall food intake and dietary variety can be limited, milk, cheese, and yogurt can be of particular importance in meeting nutrient needs, especially with the convenience of doorstep delivery.

Other Health Effects of Dairy Products

Several studies have reported an inverse association between dairy products consumption and the insulin resistance syndrome. One study reported a reduction of insulin resistance of 40% with consumption of 1 serving per day or more. However, this was observed only in men. In the CARDIA study, a reduction of 21% in insulin resistance was demonstrated among 18–30-year-old men who consumed at least one serving of dairy products per day. Similarly, results from at least 10 clinical trials show a beneficial effect of regular consumption of dairy products on cardiovascular disease risk. Taken together, these results indicate a consistent beneficial effect of milk products on risk for insulin resistance and cardiovascular disease, in addition to the already established benefits for osteoporosis. The overall effect threshold for this benefit appears to be 2 or 3 servings of dairy products per day.

The evidence for a beneficial effect of dairy products in weight management is less compelling, and mixed results have been reported. Several studies have shown a beneficial effect of calcium for weight loss, and it is possible that milk products exert their effect on body weight by being an excellent source of this nutrient. More studies are needed to clarify this potential benefit of diary products.

Yogurt and Health

Apart from its contribution to nutrient needs, the perception of yogurt as a 'healthy' food has been augmented by claims of health benefits attributed to specific live bacteria present in some yogurts, in particular *Lactobacillus acidophilus* and bifidobacteria. Both of these types of bacteria are to be found in the human gastrointestinal tract, especially in breast-fed infants, and it has been suggested that these microorganisms may be able to colonize the gut when consumed in yogurt, and protect against pathogens. It has also been speculated that they may be of benefit in a number of intestinal disorders, including those precipitated by antibiotic treatment or by diseases such as cancer and liver or kidney disease. Claims have been made that specific bacteria used in the production of a certain brand of yogurt have the potential to reduce blood levels of low-density lipoproteins (LDL). On the basis of existing research it is not possible to substantiate these various claims, although evidence is increasing and inconsistencies in the findings may in part be explained by differences in strain and species of bacterial cultures, and differences in experimental design.

There is, however, a substantial body of evidence to indicate that fermented dairy products such as yogurt are well tolerated by individuals who are lactose-intolerant. It has been suggested that this is because of the bacterial enzyme β-galactosidase (produced by the culture) in 'live' yogurt. This enzyme, which is able to digest lactose to glucose and galactose, is intracellular and hence is thought to survive gastric digestion. However, as lactose maldigesters tolerate yogurts with varying β-galactosidase activities equally well, it would seem that other factors may also be important, including rate of gastrointestinal transit of yogurt.

Intake of the types of lactic acid-producing organisms found in yogurt has also been postulated to prevent or inhibit intestinal growth of a variety of food-borne, disease-causing organisms. Most of the evidence supporting a role for cultured dairy products, or the bacteria used to make them, in controlling intestinal pathogens comes from experimental animal and *in vitro* studies. Findings are inconsistent, but various mechanisms have been put forward to explain reported protective effects. For example, the ability of lactic acid cultures to lower intestinal pH favors growth of lactic acid bacteria but provides a hostile environment for pathogens. It has also been suggested that lactic acid bacteria may produce bacteriocins, proteins with a direct antibiotic effect.

In summary, while a fairly clear case has been made for tolerance of yogurt by lactose maldigesters unable to tolerate milk, the potential benefit of yogurt (or specific types of yogurt) in protecting against pathogens, in recolonizing the gut after illness, or in lowering LDL cholesterol concentrations in the blood needs further investigation.

Hygiene and Safety Aspects

Milk, in its raw state, does not stay fresh for very long and is an ideal medium for bacteria to grow. Various types of heat treatment are used to improve the keeping quality of milk and to kill any harmful bacteria present. These techniques are pasteurization, sterilization, and ultra heat treatment, and they are also used for cream.

Pasteurization is named after the French scientist Louis Pasteur and entails the heating of milk to at least 71.7 °C for a minimum of 15 s. After heating, the milk is quickly cooled to less than 10 °C. In the UK, pasteurization accounts for over 90% of all heat-treated milk and has little effect on the taste and nutritional value of milk.

Sterilization is a more severe process, in which milk is heated to a temperature of 115–130 °C for 10–30 min and then poured into sterile plastic or glass bottles. Unopened, sterilized milk will keep for 2–3 months without refrigeration, although once opened it has to be treated in the same way as pasteurized milk and will only keep for 4–5 days in a refrigerator. Sterilized milk has a slight caramel taste because the heat 'cooks' the lactose present in milk. Sterilization also reduces the levels of the heat-labile vitamins (see above).

Ultra heat treatment is a milder form of sterilization in which the milk is held at a temperature of not less than 135 °C for at least 1 s, and is then packed into sterile cartons. Such milk will keep unrefrigerated for many months, but once opened it needs to be refrigerated and used in 4–5 days.

Cheese and yogurt

The fermentation of milk to produce cheese and yogurt are traditional processes for preserving milk's nutrients. Hard cheeses, such as Cheddar, which have a low moisture content and contain salt as a preservative, will last for many months if stored appropriately. Ideally cheese should be eaten fresh, but if properly stored it will retain its flavor for long periods. It should be wrapped in clear film or foil to prevent drying and then stored in a cool larder or refrigerator. Soft, unripened cheeses, such as cottage cheese, are highly perishable, need to be stored in the refrigerator, and have a relatively short shelf life. At low temperatures, microbiological growth will be reduced, as will enzyme action and biochemical changes that might change the flavor, color or texture of the product. Ripened soft cheeses such as Brie should also be kept refrigerated, wrapped in airtight film or aluminum foil.

Nearly all yogurt sold in the UK contains live bacteria (derived from the starter culture used to produce the yogurt). It is necessary to refrigerate the product to restrict the activity of these bacteria, to prevent development of excess acidity and impairment of flavor. At temperatures of about 5 °C, yogurt has a shelf life of about 14 days, after which time acidity levels may rise above acceptable levels. Spoiled yogurts are often referred to as 'blown.' This is because pressure has built up in the pot via the fermentation of the sugar in the yogurt by the growth of yeasts.

A small proportion of yogurts are heat treated to prolong their shelf life. As a result, they no longer contain live bacteria and do not need to be refrigerated.

See also: **Carbohydrates**: Requirements and Dietary Importance. **Food Intolerance**. **Lactation**: Dietary Requirements. **Microbiota of the Intestine**: Prebiotics; Probiotics. **Protein**: Quality and Sources.

Further Reading

Department of Health (1991) *Dietary Reference Values for Food Energy and Nutrients.* Report on Health and Social Subjects 41. London: HMSO.

Health Education Authority (1995) *Diet and Health in School Age Children.* London: HEA.

Hinds K and Gregory JR (1995) *National Diet and Nutrition Survey: Children aged $1\frac{1}{2}$–$4\frac{1}{2}$ years*, vol. 2. London: HMSO.

Holland B, Unwin ID, and Buss DH (1989) *Milk Products and Eggs*, Fourth supplement of *McCance and Widdowson's The Composition of Foods*. 4th edn. London: Royal Society of Chemistry/MAFF.

Mennen LI, Lafay L, Feskens EJM *et al.* (2000) Possible protective effect of bread and dairy products on the risk of the metabolic syndrome. *Nutrition Research* 20: 335–347.

Ministry of Agriculture, Fisheries and Food (1994) *The Dietary and Nutritional Survey of British Adults – Further Analysis.* London: HMSO.

Ministry of Agriculture, Fisheries and Food (1995) *Manual of Nutrition*, 10th edn. Reference Book 342. London: HMSO.

Ministry of Agriculture, Fisheries and Food (1995) *National Food Survey 1994.* London: HMSO.

National Dairy Council (1994) *A–Z of Dairy Products.* London: NDC.

Ruxton CHS, Kirk TR, and Belton NR (1996) The contribution of specific dietary patterns to energy and nutrient intakes in 7–8 year old Scottish schoolchildren. I: Milk drinking. *Journal of Human Nutrition and Dietetics* 9(1): 3–12.

Weaver CM (1996) Calcium and bone health. In: Buttriss J and Hyman K (eds.) *Women in Focus.* A conference held in 1995. London: National Dairy Council.

DEHYDRATION

A W Subudhi, University of Colorado at Colorado Springs, Colorado Springs, CO, USA
E W Askew, University of Utah, Salt Lake City, UT, USA
M J Luetkemeier, Alma College, Alma, MI, USA

© 2005 Elsevier Ltd. All rights reserved.

Physiological Functions of Water

After oxygen, water is the most essential nutrient needed to sustain human life. In healthy individuals, water comprises between 45 and 70% of total body weight and is responsible for connecting the diverse physiological functions of the body (**Table 1**).

Water is necessary to maintain homeostasis of the internal environment. The most obvious roles of water in the human body are to provide an aqueous medium for transport of material in blood, to dissolve and pass nutrients between blood and cells, to serve as a medium for intracellular reactions, and to transfer metabolic products for redistribution or excretion via urine. Since both the quantity of reactants and the volume of fluid in which they are dissolved influence chemical reaction rates, imbalances in hydration status can alter cellular and tissue function.

Dehydration also adversely affects the body's ability to regulate temperature. Energy transformations during digestion, absorption, and metabolism as well as muscular contraction generate heat. The heat released from the digestion of a mixed meal (thermic effect of food) equals 10–15% of the caloric content of the food ingested. Muscular contraction is dependent on the transformation of chemical energy (ATP) to mechanical energy. Nearly three-fourths of the energy used for muscular contraction is released as heat. Unless localized heat production from metabolism and muscular contraction is dissipated, the heat burden can be structurally damaging

to enzymes or other proteins. Water absorbs heat produced at the cellular level and transfers it to the surface of the skin, where it can be dissipated to the external environment (**Figure 1**).

The evaporative dissipation of heat through sweating is a two-phase, water-dependent mechanism. Water is removed from capillary blood perfusing sweat glands to produce a thin layer of sweat over the surface of the skin. Simultaneously, the water component of blood carries heat produced from cellular metabolic processes to capillary beds located near the surface of the skin. Heat is transferred by conduction to the skin surface, where it vaporizes sweat coating the skin, thus transferring body heat to the external environment. The heat of vaporization of water is 586 kcal/l (2453 kJ/l) at 20 °C. Approximately 500 ml of sweat is lost per day under average ambient environmental conditions. Such obligatory water loss occurs without visible or tactile sensations and is termed 'insensible' sweat. However, given a sufficient thermal challenge, humans are capable of producing approximately 10 l of 'sensible' sweat per day. Theoretically, if the entire 10 l of sweat was evaporated, more than 5000 kcal (20 930 kJ) of heat per day would be dissipated via the sweating mechanism. Humidity of the air and sweat that drips from the surface of

Table 1 Major physiological functions of water

Function	Example
Waste product removal	Urea excretion by kidneys
Solvent for chemical reactions	Glycolysis in the cell cytosol
Transport medium	Blood
Lubrication	Synovial fluid of joints
Shock absorber	Disks between vertebrae of spinal column
Temperature regulation	Evaporative sweat loss

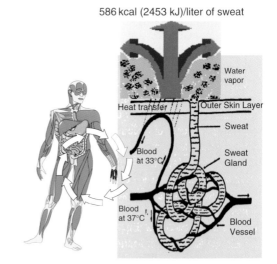

586 kcal (2453 kJ)/liter of sweat

Figure 1 Metabolic heat transfer to the skin and dissipation of heat by evaporation of sweat. The body has more than 2 million sweat glands that secrete sweat to the surface of skin. Blood-perfusing skin capillary beds transfer heat by convection to the surface of the skin. Heat is dissipated by vaporizing the water in sweat. The heat of vaporization of water at 20 °C is 586 kcal/l (2453 kJ).

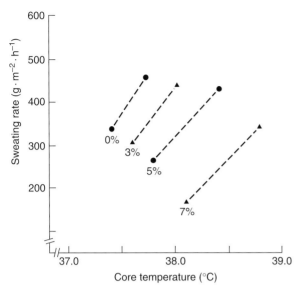

Figure 2 The influence of water loss by dehydration (hypohydration) on the sweating response to exercise following normal hydration (0%) and dehydration equal to 3, 5, and 7% of body weight. The primary stimulus for sweating is the increase in core temperature (thermal drive). Note that dehydration reduces the sweating rate at any given level of thermal drive. Hypohydration compromises exercise by reducing sweat rate and evaporative cooling and increasing body core temperature. (From Sawka MN, Young AJ, Francesconi RP *et al*. (1985) Thermoregulatory and blood responses during exercise at graded hypohydration levels. *Journal of Applied Physiology* **59**: 1394–1401, with permission.)

the skin considerably reduce the potential for evaporative heat dissipation; therefore, actual evaporative cooling is usually less than the theoretical maximum. Since water is the main component of sweat, it is not surprising that dehydration affects the sweat response. The relationship between body water loss by dehydration and the rate of sweating achievable during exercise is shown in **Figure 2**, which illustrates that dehydration reduces sweating rate at any given level of thermal drive (core temperature) during exercise. A diminished sweating response can lead to a dangerous heat buildup unless thermal strain is curtailed by other mechanisms.

Development of Dehydration

In physiological terms, dehydration is the process of progressing from the euhydrated (normally hydrated) to hypohydrated (less water than normal) state. In actual usage, dehydration means losing body water faster than it is replaced. The resultant condition is commonly referred to as the 'dehydrated state' and is associated with hypovolemia (low blood volume).

Contributing Factors

Water is lost through a variety of avenues, including urine, feces, breath, and sweat. In illness or disease, excessive diuresis, diarrhea, and/or vomiting are the main pathways of water loss. During exercise or heat exposure, sweating is the primary mechanism for dehydration. Significant water loss may be stimulated by cold- or altitude-induced diuresis. Additionally, some prescription drugs and over-the-counter herbal products have diuretic effects that exacerbate water loss. Under normal conditions, the body regulates its water contents tightly over a 24-h period (approximately ±200 ml); however, over short periods, water loss can significantly exceed water gain (**Figure 3**).

Body Fluid Balance

Body water losses are rapidly reflected in blood. Volume and electrolyte changes in response to decreased blood water content (increased osmolality) trigger the hypothalamus to stimulate antidiuretic hormone (ADH) release from the posterior lobe of the pituitary gland. ADH acts on the kidney to increase tubular water resorption and maintain plasma volume. Decreased plasma volume also

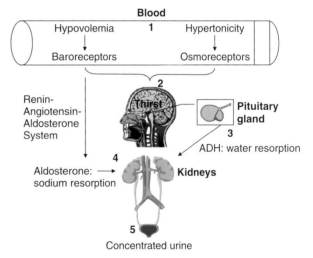

Figure 3 Water and sodium physiology: mechanisms controlling body water gain and loss. As water is lost from the body via sweat, urine, respiration, and feces, (1) plasma osmolality increases and plasma volume decreases with water loss. (2) The increase in osmolality acts on the 'thirst center' in the hypothalamus to secrete ADH and stimulates the conscious desire for water. (3) The release of ADH from the pituitary gland increases tubular resorption of water by the kidney. (4) Aldosterone is formed via a series of reactions involving renin, which is released from the adrenal cortex in response to decreased blood pressure, and a plasma protein, angiotensingen. Aldosterone promotes sodium resorption by the kidney to maintain plasma volume. (5) These events conserve water and result in the production of concentrated urine.

results in a complex series of events resulting in the release of renin from the kidneys and the subsequent formation of angiotensin II and the minerocorticoid, aldosterone. Angiotensin II is a potent vasoconstrictor and stimulator of thirst. Aldosterone promotes sodium resorption, which allows the blood to retain more water. The net result of these regulatory mechanisms is concentrated urine and maintenance of plasma volume, provided that exogenous fluid intake increases proportionally. If fluid intake is not increased, dehydration will still result.

Thirst

Thirst is not a good short-term regulator of fluid balance. Humans frequently lose up to 2% of their body weight as water before the thirst mechanism is activated. The actual point at which the thirst mechanism is activated varies considerably between individuals. Some athletes are closely attuned to their anticipated fluid needs and develop the habit of drinking before they become dehydrated. However, the majority of individuals do not feel compelled to drink until they have become moderately dehydrated, even though fluids may be available. These individuals are called 'voluntary dehydrators.' Voluntary dehydrators frequently replace only approximately two-thirds of their short-term fluid losses.

Pathophysiology of Dehydration

Dehydration and Human Performance

Natives of desert regions have, over the years, habituated to being chronically dehydrated. A study of the desert inhabitants found that they had a curtailed thirst drive that was associated with excretion of low volumes of concentrated urine and a high incidence of kidney disease (kidney stones). When additional water intake (approximately twice normal) was ingested in a subsample of this population, they were able to exercise 10% longer in the desert environment, presumably due to improved thermoregulation. The results of this and other studies illustrate that humans probably do not adapt to dehydration but can become used to a mild chronic dehydration due to inadequate fluid intake. This is not a true physiological adaptation since there are negative health and performance effects associated with chronic dehydration.

Body Water Deficits

When fluid intakes are insufficient to maintain normal body water content (approximately 60% for males and 50–55% for females), deficits arise

in all fluid compartments, with the reduction in plasma volume being of particular concern. Dehydration decreases plasma volume and increases tonicity. Plasma hypertonicity signals the circulatory system to conserve plasma volume for internal organs at the expense of skin blood flow. Reduction in skin blood flow decreases evaporative cooling. Additionally, decreased plasma volume reduces stroke volume and cardiac output, which impairs cooling capacity and exercise performance. The effects of dehydration on heart rate, body temperature, and endurance are shown in **Figure 4**. Consuming water to replace sweat loss while cycling for 6 h at 55% VO_2 max in the heat was associated with lower heart rates and core temperatures compared to a trial in which no water was ingested. The increase in heart rate while cycling without water replacement is a compensatory mechanism to maintain cardiac output in response to reduced plasma volume. Elevated core temperatures in cyclists not consuming water

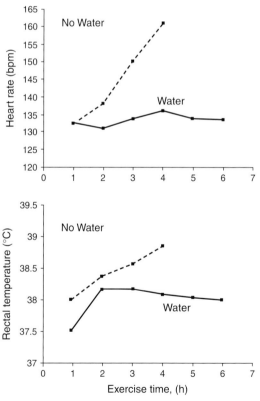

Figure 4 Consequences of consuming or not consuming water during cycle ergometer work (50% VO_2 max, 30 °C, 50% relative humidity). Subjects drank water to replace that lost during exercise (water group) or did not drink during exercise (no water group). Note that the no water group could not exercise as long as the water group. (Adapted from Barr SI, Costill DL and Fink WJ (1991) Fluid replacement during prolonged exercise: Effects of water, saline, or no fluid. *Medicine and Science in Sports and Exercise* **23**: 811–817.)

resulted from reduced skin blood flow and ultimately forced the cessation of exercise.

Dehydration and Heat Illness

If water loss due to sweating is not replaced during exercise, plasma volume and sweat rate will be decreased (**Figure 2**). The combination of reduced peripheral blood flow for heat exchange and reduced sweat volume for evaporative cooling leads to an overall reduction in the ability to dissipate heat.

The consequence of impaired heat dissipation is hyperthermia. Without evaporative cooling, human core temperatures can elevate ~5 °C/h during moderate intensity work. Heat production is proportional to the intensity and duration of work, ranging from ~75 kcal/h (314 kJ) at rest to ~300 kcal/h (1256 kJ) during moderate exercise and ~600 kcal/h (2512 kJ) for maximal sustained work. Brief periods of intense exercise can generate heat at the rate of ~900 kcal/h (3768 kJ).

Hyperthermia can lead to serious or even life-threatening heat injury if left unchecked. Heat injury can result if the rate of heat production is greater than the rate of cooling. When fluid losses are not replaced during activity, heat dissipation mechanisms are compromised. The buildup of heat in blood and tissues adversely affects various physiological systems. Minor heat injury syndromes include prickly heat (skin rash resulting from plugged sweat glands), heat syncope (light headedness due to pooling of blood in the extremities), and heat cramps (muscle cramps related to electrolyte loss). These heat illnesses are of concern but not life-threatening. Major hyperthermia syndromes involving dehydration are heat exhaustion and heat stroke. Conversely, overhydration (replacing large volumes of fluid loss) without sodium provision can, in certain instances, lead to an overdilution of blood sodium (hyponatremia). The symptoms of hyponatremia are similar to those of other forms of heat illness, but the treatment is critically different.

Heat exhaustion   Two types of heat exhaustion can be distinguished: water depletion (inadequate consumption of water) and salt depletion (loss of large volumes of sweat that are replaced without adequate sodium intake). Heat exhaustion usually occurs on a continuum somewhere between these two extremes. During heat exhaustion, thermoregulatory mechanisms cannot dissipate heat effectively, primarily because of reduced skin blood flow. People who are unacclimatized to the heat or not in good physical condition are more susceptible to heat exhaustion. Symptoms vary but usually include a temperature of less than 39.5 °C, malaise, weakness, fatigue, headaches, anorexia, nausea, vomiting, diarrhea, and muscle cramps. Although irritability, anxiety, and impaired judgment may be present, the subject is usually alert and capable of responding to questions. If left untreated, heat exhaustion can progress to heat stroke.

Heat stroke   Heat stroke is less common than heat exhaustion but is much more serious. Heat stroke is a life-threatening disorder that requires immediate medical treatment. Two forms of heat stroke are generally classified as exertional or classical. Exertional heat stroke generally occurs in young subjects working too hard for too long in the heat. Classical heat stroke is associated with environmental heat waves and primarily afflicts the very young, very old, poor, and debilitated. The pathophysiology of heat stroke involves failure of the body's thermoregulatory mechanisms following a severe heat overload. As core temperature elevates, cell function deteriorates culminating in massive cell damage. Dehydration is often a contributing factor to heat stroke, but the basic pathophysiology is uncontrolled heat overload. Core temperature is higher than that seen in heat exhaustion, generally 41 or 42 °C. Core temperatures higher than 39.5 °C reduce the function of motor centers in the brain and subsequently the ability to recruit motor units required for muscular activity. Extertional heat stroke is characterized by cessation of sweating, hot and dry skin, physical deterioration, confusion, collapse, and seizure. Rhabdomyolysis (muscle fiber destruction) may result from exertional heat stroke. In one reported case, an accelerated rhabdomyolysis resulting from exertional heat stroke occurred during an 8-km fun run when the ambient temperature was higher than 37 °C. This unfortunate runner collapsed with a rectal temperature of 42 °C and suffered acute renal failure as a consequence of an impaired immune system, infection, and decreased clotting ability. He eventually recovered, but it was necessary to amputate one of his legs that became infected following the rhabdomyolysis.

Other Consequences of Dehydration

There are other physiological consequences of dehydration that are not as serious as heat illness but can contribute to decreased performance capacity. Dehydration impairs thermoregulation in both hot and cold environments. Metabolic heat production in the cold may be less efficient in dehydrated individuals. The mechanism is not well understood, but it may involve a concomitant reduction in energy intake, decrease in resting metabolic rate, impaired shivering response, impaired vasodilation/constriction response, or a combination of these factors. Dehydration also blunts appetite, which in turn may elicit energy and thermoregulatory defects.

Management of Dehydration

Identifying Types of Dehydration

Although prevention is the best management strategy for dehydration, water imbalances may also be treated after the recognition of dehydration by replacement of appropriate fluids, such as water or water containing electrolytes. Dehydration usually occurs along a continuum of fluid and electrolyte loss. The ratio of water to electrolyte loss determines the type of dehydration present. A convenient classification of types of dehydration, their characteristics, and how to treat them is shown in **Table 2**.

It should be noted that hypotonic dehydration is the result of treating isotonic dehydration with nonelectrolyte-containing fluids and can lead to a potentially dangerous condition know as hyponatraemia (low blood sodium). This may be a particular problem in the case of 'overzealous hydrators' such as athletes who overcompensate for sweat losses. Hypotonic dehydration is also seen in infants and children who may be afflicted with gastrointestinal disturbances such as diarrhea, stomach flu, or acute gastroenteritis if water alone is used to hydrate. The American Academy of Pediatrics has published guidelines for oral rehydration therapy of infants and children younger than 5 years old with acute gastroenteritis. **Table 3** gives the Academy's guidelines for the

Table 2 Types of dehydration

Mild hypovolemia
Fluid intake is insufficient to meet needs, 2–5% body weight loss, yellow urine, dry lips, reduced skin elasticity
Many people are chronically hypovolemic in outdoor environments
Simply need to be reminded to drink, easily corrected by fluids and consuming food

Hypertonic dehydration (hypernatremic dehydration)
Body water losses greater than sodium losses, elevated blood osmolality and hypernatremia
May be accompanied by fever, profuse sweating, and/or evaporative water loss
Acute weight loss; person eats but does not drink
Treatment is provided by additional fluids (water is best)

Isotonic dehydration
Body loses equal amounts of water and sodium from routes other than sweating
Gastrointestinal fluid loss—vomiting, diarrhea
Blood electrolytes normal
Acute weight loss, tachycardia, orthostatic hypotension
Treat by replacing lost fluid *and* electrolytes or hypotonic dehydration may develop

Hypotonic dehydration (dilutional hyponatremia)
Can develop when isotonic dehydration is treated with only water
Hypotonic dehydration can occur anytime the body sodium loss exceeds water loss (e.g., sodium-restricted diets, diuretic use, overzealous hydrators, fluid replacement with only water following repeated vomiting and diarrhea)

assessment of dehydration. An algorithm for the treatment and hydration of children with acute diarrhea is shown in **Figure 5**.

Clinical standards for assessing dehydration in adults have not been well established. Measurements of plasma osmolarity and urine-specific gravity and osmolality can be used to assess relative dehydration if baseline (euhydrated) values are known. However, due to significant interindividual variation, the use of absolute specific gravity

Table 3 Guidelines for the assessment of dehydration[a]

Variable	Dehydration		
	Mild, 3–5%	*Moderate, 6–9%*	*Severe, >9%*
Blood pressure	Normal	Normal	Normal to reduced
Quality of pulses	Normal	Normal or slightly decreased	Moderately decreased
Heart rate	Normal	Increased	Increased, severe cases bradycardia
Skin turgor	Normal	Decreased	Decreased
Fontanelle	Normal	Sunken	Sunken
Mucous membranes	Slightly dry	Dry	Dry
Eyes	Normal	Sunken orbits	Deeply sunken orbits
Extremities	Warm, normal capillary refill	Delayed capillary refill	Cool, mottled
Mental status	Normal	Normal to listless	Normal to lethargic or comatose
Urine output	Slightly decreased	<1 ml/kg/h	≪1 ml/kg/h
Thirst	Slightly increased	Moderately increased	Very thirsty or too lethargic to indicate

[a]The percentages of body weight loss and their corresponding categorization sometime vary depending on the author.
From the American Academy of Pediatrics (1996) based on Duggan *et al.* (1992) Reproduced by permission of *Pediatrics* and the American Academy of Pediatrics.

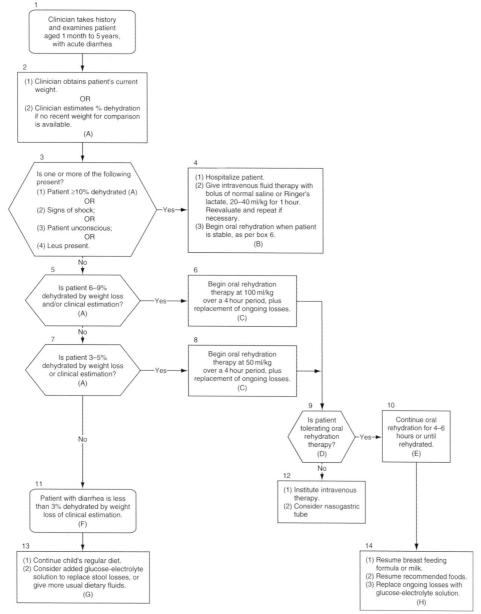

Figure 5 Algorithm for children with dehydration from acute diarrheal disease. The letters at the bottom of the decision boxes refer to the following: (A) See **Table 3** for guidance in the assessment of the degree of dehydration. (B) Restoration of cardiovascular stability is critical and is accomplished by giving bolus i.v. therapy. In the patient who does not respond, consider the possibility of an underlying disorder. When the patient is in stable condition and has achieved satisfactory mental status, oral rehydration therapy (ORT) can be implemented. (C) Solutions containing 45–90 mmol/l sodium should be given in a volume of 100 ml/kg for moderate dehydration and 50 ml/kg for mild dehydration. Giving the child these volumes requires patience and persistence, and progress must be monitored frequently. (D) Intractable, severe vomiting, unconsciousness, and ileus are contraindications to ORT. Persistent refusal to drink may require a trial of i.v. therapy. (E) The rehydration phase usually can be completed in 4 h; reevaluation should occur every 1 or 2 h. See referenced text for guidance to decide when rehydration has been achieved. (F) The type and intensity of therapy will vary with the individual clinical situation. (G) Often, a child has diarrhea but remains adequately hydrated. The parent can be reassured but should be taught to assess hydration and to identify a worsening condition. If the stool output remains modest, ORT may not be required if early, age-appropriate feeding is instituted and increased consumption of usual dietary fluids is encouraged. More significant stool losses can be replaced with an oral rehydrating solution at the rate of 10 ml/kg for each stool. (H) Breast-feeding should be resumed. Nonlactose formula, milk-based formula, or milk may be given, although a small percentage of children will not tolerate lactose-containing fluids. Lactose-containing solutions seem to be tolerated better when combined with complex carbohydrates in weaned children. Children who are eating foods may resume eating, although certain foods are tolerated better than others. Recommended foods include complex carbohydrates (rice, wheat, potatoes, bread, and cereals), lean meats, yogurt, fruit, and vegetables. Avoid fatty foods and foods high in simple sugars (including juices and soft drinks). Supplement feeding with an oral electrolyte solution, 10 ml/kg for each diarrheal stool and the estimated amount vomited for each emesis. (From American Academy of Pediatrics (1996) Practice parameter: The management of acute gastroenteritis in young children. *Pediatrics* **97**: 1–22, with permission.)

and osmolarity values for the diagnosis of dehydration remains questionable. Monitoring urine color has been suggested as a noninvasive way to measure hydration status, where light, pale yellow urine generally indicates a favorable hydration status. Assessing urine color may be a simple method to assess hydration status, but it can also be artificially influenced by dietary intake (i.e., nutritional supplements). Acute change in body weight is the most common and practical method used to assess hydration status. It is assumed that short-term body weight loss is primarily the result of water loss.

Treating Different Types of Dehydration

In the majority of simple, nonsevere dehydration cases, plain water is an adequate rehydration solution. However, there are instances (e.g., children younger than 5 years of age dehydrated by vomiting and diarrhea) when water containing sodium and potassium is the proper hydrating agent. The most effective way of preventing and treating mild to moderate dehydration in infants and children with acute diarrhea is the oral administration of oral rehydration solutions (ORSs). There are a number of commercially available ORSs. These solutions are designed to replace fluid and electrolytes when both water and food intake have been restricted or compromised by diarrheal disease. The World Health Organization recommends the ORS shown in **Table 4** for individuals afflicted with diarrheal disease and vomiting. Oral modes of fluid and electrolyte administration are always preferred in mild (3–5%) to moderate (6–9%) dehydration; however, intravenous fluids may be required in cases of severe dehydration (>9%) and vomiting or if the patient is in a comatose state. When i.v. fluids are administered, 0.45% saline with 5% dextrose is an effective hydrating agent.

In most instances involving heavy sweating, plain water containing 1.25 g of NaCl per liter is a suitable rehydration solution. Increasing the concentration of NaCl to 5 or 6 g per liter may promote the rate of rehydration but may not be palatable for some individuals. Most commercial sports drinks contain 1.2–1.8 g NaCl per liter and are also good rehydration solutions, especially when both fluid and electrolytes have been lost through sweating. Fruit juices can also provide fluid, energy, and electrolytes (e.g., fresh orange juice contains approximately 10 mg of sodium and 2000 mg of potassium per liter) but may be too concentrated and delay gastric emptying. Diluting fruit juices 1:3 with water may yield a more appropriate rehydration solution. The inclusion of carbohydrate in the rehydration solution provides energy for the intestinal sodium pump, which facilitates sodium transport across the intestinal cell wall into the blood, where it in turn exerts a positive osmotic effect on water absorption from the gut. Glucose and electrolyte sports beverages are useful rehydration solutions for sporting activities but are not a good choice for children with diarrhea since these beverages have lower electrolyte and higher carbohydrate concentrations than recommended.

Groups at Risk for Dehydration

Predisposing Factors for Heat Illness

Certain segments of the population are at greater risk for dehydration and subsequent heat illness than others (**Table 5**). The predisposing factors for dehydration and heat illness in these populations are obesity (extra exertion, heat production, and sweating are required to move a larger mass), insufficient heat acclimation (associated with reduced sweating and evaporative cooling and increased cardiovascular and renal stress), socioeconomic barriers to cooling methods (fans, air conditioners, etc.), pyrexial illness (fever), drug and alcohol abuse (interferes with fluid balance and thermoregulation), physical work in environments that contribute to dehydration (heat: sweating; cold: respiratory water loss and diuresis; altitude: respiratory water loss and

Table 4 Composition of recommended WHO/UNICEF oral rehydration solution

Solute	Content (mmol l^{-1})
Glucose	75
Sodium	75
Chloride	65
Potassium	20
Citrate	10
Total osmolarity	245

Table 5 Dehydration and heat illness: Populations at risk

Elderly
Poor
Young children
Obese people
Alcoholics
People afflicted with respiratory, cardiovascular, cerebrovascular, renal, or diarrheal disease
Athletes and outdoor workers

diuresis), and athletic competition and training (if athletes do not replace sweat loss). Even athletes who make a conscious attempt to drink during exercise only ingest approximately 300–500 ml fluid per hour; fluid loss through sweating (500–1000 ml/h) can easily surpass this intake of fluid.

Elderly and Children

The very young and the very old are two populations especially susceptible to dehydration. Children have less surface area-to-mass ratio for evaporative cooling and are less inclined to replace fluids; thus, they are less efficient thermoregulators than adults when exposed to high environmental temperatures. In the United States, approximately 9% of all hospitalizations of children younger than 5 years of age are due to diarrhea.

Aging is associated with decreased thirst, sweating, and renal responses that place the elderly at high risk during periods of extreme shifts in environmental temperature. Dehydration is a common cause for hospitalization and death in the aged population. Statistics from a 1991 U.S. survey of Medicare recipients revealed that almost half of the Medicare beneficiaries hospitalized for dehydration died within 1 year of admission. Older men and women may have a higher osmotic operating point (the point at which the thirst sensation is triggered), which may contribute to hypovolemia. Certain behavioral factors may also influence drinking patterns in older adults who may wish to avoid the physical difficulty associated with trips to the bathroom. Besides contributing to an increased risk for hyperthermia, dehydration also alters the effective dosage of medications through plasma volume changes, leading to further medical complications in the elderly. Dehydration in the elderly often accompanies or results from clinical conditions and/or medications.

Prevention of Dehydration

Dehydration resulting from nondisease causes can be easily prevented provided that people are inclined to drink and have access to cool, safe sources of fluids. Drink flavoring, beverage temperature, and sodium chloride content are important promoters of fluid intake in active children. Education of athletic coaches, the general public, and health care providers is necessary to increase

Table 6 Fluid replacement: Summary of recommendations of the American College of Sports Medicine

It is recommended that individuals consume a nutritionally balanced diet and drink adequate fluids during the 24-h period before an event, especially during the period that includes the meal prior to exercise, to promote proper hydration before exercise or competition.

It is recommended that individuals drink about 500 ml of fluid about 2 h before exercise to promote adequate hydration and allow time for excretion of excess ingested water.

During exercise, athletes should start drinking early and at regular intervals in an attempt to consume fluids at a rate sufficient to replace all the water lost through sweating, or consume the maximal amount that can be tolerated.

During exercise lasting less than 1 h, there is little evidence of physiological or physical performance differences between consuming a carbohydrate–electrolyte drink and plain water.

Inclusion of sodium (0.5–0.7 g per liter of water) in the rehydration solution ingested during exercise lasting longer than 1 h is recommended since it may be advantageous in enhancing palatability, promoting fluid retention, and possibly preventing hyponatremia in certain individuals who drink excessive quantities of fluid. There is little physiological basis for the presence of sodium in an oral rehydration solution for enhancing intestinal water absorption as long as sodium is sufficiently available from the previous meal.

From the American College of Sports Medicine (1996) Position stand on exercise and fluid replacement. *Medicine and Science in Sports and Exercise* **28**: i–vii.

awareness of the importance of proper hydration. The American College of Sports Medicine has issued a set of guidelines for fluid replacement (**Table 6**).

Simple methods, such as recording body weight before and after exercise to determine fluid loss and observing the color of urine or the turgidity of skin, can be useful for monitoring hydration status. The simplest insurance against dehydration is to consume fluids prior to and during physical activity or heat exposure to match water loss. The amount of fluid needed to maintain a favorable hydration status is variable between individuals but often necessitates drinking in the absence of thirst. Excess fluid consumption is rarely a problem. However, caution should be used to avoid dilutional hyponatraemia from overzealous hydration. Humans can acclimate to work in a hot environment and enhance their ability to thermoregulate and conserve fluid, but they cannot adapt to dehydration. Acute dehydration can decrease physical performance and thermoregulation ability and increase the risk for heat illness. Chronic dehydration can reduce metabolic and thermoregulatory efficiency and increase predisposition to kidney disease. The deleterious effects of dehydration on physiological function are summarized in **Figure 6**.

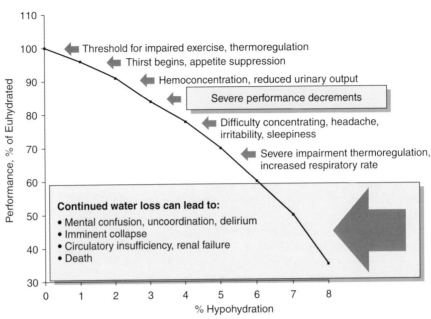

Figure 6 Progressive physiological effects of dehydration on physical performance and pathophysiology of hypohydration. The onset, magnitude, and severity depend on the workload, level of physical fitness, ambient temperature, relative humidity, and degree of heat accumulation of the individual. (From Askew EW (1996) Water. In: Ziegler EE and Filer LJ Jr (eds.) *Present Knowledge in Nutrition*, pp. 98–108. Washington, DC: ILSI Press, with permission.)

See also: **Children**: Nutritional Requirements. **Diarrheal Diseases**. **Electrolytes**: Acid-Base Balance; Water–Electrolyte Balance. **Infants**: Nutritional Requirements. **Older People**: Nutritional Requirements; Nutrition-Related Problems. **Sodium**: Physiology. **Thirst**.

Further Reading

American Academy of Pediatrics (1996) Practice parameter: The management of acute gastroenteritis in young children. *Pediatrics* **97**: 1–22.

American College of Sports Medicine (1996) Position stand on exercise and fluid replacement. *Medicine and Science in Sports and Exercise* **28**: i–vii.

Askew EW (1996) Water. In: Ziegler EE and Filer LJ Jr (eds.) *Present Knowledge in Nutrition*, pp. 98–108. Washington, DC: ILSI Press.

Askew EW (1997) Nutrition and performance in hot, cold and high altitude environments. In: Wolinski I (ed.) *Nutrition in Exercise and Sport*, 3rd edn., pp. 597–619. Boca Raton, FL: CRC Press.

Burke LM and Hawley JA (1997) Fluid balance in team sports. Guidelines for optimal practices. *Sports Medicine* **24**: 38–54.

Buskirk ER and Puhl SM (1996) *Body Fluid Balance*. Boca Raton, FL: CRC Press.

Hawley JA, Dennis SC, and Noaks TD (1995) Carbohydrate, fluid, and electrolyte requirements during prolonged exercise.

In: Kies CV and Driskell JA (eds.) *Sports Nutrition: Minerals and Electrolytes*. Boca Raton, FL: CRC Press.

Kenney L and Chiu P (2001) Influence of age on thirst and fluid intake. *Medicine and Science in Sports Exercise* **33**: 1524–1532.

Murray R (1995) Fluid needs in hot and cold environments. *International Journal of Sports Nutrition* **5**: S62–S73.

Noaks TD (1998) Fluid and electrolyte disturbances in heat illness. *International Journal of Sports Nutrition* **19**: S146–149.

Rolls BJ (1998) Homeostatic and non-homeostatic controls of drinking in humans. In: Arnaud MJ (ed.) *Hydration throughout Life*, pp. 19–28. Montrouge, France: John Libbey Eurotext.

Sawka MN, Latzka WA, and Montain SJ (2000) Effects of dehydration and rehydration on performance. In: Maughan RJ (ed.) *The Encyclopedia of Sports Medicine. Vol. VII: Nutrition in Sport*, pp. 216–225. Oxford: Blackwell Science.

Sawka MN, Montain SJ, and Latzka WA (2001) Hydration effects on thermoregulation and performance in the heat. *Comparative Biochemistry and Physiology Part A: Molecular & Integrative Physiology* **128**: 679–690.

Shirreffs SM and Maughan RJ (2000) Rehydration and recovery of fluid balance after exercise. *Exercise and Sport Science Reviews* **28**: 27–32.

Wilk BS, Kremler H, and Barr-Or O (1998) Consistency in preventing voluntary dehydration in boys who drink a flavored carbohydrate-NaCl beverage during exercise in the heat. *International Journal of Sports Nutrition* **8**: 1–9.

DENTAL DISEASE

R C Cottrell, The Sugar Bureau, London, UK

© 2005 Elsevier Ltd. All rights reserved.

Introduction

A number of dental diseases are among the most common diseases that are influenced by diet. Dental decay (caries) is experienced to some degree by most people at some time in their lives; dental erosion is thought to be an increasing problem, although data on prevalence are scarce, and dental-enamel defects are still an issue in some communities. Bacterial gum disease, while also common, is not known to be influenced by diet.

Enamel Defects

The structural integrity of the hard tissues in the mouth is influenced by the nutritional status of the mother during fetal development and by that of the child during the early years, when the permanent teeth are being formed (especially important are adequate availabilities of calcium and vitamin D). An excessive intake of fluoride during the period when the enamel of the primary or secondary teeth is being formed will lead to the characteristic defect of fluorosis. Except in rare circumstances, when the intake of fluoride is very high, this condition is usually minor, with no functional significance, and is visible only on professional inspection.

Dental Caries, Erosion, and Gum Disease

Once the teeth have erupted, they may be subject to three main conditions, all of which may threaten their survival: dental caries, tooth wear, and gum disease. Inappropriate dietary habits are a necessary contributing factor to the development of dental caries and may contribute, in part, to tooth wear by causing acid erosion. In contrast, diet has no effect on the common forms of gum disease.

Etiology of Caries

The causes of dental caries and factors influencing their formation have been the subject of research for more than 100 years. The importance of oral bacteria was discovered well before the specific influence of sugars derived from the diet became known in around 1950. While the protective effect of fluoride has also been known for more than 50 years, the mechanism of this effect is still a subject of debate.

Different approaches have been used to try to understand the caries process. Experimental studies have either induced clinically apparent caries or attempted to model the early stages of caries. Ethical limitations on studies that might cause caries in humans and increasing resistance to animal experimentation have stimulated a great deal of imaginative recent work with laboratory modelling.

Direct studies of caries induction are rarely conducted nowadays. But, in the past, important evidence in this field has come from experiments in which caries were induced in laboratory animals and, in one important instance, from a similar experiment in human subjects. The animal experiments are now regarded with some suspicion, since the information gained cannot be readily interpreted in terms of human risk. The animals used differ appreciably from their human counterparts in the structure of their teeth, their way of eating, and other factors such as saliva and oral bacterial populations. These animal experiments have been useful, however, in establishing that all fermentable carbohydrates are capable of inducing caries under appropriate conditions.

A key human experiment was conducted in the 1950s, before it was entirely clear that sugar is capable of causing caries. It was important in that it demonstrated conclusively that the consumption of a large amount of sugar does not necessarily have a discernable influence on caries risk, provided it is eaten at mealtimes, whereas frequent consumption of quite small amounts of sugar had a marked influence. Subjects given $340\,g\,day^{-1}$ of sugar at meal times showed no increase in caries incidence, while subjects given $50\,g\,day^{-1}$ or $100\,g\,day^{-1}$ between meals showed an increase. Typical European intakes of sugar are less than $100\,g\,day^{-1}$.

The subjects in this study had little or no oral hygiene and no access to fluoride. It can therefore be readily concluded that the amount of sugar consumed in the diet, even in countries with high consumption, is unlikely to influence caries risk, especially with the regular use of fluoride toothpaste for oral hygiene. Whether frequent consumption of sugar will influence caries risk in an individual who cleans his or her teeth regularly with a fluoride toothpaste is more controversial. But, given the current state of knowledge, it seems unwise to assume that any dietary behavior would be safe, however outlandish. The current fashion of eating and drinking perpetually and of sipping sugar-containing drinks from a can over long periods seems designed to cause caries and cannot be recommended.

Research into the causes of dental caries has addressed a number of questions. These include why there are large differences in the disease experience of individuals within the same population or even family group, why the prevalence and severity of the disease are so different in different populations, and why these can change so dramatically with time. Entirely satisfactory answers to these questions are still being sought, but much has been learned over the last 100 years about the contributing factors and protective measures that determine the likelihood of this disease developing. This knowledge has been synthesized into the currently held view that clinically significant caries will develop only when a number of circumstances occur simultaneously. Inappropriate dietary habits (frequent consumption of sugars or starches) will allow the selective proliferation of bacteria attached to the tooth surface that are capable of metabolizing sugars to organic acids (especially lactic acid). These acids will facilitate dissolution of the tooth enamel whenever their production is sufficient to lower the local pH below a critical level. The presence of saliva or of other components of the food matrix will influence the pH attained and also the rate at which mineral is lost from the tooth surface.

The formation of dental caries is not, however, a simple unidirectional process of demineralization. Some tooth mineral may be removed almost every time something is eaten or drunk, but this loss will generally be made good by the subsequent accretion of mineral from saliva. Thus, a cavity develops only when the balance of repeated cycles of demineralization and remineralization results in localized overall mineral loss. It is for this reason that caries are most likely to occur at sites where food residues are likely to be trapped and access for saliva is limited (for example, between two closely abutting teeth).

The presence of fluoride not only radically alters both demineralization and remineralization but may also inhibit the activity of the acid-generating bacteria. To date, the most effective methods of reducing the incidence of dental caries have involved the use of fluoride either (at low concentrations) in community water supplies or (at higher concentrations) in toothpaste.

Caries-Causing Bacteria

The surfaces of all teeth are normally covered with a biofilm (plaque) composed of a range of bacterial species embedded in a sticky organic material produced by the metabolic activity of specialized bacteria. Colonization of the surfaces of the teeth starts as soon as they erupt in a baby's mouth (from about 6 months of age) and continues throughout life. There is evidence to suggest that the initial colonization of a baby's teeth with cariogenic bacteria may arise by infection from the mother's mouth. The common practice of sampling the food in a baby's dish, to check that it is not too hot, using the same spoon that is to be used to feed the baby may be a particularly effective way of transferring bacteria from carer to baby. Brushing the teeth with a toothbrush will remove part, but not all, of this film and its accompanying bacterial population. Many of the bacteria present are harmless, but a number of species are capable both of metabolically converting carbohydrates to acids (acidogenic bacteria) and of continuing to be metabolically active when the local pH has become too acid for most bacteria to tolerate. It is these bacteria that cause caries.

Fermentable Carbohydrate

Acidogenic bacteria metabolize (ferment) simple sugars (glucose, fructose, sucrose, lactose, and maltose) to acids. Sugars may be present as a result of their direct consumption or as a result of the enzymatic breakdown of starches within the mouth by salivary amylase. Thus, a substantial proportion of a typical diet will contain a source of fermentable carbohydrate, and many, if not all, eating and drinking occasions will give these bacteria one of these metabolic precursors. The more frequently an individual consumes carbohydrate, the more the acidogenic bacteria thrive and other, less acid tolerant, bacteria are disadvantaged.

A wide variety of foods contain carbohydrate that is capable of giving rise to acids as a result of bacterial metabolism (fermentation) within dental plaque. Of the common dietary sugars, sucrose, fructose, and glucose are found in fruit and fruit juices, soft drinks, jams, honey, chocolate and other confectionary, and an immense variety of composite foods and drinks. Lactose arises naturally in milk and milk products but is also widely used as an ingredient in its own right by the food industry.

Starches are also classed as fermentable carbohydrates because they are partially broken down by amylase in saliva during chewing to maltose and glucose. Residues of starchy foods are frequently caught between the teeth and in the fissures of the molar teeth, where they may be broken down to sugars over long periods. Measurements of the pH of plaque following the ingestion of starches have suggested that the depression of pH may be as great as and last even longer than that produced by some sources of sugars, such as drinks, because of slow clearance. Highly processed starchy products, such as heat- and pressure-processed extruded snacks, are likely to be more readily converted to sugars than less processed starchy foods, such as bread.

Clearly, the wide range of individual dietary choices and eating habits may influence the risk of developing caries. The physical characteristics of fermentable carbohydrates will affect the rate at which they are cleared from specific sites in the dentition. Foods that are inclined to remain for long periods in stagnation sites (for example, between the teeth), such as toffees or raisins, are likely to give rise to a greater local fall in pH than are those that are rapidly cleared, such as chocolate. Clearance rates are also influenced by the increase in salivary flow that is stimulated by eating or drinking. When salivary flow is greater, for example after consuming a strongly flavored food, clearance will be faster and demineralization is likely to be less than that after consuming a bland food.

Susceptible Sites

Dental caries are more likely to occur at stagnation sites between teeth or in the fissures of molar teeth. Plaque will accumulate in these sites, where it is less likely to be disturbed by tooth brushing. At the same time, the protective buffering of saliva and the remineralization that arises from its mineral content are attenuated by the inaccessibility of such sites, while food debris is retained for longer periods. The reduction of salivary flow during sleep makes food debris remaining in these sites at night particularly damaging to the teeth.

Experimental Models of the Caries Process

Because direct manipulation of the caries process in human subjects is impossible for ethical reasons, a number of techniques have been developed that provide insights without risking clinical damage to the teeth of experimental subjects. Much of the earlier work relied on measurements of the change in plaque pH that followed a single consumption episode of a food or drink containing a source of fermentable carbohydrate. This approach provides an indication of the potential cariogenic challenge of these exposures and addresses the fundamental question of whether pH falls to a level that is expected to give rise to demineralization of the tooth enamel. Plaque pH measurements have thus been used to assess whether a food or drink may be considered safe for teeth. But this technique does not provide any information on the influence of the repair processes that follow exposure to a demineralizing challenge.

Approaches that provide an insight into the balance of demineralization and remineralization episodes over a period of time with naturalistic eating and drinking circumstances have now become more commonly used. These involve placing an enamel sample within a subject's dentition and carefully assessing any changes in the surface of this sample over a period of time. Particular cariogenic challenges can be applied, but, because they are continued for only a limited period of time, the subject's own teeth will not be appreciably affected. In many cases, the enamel sample is not cleaned with fluoride toothpaste, whereas the subject's own teeth are so protected (the additional enamel sample being removed while the teeth are brushed).

These models have provided useful information not only on the relative cariogenic potential of different foods and drinks but also on the protective effects of fluoride toothpaste (even though it may not be applied directly to the enamel sample) and on the influence of stagnation sites on caries risk with different dietary practices. Useful indications of answers to important public-health questions are beginning to emerge from this kind of research, such as the number of exposures to fermentable carbohydrate that can be tolerated without appreciable risk to the teeth, and the influence of fluoride toothpaste use on this number.

Etiology of Tooth Wear

The enamel surfaces of the crowns of the teeth may be damaged by wear arising from abrasion, attrition, or erosion. Abrasion can arise from the action of rubbing a hard substance across the surfaces of the teeth, for example when brushing too vigorously with a hard toothbrush. Attrition involves one tooth surface wearing down because of contact with another. A third form of wear involves the direct erosive action of acids present in foods (such as yoghurt or pickles) or drinks (especially citrus fruit juices). No bacterial metabolism is required for these processes to occur. It is unclear, however, whether the apparent increase in the prevalence of clinically apparent erosion of the teeth is the result of dietary habits or of some other factor. Only recently have dental-health surveys assessed this problem specifically, so it is possible that it has been noticed more, rather than actually occurring more, in these later surveys. It is also not always possible to distinguish acid erosion from other causes of tooth wear, such as over-vigorous tooth brushing. In addition, a common source of acid erosion is not dietary but arises from the regurgitation of the extremely acidic contents of the stomach. This is often seen in young children and, in adults, may be a presenting symptom of bulimia nervosa as a result of repeated vomiting.

Etiology of Gum Disease

Gum disease arises as a result of bacterial infection of the gums, especially at the tooth margins. It is often assumed that excessive accumulation of plaque, arising from inappropriate dietary habits, is a factor in this condition, but there is little evidence for any material influence of diet. The milder forms of gum disease are extremely common in all populations. More severe disease is the most frequent cause of tooth loss in older people. The best form of protection from gum disease is regular tooth brushing.

Protection from and Prevention of Dental Caries

Variations among individuals, and with time, will arise as a result of differences in acid generation from sugars at different localities within the dentition. These variations may be influenced by changing dietary habits and by the extent of the colonization of the relevant tooth surface by acidogenic bacteria. They may also be affected by changes in saliva flow, for example as a result of the use of certain medications or radiotherapy.

These factors may provide a reasonable explanation for many of the differences in caries experience observed between individuals and populations and between different locations within an individual's dentition. They do not explain the dramatic reduction in caries prevalence seen throughout the developed world in the last 30 years. There is no doubt that this improvement has been caused by the introduction of fluoride toothpaste.

Fluoride

Fluoride has provided the great success story in dental public health in the last 30 years. There are two main routes of delivery: water and toothpaste. Both are, in effect, dietary modifications.

The observation that tooth decay was less common in communities whose water supplies naturally contained low concentrations of fluoride led to the introduction of appropriate concentrations of fluoride into many public water supplies that did not naturally contain it. The prevalence of dental caries appeared to fall by between 20% and 50% as a result of this simple public-health measure.

There have been many thorough studies of the general health of populations receiving fluoridated water, which have found no credible evidence of adverse affects, except in a few areas where the fluoride content of the water is naturally very much higher than the level used for caries prevention. Despite vocal opposition to what is seen by some as compulsory medication of the population, many countries (for example, the USA and Ireland) still use this approach widely. Some, however, such as The Netherlands, have discontinued the practice.

Even greater improvements in dental health have followed the introduction of fluoridated toothpastes. The benefits seen at the population level from this innovation have been far greater than those predicted by the controlled clinical trials that preceded the widespread sale of fluoridated toothpastes to the public. Improvements of greater than 60% have been common. Interestingly, caries rates in The Netherlands continued to fall after the discontinuation of fluoridated water supplies, probably as a result of intense dental-health education of the population about the value of regular brushing with fluoridated toothpaste. In contrast, the abandonment of water fluoridation in the UK region of Anglesey was followed by a sharp rise in caries incidence.

A Practical Approach to the Prevention of Caries

The success of fluoridated toothpaste in preventing dental caries has resulted in a change in professional approaches to prevention. Instead of focusing simply on attempts to reverse the main causative factors, attention is now centered on exploiting protective influences. The interaction of the three main causative factors is illustrated in **Figure 1**. Numerous attempts to change the impact of any of these influences on caries have proved ineffective, except, perhaps, under the most extreme situations, such as during war time.

In contrast, exploiting the protective potentials of fluoride, tooth brushing, and salivary stimulation have proved successful. **Figure 2** illustrates the roles of these factors in comparison with the

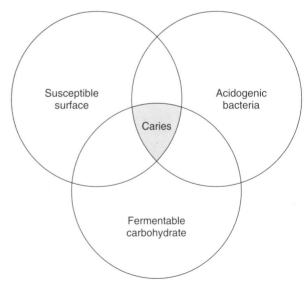

Figure 1   Interacting factors causing tooth decay.

Window of risk

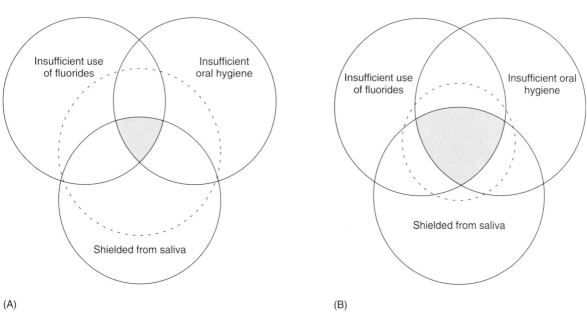

Figure 2 A new model to explain and guide caries prevention. The local factors – insufficient use of fluorides, insufficient oral hygiene, and protection from saliva – form a 'window of risk' through which the circle of cariogenic food (shown dashed) can be seen in the background. (A) In this example it is clear that it would be impossible to reduce the food circle to such an extent that the window is not completely filled (less caries risk). (B) If oral hygiene and, concomitantly, fluoride supply are neglected (large window of risk), a reduction in the burden of cariogenic food could reduce the caries risk. Reproduced with permission from van Loveren CM and Duggal MS (2001) The role of diet in caries prevention. *International Dental Journal* **51**: 399–406.

pervasive challenge of diet. Where a tooth site is shielded from saliva (stagnation site) and oral hygiene and the availability of fluoride are insufficient it is likely that a dietary modification of sufficient magnitude could exert some influence on the final outcome. But where these protective factors are adequate it is highly unlikely that dietary variations will exert any material effect. These predictions are borne out by epidemiological observations. In most developed countries, where fluoride use is adequate, wide variations in dietary exposure to fermentable carbohydrates between individuals are not accompanied by predictable differences in caries experience.

Epidemiology

Studies of Risk Factors

A large number of observational epidemiological studies have been conducted that have attempted to show associations between caries experience and one, or several, of the known risk factors. The large majority of these studies have been of poor design, examining insufficient numbers of subjects and ignoring important confounding influences. Many have been cross-sectional in design and have sought to draw

conclusions about the causes of caries by assessing the dietary and other habits of subjects at the same time as measuring their caries experience. Such a study design is somewhat unsatisfactory for this purpose.

The few longitudinal studies in the scientific literature are equally weakened by poor data on dietary habits and, in some cases, idiosyncrasies in caries assessments. Taken together, these studies provide scant evidence about the relative importance of the different etiological factors. It is fortunate that more convincing evidence is available from experimental studies.

National Trends in Caries Prevalence

Data on the prevalence of dental caries within populations are nowadays very reliable as they are collected to internationally recognized standards. Surveys of 12-year-old children are carried out in most countries, and the data are collated by the World Health Organization (see **Table 1**). In contrast, data for adults are scarcer.

The general picture emerging from the repetition of these national surveys is clear. In many countries the prevalence of caries is falling, often dramatically. In poorer countries this is unlikely to be the case, and, even within the richest countries, the dental-health experience of the economically disadvantaged

Table 1   Prevalence of caries by region; the table shows the mean number of teeth with decay experience in 12-year-old children

Lowest DMFT	Country	Year of Survey	Highest DMFT	Country	Year of Survey
Europe					
0.9	Denmark	2001	7.3	Romania	1998
	The Netherlands	1992			
	Switzerland	2000			
	UK	2000			
Americas					
0.9	Belize	1999	8.1	Guatemala	1987
Africa					
0.3	Tanzania	1994	4.9	Mauritius	1993
	Togo	1986			
	Rwanda	1993			
Southeast Asia					
0.86	India	1993	3.0	North Korea	1991
Eastern Mediterranean					
0.9	Djibouti	1990	3.3	Jordan	1995
	Pakistan	1999			
Western Pacific					
0.6	South Korea	1972	4.9	Brunei Darussalam	1994
0.8	Australia	1999			
	Hong Kong	2001			

DMFT, decayed, missing, or filled permanent teeth.
Data obtained from the WHO Oral Health Country Profile Programme, WHO Collaborating Centre (website http:/www.whocollab. odont.lu.se/index.html).

is significantly poorer than that of those with a higher socioeconomic position. In many countries there is evidence that inequalities in dental health between the rich and the poor have widened.

Attempts to account for these trends are hampered by the unreliability of data on factors that are likely to attenuate caries risk. All assessments of these factors rely on people (often children) accurately remembering and reporting aspects of their everyday behavior, such as whether they clean their teeth and how often and what they have eaten and drunk and when. These data are subjective and notoriously unreliable. More secure conclusions about factors

that have influenced caries rates must therefore come from more objective data (see below).

Fluoride Toothpaste

The effect, at a population level, of the introduction and widespread availability of fluoride toothpaste is clear. **Figure 3** shows the falls in caries incidence in 5-year-old and 12-year-old children in the UK seen in successive national representative surveys. A similar picture has been seen in Denmark (**Figure 4**). Fluoride toothpaste was introduced onto the UK market in around 1976 and rapidly became universal. The falls

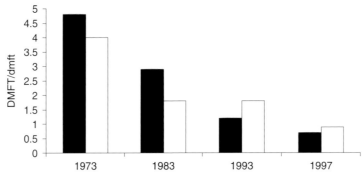

Figure 3   The change in the average decay experience of children in the UK. DMFT (decayed, missing, and filled permanent teeth) in 12-year-olds (filled bars) and dmft (decayed, missing, and filled primary teeth) in 5-year-olds (open bars). Data from OPCS (1973–1993) and NDNS (1997).

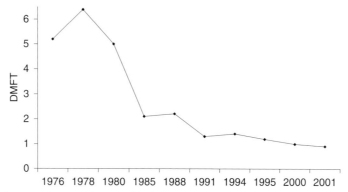

Figure 4 The change in caries experience of 12-year-old children in Denmark. DMFT, decayed, missing, or filled permanent teeth. Data obtained from WHO Collaborating Centre.

in caries prevalence seen at the next survey date (1983) exceeded expectations, based on earlier clinical trials, and led many experts to predict that no further fall would occur. In the event, an even greater decline was seen among 12-year-olds at the next decennial survey (1993). The caries prevalence among 5-year-olds appeared to have reached a plateau by 1993, but later data suggests that further falls in both age groups may have occurred. Regrettably, the self-reported use of fluoride toothpaste (almost certainly an overestimate of actual use) is still not universal, even among children in comfortable socioeconomic conditions.

The variation in caries experience with family income is illustrated for the UK in **Figure 5**. A clear gradient exists, with the poorest dental health seen in the lowest-income families. Trend data indicates that the greatest improvements have occurred among higher-income families and the least among those at the other end of the socioeconomic scale. The reasons for these differences are not entirely clear, but oral hygiene and the use of fluoride toothpaste appear to be important. Evidence of gum

disease (an indicator of oral hygiene) is more common among poorer children.

Diet

Attempts to attribute the recent changes in caries prevalence to improvements in dietary habits have been unconvincing. Apart from the difficulty in determining what people are eating and drinking with any accuracy, data on when food and drink have been consumed are needed to assess the overriding dietary influence of frequency of exposure of the teeth to fermentable carbohydrate. These data are rarely collected in surveys and are then of uncertain reliability. All dietary surveys are seriously hampered by the unreliability of the subjective reporting of dietary habits by those surveyed.

The use of nationally aggregated data (such as food-supply data) is hardly more useful, since a large proportion (up to 50%) of the food available for consumption is never actually eaten. Nonetheless, some experts have pointed to changes in caries prevalence following dramatic changes in food supply as evidence of the practical utility of dietary

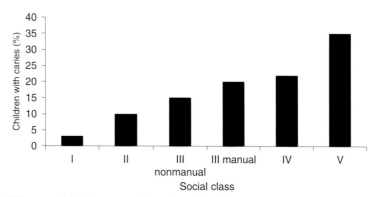

Figure 5 Percentage of children aged 1.5–4.5 years with caries across social-class groups in the UK, calculated from data presented in Hinds and Gregory (1995). Social class I has the highest income, social class V has the lowest.

manipulation as a means of reducing the remaining burden of this disease. The weakness of this argument is that predictable changes in caries prevalence at a population level have rarely been seen except under conditions of extreme dietary change, such as during war time. These changes all occurred before the advent of the widespread use of fluoride. When the food supply of fermentable carbohydrates is severely restricted, changes in the frequency of consumption may occur to a degree that is sufficient to alter caries risk when fluoride is not used. Where fluoride toothpaste and oral hygiene are adequate, even such extreme changes in diet are unlikely to alter caries experience materially. In addition, attempts to use dietary manipulation to reduce the risk of caries in free-living populations have proved unsuccessful.

Other Factors Affecting the Epidemiology of Caries

The influence of other factors that might be expected to have a bearing on caries experience has proved difficult to establish for practical reasons. These include the susceptibility of particular sites within the dentition or in an individual's mouth and local salivary flow rates. Both of these factors are known to be strongly influenced by genetic inheritance. The morphology of the teeth and, especially, the depth and shape of the fissures on the surfaces of the molar teeth are strongly heritable. It is generally difficult to predict, in advance of caries developing, which sites will be particularly susceptible. But one successful preventative approach has been to identify children with deep fissures in their molar teeth at an early age and offer prophylactic treatment in the form of sealants. This addresses the most common site of early childhood caries (the molars) and targets those children most at risk because of unfavorable tooth morphology.

The rate of salivary flow, both at rest and when stimulated by eating or drinking, is also known to be a crucial influence on risk. Patients who have had a salivary duct removed for any reason have a far higher risk of caries than those with normal function. Some people have low salivary flow rates and, again, have a greater risk. Older people are inclined to suffer from a dry mouth, and a number of medications reduce salivary flow.

Epidemiological studies to assess the importance of salivary flow rates in altering the risk of caries have not been carried out because of the practical difficulty of measuring this factor. But the stimulation of salivary flow that accompanies chewing has been successfully exploited to reduce caries risk in experimental studies using chewing gum (usually sugar-free). Reductions in caries incidence were seen when subjects were encouraged to chew the gum, especially between and immediately after meals, while continuing their normal regular oral-hygiene practices. Convincing evidence of an effect at the population level, however, is awaited.

See also: **Calcium**. **Carbohydrates**: Resistant Starch and Oligosaccharides. **Fructose**. **Galactose**. **Glucose**: Chemistry and Dietary Sources. **Sucrose**: Dietary Sucrose and Disease. **Vitamin D**: Rickets and Osteomalacia.

Further Reading

Beighton D (2004) The complex microflora in high risk individuals and groups and its role in the caries process. *Community Dentistry and Oral Epidemiology* 32: In Press.

Bratthall D, Hansel Petersson G, and Sundberg H (1996) Reasons for the caries decline: what do the experts believe? *European Journal of Oral Science* 104: 416–422.

Curzon MEJ and Hefferen JJ (2001) Modern methods for assessing the cariogenic and erosive potential of foods. *British Dental Journal* 191: 41–46.

Duggal MS, Toumba KJ, Amaechi BT *et al.* (2000) Enamel demineralization *in situ* with varying frequency of carbohydrate consumption with and without fluoride toothpaste. *Journal of Dental Research* 80: 1721–1724.

Food and Agriculture Organization (1998) *Carbohydrates in Human Nutrition*. FAO Food and Nutrition Paper 66. Rome: FAO.

Gibson S and Williams S (1999) Dental caries in pre-school children: associations with social class, toothbrushing habit and consumption of sugars and sugar-containing foods. Further analysis of the national diet and nutrition survey of children aged 1.5–4.5 years. *Caries Research* 33: 101–113.

Gustaffson BE, Quensel CE, Lanke LS *et al.* (1954) The Vipeholm dental caries study: the effect of different levels of carbohydrate intake on caries activity in 436 individuals over five years. *Acta Odontica Scandanavica* 11: 232–365.

Hausen H (2003) Fluoride toothpaste prevents caries. *Evidence Based Dentistry* 4: 28.

Hinds K and Gregory JR (1995) *National Diet and Nutrition Survey: Children Aged 1.5–4.5 Years*. vol. 2. Report of the Dental Survey. London: HMSO.

Marquis RE, Clock SA, and Mota-Meira M (2003) Fluoride and organic acids as modulators of microbial physiology. *FEMS Microbiology Reviews* 26: 493–510.

Reich E (2001) Trends in caries and periodontal health epidemiology in Europe. *International Dental Journal* 51: 392–398.

van Loveren CM and Duggal MS (2001) The role of diet in caries prevention. *International Dental Journal* 51: 399–406.

Woodward M and Walker ARP (1994) Sugar consumption and dental caries: evidence from 90 countries. *British Dental Journal* 176: 297–302.

World Health Organization (1994) *Fluorides and Oral Health*. WHO Technical Report Series 846. Geneva: WHO.

DIABETES MELLITUS

Contents
Etiology and Epidemiology
Classification and Chemical Pathology
Dietary Management

Etiology and Epidemiology

J Sudagani and G A Hitman, Queen Mary's, University of London, London, UK

© 2005 Elsevier Ltd. All rights reserved.

Introduction

Diabetes mellitus is a chronic metabolic disorder characterized by disturbance in glucose metabolism leading to a state of hyperglycemia and is associated with microvascular and macrovascular complications in the long term. Diabetes is the leading cause of noncommunicable diseases worldwide and it is true to say that diabetes has reached epidemic proportions in certain parts of the world and in certain ethnic groups. This has widespread implications for health resources.

Diabetes mellitus is an etiologically and clinically heterogenous group of disorders that share hyperglycemia in common. The two main types of diabetes, type 1 diabetes (T1D) and type 2 diabetes (T2D), are quite distinct from each other in their etiology and epidemiology. T2D is the most common form of diabetes worldwide accounting for 90% of cases globally and affecting approximately 4% of the world's adult population. Type 1 diabetes is an autoimmune disease that results in insulin deficiency. Both T1D and T2D are distinct from 'other causes of diabetes' as defined by the etiological classification of the World Health Organization (WHO); we will not comprehensively review the many types of diabetes but illustrate it with maturity onset diabetes of the young (MODY) and fibrocalculous pancreatic diabetes (FCPD). Gestational diabetes is the fourth category defined by the WHO.

Type 1 Diabetes

Worldwide Prevalence

In 1997 there were 11.5 million people with T1D in the world; this figure is expected to rise to 23.7 million in the year 2010. These increasing figures will have most impact in Asia, where there are currently 4.5 million people with T1D, and this is expected to rise to 12 million by the year 2010. One of the best incidence studies has come from Europe as part of a European collaboration, where the highest incidence of T1D is found in Finland and the lowest rates in Romania (**Table 1**). The incidence of T1D follows a north–south gradient, with the notable exception of Sardinia. The figures from countries such as India are less precise, although one study in Chennai suggested an incidence equivalent to that found in Southern European countries. These different rates of T1D are likely to reflect both the genetic background of individual countries and differences in exposure to environmental agents. In recent years,

Table 1 Extremes of incidence of childhood type 1 diabetes mellitus in different ethnic groups

Higher	Incidence[a]	Lower	Incidence[a]
Sardinia	35–40	Venezuala	0–5
Finland	35–40	Peru	0–5
Sweden	25–30	China	0–5
Canada	20–25	Paraguay	0–5
Norway	20–25	Mauritius	0–5
UK	15–25	Chile	0–5
NewZealand	10–25	Japan	0–5
Portugal	5–20	Barbados	0–5

[a]Age standardized incidence (per 100,000 per year) of type 1 diabetes in children <14 years of age.
Data from Karvonen M, Viik-Kajander M, Moltchanova E *et al* (2000) Incidence of childhood type 1 diabetes worldwide. Diabetes Care **23**: 1516–1526.

the incidence of T1D has been increasing in several different countries. These changes must reflect environmental influences.

Etiology

Type 1 diabetes is due to autoimmune destruction of insulin-secreting pancreatic β cells of islets of Langerhans. T1D typically occurs in young individuals with an age of onset of less than 40 years. The autoimmune reaction is likely to be triggered by an environmental agent *in utero* or in very early life (**Figure 1**). The earliest markers of β cell destruction are the appearance of autoantibodies to glutamic acid decarboxylase(GAD), islet cells, and insulin. Autoantibodies have been detected 10–15 years before the onset of disease and, furthermore, have been known to disappear without T1D occurring in a few individuals. One to two years before onset of the disease, evidence of β cell impairment can be detected, initially evidenced by a reduction in the first phase of insulin response to intravenous glucose and in the later stages by an abnormal oral glucose tolerance. In contrast to the slow β cell destruction, the onset of T1D is acute and is usually measured in weeks. At this stage in the etiological process, it is likely that 70% of β cells have been destroyed and those remaining are inhibited by the action of cytokines.

There is a subgroup of patients who develop diabetes in adult life and do not require insulin during the first few years after diagnosis; they have an autoimmune component to their disease with positive GAD and islet cell antibodies. This condition is named latent autoimmune diabetes (LADA). There are several common features between T1D and LADA, including T cell insulitis, islet antibody positivity, and high rates of HLA DR3 and DR4. The prevalence of LADA in newly diagnosed diabetics

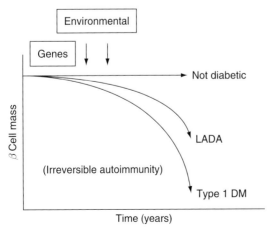

Figure 1 The etiology of type 1 diabetes mellitus. DM, diabetes mellitus; LADA, latent autoimmune diabetes.

has been shown to range from 2.8% to 22.3% in different studies depending on the markers used and characteristics of the patients. Although these patients present with type 2 diabetes, they have been shown to progress to insulin dependency especially if the diabetes is diagnosed at a younger age and the patient is not overweight. Therefore, there may be a role for measuring GAD antibody in newly diagnosed patients with type 2 diabetes to identify the LADA subgroup especially in the younger age groups. This group of patients is now classified as type 1 diabetes by the new WHO classification.

Genetics

Type 1 diabetes is a multifactorial disease with both genetic and environmental components. The largest genetic contribution to T1D is determined by genes in the major histocompatibility complex (MHC) located to the short arm of chromosome 6 (IDDM1-HLA, 6p21). Initial associations between T1D and the MHC were described for the HLA class I antigens A1-B8 and B15. With advent of HLA class II serology, closer associations were found with HLA-DR with an increased frequency of DR3 and DR4 and a decreased frequency of DR2 in T1D subjects. At the population level the strongest genetic association with T1D is with HLA-DQ alleles. This is best defined by DNA typing of HLA-DQ1, DQB1, and DRB1. However, due to the strong linkage disequilibrium between these loci it has been very difficult to study the effect of individual HLA-DQ or HLA-DR genes separately. For the individual, susceptibility is best defined by allelic combinations of MHC genes located to all three major regions (classes I, II, and III) called HLA haplotypes. Haplotypes occur because of strong linkage disequilibrium observed in the MHC whereby the combinations of alleles are seen more frequently than would be expected by their individual gene frequencies. An example of a haplotype would be A2, Cw1, B56, TNFa6, DRB1*401, DQA1*0301, DQB1*0302. The haplotypes are likely to relate to functional groups of genes involved in the etiology of T1D. Thus, the critical residues of DR and DQ, accounting for the disease association with T1D, are located in the antigen-binding cleft of the HLA molecule and are likely to influence the binding of antigenic peptides for subsequent presentation to T helper cells. Similarly, polymorphism of the HLA class I molecules are likely to relate to antigen presentation to cytotoxic T cells, and polymorphisms of tumor necrosis factor (TNF) have been associated with differing TNF responses to mitogenic stimulation.

The MHC accounts for approximately 40% of the genetic component to T1D. Evidence from genome scans and candidate gene studies indicates the existence of a large number of putative non-MHC genes contributing to the etiology of T1D, although all of comparatively small effect compared to the MHC. The most reproducible T1D associations have been found with the insulin gene, cytotoxic T lymphocyte antigen 4 gene (CTLA4), and the vitamin D receptor. An association between the insulin gene (located on chromosome 11p15.5; INS), and T1D was described in the 1980s and subsequently confirmed by linkage studies. The INS locus on chromosome 11p15.5 contains a major polymorphism 5′ to the transcription site, which is a variable number of tandem repeats (VNTR) region. One functional hypothesis to explain the association between the insulin gene and T1D is that 'hypersecretors' of insulin determined by the disease-associated polymorphism might induce thymic tolerance to insulin, thus providing protection from the autoimmune reaction. A recent study showed association of the T-cell regulatory gene CTLA4 with susceptibility to autoimmune disease, including type 1 diabetes. CTLA4 (gene located on chromosome 2q33) plays an important role in the counter-regulation of CD28 T cell antigen receptor activation of T cells. In the mouse model of T1D, susceptibility was also associated with variation in CTLA4 gene splicing with reduced production of a splice form encoding a molecule lacking the CD80/CD86 ligand-binding domain. There are associations reported between vitamin D receptor gene polymorphisms and type 1 diabetes. The VDR gene is located on chromosome 12q and polymorphisms of the VDR gene may be related to T-cell-mediated autoimmune destruction of β cells of pancreas. Vitamin D compounds suppress T cell activation and significantly repress the development of insulitis and diabetes in the nonobese diabetic (NOD) mouse, a mouse model of human type 1 diabetes. Results from other candidate gene studies and a 'total genome' analysis have identified at least another 19 chromosomal regions that may be involved in pathogenesis of the disease. The finding that so many genes are involved in T1D raises the possibility that there are several disease processes that might lead to β cell destruction. Furthermore, evidence is still emerging that the genetic susceptibility to T1D is graded both within and among populations.

Environmental Factors

Environmental factors play a significant part in the etiology of T1D and have been implicated in both initiation and progression of β cell damage. The majority of evidence points to the effects of viruses and/or dietary factors as etiological agents.

Many viruses have been implicated in the pathogenesis of T1D; they may have a direct effect on β cells by infection and cell lysis, or alternatively they may act as triggers to the autoimmune process. Among the viruses that have been implicated in humans are coxsackie A, coxsackie B, rubella, cytomegalovirus, mumps, and Epstein-Barr viruses. The enteroviruses (Coxsackie A, Coxsackie B, and Echovirus) are the most commonly associated viruses with diabetes and serve as a major trigger for T1D in the young possibly by induction of islet cell antibodies. The evidence for viral involvement in type 1 diabetes came from several sources, including anecdotal case reports, epidemiological studies, seasonal incidence studies, and animal models. There is data to support the theory that enterovirus infection either accompanies or precedes the development of T1D in young people in many instances.

Coxsackie B was first implicated in the early 1970s by Gamble, who found an increased titer of coxsackie B antibodies in newly diagnosed T1D patients. More recently, coxsackie virus has been identified in very young onset type 1 diabetes (in patients under 5 years of age) using the polymerase chain reaction. Furthermore, when the coxsackie virus was sequenced, although it had extensive homology to coxsackie virus B4, there was some unique sequence variation indicating an T1D variant. There have also been many anecdotal reports of coxsackie B virus causing T1D, presumably by a direct cytolytic effect on β cells. A previously fit child died in diabetic ketoacidosis 3 days after a flu-like illness. At, necropsy, there was an extensive lymphocytic infiltration into the β cells of pancreas and coxsackie B4 was found in the child's serum. This virus was extracted from the pancreas and, when used to infect mice, led to diabetes.

There is a high incidence of T1D among patients with the congenital rubella syndrome. Clearly, this results from an *in utero* infection, but the diabetes that ensues is indistinguishable from the primary type 1 diabetes: the disease presents in the second decade of life, the onset is preceded by islet cell antibodies, and the genetic predisposition is defined by the same HLA association as T1D. This is likely to be a good example of a virus triggering the immune process.

Dietary factors have also been implicated in the development of T1D. Among the dietary factors indirectly linked to either susceptibility or protection to T1D are cows' milk protein (including bovine serum albumin and β-lactoglobulin), β-cell-toxic drugs (alloxan, streptozotocin, rodenticides), dietary toxins (in particular nitroso-containing compounds), and others such as coffee and sugar. There is an interesting interplay between vitamin D, vitamin D receptor (VDR), and association with T1D as discussed earlier. The contribution of vitamin D as a potent modulator of the immune system is well recognized. The main sources of vitamin D are ergocalciferol and cholecalciferol found in dietary sources and cholecalciferol produced in the skin by ultraviolet radiation of 7-dehydrocholesterol. Vitamin D deficiency in infancy and VDR polymorphisms may be risk factors for T1D. In nonobese diabetic (NOD) mice, long-term treatment with high doses of vitamin D_3 reduced the incidence of diabetes by changing the cytokine balance at the local pancreatic lesion.

The Future

The working out of the complete genetic basis of type 1 diabetes will lead to a better understanding of disease pathogenesis and, through studies of genetic and environmental interaction, direct evidence of environmental factors. T1D may be the first multifactorial disease to benefit from primary prevention of both insulitis (before immune process has been initiated) and of T1D (once autoantibodies have been detected). In the Diabetes Prevention Trial, low-dose insulin was administered to persons with high risk of T1D as ascertained by family history, islet antibodies, and HLA typing. It was concluded that low-dose insulin does not delay or prevent the onset of T1D. In a European study (European Nicotinamide Diabetes Intervention Trial, ENDIT) high-dose nicotinamide was used to protect the β cells in high-risk individuals for type 1 diabetes; unfortunately this trial also failed to show benefit on active treatment. However, 90% of type 1 diabetes patients do not have a family history of type 1 diabetes. The approach in this latter group might be to identify the genetically susceptible by the use of genetic markers and then test for autoantibodies. If the latter subjects are autoantibody positive then intervention may be considered in the future. The sensitivity and specificity that would be required for such sequential testing would depend on how safe the proposed intervention would be.

Type 2 Diabetes

Worldwide Prevalence

Type 2 diabetes is one of the most common noncommunicable diseases in the world with an estimated 147.2 million people suffering from this disorder; by 2010 this figure is expected to reach 212.9 million. Furthermore, it has been predicted that by the year 2010 over half the people with T2D will be living in Asia. This trend is likely to be due to increasing urbanization and industrialization. According to WHO estimates the figure is likely to double by the year 2025. The prevalence of T2D varies widely from the highest in Pima Indians (almost half of the population affected) to the lowest in Rural Africa (1%). As with T1D, the incidence of diabetes in different countries is likely to reflect the different genetic architecture as well as the differing environment. A good example is afforded by the population of Nauru. In full-blooded Nauruans over the age of 60 years the prevalence of T2D is 83%, whereas in those with genetic admixture as adduced by HLA typing the prevalence is 17%; this clearly reflects the genetic component. However, the rapid increase of T2D in the world in the last few decades, and the rise and a recent decrease in prevalence of T2D in the Nauruan community, can only be ascribed to environmental factors. This illustrates the multifactorial nature of T2D, with strong genetic and environmental contributions.

Etiology

Type 2 diabetes is a multifactorial disease with genetic and environmental factors playing a key role in its pathogenesis. Central to the etiology is a defect in insulin action, hepatic glucose output, and insulin secretion. Although insulin resistance is frequently the first detectable abnormality in the progression of T2D, insulin resistance by itself does not cause the disease, which is only manifested when there is a coexisting insulin secretory defect. T2D typically occurs in middle-aged and elderly people but there is an increasing trend of T2D occurring in young individuals. The main question yet to be answered is whether T2D is one disorder or a group of disorders with hyperglycemia as the end point in disease pathogenesis. Insulin resistance is common to several other disorders, including ischemic heart disease, hypertension, dyslipidemia, central obesity, and coagulation defects; the clustering of these disorders is known as the metabolic syndrome or the insulin resistance syndrome. The interface of T2D with obesity is a complex one, highlighted by the discovery of leptin and adiponectin. The cause of obesity and T2D in the ob mouse is a mutation of the *ob* gene. With administration of the ob gene protein (leptin) the ob mouse decreases its food consumption and increases exercise, leading to a dramatic weight loss; if given early enough it will also prevent diabetes. In contrast, common human obesity is associated with increased leptin levels, and which have been found to correlate with hyperinsulinemia. The newly discovered protein adiponectin signals adipose tissue mass; reduced levels are found in obese subjects and there is an important interplay between adiponectin, insulin resistance, T2D, and atherosclerosis. Ghrelin is a gut hormone that is a signal of satiety and therefore has a direct effect on obesity. In the obese subject with T2D, there may be interplay between leptin, adiponectin, ghrelin, and insulin, contributing to insulin resistance and the metabolic syndrome.

Genetics

Type 2 diabetes is a complex disease and the heterogeneity both at the phenotypic and pathophysiological level indicates that the genetic component is likely to be heterogeneous with no single locus accounting for the disease. There are many strands of evidence to support a strong genetic component to T2D; these include a near 100% concordance in identical twins, familial clustering, genetic admixture and migration studies, complex segregation analysis, and the detection of gene variants leading to diabetes including the identification of genes responsible for human monogenic diabetes (MODY – see below).

Many groups worldwide have completed the first stages of genome scans for genes that predispose an individual to T2D. Currently, a large international research effort is being directed to those diabetes-associated linkage peaks that are overlapping in several genome scans; specifically on chromosomes 1, 12, and 20. One genome scan has been taken to completion with the identification of the calpain10 gene (located to chromosome 2q37) as a major susceptibility gene in Mexican-Americans. The majority of subsequent studies have confirmed an association between calpain10 and T2D as well as insulin action, insulin secretion, endothelial function, and aspects of adipose metabolism. This putative diabetes susceptibility gene encodes a ubiquitously expressed member of the calpain-like cysteine protease family, calpain-10. Functional studies would suggest a role in insulin secretion, insulin action, and adipocyte metabolism. For instance, reduced levels of calpain10 have been found in skeletal muscle associated with disease-associated polymorphisms and inhibition of calpain affects insulin secretion and translocation of glucose transporter-4 in an adipocyte cell line.

A large number of candidate genes have been studied in T2D. Only a few have produced consistent results, i.e., the genes for the insulin receptor substrate-1, insulin, *KCNJ11*, peroxisome proliferator-activated receptor gamma (*PPARγ*), and are critically dependent on the power of individual studies. Insulin receptor substrate 1 (*IRS-1*) is a protein involved in insulin signaling. After insulin binds to its insulin receptor, it stimulates autophosphorylation of its β chain, which, in turn, leads to phosphorylation of several multisite insulin receptor substrate (*IRS*) docking proteins including *IRS-1*. This then generates one of the signals for insulin action. Several variants of *IRS-1* have been detected, one of which (due to the substitution of a glycine for arginine at position 972 (G972R) in the molecule) is associated with insulin resistance, but only in the presence of obesity. This is a good example of a gene variant that is common in the population (at least 8% in the white population) and will only lead to disease in association with other contributing factors for diabetes. Recently a meta-analysis has confirmed the role of the G972R variant in T2D with an odds ratio of 1.25.

KCNJ11 encodes *Kir6.2*, which is an essential subunit of the pancreatic β cell potassium ATP (K_{ATP}) channel. Rare mutations of this locus lead to the monogenic syndrome of familial hyperinsulinemia, confirming the important role of *KCNJ11* in insulin secretion. Although there are a large number of rare variants of the *KCNJ11* gene only one common variant (E23K) has been associated with T2D, although by no means consistently in all studies. It is likely that the studies mentioned above were underpowered as a meta-analysis, that additionally included a large new study, has demonstrated a significant odds ratio for T2D of 1.23. However, it should be borne in mind that the E23K variant does not change protein function and therefore it is unlikely to be the predisposing mutation.

The *PPARγ* gene is mainly expressed in adipose tissue and is the target of the thiazolidinedione class of drugs used to treat T2D by improving insulin action and secretion. In man, rare mutations of *PPARγ* are associated with a monogenic syndrome of severe insulin resistance, T2D, and hypertension. In contrast, a common amino acid polymorphism (Pro12Ala) in *PPARγ* has been shown to be associated with a increased risk of typical T2D, confirmed by a meta-analysis with an odds ratio for diabetes of 1.25 for the common proline allele. Furthermore, a gene nutrient interaction has been demonstrated with an important interaction of the Pro12Ala variant and the ratio of dietary polyunsaturated fat to saturated fat in the diet. *PPARγ* is a nuclear receptor, which upon activation stimulates the transcription of genes responsible for growth and differentiation of adipocytes. This clearly indicates a role for *PPARγ* in fat cell biology and pathophysiology of obesity, diabetes, and insulin resistance.

One of the first candidate genes to be studied in T2D was the insulin gene with an association described with the class 3 allele. As mentioned in the section on the genetics of T1D the insulin gene hypervariable region is a determinant of insulin secretion. Although consistent associations were found of the insulin gene and T1D, this was not the case for T2D. However, the earlier T2D studies were very much underpowered and the controls and patients not well matched. Using a family-based design the association between T2D and the class 3 allele has been confirmed demonstrating paternal but not maternal transmission. This is in keeping with the fact that the insulin/insulin growth factor II gene locus is maternally imprinted. In addition to the importance of adequately powered studies, the paternal transmission is likely to be another explanation for variable results in a case–control study design, emphasizing the importance of family-based designs as an additional strategy in association studies. The insulin/insulin growth factor II gene locus is a determinant of fetal and postnatal growth, which is also an important factor in susceptibility to T2D.

Environmental Factors

Evidence of a strong environmental element to T2D has come from the studies of Barker and Hales. In a number of separate studies, a strong relationship of the development of glucose intolerance and other associated factors of the insulin resistance syndrome with low birth weight or thinness at birth has been demonstrated. Furthermore, these associations are not confined to those with growth retardation *in utero* but extend to the whole range of birth weights. As a consequence of these epidemiologic studies, the 'thrifty phenotype' hypothesis has been proposed, whereby nutritional deficiencies *in utero* lead to poor fetal and infant growth and the subsequent development of T2D in later life, especially when combined with obesity due to excess food intake and lack of physical activity. These changes are recognized to be due to insulin resistance, which is favorable for survival in the immediate postnatal period but plays a significant role in the progression to T2D and metabolic syndrome, and to a certain extent insulin secretion. While there is much discussion regarding this hypothesis, it illustrates the importance of environmental factors in early life, which might prime the fetus for T2D in later life.

Dietary factors and physical inactivity undoubtedly affect the progression of abnormal glucose tolerance to diabetes in a genetically predisposed individual. The best way to lower the risk of diabetes is to lead a healthy life style by eating a healthy balanced diet, engaging in regular physical activity, and balancing the energy intake with energy expenditure. Indeed, recent evidence would suggest that the adoption of a healthy life style in high-risk subjects can decrease the risk of developing T2D by 60%. There is a close relationship between diabetes and obesity, especially when the latter has central distribution. Apart from obesity, several other nutritional factors affect glucose metabolism and the risk of T2D. Current evidence suggests an association between different types of fats and carbohydrates and insulin resistance and T2D. Diets rich in saturated fats are associated with insulin resistance; a multicentre study in a group of healthy individuals showed that a diet high in saturated fat decreased insulin sensitivity compared with a diet high in monounsaturated fat with the same total fat content. Prospective and cross-sectional studies suggest a role of specific types of fat rather than the total fat content in the development of T2D, where high intake of vegetable oils, oils consisting primarily of polyunsaturated fat, was associated with reduced risk of developing diabetes and a positive association between saturated fat and hyperglycemia or glucose intolerance. In a 20-year follow-up of the Finnish and Dutch cohorts of the Seven Countries Study, it was found that a high intake of fat (in particular saturated fatty acids) contributed to the risk of glucose intolerance and T2D. Dietary carbohydrates are classified into simple or complex carbohydrates depending on their chemical structure. The traditional view is that simple carbohydrates be avoided and substituted with complex (starchy) carbohydrates to reduce postprandial glucose response, but this has been challenged by various studies that recognized that starchy foods such as baked potatoes and white bread produce even higher glycemic responses than simple sugars. Glycemic index (GI) was developed to quantify the different glycemic responses induced by different carbohydrate foods. A low GI diet with a greater amount of fiber and minimally processed whole-grain products seems to improve glycemic and insulin responses and lowers the risk of T2D. This shows that dietary recommendations to prevent and manage diabetes should focus more on the quality of fat and carbohydrate than the quantity alone.

A number of environmental toxins have been shown to cause diabetes in humans, including nitrosated compounds, as well as streptozotocin, the rat poison Vacor, and foods such as smoked mutton; depending on the amount consumed they could lead to either T1D or T2D, presumably dependent on the amount of direct β cell destruction. It has also been proposed that vitamin D might modulate the diabetic process. Vitamin D deficiency has been shown to reduce insulin secretion. In a UK study of Bangladeshi subjects living in east London who were particularly prone to vitamin D deficiency, vitamin D levels were found to be low in those most at risk of diabetes. Furthermore, there was a correlation between vitamin D levels and 30 min oral glucose tolerance test, blood glucose, insulin, and C-peptide levels.

The Future

Research into the identification of genes involved in T2D is beginning to lead to insights into the pathogenesis of this common condition. With knowledge of the precise biochemical variants involved in disease pathogenesis, we will be in a better position to classify the disease and design more rational therapeutic maneuvers to prevent and ameliorate this condition. Research also needs to be directed at the gene–environment interaction, as this will indicate the appropriate population strategies to combat the increasing incidence of this common noncommunicable disease. Recently, life style interventions (healthy diet and exercise) have demonstrated significant reduction in onset of diabetes in high-risk individuals for T2D. In the future genetic profiling might be used to identify those likely to respond to such strategies including pharmacological treatment.

Other Types of Diabetes

Maturity Onset Diabetes of the Young (MODY)

MODY are a group of monogenic disorders inherited in an autosomal dominant pattern. MODY is characterized by early onset (usually before the age of 25 years) of T2D β cell dysfunction and there being a family history (at least two generations) of early onset diabetes. The defect is in insulin secretion due to mutations in the glucokinase and β cell transcription factor genes (**Table 2**). Hepatocyte nuclear factors *(HNF) 1α, 1β,* and *4α,* insulin promoter factor *(IPF1),* and neurogenic differentiation-1 *(NEUROD1)* play an important role in the normal development and function of the β cells of the pancreas. In the UK mutations in *HNF1α* is the commonest cause of MODY accounting for 63% of cases, followed by mutations in the glucokinase gene (20% of cases). The clinical presentation and progression of diabetes is

Table 2 Maturity onset diabetes of the young

MODY subgroup	Gene	Chromosome	MODY frequency
MODY1	HNF4α	20q	Rare
MODY2	GCK	7p	10–65%
MODY3	HNF1α	12q	20–75%
MODY4	IPF1	13q	Rare
MODY5	HNF1β	17q	Rare
MODY6	NEUROD1	2q	Rare

different among patients with mutations of glucokinase, *HNF1α,* and *HNF1β.* Subjects with glucokinase mutations are frequently asymptomatic but can be identified when diagnosed with gestational diabetes or with a milder form of diabetes, which is frequently treated with diet alone and is not associated with the complications of diabetes. In contrast subjects with *HNF1α* mutations are more like lean patients with T2D with susceptibility to microvascular complications and progressive loss of β cell function exacerbated by increasing body mass index. In comparison to patients with T2D, subjects with *HNF1α* mutations are very sensitive to sulfonylurea treatment as might be predicted from the genetic defect. Finally, patients with *HNF1β* mutations in addition to T2D have renal cysts that may lead to renal failure and hence such patients are more frequently found in the renal clinic.

Gestational Diabetes

Gestational diabetes (GDM) is defined as glucose intolerance first recognized in pregnancy. This therefore, excludes those women with either type 1 diabetes or type 2 diabetes diagnosed before conception. GDM is a relatively common occurrence in pregnancy affecting 1–14% in White European and North American populations and higher in certain ethnic groups such as South Asian and Afro-Caribbean populations.

GDM increases the risk to both mother and fetus although the levels of maternal glycemia that leads to an adverse outcome are not well defined. Furthermore, there is controversy as to who should be screened in pregnancy and the best available diagnostic test that has high sensitivity and specificity and the timing of the test during gestation. This is reflected in the lack of international agreement on diagnostic criteria ranging from the WHO critieria to a more pragmatic approach based on fasting and post prandial glucose levels. Those at particular risk for GDM are ethnic groups with a high prevalence of diabetes, women with a previous history of delivering large babies, a family history of diabetes, obesity, older women and multiparous women.

Pregnancy is associated with an increase in insulin resistance and an increase in hormones with actions opposing insulin (i.e. cortisol, progesterone, growth hormone and human placental lactogen). GDM develops at a time when the beta cell reserve cannot cope with the prevailing state of insulin resistance. Therefore by definition after pregnancy when the insulin resistance reduces, then the subject becomes normoglycemic. However, GDM can be considered a pre-diabetic condition with an increased future risk of developing type 2 diabetes during their lifetime approaching 20–50%. The treatment of GDM consists of maintaining strict glycemic control. If dietary intervention fails to achieve normoglycemia, the treatment of choice is insulin.

The maternal risk due to GDM include increased risks in pregnancy, accelerated fetal growth leading to macrosomia and increased rates of caesarian section. The fetal risks include stillbirth, congenital malformations, shoulder dystocia, birth trauma and the risk of neonatal hypoglycemia and calcium and bilirubin disturbances in the neonatal period. There is also an increased risk of the child subsequently becoming obese and developing diabetes in adult life as a result of *in utero* hyperglycemia.

Fibrocalculous Pancreatic Diabetes

In tropical countries there is a form of nonalcoholic chronic pancreatitis characterized by pancreatic exocrine and endocrine insufficiency and associated with pancreatic calcification. This disease, tropical calcific pancreatitis, affects young individuals who are malnourished and present with abdominal pain, extreme emaciation characteristic of protein-energy malnutrition, glucose intolerance, and at a later stage diabetes. The diabetic stage of the illness is referred to as fibrocalcific pancreatic diabetes (FCPD). Several reports of FCPD have been reported from the tropical countries and many cases have been reported from the Indian subcontinent. The pathogenesis of the disease is still unclear and is attributed to various possible causes – malnutrition, cassava toxicity, oxidant stress due to micronutrient deficiency, genetic and environmental factors. Recently, a study showed the N34S variant of the *SPINK1* trypsin inhibitor gene as a susceptibility gene for FCPD in the Indian subcontinent. Although by itself it is not sufficient to cause FCPD, it indicates the role of gene–environment interaction in the pathogenesis of diabetes.

Patients with FCPD are at risk of long-term diabetic complications and require insulin to control their hyperglycemia. Given the underlying problem of malnutrition they benefit from high calorie intake, especially the protein content. There is a need for further investigation into the roles of nutritional, environmental, and genetic factors to establish the etiopathogenesis of this illness.

See also: **Diabetes Mellitus**: Classification and Chemical Pathology; Dietary Management. **Glucose**: Metabolism and Maintenance of Blood Glucose Level. **Obesity**: Complications. **World Health Organization**.

Further Reading

Altshuler D, Hirschhorn JN, Klannemark M *et al.* (2000) The common PPARgamma Pro12Ala polymorphism is associated with decreased risk of type 2 diabetes. *Nature Genetics* **26**: 76–80.

Amos AF, McCarty DJ, and Zimmet P (1997) The rising global burden of diabetes and its complications: estimates and projections to the year 2010. *Diabetes in Medicine* **14**(supplement) 5: S1–85.

Feskens EJ, Virtanen SM, Rasanen L *et al.* (1995) Dietary factors determining diabetes and impaired glucose tolerance. A 20-year follow-up of the Finnish and Dutch cohorts of the Seven Countries Study. *Diabetes Care* **18**: 1104–1112.

Forrest JM, Menser MA, and Harley JD (1969) Diabetes mellitus and congenital rubella. *Pediatrics* **44**: 445–447.

Frayling TM, Evans JC, Bulman MP *et al.* (2001) beta-cell genes and diabetes: molecular and clinical characterization of mutations in transcription factors. *Diabetes* **50**(supplement 1): S94–100.

Gloyn AL, Weedon MN, Owen KR *et al.* (2003) Large-scale association studies of variants in genes encoding the pancreatic beta-cell KATP channel subunits Kir6.2 (KCNJ11) and SUR1 (ABCC8) confirm that the KCNJ11 E23K variant is associated with type 2 diabetes. *Diabetes* **52**: 568–572.

Hales CN and Barker DJ (1992) Type 2 (non-insulin-dependent) diabetes mellitus: the thrifty phenotype hypothesis. *Diabetologia* **35**: 595–601.

Hassan Z, Mohan V, Ali L *et al.* (2002) SPINK1 is a susceptibility gene for fibrocalculous pancreatic diabetes in subjects from the Indian subcontinent. *American Journal of Humam Genetics* **71**: 964–968.

Horikawa Y, Oda N, Cox NJ *et al.* (2000) Genetic variation in the gene encoding calpain-10 is associated with type 2 diabetes mellitus. *Nature Genetics* **26**: 163–175.

Hyoty H and Taylor KW (2002) The role of viruses in human diabetes. *Diabetologia* **45**: 1353–1361.

Mohan V, Premalatha G, and Pitchumoni CS (2003) Tropical chronic pancreatitis: an update. *Journal of Clinical Gastroenterology* **36**: 337–346.

Pociot F and McDermott MF (2002) Genetics of type 1 diabetes mellitus. *Genes and Immunology* **3**: 235–249.

Ramachandran A, Snehalatha C, Kapur A *et al.* (2001) High prevalence of diabetes and impaired glucose tolerance in India: National Urban Diabetes Survey. *Diabetologia* **44**: 1094–1101.

Tuomilehto J and Lindstrom J (2003) The major diabetes prevention trials. *Current Diabetes Reports* **3**: 115–122.

Zimmet P, Alberti KG, and Shaw J (2001) Global and societal implications of the diabetes epidemic. *Nature* **414**: 782–787.

Classification and Chemical Pathology

K C McCowen, Beth Israel Deaconess Medical Center and Harvard Medical School, Boston, MA, USA
R J Smith, Brown Medical School, Providence, RI, USA

© 2005 Elsevier Ltd. All rights reserved.

Diabetes mellitus is a common, serious metabolic disorder with diverse causes and multiple complications. In this article, the definition and classification are discussed and diagnostic criteria outlined. Subsequently, an overview of the physiology of normal blood glucose homeostasis and normal insulin action leads to consideration of the pathophysiologic events that occur in uncontrolled diabetes.

Definition

Diabetes mellitus is a chronic disorder that results from a deficiency of the hormone insulin. This occurs either because of an absolute decrease in the amount of insulin produced by the β cells of the islets of Langerhans in the pancreas or because of a relative deficiency of insulin in patients whose tissues are resistant to the hormone. The hallmark of untreated diabetes mellitus is elevated blood glucose concentrations. Frequently, there are associated disturbances of fat and protein metabolism. In addition to reversible acute metabolic abnormalities resulting from inadequate effects of insulin, long-term diabetes is often characterized by the development of irreversible complications that include damage to the kidney, retina, nervous system, and both large and small blood vessels.

The diagnosis of diabetes mellitus is based on the existence of hyperglycemia alone and does not require the presence of any of the associated metabolic or systemic complications. Although patients with diabetes mellitus exhibit a characteristic pattern of metabolic abnormalities and long-term complications, this disease state results from multiple underlying causes that include genetic as well as environmental influences and also certain pancreatic or hormonal conditions.

Diagnostic Criteria

Random Plasma Glucose Determination

In the presence of symptoms of hyperglycemia, a random plasma glucose >11.1 mmol/l is consistent with a diagnosis of diabetes in an ambulatory patient. Classic symptoms of hyperglycemia include thirst, polydipsia, polyuria, and unexplained weight loss.

Fasting Plasma Glucose Determination

Nondiabetic individuals have fasting plasma glucose levels below 5.6 mmol/l. The diagnosis of diabetes mellitus can be made when fasting plasma glucose levels are significantly elevated (>7.0 mmol/l) on at least two occasions. Fasting glucose below 7.0 mmol/l but above 5.6 mmol/l, although not normal, does not meet the criteria for definite diagnosis and is classified as impaired fasting glucose. Although not absolutely predictive of diabetes, individuals with impaired fasting glucose progress to overt diabetes at a rate of approximately 5% per year. Plasma or serum measurements are generally more reliable than whole blood glucose determinations (in which the normal range is lower) because they are independent of the hematocrit and are appropriate for accurate, automated analysis. For accurate measurement, blood samples must be put into tubes containing sodium fluoride (which prevents glycolysis) or be centrifuged within 30 min to remove cells. Fasting plasma glucose is considered the desired method to diagnose diabetes because of its simplicity and reproducibility.

Oral Glucose Tolerance Test

In the absence of an obvious elevation in fasting or random plasma glucose levels, the diagnosis of diabetes mellitus can be made with an oral glucose tolerance test (OGTT). This involves, for the nonpregnant adult, the ingestion of a solution containing 75 g of glucose over 5 min, with a measurement of baseline and 2-h plasma glucose. The criteria used to diagnose diabetes are listed in **Table 1**. The diagnosis can be made if the fasting glucose exceeds 7.0 mmol/l or the 2-h value exceeds 11.1 mmol/l. People with impaired glucose tolerance have normal fasting values but 2-h post-glucose load values above 7.8 mmol/l.

Table 1 Oral glucose tolerance test criteria for diabetes in nonpregnant adults (75 g glucose load)

	Venous plasma glucose (mmol/l)
Diabetes	
Fasting	>7.0
2-h	>11.1
Impaired glucose tolerance	
2-h	7.8–11.1
Impaired fasting glucose	
Fasting	5.6–6.9
2-h	<7.8

The standard OGTT must be performed under certain conditions for the previous thresholds to apply. Subjects need to ingest at least 200 g carbohydrates per day during the 3 days preceding the test, fast overnight (>8 h), not smoke on the day of the test, and have the test performed in the morning. Because glucose tolerance is reduced by bed rest and stressors such as recent surgery or burn injury, subjects must be ambulatory and have been so for at least 1 month prior to the test. Despite this standardization, results are not always precisely reproducible, even in the same person, which may relate in part to variable rates of absorption of glucose from the small intestine. For this reason, elevated fasting glucose is a more reliable diagnostic criterion. In children, if an OGTT is performed, the amount of glucose to be ingested should be determined by body weight (i.e., 1.75 g/kg ideal body weight).

Controversy has existed with regard to proper methods of diagnosis of diabetes in pregnancy. The National Diabetes Data Group (NDDG) of the National Institutes of Health recommends screening between 24 and 28 weeks with a 50 g oral glucose load test. No special preparations are required for this test, and fasting is unnecessary. Blood glucose is measured once only, after 1 h. Women with values above 7.8 mmol/l are evaluated with a full OGTT with a glucose load of 100 g. Clearly, use of a lower threshold (e.g., 7.2 mmol/l) minimizes the occurrence of false-negative tests. Opponents of the use of a lower threshold note that only the milder cases of diabetes in pregnancy are missed using the 7.8 mmol/l criteria to proceed to full OGTT. The NDDG criteria for diagnosis are listed in **Table 2**. The original data used in the determination of normal plasma glucose values during pregnancy have been reevaluated taking into account changes in the methodology for glucose measurement, which led to the American Diabetes Association using even lower threshold values on the 100 g OGTT to diagnose diabetes (**Table 2**, revised criteria). Controversy exists as to which set of values should be used, and cost-effectiveness evaluations of the different criteria are pending.

Table 2 Criteria for the diagnosis of gestational diabetes (100 g glucose load)

	Venous plasma glucose (mmol/l)	
	National Diabetes Data Group	Modified criteria
Fasting	>5.8	>5.3
1 h	>10.6	>10.0
2 h	>9.2	>8.6
3 h	>8.1	>7.8

The World Health Organization proposes that the test and criteria for gestational diabetes should be the same as for nonpregnant adults, with the exception that individuals fitting the category of impaired glucose tolerance be treated the same as diabetics because of the potentially harmful effects of hyperglycemia on the fetus.

Glycosuria

Glycosuria may indicate the presence of diabetes, but it is not diagnostic, nor does the absence of glycosuria exclude diabetes. In individuals with a low renal threshold, glucose may be present in the urine in the absence of hyperglycemia. Such "renal glycosuria" is particularly common during the later stages of pregnancy and in some renal tubular disorders. The excretion of other sugars, such as lactose (more common during pregnancy) or fructose, galactose, or xylose (people with inborn errors of metabolism), can yield false-positive results through cross-reactivity in the testing method unless glucose-specific test strips are used. In patients with compromised renal perfusion or function, glycosuria may be absent despite significant hyperglycemia.

Glycosylated Hemoglobin

Glycohemoglobin is formed when a ketoamine reaction occurs between glucose and the N-terminal amino acid of the β chain of hemoglobin. The amount of glycohemoglobin generated is proportional to the mean blood glucose during the 8–10 weeks before the test. Thus, the glycohemoglobin level is a useful indicator of long-term blood glucose control. This is not a useful test for diagnosing diabetes, however, since the normal range is broad, the test is not well standardized between laboratories, and it can be affected by conditions that alter the life span of the red blood cell.

Classification

A new classification system for diabetes mellitus was developed in 1997, which divides patients into four major groups and a number of subgroups, as shown in **Table 3**. It is probable that these categories will be further refined as knowledge of the underlying etiologies of various forms of diabetes progresses.

I. Type 1 Diabetes Mellitus

This form of diabetes is defined by insulin deficiency due to destruction of the β cells of the pancreas. It was formerly designated "insulin-dependent diabetes," but efforts are being made to eliminate this name because many patients with other types of

Table 3 Classification of diabetes mellitus[a]

I. Type 1 diabetes (formerly designated insulin-dependent diabetes)
  A. Autoimmune
  B. Idiopathic
II. Type 2 diabetes (formerly designated non-insulin-dependent diabetes)
III. Secondary diabetes
  A. Genetic defects of β cell function (e.g., maturity onset diabetes of youth)
  B. Genetic defects of insulin action pathway
  C. Exocrine pancreatic disease
  D. Endocrinopathies (e.g., Cushing's syndrome and acromegaly)
  E. Drugs or chemicals
  F. Infections (e.g., congenital rubella)
  G. Other genetic syndromes (e.g., Down's and Klinefelter's syndromes)
IV. Gestational diabetes

[a]Classification proposed by the Expert Committee on the Diagnosis and the Classification of Diabetes Mellitus under the sponsorship of the American Diabetes Association (*Diabetes Care* **27**: S5–S10, 2004).

diabetes also require insulin for adequate control. The predominant cause is believed to be an autoimmune attack against the insulin-producing β cells within the islets of Langerhans (diabetes type 1A). At the time of diagnosis, most patients demonstrate antibodies to certain pancreatic autoantigens, which include antibodies to islet cell cytoplasmic components, glutamic acid decarboxylase, insulin, and tyrosine phosphatases IA-2 and IA-2β. Such autoantibodies, when present, help to confirm the diagnosis. This disease also has strong HLA antigen associations, which may either predispose to or protect from the development of diabetes. In a minor subset of patients classified as idiopathic type 1 diabetes (type 1B), the presentation and clinical course is similar to autoimmune type 1A diabetes, but all tests for autoimmune markers are negative.

Early diagnosis of autoimmune diabetes Type 1 diabetes has a variable presymptomatic phase that may extend for several years, during which time it is possible to make a diagnosis. This form of diagnostic testing is reserved for research purposes because the disease is not sufficiently common to warrant widespread screening strategies and because practical methods for preventing the progression to overt diabetes are not available. Because type 1 diabetes is occasionally familial, screening of individuals with strong family histories can be performed by measuring levels of the specific pancreatic autoantigens described previously; subjects with high titers of antibodies who possess unfavorable HLA subtypes,

indicating significant risk of later development of diabetes, may then undergo intravenous glucose tolerance testing with quantitation of the insulin response. Diminution of the early phases of insulin release can be seen even years before the onset of symptoms of disease. Currently, such diagnosis is important only to enable participation in clinical trials of diabetes prevention.

II. Type 2 Diabetes Mellitus

This is a heterogeneous disorder in which there is both resistance to the action of insulin and relative insulin insufficiency. In contrast to type 1 diabetes, endogenous insulin secretion is at least partially preserved and thus most patients are not insulin dependent for acute survival (hence the former name, non-insulin-dependent diabetes). The circulating insulin levels are adequate to protect these patients from ketosis, except during periods of extreme stress. Some patients in this category can be treated with oral agents (sulfonylureas, metformin, and thiazolidinediones), but many are managed with insulin because their pancreases are unable to produce sufficient insulin to overcome their tissue insulin resistance. Obesity is a frequent contributing factor to the insulin resistance in this disorder.

Occasionally, it is difficult to determine whether a patient has type 1 or type 2 diabetes. This is particularly likely in a nonobese person older than 35 years of age who has never had significant ketosis but who has been treated with insulin. Unfortunately, there is no completely reliable diagnostic test. Measurement of autoantibodies in such people may not be helpful because patients with type 1 diabetes lose these markers with time. Several studies have shown that the plasma C-peptide level is a good discriminator between the two forms of diabetes. C-peptide is released during processing of proinsulin to insulin and, thus, is an indicator of endogenous insulin secretion. Values higher than 0.6 nmol/l, either basal or following provocation with a 1 mg glucagon stimulus, indicate sufficient residual insulin secretion for a person to be considered in the type 2 diabetes class.

III. Secondary Diabetes Mellitus/Other Specific Types

This broad category includes multiple disorders that are associated with either extensive pancreatic destruction or significant insulin resistance. Secondary diabetes as a consequence of decreased insulin production can occur following pancreatectomy, chronic pancreatitis, cystic fibrosis, or hemochromatosis. In the absence of pancreatic damage, secondary diabetes can result from extreme insulin resistance induced by glucocorticoids (Cushing's syndrome); growth hormone (acromegaly); adrenergic hormones (pheochromocytoma); other medical conditions, such as uremia, hepatic cirrhosis, or polycystic ovary syndrome; or medications (diuretics or exogenous glucocorticoids).

Included in this category of secondary diabetes are patients who appear to have type 2 diabetes but in whom monogenic molecular defects in either the glucose-sensing or insulin action pathways have been defined. The best established molecular defects are mutations in the gene coding for the enzyme glucokinase, which has a role in the sensing of glucose by the β cell. Individuals with this autosomal dominant condition usually develop mild diabetes in early adulthood or adolescence. Hence, the condition is known as maturity onset diabetes of the young (MODY). Several other types of MODY have been defined, due to gene defects in β cell transcription factors. Rare causes of diabetes secondary to insulin resistance include various inborn errors of metabolism (e.g., insulin receptor mutations or type 1 glycogen storage disease), chromosomal abnormalities such as Down's and Turner's syndrome, and muscle diseases (e.g., myotonic dystrophy).

IV. Gestational Diabetes Mellitus

This disorder, which is defined as hyperglycemia first detected during pregnancy, occurs in 2–5% of pregnant women. Often, one cannot determine whether glucose intolerance antedated the pregnancy or whether hyperglycemia was provoked by the hormonal milieu associated with pregnancy. Hyperglycemia remits postpartum in 90% of women with gestational diabetes, but these women are at increased risk for subsequent development of diabetes, which is usually type 2. Although most cases of this form of diabetes are detected by blood glucose screening performed as a routine procedure early in the third trimester, the current recommendation is that universal screening is probably unwarranted. A woman younger than age 25 years, of normal body weight, without a family history of diabetes or a personal history of poor pregnancy outcome, and from an ethnic group with low rates of diabetes is at sufficiently low risk of gestational diabetes that glucose testing can be omitted. In contrast, women with clinical features associated with a high risk of gestational diabetes (obesity, positive family history, persistent glycosuria, and prior gestational diabetes) should be screened as early in the pregnancy as is feasible.

In women who have documented gestational diabetes, a follow-up glucose tolerance test should be performed 6 weeks postpartum unless overt diabetes is evident.

Other Abnormalities of Glucose Tolerance

Impaired glucose tolerance This is a condition defined by oral glucose tolerance testing and includes nonpregnant individuals with normal fasting blood glucose but modestly elevated postprandial glucose. People with impaired glucose tolerance are at a high risk for subsequent development of diabetes, usually type 2 (approximately 5% per year). Thus, impaired glucose tolerance is a stage in the evolution of diabetes. Until overt diabetes develops, people with impaired glucose tolerance are not believed to have elevated risk of microvascular complications of diabetes. However, impaired glucose tolerance is associated with an increased risk of cardiovascular disease.

Impaired fasting glucose Some patients will have abnormal elevations in fasting plasma glucose, even though 2 h post-glucose challenge values are normal. These people are also at increased risk of developing diabetes, although diabetes incidence rates are highly variable between different populations. Fasting glucose is defined as impaired in the range 5.6–7.0 mM. Until recently, impaired fasting glucose was defined as 6.1–7.0 mM, and the change was recommended by the American Diabetes Association to align better with the category of impaired glucose tolerance discussed previously. However, people in this category who have normal postprandial glycemia, or normal 2-h post-challenge glucose values, have a lower risk of cardiovascular disease than people with impaired glucose tolerance.

Stress hyperglycemia This denotes an individual who is frankly hyperglycemic (>7.8 mmol/l) under conditions of intercurrent illness or during treatment with medications that provoke diabetes. Such people may revert to normal glucose tolerance following removal of the stress. Although not an official category of diabetes, such abnormal glucose values in hospitalized patients cannot be ignored since there is strong evidence that treatment to normoglycemia significantly lowers mortality, at least for patients with acute myocardial infarction or with critical illness in an intensive care unit. Precipitants of stress hyperglycemia are listed in **Table 4**.

Table 4 Risk factors for the development of stress hyperglycemia in critical illness

Factor	Major mechanism
Preexisting diabetes mellitus	Insulin deficiency (relative or absolute)
Infusion of catecholamine pressors	Insulin resistance
Glucocorticoid therapy	Insulin resistance
Obesity	Insulin resistance
Increasing APACHE score	Higher counterregulatory hormone levels
Older age	Insulin deficiency
Excessive dextrose administration	Glucose removal rates overwhelmed in the face of ongoing hepatic glucose production
Pancreatitis (acute and chronic)	Insulin deficiency
Sepsis	Insulin resistance
Hypothermia	Insulin deficiency
Hypoxemia	Insulin deficiency
Uremia	Insulin resistance
Cirrhosis	Insulin resistance

APACHE, Acute Physiology and Chronic Health Evaluation.

Pathophysiology of Diabetes

Physiology of Normal Blood Glucose Regulation

The metabolic fate of ingested glucose is determined by the interplay of multiple hormones. Insulin is of major importance in this homeostasis, but glucagon, glucocorticoids, catecholamines, and growth hormone also have significant effects that are interactive with insulin. Glucose ingested with a meal or derived from the digestion of other dietary carbohydrates is rapidly absorbed by the small intestine. It is carried first to the liver by the portal vein, where a substantial portion (30–70%) is removed; the remainder enters the peripheral circulation, where regulated insulin secretion and target tissue responses to insulin contribute to glucose clearance and control of blood glucose levels (**Figure 1**).

Following a meal, insulin is secreted from pancreatic β cells in response to increased circulating glucose concentrations. This direct effect of glucose on β cells is augmented by neural (vagal) and hormonal factors of intestinal origin (e.g., glucose-dependent insulinotropic peptide, cholecystokinin, and glucagon-like peptide 1), such that the insulin secretory response to oral glucose greatly exceeds the response to an equivalent intravenous glucose infusion.

The overall effect of the increase in insulin levels in parallel with increased glucose entry to the circulation is promotion of the net removal of glucose by the liver and stimulation of glucose transport into muscle and adipose tissue, where it is consumed as a metabolic fuel or stored. Insulin also inhibits the catabolism of the alternative energy sources, fat and protein. This is an appropriate response to the abundance of circulating nutrients that occurs after meals. During fasting, insulin levels are low, these processes are reversed, and stored fuel is made available to all tissues.

Liver Glucose enters the liver by facilitated (carrier-mediated) diffusion driven by the concentration gradient that exists in the fed state. A portion of the glucose taken up by the liver is metabolized via glycolytic pathways to produce ATP. A substantial amount is transformed into glycogen and stored. The maximal storage capacity of the liver is approximately 100 g glycogen (400 kcal). The specific molecular effects of insulin in the fed state lead to altered activities of enzymes that trap glucose inside the hepatocyte, promote glycolysis, and enhance glycogen synthesis (**Figure 1**). Insulin also inhibits enzymes important for both glycogenolysis and gluconeogenesis and thus shuts off hepatic glucose production. A portion of the glucose entering the liver is converted into triglyceride and exported to the adipocyte for storage.

Skeletal muscle In skeletal muscle, insulin directly stimulates glucose uptake, which is the rate-limiting step for muscle clearance of glucose. This appears to occur predominantly by causing the rapid translocation of glucose transporters (in particular the Glut-4 transporter) from an as yet undefined intracellular site to the muscle cell surface. Insulin also stimulates glycolysis and the net formation of glycogen in muscle. Even at low insulin concentrations, however, a rise in ambient glucose stimulates substantial glucose clearance by muscle, probably via the Glut-1 transporter. Glycogen stores in muscle (500–600 g glycogen in a 70 kg human) serve as a rapidly mobilized energy source during exercise but do not directly support blood glucose concentrations in the fasted state because muscle lacks the enzyme glucose-6-phosphatase, which is needed for release of free glucose to the circulation. Insulin-stimulated amino acid entry into muscle enhances insulin stimulatory effects on protein synthesis and decreases the availability of circulating amino acids as substrates for hepatic gluconeogenesis. Muscle proteolysis, which yields amino acid precursors that contribute to hepatic gluconeogenesis in the fasted state, is inhibited by insulin.

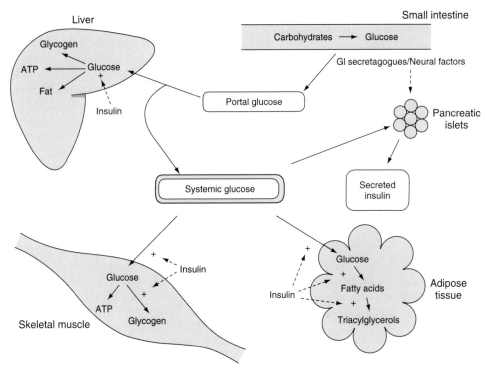

Figure 1 Insulin effects on glucose homeostasis in the fed state.

Adipose tissue In adipose tissue, insulin stimulates glucose uptake via the Glut-4 transporter, providing substrate for energy generation and glycerol synthesis. Even more important effects of insulin in adipose tissue are inhibition of lipolysis and stimulation of FFA uptake and triglyceride synthesis. This limits the availability of fat-derived fuels for other tissues and indirectly contributes to the lowering of blood glucose by favoring glucose utilization in multiple tissues.

From this brief overview, it can be seen that the rise in insulin following a meal has multiple tissue-specific actions that serve to lower blood glucose, prevent hyperglycemia, and inhibit the mobilization of alternative metabolic fuels. Many of the metabolic abnormalities that develop acutely in uncontrolled diabetes can be explained by the loss of these actions of insulin.

Pathophysiology of Uncontrolled Diabetes

Uncontrolled diabetes mellitus occurs when circulating insulin levels are inadequate to lower elevated blood glucose concentrations. This condition includes a spectrum of metabolic abnormalities that range from the effects of mild insulin deficiency (i.e., hyperglycemia) to the effects of marked and prolonged insulinopenia (i.e., ketoacidosis and fluid and electrolyte depletion). Diabetic ketoacidosis,

which is the most severe acute manifestation of insulin deficiency, is almost entirely restricted to patients with type 1 diabetes, or those with severe pancreatic disease of other etiologies. In people without absolute insulin deficiency, although the combination of significant insulin resistance and relatively low levels of insulin can result in significant hyperglycemia, ketone body production sufficient to cause ketosis and metabolic acidosis does not occur. Even low levels of insulin, such as are typically present in type 2 diabetes, suffice to restrain lipolysis and limit the availability of free fatty acid precursors for ketone body formation. Otherwise, many of the derangements seen in uncontrolled diabetes are common to all forms of diabetes.

The pathophysiologic events that affect blood glucose levels in states of mild-to-moderate insulin deficiency are classified into two broad categories. First, the normal pathways for glucose clearance after a meal are ineffective; second, body fuel stores are broken down with release of other substrates that lead to inappropriate synthesis of more glucose. These events are brought about by insulinopenia and often are further promoted by the relative abundance of the counterregulatory hormones, glucagon, catecholamines, and, to a lesser extent, cortisol and growth hormone. In addition, hyperglycemia further inhibits pancreatic β cell insulin secretion, compounding the problem ("glucose toxicity").

Following the ingestion of a meal, a substantial portion of the glucose absorbed into the portal circulation is removed by the liver, where it is stored as glycogen, converted to lipid, or consumed via energy-generating pathways. Each of these processes is decreased by insulin deficiency, resulting in increased entry of absorbed glucose to the systemic circulation. Skeletal muscle represents the main tissue site for removal of circulating blood glucose following a meal. In diabetes, insulin deficiency leads to a marked decrease in activity of the Glut-4 glucose transporter largely as a consequence of decreased insulin-stimulated Glut-4 localization to the surface membranes. This decreases the normal postmeal flux of glucose into skeletal muscle. In addition, glucose that does enter muscle is metabolized inefficiently in the absence of insulin. Other insulin-sensitive tissues, such as adipose tissue and myocardium, are affected in a similar manner, with consequent reduction in both glucose uptake and metabolism, although their contribution to glucose clearance is quantitatively less than that of muscle.

In postabsorptive or fasted states, hyperglycemia in uncontrolled diabetes does not resolve and often worsens (**Figure 2**). Abnormally low insulin concentrations lead to an exaggeration of metabolic responses that normally serve to protect against the development of hypoglycemia during fasting. These responses to low insulin and elevated counterregulatory hormones include, initially, the conversion of stored glycogen to glucose. Simultaneously, the hepatic enzymes involved in gluconeogenesis are activated, which results in glucose production from such carbon sources as lactate and pyruvate (by-products of muscle glycolysis), amino acids (from muscle protein breakdown), and glycerol (derived from adipocyte triglyceride stores). With persistent insulin deficiency, glycogen stores are depleted, and hepatic gluconeogenesis becomes the most important contributor to the increasing hyperglycemia. Meanwhile, body stores of protein and fat are being depleted in the futile synthesis of new glucose that cannot be used efficiently and serves to aggravate the existing hyperglycemia.

Excessive glucose accumulation in the circulation and in the extracellular space leads to the movement of water out of cells to maintain osmotic balance, causing intracellular dehydration. The high filtered load of glucose at the renal glomerulus overwhelms the reabsorptive capacity of the renal tubule, and an osmotic diuresis results. Ultimately, this leads not only to water loss along with the glucose but also to excess excretion of potassium, sodium, magnesium, calcium, and phosphate in the urine. The magnitude of the total body electrolyte loss depends on the duration and severity of the hyperglycemia.

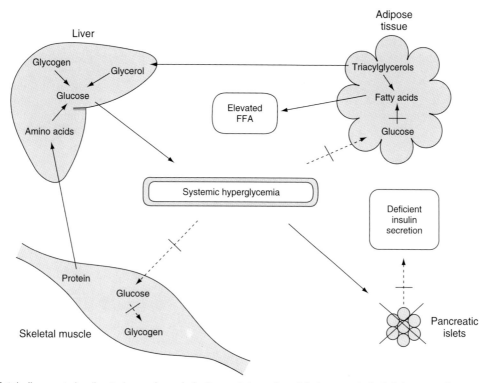

Figure 2 Metabolic events leading to hyperglycemia in the postabsorptive state in uncontrolled diabetes mellitus.

The main symptoms with moderate insulin deficiency are polyuria and consequent thirst and polydipsia. With more severe and prolonged insulin deficiency, loss of large quantities of glucose in the urine can lead to weight loss. If hyperosmolarity is not compensated by an adequate increase in water intake, patients can develop altered mental status and obtundation. In elderly patients with type 2 diabetes, this sequence can lead to the life-threatening state of nonketotic hyperosmolar coma.

In type 1 diabetes, the clinical picture of poor control differs from that described previously in that insulin deficiency is more severe (**Figure 3**). Glucose uptake by muscle is diminished, and glucose production by the liver is augmented. Marked insulinopenia, however, also leads to rapid, uncontrolled lipolysis. Triglyceride breakdown results in accelerated release of free fatty acids and glycerol. The increased delivery of glycerol from adipose tissue to the liver further promotes hepatic gluconeogenesis. In the absence of insulin, the liberated free fatty acids are taken up by the liver and converted at an accelerated rate to ketone bodies (β-hydroxybutyric acid, acetoacetic acid, and acetone).

In the fasting state in nondiabetic individuals, ketone bodies are metabolized under the influence of even low levels of insulin as a source of energy, particularly in skeletal and cardiac muscle. In extreme insulin deficiency states, ketone body utilization is inhibited at the same time that synthesis is increased. With increasing duration of insulinopenia, the ketoacid levels in the bloodstream rise. Ketones, like glucose, spill into the urine, either as free acids or, depending on the pH, as sodium or potassium salts, worsening the osmotic diuresis and electrolyte deficiency. Eventually, the blood buffering capacity for acid is overwhelmed and systemic acidemia occurs. Acidemia has a deleterious effect on all cell membranes and many cellular functions and, when severe, can cause arrhythmias, cardiac depression, and vascular collapse. In combination with the previously described hyperosmolarity and dehydration, diabetic ketoacidosis is a life-threatening situation.

In summary, poor control can lead to dangerous metabolic consequences and, occasionally, death. A primary goal of therapy is insulin replacement, which is needed to reverse the production of glucose and ketoacids by the liver, to promote muscle glucose and ketone body uptake, and to inhibit further breakdown of fat and protein. An equally important goal of therapy should be the replenishment of lost extracellular and intracellular fluids and electrolytes.

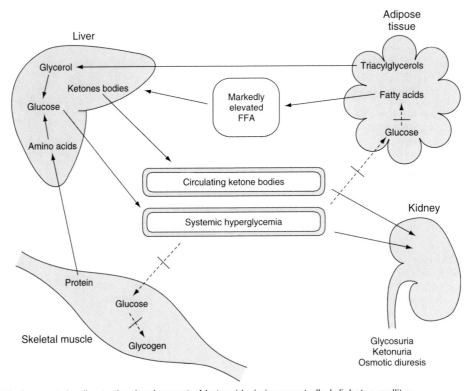

Figure 3 Metabolic events leading to the development of ketoacidosis in uncontrolled diabetes mellitus.

See also: **Diabetes Mellitus**: Etiology and Epidemiology; Dietary Management. **Glucose**: Chemistry and Dietary Sources; Metabolism and Maintenance of Blood Glucose Level; Glucose Tolerance. **Liver Disorders**.

Further Reading

Arner P (1996) Regulation of lipolysis in fat cells. *Diabetes Reviews* 4: 450–463.

Coustan DR and Carpenter MW (1998) The diagnosis of gestational diabetes. *Diabetes Care* 21(supplement 2): B5–B8.

Deerochanawong C, Putiyaun C, Wongsuryat M, Serirat S, and Jinayon P (1996) Comparison of National Diabetes Data Group and World Health Organization criteria for detecting gestational diabetes mellitus. *Diabetologia* 39: 1070–1073.

Delaney MF, Zisman A, and Kettyle WM (2000) Diabetic keto-acidosis and hyperglycemic hyperosmolar nonketotic syndrome. *Endocrinology and Metabolism Clinics of North America* 29(4): 683–705.

Dinneen S, Gerich J, and Rizza R (1992) Carbohydrate metabolism in non-insulin-dependent diabetes mellitus. *New England Journal of Medicine* 327: 707–713.

Expert Committee on the Diagnosis and Classification of Diabetes Mellitus (1997) Report of the Expert Committee on the Diagnosis and Classification of Diabetes Mellitus. *Diabetes Care* 20: 1183–1197.

Expert Committee on the Diagnosis and Classification of Diabetes Mellitus (2003) Follow up report on the diagnosis of diabetes mellitus. *Diabetes Care* 26: 3160–3167.

Foster DW and McGarry JD (1983) The metabolic derangements and treatment of diabetic ketoacidosis. *New England Journal of Medicine* 309: 159–169.

Genuth S, Alberti KG, Bennett P *et al.* Expert Committee on the Diagnosis and Classification of Diabetes Mellitus (2003) Follow-up report on the diagnosis of diabetes mellitus. *Diabetes Care* 26(11): 3160–3167.

Kuzuya T and Matsuda A (1997) Classification of diabetes on the basis of etiologies versus degree of insulin deficiency. *Diabetes Care* 20: 219–220.

Malmberg K, Ryden L, Efendic S *et al.* (1995) Randomized trial of insulin-glucose infusion followed by subcutaneous insulin treatment in diabetic patients with acute myocardial infarction (DIGAMI study): Effects on mortality at 1 year. *Journal of the American College of Cardiology* 26(1): 57–65.

McCance D, Hanson R, Pettitt D *et al.* (1997) Diagnosing diabetes mellitus—Do we need new criteria? *Diabetologia* 40: 247–255.

McCowen KC, Malhotra A, and Bistrian BR (2001) Stress-induced hyperglycemia. *Critical Care Clinics* 17(1): 107–124.

Mitchell GA, Kassovska-Bratinova S, Boukaftane Y *et al.* (1995) Medical aspects of ketone body metabolism. *Clinical and Investigative Medicine* 18: 193–216.

National Diabetes Data Group (1979) Classification and diagnosis of diabetes mellitus and other categories of glucose intolerance. *Diabetes* 28: 1039–1057.

Tchobroutsky G (1991) Blood glucose levels in diabetic and non-diabetic subjects. *Diabetologia* 34: 67–73.

van den Berghe G, Wouters P, Weekers F *et al.* (2001) Intensive insulin therapy in the critically ill patients. *New England Journal of Medicine* 345(19): 1359–1367.

Dietary Management

C D Saudek, Johns Hopkins University School of Medicine, Baltimore, MD, USA
S H Oh, Johns Hopkins General Clinical Research Center, Baltimore, MD, USA

© 2005 Elsevier Ltd. All rights reserved.

The successful treatment of diabetes mellitus starts with a sound diet, although the specifics of the diet vary depending on the kind of diabetes being treated and the individual circumstances. Individualization is the hallmark of medical nutrition therapy in diabetes. Since approximately 90% of all people with diabetes have type 2, and approximately 80% of them are obese, weight reduction is often the main therapeutic goal. Many also need treatment of comorbidities such as hypertension or dyslipidemia. People with type 1 diabetes, on the other hand, usually require far more attention to exactly how much carbohydrate they ingest and exactly how their intake matches their insulin dose and activity level. In all cases, education of the patient by a trained nutritionist is essential. Diabetes is rarely well controlled unless patients have at least a basic understanding of what they should eat and why.

Overall Objectives in the Management of Diabetes

Control of Blood Glucose Level

A first and very basic goal of diabetes care is to eliminate the symptoms of hyperglycemia. Treatment is inadequate if the person remains polyuric, thirsty, or continues to lose weight from hyperglycemia. To cause symptoms, however, hyperglycemia usually must average more than 11 mM (200 mg/dl). Since blood glucose in the 7–11 mM (125–200 mg/dl) range is distinctly abnormal and does cause long-term diabetic complications, freedom from symptoms is only the beginning of adequate therapy.

Irrefutable evidence exists that better control of blood glucose concentration reduces the risk of developing long-term complications from diabetes. This is especially true of microvascular complications such as retinopathy (eye disease), nephropathy (kidney disease), and nerve damage in both type 1 and type 2 diabetes. Control of blood glucose also reduces the risk of macrovascular disease (heart disease, stroke, and peripheral vascular disease), although the contribution of blood glucose to these complications is less strong.

Carbohydrate ingestion (rather than fat or protein) is the main determinant of postmeal blood glucose level.

Dietary intake, oral medications, insulin, exercise, and stress all contribute to blood glucose levels in the person with diabetes and must be understood when establishing and implementing medical nutrition therapy.

To determine the efficacy of treating glycemia, blood glucose must be monitored. There are two ways to assess diabetic control: self-monitoring of blood glucose (SMBG) laboratory monitoring of hemoglobin A1c (HbA1c). SMBG, done by obtaining a drop of blood and using a small, handheld meter, measures the blood glucose at the time the measurement is taken. It may be done as often as six to eight times per day or as infrequently as several times per week. The HbA1c is a laboratory test that reflects glycemic control during the previous 60–90 days and should be done every 3–6 months. Target HbA1c is generally considered to be <6.5–7% when the upper limit of normal is <6%.

Prevention or Control of Comorbidities

Morbidity and mortality among people with diabetes are rarely due to acute hyperglycemia or diabetic ketoacidosis. Rather, the long-term complications are either specific to diabetes (e.g., diabetic retinopathy or nephropathy) or accelerated by diabetes (e.g., atherosclerosis). Diabetes significantly increases the risk of coronary artery, cerebrovascular, and peripheral vascular disease, with these cardiovascular complications accounting for approximately 80% of deaths in diabetes. Prudent dietary management of diabetes therefore requires consideration of what can be done to prevent or control the various comorbidities of this disease. For example, all people with diabetes should be on a diet that minimizes the risk of atherosclerosis. At the first clinical sign of hypertension, dietary methods should be implemented to lower blood pressure.

Minimum Intrusion on Quality of Life

To people with diabetes, the 'diabetic diet' can be a fearsome thing, often made worse by the way it is presented. Many modern dieticians refuse even to use the word 'diet' since it conjures up so many bad associations, preferring 'nutrition plan' or 'medical nutrition therapy.' Most patients will not totally abandon their dietary habits of a lifetime, forgoing favorite ethnic flavors and socially accepted foods. Rather, the prescribed diet that intrudes least on a person's quality of life is the most successful nutrition plan. Expert professionals can identify exactly what changes are required and what favorite dishes, spices, or food groups can be built into a good nutrition prescription.

Dietary Approaches to Diabetes

Principles of Dietary Management of Diabetes

Assessment The first step for planning an appropriate nutrition plan is a full assessment of the diabetic patient. Topics covered in the nutritional assessment are included in **Table 1**.

Individualization Individualization is a cardinal principle of medical nutrition therapy for diabetes, facilitating individual lifestyle and behavior changes that will lead to improved metabolic control. Since no one diet fits all, the standard, printed diabetic diet is inadequate. Rather, people with diabetes need to consult a person trained in dietetics, one able to develop and teach an individualized nutritional prescription. **Table 2** indicates the range of goals that may need accommodation among different people with diabetes.

Developing the diabetes nutrition plan With the emphasis on individualization, the meal plan is driven by the diagnosis, pharmacologic treatment, lifestyle, and treatment goals. Important consideration is given to dietary preferences, socioeconomic factors, and the patient's ability to understand and implement instructions. Some patients will need instruction on fine points such as carbohydrate counting; others will benefit from the crudest of prescriptions, such as advice to stop buying concentrated sweets or frequenting fast-food restaurants.

Total energy intake The total energy requirement to maintain constant body weight may be calculated using the Harris–Benedict equation, taking into consideration the patient's activity level. The weight-maintaining requirement is then adjusted according to the therapeutic objective—to accomplish weight loss, maintenance of weight, or weight gain. Examples of how to make these calculations are shown in **Table 3**. Specific conditions such as childhood growth and development, pregnancy, malabsorption, or existing nutritional deficiencies are beyond the scope of this article.

Distribution of energy intake Distribution of carbohydrate, protein, and fat into the total energy target also depends on individual needs and therapeutic objectives. Most guidelines recommend that carbohydrate intake represent up to 50–60% of total energy, protein 15–20%, and fat 20–35%. Another approach groups carbohydrate and monounsaturated fats, recognizing that saturated fat should be restricted. This approach suggests that carbohydrate and monounsaturated fat should together account for 60–70% of energy intake.

Table 1 The Nutritional Assessment

Diet history/nutrition information—can be obtained using dietary assessment tools such as 24-h recalls, food records, food frequency questionnaires, or dietary intake interviews

Meal patterns: Usual distribution of meals and snacks throughout the day, including variations from day to day, weekdays versus weekends, skipped meals, and external influences such as work, school, travel, vacations, and holidays

Food choices: Types and amounts of foods consumed at meals and snacks

Nutritional adequacy: Dietary excess or deficiency; also considers overall dietary balance

Beliefs or misconceptions: Fears or misconceptions of a 'strict' diabetic diet or about certain foods; can also include certain religious beliefs or ethnic beliefs about foods

Personal information

Age, gender, socioeconomic status, ethnicity, occupation, education, and literacy level

Ability and willingness to change (stages of change)

Emotional and mental state if distressed by a new diagnosis of diabetes or other health complications related to diabetes

External stressors that may interfere with compliance

Smoking or drug history

Exercise or activity schedule

Clinical information

Type of diabetes and treatment, such as with insulin, oral hypoglycemic drugs, or diet alone

Physical activity, body weight, and blood pressure

Lab results, A1C, and lipid profile

Other medical conditions

Education

Diabetes education should be an ongoing interactive process between patient and health professional and cannot be given in a single session

Individualism is key to successful nutritional management

Most important aspect is to match the type and level of information to individual needs and abilities

Important to provide written information summarizing key messages that patient can take home and refer to later

Follow-up and monitoring progress

Follow-up and review of progress essential

Frequency will depend on type of treatment, glycemic control, and patient's ability to meet goals

Consider if specific dietary targets have been achieved and/or reasons why targets have not been met and what barriers need to be overcome

Consider acceptability of dietary changes and impact on patient's quality of life

Clinical picture should examine glycemic control, lipid profiles, weight changes, and blood pressure

---

Adapted from Conner H *et al.* Nutrition Subcommittee of the Diabetes Care Advisory Committee of Diabetes UK (2003) The implementation of nutritional advice for people with diabetes. *Diabetic Medicine* **20**(10): 786–807.

Even these broad goals are the subject of considerable controversy, with some experts recommending a lower carbohydrate intake and higher fat intake, particularly of monounsaturates. A common mistake is for the patients to think they have a diet low in both carbohydrate and fat without being low in total energy intake. It is unlikely that a person's dietary protein intake will exceed 15–30% of all energy consumed; therefore, 70–85% of intake is generally distributed between fat and carbohydrate.

Distribution of energy intake throughout the day may vary, too. Insulin-requiring diabetic patients, for example, may need a more evenly distributed energy intake, even including a bedtime snack to avoid hypoglycemia. This would not necessarily be indicated for someone with type 2 diabetes trying to lose weight, although weight-reducing diets are generally considered more effective if the total energy intake is spread more or less evenly throughout the day so that the patient does not build up a hunger and gorge late in the day. One report of Muslims observing daytime fasting during Ramadan found that more than half did not lose weight, suggesting a major redistribution of caloric intake to nighttime hours. A significant increase in hypoglycemia occurred during the days of Ramadan. Reduced energy intake for prolonged periods is most dangerous for patients taking insulin, but it may also be significant in those taking oral hypoglycemic agents such as sulfonylureas.

The utility of exchange lists There has been a shift on the part of patients and some health professionals away from the use of formal 'exchange lists' for meal planning. The traditional exchanges estimate not only carbohydrate but also certain proportions of fat and protein in similar foods. Food labels make the calculation of specific fat and carbohydrate content easier. The trend, therefore, is to emphasize the carbohydrate and fat awareness by teaching them directly rather than lumping mixed foods together in exchanges.

Gastroparesis An extremely difficult challenge is posed by the patient with diabetic gastroparesis. This

Table 2 Cases illustrating the variable clinical issues affecting people with diabetes and the resulting diversity of their nutritional needs

Type of diabetes	Type 1	Type 1	Type 2	Type 2
Age (years)	14	38	56	76
Duration of DM (years)	6	26	6	6
BMI	18	23	27	34
Physical activity	Vigorous	Moderate	Mild	Minimal
Prone to hypoglycemia	Yes	Yes	Yes	No
Prone to hyperglycemia	Yes	Yes	Yes	Yes
Blood lipids	Normal	Normal	High LDL cholesterol	High TG, Low HDL
Blood pressure	Normal	High	Normal	High
Dietary preferences	Likes sweets, snacks	Healthy, little carb awareness	Spicy foods, irregular meals	Fried foods, sweets
Pharmacologic therapy	Multiple-dose insulin	Multiple-dose insulin	Oral agents plus insulin	Oral agents
Life expectancy without diabetes	66 years more	44 years more	26 years more	8 years more
Major nutritional considerations	Adequate caloric intake for growth (see **Table 3**)	Stabilize carb intake, count carbs	Mildly hypocaloric (see **Table 3**)	Low salt, high vegetable for hypertension (DASH diet)
	Recognize carb portions, regularize carb intake	Low salt, high vegetable for hypertension (DASH diet)	Hypolidemic (low saturated fat)	Hypolipemic diet (low saturated fat)
	Avoid excess concentrated sweets		Regularity of meals, consistency of carb and fat intake	Moderately hypocaloric
	Learn factors causing hypoglycemia			Control of dietary carb, especially high-energy concentrated sweets
	Healthy heart diet			

BMI, body mass index; DM, diabetes mellitus; HDL, high-density lipoprotein; LDL, low-density lipoprotein.

condition, a severe autonomic neuropathy reducing gastric motility and gastric emptying time, is often difficult to diagnose by standardized testing, such as gastric emptying studies. Gastroparesis typically causes early satiety, nausea, vomiting, and abdominal pain, with markedly variable food ingestion. Along with pharmacologic management and good glycemic control, the dietary prescription should include small, frequent feeding as tolerated, but the condition can progress to the point that any oral intake is difficult, and tube feeding or a gastrostomy is required. Fortunately, diabetic gastroparesis tends to wax and wane in severity.

Glycemic control and weight gain Research studies have repeatedly found that when a patient with poor glycemic control achieves good glycemic control, there is a strong, almost inevitable, tendency to gain weight. This may simply be due to the retention of energy that was previously lost in the urine as glucosuria, but the patient should be warned of the likelihood of gaining weight when poor diabetic control is adequately treated. As for quitting smoking, the health benefit of glycemic control far outweighs the risk of weight gain.

Nutritional instruction To achieve a stable, healthy diet, the following key educational issues must be

considered (adapted from Franz M, Krosnick A, Maschak-Carey BJ *et al.* (1986) *Goals for Diabetes Education*. Chicago: American Diabetes Association):

Survival skills
  Relation of food to insulin and activity
  Importance of good nutrition in the control of blood glucose and lipid levels
  Necessity of maintaining normal weight
  Types and amounts of food in meal plan
  Modification of food intake during brief illnesses
In-depth counseling
  Meal planning
  Types of nutrients, their functions, relation to insulin, and effect on blood glucose and lipid levels
  Caloric level of meal plan and percentages of carbohydrate, protein, and fat
Food sources of fiber
Importance of reducing total fat, saturated fat, and cholesterol in the diet
Relation of sodium to hypertension
Proper serving sizes
Changes in food intake based on activity level
Eating out and special occasions
Label reading and grocery shopping
Use of sweeteners, alcohol, and 'dietetic' foods
Food modifications for other disorders
Incorporation of favorite recipes

Table 3 Sample calculations of energy requirement in differing circumstances using the Harris–Benedict formula to determine caloric requirements for children and adults

Caloric requirements = basal metabolic rate × activity factor × injury factor

Basal metabolic rate (BMR)

For men: BMR = 66 + [13.7 × wt (kg)] + [5 × ht (cm)] − [6.8 × age (years)]

For women: BMR = 655 + [9.6 × wt (kg) + [1.8 × ht (cm)] − [4.7 × age (years)]

Multiply by the following factors:

Activity factors

1. Sedentary (little or no exercise): BMR × 1.2
2. Lightly active (light exercise/sports 1–3 days/week): BMR × 1.375
3. Moderately active (moderate exercise/sports 3–5 days/week): BMR × 1.55
4. Very active (hard exercise/sports 6–7 days/week): BMR × 1.725
5. Extra active (very hard daily exercise/sports and physical job or 2X day training): BMR × 1.9

Injury factors (not used for healthy individuals)

1. Generalized stress: 1.1–1.2
2. Surgery (minor): 1.1–1.5
3. Infection: 1.2–1.5
4. Trauma: 1.14–1.37
5. Cancer: 1.2

For weight loss, use the above calculated formula for caloric requirements and subtract by 500 calories:

Caloric requirements − 500 calories/day = modified calorie requirements

This is for a recommended 0.5–1 pound of weight loss per week

Special aspects: Type 2 diabetes There are two pathophysiologic mechanisms underlying type 2 diabetes: The body's cells are resistant to the action of insulin, and the pancreas is unable to secrete enough insulin to overcome that resistance. Although it is not entirely clear which of these processes occurs first, and although the balance of the two may vary from case to case, the most common cause of insulin resistance is overweight or obesity. Unfortunately, much evidence has shown that people of Asian ethnicity are especially prone to obesity-related type 2 diabetes even when their body weight, by Western standards, is normal. Japanese Americans, for example, show an increase risk of diabetes if their body mass index (BMI) increases to only 24. This excessive risk with even mild degrees of excess body weight may explain the marked rise in diabetes when previously undernourished populations begin to have adequate nutrition. In this sense, diabetes is a disease of prosperity.

Major objectives Approximately 95% of all people with diabetes have type 2, and the major increase in the prevalence of diabetes in recent years is almost entirely accounted for by increase in body weight. It cannot be overemphasized that medical nutrition therapy of type 2 diabetes should address normalization of body weight. In most cases, the focus is on reducing dietary intake of saturated fat and increasing energy expenditure through exercise. By reducing body weight, insulin resistance is reduced, making the patient's endogenous insulin more effective. Given that approximately 85% of people with type 2 diabetes die of cardiovascular cause, the second emphasis of medical nutrition therapy for type 2 diabetics must address dyslipidemia and blood pressure.

Hypoenergetic diets are remarkably effective in controlling hyperglycemia. Indeed, blood glucose levels improve, often dramatically, as soon as a low-energy diet is started, apparently by reducing hepatic glucose production. The correction of insulin resistance is more closely correlated with actual weight loss, which takes much longer. The best strategy for accomplishing and maintaining weight loss is unclear and may vary from person to person depending on the different factors involved, such as willingness to change and other lifestyle behaviors. Dosages of antidiabetic drugs may have to be altered as the person loses weight.

Persistent insulin resistance in type 2 diabetes, together with deteriorating pancreatic insulin secretion over time, means that many people with type 2 diabetes eventually require exogenous insulin therapy. This does not change the diagnosis to type 1 diabetes, which is a disease of entirely different pathogenesis. Because of the insulin resistance, people with type 2 diabetes taking insulin often need high doses, often 50–100 units per day or higher. Insulin requirements will predictably be less when energy intake is reduced.

Recently, in Western societies, many overweight teenagers have presented with type 2 diabetes. It can no longer be assumed that children with diabetes have type 1. Indeed, some reports find that half of all teenagers with diabetes have type 2, a marked shift from prior years. Furthermore, nutrition therapy for children with diabetes must be designed with a clear understanding of what type of diabetes they have. In cases of obesity-related type 2, calorie restriction may be indicated.

Coexisting risk factors Obesity, dyslipidemia, and hypertension are especially prevalent in type 2 diabetes. The constellation of comorbidities has been called metabolic syndrome, 'syndrome X,' or the insulin resistance syndrome (**Table 4**), and some investigators believe that insulin resistance is the primary lesion. Whatever the pathophysiologic mechanisms, it is clear that dyslipidemia and hypertension must be sought and aggressively treated if

Table 4 The Metabolic Syndrome

Three or more of the following components:
   Central obesity as measured by waist circumference
      Men: >102 cm (40 in.)
      Women: >88 cm (35 in.)
   Fasting blood triglycerides ≥1.69 mmol/l (150 mg/dl)
   Blood HDL cholesterol
      Men: <1.04 mmol/l (40 mg/dl)
      Women: <1.29 mmol/l (50 mg/dl)
   Blood pressure ≥130/85 mmHg
Fasting glucose ≥6.1 mmol/l (110 mg/dl)

present. In fact, most evidence suggests that the management of coexisting risk factors, particularly hypertension, dyslipidemia, and smoking, is more important than the treatment of hyperglycemia in preventing morbidity and mortality.

Special aspects: Type 1 diabetes With type 1 diabetes, there is essentially no endogenous insulin secretion, due to autoimmune destruction of the insulin-producing beta cells of the pancreas. This lack of an essential hormone for life means that insulin must be injected, often multiple times daily. Furthermore, the replacement of a very finely tuned normal insulin secretory mechanism, which provides insulin precisely 'on demand,' cannot be well reproduced by injections, explaining the glycemic lability of type 1 diabetes.

Major objectives Generally, the treatment objective in type 1 diabetes is stabilization of glycemic control in an acceptable range, control of other risk factors, and thus avoidance of long-term complications. This requires close attention not only to diet but also to its interrelationships with insulin dose and timing, activity, stress, and other life factors. In fact, despite the best efforts, almost all people with type 1 diabetes are prone to wide swings of blood glucose, sometimes from 2.8 to 17 mmol/l (50–300 mg/dl) or more during a day.

To control the intrinsic 'brittleness' of type 1 diabetes, the individual needs to learn to stabilize dietary intake, making it as reproducible as possible. If carbohydrate, in particular, varies significantly from day to day and meal to meal, the person must learn to adjust insulin doses to match the changed intake. Carbohydrate counting helps stabilization of the diet or adjustment in insulin doses. It is useful for the nutritionist to understand the various insulin regimens that people with type 2 diabetes are given. Several different typical regimens, with comments on the dietary implications, are shown in **Figure 1**.

In addition to carbohydrate awareness, dietary fat intake should be taken into consideration. Dietary fat is often the main determinant of serum lipids and

contributes significantly to total energy intake and thus body weight. It also delays gastric emptying, prolonging the glycemic response to dietary carbohydrate.

Very few people continue to measure and weigh foods, but weighing is a useful tool during the instruction phase. Ultimately, people with type 1 diabetes should become proficient in estimating the carbohydrate content of food so that their food selection becomes second nature.

Energy intake distribution will depend on the type of insulin, the number of injections, and the glycemic targets (very tight blood glucose control or not as tight). Often, small changes in food ingestion can make a significant difference. If, for example, a patient tends to develop hypoglycemia at approximately noon, the skillful dietitian can either emphasize the necessity of eating lunch regularly before noon or suggest the patient consume some of the lunch carbohydrates as an 11 AM snack. These changes may eliminate the need to change insulin dose.

Especially with intensive insulin therapy (three or four daily injections or an external insulin pump), there is some flexibility in the timing of the meals but also a need for more accurate assessment of meal content. Some patients will learn their own ratio of grams of carbohydrate to insulin dose necessary to maintain blood glucose in a good range.

Eating disorders pose a serious problem to the management of type 1 diabetes. Presumably because people with diabetes are often diet conscious, the prevalence of eating disorders is surprisingly high among teenagers with diabetes. The problem is especially dangerous because young people may skip insulin injections in order to induce glucosuria, a sort of 'metabolic purging.' These conditions clearly require prompt professional help.

Growth and development The total daily energy intake of a person with type 1 diabetes should be calculated to maintain normal growth and development in a child and normal weight in an adult. Examples of these calculations are provided in **Table 3**. Since most people with type 1 diabetes are not overweight, most do not need low-energy diets. Indeed, underfeeding is a poor way to maintain blood glucose control. The energy needed to establish and maintain normal weight should be matched with the insulin needed to control glycemia. There is no need for a thin or normal-weight person with type 1 diabetes to be perpetually hungry.

Special aspects of dietary management of other types of diabetes Other types of diabetes include those with relatively well-recognized etiologies, such as

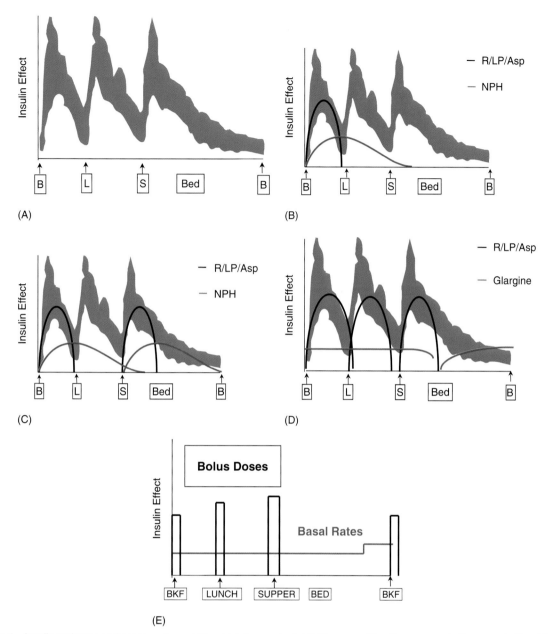

Figure 1 Insulin regimens and notes on the nutritional intake required. (A) The normal insulin response to three meals (breakfast (B), lunch (L), and supper (S)). Note that insulin increases sharply after ingestion of a carbohydrate-containing meal, declining to baseline within several hours. (B) When a combination of short-acting and intermediate-acting insulin is given only at breakfast, the normal response to breakfast is reproduced and the intermediate-acting insulin 'covers' lunch. It is important that the patient ingest a regular breakfast and lunch in order to avoid hypoglycemia from the insulin present at these times. (C) When a combination of short-acting and intermediate-acting insulin is given at breakfast and supper, there is better 'coverage' of the supper meal, but the intermediate-acting insulin peaks near bedtime and the middle of the night, so a bedtime snack may be necessary. (D) A more intensive regimen provides insulin as a 'basal' dose at bedtime, lasting the full 24 h, and short-acting insulin with every meal, for a total of four doses per day. The regimen usually requires patients to monitor their own blood glucose before each meal to adjust their short-acting dose to both the amount of carbohydrate to be ingested and the blood glucose level at the time. The regimen does provide more flexibility of meal timing. (E) Use of an external insulin pump infuses insulin at a precise basal rate, and the patient signals the pump to deliver bolus doses of insulin with each meal. As with D, regular monitoring is required as well as accurate understanding of the content of the meal to be ingested. Basal rate can be adjusted, for example, to avoid nighttime hypoglycemia, and there is flexibility of when meals are eaten.

pancreatectomy-induced diabetes, diabetes due to pancreatitis, cystic fibrosis, iron infiltration of the pancreas (hemochromatosis), or rare syndromes of insulin resistance.

Pancreatitis may be secondary to severe hypertriglyceridemia (triglyceride content >1100 mmol/l (1000 mg/dl)). In this case, a very low-fat diet is often indicated. When there is widespread destruction of pancreatic cell mass, as with cystic fibrosis, pancreatectomy, or extensive cancer, the exocrine as well as endocrine functions are affected, leading to malabsorption and impaired glucagon secretion. Malabsorption causes steattorhea and may require pancreatic enzyme replacement to avoid marked variability in carbohydrate as well as fat absorption. Lack of the hormone glucagon increases the risk of severe hypoglycemia after insulin administration since there is less counterregulatory ability to raise blood glucose levels after mild hypoglycemia.

Effects of Ingested Nutrients on Blood Glucose

Carbohydrate

Carbohydrate ingestion causes blood glucose to increase. In people without diabetes, the normal increase in blood glucose is approximately 0.5–2.8 mmol/l (10–50 mg/dl) above baseline, returning to baseline within 1–3 h. The pancreatic hormonal response to dietary carbohydrate mediates the return to normal. Insulin is the central mediator of energy metabolism. The basics of insulin-dependent energy metabolism in the fed and the fasting states are depicted in **Figure 2**.

Although carbohydrate intake plays the major role in postprandial blood glucose, there are other factors to consider. The diet is not the only source of glucose in blood; hepatic gluconeogenesis maintains blood glucose in the absence of dietary intake. For example, when a person is ill and dietary intake is curtailed, it would be a mistake to stop insulin administration since hepatic glucose production may in fact be increased. Sick-day instruction is essential for people with diabetes so that they do not simply stop their treatment if they are not eating well. Pharmacologic therapies (insulin or oral agents), of course, also affect blood glucose.

A long-standing debate has surrounded the optimal proportion of intake from carbohydrate, fat, and protein. People with diabetes, especially when insulin is administered, will discover that if they hold back carbohydrate their blood glucose does not increase as much. Holding back carbohydrate, however, unless the diet is hypocaloric, inevitably leads to a high-fat diet, and carbohydrate restriction leaves insulin with no substrate to act on. In our experience, this can cause blood glucose levels to be more unstable, susceptible to swings of hypoglycemia and hyperglycemia. We support the recommendation of most professional guidelines that carbohydrate should make up a substantial percentage (50–60%) of total nutrient intake.

Two areas of controversy and of nutrition research deserve special attention: the glycemic response to oral sucrose (concentrated sweets) versus complex carbohydrates and the so-called 'glycemic index.'

Sucrose versus complex carbohydrate Careful metabolic studies suggest that, gram for gram, sucrose does not increase blood glucose more than complex carbohydrates, either acutely or over a matter of weeks. In these studies, sucrose was isoenergetically substituted for other carbohydrates, mostly under carefully defined research ward conditions in which precise substitutions can be made. Since complex carbohydrates and sucrose are both digested to monosaccharides before they are absorbed, it is not unexpected that each should cause the same glycemic excursion if administered in the same number of grams. It does run counter, however, to the traditional advice that people with diabetes should avoid concentrated sweets.

A number of organizations have cited these research studies in support of a recommendation that allows ingestion of concentrated sweets. The caveat, in the words of the American Diabetes Association, is that "sucrose should be substituted for other carbohydrate sources in the food/meal plan." In our view, there is a practical fallacy in this recommendation: People are unlikely to substitute sucrose for complex carbohydrates in equal amounts. Due simply to taste, concentrated sweets are likely to be taken in far greater quantity than the more filling and less sweet starches. Thus, in reality, people who routinely eat concentrated sweets are likely to have greater and less predictable glycemic excursions than those who stick to complex carbohydrates. There is also the significant risk that excess concentrated sweet intake will cause weight gain (as well as dental caries). However, if a person with diabetes can include a fixed amount of concentrated sweet in his or her diet and can demonstrate that his or her diabetes is well controlled and the postmeal glycemia is not excessive, there is no reason to deny the person the sweet.

Glycemic index The glycemic index (GI) is defined as the area under the 2-h curve of blood glucose after the ingestion of a set amount of carbohydrate compared to ingestion of the same amount of carbohydrate from a reference food (white bread or glucose). The GI is expressed as a percentage of the standard food value:

$$\text{Glycemic index} = \frac{\text{Area under the curve of test food}}{\text{Area under the curve of standard food}} \times 100$$

The glycemic load (GL) is an additional measure in which the amount of carbohydrate in a typical

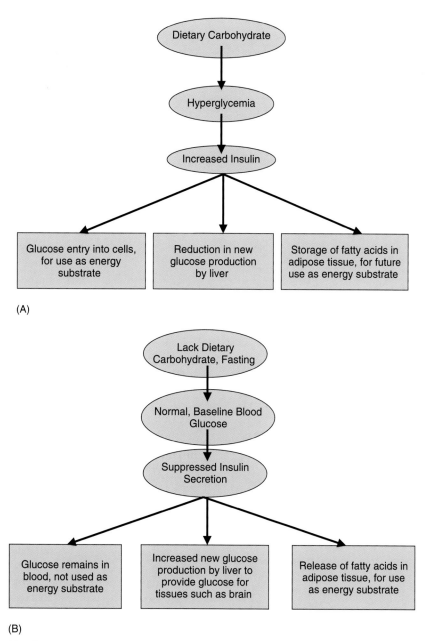

Figure 2 Influence of insulin on basic energy metabolism. (A) With dietary carbohydrate intake, hyperglycemia induces insulin secretion that acts to enhance glucose entry into cells for utilization as metabolic fuel. Simultaneously, insulin decreases new glucose production in the liver, since dietary glucose is already available, and stores excess caloric intake in adipose tissue as fat. (B) With lack of dietary carbohydrate, as in fasting, the reverse occurs: With lower blood glucose, insulin secretion is suppressed. This minimizes entry of glucose into cells but stimulates enough new glucose production from the liver to provide for obligate glucose using tissues such as the brain. Meanwhile, low insulin concentration promotes fatty acid release from adipose tissue to serve as an alternate fuel for metabolism.

portion is taken into account. **Table 5** provides examples of foods high and low in GI and GL. These indices have been calculated for more than 500 different carbohydrates, and values are readily available on the Internet. A number of factors in addition to the reported GI and GL actually affect the blood glucose response to meals, however, because mixed meals are ingested in everyday living. Among these are the fat and fiber content of the

meal, type of cooking, the patient's absorptive rate, and micronutrient content.

In our opinion, the concept of the GI is valid in a research sense: Certain carbohydrates, gram for gram, do raise blood glucose levels more, or with different glycemic patterns, than others. However, we believe that basing nutrition plans on the GI and the GL of foods is usually too much of a burden for people with diabetes, who have to closely monitor

Table 5 Examples of foods high and low in glycemic index (GI) and glycemic load (GL)[a]

	GI	Serving size (g)	GL
Low GI/low GL			
Apple, NS (USA)	40	120	6
Oranges (Sunkist, USA)	48	120	5
Healthy Choice hearty 7-grain bread (USA)	55 ± 6	30	8
Ice cream, premium, French Vanilla—16% fat (Australia)	38 ± 3	50	3
Kidney beans (USA)	23	150	6
Pizza, Super Supreme, thin and crispy—13.2% fat, Pizza Hut (Australia)	30 ± 4	100	7
Low GI/high GL			
Barley (*Hordeum vulgare*) (India)	43 ± 6	150	26
High GI/low GL			
Watermelon, raw (Australia)	72 ± 13	120	4
White wheat flour bread	70	30	10
High GI/high GL			
Cornflakes (Kellogg's, USA)	92	30	24
Bagel, white, frozen (Lenders, Canada)	72	70	25
White rice, type NS, boiled 13 minutes (Italy)	102	150	31

[a]High GI is considered >70 and low <55. High GL is considered >20 and low <10.
Adapted from Foster-Powell K, Holt SH, and Brand-Miller JC (2002) International table of glycemic index and glycemic load values. *American Journal of Clinical Nutrition* **76**(1): 5–56.

the total amount of carbohydrates. It is more practical to encourage people to learn their own glycemic response to different foods from experience. They may learn, for example, that far more insulin is needed before eating pizza or a bagel; they may learn to avoid certain deserts. A general awareness of what preferred foods, in what amounts, raise blood glucose may be more practical than memorizing GI or GL.

Protein

Since the classic experiments by Benedict in the 1910s, it has been known that protein ingestion causes hyperglycemia and glucosuria. The effect of protein ingestion on blood glucose, however, is far less pronounced than the effect of carbohydrate ingestion. A rule of thumb is that a gram of protein raises blood glucose approximately one-third as much as a gram of carbohydrate. In most diets, approximately 50–100 g protein is ingested per day, compared to approximately 200–300 g carbohydrate. Therefore, protein is a calorically less significant part of the diet and far less important in regulating blood glucose. In people with type 2 diabetes, protein does not slow the postprandial absorption of carbohydrate. The same cannot be said about dietary fat.

Fat

Dietary fat has little, if any, immediate effect on blood glucose concentration because the constituent fatty acids do not produce new glucose and the glycerol moieties are insignificant in their contribution to blood glucose. However, there is considerable evidence that circulating free fatty acids promote gluconeogenesis and hyperglycemia. In a normal overnight fast this is good: Fatty acids help maintain normoglycemia. However, in uncontrolled diabetes, when fatty acids can be very high, they significantly worsen hyperglycemia. This has been referred to as 'fat toxicity.'

Fat ingestion slows gastric emptying. The delayed delivery of carbohydrate to the circulation can cause a late, slow postprandial rise in blood glucose, although people who do not self-monitor frequently are unlikely to be aware of this effect of dietary fat.

Nonnutritive Sweeteners

Sweeteners are important to the quality of life of people with diabetes. An essential distinction is to differentiate those with from those without significant energy content. **Tables 6** and **7** provide many of the available nonnutritive and nutritive sweeteners. The nonnutritive sweeteners have no or virtually no energy content, and they can be consumed without concern about their effect on blood glucose.

Table 6 Nonnutritive sweeteners

Type	US brand names	kcal/g	Description
Saccharin	Sweet and Low, Sweet Twin, Sweet 'N Low Brown, Necta Sweet	0	200–700 times sweeter than sucrose; noncarcinogenic and produces no glycemic response
Aspartame	Nutrasweet, Equal, Sugar Twin (blue box)	4	160–220 times sweeter than sucrose; noncarcinogenic and produces limited glycemic response
Acesulfame-K	Sunett, Sweet & Safe, Sweet one	0	200 times sweeter than sucrose; noncarcinogenic and produces no glycemic response
Sucralose	Splenda	0	600 times sweeter than sucrose; noncarcinogenic and produces no glycemic response

Table 7 Polyols and novel sugar sweeteners

Type	kcal/g	Description
Monosaccharide polyols or novel sugars		
Sorbitol	2.6	50–70% as sweet as sucrose; some people experience a laxative effect from a load ≥50 g
Mannitol	1.6	50–70% as sweet as sucrose; some people experience a laxative effect from a load ≥20 g
Xylitol	2.4	As sweet as sucrose
Erythritol	0.2	60–80% as sweet as sucrose; also acts as a flavor enhancer, formulation aid, humectant, stabilizer and thickener, sequestrant, and texturizer
Disaccharide polyols or novel sugars		
Isomalt	2	45–65% as sweet as sucrose; used as a bulking agent
Lactitol	2	30–40% as sweet as sucrose; used as a bulking agent
Maltitol	2.1	90% as sweet as sucrose; used as a bulking agent
Polysaccharide polyols		
HSH	3	25–50% as sweet as sucrose; other names include hydrogenated starch hydrolysates and maltitol syrup

Adapted with permission from the Journal of the American Diabetic Association Position Paper: Use of Nutritive and Nonnutritive Sweetners.

Many 'diet' sweeteners, such as sorbitol or fructose-based snacks, do cause at least some degree of hyperglycemia. Sugar alcohols (polyols) such as sorbitol, mannitol, and xylitol are classified as hydrogenated monosaccharides, hydrogenated disaccharides, and oligosaccharides. They do contain calories, but because they are only partially absorbed in the small intestine, they have a reduced energy value per gram. Excessive use of sugar alcohols has laxative effects and can cause diarrhea.

It is important for people with diabetes to understand clearly these distinctions because many calories can be ingested with foods labeled as 'diet' under the false assumption that they are without effect on blood glucose.

Trace Elements

There has been recurrent interest in whether such trace elements as chromium, potassium, magnesium, vanadium, and zinc affect blood glucose control in diabetes. It would obviously be attractive if simple oral supplements could facilitate normoglycemia. The evidence, though, is slim and unconvincing that supplementation of any of these trace elements has a beneficial effect except when there is a true deficiency. Such deficiency may occur in an undernourished setting, in the elderly with poor dietary intake, or in certain strict vegetarian diets.

The same conclusion can be reached regarding vitamin supplementation: It is indicated when vitamin deficiency is suspected or likely. For example, populations such as the elderly, those pregnant or lactating, strict vegetarians, or those on a calorie-restricted diet supplementation may require vitamin supplements. Folate supplementation is well documented to improve the outcome of pregnancy, with or without diabetes. However, there is no clear evidence that supplementation is helpful for those eating an adequate diet.

Antioxidants such as vitamins C, E, or A and α-lipoic acid are the object of intensive research. It is unclear whether or which of these actually prevent long-term complications of diabetes, but the literature should be monitored. Vitamins B_1, B_6, and B_{12} are sometimes used to treat diabetic peripheral neuropathy, but without much supporting evidence of benefit. On the other hand, calcium supplementation is indicated, particularly in the elderly, if daily intake is less than 1.0–1.5 g.

In summary, evidence is weak that vitamin or trace element deficiencies occur due to diabetes. Supplementation in more normal circumstances has little or no role in the control of diabetes, and general nutritional guidelines for vitamins and trace elements should be followed.

Major Nonnutrient Factors That Regulate Blood Glucose

No element of diabetes management exists in a vacuum, so it is essential to consider how dietary therapy interacts with other elements of management. Most prominent are insulin, oral hypoglycemic agents, activity, and stress.

Insulin

As two major types of diabetes (1 and 2) differ, so the use of insulin differs for each. As described earlier, in type 1 diabetes the insulin doses must be closely matched to the meals ingested. Too much insulin or too little ingested carbohydrate can cause serious hypoglycemia. Frequently, patients are on intensive insulin regimens, sometimes four doses per day, and sometimes using an insulin pump. People with well-controlled type 1 diabetes have usually learned to pay close attention to their carbohydrate intake, recognize portion sizes, or even count grams of carbohydrate. They often adjust insulin dose or carbohydrate intake, but this can be done effectively only if they have a good, quantitative understanding of both. Meals skipped or eaten late can be a problem.

Intensive insulin regimens may involve the use of an insulin pump or insulin doses based on a 'sliding scale.' Ordinarily, sliding scales are developed for the patient based on the self-monitored blood glucose at the time of the meal. For higher blood glucose levels, more short-acting insulin is administered. In more intensive regimens, often with insulin pump use, the amount of insulin delivered is also adjusted depending on both blood glucose level at the time and the carbohydrate to be ingested. To be safe and effective, this self-adjusted fine-tuning of insulin dose requires considerable knowledge of diet as well as insulin.

Examples of sliding scales are provided in **Table 8**. Some people, particularly those with intensive insulin regimens, learn to adjust their insulin dose according to both the blood glucose at the start of a meal and the estimated amount that a unit of insulin will reduce their blood glucose. Examples are provided in **Table 9**. Also, although nutritionists do not usually prescribe changes in insulin dosage, it is useful to know the various types of insulin available (**Table 10**) and patterns of insulin action (**Figure 1**).

With type 2 diabetes, since there is usually some insulin secreted on demand from the pancreas and considerable resistance to insulin, dietary intake may not have to be so precisely regulated according to insulin dose. There is a risk of hypoglycemia but it is usually less than that seen in type 1 diabetes. As discussed previously, the nutritional emphasis is usually on reducing the caloric intake, with careful control of fat as well as carbohydrate.

Oral Antidiabetic Agents

Oral antidiabetic agents are not insulin; insulin is delivered only by injection or infusion. The variety of agents in use has escalated dramatically in recent years, so it is worth knowing how the various classes act and how they may interact with diet.

Sulfonylureas (e.g., glyburide, glimepiride, and glipizide) commonly act by stimulation of pancreatic insulin secretion. They therefore can cause hypoglycemia if taken in excess or without normal food intake.

The other most popular oral agent is metformin, which does not stimulate insulin secretion and therefore should not cause hypoglycemia by itself. Metformin can cause bloating and diarrhea, but it can also be mildly weight reducing in conjunction with diet.

The drugs called thiazolidinediones (TZDs), pioglitazone and rosiglitazone, improve insulin sensitivity but do not by themselves cause hypoglycemia. TZDs can, however, cause fluid retention and weight gain, so they are sometimes counterproductive in someone trying to lose weight.

Finally, a class of drugs called α-glucosidase inhibitors (acarbose and miglitol) inhibit digestion and absorption of carbohydrate. They do not cause hypoglycemia, but they may interfere with the treatment of hypoglycemia by oral carbohydrate.

Physical Activity

The effects of exercise on blood glucose levels are complex and sometimes unpredictable. Although moderate, extended aerobic exercise generally causes progressive lowering of blood glucose, intense exercise may transiently increase the blood glucose. We generally recommend modification of diet to accommodate exercise, rather than changing the dose of

Table 8 Examples of sliding scale insulin doses based on blood glucose level at the time of the meal[a]

Meal	Blood glucose (mmol/l)	<3.33	3.33–6.7	6.8–8.3	8.4–11.1	11.2–13.9	14–16.7	>16.7
	Blood glucose (mg/dl)	<60	60–120	121–150	151–200	201–250	250–300	>300
Breakfast	NPH/regular	8/0	8/4	8/5	8/6	10/7	10/8	10/9
Lunch	Regular	0	2	3	4	5	6	7
Supper	Regular	2	4	6	7	8	9	10
Bedtime	NPH/regular	6/0	6/0	7/0	7/0	8/0	8/2	8/3

Example: Prebreakfast blood glucose 10 mmol/l (180 mg/dl): Take 8 units NPH + 6 units regular.

[a]Each patient will have individual insulin requirements and needs. Longer acting insulin (such as glargine) may be used at bedtime, and faster acting insulins (such as lispro or aspart) may be used premeal.

Table 9 Examples of mealtime insulin dose based on blood glucose level *and* amount of carbohydrate to be ingested[a]

Short-acting or fast-acting insulin dose

'Correction factor': 1 unit per 2.8 mmol/l (50 mg/dl) >5.5 mmol/l (100 mg/dl)

plus

'Meal factor': 1 unit per 15 g carbohydrate

Example: Before ingesting a meal estimated to have 45 g of carbohydrate, the blood glucose is measured to be 150. Insulin dose would be 1 unit (for the blood glucose) + 3 units (for the carbohydrate) = 4 units.

[a]Both the correction factor and the meal factor will vary from patient to patient. Long acting insulins are used in addition to these prandial doses.

insulin or oral agents, since the duration and intensity of exercise may be unpredictable. Trained athletes or 'weekend warriors' often learn to take extra carbohydrate before a strenuous workout rather than anticipating exercise by reducing the morning insulin dose. They also learn that the time of greatest hypoglycemic risk may be 6–12 h after exercise.

Stress

Stress in normal life is difficult to quantify or study, but the usual experience is that diabetic control deteriorates under stress. This makes sense, considering the hyperglycemic effects of 'fight or flight' hormones such as adrenaline (epinephrine) and cortisol. However, it is likely that the main problem for people under unusual stress is less hormonal than behavioral—simply neglecting their diet or eating as a stress reliever. Therapists may be most effective by reminding patients to maintain their normal diet even when experiencing emotional stress.

Dietary Prevention and Management of Comorbidities

Accelerated Atherosclerosis

Essentially the same nutritional approaches to the prevention of atherosclerosis apply whether or not a person has diabetes. However, they are even more important for the patient with diabetes since hyperglycemia is a risk factor, and most people with diabetes die of atherosclerotic cardiovascular disease. Therefore, anyone with diabetes should follow a 'heart healthy' diet that focuses on lowering low-density lipoprotein (LDL) cholesterol level, which is a major contributor to the progression of atherosclerosis. Total fat intake can be held to 25–35% of total calories, less than 7% saturated fat and the remainder divided between monounsaturated fat and polyunsaturated fats. The recommendation allows for increased intake of unsaturated fats in place of carbohydrates in people with diabetes. In addition to the antiatherosclerotic diet, there should be routine screening for other specific risk factors, notably hypertension and dyslipidemia. If found, these risk factors, which are even more dangerous in diabetes, should be vigorously treated.

Dyslipidemia

If the dyslipidemia is predominantly elevation of LDL cholesterol, then dietary manipulations are no different in diabetes from those used to treat hypercholesterolemia generally: Low intakes of saturated fat and cholesterol are indicated, with cholesterol-lowering medications (usually statins) given as needed. Target goals for LDL cholesterol are <100 mg/dl, and there have been recommendations to lower LDL

Table 10 Types of available insulin by onset, peak, and duration of action

Category	Insulin type	Approximate onset	Approximate peak	Approximate duration
Fast acting	Aspart	5–10 minutes	1–3 h	3–5 h
	Lispro	<15 minutes	0.5–1.5 h	2–4 h
Rapid acting	Regular	0.5–1 h	2–3 h	3–6 h
Intermediate acting	NPH	2–4 h	4–10 h	10–16 h
	Lente	3–4 h	4–12 h	12–18 h
Long acting	Glargine	1.1 h	?	24 h
	UltraLente	6–10 h	18–20 h	20–24 h

Premixes

50/50: 50% NPH, 50% regular

70/30: 70% NPH, 30% regular

Mix 70/30: 70% aspart–protamine suspension (e.g., NPH), 30% aspart

75/25: 75% lispro–protamine suspension (e.g., NPH), 25% lispro

[a]Onset, peak, and duration will vary for each individual. Based on American Diabetes Association (2004) *Diabetes Forecast, Resource Guide*. Alexandria, VA: American Diabetes Association.

cholesterol to as low as <70 mg/dl if there are other risk factors for coronary artery disease.

Hypertriglyceridemia, on the other hand, is the more common dyslipidemia in diabetes, and especially it is dangerous when it is associated with low levels of high-density lipoprotein cholesterol. Insulin–glucose homeostasis is intrinsically and complexly related to triglyceride metabolism. Insulin stimulates both very low-density lipoprotein–triglyceride synthesis in the liver and its clearance via lipoprotein lipase in the periphery.

In extreme cases, reduced chylomicron clearance causes 'diabetic lipemia,' characterized by chylomicronemia and extreme hypertriglyceridemia. More moderate levels of hypertriglyceridemia, on the other hand, are considered to be due to overproduction of hepatic (endogenous) lipid under the influence of hyperinsulinism and peripheral insulin resistance.

Compounding the confusion is the phenomenon of 'carbohydrate induction of hypertriglyceridemia.' Most normal people switched isoenergetically from a low- to a high-carbohydrate diet (i.e., with less dietary fat) will actually increase their fasting triglyceride level. This carbohydrate induction of hypertriglyceridemia may be transient, lasting only a few weeks.

For the person with diabetes, treatment of hypertriglyceridemia begins with optimization of blood glucose control and a diet designed to achieve normal body weight. Weight reduction is often very effective.

If hypertriglyceridemia persists, evidence favors the use of monounsaturated fats when dietary fat increases. Since hypertriacylglyceridemia is sometimes associated with excess alcohol, reducing the amount consumed may be effective. For the unusual condition of fasting chylomicronemia, with triglyceride levels remaining over approximately 11 mmol/l (1000 mg/dl), a low-fat diet is necessary to avoid exacerbating the situation by adding dietary fat and precipitating pancreatitis from the chylomicronemia.

If pharmacologic treatment is necessary to treat hypertriglyceridemia, a fibric acid derivative, such as gemfibrazol or fenofibrate, or nicotinic acid should be used. Statins are usually the first drug of choice when LDL cholesterol is also elevated.

Hypertension

The current nutritional management of hypertension focuses on reducing dietary sodium intake and weight reduction, as well as the recently proven 'DASH' diet. There has been long-standing evidence that in both normal and hypertensive people, a reduction in sodium intake lowers blood pressure. The DASH diet was shown to be effective in a large trial of dietary intervention. It is a fruit and vegetable diet, with balanced consumption of foods emphasizing high fiber, grains, and low-fat dairy products. Potassium, magnesium, and fiber replace some snacks and sweets.

Modest amounts of weight loss and increased activity are also beneficial for the person with hypertension. Thus, overweight and obese individuals should be encouraged to lose weight as part of their medical therapy. In diabetes, ACE inhibitors or ARBs (Angrotensin Receptor Blockers) are usually the first line of medication used when diet and exercise are not effective in controlling blood pressure. Frequently, additional antihypertensives must be added.

Renal Disease

Nutritional therapy of established diabetic nephropathy continues to be studied. In both type 1 and type 2 diabetes, persistent microalbuminuria is a strong predictor of gross proteinuria and developing nephropathy. Evidence suggests that microalbuminuria actually reverses in many cases, but gross proteinuria (over approximately 300 mg/24 h) in most cases eventually progresses to end-stage renal disease. Therefore, treatment focuses on reversing or at least retarding the progression of nephropathy. In recent years, the nutrition recommendation has been to lower dietary protein intake to 0.8–1.0 g/kg of body weight per day for patients with microalbuminuria. For people with overt nephropathy, reducing dietary protein intake to 0.8 g/kg of body weight per day may slow the progression of nephropathy. Protein restriction should not be attempted if serious protein loss from nephrotic-range proteinuria has reduced total serum albumin concentration, in which case it is agreed that a low-protein diet is not indicated. In fact, a large study of the dietary treatment of kidney disease in nondiabetic subjects did not support the value of protein restriction in slowing progression of kidney damage.

The best documented therapies for proteinuria and reducing nephropathy are improved glycemic control and reduction of blood pressure using ACE inhibitors or ARBs. Cessation of smoking is also of established benefit.

Conclusions

Medical nutrition therapy is essential to all people with diabetes, of whatever type or severity. A healthy diet should contain important components, including foods containing carbohydrates from whole grains, fruits, vegetables, vitamins, and low-fat dairy products. Although blood glucose control and management of coexisting risk factors are overall goals, the implementation of dietary management is a highly complex and individualized process. Principles of medical nutrition therapy that generally apply to all diabetes, and specific features that apply to the various types of diabetes, have been discussed; but it must be emphasized that good nutritional management requires the close interaction of each individual patient with a knowledgeable expert in dietetics.

See also: **Carbohydrates**: Chemistry and Classification; Regulation of Metabolism. **Diabetes Mellitus**: Etiology and Epidemiology; Classification and Chemical Pathology. **Glucose**: Metabolism and Maintenance of Blood Glucose Level. **Obesity**: Complications. **Sucrose**: Nutritional Role, Absorption and Metabolism; Dietary Sucrose and Disease. **Weight Management**: Approaches.

Further Reading

American Diabetes Association (2004) Position statement: Nutrition principles and recommendations in diabetes. *Diabetes Care* 27(supplement 1): S36–S46.

Connor H, Annan F, Bunn E et al. Nutrition Subcommittee of the Diabetes Care Advisory Committee of Diabetes UK (2003) The implementation of nutritional advice for people with diabetes. *Diabetic Medicine* 20(10): 786–807.

Eyre H, Kahn R, and Robertson RM (2004) Preventing cancer, cardiovascular disease, and diabetes: A common agenda for the American Cancer Society, the American Diabetes Association, and the American Heart Association. American Cancer Society, the American Diabetes Association, and the American Heart Association Collaborative Writing Committee. *Diabetes Care* 27(7): 1812–1824.

Franz MJ, Bantle JP, Beebe CA et al. (2002) Evidence based nutrition principles and recommendations for the treatment and prevention of diabetes and related complications [Technical review]. *Diabetes Care* 25: 148–198.

DIARRHEAL DISEASES

A Baqui, R Heinzen, M Santosham and R Black, Johns Hopkins Bloomberg School of Public Health, Baltimore, MD, USA

© 2005 Elsevier Ltd. All rights reserved.

Global Burden of Diarrhea and Epidemiological Trends

Diarrheal illnesses in young children are among the leading causes of morbidity and mortality in developing countries. Diarrhea is an important cause of morbidity in developed countries as well. In developing countries, children younger than 5 years old suffer 3–10 episodes of diarrhea per year, whereas in developed countries young children have on average 1 or 2 diarrheal episodes per year. The advent of oral rehydration therapy (ORT) and its use in the past three decades have dramatically reduced the case fatality rate for diarrhea. However, globally the estimated 3 billion annual episodes of diarrhea account for approximately 2 million deaths in children younger than 5 years old. The majority of diarrhea-related mortality occurs in developing countries and the highest rates of diarrhea occur among infants with malnutrition. The case fatality rate is highest among children 6 months to 1 year old. The primary reason is that for most children this is the period when the immune system is not yet fully matured and the maternal antibodies are reduced. In addition, they may receive contaminated foods to complement breast-feeding, and they begin to crawl, potentially to areas where they may have direct contact with human or animal feces.

Although dehydration is the most direct effect of diarrhea, there are many adverse and potentially fatal nutritional consequences when proper nutritional management is not followed. This article provides an overview of the epidemiology of diarrheal diseases, including the interaction of diarrhea and malnutrition, and discusses the treatment of diarrhea, including fluid therapy and dietary management to minimize the nutritional cost of diarrhea.

Diarrhea–Malnutrition Interaction

Diarrheal illnesses are more common, last longer, are clinically more severe, and are more likely to have a fatal outcome for impoverished children in less developed countries because of a complex interaction between infection, protein-energy malnutrition, and micronutrient deficiencies. Diarrhea and malnutrition have a bidirectional relationship in which malnutrition increases the incidence and duration of diarrhea and, conversely, diarrhea exerts a negative effect on nutritional status.

Malnourished children have defects in cell-mediated immune functions and a decrease in IgA-containing cells in the jejunal mucosa. Malnutrition produces morphological and functional changes in virtually all organs. Changes in the intestine include thinning of the gut epithelium, marked flattening and broadening of villi, extensive infiltration of the lamina propria, and diminished secretion of gastric acid. These changes lead to an increased risk of diarrhea. The risk of developing diarrhea may be predicted by a child's ability to respond to skin test antigens. This effect of impaired cellular immunity is independent of age and nutritional status. Studies have shown that patients with a variety of viral and bacterial infections, such as measles, influenza, tuberculosis, and streptococcal infections, develop impaired cell-mediated immunity (anergy). Anergy or reduced responsiveness may also be associated with single nutrient deficiency, such as deficiency of vitamin A, zinc, pyridoxine, folic acid, and iron. Therefore, it may be possible that in an otherwise healthy child, infection or micronutrient deficiencies induce immunodeficiency may increase susceptibility to diarrhea and other infections and lead to a vicious cycle of repeated infections, anergy, and deteriorating nutritional status.

Diarrheal diseases have generally been noted to have an adverse effect on growth of underprivileged children in developing countries. Community-based prospective studies in developing countries have consistently demonstrated a significant negative effect of diarrhea on short-term weight gain, but studies on the effect on short-term height gain are less consistent. On the contrary, some investigators have concluded that the effect of diarrhea on growth is transient and that efforts to control diarrhea are unlikely to improve children's nutritional status. One possible explanation for the discrepant findings is the heterogeneity of diarrheal illnesses. Most studies that have examined the effect of diarrhea on growth have considered diarrhea as a single entity. Studies that have examined the effect of diarrhea on growth by type of diarrheal illness have suggested that certain etiological (e.g., *Shigella* spp.) and clinical-type (dysentery) illnesses are associated with significant growth retardation. It has been estimated that diarrheal illnesses account for 10–80% of growth retardation in the first few years of life, with the magnitude of effect possibly modified by other factors, such as etiology and clinical type, the source and adequacy of dietary intake, treatment and feeding practices during and following illness, and the opportunity for catch-up growth after illness. A cohort study conducted in Bangladesh observed that dysentery had the most deleterious consequences on both ponderal and linear growth, although other types of diarrhea showed a similar but relatively less pronounced negative effect on growth. Losses of approximately 0.5 kg in annual weight gain and 1.25 cm in annual height gain were associated with dysentery in children <5 years old in this population.

Understanding the mechanisms of diarrhea-induced undernutrition and appropriate treatment of diarrhea is important for the immediate illness and also for the long-term well-being of children. Approximately 10% of diarrheal episodes result in persistent diarrhea lasting more than 2 weeks. These infants need specialized treatment in addition to rehydration therapy, such as antibiotics for concurrent infections, micronutrients, and careful dietary management. In many settings, up to 50% of diarrhea-associated deaths occur in children with malnutrition-associated persistent diarrhea.

Clinical Types and Etiology of Diarrhea

Since nutritional costs of diarrhea vary by etiology and clinical type, a discussion of different types of diarrhea is pertinent. Diarrheal episodes can be classified based on clinical presentation as inflammatory (dysentery) and noninflammatory (nondysentery) diarrhea. Therefore, the clinical presentation of diarrheal illnesses may suggest a causative diagnosis. Diarrheal episodes can also be classified based on duration as acute (<14 days) and persistent (≥14 days) diarrhea. The diarrhea is generally due to either infectious or noninfectious causes. This article focuses on infectious diarrhea. Pathogens that cause infectious diarrhea include bacteria, viruses, and parasites (**Table 1**).

Most diarrheal episodes are acute. Occasionally, they become prolonged, leading to a vicious cycle of malabsorption, malnutrition, and failure to thrive. Noninfectious diarrhea tends to be persistent because it is often due to a chronic health problem. However, most persistent diarrhea is due to infection or is a sequeale of infection. Infections can lead to persistent diarrhea in the following situations: (i) Some pathogens cause chronic symptoms, usually parasites but sometimes bacteria; (ii) immunosuppressed individuals, such as those with human immunodeficiency virus (HIV) infection, cannot effectively clear pathogens and can develop persistent diarrhea; and (iii) at times the infection clears, but people develop chronic symptoms, such as irritable bowel syndrome, with diarrhea. If the diarrhea is persistent, it can cause dehydration, malnutrition, and systemic infections. Diarrhea in combination with a severe case of malnutrition (e.g., marasmus and kwashiorkor) is very dangerous and can lead to

Table 1 Infectious causes of diarrhea

Bacterial
Shigella species
Salmonella
Campylobacter jejuni
Enteroadherent *Escherichia coli*
Enteroinvasive *Escherichia coli*
Enterohemorrhagic *Escherichia coli*
Yersinia enterocolitica
Staphylococcus aureas
Bacillius cereus
Vibrio cholerae non-O group 1
Vibrio parahaemolyticus
Listeria monocytogenes
Aeromonas hydrophilia
Plesliomonas shigelloides

Viruses
Rotavirus
Norovirus
Enteric adenovirus
Calcivirus
Astrovirus
Coronavirus
Cytomegalovirus

Parasites
Giardia lamblia
Entamoeba histolytica
Cryptosporidium
Cyclospora
Isospora belli
Microsporidia
Strongyloides

Food poisoning
Staphylococcus aureus
Clostridium perfringens
Bacillus cereus

Drugs, especially antibiotic induced
Clostridium difficile

systematic infections and death. Although many different mechanisms may contribute to persistent diarrhea, the result is a similar pathophysiologic syndrome of mucosal atrophy, inflammation, and malabsoption. Therapeutic efforts should concentrate on nutritional rehabilitation.

Factors Influencing Nutritional Decline in Diarrhea

Factors that influence a nutritional decline during a period of diarrhea include reduced food intake, diminished nutrient absorption due to malabsorption of macro- and micronutrients and shorter intestinal transit time, direct loss of protein and other nutrients, and an increase in the body's demand for nutrients. In addition, diarrhea of infectious origins causes cytokine-induced malnutrition, which results from the action of proinflammatory cytokines such as tumor necrosis factor and interleukin-1, -6, and -8.

Food Intake during Diarrhea

Food intake during diarrhea is often reduced due to poor appetite (anorexia), vomiting, deliberate withholding of food, and inappropriate dietary supplementation with diluted food items. Diarrhea can also be associated with fever. Both fever and anorexia have clear effects on the nutritional status of the host. An increase in body temperature of 1 °C causes an increase in the basal metabolic rate of 12–23%. Although the reason for anorexia is not clear, its effect can be important. In a controlled study in Bangladesh, 41 hospitalized children with acute diarrhea consumed only about half of the total calories consumed by healthy children despite an educational intervention.

Malabsorption of Nutrients

Malabsorption in diarrheal illness may result from the epithelial destruction by the pathogen. Diminished nutrient absorption often begins during acute diarrhea. At this time, the body is less able to absorb needed macronutrients, including fats and proteins, as well as some carbohydrates. This is most severe in undernourished children who suffer from persistent diarrhea due to damage to the gut epithelium. When the gut is damaged, food is not properly digested or absorbed. The causes of insufficient nutrient absorption include diminished concentration of bile acids, which are used for fat absorption; damaged epithelial cells, which provide the absorptive surface on the bowel; and a deficiency of disaccharides due to damaged microvilli, which normally produce the needed enzymes. In symptomatic rotavirus infection, the most common cause of acute severe diarheal illness worldwide, there is a 42% decrease in the absorption of nitrogen and fat, a 48% decrease in absorption of carbohydrates, and a 55% decrease in the total carbohydrate absorption. Malabsoption is more severe in both ETEC and shigella diarrhea. In shigellosis, loss of protein and vitamin A is sizeable. Giardiasis leads to malabsorption of vitamin A. A large amount of zinc is lost in diarrhea, usually resulting in a negative net zinc balance during the illness.

Increased Demand for Nutrients

During episodes of diarrhea, the body requires more nutrients than normal. This is due to the need to repair the damage to the gut epithelium, the increased metabolic demand on the body made by a fever, and, during dysentery, the need to replace serum protein lost by exudation through the damaged intestinal mucosa.

Management of Diarrhea

An invariable accompaniment of diarrhea, particularly persistent diarrhea, is protein-energy malnutrition. However, dehydration is the most immediate complication of diarrhea. Clinical management of acute diarrhea includes four major components: (i) replacement of fluid and electrolyte losses, (ii) zinc therapy, (iii) antimicrobial therapy when indicated, and (iv) continued feeding to supply a sufficient quantity of nutrients to meet both the patient's usual maintenance requirement and the increased needs imposed by infection and malabsoption.

Fluid Therapy

The majority of the diarrhea-associated deaths result from dehydration. Parents should be encouraged to increase fluid intake as soon as diarrhea begins and to give oral rehydration solution if available. Children presenting with diarrhea should be assessed for dehydration. Thirst is an early sign of dehydration in a child. Other signs are mucosal dryness (e.g., dry mouth), sunken eyes, and loss of skin turgor. The coexistence of fever or vomiting exacerbates dehydration. The World Health Organization (WHO) guidelines classify dehydration into two categories—some dehydration and severe dehydration. Weight loss is the main clinical index of degree of dehydration. A vast majority of children with diarrhea present with some dehydration or no clinical signs of dehydration. The cornerstone of treatment for these children is oral rehydration solution (ORS) containing glucose or sucrose and electrolytes. ORS is effective but it must start as soon as diarrhea starts. In children with some dehydration, approximately 100 ml/kg of body weight of ORS should be given within 4 h. Ongoing stool losses should be replaced with ORS. Rehydration and maintenance of hydration in a vomiting child is feasible using ORS by giving small amounts frequently. Severe dehydration is a medical emergency that requires immediate intravenous fluid replacement, and children should preferably be hospitalized. Patients presenting with severe dehydration should receive 40 ml/kg body weight of Ringers lactate or similar intravenous solutions over a 4-h period. ORS should be given as soon as the child is able to drink.

Regardless of etiology, watery diarrhea requires fluid and electrolyte replacement. For more than three decades, an ORS containing 90 mmol/l of sodium and 111 mmol/l of glucose was used throughout the world. This solution has been credited with saving millions of lives. WHO and UNICEF have recommended the use of a new reduced osmolarity ORS formulation consisting of 75 mmol/l of sodium and 75 mmol/l of glucose and total osmolarity of 245 mOSm/l. This recommendation was made on the basis of studies that have demonstrated that the reduced osmolarity ORS was at least as efficacious as the standard ORS containing 90 mmol/l of sodium and an osmolarity of 311/l. In addition, in a meta-analysis, the reduced osmolarity ORS was shown to decrease the need for unscheduled intravenous therapy by 33%, the stool output was reduced by 20%, and the incidence of vomiting was reduced by 30%. However, there is concern that this low osmolar ORS may lead to asymptomatic and symptomatic hyponatremia in adults with severe diarrhea. This issue needs to be evaluated in large-scale effectiveness trials. Despite the proven efficacy of ORS, only approximately 20% of children receive appropriate ORS therapy during diarrheal episodes. The barriers to use of ORS include lack of knowledge of the importance of rehydration therapy, lack of access to ORS, and the perception that ORS is not a medicine since it does not stop the diarrhea.

The management of a child with persistent diarrhea is often difficult due to other related heath issues. These children are more likely to be severely undernourished due to micronutrient and protein-energy malnutrition as well as more prone to systematic infections. Due to the systematic infections, appropriate antibiotic therapy is needed.

Dietary Management of Diarrhea, Including Persistent Diarrhea

Data suggest that continued feeding during diarrhea is generally well tolerated and it minimizes the nutritional cost associated with diarrhea. A child should receive the same type of food during an episode of diarrhea as when the child is healthy. Feeding is usually tolerated, with the occasional exception of lactose intolerance. A small subgroup of children exclusively receiving nonhuman milk may have a higher rate of complications. These children should be closely supervised and provided with alternatives if needed. Full feedings will help to minimize growth faltering and a decline in nutritional status. Growth faltering may still occur, especially in severely undernourished children, due to poor nutrient absorption.

Importance of Continued Breast Feeding

Breast feeding should be continued for as long as the child can tolerate it during episodes of acute diarrhea as well as during persistent diarrhea. It is normally well tolerated during such episodes and has been shown to reduce stool output and decrease the duration of the illness compared to those of non-breast-fed children.

Milk Intolerance: Lactose Intolerance

The majority of children can tolerate lactose during a diarrheal episode. A small proportion of children with diarrhea may not be able to digest lactose and are therefore not tolerant of milk- and lactose-containing formulas. This is more likely to occur among young children who only receive animal milk or formula in their diet and who have persistent diarrhea, and it rarely occurs in children on a diet of breast milk. In a lactose-intolerant child, milk- and lactose-containing formulas result in a significant increase in stool output. Stool output reduces dramatically when the milk- or lactose-containing formula is stopped. The warning signs of lactose intolerance include deterioration of the child's clinical condition, signs of dehydration, and an increase in the stool volume when milk feedings are given. However, only when the child is not gaining weight, eating less, and not fully alert is this a real cause for concern. This condition can be managed by continuing breast feeding. If the child is not yet in the weaning period but takes animal milk, yogurt or diluted milk (equal water and milk) or soy milk can be used as a substitute given in small feedings. The child should be taken to a health care provider if the condition does not improve in 2 days.

If the child eats soft or solid foods, the lactose in the diet should be substituted in the same manner as for the infant (with diluted milk or soy milk) but mixed with cooked cereals and vegetables. If this does not improve the condition of the child, all animal milk should be excluded from the diet, and protein- and energy-rich foods such as finely ground chicken should be given. The treatment should be continued for a few days after the cessation of the diarrhea, when the milk is slowly replaced in the diet.

Soft or Solid Food, Energy Density of Diet, and Protein and Energy Requirements

A child's diet during the period of diarrhea should not be drastically different from his or her normal healthy diet. Therefore, for children who are currently breast-feeding, they should continue to do so, and for children who are in the weaning period and have a mixed diet, they should continue to have a mixed diet of soft or solid food. If the child on a mixed diet is dehydrated, his or her soft and solid

foods should be temporarily stopped for a period of approximately 4 h when he or she rehydrates. However, it should then be resumed. For children who are in the weaning stages, WHO recommends small, frequent feedings (six or more times a day) to increase nutrient absorption. The type of food should be energy rich, low in bulk, locally available, and nutritious. The diet should contain complementary protein sources and easily digestible fats, and complex carbohydrates should be avoided. All the foods should be well cooked. Easily digestible staple foods that can be easily mashed include rice, corn, potatoes, and noodles. These staple foods should be mixed with vegetables as well as sources of protein if possible. It is also important to ensure adequate rehydration. In addition, the consumption of fresh fruit juices and mashed bananas is highly encouraged because they provide a good source of potassium.

Feeding during the Convalescent Period

The convalescent period is the recovery period for the body during which the child's diarrhea has stopped but the body has not yet fully recovered to its initial condition. During the first few weeks, the child's appetite will be returning and the child may consume up to twice as much as usual. This is a necessary part of the process because even if the child was fully fed during diarrhea, he or she most likely did not absorb sufficient nutrients. During this time, the child's nutritional state should return to at least the level before the child became ill. The desired energy intake ranges from 100 to 160 J/kg per day, which is achieved with a high-energy, low-bulk, and low-viscosity diet. This is needed for a catch-up growth period and rapid nutritional recovery.

Supplementation with Micronutrients

ORT reduces mortality from dehydrating diarrhea, but it does not decrease the duration of episodes or their consequences, such as malnutrition. In addition, adherence to recommendations regarding ORT in children is poor because caregivers want to reduce the duration of illness. This often leads to use of antibiotics and other treatment of no proven value. In addition, there are indications that knowledge and use of appropriate home therapies, including ORT, to manage diarrhea successfully may be declining in some countries. The limitations of ORT and continued high diarrhoeal morbidity, mortality, and associated malnutrition led to a search for adjunct therapies. Zinc and vitamin A are essential to repair the intestinal mucosa and boost immunological responses. These supplements should be given during periods of diarrhea.

Zinc

Based on the results of a large number of randomized controlled trials that have demonstrated the therapeutic benefits of zinc supplementation during diarrhea, WHO and UNICEF have recommended the use of zinc supplementation at a dose of approximately 2 RDAs per day (10–20 mg) for 10–14 days. This strategy has the advantage of having a good delivery mechanism (i.e., during the delivery of ORS packets). The effectiveness of different delivery strategies is being evaluated in large-scale trials.

A study from India evaluated the efficacy of zinc-fortified ORS and reported that zinc–ORS was moderately efficacious in reducing the severity of acute diarrhea. If these results are confirmed by other studies, this strategy has the advantage of reducing the need to deliver the zinc supplementation separate from the ORS packets. However, it will probably result in increased cost of ORS production and not all countries will be able to rapidly scale up the production of zinc–ORS in the near future. Additional potential disadvantages of this strategy are that coverage with ORS is low, ORS is usually needed only for 2 or 3 days, and the volume of ORS taken is generally low. Therefore, it will be difficult to ensure adequate zinc intake.

Vitamin A

The body's ability to absorb vitamin A during diarrhea is reduced, which may lead to acute vitamin A deficiency. Repeated episodes may lead to blindness and signs of xerophthalmia. If these are recognized, 200 000 units of vitamin A should be orally administered to children (100 000 units for infants). There should be two subsequent doses, one the following day and another in 4 weeks. In areas where vitamin A deficiency is a problem, any foods that are rich in carotene should be administered (including dark leafy vegetables and yellow or orange fruits and vegetables). Vitamin A deficiency is most common among severely undernourished children and among children who have recently recovered from the measles.

Medications

Antimicrobials and antiparasitics should not be regularly used. Most episodes do not benefit from these treatments, with the following exceptions: in suspect cases of cholera, in cases of persistent diarrhea when cysts or trophozoites of Giardia are identified in the feces, and antibiotics that are effective for Shigella are only used for cases of dysentery (blood in the stool).

Management of Diarrhea in Children with Severe Malnutrition

Children who are severely undernourished and have diarrhea often have other infections. Infections can cause hypothermia as opposed to fever. An appropriate antibiotic should be give if an infection is identified.

Assessment of Dehydration in a Severely Malnourished Child

Children who are severely undernourished have different, unreliable signs and symptoms to assess the status of their hydration. For example, children with marasmus have poor skin elasticity even though they are not dehydrated, and sunken eyes are also not a reliable sign. Irritability in these children may be a sign of systemic infection rather than dehydration. The skin of children with kwashiorkor, on the other hand, may appear to be normal even if they are dehydrated. These children generally have apathetic attitudes. Undernourished children do not readily cry, so determining the absence of tears is also a challenge. Signs that prove to be more indicative to the status of a child's level of hydration include cool and clammy extremities, eagerness to drink, dry mouth and tongue, and a weak radial pulse.

Rehydration

Severely undernourished children should be hospitalized. ORS should be started as soon as possible. A standard ORS treatment with additional potassium should be given orally (preferred method) or using a nasogastric tube. An intravenous solution should be avoided since fluid overload may potentially cause heart failure and increase the risk of septicemia. By dissolving 7.5 g of potassium chloride in 100 ml of water, it is possible to prepare 1 mmol of potassium per milliliter of solution. Every 24 h, 4 ml/kg body weight should be given, mixed with food, for 14 days.

Feeding

Children with marasmus must limit their food intake to approximately 110 kcal/kg/day for the first week. On the other hand, children with kwashiorkor must begin a slow feeding treatment starting as low as 50 kcal/kg/day and work their way up to approximately 110 kcal/kg/day after approximately 1 week. This can be a difficult task since these children are often apathetic and have severe anorexia. The initial diets of all severely undernourished children must be given in small, frequent (every 2 h day and night), semiliquid doses. An example of an initial diet packet is 8 g skim milk powder, 6 g vegetable oil, 5 g sugar, and 100 ml water to make a high-energy (100 kcal/100 ml) meal with additional minerals, including 60 mg iron, 100 mg folic acid, and 200 000 units of vitamin A and vitamins B (complex), C, and D.

Conclusion

Diarrhea, a disease of fluid and electrolyte imbalance, is an important worldwide cause of morbidity and mortality among infants and children, especially in developing countries. However, it is also very much a nutritional disease. This is primarily because during periods of diarrhea, nutrient intake and absorption are dramatically decreased, which results in undernutrition even when sufficient food is available. The losses of nutrients affect growth rates, and where diarrhea occurs frequently the child may not grow properly. This is a cyclical pattern in that undernourishment in children makes them more prone to diarrhea. Their immune systems are less robust and the episodes affect them more than well-nourished children. Undernourishment and diarrhea can be a fatal combination that can result in a vicious cycle. This cycle requires intervention, sometimes at a treatment center if the case is severe enough. Therefore, is a matter of not only replacing the fluids and electrolytes but also of managing good feeding practices at all times before, during, and after the illness.

Sixty percent of the 10 million deaths among children younger than 5 years old are associated with malnutrition. Approximately 2 million of the deaths are due to diarrhea. Repeated episodes of diarrhea result in malnutrition, which in turn puts the child at an increased risk of recurrent infections, including diarrhea. To break this cycle, diarrheal episodes should be managed with appropriate fluid and nutritional therapy.

See also: **Colon**: Disorders; Nutritional Management of Disorders. **Lactose Intolerance**. **Malnutrition**: Primary, Causes Epidemiology and Prevention; Secondary, Diagnosis and Management. **United Nations Children's Fund**. **Vitamin A**: Biochemistry and Physiological Role. **World Health Organization**. **Zinc**: Deficiency in Developing Countries, Intervention Studies.

Further Reading

Ahmed T, Ali M, Ullah MM *et al.* (1999) Mortality in severely malnourished children with diarrhoea and use of a standardised management protocol. *Lancet* 353(9168): 1919–1922.

Alam DS, Marks GC, Baqui AH *et al.* (2000) Association between clinical type of diarrhea and growth of children younger than 5 years old in rural Bangladesh. *International Journal of Epidemiology* 29(5): 916–921.

Baqui AH, Black RE, Arifeen SE *et al.* (2002) Community randomized trial of zinc supplementation started during diarrhoea reduces morbidity and mortality in Bangladeshi children. *British Medical Journal* 325(7372): 1059.

Baqui AH, Black RE, Sack RB *et al.* (1993) Malnutrition, cell-mediated immune deficiency and diarrhoea: A community-based longitudinal study in rural Bangladeshi children. *American Journal of Epidemiology* 137(3): 355–365.

Baqui AH, Sack RB, Black RE *et al.* (1992) Enteropathogens associated with acute and persistent diarrhoea in rural Bangladeshi children. *Journal of Infectious Disease* 166: 792–796.

Baqui AH, Sack RB, Black RE *et al.* (1993) Cell-mediated immune deficiency and malnutrition are independent risk factors for persistent diarrhea in Bangladeshi children. *American Journal of Clinical Nutrition* 58: 453–458.

Baqui AH, Zaman K, Persson LA *et al.* (2003) Simultaneous weekly supplementation of iron and zinc is associated with lower morbidity due to diarrhea and acute lower respiratory infection in Bangladeshi infants. *Journal of Nutrition* 133(12): 4150–4157.

Black RE, Morris SS, and Bryce J (2003) Where and why are 10 million children dying every year? *Lancet* 361(9376): 2226–2234.

Brown KH (2003) Diarrhea and malnutrition. *Journal of Nutrition* 133(1): 328S–332S.

Kosek M, Bern C, and Guerrant RL (2003) The global burden of diarrhoeal disease, as estimated from studies published between 1992 and 2000. *Bulletin of the World Health Organization* 81(3): 197–204.

Lutter CK, Habicht J-P, Rivera JA *et al.* (2004) *Clinical Management of Acute Diarrhoea*, WHO/UNICEF Joint Statement (WHO/FCH/CAH/04.7). New York: United Nations Children's Fund/World Health Organization.

Rahman MM, Vermund SH, Wahed MA *et al.* (2001) Effect of simultaneous zinc and vitamin A supplementation on diarrhoea and acute lower respiratory infection in Bangladeshi children: A randomized double-blind placebo controlled trial. *British Medical Journal* 323: 314–318.

Schrimshaw NS (2003) *Nutrition and Diarrhoea: Fifty Years Experience. Keynote Lecture 1, Nutrition and Diarrhoea.* Presented at the 10th Asian Conference on Diarrhoeal Diseases and Nutrition (ASCODD), December 7–9, Abstract Book, ICDDR, B, Dhaka.

Thapar N and Sanderson IR (2004) Diarrhoea in children: An interface between developing and developed countries. *Lancet* 363(9409): 641–653.

World Health Organization (2000) *IMCI Model Handbook*, WHO/FCH/CAH/00.12. Geneva, WHO.

DIETARY FIBER

Contents
Physiological Effects and Effects on Absorption
Potential Role in Etiology of Disease
Role in Nutritional Management of Disease

Physiological Effects and Effects on Absorption

I T Johnson, Institute of Food Research, Norwich, UK

© 2005 Elsevier Ltd. All rights reserved.

Introduction

It has long been recognized that both animal feedstuffs and human foods contain poorly digestible components, which do not contribute to nutrition in the classical sense of providing essential substances or metabolic energy. With the development of scientific approaches to animal husbandry in the nineteenth century, the term 'crude fiber' was coined to describe the material that remained after rigorous nonenzymic hydrolysis of feeds. During the twentieth century, various strands of thought concerning the virtues of 'whole' foods, derived from plant components that had undergone only minimal processing, began to converge, leading eventually to the dietary fiber hypothesis. Put simply, this states that the nondigestible components of plant cell walls are essential for the maintenance of human health.

In the early 1970s the physician and epidemiologist Hugh Trowell recognized that the crude fiber figures available at the time for foods had little physiological significance and were of no practical value in the context of human diets. He was amongst the first to use the term dietary fiber to describe the 'remnants of plant cell walls resistant to hydrolysis (digestion) by the alimentary enzymes of man.' This definition was later refined and given the more quantitative form: "The sum of lignin and the plant polysaccharides that are not digested by the endogenous secretions of the mammalian digestive tract." This definition paved the way for the development of analytical methods that could be used to define the fiber content of human foods. Broadly, these techniques are based on enzymic removal of the digestible elements in food, followed by either gravimetric analysis of the residue ('Southgate' and Association of Analytical Chemists (AOAC) methods), which results in the retention of some undigested starch, or chemical analysis ('Englyst' method), which enables a more precise separation of starch from the structural polysaccharides of the cell wall. In the latter case, the cell wall components are defined as 'nonstarch polysaccharides' (NSP). Whatever analytical approach is used, both 'dietary fiber' and nonstarch polysaccharides are shorthand terms for large and complex mixtures of polysaccharides. The components of such mixtures vary widely among foods and they often share few properties other than resistance to digestion in the small intestine. A summary of the main types of plant cell polysaccharides contained in the general definition of dietary fiber is given in **Table 1**.

In recent years this problem has been made more complex in some ways because of the explosion of interest in functional foods for gastrointestinal health. These often contain high levels of novel oligo- and polysaccharides, which might perhaps be regarded as analogs of dietary fiber. Fructose oligosaccharides, which are nondigestible but highly fermentable, are now often added to foods as prebiotic substrates for the colonic microflora. Such materials may not fit the original definition of dietary fiber, but it is certainly not helpful to exclude them from the contemporary concept, which needs to expand to accommodate modern developments.

The presence of large undigested cell wall fragments, finely dispersed particulates, or soluble polysaccharides can alter physiological processes

Table 1 Major components of dietary fiber

Food source	Polysaccharides and related substances
Fruits and vegetables	Cellulose, xyloglucans, arabinogalactans, pectic substances, glycoproteins
Cereals	Cellulose, arabinoxylans, glucoarabinoxylans, β-D-glucans, lignin, and phenolic esters
Legume seeds	Cellulose, xyloglucans, galactomannans, pectic substances
Manufactured products	Gums (guar gum, gum arabic), alginates, carrageenan, modified cellulose gums (methyl cellulose, carboxymethyl cellulose)

throughout the gut. The effects of different fiber components depend upon their varied physical and chemical properties during digestion, and also upon their susceptibility to degradation by bacterial enzymes in the colon. The complex nature of the various substances covered by the general definition of dietary fiber means that a single analytical value for the fiber content of a food is a poor guide to its physiological effects. This article will review the main mechanisms of action of resistant polysaccharides in the alimentary tract and their implications for human health.

Sources and Types of Dietary Fiber

The main sources of dietary fiber in most Western diets are well characterized, and high-quality data are available for both food composition and dietary intakes. This is not always true for diets in developing countries, however, and this problem bedevils attempts to investigate the importance of fiber by making international comparisons of diet and disease. Another problem is that different analytical approaches give slightly different values for the dietary fiber content of foods, and do not reflect the physical and chemical properties of the different polysaccharide components. The use of enzymic hydrolysis to determine the 'unavailable carbohydrate' content of foods was refined by Southgate, and his technique was used for the 4th edition of the UK standard food tables, *The Composition of Foods* published in 1978. The 6th edition, published in 2002, contains values for nonstarch polysaccharides, derived using the Englyst technique, but recommends use of AOAC methods for food labeling purposes. A comparison of values for nonstarch polysaccharides and dietary fiber values obtained by the AOAC method is given in **Table 2**.

Table 2 A Comparison of values for nonstarch polysaccharides and dietary fiber

Food source	Nonstarch Polysaccharides (Englyst method)	Total dietary fiber (AOAC method)
White bread	2.1	2.9
Brown bread	3.5	5.0
Wholemeal bread	5.0	7.0
Green vegetables	2.7	3.3
Potatoes	1.9	2.4
Fresh fruit	1.4	1.9
Nuts	6.6	8.8

Data modified from McCance and Widdowson's (2002) *The Composition of Foods*, 6th Edition, Cambridge: Royal Society of Chemistry.

In the UK about 47% of dietary fiber is obtained from cereal products, including bread and breakfast cereals. The level of cell wall polysaccharides in a product made from flour depends on the extraction rate, which is the proportion of the original grain present in the flour after milling. Thus a 'white' flour with an extraction rate of 70% usually contains about 3% NSP, whereas a 'wholemeal' flour with an extraction rate of 100% contains about 10% NSP. The terms 'soluble' and 'insoluble' fiber have been coined in order to partially overcome the problem of the lack of correspondence between the total analytical value for fiber and the physical properties of the measured polysaccharides. By adopting the Englyst technique for the separation and chemical analysis of nonstarch polysaccharides it is possible to specify both the soluble and insoluble fiber content of foods. Some representative values for soluble and insoluble fiber in cereal foods are given in **Table 3**, and those for fruits and vegetables, which provide a further 45% of the fiber in UK diets, are given in **Table 4**.

Fiber in the Digestive Tract

The primary function of the alimentary tract is to break down the complex organic macromolecules of which other organisms are composed into smaller molecules, which can then be selectively absorbed into the circulation by specialized mucosal epithelial

Table 3 Soluble and insoluble nonstarch polysaccharides in some cereal products and nuts

Food source	Nonstarch polysaccharides (g per 100 g fresh weight)		
	Total NSP	Soluble NSP	Insoluble NSP
Sliced white bread	1.5	0.9	0.6
Sliced brown bread	3.6	1.1	2.5
Wholemeal bread	4.8	1.6	3.2
Spaghetti	1.2	0.6	0.6
Rye biscuits	11.7	3.9	7.8
Cornflakes	0.9	0.4	0.5
Crunchy oat cereal	6.0	3.3	2.7
Walnuts	3.5	1.5	2.0
Hazelnuts	6.5	2.5	4.0
Peanuts	6.2	1.9	4.3
Brazil nuts	4.3	1.3	3.0

Data modified from Englyst HN, Bingham SA, Runswick SS, Collinson E, and Cummings JH (1989) Dietary fibre (non-starch polysaccharides) in cereal products. *Journal of Human Nutrition and Dietetics* **2**: 253–271 and Englyst HN, Bingham SA, Runswick SS, Collinson E, Cummings JH (1989) Dietary fibre (non-starch polysaccharides) in fruit vegetables and nuts. *Journal of Human Nutrition and Dietetics* **1**: 247–286.

Table 4 Soluble and insoluble nonstarch polysaccharides in some vegetables and fruits

Food source	Nonstarch polysaccharides (g per 100 g fresh weight)		
	Total NSP	Soluble NSP	Insoluble NSP
Apples (Cox)	1.7	0.7	1.0
Oranges	2.1	1.4	0.7
Plums	1.8	1.2	0.6
Bananas	1.1	0.7	0.4
Potatoes	1.1	0.6	0.5
Sprouts	4.8	2.5	2.3
Peas (frozen)	5.2	1.6	3.6
Carrots	2.5	1.4	1.1
Courgettes	1.2	0.6	0.6
Runner beans	2.3	0.9	1.4
Baked beans	3.5	2.1	1.4
Tomato	1.1	0.4	0.7
Lettuce	1.2	0.6	0.6
Onion	1.7	0.9	0.8
Celery	1.3	0.6	0.7

Data modified from Englyst HN, Bingham SA, Runswick SS, Collinson E, and Cummings JH (1989) Dietary fibre (non-starch polysaccharides) in fruit vegetables and nuts. *Journal of Human Nutrition and Dietetics* 1: 247–286.

cells. Food is conveyed progressively through the alimentary tract, stored at intervals, and broken down mechanically as required, by a tightly controlled system of rhythmic muscular contractions. The digestive enzymes are released into the lumen at the appropriate stages to facilitate the decomposition of carbohydrates, proteins, and complex lipids. By definition, the polysaccharides that comprise dietary fiber are not digested by endogenous enzymes, though they are often fermented to a greater or lesser degree by bacterial enzymes in the large intestine.

The Mouth and Pharynx

The earliest stages of digestion begin in the mouth, where food particles are reduced in size, lubricated with saliva, and prepared for swallowing. The saliva also contains the digestive enzyme salivary amylase, which begins the hydrolysis of starch molecules. Cell wall polysaccharides are an important determinant of food texture, and they exert an indirect effect on the degree of mechanical breakdown of plant foods prior to swallowing. Hard foods tend to be chewed more thoroughly than soft ones, and hence the presence of dietary fiber in unrefined foods may begin to regulate digestion at a very early stage.

The Stomach

The first delay in the transit of food through the digestive tract occurs in the stomach, where large food fragments are further degraded by rigorous muscular activity in the presence of hydrochloric acid and proteolytic enzymes. The need to disrupt and disperse intractable food particles and cell walls appears to delay the digestive process significantly. For example, the absorption of sugar from whole apples is significantly slower than from apple juice. Similarly, the rate at which the starch is digested and absorbed from cubes of cooked potato has been shown to be much slower when they are swallowed whole than when they are chewed normally. Thus, simple mechanical factors can limit the rate at which glucose from carbohydrate foods enters the circulation.

The Small Intestine

The small intestine is the main site of nutrient absorption, and it is in fact the largest of the digestive organs in terms of surface area. The semi-liquid products of gastric digestion are released periodically into the duodenum, and then propelled downstream by peristaltic movements, at about 1 cm per minute. The hydrolysis of proteins, triglycerides, and starch continues within the duodenum and upper jejunum, under the influence of pancreatic enzymes. The final stages of hydrolysis of dietary macromolecules occur under the influence of extracellular enzymes at the mucosal surface. The released products are absorbed into the circulation, along with water and electrolytes, via the specialized epithelial cells of the intestinal villi. Muscular activity in the small intestinal wall, together with rhythmic contractions of the villi, ensures that the partially digested chyme is well stirred. In adults, the first fermentable residues from a meal containing complex carbohydrates enter the colon approximately 4.5 h after ingestion. When a solution containing indigestible sugar is swallowed without food it reaches the colon about 1.5 h earlier than when the same material is added to a solid meal containing dietary fiber. The presence of solid food residues slows transit, probably by delaying gastric emptying and perhaps also by increasing the viscosity of the chyme so that it tends to resist the peristaltic flow. Soluble polysaccharides such as guar gum, pectin, and β-glucan from oats increase mouth to cecum transit time still further.

In creating the dietary fiber hypothesis, Trowell's principal interest was its role in the prevention of metabolic disorders. In particular, he believed that dietary fiber was a major factor in the prevention of diabetes mellitus, which, he argued, was probably unknown in Western Europe prior to the introduction of mechanized flour milling. In earlier times the near-universal consumption of unrefined carbohydrate foods would have ensured that intact indigestible cell wall polysaccharides were present throughout the upper alimentary tract during digestion. This, according to Trowell and others, favored slow absorption of glucose, which in turn placed less strain upon the ability of the pancreas to maintain glucose homeostasis. There is no doubt that type 2 diabetes has become more common in Western countries as prosperity, and an excess of energy consumption over expenditure, has grown. It is not established that rapid absorption of glucose due to consumption of refined starches is a primary cause of diabetes, but the control of glucose assimilation is certainly a key factor in its management. Cell wall polysaccharides influence the digestion and absorption of carbohydrates in a variety of ways, and are a major determinant of the 'glycemic index,' which is essentially a quantitative expression of the quantity of glucose appearing in the bloodstream after ingestion of a carbohydrate-rich food. To calculate the index, fasted subjects are given a test meal of the experimental food containing a standardized quantity of carbohydrate. The change in concentration of glucose in the blood is then measured over a period of time. The ratio of the area under the blood-glucose curve in response to the test meal to that produced by an equal quantity of a standard reference food is then calculated and expressed as a percentage. When glucose is used as the standard, most complex starchy foods have glycemic indices lower than 100%.

The physical resistance of plant cell walls during their passage through the gut varies considerably from one food to another. Cell walls that remain intact in the small intestine will impede the access of pancreatic amylase to starch. This is particularly true of the cells of legume seeds, which have been shown to retain much of their integrity during digestion. Legume-based foods such as lentils and chilli beans have glycemic indices that are amongst the lowest of all complex carbohydrate foods. Even when enzymes and their substrates do come into contact, the presence of cell wall polysaccharides may slow the diffusion of hydrolytic products through the partially digested matrix in the gut lumen. These effects of dietary fiber on carbohydrate metabolism emphasize once more that physiological effects cannot be predicted from simple analytical values for total fiber, because they are consequences of cellular structure, rather than the absolute quantity of cell wall polysaccharides within the food.

Many studies on postprandial glycemia have been conducted using isolated fiber supplements such, as pectin or guar gum added to glucose testmeals or to low-fiber sources of starch. They demonstrate that, contrary to Trowell's original hypothesis, wheat bran and other insoluble cell wall materials have little effect on glucose metabolism. However, certain soluble polysaccharides, such as guar gum, pectin, and oat β-glucan, which form viscous solutions in the stomach and small intestine, do slow the absorption of glucose. Highly viscous food components may delay gastric emptying and inhibit the dispersion of the digesta along the small intestine, but the primary mechanism of action appears to be suppression of convective stirring in the fluid layer adjacent to the mucosal surface. The rapid uptake of monosaccharides by the epithelial cells tends to reduce the concentration of glucose in this boundary layer, so that absorption from the gut lumen becomes rate-limited by the relatively slow process of diffusion. The overall effect is to delay the assimilation of glucose and hence suppress the glycemic response to glucose or starchy foods in both healthy volunteers and in people with diabetes. A similar mechanism probably inhibits the reabsorption of cholesterol and bile salts in the distal ileum and this may account for the ability of some viscous types of soluble dietary fiber such as guar gum and β-glucan to reduce plasma cholesterol levels in humans.

One of the main reasons for developing analytical methods to distinguish between soluble and insoluble components of dietary fiber was to provide a means of assessing the capacity of fiber-rich foods to influence carbohydrate and lipid metabolism. There is evidence that diets that provide 30–50% of their fiber in the form of soluble polysaccharides are associated with lower cholesterol levels and better glycemic control than diets that contain mostly insoluble fiber. Several officially recognized sets of guidelines for patients with impaired glucose metabolism and its complications (syndrome X) now specifically recommend a high intake of carbohydrate foods that are rich in soluble fiber.

Some of the interactions between cell wall polysaccharides and other food components in the small intestine are much more specific. There has been considerable interest over a number of years in the possibility that the polysaccharides and complex phenolic components of cell walls contain polar groups that could interact with and bind ionized species in the gastrointestinal contents, thereby reducing their availability for absorption. Intraluminal binding of heavy metals, toxins, and carcinogens might be a valuable protective mechanism, but binding of micronutrients could seriously compromise nutritional status.

Interactions of this type can be shown to occur *in vitro*, and studies with animals and human ileostomists suggest that charged polysaccharides such as pectin can displace cations into the colon under experimental conditions. However, there is little objective evidence that dietary fiber *per se* has much of an adverse effect on mineral metabolism in humans. Indeed, highly fermentable polysaccharides and fructose oligosaccharides have recently been shown to promote the absorption of calcium and magnesium in both animal and human studies. The mechanism for the effect is not entirely clear, but it is probably a consequence of fermentation acidifying the luminal contents of the colon and enhancing carrier-mediated transport of minerals across the colonic mucosa.

In unprocessed legume seeds, oats, and other cereals phytate (myo-inositol hexaphosphate) is often present in close association with cell wall polysaccharides. Unlike the polysaccharides themselves, phytate does exert a potent binding effect on minerals, and has been shown to significantly reduce the availability of magnesium, zinc, and calcium for absorption in humans. Phytate levels in foods can be reduced by the activity of endogenous phytase, by hydrolysis with exogenous enzymes, or by fermentation. Dephytinized products may therefore be of benefit to individuals at risk of suboptimal mineral status. However, there are indications from animal and *in vitro* studies that phytate is an anticarcinogen that may contribute to the protective effects of complex fiber-rich foods. The overall significance of phytate in the diet therefore requires further assessment in human trials.

The Large Intestine

Microorganisms occur throughout the alimentary tract but in healthy individuals their numbers and diversity are maintained within strict limits by the combined effects of intraluminal conditions, rapid transit, and host immunity. The colon and rectum, however, are adapted to facilitate bacterial colonization, and the typical adult human colonic microflora has been estimated to contain about 400 different bacterial species. The largest single groups present are Gram-negative anaerobes of the genus *Bacteroides*, and Gram-positive organisms including bifidobacteria, eubacteria, lactobacilli, and clostridia. However, a large proportion of the species present cannot be cultured *in vitro* and are very poorly characterized.

The proximal colon, which receives undigested food residues, intestinal secretions, and the remnants of exfoliated enterocytes from the distal ileum, contains around 200 g of bacteria and substrates in a semiliquid state. These conditions are ideal for

bacterial fermentation. Most of the bacteria of the human colon utilize carbohydrate as a source of energy, although not all can degrade polysaccharides directly. Many that are ultimately dependent upon dietary carbohydrate residues for energy are adapted to utilize the initial degradation products of the polysaccharide utilizers, rather than the polymers themselves. It has been estimated that somewhere between 20 and 80 g of carbohydrate enter the human colon every day, about half of which is undigested starch. Around 30 g of bacteria are produced for every 100 g of carbohydrate fermented.

Apart from dietary fiber, there are three major sources of unabsorbed carbohydrate for the colonic microflora. Perhaps the most important is resistant starch, which consists of retrograded starch polymers and starch granules enclosed within intact plant cell walls. Nondigestible sugars, sugar alcohols, and oligosaccharides such as fructooligosaccharides and galactooligosaccharides occur only sparingly in most plant foods, but they are now of great commercial interest because they can be used as prebiotics to selectively manipulate the numbers of bifidobacteria in the human colon. Endogenous substrates including mucus are also important for the colonic microflora. Mucus is an aqueous dispersion of a complex group of glycoproteins containing oligosaccharide side-chains, which are a major source of fermentable substrates. Even when the colon is surgically isolated and has no access to exogenous substrates it still supports a complex microflora.

The beneficial effects of dietary fiber on the alimentary tract were emphasized by another of the founders of the dietary fiber hypothesis, Denis Burkitt, who based his arguments largely on the concept of fecal bulk, developed as a result of field observations in rural Africa, where cancer and other chronic bowel diseases were rare. His hypothesis was that populations consuming the traditional rural diets, rich in vegetables and cereal foods, produced bulkier, more frequent stools than persons eating the refined diets typical of industrialized societies. Chronic constipation was thought to cause straining of abdominal muscles during passage of stool, leading to prolonged high pressures within the colonic lumen and the lower abdomen. This in turn was thought to increase the risk of various diseases of muscular degeneration including varicose veins, hemorrhoids, hiatus hernia, and colonic diverticulas. Colorectal neoplasia was also thought to result from infrequent defecation, because it caused prolonged exposure of the colonic epithelial cells to mutagenic chemicals, which could initiate cancer. Burkitt's overall hypothesis for the beneficial effects of fecal bulk has never really been refuted, and epidemiological evidence continues to support a protective role of fiber against colorectal cancer, particularly within Europe. However, the origins of intestinal neoplasia are now known to be far more complex than Burkitt was able to envisage, and there is little evidence to suggest a direct causal link between chronic constipation and colorectal cancer. Indeed, in one recent prevention trial, the risk of recurrence of colorectal polyps was slightly increased by prolonged supplementation with a bulk laxative based on one specialized source of cell wall polysaccharides.

Whatever the relationship to disease, it is certainly true that the consumption of dietary fiber is one major determinant of both fecal bulk and the frequency of defecation (bowel habit). However, the magnitude of the effect depends upon the type of fiber consumed. Soluble cell wall polysaccharides such as pectin are readily fermented by the microflora, whereas lignified tissues such as wheat bran tend to remain at least partially intact in the feces. Both classes of dietary fiber can contribute to fecal bulk but by different mechanisms. The increment in stool mass caused by wheat bran depends to some extent on particle size, but in healthy Western populations it has been shown that for every 1 g of wheat bran consumed per day, the output of stool is increased by between 3 and 5 g. Other sources of dietary fiber also favor water retention. For example, isphagula, a mucilaginous material derived from *Psyllium*, is used pharmaceutically as a bulk laxative. Soluble polysaccharides such as guar and oat β-glucan are readily fermented by anaerobic bacteria, but solubility is no guarantee of fermentability, as is illustrated by modified cellulose gums such as methylcellulose, which is highly resistant to degradation in the human gut. Fermentation reduces the mass and water-holding capacity of soluble polysaccharides considerably, but the bacterial cells derived from them do make some contribution to total fecal output. Thus, although all forms of dietary fiber are mild laxatives, the single analytical measurement of total fiber content again provides no simple predictive measure of physiological effect.

Although fermentation of fiber tends to reduce its effectiveness as a source of fecal bulk, it has other very important benefits. The absorption and metabolism of short-chain fatty acids derived from carbohydrate fermentation provides the route for the recovery of energy from undigested polysaccharides. Butyrate functions as the preferred source of energy for the colonic mucosal cells, whilst propionate and acetate are absorbed and metabolized systemically. There continues to be much debate about the importance of butyrate for the colon. *In vitro*, butyrate causes differentiation of tumor cells, suppresses cell division, and induces programed cell death (apoptosis). These effects are thought likely to suppress the development of cancer, but it is not yet entirely clear whether they also occur in the intact intestine. Research continues on the importance of butyrate and other short-chain fatty acids for human health.

The other major breakdown products of carbohydrate fermentation are hydrogen, methane, and carbon dioxide, which together comprise flatus gas. Excess gas production can cause distension and pain in some individuals, especially if they attempt to increase their fiber consumption too abruptly. In most cases, however, extreme flatus is probably caused more by fermentation of oligosaccharides such as stachyose and verbascose, which are found principally in legume seeds, rather than the cell wall polysaccharides themselves.

Conclusion

Several decades of research have confirmed that cell wall polysaccharides modify physiological mechanisms throughout the alimentary tract. Delayed absorption of glucose and lipids in the small intestine makes an important contribution to metabolic control in type 2 diabetes, and certain types of hypercholesterolemia, respectively. Any loss of carbohydrates to the colon will lead to increased fermentative activity, and through this pathway, most of the unabsorbed energy will be recovered as short-chain fatty acids. Unfermented cell wall polysaccharides and increased bacterial mass contribute to fecal bulk. All these established physiological effects, coupled with the possibility of using oligosaccharides as prebiotics to modify the colonic microflora, have greatly stimulated interest in nondigestible carbohydrates amongst food manufacturers and consumers in the past few years. There is little to suggest that conventional sources of fiber compromise micronutrient metabolism in otherwise healthy individuals, but the possibility of this and other adverse effects needs to be considered, as the use of novel polysaccharides as sources or analogs of dietary fiber, both for conventional products and for functional foods, continues to expand.

See also: **Cancer**: Epidemiology and Associations Between Diet and Cancer. **Carbohydrates**: Resistant Starch and Oligosaccharides. **Cereal Grains**. **Colon**: Disorders. **Diabetes Mellitus**: Etiology and Epidemiology; Classification and Chemical Pathology; Dietary Management. **Dietary Fiber**: Potential Role in Etiology of Disease; Role in Nutritional Management of

Disease. **Functional Foods**: Health Effects and Clinical Applications; Regulatory Aspects.

Further Reading

Bell S, Goldman VM, Bistrian BR, Arnold AH, Ostroff G, and Forse RA (1999) Effect of beta-glucan from oats and yeast on serum lipids. *Critical Reviews in Food Science and Nutrition* **39**: 189–202.

Burkitt DP and Trowell HC (eds.) (1975) *Refined Carbohydrate Foods: Some Implications of Dietary Fibre*. London: Academic Press.

Englyst HN, Bingham SA, Runswick SS, Collinson E, and Cummings JH (1989) Dietary fibre (non-starch polysaccharides) in cereal products. *Journal of Human Nutrition and Dietetics* **2**: 253–271.

Englyst HN, Bingham SA, Runswick SS, Collinson E, and Cummings JH (1989) Dietary fibre (non-starch polysaccharides) in fruit vegetables and nuts. *Journal of Human Nutrition and Dietetics* **1**: 247–286.

Englyst HN, Bingham SA, Runswick SS, Collinson E, and Cummings JH (1989) Dietary fibre (non-starch polysaccharides) in fruit vegetables and nuts. *Journal of Human Nutrition and Dietetics* **1**: 247–286.

Food Standards Agency (2002) *McCance and Widdowson's The Composition of Foods*, 6th summary edn Cambridge: The Royal Society of Chemistry.

Johnson IT and Southgate DAT (1994) *Dietary Fibre and Related Substances*. London: Chapman Hall.

Kushi LH, Meyer KA, and Jacobs Jr DR (1999) Cereals legumes and chronic disease risk reduction: Evidence from epidemiologic studies. *American Journal of Clinical Nutrition* **70**: 451S–458S.

McCance and Widdowson's (2002) *The Composition of Foods*, 6th Edition, Cambridge: Royal Society of Chemistry.

Nutrition Society (2003) Symposium on "Dietary Fibre in Health and Disease". *Proceedings of the Nutrition Society* **62**: 1–249.

Scholz-Ahrens KE and Schrezenmeir J (2002) Inulin, oligofructose and mineral metabolism – experimental data and mechanism. *British Journal of Nutrition* **87**(suppl 2): S179–186.

Southgate DAT (1992) *Determination of Food Carbohydrates*, 2nd edn. London: Elsevier Applied Science Publishers.

Potential Role in Etiology of Disease

D L Topping and **L Cobiac**, CSIRO Health Sciences and Nutrition, Adelaide, SA, Australia

© 2005 Elsevier Ltd. All rights reserved.

Noninfectious diseases cause much morbidity and mortality in developed countries in Europe, the Americas, Asia, and Australasia. They are expected to increase due to an alarming increase in obesity, with its attendant risk of diabetes, coronary heart disease (CHD), and some cancers. Equally important, they are becoming an issue in developing countries through greater affluence. In every case, they have serious negative socioeconomic impacts, and their prevention through appropriate dietary and lifestyle change is the optimal strategy to minimize personal and community costs. This strategy is believed to have contributed substantially to economic growth in countries where it has been applied.

Obesity is a fairly visible problem that tends to overshadow other considerations. Energy intake in excess of expenditure is the root cause of obesity, and dietary carbohydrates are implicated specifically in the development of overweight. Exclusion of carbohydrates is attracting attention as a weight control strategy but this ignores the fact that digestible carbohydrates (including starch) provide the same amount of energy per gram as protein and less than 45% of the energy of fat and 60% of the energy of alcohol. Furthermore, it overlooks the many early comparative population studies that showed that several low-risk groups ate high-starch diets compared to high-risk populations that consumed processed foods high in refined carbohydrates and fat and low in fiber. With time, dietary fiber (rather than the whole diet) received specific attention, and many studies were conducted on the health benefits. This may have contributed to some of the current lack of clarity of the role of fiber and complex carbohydrates in health promotion. It may be compounded by the inadequacy of population data linking fiber (and also starches) to disease processes for important conditions such as colorectal cancer. Only recently have good population data emerged for a protective role for fiber in this condition. This is in marked contrast to the well-established therapeutic and preventive action of fiber in constipation and diverticular disease. Furthermore, it is critical to determine what is meant by the term 'dietary fiber' because other food components may contribute to the major effects ascribed to fiber. This is important when considering the apparent protection conferred by whole grains against disease risk, especially because a health claim is permitted in the United States for their consumption.

Associations between Dietary Fiber and Disease Processes

The early population studies of Walker, Burkitt, and Trowell in Africa in the 1950s showed that serum cholesterol concentrations were low in South African Bantus (at low risk of CHD) who consumed a diet apparently high in fiber and low in fat. Additionally, colon cancer was virtually unknown among the latter, in contrast to white South Africans. Dietary fiber was known to resist digestion by human intestinal enzymes, which helped to explain the greater fecal bulk seen with higher fiber intakes. This was thought to lower colonic exposure to carcinogens through a simple dilution effect with fiber consumption. Subsequently, it was suggested that diabetes may be related to a deficiency of fiber in the diet whereas other epidemiological studies have shown associations between more dietary fiber consumption and lower risk of some of the hormone-dependent cancers (prostate and breast). Many of these observational population studies are limited by their reliance on reported food intakes which may be compromised in turn by food compositional data because the latter can be limited by the analytical methodology used. Multinational comparisons may be affected by the fact that food sources and processing vary between countries. There are other potential confounders. For example, diets high in fiber-rich foods may contain other protective agents (e.g., phytoestrogens folate and antioxidants) that could be the actual mediators of protection. Finally, some of the experimental studies and human interventions, especially in colorectal cancer, have given ambiguous or negative outcomes due to limitations of study design.

Dietary Fiber, Complex Carbohydrates, and Health Outcomes: A Need for Fiber Equivalents?

Technology has proved to be a significant issue in human fiber research. Early studies were limited by the relatively simple analytical methods then current. These were designed to measure the fiber components of forage consumed by important ruminant farm animals. Forage foods are high in insoluble polysaccharides and contain lignin (which is not a carbohydrate but a complex polyphenolic ether) and look 'fibrous,' so dietary fiber was equated with roughage and was defined as "those structural and exudative components of plants that were resistant to digestion by human gut enzymes." The methods used initially were quite severe and, with increasing sophistication of analytical methodology (notably chromatography), it became apparent that lignin was only a minor component of fiber compared with nonstarch polysaccharides (NSPs). Technological advances have revealed the importance of fractions such as soluble NSPs. As their name suggests, these dissolve in water but not necessarily under gut conditions. Fiber was then redefined as NSPs plus

lignin, which has moved the concept of away from the roughage model. Recently, there has been a further substantial revision of the view of what exactly constitutes dietary fiber with the emerging recognition of the contribution of resistant starch (RS) and oligosaccharides (OSs) to 'fiber' action. It was thought that all of dietary starch consumed in cooked foods was digested in the human small intestine. It is becoming clear that this is not so, and that a substantial fraction of ingested starch, RS, escapes from the small intestine and enters the colon of healthy humans. In terms of the dietary polysaccharides entering that viscus, RS may exceed NSPs in quantity and in the range of its actions. Indeed, some populations that were thought to consume high-fiber diets actually eat less than higher risk groups. An example is the native Africans studied by Burkitt and colleagues who eat unrefined diets based on maize but in fact eat less fiber than the high-risk whites.

Unlike NSPs (which are intrinsically resistant to human digestive enzymes), RS is influenced greatly by physiological and physical factors. Thus, raw starches are highly resistant and gelatinized starches (cooked in the presence of water) are much more digestible due to hydration and the loss of granular structure. However, cooling of cooked starchy foods leads to the generation of RS through retrogradation (which is a realignment of the polysaccharide chains). Other factors, including the relative proportions of amylose and amylopectin and the presence of other food components such as NSPs and lipids, influence RS. High-fiber foods tend to be higher in RS, whereas fats can form complexes with starch that resist digestion. Mastication, transit time, and gender can influence the amount of RS, which means that purely chemical determinations probably give an underestimate of the quantity of starch entering the large bowel. Physical breakdown of foods (especially whole grains) may be particularly important because access to upper intestinal digestive enzymes is limited in large particles, especially in the presence of NSPs. RS has been classified into four types based on the main factors that influence its presence, including physical inaccessibility, cooking, and retrogradation (RS types RS_{1-3}). Of particular interest is the emergence of chemically modified starches (RS_4) as RS because these are used widely in food processing.

In the large bowel NSPs and RS are fermented by the microflora, yielding metabolic end products, principally short-chain fatty acids (SCFAs), which may mediate some of the health benefits ascribed to the carbohydrates. Undigested protein (resistant protein) and other nondigested carbohydrates (e.g., OSs) also contribute to large bowel fermentation. These nondigested fractions contribute to dietary fiber via fermentation and could be considered in net dietary fiber intake. This problem could be overcome relatively easily by classifying them (and other non-NSP carbohydrates) as fiber equivalents in which their actions are compared against an agreed standard. This is similar to the situation with other nutrients such as vitamin A, where retinol equivalents include carotenoids, which are retinol precursors. It follows that classifications based on chemical composition alone appear to be quite inadequate if one considers as improved health and diminished disease risk as the most important issues.

Dietary Fiber and the Etiology of Coronary Heart Disease

Population Studies

Consumption of unrefined plant foods has been related to lower risk of CHD for some time, but the hypothesis that dietary fiber (i.e., NSP) intake could protect directly against the disease is relatively recent. The suggestion has been supported by a number of epidemiological studies linking higher intakes with lower risk. Vegetarians who consume more plant foods tend to have lower plasma lipids and blood pressure than age- and gender-matched omnivores. However, the strongest evidence derives not from these studies but from a number of very large cohort studies in several countries showing a consistent protective effect of whole grain consumption and CHD risk. Whole grain cereal consumption has been related to substantially lower risk of CHD in both men and women. The evidence for the latter is considered to be sufficiently strong for the US Food and Drug Administration to permit a health claim for consumption of whole grain cereal foods and lowering of the risk of CHD. Similar claims are being considered in Europe. However, these relationships are a long way from proving a specific protective effect of dietary fiber. A study of the relationship of long-term intake of dietary fiber by 68 782 women showed a substantial lowering of relative risk of 0.53 for women in the highest quintile of fiber consumption (22.9 g/day) compared with the lowest (11.5 g/day). These intakes are low compared to those recommended by health authorities. Nevertheless, they do support the view that fiber is protective against CHD. Only the effect of cereal fiber was significant; that of fruits and vegetables was not. However, they leave unanswered the question of the relationship of other contributors to the effects of dietary fiber (e.g., RS) and CHD risk.

Potential Mechanisms Indicating a Role in the Etiology of Coronary Heart Disease

The mechanism for risk reduction and the fiber components responsible need resolution. Elevated plasma total and low-density lipoprotein (LDL) cholesterol concentrations are established risk factors for coronary morbidity and mortality. There are abundant human and animal data showing that diets high in soluble fiber lower plasma cholesterol. One population study has shown a significant negative relationship between viscous (soluble) fiber intake and carotid artery atherogensis as measured by intima–media thickness. This association was significant statistically even though average fiber intakes were not particularly high. When dietary fiber intakes have been related to measures of actual disease outcomes, the evidence is less convincing. A protective effect is often observed on univariate analyses, but once confounding variables are added, dietary fiber intake tends not to be a significant independent predictor of risk for developing CHD. However, in one 12-year follow-up study of men and women, a 6-g increase in daily dietary fiber intake was associated with a 25% reduction in the risk of developing CHD. The most likely direct protective role for dietary fiber in CHD etiology is through plasma lipid lowering. The effect appears to be specific for plasma total and LDL cholesterol, and, possibly, triacylglycerols (TAG). Of the main fiber components, soluble NSPs seem to be effective, but insoluble NSPs and RS (and probably OSs) are not. Indeed, it appears that some insoluble NSP preparations, such as wheat bran, may raise plasma cholesterol slightly. There is good evidence from animal and human studies to support a hypocholesterolemic effect of soluble NSPs either in enriched plant fractions (e.g., oat bran) or as natural (e.g., pectins and guar gum) or synthetic isolates (e.g., hydroxypropylmethylcellulose). The magnitude of the effect varies with dose, but reductions of approximately 5–10% at intakes of 6–12 g of NSPs/day appear to be reasonable. This lowering response approaches that seen with certain drugs, such as cholestyramine, used to manage hypercholesterolemia. Some studies have also shown a reduction in TAGs with soluble fibers such as oat bran. However, it is important to recognize that many of the demonstrations of plasma cholesterol lowering by soluble fiber products are against insoluble NSPs such as wheat bran.

There are several hypotheses to explain the NSP action on plasma cholesterol, including enhanced bile acid and neutral sterol excretion, the slowing of fat and cholesterol absorption and direct inhibition of hepatic cholesterol synthesis by propionate formed by large bowel fermentation of NSPs. Whole body cholesterol homoeostasis represents a balance between influx and loss. Cholesterol influx can come from dietary intake and *de novo* synthesis. Losses occur through the sloughing of epithelial cells and through the fecal excretion of nonabsorbed dietary cholesterol and biliary steroids (bile acids and neutral sterols). Bile acids are generally recovered in the ileum, and those that are not absorbed are excreted in the feces. Any increase in bile acid excretion leads to enhanced hepatic uptake of cholesterol and its conversion to bile acids with a consequent depletion of the plasma cholesterol pool.

It was initially thought that fiber could bind some bile acids selectively, in a similar manner to cholestyramine, an ion exchange resin that binds bile acids. Bile acid binding *in vitro* by insoluble fiber preparations appears to be an artefact. Cholestyramine is strongly charged, whereas most NSPs with cholesterol-lowering potential are neutral or even acidic (e.g., pectins). Neutrality is not consistent with ionic binding and uronic acid residues would repel bile acids at the pH of the small intestine. The property that appears to mediate the increased steroid excretion is the viscosity in solution. Most (but not necessarily all) NSPs that lower cholesterol form viscous solutions in water. Presumably, bile acids are lost from the ileum through a form of entrapment in a viscous gel. This would also contribute to the loss of cholesterol and the slower digestion of fat seen with ingestion of NSPs. Abundant animal and human data show that feeding soluble NSPs increases fecal steroid excretion. However, the major problem with these relationships is that although soluble fibers may lower plasma cholesterol, the strongest evidence of a protective effect is for insoluble fibers which do not lower plasma cholesterol. It may be that other components in the grain are actually mediating the effect and fiber is the surrogate marker for their intake.

Dietary Fiber and the Etiology of Cancers—Colon and Rectum

Population Studies

This is one long-standing association that has been surprisingly problematic. Early studies on native Africans who consumed an unrefined diet showed them to have a very low incidence of this cancer.

Although subsequent studies have shown a negative association between greater fiber intake and lowered risk, it has proved to be relatively weak. Indeed, in one US study there was no real association between fiber intake and cancer susceptibility. Some of the loss of significance seen in this evaluation may reflect the lack of allowance for confounding variables. For example, in a 6-year follow-up of women, the association between low fiber intake and the incidence of colon cancer disappeared after adjustment was made for meat intake. In another study of men, low fiber intake was an independent risk factor for the incidence of adenomatous polyps during a 2-year follow-up period.

Fruit and vegetable fiber has been consistently associated with a lower risk of colon cancer, but the relationship with cereal fiber is less clear. However, whole grain cereals appear to be protective—a further anomaly in the relationships between plant foods and disease risk. These discrepancies may be in the process of resolution. First, it seems that the early observational data were confounded by the analytical technologies available, and the perception that native populations consuming unrefined diets had high fiber intakes is incorrect. It seems likely that they ate relatively little fiber but had high intakes of RS. Population studies have shown a protective effect of apparent RS intake and colorectal cancer risk. The word 'apparent' is pivotal because there is currently no accepted method for RS determination and thus, there are no reliable data on dietary intakes. There are also issues regarding the intakes of dietary fiber and cancer risk. Part of the problem inherent in the study of colonic cancer is that, in contrast to CHD (in which there are easily measurable risk markers such as plasma cholesterol that can be modified by diet), the only indices for colon cancer are not easily measurable: the appearance of aberrant crypts, adenomatous polyps, or the disease itself. Hitherto, animal studies have largely been confined to rodents treated with chemical carcinogens (usually dimethylhydrazine), and they suggest that dietary fiber from wheat bran and cellulose may afford greater protection against the development of colon cancer when associated with a low-fat diet compared with soluble NSPs. These data stand in contrast to observational studies but are supported by interventions in humans with familial adenomatous polyposis. These people are at genetically greater risk of colonic cancer and represent one means of assessing risk modification through dietary intervention and monitoring polyp size and frequency through colonoscopy. In the Australian

Polyp Prevention Trial, subjects consumed 25 g of wheat bran per day and there was a decrease in dysplasia and total adenoma surface area when the diet was also low in fat. This supports epidemiological studies that show that increased fat and protein intakes increase risk. Other prevention trials have examined the effects of increasing fiber intake on the recurrence of polyps following a polypectomy. In a Canadian study of 201 men and women, a high-fiber, low-fat diet protected against polyp recurrence in women but in men there was actually an increase. A third trial examined the effects of diet on the prevalence of rectal polyps in 64 people with familial polyposis coli who had a total colectomy. Those who received and actually took the high-fiber (22.5 g fiber as a breakfast cereal) showed a reduction in polyps. These data are not conclusive but are reasonably consistent with overall knowledge.

Complex Carbohydrates and Colorectal Cancer

An obvious factor for the inconsistent results of the effect of different intakes of dietary fiber on colorectal cancer is the variation in the analytical methodology used in different studies. There is also increasing evidence that total dietary complex carbohydrates may be as important as fiber. Analysis of stool weight from 20 populations in 12 countries showed that larger stools were correlated with a lower incidence of colon cancer. Intakes of starch and dietary fiber (rather than fiber alone) were the best dietary correlates with stool weight. A subsequent meta-analysis showed that greater consumption of starch (but not of NSPs) was associated with low risk of colorectal cancer in 12 populations. The examination also showed that fat and protein intakes correlated positively with risk. This meta-analysis is probably the first of its kind to suggest a protective role for starch in large bowel cancer and underscores the need to consider complex carbohydrates as fiber equivalents and not just as NSPs and starch. The need for better information on dietary intake data and risk is underscored by the data from the European Prospective Investigation of Cancer and Nutrition, which showed a substantial reduction in risk with increasing fiber intake. This multinational study is important because it has sufficient power (expressed as a range of fiber intakes and individuals observed) to give confidence in the observations. Follow-up of 1 939 011 person-years throughout 10 countries showed that a doubling of fiber intake from foods could reduce risk by 40%.

Potential Mechanisms Indicating a Role in the Etiology of Colorectal Cancer

Colorectal tumorigenesis is a multistep process. These steps involve a number of genetic alterations that convert a normal epithelium to a hyperproliferative state and then to early adenomas, later adenomas, and, finally, frank carcinoma and metastasis. Fiber may, and probably does, play a role in all of these stages, and several mechanisms have been proposed by which it could play a role in the etiology of the disease (Table 1).

A number of agents may induce genetic damage in the colonocyte, including mono- and diacylglycerols, nonesterified fatty acids, secondary bile acids, aryl hydrocarbons and other pyrrolytic products of high-temperature cooking, and ammonia and amines and other products of large bowel bacterial protein degradation. One of the simplest protective mechanisms for dietary fiber is purely physical. By increasing fecal bulk, fiber could produce a more rapid transit time as well as act as a diluent and thus reduce exposure to potential mutagenic agents. It is also possible that fiber components could bind mutagens. However, because this appears to be unlikely for bile acids, the same may apply to other carcinogens.

Table 1 Effects of dietary fiber and resistant starch that could impact on the etiology of colorectal cancer

Increased stool bulk (mainly insoluble NSPs)
Decreases transit time, minimizing contact between colonocytes and luminal carcinogens
Reduces exposure through dilution of carcinogens

Binding of bile acids and other potential carcinogens (mainly insoluble NSPs)
Lowers free concentrations of mutagens

Modifying fecal flora and increasing bacterial numbers (soluble and insoluble NSPs and RS)
Decreases secondary bile acids, which are potential carcinogens
Lowers colonic NH_3 (a cytotoxic agent) by fixing nitrogen in the bacterial mass

Lowering fecal pH through SCFA production (NSPs but mainly RS)
Inhibits growth of pH-sensitive, potentially pathogenic species, which may degrade food constituents, and endogenous secretions to potential carcinogens
Lowers absorption of toxic alkaline compounds (e.g., amines)
Lowers solubility of secondary bile acids

Fermentation to SCFAs (NSPs but mainly RS)
Depending on source, raises butyrate which is a preferred substrate for normal colonocytes, and (in vitro) promotes a normal cell phenotype, retards the growth of cancer cells, and facilitates DNA repair

NSPs, nonstarch polysaccharides; RS, resistant starch; SCFAs, short-chain Fatty acids.

Production of SCFAs by the resident microflora induces a number of general changes in the colonic environment, including a lowering of pH. Case–control studies show that pH is higher in patients with cancer compared to controls but this may reflect altered dietary habits rather than long-term risk. However, at lower pH, basic toxins are ionized while secondary bile acids are less soluble so that the absorption of both would be reduced. The activities of both of the enzymes 7α-dehydroxylase and glucuronidase are decreased at lower pH. These changes would diminish the conversion of primary to secondary bile acids and the hydrolysis of glucuronide conjugates, respectively and thus limit their carcinogenic potential. However, there is consensus that the effects of SCFAs may be rather more specific and mediated through one acid—butyrate. Butyrate is a preferred substrate for normal colonocytes and numerous studies in vitro have shown that it has several actions that promote a normal cell phenotype. Cell studies show that butyrate induces hyperacylation of histones, leading to downregulation of gene expression and arrest of proliferation. Other actions include DNA hypermethylation which would have similar effects on tumor cell growth. Butyrate also has favorable effects on apoptosis so that a normal program of cell death is maintained. One marker of a differentiated colonocyte is its ability to produce alkaline phosphatase and butyrate is a powerful promoter of alkaline phosphatase in vitro. There is reciprocal downregulation of various oncogenes in colorectal cancer cell lines. These data are very promising for a direct role of butyrate in protecting against colonic cancer but there is an emerging paradox. In the presence of butyrate, there is either increased proliferation or no effect in normal cells but the proliferation of neoplastic cells is reduced. The differentiation of the normal cells is unchanged or suppressed with butyrate but is induced in cancer cells. These differing effects may be explained by neoplastic alterations (perhaps as a result of mutations in oncogenes) in cell signal systems.

It must be emphasized that none of the effects of butyrate in vitro have been duplicated in vivo, but they are of great promise and supportive evidence continues to accumulate. This is especially true for RS which appears to produce relatively more butyrate than other nondigestible carbohydrates. However, consideration may also need to be given to the existence of interindividual differences in the fermentative capacity of the microflora, the fact that RS from different sources may be fermented to different extents, and the actual colonic site at which fermentation takes place (i.e., whether in the proximal or distal colon).

Inter alia, the data suggest that protection against colorectal cancer is due to several mechanisms and that these can interact. One factor of considerable importance is the issue of overweight which is an independent risk factor for colorectal cancer. Obesity may have to be taken into account much more than has been the case in earlier studies. It appears that some of the effect may be mediated through raised plasma insulin and insulin-like growth factors (which may well be influenced by dietary carbohydrates).

Dietary Fiber and the Etiology of Hormone-Dependent Cancers

Population Studies

Cancers of the breast, endometrium, ovary, and prostate fall into the hormone-dependent classification. An association between hormonal status and cancer risk arose from observations of oestrogen deprivation and breast cancer and testosterone deprivation and prostate cancer. Nutritional influences on breast cancer have been studied extensively and several (but not all) studies show diminished risk with greater intakes of dietary fiber. The situation for other cancers, especially prostate cancer, appears to be rather unclear, but given the commonality of the proposed protective mechanisms, it is reasonable to expect that some linkage may be found. Male vegetarians have been reported to have lower testosterone and oestradiol plasma concentrations compared to omnivores, and inverse correlations of testosterone and oestradiol with fiber intake have been reported.

Potential Mechanisms Indicating a Role in the Etiology of Hormone-Dependent Cancers

There are many published studies that have produced mixed and inconsistent results on the potential mechanisms involved. Dietary fiber could act by reducing circulating concentrations of oestrogen and testosterone. Such an effect would not be unexpected in view of the fact that soluble NSPs can increase bile acid and neutral steroid excretion and fecal steroid outputs are higher in vegetarians than in omnivores. However, one anomaly is the finding that wheat bran (which does not enhance biliary steroid excretion) lowers circulating and urinary oestrogens. It is possible that fiber acts rather differently on hormones than on bile acids and neutral sterols. For example, the colonic flora may be modified so as to increase deconjugation of the sex hormone precursors or their conversion to other metabolites. Direct binding of sex hormones is possible but is subject to the same concerns as were raised for cholesterol reduction. In addition, it is possible that other components in, or associated with, fiber (phytooestrogens or antioxidants) may be responsible for any observed protective effect. Soy phytooestrogens are believed to play a role in lowering the risk of breast cancer in Asian populations. Lycopenes are antioxidant carotenoids from tomatoes, and their intake has been correlated with a lower risk of prostate cancer.

Dietary Fiber, Obesity, and the Etiology of Diabetes

In 1975, Trowell suggested that the etiology of diabetes might be related to a dietary fiber deficiency. This is supported by several key pieces of evidence. Vegetarians who consume a high-fiber lacto-ovo vegetarian diet appear to have a lower risk of mortality from diabetes-related causes compared to nonvegetarians. Consumption of whole grain cereals is associated with a lower risk of diabetes. Importantly, the same dietary pattern appears to lower the risk of obesity, itself an independent risk factor in the etiology of type 2 diabetes. Obesity is emerging as a problem of epidemic proportions in affluent and developing countries. Consumption of whole grain cereal products lowers the risk of diabetes. A report showed that in 91 249 women questioned about dietary habits in 1991, greater cereal fiber intake was significantly related to lowered risk of type 2 diabetes. In this study, glycemic index (but not glycemic load) was also a significant risk factor, and this interacted with a low-fiber diet to increase risk. These results provide epidemiological evidence of a role of fiber in the etiology of diabetes.

Potential Mechanisms Indicating a Role in the Etiology of Diabetes

It can be hypothesized that a reduction in the general and postprandial glycemic and insulinemic response may delay the development of insulin resistance and thus the development of diabetes (NIDDM) although there is very little direct evidence to support this hypothesis. However, diets high in both carbohydrate and dietary fiber have been reported to improve insulin sensitivity. Much of the research in this area has studied the effect of dietary fiber on the management rather than the prevention or etiology of diabetes.

There is good evidence that diminished glucose absorption lowers the insulin response to a meal.

The action of fiber in this regard may be through slowing the digestion of starch and other nutrients. It seems that soluble fiber may play a role because large amounts of soluble dietary fiber have been shown to reduce postprandial glucose concentration and insulinemic responses after a single meal in both normal and diabetic subjects. However, the effect appears to be dependent on viscosity rather than on solubility *per se*. The very viscous gum, guar gum, gum tragacanth, and oat gum are all very effective whereas psyllium and some pectins are less viscous and less effective. One suggested mechanism for reducing the glycemic response is an impairment in the convective movement of glucose and water in the intestinal lumen due to the formation of a viscous gel: Glucose is trapped in the gel matrix, such that there is less movement toward the absorptive brush border of the surface of the intestinal wall and the glucose needs to be squeezed out by the intestinal motor activity of the intestine. However, other factors may also be important. There may be some impairment in digestive activity in the lumen, an alteration in hormonal secretion by cells in the gut mucosa, and a reduced gut motility that delays transit time. In the case of whole grains, there is scope for the fiber to interfere with the physical accessibility of starch to small intestinal α-amylase. Clearly, there is also potential for foods of low glycemic index to be high in RS and this does seem to be the case. A specific instance is a novel barley cultivar that exhibits both characteristics. It should be noted that there are reports of a second meal effect (i.e., the dietary fiber ingested at one meal can affect the glucose rise after the subsequent meal). The mechanism for this is unknown.

A Role for Fiber in the Etiology of Other Diseases?

Although much of the earlier observational studies in native African populations were wide ranging, most attention has subsequently focused on CHD and cancer. Probably this is a reflection of the socioeconomic importance of these conditions in economically developed societies. However, fiber has a role in the prevention and management of other conditions, but much of the relevant information has come from interventions, not from case–control or cross-sectional studies.

Constipation, diverticular disease, and laxation
Unquestionably, fiber is of direct benefit in relieving the symptoms of constipation and diverticular disease but there is little information about its role in the etiology of these conditions. Numerous

interventions have shown that foods high in insoluble NSPs (e.g., certain cereal brans) and some soluble NSP preparations (e.g., psyllium) are very effective at controlling constipation and diverticular disease and enhancing laxation. The actual effect can vary with source. Wheat bran increases undigested residue, and fiber from fruits and vegetables and soluble polysaccharides tend to be fermented extensively and are more likely to increase microbial cell mass. Some NSP (and OS) preparations retain water in the colon. The physical form of the fiber is also important: Coarsely ground wheat bran is a very effective source of fiber to increase fecal bulk, whereas finely ground wheat bran has little or no effect and may even be constipating. RS appears to be a mild laxative and seems to complement the laxative effects of NSPs. The effective dose appears to be approximately 20–30 g of total fiber/day consumed either in food or as a supplement. In addition, animal studies show that NSPs and RS appear to prevent colonic atrophy seen in low-fiber diets. The mechanism of action appears to be greater fecal bulking and fermentation and the generation of SCFAs, which is necessary to prevent atrophy.

Diarrhea Colonic SCFA absorption stimulates fluid and electrolyte uptake in the colon and thus can assist in reducing diarrhea. Complex carbohydrates may also play a role in modifying the colonic microflora thus reducing the number of pathogens. An etiological role for fiber is unknown, but there is good evidence that RS can act to minimize the fluid losses that occur in serious conditions such as cholera.

Inflammatory bowel diseases (colitis and Crohn's disease) Clearly, inflammatory conditions have an immune component. In the case of Crohn's disease, there appears to be no established therapeutic or etiological role for fiber. The situation is slightly different for distal ulcerative colitis, in which fiber intake seems unrelated to incidence. However, rectal infusion of SCFAs (especially butyrate) has been reported to lead to remission, so it appears that either the generation of these acids or their delivery to the distal colon may be the issue.

See also: **Cancer**: Epidemiology and Associations Between Diet and Cancer. **Cereal Grains**. **Colon**: Disorders; Nutritional Management of Disorders. **Coronary Heart Disease**: Prevention. **Diabetes Mellitus**: Etiology and Epidemiology. **Diarrheal Diseases**. **Dietary Fiber**: Physiological Effects and Effects on Absorption. **Food Safety**: Bacterial Contamination. **Obesity**: Prevention. **Vegetarian Diets**.

Further Reading

Baghurst PA, Baghurst KI, and Record SJ (1996) Dietary fibre, non-starch polysaccharides and resistant starch—A review. *Food Australia* 48(supplement): S3–S35.

Bingham SA, Day NE, Luben R et al. European Prospective Investigation into Cancer and Nutrition (2003) Dietary fibre in food and protection against colorectal cancer in the European Prospective Investigation into Cancer and Nutrition (EPIC): An observational study. *Lancet* 361: 1496–1501.

Ellis PR, Rayment P, and Wang Q (1996) A physico-chemical perspective of plant polysaccharides in relation to glucose absorption, insulin secretion and the entero-insular axis. *Proceedings of the Nutrition Society* 55: 881–898.

Giovannucci E (2001) Insulin, insulin-like growth factors and colon cancer: A review of the evidence. *Journal of Nutrition* 131(supplement 3): 109S–120S.

Olson BH, Anderson SM, Becker MP et al. (1997) Psyllium-enriched cereals lower blood total cholesterol and LDL cholesterol, but not HDL cholesterol in hypercholesterolemic adults: Results of a meta-analysis. *Journal of Nutrition* 127: 1973–1980.

Richardson DP (2003) Whole grain health claims in Europe. *Proceedings of the Nutrition Society* 62: 161–169.

Schulze MB, Liu S, Rimm EB et al. (2004) Glycemic index, glycemic load, and dietary fiber intake and incidence of type 2 diabetes in younger and middle-aged women. *American Journal of Clinical Nutrition* 80: 243–244.

Slavin JL (2000) Mechanisms for the impact of whole grain foods on cancer risk. *Journal of the American College of Nutrition* 19: 300S–307S.

Stamler J, Caggiula AW, Cutler JA et al. (1997) Dietary and nutritional methods and findings: The Multiple Risk Factor Intervention Trial (MRFIT). *American Journal of Clinical Nutrition* 65(1 supplement): 183S–402S.

Topping DL and Clifton PM (2001) Short-chain fatty acids and human colonic function: Roles of resistant starch and nonstarch polysaccharides. *Physiological Reviews* 81: 1031–1064.

Topping DL, Morell MK, King RA et al. (2003) Resistant starch and health – *Himalaya* 292, a novel barley cultivar to deliver benefits to consumers. *Starch/stärke* 53: 539–545.

Truswell AS (2002) Cereal grains and coronary heart disease. *European Journal of Clinical Nutrition* 56: 1–14.

Wu H, Dwyer KM, Fan Z et al. (2003) Dietary fiber and progression of atherosclerosis: The Los Angeles Atherosclerosis Study. *American Journal of Clinical Nutrition* 78: 1085–1091.

Role in Nutritional Management of Disease

A R Leeds, King's College London, London, UK

© 2005 Elsevier Ltd. All rights reserved.

Introduction

Dietary Fiber was an unknown phrase to all but a handful of individuals in the early years of the 1970s when a wide range of potential therapeutic applications were suggested by Hugh Trowell, Denis Burkitt, and Alexander Walker. Twenty-five years later there can hardly be an ordinary mortal who has not heard the term, though he may not be able to define it. In some cases the claims remain largely unsubstantiated but in three areas, hyperlipidemia, diabetes, and bowel function, there is sufficient evidence to allow dietary advice to be given.

Hyperlipidemia

Some forms of dietary fiber lower blood lipids, notably total cholesterol and low-density lipoprotein (LDL) cholesterol. The earliest observations on fiber preparations and blood lipids date from the mid 1930s when there was a fairly extensive investigation of the effects of pectin (polygalacturonic acid). The next period of investigation dates from 1974 when extracted and purified dietary fiber preparations such as guar gum – a glucomannan – were tested in normal subjects, diabetics, and hyperlipidemic subjects and were found to lower blood cholesterol when given in sufficient quantities. In very large doses these materials increase fecal excretion of fat and sterol compounds and would be expected to reduce the body bile salt pool. Subsequent work has shown that at lower doses preparations of soluble dietary fiber have a mild cholestyramine-like effect: they bind bile salts rendering them unavailable for reabsorption in the terminal ileum, thus interfering with the normal entero-hepatic cycle of bile salts and depleting the bile salt pool. Total and LDL cholesterol fall as cholesterol is diverted for the resynthesis of lost bile salts. There have been few direct clinical applications of the early experimental work on pectin and guar gum. No pectin compounds have been developed commercially, but there are a few pharmaceutical preparations of guar gum presented primarily as adjuncts to dietary therapy in diabetes rather than for lipid lowering. Dietetic food products containing guar gum have been developed, again for use in controlling diabetes.

Preparations of soluble dietary fiber have been shown to lower blood cholesterol whereas most preparations of predominantly insoluble fiber, such as wheat bran, have little or no effect. The major food sources of soluble fiber are oats, beans, lentils, rye, and barley, and these foods have naturally become the subject of investigations. The addition of oats to the diet in normolipidemic and hyperlipidemic subjects following either their normal diets or where pretreated with low-fat diets has been the subject of extensive research. In sufficient quantity oats, oat products, and oat β-glucan (providing at least 3 g oat β-beta glucan per day) lower blood total cholesterol and LDL cholesterol (usually by 5–10%) while leaving triglycerides and HDL cholesterol largely unchanged. A sufficiently large number of good-quality studies have now been done on oats that the Food and Drug Administration (FDA) has allowed the first ever food-specific health claim: "Soluble fiber from oatmeal, as part of a low saturated fat, low cholesterol diet, may reduce the risk of heart disease." Products that are labeled with this claim must provide at least 0.75 g of soluble fiber (as β-glucan) per serving. When considering the above claim the FDA reviewed 37 studies and found that a sufficient number provided convincing evidence of efficacy. An earlier meta-analysis of some of those trials had shown that the efficacy of oats and oat products was influenced by the initial values of blood cholesterol in the subjects: patients with high starting values (over 6.7 mmol per liter total cholesterol) showed the greatest reductions when treated with oats, while healthy young subjects with low–normal starting values showed little response. There was a dose effect: food products providing more than 3 g soluble fiber per day had a greater blood cholesterol lowering effect than diets that provided less than 3 g per day.

Other soluble fiber-containing products have been shown to lower blood cholesterol. Recent extensive studies on psyllium (*Plantago ovata*) presented both as a pharmaceutical preparation and as a food product (a ready to eat breakfast cereal) have shown blood cholesterol-lowering properties where the dose–effect relationship is such that a useful additional therapeutically meaningful lipid-lowering effect can be achieved by prescribing a daily portion of psyllium-fortified breakfast cereal. Products of this type are now marketed in the US and Australia, and the US FDA has now allowed a food specific health claim for psyllium.

There is also a small literature on the effects of beans on blood lipids and the findings of a blood cholesterol-lowering effect are as expected.

Virtually all of the reports of the effects of soluble fiber products on blood lipids report lowering effects on total cholesterol and LDL cholesterol without any effect on HDL cholesterol or triglycerides – this contrasts with the effects of some drugs that may cause slight rises of triglycerides and falls of HDL cholesterol. The relationship between lowering of blood cholesterol and lowering of risk of heart disease is now generally accepted and a proven lipid-lowering effect is taken to mean a beneficial effect on risk of coronary heart disease. This means that in clinical practice it is perfectly reasonable to include advice on use of foods high in soluble dietary fiber in a lipid-lowering diet, and perfectly proper to emphasize the benefits of oats and oat products. Generally, a high-soluble-fiber diet is more acceptable when the soluble fiber is drawn from smaller quantities of a larger range of foods; thus the diet includes beans, lentils, rye breads, and barley as well as generous use of oats. A range of foods containing mycoprotein and fungal mycelial cell walls (chitin) may also help to lower blood cholesterol.

Diabetes

Diabetes mellitus is characterized by either an absolute or relative lack of insulin, which has short-term and long-term consequences. Diabetic people may develop both microvascular complications (mainly affecting the eyes, kidneys, and nerves) and macrovascular complications (essentially accelerated development of atherosclerosis presenting mainly as heart attack and peripheral vascular disease). Medical management aims to replace the insulin, or modulate its production or efficacy using oral (hypoglycemic) drugs, in a metabolic environment enhanced by good control of diet and body composition. Medical management also aims to achieve early detection of complications and other risk factors for cardiovascular disease by regular testing of blood and urine biochemical variables and blood pressure and by regular physical examination of the eyes, neurological, and cardiovascular systems.

Control of dietary energy intake (in relation to the varying demands for growth, maintenance, physical activity, etc.) remains the key feature of dietary control affecting metabolic fluxes, blood glucose levels, and body weight. Views on the appropriate proportional sources of energy from fat, carbohydrate, and protein have changed enormously over the last century from seriously energy-restricted high-fat diets (with percentage energy from fat as high as 70% raising some doubts about the level of compliance) through to very high-carbohydrate diets (sometimes 60–65% energy from carbohydrate) used in specialist centers in the US. Today, for most diabetic patients in most countries the target is to achieve 50–55% energy from carbohydrate sources. Prior to the 1970s, when the move towards high-carbohydrate diets began, the high fat content of the diet along with less tight blood glucose (and urine glucose) control than is customary today was partly responsible for the high relative mortality from cardiovascular disease seen among diabetic patients. At that time young male diabetics were up to nine times more likely to die from heart attack than matched nondiabetic individuals. Reduction of fat in the diet and achievement of an optimal distribution from saturated, monounsaturated, and polyunsaturated sources (<10%, 10–20%, and no more than 10%, respectively, for patients with diabetes in the UK) remain a major aspect of dietary management of diabetic people in order to reduce the risk of developing coronary heart disease.

Control of blood glucose is critical in order to achieve avoidance of prolonged periods of hyperglycemia, which is associated with glycation of proteins and the risk of development of microvascular complications, and avoidance of hypoglycemia with its attendant risks of coma. In day-to-day practice, the avoidance of hypoglycemia is very important to patients and any new method of achieving normalization of blood glucose profiles is an advance. Dietary fiber offered such an advance from the mid 1970s when some forms (notably isolated polysaccharides such as guar gum, a glucomannan, and pectin, polygalacturonic acid) were shown to reduce the area under the blood glucose and insulin curves after acute test meals. Subsequent long-term (6-week) clinical trials showed that diets high in foods containing soluble dietary fiber, such as beans, oats, and barley, were more effective in reducing the area under the 24-h blood glucose profiles than diets containing more high-fiber foods based on wheat products.

Research in this area led David Jenkins to describe (in 1981) the concept of the 'glycemic index' (GI) which is a numerical expression of the ability of a food to raise blood glucose levels. In practice it is measured by comparing the blood glucose response to a 50-g carbohydrate portion of food with the response to 50 g glucose (in some papers the comparison is with a 50-g carbohydrate portion of bread). The dietary fiber (especially soluble fiber) content of a food slows down the rate of digestion and absorption of starch in foods giving flatter blood glucose responses and a lower GI; however, the structure of the starch (whether amylose or amylopectin) influences its rate of degradation and the extent to which the starch granules are hydrated by processing (including cooking) is also important. The physical structure of the food (particularly the extent to which plant cells are intact), the presence of fat, which may slow gastric emptying, and the presence of some 'antinutrient' substances may all influence the GI. Low-GI diets have been shown in many clinical trials to improve important variables that are secondary indicators of blood glucose control, and to reduce blood lipids. Low-GI diets may be particularly helpful to patients who are frequently troubled by episodes of hypoglycemia though adequate proof of this is still awaited. Low-GI diets are not just relevant to treatment of diabetes but have been shown in two large-scale epidemiological surveys published in 1997 to result in a significant reduction in the risk of development of maturity onset (type 2) diabetes in middle-aged American men and women. Thus, there is good reason to believe that there should be greater emphasis on the GI of diabetic diets and the fiber content, as well as emphasis on GI for those at risk of developing diabetes, especially the older obese person. Expert committees in many developed countries of the world have set target values for dietary fiber intake for diabetic patients (e.., the American Diabetes Association (ADA) recommends 20–35 g day^{-1} total dietary fiber by the AOAC method) and many, especially the Australian Diabetes Association and with the notable exception of the ADA, have recommended an increase in low-GI foods. In 2003 even Diabetes UK (the UK Diabetes Association) noted that there might be merit in taking account of GI in dietary management for those with diabetes. Some physicians believe that the GI of foods is too complex an issue for patients to grasp, but in essence simply requires a partial substitution of bread and potatoes with pasta products, an increased use of high-fiber breakfast cereals including oats, increased use of beans and lentils, and emphasis on the use of temperate fruits (e.g., apples and pears).

Obesity (body mass index (weight in kilograms divided by height in meters squared) in excess of 30 kg m^{-2}) is becoming more prevalent in developing countries and attracts an increased risk of the development of diabetes mellitus; a high proportion of established type 2 diabetics are obese and overweight. In the popular diet book 'The F-Plan Diet,' published in 1982, Audrey Eyton claimed that dietary fiber would help people lose weight by a number of mechanisms including reducing the efficiency of dietary energy absorption and by making people feel full for longer after meals thus having an overall effect on reducing food intake. At the time of publication these ideas were hypothetical - subsequent investigation has shown that increasing fiber intake two- or threefold by a variety of dietary changes can increase fecal energy losses by 75–100 kcal day^{-1}. Studies on the effects of dietary fiber on postprandial satiety where experimental meals are carefully designed to differ little except for fiber content have given variable results. However, there is a clear effect of fiber on chewing (the number of chews necessary to eat the same energy equivalent of food) where high- and low-fiber types of commonly consumed foods are eaten and this may have an important satiating effect. Clinical trials of high-fiber weight loss regimens have given variable results. Double-blind placebo-controlled trials using pressed barley fiber and pectin tablets compared to a starch control have been undertaken in Scandinavia and have demonstrated statistically significantly greater weight losses in the fiber-treated groups up to 26 weeks of treatment. It seems reasonable to conclude that under some conditions the right kind of high-fiber diet can facilitate weight loss, but may not always do so.

Diabetic people are more likely to have dyslipidemia than nondiabetic people. When control of diabetes is lost, patients may demonstrate gross hypertriglyceridemia due to increased production of very-low-density lipoprotein (VLDL) particles in the liver as a consequence of the increased flux of free fatty acids from the peripheral tissues. At the same time total and LDL cholesterol may be raised. Improvement in diabetic control often achieves normalization of blood lipids, but where hyperlipidemia persists there may be a place for use of dietary fiber, especially soluble fiber, and especially oat β-glucan-containing foods as an adjunct to dietary and pharmacological therapy (see above).

Bowel Disorders

Denis Burkitt first suggested a role for dietary fiber in bowel disorders in 1971. In the intervening period understanding of the normal physiology and pathophysiology of the colon have improved enormously. During the same period methods of analysis have been refined and a distinction is drawn between dietary fiber (as determined by the AOAC gravimetric method) and nonstarch polysaccharide (NSP; determined by GLC analysis of component sugars), and starch not digested in the small gut is now defined as being resistant. Three types of resistant starch have been described. These advances in analysis have helped physiologists appreciate the contributions of various substrates to colonic fermentation and stool bulking.

The intake of dietary fiber (nonstarch polysaccharides) is directly related to the amount of wet stool passed each day in large population groups. An average wet stool weight for the UK is about $105\,g\,day^{-1}$, which corresponds roughly to a nonstarch polysaccharide (Englyst method) intact of $12.5\,g\,day^{-1}$. Nearly half of the members of groups studied in the UK have stool weights of less than $100\,g\,day^{-1}$ below which complaints of constipation are common. Stool weight has been shown to be clearly inversely related to colon cancer incidence in population groups: a mean daily stool weight of $105\,g$ corresponding to a relatively high population colon cancer incidence of about 22 per 100 000 per annum. An incidence rate of 11 per 100 000 per annum corresponds to a mean daily stool weight of about $175\,g\,day^{-1}$. This information was used as the numerical basis for calculating the UK's dietary reference value (DRV) for nonstarch polysaccharide (NSP) in the late 1980s. In the UK the population is urged to increase NSP intake by 50% to a population averageof $18\,g\,day^{-1}$ in order to shift the distribution of wet stool weight upwards.

Constipation is generally considered to be infrequent opening of the bowels with straining to pass stools (less than three defecations per week and straining and or the passing of hard stools in more than one in four defecations). Constipation is sometimes caused by other specific disease of either an endocrine nature (e.g., myxoedema – reduced thyroid function) or physical obstructive nature (e.g., colon cancer). Where constipation has developed recently in a previously nonconstipated individual over the age of 40 years colon cancer must be excluded as the cause of the change of bowel habit. In the absence of evidence that the constipation is secondary it is probably due to dietary and life-style factors. The mucosa of the lower colon has a great capacity to desiccate its contents. If the call to stool does not occur or is ignored residual material drys out and individual fecal pellets become smaller. There is experimental evidence to suggest that greater abdominal pressures are needed to expel pellets that are 1 cm in diameter than those that are 2 cm in diameter. Thus, factors that result in the call to stool being ignored, like not allowing sufficient time for defecation after a stimulus such as breakfast or the walk to the station or being unprepared to defecate anywhere except at home (a common characteristic consistent with mammalian behavior), are likely to cause constipation. Simple solutions include going to bed earlier and getting up earlier in the morning, and finding another acceptable location for defecation at the workplace. Increasing fiber in the diet, most easily achieved by making breakfast a high-fiber meal with either high-fiber breakfast cereals or high-fiber breads, will increase stool bulk, shorten transit time (the time for a marker to pass from the mouth and be passed in the stool), and alleviate symptoms in many cases. The importance of exercise in maintaining normal colon function is gradually being recognized – the importance of brisk walking should not be underestimated. However, some specific types of simple constipation have been identified which do not necessarily respond to high-fiber diets. Grossly prolonged transit times reflecting seriously slow colonic motility has been seen particularly in young women and do not respond well to high-fiber diets, and some 'outflow abnormalities,' which sometimes have a basis in abnormal rectal conformation, may also not respond.

Diverticular disease of the colon, characterized by the development of protrusions of mucosa through the bowel wall, is common and usually asymptomatic. It has been shown to be less likely to develop in those following a high-fiber diet, and once acquired can be managed, in many cases, by ensuring an adequate amount of fiber in the diet. Experimentally, various fiber supplements and 'bulking agents' have been shown to reduce the abnormally high peak intracolonic pressures that are characteristic of diverticular disease. Sometimes $10–20\,g$ of coarse wheat bran as a supplement is all that is required, but some patients develop flatulence and distension at least initially. Other fiber supplements such as ispaghula husk (psyllium) may be as effective, without the initial adverse side effects. Sometimes, simple dietary changes to achieve an adequate total daily intake of dietary fiber particularly from wheat-based foods are effective. Diverticulitis (inflammation of the diverticula) is a complication requiring medical management, which will usually include a short period of abstention from food. Many patients remain largely without symptoms once the right 'fiber' regimen has been determined.

The irritable bowel syndrome (IBS) is a 'functional' disorder of the bowel, which is said to affect up to 15% of the population and is characterized by some, but not necessarily all, of a range of symptoms including abdominal pain relieved by constipation, alternating diarrhea and constipation, recurrent abdominal pain, and urgent or frequent defecation. An important part of management is the exclusion of other serious organic disease such as inflammatory bowel diseases. In IBS the gut is abnormally sensitive to distension, and symptoms may be related to or exacerbated by external emotional events. The role of high-fiber diets in IBS has been investigated and not surprisingly is only of benefit in some cases: in those patients in whom the predominant feature is constipation. In some patients high-fiber diets may make their symptoms worse.

In inflammatory bowel disease (IBD) high fiber diets have no special part to play in the management of Crohn's disease where enteral feeding (with formula low-residue, low-fiber preparations) is especially beneficial where there is acute extensive small bowel disease. In ulcerative colitis specific dietary advice is usually unnecessary though fiber supplements may be of benefit in patients whose disease is limited to proctitis (inflammation of the rectum).

The treatment of newly diagnosed colon cancer does not include diet therapy, but treatment of those at increased risk of developing colon cancer by dietary and other means will become increasingly common as more information about the effects of high fiber diets and supplements on colon function becomes available. The critical step in the adenoma-carcinoma sequence in the human large bowel is the enlargement of the small adenoma (which has a low risk of malignant transformation) to a large adenoma (which has a high risk of malignant transformation); dietary factors, including low amounts of fiber in the diet, enhance adenoma growth. Bile acids are strongly linked to adenoma growth and bile acid concentrations in the colon are influenced by dietary fat and dietary fiber. Other effects of fiber may also be protective: bulking the stool and accelerating material through the colon, and provision of substrate for fermentation particularly with production of butyrate, which may have antineoplastic properties. However, despite a great deal of epidemiological and experimental work the potential role of dietary fiber in modulating the risk of colon cancer remains controversial.

See also: **Cereal Grains**. **Cholesterol**: Factors Determining Blood Levels. **Colon**: Nutritional Management of Disorders. **Diabetes Mellitus**: Etiology and Epidemiology; Classification and Chemical Pathology; Dietary Management. **Dietary Fiber**: Physiological Effects and Effects on Absorption; Potential Role in Etiology of Disease. **Glucose**: Metabolism and Maintenance of Blood Glucose Level. **Glycemic Index**. **Hyperlipidemia**: Overview; Nutritional Management. **Lipids**: Chemistry and Classification. **Lipoproteins**.

Further Reading

Committee on Medical Aspects of Food Policy (1991) *Dietary Reference Values for Food Energy and Nutrients for the United Kingdom: Non Starch Polysaccharides*, pp. 61–71. London: HMSO.

Cummings JH (1997) *The Large Intestine in Nutrition and Disease. Danone Chair Monograph*. Brussels: Institute Danone.

Diabetes UK Dietary Guidelines (2003) The implementation of nutritional advice for people with diabetes. *Diabetic Medicine* 20: 786–807.

Food and Agriculture Organization (1998) *Carbohydrates in Human Nutrition*. FAO Food and Nutrition Paper 66. Rome: FAO.

Jenkins DJA *et al.* (2003) The garden of Eden – plant based diets, the genetic drive to conserve cholesterol and its implications for heart disease in the 21st century. *Comparative Biochemistry and Physiology Part A* **136**: 141–151.

Relevant Websites

http://www.fda.gov – FDA health claim for psyllium on reducing risk of heart disease.

http://www.cfsan.fda.gov – FDA health claim for soluble fiber from whole oats and risk of coronary heart disease.

http://www.jhci.org.uk – JHCI final health claim for whole-grain foods and heart health.

http://www.jhci.org.uk – JHCI generic health claim for whole oats and reduction of blood cholesterol.

ISBN 0-12-150110-8

9 780121 501105